FOUNDATIONS *for* POPULATION HEALTH
in COMMUNITY/PUBLIC HEALTH NURSING

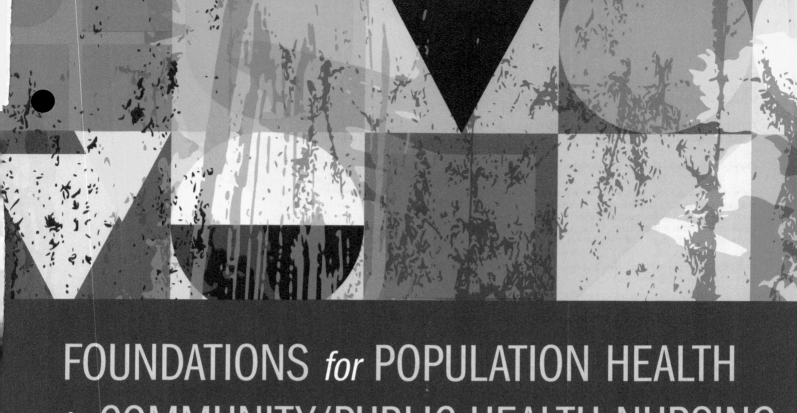

FOUNDATIONS *for* POPULATION HEALTH *in* COMMUNITY/PUBLIC HEALTH NURSING

SIXTH EDITION

MARCIA STANHOPE, PhD, RN, FAAN
Education and Practice Consultant and
  Professor Emerita
College of Nursing
University of Kentucky
Lexington, Kentucky

JEANETTE LANCASTER, PhD, RN, FAAN
Sadie Heath Cabiness Professor and Dean
  Emerita
School of Nursing
University of Virginia;
Associate, Tuft & Associates, Inc.
Charlottesville, Virginia

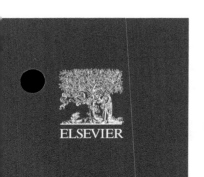

ELSEVIER

Elsevier
3251 Riverport Lane
St. Louis, Missouri 63043

FOUNDATIONS FOR POPULATION HEALTH IN COMMUNITY/PUBLIC
HEALTH NURSING, SIXTH EDITION

ISBN: 978-0-323-77688-2

Notice

Practitioners and researchers must always rely on their own experience and knowledge in evaluating and
using any information, methods, compounds or experiments described herein. Because of rapid advances
in the medical sciences, in particular, independent verification of diagnoses and drug dosages should
be made. To the fullest extent of the law, no responsibility is assumed by Elsevier, authors, editors or
contributors for any injury and/or damage to persons or property as a matter of products liability,
negligence or otherwise, or from any use or operation of any methods, products, instructions, or ideas
contained in the material herein.

Previous editions copyrighted 2018, 2014, 2010, 2006, and 2002

Library of Congress Control Number: 2021934549

Content Strategist: Heather Bays-Petrovic
Senior Content Development Manager: Lisa P. Newton
Senior Content Development Specialist: Tina Kaemmerer
Publishing Services Manager: Julie Eddy
Senior Project Manager: Rachel E. McMullen
Design Direction: Brian Salisbury

Printed in the United States of America

Last digit is the print number: 9   8   7   6   5   4   3   2   1

MARCIA STANHOPE, PhD, RN, FAAN

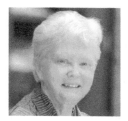

Marcia Stanhope is currently an education consultant; an Associate with Tuft and Associates Search Firm, Chicago, Illinois; and Professor Emerita at the University of Kentucky, College of Nursing, Lexington, Kentucky. In recent years she was a co-developer of the Doctorate of Nursing Practice (DNP) program and co-director of the first DNP program nationally, which began at the University of Kentucky. While at the University of Kentucky, she received the Provost Public Scholar award for contributions to the communities of Kentucky. She was also appointed to the Good Samaritan Endowed Chair in Community Health Nursing by the Good Samaritan Foundation, Lexington, Kentucky. She has practiced public health, community, and home health nursing; has served as an administrator and consultant in home health; and has been involved in the development of a number of nurse-managed centers. She has taught community health, public health, epidemiology, primary care nursing, and administration courses. Dr. Stanhope was the former Associate Dean and formerly directed the Division of Community Health Nursing and Administration in the College of Nursing at the University of Kentucky. She has been responsible for both undergraduate and graduate courses in population-centered, community-oriented nursing. She has also taught at the University of Virginia and the University of Alabama, Birmingham. Her presentations and publications have been in the areas of home health, community health and community-focused nursing practice, nurse-managed centers, and primary care nursing. Dr. Stanhope holds a diploma in nursing from the Good Samaritan Hospital, Lexington, Kentucky, and a bachelor of science in nursing from the University of Kentucky. She has a master's degree in public health nursing from Emory University in Atlanta and a PhD in nursing from the University of Alabama, Birmingham. Dr. Stanhope is the co-author of four other Elsevier publications: *Handbook of Community-Based and Home Health Nursing Practice, Public and Community Health Nurse's Consultant, Case Studies in Community Health Nursing Practice: A Problem-Based Learning Approach,* and *Foundations of Community Health Nursing: Community-Oriented Practice.*

Recently Dr. Stanhope was inducted into the University of Kentucky College of Nursing Hall of Fame and was named an outstanding alumna of the University of Kentucky.

JEANETTE LANCASTER, PhD, RN, FAAN

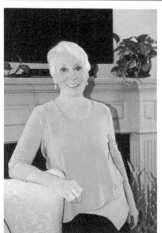

Jeanette Lancaster is a Professor and Dean Emerita at the University of Virginia, where she served as Dean for 19 years and remained on the faculty an additional 4 years. She served as a Visiting Professor at the University of Hong Kong from 2008–2009, where she taught undergraduate and graduate courses in public health nursing and worked on a number of special projects, including the development of a doctoral program. She also served as a visiting professor at Vanderbilt University and taught and delivered talks in Hong Kong and Taiwan. Dr. Lancaster taught public health courses on Semester at Sea in both 2013 and 2014. She works as an Associate with Tuft & Associates, Inc. an executive search firm. She has practiced psychiatric nursing and taught both psychiatric and public health nursing courses, as well as courses in nursing management. She taught at Texas Christian University; directed the community health master's program; and served as director of all master's programs at the University of Alabama in Birmingham. She was Dean of the School of Nursing at Wright State University in Dayton, Ohio before going to the University of Virginia in 1989. Dr. Lancaster is a graduate of the University of Tennessee Health Sciences Center, Memphis. She holds a master's degree in psychiatric nursing from Case Western Reserve University and a doctorate in public health from the University of Oklahoma. Dr. Lancaster authored the Elsevier publication *Nursing Issues in Leading and Managing Change* and is co-author with Dr. Marcia Stanhope of *Foundations for Population Health in Community/Public Health Nursing.* She received outstanding alumni awards from the University of Tennessee Health Sciences Center and the Frances Payne Bolton School of Nursing at Case Western Reserve University and an honorary Doctor of Humane Letters from SUNY Downstate Medical Center's College of Nursing and Related Health Sciences.

I am dedicating this edition of *Foundations* to the memory of my beloved aunt, Betty Lamb. She has been my touchstone to the family and has been my friend and supporter for many years. I do miss her. Also to my Aunt Ruby, who was an integral part of my life from birth. I have also enjoyed the friendship, support, and fun times with my closest friends and colleagues Joann Brashear, Nancy D. Hazard, Carolyn A. Williams, and Jeanette Lancaster, as well as many others through my life and career. I have benefited from the closeness I have shared with their husbands and the children, who are now grown and making their contributions to life, Ronn and Larry Brashear, John B. Hazard, and Anne Hazard Hoblik. Fun with Dusty, Buster, Lilbeth, Clem and Chip, Freckles, Simon, and the Phynx, as well as A.D., L.B., L.O., F.C., P.B., O.B & O.J, has been interesting and challenging for many years.

Marcia Stanhope

I dedicate this edition to my new COVID-inspired rescue cats: Loki and Arlo. They are 8-year-old brothers who have great fun walking across my keyboard when I am working on chapters. Of course, their exercise often causes difficulty since they alter the page on which I am working. Perhaps they have learned a little about public health nursing in their computer travels.

Jeanette Lancaster

We wish to thank the Public Health nurses who work daily to improve the health of populations and to faculty who assist students to understand the importance of population-level health care. Our special thanks to the Elsevier team who make our contributions possible, especially Heather Bays-Petrovic, Tina Kaemmerer, and Rachel McMullen and her staff. A very special thanks to our contributors in *PHN 10* for their outstanding work developing the text content, which supports the updates for *Foundations*, and to Lisa Pedersen Turner, PhD, RN, PHCNS-BC, who has worked with us through several editions of the text. The contributions of this talented group of people make our work easier.

Marcia Stanhope and Jeanette Lancaster

CONTRIBUTORS

We gratefully acknowledge the following individuals who wrote chapters for the 10th edition of *Public Health Nursing*, on which the chapters in this book are based.

Swann Arp Adams, MS, PhD
Associate Professor
College of Nursing
University of South Carolina
Columbia, South Carolina

Mollie E. Aleshire, DNP, MSN, FNP-BC, PPCNP-BC, FNAP
Associate Professor
School of Nursing
University of North Carolina at Greensboro;
Family and Pediatric Nurse Practitioner
Greensboro, North Carolina

Jeanne L. Alhusen, PhD, CRNP, RN, FAAN
Associate Professor and Assistant Dean for Research
School of Nursing
University of Virginia
Charlottesville, Virginia

Kacy Allen-Bryant, PhD(c), MSN, MPH, RN
Lecturer
College of Nursing
University of Kentucky
Lexington, Kentucky

Debra Gay Anderson, PhD, PHCNS-BC
Associate Dean for Research
College of Nursing
South Dakota State University
Brookings, South Dakota

Amber M. Bang, RN, BSN
Registered Nurse
Grants Pass, Oregon

Whitney Rogers Bischoff, DrPH, MSN, BSN
Associate Professor
Nursing
Texas Lutheran University
Seguin, Texas

Kathryn H. Bowles, RN, PhD, FAAN
van Ameringen Professor in Nursing Excellence
School of Nursing
University of Pennsylvania
Philadelphia, Pennsylvania;
Director of the Center for Home Care Policy and Research
Visiting Nurse Service of New York
New York, New York

Hazel Brown, DNP, RN
Chief Nursing Officer
Nursing Administration
Cayman Islands Health Services Authority
George Town, Grand Cayman
Cayman Islands

Angeline Bushy, PhD, RN, FAAN
Professor, Bert Fish Chair
College of Nursing
University of Central Florida
Orlando, Florida

Jacquelyn C. Campbell, PhD, RN, FAAN
Professor
Anna D. Wolf Chair
National Program Director, Robert Wood Johnson Foundation Nurse Faculty Scholars
Department of Community-Public Health
The Johns Hopkins University
Baltimore, Maryland

Catherine Carroca, MSN, RN
Assistant Professor
School of Nursing
Massachusetts College of Pharmacy and Health Sciences
Worcester, Massachusetts

Ann H. Cary, PhD, MPH, RN, FNAP, FAAN
Dean
School of Nursing and Health Studies
University of Missouri Kansas City
Kansas City, Missouri

Laura H. Clayton, PhD, RN, CNE
Professor
Department of Nursing Education
Shepherd University
Shepherdstown, West Virginia

Erin G. Cruise, PhD, RN
Associate Professor
School of Nursing
Radford University
Radford, Virginia

Lois A. Davis, RN, MSN, MA
Public Health Clinical Instructor
College of Nursing
University of Kentucky
Lexington, Kentucky

Sharon K. Davis, DNP, APRN, WHNP-BC
Clinical Assistant Professor
Nursing
University of Tennessee
Knoxville, Tennessee

Cynthia E. Degazon, RN, PhD
Professor Emerita
School of Nursing
Hunter College
New York, New York

Janna Dieckmann, PhD, RN
Associate Professor
School of Nursing
University of North Carolina at Chapel Hill
Chapel Hill, North Carolina

Sherry L. Farra, PhD, RN, CNE, CHSE, NDHP-BC
Associate Professor
Nursing
Wright State University
Dayton, Ohio

Mary E. Gibson, PhD, RN
Associate Professor
Nursing
University of Virginia
Charlottesville, Virginia

Mary Kay Goldschmidt, DNP, MSN, RN, PHNA-BC
Assistant Professor
Family and Community Health
Virginia Commonwealth University School of Nursing;
Co-director
PIONEER NEPQR Grant
Health Resources and Services Administration
Washington, DC

Monty Gross, PhD, MSN, RN, CNE, CNL
Senior Nurse Leader for Professional Development
Nursing Administration
Health Services Authority
George Town, Grand Cayman
Cayman Islands

Gerard M. Jellig, EdD
School Principal/Leader
KIPP DC WILL Academy
Washington, DC

Tammy Kiser, DNP, RN
Assistant Professor of Nursing
School of Nursing
James Madison University
Harrisonburg, Virginia

Andrea Knopp, PhD, MPH, MSN, FNP-BC
Nurse Practitioner Program Coordinator, Associate Professor
School of Nursing
James Madison University
Harrisonburg, Virginia

Candace Kugel, BA, MS, FNP, CNM
Clinical Specialist
Migrant Clinicians Network
Austin, Texas

Roberta Proffitt Lavin, PhD, FNP-BC, FAAN
Professor and Executive Associate Dean of Academic Programs
College of Nursing
University of Tennessee
Knoxville, Tennessee

Susan C. Long-Marin, DVM, MPH
Epidemiology Manager
Public Health
Mecklenburg County
Charlotte, North Carolina

Karen S. Martin, RN, MSN, FAAN
Health Care Consultant
Martin Associates
Omaha, Nebraska

Mary Lynn Mathre, RN, MSN, CARN
President and Co-founder
Patients Out of Time
Howardsville, Virginia

DeAnne K. Hilfinger Messias, PhD, RN, FAAN
Professor
College of Nursing and Women's and Gender Studies
University of South Carolina
Columbia, South Carolina

Emma McKim Mitchell, PhD, MSN, RN
Assistant Professor
Department of Family, Community & Mental Health Systems
University of Virginia School of Nursing
Charlottesville, Virginia

Carole R. Myers, PhD, MSN, BS
Associate Professor
College of Nursing
University of Tennessee
Knoxville, Tennessee

Victoria P. Niederhauser, DrPH, RN, PPCNP-BC, FAAN
Dean and Professor
College of Nursing
University of Tennessee
Knoxville, Tennessee

Bobbie J. Perdue, RN, PhD
Professor Emerita
College of Human Ecology
Syracuse University
Syracuse, New York;
Adjunct Faculty
Jersey College of Nursing
Tampa, Florida

Bonnie Rogers, DrPH, COHN-S, LNCC, FAAN
Professor and Director
North Carolina Occupational Safety and Health Education
and Research Center
University of North Carolina
Chapel Hill, North Carolina

Cynthia Rubenstein, PhD, RN, CPNP-PC
Chair and Professor
Nursing
Randolph-Macon College
Ashland, Virginia

Barbara Sattler, RN, MPH, DrPH, FAAN
Professor
School of Nursing and Health Professions
University of San Francisco
San Francisco, California

Erika Metzler Sawin, PhD
Associate Professor
Nursing
James Madison University
Harrisonburg, Virginia

Donna E. Smith, MSPH
Epidemiology Specialist
Epidemiology Program
Mecklenburg County Health Department
Charlotte, North Carolina

Sherrill J. Smith, RN, PhD, CNE, CNL
Professor
College of Nursing and Health
Wright State University
Dayton, Ohio

Esther J. Thatcher, PhD, RN, APHN-BC
Assistant Nurse Manager
Internal Medicine
University of Virginia Health System
Charlottesville, Virginia

Anita Thompson-Heisterman, MSN, PMHCNS-BC, PMHNP-BC
Assistant Professor
School of Nursing
University of Virginia
Charlottesville, Virginia

Lisa M. Turner, PhD, RN, PHCNS-BC
Associate Professor of Nursing
Department of Nursing
Berea College
Berea, Kentucky

Connie M. Ulrich, PhD, RN, FAAN
Professor of Nursing and Bioethics
University of Pennsylvania
Philadelphia, Pennsylvania

Lynn Wasserbauer, RN, FNP, PhD
Nurse Practitioner
Strong Ties Community Support Program
University of Rochester Medical Center
Rochester, New York

Jacqueline F. Webb, DNP, FNP-BC, RN
Associate Professor
School of Nursing
Linfield College
Portland, Oregon

Carolyn A. Williams, RN, PhD, FAAN
Professor and Dean Emerita
College of Nursing
University of Kentucky
Lexington, Kentucky

Lisa M. Zerull, PhD, RN-BC
Director and Academic Liaison
Nursing
Winchester Medical Center-Valley Health System;
Adjunct Clinical Faculty
School of Nursing
Shenandoah University
Winchester, Virginia

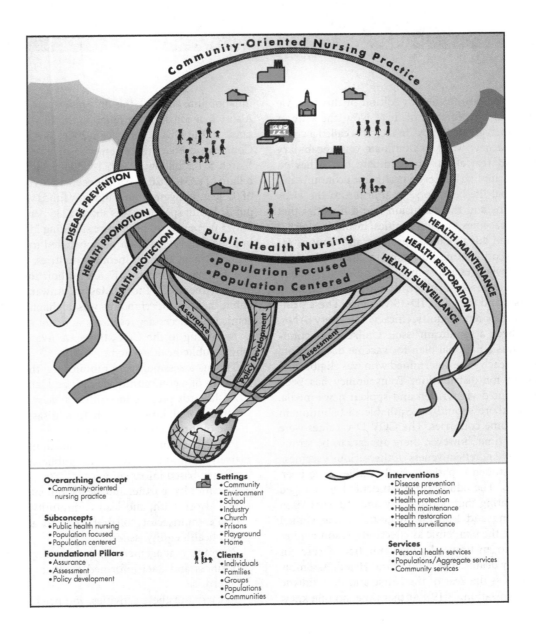

Overarching Concept
- Community-oriented nursing practice

Subconcepts
- Public health nursing
- Population focused
- Population centered

Foundational Pillars
- Assurance
- Assessment
- Policy development

Settings
- Community
- Environment
- School
- Industry
- Church
- Prisons
- Playground
- Home

Clients
- Individuals
- Families
- Groups
- Populations
- Communities

Interventions
- Disease prevention
- Health promotion
- Health protection
- Health maintenance
- Health restoration
- Health surveillance

Services
- Personal health services
- Populations/Aggregate services
- Community services

COMMUNITY NURSING DEFINITIONS

Community-Oriented Nursing Practice is a philosophy of nursing service delivery that involves the generalist or specialist public health and community health nurse providing "health care" through community diagnosis and investigation of major health and environmental problems, health surveillance, and monitoring and evaluation of community and population health status for the purposes of preventing disease and disability and promoting, protecting, and maintaining "health" to create conditions in which people can be healthy.

Public Health Nursing Practice is the synthesis of nursing theory and public health theory applied to promoting and preserving health of populations. The focus of practice is the community as a whole and the effect of the community's health status (resources) on the health of individuals, families, and groups. Care is provided within the context of preventing disease and disability and promoting and protecting the health of the community as a whole. Public Health Nursing is population focused, which means that the population is the center of interest for the public health nurse. Community Health Nurse is a term used interchangeably with Public Health Nurse.

Community-Based Nursing Practice is a setting-specific practice whereby care is provided for "sick" individuals and families where they live, work, and go to school. The emphasis of practice is acute and chronic care and the provision of comprehensive, coordinated, and continuous services. Nurses who deliver community-based care are generalists or specialists in maternal-infant, pediatric, adult, or psychiatric-mental health nursing.

When we wrote the preface to the 5th edition of this text, we said "health care is in a rapid state of flux." Now, the state of health care is in a much greater "flux." In fact, it is called a crisis. We did not expect a new word to dominate our vocabulary and its possible and real effects to dominate our behavior. COVID-19 has had crippling effects on health, the economy, and many aspects of usual life behaviors. In addition to the virus with its several strains and the confusion and difficulties that occurred in getting vaccines to communities, health is affected by unrest in the nation due to killings, protests, and demonstrations, as well as a record-setting hurricane in 2020 and subsequent flooding, and wildfires across many of the Western states.

The American Nurses Association developed five guiding principles for nurses and the COIVID-19 vaccines. These principles are: access, transparency, equity, efficacy, and safety (ANA, 2021). Access has been a significant issue. Unlike some countries, where there was a national plan for vaccine distribution, in the United States, each state determined who was eligible and the priority system for distribution. Transparency has been more fully implemented via written and spoken news media. Equity means that there should be equitable distribution in more than high income countries. The COVID vaccines were developed in record time; however, there appears to be strong efficacy for the safety and effectiveness of the various vaccines.

Nurses, nursing students, patients, and families have been affected by the virus. The education of students has changed remarkably, necessitating that both faculty and students learn new ways of teaching and learning. Regrettably, the United States did not handle the pandemic as effectively as some other nations, which led to an unusually high number of cases of COVID-19 and many deaths. The 72nd World Health Assembly had designated 2020 as the Year of the Nurse and the Midwife (World Health Organization, 2019). At that time, no one knew how much attention would focus on nurses as they cared for COVID patients. This designation was intended to recognize Florence Nightingale's 200th birthday. Due to the state of the world in 2020, the Year of the Nurse and the Midwife continues through 2021.

The Trust for America's Health (TFAH.org) found a chronic pattern of underfunding of vital public health programs in its report "The Impact of Chronic Underfunding on America's Public Health System: Trends, Risks, and Recommendations" (April 2020). They concluded that this lack of underfunding puts Americans' lives at risk. This risk occurs at a time when the nation is facing the "ongoing challenges of seasonal flu, vaccine-preventable disease outbreaks, the growing number of Americans who have obesity, risks associated with vaping, rising rates of sexually transmitted infections, and the opioid and other substances misuse and suicide epidemics" (TFAH, 2020, p. 3).

The Centers for Disease Control and Prevention (CDC) is the primary driver for public health funding through its grant programs to states and larger cities. The CDC's overall budget was increased by 9 percent in 2020 from 2019; however, when taking inflation into account, this only represented a 7 percent increase. Also, when adjusting for inflation the 2020 budget was about the same as the CDC's budget in 2008. The COVID-19 crisis led Congress to enact three response bills on each of these dates: March 5: 8.3 billion; March 18: 500 million; and March 27: 4.3 billion (TFAH, 2020, p. 3). The report provides details about each of these funding programs and how funds were allocated. In 2018 public health spending was about $286 per person, and that was only 3 percent of all healthcare spending in the nation. Spending in public health has been demonstrated to have a strong return on investment in high-income countries. Specifically, in a systematic report done in 2017, the authors found a median return on investment of 14 to 1 (Masters, Anwar, Collins et al., 2017). Public health underfunding was highlighted during the pandemic when necessary resources were not available.

According to the CDC, there are five core capabilities of a robust public health system:

- Threats assessment and monitoring: the ability to track the health of a community via data and laboratory testing.
- All-hazards preparedness: the capacity to respond to emergencies of all kinds, from natural disasters to infectious disease outbreaks to bioterrorism.
- Public communication and education: the ability to effectively communicate to diverse public audiences with timely, science-based information.
- Community partnership development: the ability to harness, work with, and lead community stakeholders and to create multisector collaborations to address public health and health equity issues.
- Program management and leadership: applying the best business and data-informed practices to the public health enterprise.

To carry out these activities, you need a well-trained public health workforce, and the numbers have been declining. From 2016 to 2019 the number of state full-time or equivalent people working in public health declined from 98,877 to 91,540, and an estimated 25 percent of the public health workforce was expected to retire in 2020 (TFAH, 2020, p. 7). Also, as will be discussed in Chapter 23, social determinants of health and the creation of health equity need to be addressed to ensure an effective public health system.

Public health workers, nurses, physicians, first responders, and other essential workers have been at the forefront of appreciation from Americans. Nurses who cared for COVID-19 patients have contracted the virus, and many have lost their lives and endangered their families due to the transmission of the virus.

As discussed in Chapter 2, throughout history, public health initiatives have had significant effects on health care in the United States and around the world. However, in recent years, we have seen a continual decline in funding for public health.

What is new is the launch of *Healthy People 2030*. Since 1980, *Healthy People* editions have set measurable goals designed to improve the health and well-being of Americans. This document is published every decade following review and feedback from a diverse group of individuals and organizations. The goal is to set national objectives to address the nation's most critical health objectives. Some of the key changes in *Healthy People 2030* that differentiate it from prior versions include:

- A reduction in the number of objectives to avoid overlap and to prioritize the most critical public health issues.
- Each objective is clearly labeled as to its relationship to *Healthy People 2020* objectives as: retained, modified, related, or removed.
- There is an increased focus on health equity and the social determinants of health.
- Health literacy is a central focus as reflected in one of the document's overarching goals: "Eliminate health disparities, achieve health equity, and attain health literacy to improve the health and well-being of all." Health literacy is divided into personal health literacy and organizational health literacy.
- Personal health literacy is "the degree to which individuals have the ability to find, understand, and use information and services to inform health-related decisions and actions for themselves and others" *(Healthy People 2030)*.
- Organizational health literacy is "the degree to which organizations equitably enable individuals to find, understand, and use information and services to inform health-related decisions and actions for themselves and others" *(Healthy People 2030)*.
- There is also an increased focus on how conditions in the environment where people are born, live, learn, work, play, worship, and age affect health.
- *Healthy People 2030* groups objectives according to health conditions; health behaviors; populations; setting and systems; and social determinants of health.

Each chapter in the text has a box that gives three examples of *Healthy People 2030* objectives that relate to the content of the chapter.

Two other documents to pay attention to are *Core competencies for public health professionalism*, which was updated in June 2014 by the Council on Linkages Between Academia and Public Health Practice (phf.org/corecompetencies) and *Community/Public Health Nursing (C/PHN) Competencies* (http: www.nationalacademies.org/), which was updated in 2018 by the Quad Council Coalition (QCC) of Public Health Nursing Organizations. The QCC was founded in 1988 to address priorities for public health nursing education, practice, leadership, and research, and services as the voice for public health nursing (Quad Council Coalition Competency Review Task Force, 2018): Community/Public Health Nursing Competencies. The Quad Council Coalition of Public Health Nursing Organizations is comprised of these groups:

Association of Community Health Nurse Educators (ACHNE)
Association of Public Health Nurses (APHN)
American Public Health Association (APHA)-Public Health Nursing Section
Alliance of Nurses for Healthy Environments (ANHE).

The Future of Nursing 2020-2030: document was released in May 2020 and has a significant emphasis on health equity and the social determinants of health that affect health equity. The report also recommends that nurses achieve the highest level of nursing

education possible. See http://www.nationalalacademies.org/future-of-nursing-2020-2030.

Also, the Public Health Association defines public health nursing as "the practice of promoting and protecting the health of populations using knowledge from nursing, social, and public health sciences" (APHA, 2013). Throughout the chapters, you will find information that supports this definition as public health nurses work with individuals, families, groups, and communities to promote health and prevent illness.

The National Council of State Boards of Nursing (NCSBN) determined that the nursing process, which has been the "gold standard" to guide nursing practice for over 50 years did not necessarily use this process to make "clinical judgment." The NCSBN's definition of clinical judgment builds on and expands the nursing process. The definition of clinical judgment is "the observed outcome of critical thinking and decision-making. It is an iterative process that uses nursing knowledge to observe and assess presenting situations, identify a prioritized client concern, and generate the best possible evidence-based solutions in order to deliver safe client care" (NCSBN, 2018, p. 12). The six essential cognitive skills of clinical judgment include:

1. Recognize cues
2. Analyze cues
3. Prioritize hypotheses
4. Generate solutions
5. Take action
6. Evaluate outcomes

These six skills are consistent with the steps of the nursing process as can be seen in the following table, and these are important steps to take in public health nursing (Ignatavicius and Silvestri, 2019, developed for Elsevier).

With the onset of the COVID-19 pandemic, the need for clinical judgment has been intensified. These are important times for nurses and especially so for those who choose public health nursing.

COMPARISON OF NURSING PROCESS STEPS WITH CLINICAL JUDGMENT COGNITIVE SKILLS

Steps of the Nursing Process	Cognitive Skills for Clinical Judgment
Assessment	Recognize Cues
Analysis	Analyze Cues
	Prioritize Hypotheses
Planning	Generate Solutions
Implementation	Take Action
Evaluation	Evaluate Outcomes

(NCBSN, 2019).

These steps are integrated in chapters to help readers make their best clinical decisions.

REFERENCES

American Nurses Association: ANA member news, January 22, 2021. www.NursingWorld.org/.
American Public Health Association, Public Health Nursing Section: *The definition and practice of public health nursing: A statement of*

the public health nursing section. Washington, CD: American Public Health Section.

The Council on Linkages Between Academic and Public Health Practice: *Core competencies for public health professionals,* 2014, Washington, DC, Public Health Foundation, available at phf.org/corecompetencies.

Ignatavicius D, Silvestri L: *Developing clinical judgment in nursing: A primer,* developed for Elsevier, 2019.

Masters R, Anwar E, Collins B et al., Return on investment of public health interventions: a systematic review, *J Epidemiol Community Health,* 71(8):827-834, 2017.

National Council of State Boards of Nursing (NCSBN): *NCLEX-RN Examination: Test plan for the National Council Licensure Examination for Registered Nurses.* Chicago, IL: Author.

National Council of State Boards of Nursing (NCSBN): The clinical judgment model, *Next generation NCLEX News,* Winter: 1-6, 2019.

Quad Council Coalition Competency Review Task Force: *Community/Public Health Nursing Competences,* 2018. Author.

Trust for America's Health: *The impact of chronic underfunding on America's public health system: Trends, risks, and recommendations,* April 2020. http://www.TFAH.org.

USDHHS: *Healthy People 2030,* 2020, Retrieved October 2020 at http://www.health.gov.

World Health Organization. Year of the Nurse and Midwife 2020. Accessed February 2021 at www.WHO.int.

ORGANIZATION

The text is divided into seven sections:

- *Part 1,* **Factors Influencing Nursing in Community and Population Health,** describes the historical and current status of the health care delivery system and nursing practice in the community.
- *Part 2,* **Forces Affecting Nurses in Community and Population Health Care Delivery,** addresses specific issues and societal concerns that affect nursing practice in the community.
- *Part 3,* **Frameworks Applied to Nursing Practice in the Community,** provides conceptual models for nursing practice in the community; selected models from nursing and related sciences are also discussed.
- *Part 4,* **Issues and Approaches in Health Care Populations,** examines the management of health care and select community environments, as well as issues related to managing cases, programs, disasters, and groups.
- *Part 5,* **Issues and Approaches in Family and Individual Health Care,** discusses risk factors and health problems for families and individuals throughout the life span.
- *Part 6,* **Vulnerability: Predisposing Factors,** covers specific health care needs and issues of populations at risk.
- *Part 7,* **Nursing Practice in the Community: Roles and Functions,** examines diversity in the role of nurses in the community and describes the rapidly changing roles, functions, and practice settings.

PEDAGOGY

Each chapter is organized for easy use by students and faculty. Chapters begin with Objectives to guide student learning and assist faculty in knowing what students should gain from the content. The Chapter Outline alerts students to the structure and content of the chapter. Key Terms, along with text page references, are also provided at the beginning of the chapter to assist the student in understanding unfamiliar terminology. The key terms are in boldface within the text.

The following features are presented in most or all chapters:

HOW TO
Provides specific, application-oriented information

EVIDENCE-BASED PRACTICE
Illustrates the use and application of the latest research findings in public health, community health, and nursing

LEVELS OF PREVENTION
Applies primary, secondary, and tertiary prevention to the specific chapter content

 HEALTHY PEOPLE 2030
Selected *Healthy People 2030* objectives are integrated into each chapter

APPLYING CONTENT TO PRACTICE
Provides highlights and links chapter content to nursing practice in the community

QSEN FOCUS ON QUALITY AND SAFETY EDUCATION FOR NURSES (QSEN)
Gives examples of how quality and safety goals, competencies, objectives, knowledge, skills, and attitudes can be applied in nursing practice in the community

CASE STUDY
Real-life clinical situations help students develop their assessment and critical thinking skills

 CHECK YOUR PRACTICE
This box provides a clinical situation and asks questions to stimulate problem solving and application to practice. Some boxes integrate the Clinical Judgment in Nursing process.

PRACTICE APPLICATION

At the end of each chapter, this section provides readers with an understanding of how to apply chapter content in the clinical setting through the presentation of a case situation with questions students will want to think about as they analyze the case.

▌REMEMBER THIS!

Provides a summary in list form of the most important points made in the chapter.

TEACHING AND LEARNING PACKAGE

A website (http://evolve.elsevier.com/stanhope/foundations) that includes instructor and student materials

For The Instructor:

- Next-Generation NCLEX® (NGN) Examination–Style Case Studies for Community and Public Health Nursing

- TEACH for Nurses, which contains: Detailed chapter lesson plans containing references to curriculum standards such as QSEN, BSN Essentials and Concepts, BSN Essentials for Public Health, unique Case Studies, and Critical Thinking Activities
- Test Bank with 800 questions
- Image Collection with all illustrations from the book
- PowerPoint slides

For The Student:

- NCLEX® Review Questions, with answers and rationale provided
- Case Studies with Questions and Answers
- Answers to Practice Application Questions

CONTENTS

Public Health Nursing and Population Health

Carolyn A. Williams

OBJECTIVES

After reading this chapter, the student should be able to:

1. State the mission and core functions of public health, the essential public health services, and the quality performance standards program in public health.
2. Describe specialization in public health nursing and other nurse roles in the community and the practice goals of each.
3. Describe what is meant by population health.
4. Identify barriers to the practice of community and prevention–oriented, population-focused practice.
5. Describe the importance of the social determinants of health to the health of a population.
6. State key opportunities for nurses in public health practice.

CHAPTER OUTLINE

KEY TERMS

In the year 2019, the United States and the world began experiencing a major public health crisis, a worldwide pandemic—a newly identified coronavirus, now well known as COVID-19. A pandemic is defined as an epidemic spread over several countries or continents, usually affecting a large number of people (www.cdc.gov. retrieved August 2020). The COVID-19 pandemic is identified as one of the 10 worst pandemics to occur since 165 AD.

As the United States endures this pandemic and approaches the third decade of the 21st century, considerable public attention is being given to issues related to the availability of affordable health insurance so individuals are assured that they can have access to health care. The central features in the Patient Protection and Affordable Care Act (ACA) of 2010 are the mechanisms to increase the number of people with health insurance. Difficulties with program enrollments have occurred; however, there is good evidence that identifies progress was made with the increasing numbers of enrollment (Census Bureau, 2018).

Before the passage of the ACA, many at the national level were seriously concerned about the growing cost of medical care as a part of federal expenditures Orszag (2007) and Orszag and Emanuel (2010). The concern with the cost of medical care remains a national issue and Blumenthal and Collins (2014) argued that the sustainability of the expansions of coverage provided by the ACA will depend on whether the overall costs of care in the United States can be controlled. If costs are not controlled the resulting increases in premiums will become increasingly difficult for all—consumers, employers, and the federal government. Other health system concerns focus on the quality and safety of services, warnings about bioterrorism, and global public health threats such as infectious diseases and contaminated foods, and the current pandemic. Because of all of these factors, the role of public health in protecting and promoting health, as well as preventing disease and disability, is extremely important.

Whereas the majority of national attention and debate surrounding national health legislation has been focused primarily on insurance issues related to medical care, there are indications of a growing concern about the overall status of the nation's health. In 2013 the Institute of Medicine issued a report, *U.S. Health in International Perspective: Shorter Lives, Poorer Health* which presented some sobering information. The report concluded that "Although Americans' life expectancy and health have improved over the past century, these gains have lagged behind those in other high-income countries. This health disadvantage prevails even though the United States spends far more per person on health care than any other nation. But compared to other high-income countries the United States spends less on social services" (Bradley and Taylor, 2013). The IOM report on shorter lives and poorer health summarizes their findings with this statement, "The U.S. health disadvantage has multiple causes and involves a combination of inadequate health care, unhealthy behaviors, adverse economic and social conditions, environment factors, public policies and social values that shape those conditions."

It is time to refocus attention on public health, on the concept of population health, which is emerging as a focal point for improving the health of the population, and the opportunities for nurses to be involved in and provide leadership in population health initiatives especially as the primary need in 2020 is to slow the pandemic crisis occurring.

This chapter and others that follow in this book will present information on many factors, outlooks, and strategies related to the protection, maintenance, and improvement of the health of populations. This chapter is focused on three broad topics: public health as a broad field of practice, which is the backbone of the infrastructure supporting the health of a country, state, province, city, town, or community; population health, which can be viewed as a particularly important set of analytical strategies and approaches first used in public health to describe, analyze, and mobilize efforts to improve health in community-based populations and now being used in initiatives to improve outcomes of clinical populations; and a discussion of public health nursing and emerging opportunities for nurses practicing in a variety of settings to be engaged in community-based, population-focused efforts to improve the health of populations.

This is a crucial time for public health nursing, a time of opportunity and challenge. The issue of growing costs, together with the changing demography of the US population, particularly the aging of the population, is expected to put increased demands on resources available for health care. In addition, the threats of bioterrorism, highlighted by the events of September 11, 2001, and the anthrax scares, will divert health care funds and resources from other health care programs to be spent for public safety. Also important to the public health community is the emergence of modern-day globally induced infectious diseases that result in pandemics and epidemics such as COVID-19, the mosquito-borne West Nile virus, the H1N1 influenza virus, the opioid epidemic, gun violence, avian influenza and other causes of mortality, many of which affect the very young. Most of the causes of pandemics and epidemics are preventable. What has all of this to do with nursing?

Understanding the importance of community-oriented, population-focused nursing practice and developing the knowledge and skills to practice it will be critical to attaining a leadership role in health care regardless of the practice setting. The following discussion explains why those who practice community- and prevention-oriented, population-focused nursing will be in a very strong position to affect the health of populations and decisions about how scarce resources will be used.

PUBLIC HEALTH PRACTICE: THE FOUNDATION FOR HEALTHY POPULATIONS AND COMMUNITIES

During the last 30 years, considerable attention has been focused on proposals to reform the American health care system. These proposals focused primarily on containing cost in medical care financing and on strategies for providing health insurance coverage to a higher proportion of the population. While it was important to make reforms in the medical insurance system, there is a clear understanding among those familiar with the history of public health and its impact that such reforms alone will not be adequate to improve the health of Americans.

Historically, gains in the health of populations have come largely from public health efforts, for example, (1) safety and adequacy of food supplies; (2) the provision of safe water; (3) sewage disposal; (4) public safety from biological threats; and (5) personal behavioral changes, including reproductive behavior. These are a few examples of public health's influence.

There is indisputable evidence collected over time that public health policies and programs were primarily responsible for increasing the average life span from 47 in 1900 to 78.6 years in 2017, an increase of approximately 60% in just over a century, through improvements in (1) sanitation; (2) clean water supplies; (3) making workplaces safer; (4) improving food and drug safety; (5) immunizing children; and (6) improving nutrition, hygiene, and housing (Fussenich,, 2019).

In an effort to help the public better understand the role public health has played in increasing life expectancy and improving the nation"s health, in 1999 the Centers for Disease Control and Prevention (CDC) began featuring information on the Ten Great Public Health Achievements in the 20th Century. The areas featured include: immunizations, moter vehicle safety, workplace safety, control of infectious diseases, safer and healtier foods, healthier mothers and babies, family planning,, drinking water flouridation,, tobacco as a health hazard, and declines in death from heart disease and stroke (CDC, 2018)

The payoff from public health activities is well beyond the money given for the effort. In 2012 only 3% (up from 1.5% in 1960) of all national expenditures supported governmental public health functions and in 2017 such expenditures remained at 3% (CMS, 2012, 2018).

Time will tell whether the gains in insurance coverage due to the ACA will stabilize or improve. What happens will have an impact on the activities of public health organizations. If the majority of the population remains covered by insurance, public health agencies will not need to provide direct clinical services, as in the past, in order to assure that those who need them can receive them. Public health organizations could refocus their efforts and emphasize community-oriented, population-focused health promotion and preventive strategies, if ways can be found to finance such efforts.

Unfortunately, the CMS data presented above clearly show that in the 5 years between 2012 and 2017 there has not been any overall increase in government funds directed to public health efforts.

Definitions in Public Health

In 1988 the Institute of Medicine published a report on the future of public health, which is now seen as a classic and influential document. In the report, public health was defined as "what we, as a society, do collectively to assure the conditions in which people can be healthy" (IOM, 1988, p. 1). The committee stated that the mission of public health was "to generate organized community efforts to address the public interest in health by applying scientific and technical knowledge to prevent disease and promote health" (IOM, 1988 p. 1; Williams, 1995).

It was clearly noted that the mission could be accomplished by many groups, public and private, and by individuals. However, the government has a special function "to see to it that vital elements are in place and that the mission is adequately addressed" (IOM, 1988, p. 7). To clarify the government's role in fulfilling the mission, the report stated that assessment, policy development, and assurance are the public health core functions at all levels of government:

- Assessment refers to systematically collecting data on the population, monitoring the population's health status, and making information available about the health of the community.
- Policy development refers to the need to provide leadership in developing policies that support the health of the population, including the use of the scientific knowledge base in making decisions about policy.
- Assurance refers to the role of public health in ensuring that essential community-oriented health services are available, which may include providing essential personal health services for those who would otherwise not receive them. Assurance also refers to making sure that a competent public health and personal health care workforce is available. Fielding (2009) made the case that assurance also should mean that public health officials should be involved in developing and monitoring the quality of services provided.

Because of the importance of influencing a population's health and providing a strong foundation for the health care system, the US Public Health Service and other groups strongly advocated a renewed emphasis on the population-focused essential public health functions and services that have been most effective in improving the health of the entire population. As part of this effort, a statement on public health in the United States was developed by a working group made up of representatives of federal agencies and organizations concerned about public health. The list of essential services presented in Fig. 1.1 represents the obligations of the public health system to implement the core functions of assessment, assurance, and policy development. The How To Box further explains these essential services and lists the ways public health nurses implement them (US Public Health Service, 1994 [updated 2008]; CDC, 2018).

Public Health Core Functions

The Core Functions Project (US Public Health Service, 1994 [updated 2008]), CDC, 2018) developed a useful illustration, the Health Services Pyramid (Fig. 1.2), which shows that population-based public health programs support the goals of providing a foundation for clinical preventive services. These services focus on disease prevention; on health promotion and protection; and on primary, secondary, and tertiary health care services. All levels of services shown in the pyramid are important to the health of the population and thus must be part of a health care system with health as a goal. It has been said that "the greater the effectiveness of services in the lower tiers, the greater is the capability of higher tiers to contribute efficiently to health improvement" (US Public Health Service, 1994 [updated 2008]). Because of the importance of the basic public health programs, members of the Core Functions

HOW TO PARTICIPATE, AS A PUBLIC HEALTH NURSE, IN THE ESSENTIAL SERVICES OF PUBLIC HEALTH

1. *Monitor health status to identify community health problems.*
   - *Participate in community assessment.*
   - *Identify subpopulations at risk for disease or disability.*
   - *Collect information on interventions to special populations.*
   - *Define and evaluate effective strategies and programs.*
   - *Identify potential environmental hazards.*
2. *Diagnose and investigate health problems and hazards in the community.*
   - *Understand and identify determinants of health and disease.*
   - *Apply knowledge about environmental influences of health.*
   - *Recognize multiple causes or factors of health and illness.*
   - *Participate in case identification and treatment of persons with communicable disease.*
3. *Inform, educate, and empower people about health issues.*
   - *Develop health and educational plans for individuals and families in multiple settings.*
   - *Develop and implement community-based health education.*
   - *Provide regular reports on health status of special populations within clinic settings, community settings, and groups.*
   - *Advocate for and with underserved and disadvantaged populations.*
   - *Ensure health planning, which includes primary prevention and early intervention strategies.*
   - *Identify healthy population behaviors and maintain successful intervention strategies through reinforcement and continued funding.*
4. *Mobilize community partnerships to identify and solve health problems.*
   - *Interact regularly with many providers and services within each community.*
   - *Convene groups and providers who share common concerns and interests in special populations.*
   - *Provide leadership to prioritize community problems and development of interventions.*
   - *Explain the significance of health issues to the public and participate in developing plans of action.*
5. *Develop policies and plans that support individual and community health efforts.*
   - *Participate in community and family decision-making processes.*
   - *Provide information and advocacy for consideration of the interests of special groups in program development.*
   - *Develop programs and services to meet the needs of high-risk populations as well as broader community members.*
   - *Participate in disaster planning and mobilization of community resources in emergencies.*
   - *Advocate for appropriate funding for services.*
6. *Enforce laws and regulations that protect health and ensure safety.*
   - *Regulate and support safe care and treatment for dependent populations such as children and frail older adults.*
   - *Implement ordinances and laws that protect the environment.*
   - *Establish procedures and processes that ensure competent implementation of treatment schedules for diseases of public health importance.*
   - *Participate in development of local regulations that protect communities and the environment from potential hazards and pollution.*
7. *Link people to needed personal health services and ensure the provision of health care that is otherwise unavailable.*
   - *Provide clinical preventive services to certain high-risk populations.*
   - *Establish programs and services to meet special needs.*
   - *Recommend clinical care and other services to clients and their families in clinics, homes, and the community.*
   - *Provide referrals through community links to needed care.*
   - *Participate in community provider coalitions and meetings to educate others and to identify service centers for community populations.*
   - *Provide clinical surveillance and identification of communicable disease.*
8. *Ensure a competent public health and personal health care workforce.*
   - *Participate in continuing education and preparation to ensure competence.*
   - *Define and support proper delegation to unlicensed assistive personnel in community settings.*
   - *Establish standards for performance.*
   - *Maintain client record systems and community documents.*
   - *Establish and maintain procedures and protocols for client care.*
   - *Participate in quality assurance activities such as record audits, agency evaluation, and clinical guidelines.*
9. *Evaluate effectiveness, accessibility, and quality of personal and population-based health services.*
   - *Collect data and information related to community interventions.*
   - *Identify unserved and underserved populations within the community.*
   - *Review and analyze data on health status of the community.*
   - *Participate with the community in assessment of services and outcomes of care.*
   - *Identify and define enhanced services required to manage health status of complex populations and special risk groups.*
10. *Research for new insights and innovative solutions to health problems.*
    - *Implement nontraditional interventions and approaches to effect change in special populations.*
    - *Participate in the collecting of information and data to improve the surveillance and understanding of special problems.*
    - *Develop collegial relationships with academic institutions to explore new interventions.*
    - *Participate in early identification of factors that are detrimental to the community's health.*
    - *Formulate and use investigative tools to identify and impact care delivery and program planning.*

Project argued that all levels of health care, including population-based public health care, must be funded or the goal of health of populations may never be reached.

Several new efforts to enable public health practitioners to be more effective in implementing the core functions of assessment, policy development, and assurance have been undertaken at the national level.

In 1997 the Institute of Medicine published *Improving Health in the Community: A Role for Performance Monitoring* (IOM, 1997) to highlight how a performance monitoring system could be developed and used to improve community health. The outcomes of the work were:

- the Community Health Improvement Process (CHIP), a method for improving the health of the population on a community-wide basis brought together key elements of the public health and personal health care systems in one framework,
- the development of a set of 25 indicators that could be used in the community assessment process to develop a community health profile (Box 1.1), and
- a set of indicators for specific public health problems that could be used by public health specialists as they carry out their assurance function and monitor the performance of public health and other agencies.

PUBLIC HEALTH IN AMERICA

Vision: Healthy people in healthy communities

Mission: Promote physical and mental health and prevent disease, injury, and disability

Public health
- Prevents epidemics and the spread of disease
- Protects against environmental hazards
- Prevents injuries
- Promotes and encourages healthy behaviors
- Responds to disasters and assists communities in recovery
- Ensures the quality and accessibility of health services

Essential public health services by core function *Assessment*
1. Monitor health status to identify community health problems
2. Diagnose and investigate health problems and health hazards in the community

Policy Development
3. Inform, educate, and empower people about health issues
4. Mobilize community partnerships to identify and solve health problems

5. Develop policies and plans that support individual and community health efforts

Assurance
6. Enforce laws and regulations that protect health and ensure safety
7. Link people to needed personal health services and assure the provision of health care when otherwise unavailable
8. Assure a competent public health and personal health care workforce
9. Evaluate effectiveness, accessibility, and quality of personal and population-based health services

Serving All Functions
10. Research for new insights and innovative solutions to health problems

---

Fig. 1.1 Public Health in America. (From US Public Health Service: The Core Functions Project, Washington, DC, 1994/update 2000, DC, Office of Disease Prevention and Health Promotion. Update 2008, CDC, 2019.)

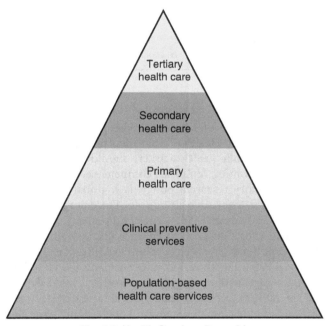

Fig. 1.2 Health Services Pyramid.

In 2000 the CDC established a Task Force on Community Preventive Services (CDC, 2014). The result was *The Community Guide: What Works to Promote Health*, a versatile set of resources available electronically at www.thecommunityguide.org (accessed September 15, 2020) that can be used for a community-level approach to health improvement and disease prevention. A particularly useful interactive internet-based resource available on the CDC website is the *Community Health Improvement Navigator* which outlines a process to identify and address the health needs of the community (accessed at CDC.gov, September 15, 2020).

Core Competencies of Public Health Professionals

To improve the public health workforce's abilities to implement the core functions of public health and to ensure that the workforce has the necessary skills to provide the 10 essential services listed in Fig. 1.1, a coalition of representatives from 17 national public health organizations (the Council of Linkages) began working in 1992 on collaborative activities to "assure a well-trained, competent workforce and a strong, evidence-based public health infrastructure" (US Public Health Service, 1994 [updated 2008) (updated by the Council on Linkages, 2010/2014). The 72 Competencies are divided into 8 categories (Box 1.2). In addition, each competency is presented at three levels (tiers), which reflect the different stages of a career.

- Tier 1 applies to entry-level public health professionals without management responsibilities.
- Tier 2 competencies are expected in those with management and/or supervisory responsibilities.
- Tier 3 is expected of senior managers and/or leaders in public health organizations.

It is recommended that these categories of competencies be used by educators for curriculum review and development and for workforce needs assessment, competency development, performance evaluation, hiring, and refining of the personnel system job requirements (www.phf.org/programs/corecompetencies/).

BOX 1.1   Indicators Used to Develop a Community Health Profile

Sociodemographic Characteristics
- Distribution of the population by age and race/ethnicity
- Number and proportion of persons in groups such as migrants, homeless, or the non–English speaking, for whom access to community services and resources may be a concern
- Number and proportion of persons aged 25 and older with less than a high school education
- Ratio of the number of students graduating from high school to the number of students who entered ninth grade 3 years previously
- Median household income
- Proportion of children less than 15 years of age living in families at or below the poverty level
- Unemployment rate
- Number and proportion of single-parent families
- Number and proportion of persons without health insurance

Health Status
- Infant death rate by race/ethnicity
- Numbers of deaths or age-adjusted death rates for motor vehicle crashes, work-related injuries, suicide, homicide, lung cancer, breast cancer, cardiovascular diseases, and all causes, by age, race, and sex as appropriate
- Reported incidence of AIDS, measles, tuberculosis, and primary and secondary syphilis, by age, race, and sex as appropriate
- Births to adolescents (ages 10–17) as a proportion of total live births
- Number and rate of confirmed abuse and neglect cases among children

Health Risk Factors
- Proportion of 2-year-old children who have received all age-appropriate vaccines, as recommended by the Advisory Committee on Immunization Practices
- Proportion of adults aged 65 and older who have ever been immunized for pneumococcal pneumonia; proportion who have been immunized in the past 12 months for influenza
- Proportion of the population who smoke, by age, race, and sex as appropriate
- Proportion of the population aged 18 and older who are obese
- Number and type of US Environmental Protection Agency air quality standards not met
- Proportion of assessed rivers, lakes, and estuaries that support beneficial uses (e.g., approved fishing and swimming)

Health Care Resource Consumption
- Per capita health care spending for Medicare beneficiaries—the Medicare-adjusted average per capita cost (AAPCC)

Functional Status
- Proportion of adults reporting that their general health is good to excellent
- Average number of days (in the past 30 days) for which adults report that their physical or mental health was not good

Quality of Life
- Proportion of adults satisfied with the health care system in the community
- Proportion of persons satisfied with the quality of life in the community

BOX 1.2   Categories of Public Health Workforce Competencies

- Analytic/assessment
- Policy development/program planning
- Communication
- Cultural competency
- Community dimensions of practice
- Basic public health sciences
- Financial planning and management
- Leadership and systems thinking

Compiled from Centers for Disease Control and Prevention: Genomics and disease prevention: Frequently asked questions, 2010. http://www.cdc.gov. Accessed January 11, 2011; Centers for Disease Control and Prevention: Genomics and disease prevention.

A coalition of public health nursing organizations initially called the Quad Council developed descriptions of skills to be attained by public health nurses for each of the public health core competencies. Skill levels are specified and have been updated for nurses by the Quad Council Coalition (QCC) in three tiers:
- Tier 1: the generalist/public health staff nurse
- Tier 2: the public health staff nurse with an array of program implementation, management, and supervisory responsibilities including clinical services, home visiting, community-based and population-focused programs
- Tier 3: the public health nurse at an executive or senior management level and leadership levels in public health or community organizations (Quad Council Coalition, 2018). (See Appendix C.3 for the Public Health Nursing Core Competencies.)

Quality Improvement Efforts in Public Health

In 2003, the Institute of Medicine released a report, "Who Will Keep the Public Healthy?" that identified eight content areas in which public health workers should be educated—informatics, genomics, cultural competence, community-based participatory research, policy, law, global health, and ethics—in order to be able to address the emerging public health issues and advances in science and policy.

Two broad efforts designed to enhance quality improvement efforts in public health have been developed within the last 20 years: The National Public Health Performance Standards (NPHPS) Program and the accreditation process for local and state health departments. The NPHPS "provide a framework to assess capacity and performance of public health systems and public health governing bodies." The program is "to improve the practice of public health, the performance of public health systems, and the infrastructure supporting public health actions" (CDC, 2018b). The performance standards set the bar for the level of performance that is necessary to deliver essential public health services. Four principles guided the development of the standards. First, they were developed around the 10 Essential Public Health Services. Second, the standards focus on the overall public health system rather than on single organizations. Third, the standards describe an optimal level of performance. Fourth, they are intended to support a process of quality improvement.

States and local communities seeking to assess their performance can access the Assessment Instruments developed by the program and other resources such as training workshops, on-site training, and technical assistance to work with them in conducting assessments (CDC, 2018b).

After this process is completed, the state and local health departments can voluntarily apply to the Public Health Accreditation Board located in Alexandria, Virginia, for recognition as an accredited health department.

Public Health 3.0

Public Health 3.0 as described by DeSalvo, Wang, Harris et al. (2017) represents an effort to build on the past and put forth "a new era of enhanced and broadened public health practice that goes beyond traditional public department functions and programs" (p. 4). Key features of the Public Health 3.0 agenda are: (1) to focus on prevention at the total population level or community-wide prevention; (2) to improve the social determinants of health; and (3) to engage multiple sectors and community partners to generate collective impact. To accomplish the stated goals a major recommendation is that "Public health leaders should embrace the role of Chief Health Strategists for their communities—working with all relevant other community leaders."

The Public Health 3.0 initiative represents a Call to Action for Public Health to regenerate and refocus to meet the challenges of the 21st century that emerged after the growing recognition that there are troubling indicators regarding the health of Americans. For example, the Centers for Disease Control reported in 2014 that the historical gains in longevity had plateaued for 3 years in a row (Murphy, Kkochanek, Arias, 2014). It is important to note that more recent data discussed by Woolf in an editorial in the *British Journal of Medicine* (2018) shows that life expectancy in the United States is actually beginning to decline. Other data have shown wide variations in life expectancy between those with the highest incomes and lowest incomes in some communities while the variation was small in others (Murphy 2014). Researchers (Chapman, Kelley, Woolf, 2015–2016, VCU Center on Society and Health, 2018) have shown that life expectancy can vary by up to 20 years in areas only a few miles apart. Such information suggests that more attention needs to be given to the environments in which people live, work, play, and age and requires community-based interventions. In discussing Public Health 3.0, DeSalvo, Wang, Harris, et al. argue that in dealing with the challenges presented by such disturbing population data an approach that goes beyond health care is called for and requires community-based interventions. These factors that influence an individual's health and well-being are now commonly referred to as the social determinants of health. They include housing, transportation, safe environments, access to health foods, economic development, and social support.

Other factors that require interventions are life expectancy rates, policy changes in payment approaches, moving away from episodic nonintegrated care toward value-based approaches, and more emphasis on partnerships to address community health problems.

Population Health

Kindig and Stoddard are credited with publishing the first formal definition of *Population Health in the American Journal of Public Health* in 2003. Their definition is: "the health outcomes of a group of individuals, including the distribution of such outcomes with the group" (p. 1).

With the growing popularity and usage of the term "population health" has come confusion about the meaning of the term. Some of this confusion can be resolved by being descriptive about the type of population whose health is being considered. For example, those in public health primarily focus on community-based populations defined in geographic terms, such as those residing in a particular country, state, county, city, or a specific community, whereas those working in a health care institution such as a hospital or health care system may define the population as those who are receiving or did receive care in their system or institution, which would constitute a clinical population.

Although the health of community-based populations has historically been the focus of public health practice, specifically defined populations of patients/clients, potential or actual are increasingly becoming a focus of the "business" of managed care. This has resulted in managed care executives, program managers, and others associated with health care organizations joining public health practitioners in becoming population oriented. This focus on clinical populations can be described as *Population Health Management*. A population-focused approach to planning, delivering, and evaluating various interventions is increasingly being used in an effort to achieve better outcomes in the population of interest and has never been more important whether in the clinical practice or community setting.

The concept of population health is relevant to populations defined in a variety of ways beyond those in a geographic jurisdiction or those receiving care from a particular care facility and can be applied to various groups such as workers/employees and students in a school setting. In order to be clear about what population is being considered by indicating that a specific population should be identified and to focus on the health of the population rather than the many factors responsible for that health, Williams proposed in a presentation at the spring 2018 meeting of the Association of Community Health Nursing Educators (ACHNE) the following definition which is adapted from Kindig and Stoddard:

Population Health is the health status of a defined population of individuals, including the distribution of health status within the group (Williams, 2020. Explore the two definitions and debate the similarities and differences in the definitions.

In view of all of the activity and "buzz" around the concept of population health, it appears that *population health could also be seen as an emerging field within the health sciences which includes ways of defining health status, determinants of the population's health, policies and interventions that link those factors, and biostatistical and analytical strategies and approaches to describe, analyze, and mobilize collaborative, interdisciplinary, and cross-sector efforts to improve health in a defined population.*

The idea of looking at the health of populations is not new. Epidemiologists have been doing this for many years but what is different now and makes the effort much more feasible, practical, and useful is the use of technology in gathering, processing, analyzing, displaying, and sharing the data. In the not-too-distant past it was necessary to rely on very basic hand counts or paper records which were processed by hand and involved the investment of much time and a considerable lag between when the data were originally obtained and when they could be available for decision making. With the development of information technology—computers, handheld devices, and amazing software—it is now becoming increasingly possible to look at population health data in ways that are practical, useful, and actionable.

Examples of Publicly Accessible Electronic Databases for Assessment of Population Health at the National, State, and County Level

The availability of interactive databases has made it more feasible for public health practitioners and others to have access to population health data that they can actually use to understand what is happening in their state and community. Two such databases are *Healthy People 2030* and *County Health Rankings*.

Healthy People focuses on national-level data but on some of the areas examined, state-level data are available.

Healthy People 2030 (www.healthypeople.gov/2030):
- Includes evidence-based objectives organized into user-friendly topics
- Provides resources and data to help health professionals and others address public health priorities and monitor progress toward achieving objectives
- Has an increased focus on health equity and the social determinants of health.

In the document there are five topic areas with 355 national objectives to be reached over the period of 10 years (from 2020 to 2030). The framework includes foundational principles, overarching goals, plan of action, and history and context.

A very important part of the *Healthy People* initiative is the identification of recommended evidence-based interventions that can be used to address each of the objectives. In January of 2017, a Midcourse Review of data on progress toward the 2020 goals became available. This review served to influence the development of the goals and objectives for *Healthy People 2030*.

The County Health Rankings and Roadmaps (www.county-healthrankings.org) is an interactive database that provides information at the state and county level on Health Outcomes (length of life and quality of life); Health Factors (health behaviors—tobacco use, diet and exercise, alcohol and drug use, and social activity); Clinical Care (access to care and quality of care); Social and Economic Factors (education, employment, income, family and social support, and community safety); and Physical Environment (air and water quality, and housing and transit). In addition, there is a searchable database of evidence-informed policies and programs (roadmaps) that can make a difference. Other features are the Action Center, which helps users to move from data to action at the community level; a Partner Center, which helps users identify possible partners and provides tips for engaging them; and Community Coaches, who can provide guidance to local communities to assist them in their efforts to make change. The user of the website can compare data on a given county with other counties in their state, with data at the state level, and with counties in other states. This website is a collaboration between the Robert Wood Johnson Foundation and the University of Wisconsin Population Health Institute and can be assessed at www.county-healthrankings.org

PUBLIC HEALTH NURSING AS A FIELD OF PRACTICE: AN AREA OF SPECIALIZATION

Most of the preceding discussion has been about the broad field of public health. Now attention turns to public health nursing. What is public health nursing? Is it really a specialty, and if so, why? It can be argued that public health nursing is a specialty because it has a distinct focus and scope of practice, and it requires a special knowledge base. The following characteristics distinguish public health nursing as a specialty:
- *It is population focused.* Primary emphasis is on populations whose members are free-living in the community as opposed to those who are institutionalized.
- *It is community oriented.* There is concern for the connection between the health status of the population and the environment in which the population lives (physical, biological, sociocultural). There is an imperative to work with members of the community to carry out core public health functions.
- *There is a health and preventive focus.* The primary emphasis is on strategies for health promotion, health maintenance, and disease prevention, particularly primary and secondary prevention.
- *Interventions are made at the community or population level.* Target populations are defined as those living in a particular geographic area or those who have particular characteristics in common and political processes are used as a major intervention strategy to affect public policy and achieve goals.
- *There is concern for the health of all members of the population/community, particularly vulnerable subpopulations.*

In 1981 the public health nursing section of the American Public Health Association (APHA) developed *The Definition and Role of Public Health Nursing in the Delivery of Health Care* to describe the field of specialization (APHA, 1981). This statement was reaffirmed in 1996 (APHA, 1996). In 1999 the American Nurses Association (ANA), with input from three other nursing organizations—the Public Health Nursing Section of the APHA, the Association of State and Territorial Directors of Public Health Nursing, and the Association of Community Health Nurse Educators—published the *Scope and Standards of Public Health Nursing Practice* (Quad Council, 1999 [revised 2005]). In that document, the 1996 definition was supported. Since 1999 the scope and standards have been revised twice. In the latest version, public health nursing continues to be defined as "the practice of promoting and protecting the health of populations using knowledge from nursing, social, and public health sciences" (APHA, 1996; Quad Council, 1999 [revised 2005], 2011) but the following statement was added in 2011: "Public Health Nurses engage in population-focused practice, but can and do often apply the Council of Linkages concepts at the individual and family level" (see Quad Council, 2011, p. 9). In 2018 the Quad Council Coalition(QCC) of Public Health Nursing Organizations, which is comprised of the Alliance of Nurses for

Healthy Environments (AHNE), the Association of Community Health Nursing Educators (ACHNE), the Association of Public Health Nurses (APHN), and the American Public Health Association—Public Health Nursing section (APHA—PHN), published an updated set of competencies for Community/Public Health Nurses (Quad Council Coalition, 2018) and adopted the APHA——PHN's 2013 definition of Public Health Nursing which is "The practice of promoting and protecting the health of populations using knowledge from nursing, social, and public health sciences. Public health nursing is a specialty practice within nursing and public health. It focuses on improving *population health* by emphasizing prevention and attending to multiple determinants of health. Often used interchangeably with community health nursing, this nursing practice includes advocacy, policy development, and planning, which addresses issues of social justice" (APHA—PHN, 2013).

Educational Preparation for Public Health Nursing

Targeted and specialized education for public health nursing practice has a long history. In the late 1950s and early 1960s, before the integration of public health concepts into the curriculum of baccalaureate nursing programs, special baccalaureate curricula were established in several schools of public health to prepare nurses to become public health nurses. Today it is generally assumed that a graduate of any baccalaureate nursing program has the necessary basic preparation to function as a beginning staff public health nurse.

Since the late 1960s, public health nursing leaders have agreed that a specialty in public health nursing requires a master's degree. In the future, a Doctor of Nursing Practice (DNP) degree will probably be expected since the American Association of Colleges of Nursing has proposed the DNP should be the expected level of education for specialization (Box 1.3) in an area of nursing practice (AACN, 2004, 2006).

The ACHNE reaffirmed the results of the 1984 Consensus Conference on the Essentials of Public Health Nursing Practice and Education sponsored by the USDHHS Division of Nursing (ACHNE, 2003; USDHHS, 1985). The educational requirements were reaffirmed by ACHNE (2009) and in the revised *Scope and Standards of Public Health Nursing Practice* and include both clinical specialists and nurse practitioners who engage in population-focused care as advanced practice registered nurses in public health (Quad Council, 1999 [revised 2005]). The latest iteration of the *Scope and Standards of Practice for Public Health Nursing* was published by the ANA in 2013 (ANA, 2013).

Population-Focused Practice Versus Practice Focused on Individuals

A key factor that distinguishes public health nursing from other areas of nursing practice is the focus on populations, a focus historically consistent with public health philosophy and a cornerstone of population health. Box 1.4 lists principles on which public health nursing is built. Although public health nursing is based on clinical nursing practice, it also incorporates the population perspective of public health. It may be helpful here to define the term *population*.

A population, or aggregate, is a collection of individuals who have one or more personal or environmental characteristics in common. Members of a community who can be defined in terms of geography (e.g., a county, a group of counties, or a state) or in terms of a special interest or circumstance (e.g., children attending a particular school) can be seen as constituting a population. Often there are subpopulations or high-risk groups within the larger population, such as high-risk infants under the age of 1 year, unmarried pregnant adolescents, or individuals exposed to a particular event such as a chemical spill. In population-focused community-based practice, problems are defined (by assessments or diagnoses), and solutions (interventions), such as policy development or providing a particular preventive service, are implemented for or with a

---

BOX 1.3   Areas Considered Essential for the Preparation of Specialists in Public Health Nursing

- Epidemiology
- Biostatistics
- Nursing theory
- Management theory
- Change theory
- Economics
- Politics
- Public health administration
- Community assessment
- Program planning and evaluation
- Interventions at the aggregate level
- Research
- History of public health
- Issues in public health

From Consensus Conference on the Essentials of Public Health Nursing Practice and Education, Rockville, MD, 1985, US Department of Health and Human Services, Bureau of Health Professions, Division of Nursing.

BOX 1.4   Eight Principles of Public Health Nursing

1. The client or "unit of care" is the population.
2. The primary obligation is to achieve the greatest good for the greatest number of people or the population as a whole.
3. The processes used by public health nurses include working with the client(s) as an equal partner.
4. Primary prevention is the priority in selecting appropriate activities.
5. Selecting strategies that create healthy environmental, social, and economic conditions in which populations may thrive is the focus.
6. There is an obligation to actively reach out to all who might benefit from a specific activity or service.
7. Optimal use of available resources to assure the best overall improvement in the health of the population is a key element of the practice.
8. Collaboration with a variety of other professions, organizations, and entities is the most effective way to promote and protect the health of the people.

From Quad Council of Public Health Nursing Organizations: Scope and standards of public health nursing practice, Washington, DC, 1999, revised 2005, 2007, 2013 with the American Nurses Association

defined population or subpopulation (examples are provided in the Levels of Prevention Box). In other nursing specialties, the diagnoses, interventions, and treatments are usually carried out at the individual client level. However, with the adoption of population health strategies by those working with clinical populations—Population Health Management—this is beginning to change. Specifically, in some clinical settings population health management efforts are being developed in which patients with a common set of problems or conditions are defined as a population and a defined set of services are offered to the entire population, or a specific set of services are offered to those at varying levels of risk.

LEVELS OF PREVENTION

Examples in Public Health Nursing

Primary Prevention

Using general and specific measures in a population to promote health and prevent the development of disease (incidence) and using specific measures to prevent diseases in those who are predisposed to developing a particular condition.

Example: The public health nurse develops a health education program for a population of school-age children that teaches them about the effects of smoking on health.

Secondary Prevention

Stopping the progress of disease by early detection and treatment, thus reducing prevalence and chronicity.

Example: The public health nurse develops a program of toxin screenings for migrant workers who may be exposed to pesticides and refers for treatment those who are found to be positive for high levels.

Tertiary Prevention

Stopping deterioration in a patient, a relapse, or disability and dependency by anticipatory nursing and medical care.

Example: The public health nurse provides leadership in mobilizing a community coalition to develop a Health Maintenance and Promotion Center to be located in a neighborhood with a high density of residents with chronic illnesses and few health education and appropriate recreation resources. In addition to educational programs for nutrition and self-care, physical activity programs such as walking groups are provided.

Professional education in nursing, medicine, and other clinical disciplines focuses primarily on developing competence in decision making at the individual client level by assessing health status, making management decisions (ideally *with* the client), and evaluating the effects of care. Fig. 1.3 illustrates three levels at which problems can be identified. For example, community-based nurse clinicians or nurse practitioners focus on individuals they see in either a home or a clinic setting. The focus is on an individual person or an individual family in a subpopulation (the C arrows in Fig. 1.3). The provider's emphasis is on defining and resolving a problem for the individual; the client is an individual.

In Fig. 1.3 the individual clients are grouped into three separate subpopulations, each of which has a common characteristic (the B arrows in Fig. 1.3). Public health nursing

specialists often define problems at the population or aggregate level as opposed to an individual level. Population-level decision making is different from decision making in clinical care. For example, in a clinical direct-care situation, the nurse may determine that a client is hypertensive and explore options for intervening. However, at the population level, the public health nursing specialist might explore the answers to the following set of questions:

1. What is the prevalence of hypertension among various age, race, and sex groups?
2. Which subpopulations have the highest rates of untreated hypertension?
3. What programs could reduce the problem of untreated hypertension and thereby lower the risk of further cardiovascular morbidity and mortality for the population as a whole?

Public health nursing specialists are usually concerned with more than one subpopulation and frequently with the health of the entire community (in Fig. 1.3, arrow A: the entire box containing all of the subgroups within the community). In reality, of course, there are many more subgroups than those in Fig. 1.3. Professionals concerned with the health of a whole community must consider the total population, which is made up of multiple and often overlapping subpopulations. For example, the population of adolescents at risk for unplanned pregnancies would overlap with the female population 15 to 24 years of age. A population that would overlap with infants under 1 year of age would be children from 0 to 6 years of age. In addition, a population focus requires considering those who may need particular services but have not entered the health care system (e.g., children without immunizations or clients with untreated hypertension).

Public Health Nursing Specialists and Core Public Health Functions: Selected Examples

The core public health function of *assessment* includes activities that involve collecting, analyzing, and disseminating information on both the health status and the health-related aspects of a community or a specific population. Questions such as whether the health services of the community are available to the population and are adequate to address needs are considered. Assessment also includes an ongoing effort to monitor the health status of the community or population and the services provided. As described earlier in this chapter, *Healthy People* is an excellent example of the efforts of the USDHHS to organize the goal setting, data collecting and analysis, and monitoring necessary to develop the series of publications describing the health status and health-related aspects of the US population. These efforts began with *Healthy People: The Surgeon General's Report on Health Promotion and Disease Prevention* in 1980 and continued with *Promoting Health/Preventing Disease: Objectives for the Nation, Healthy People 2000,* and *Healthy People 2010, Healthy People 2020,* and are now moving forward into the future with *Healthy People 2030* (US Department of Health, Education, and Welfare, 1979; USDHHS, 1979, 1980, 1991, 2000, 2010, 2020, and *Healthy People* 2030 retrieved at www.healthypeople.gov).

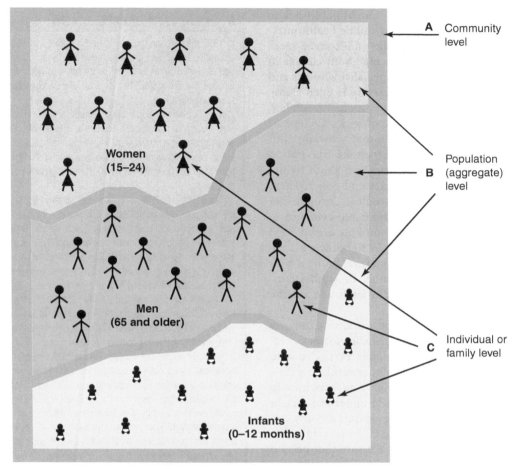

Fig. 1.3 Levels of Health Care Practice.

EVIDENCE-BASED PRACTICE

This study was a quasi-experimental pre-post design with no control group. The study sample consisted of 21 community institutions (7 hospitals, 8 YMCAs, 4 community health centers, and 2 organizations serving homeless populations). All Boston hospitals were invited to participate because they have an employee base that includes many lower-wage workers who live in the priority neighborhoods. The other settings were selected from priority neighborhoods defined as those with the highest proportion of Black and Latino residents and a disproportionate chronic disease burden. The researchers estimated that approximately 78,000 people were reached by the intervention every week.

The goal was to reduce the percentage of prepackaged foods with greater than 200 mg of sodium available at the sites, thus the outcome measure was the change in the percent of prepackaged foods with greater than 200 mg per serving from baseline to follow-up. The intervention consisted of education provided by registered dietitians to the food service directors at the sites, feedback on baseline assessment of levels of sodium in products available at each site and how they compared with other organizations in their sector, an action plan at each site for goal setting, technical assistance which included webinars on how they could support the desired changes, and educational materials to identify healthy, lower sodium options and to increase consumer awareness of the health effects associated with excess sodium. The intervention period ranged from 1 to 1.5 years.

Overall the percent of prepackaged products with greater than 200 mg of sodium decreased from 29.0% at baseline to 21.5% at follow-up (*P* = .003). Those changes were found to be due to improvements in the hospital cafeterias and kiosks. In the YMCA vending machines, the percent of high-sodium products decreased from 27.2% to 11.5% (*P* = .017). While declines were observed in the vending machines in the community health centers and the organizations serving the homeless, they were not statistically significant due to the small sample sizes. While the study has the limitation of no control group, it is difficult to know whether the changes were from the intervention or due to secular trends. However, the investigators had documented information that the sites made intentional decisions to produce the outcome. The study also is limited in not including any information on consumption behavior. The study provides information on the feasibility and modest effectiveness of a community-level intervention to increase the availability of lower sodium products in the food supply.

Nurse Use

This study indicates that there is potential to reduce the public's access to high-sodium products by providing options with less sodium which can be useful in nurse-led public policy advocacy for healthier options in vending machines in schools and public buildings.

Data from Brooks CJ, Barret J, Daly J, et al: A Community-Level Sodium Reduction Intervention, Boston, 2013–2015, *Am J Public Health* 107(12):1951–1957, December 2017.

Policy development is both a core function of public health and a core intervention strategy used by public health nursing specialists. Policy development in the public arena seeks to build constituencies that can help bring about change in public policy. A public health nursing specialist who has and continues to provide strong policy leadership is Ellen Hahn, PhD, director of the Kentucky Center for Smoke Free Policy, which is based at the University of Kentucky's College of Nursing. More information care be found at www.uky.edu/breathe/tobacco-policy/kentucky-center-smoke-free-policy. This website is a treasure trove of information about reducing exposure to tobacco through advocacy and policy. There are fact sheets, videos, and research studies. Through her research Dr. Hahn has developed considerable evidence to support important policy changes (antismoking ordinances) to reduce exposure to tobacco smoke in Kentucky, a state that has a long tradition of a tobacco culture, both in production of tobacco and in use. A number of studies conducted by Hahn and her colleagues can be found on the website identified above.

The third core public health function, *assurance*, focuses on the responsibility of public health agencies to make certain that activities have been appropriately carried out to meet public health goals and plans. This may result in public health agencies requiring others to engage in activities to meet goals, encouraging private groups to undertake certain activities, or sometimes actually offering services directly. Assurance also includes the development of partnerships between public and private agencies to make sure that needed services are available and that assessing the quality of the activities is carried out. Review the Evidence-Based Practice Box for an example.

PUBLIC HEALTH NURSING VERSUS COMMUNITY-BASED NURSING

The concept of public health should include all populations within the community, both free-living and those living in institutions. Furthermore, the public health specialist should consider the match between the health needs of the population and the health care resources in the community, including those services offered in a variety of settings. Although all direct care providers may contribute to the community's health in the broadest sense, not all are primarily concerned with the population focus—the big picture. All nurses in a given community, including those working in hospitals, physicians' offices, and health clinics, may contribute positively to the health of the community. However, the special contributions of public health nursing specialists include looking at the community or population as a whole; raising questions about its overall health status and associated factors, including environmental factors (physical, biological, and sociocultural); and *working with the community* to improve the population's health status.

Fig. 1.4 is a useful illustration of the arenas of practice. Because most nurses working in the community and many staff

 HEALTHY PEOPLE 2030

In 1979 the surgeon general issued a report that began a 30-year focus on promoting health and preventing disease for all Americans. The report, entitled *Healthy People*, used morbidity rates to track the health of individuals through the five major life cycles of infancy, childhood, adolescence, adulthood, and older age.

In 1989 *Healthy People 2000* became a national effort of representatives from government agencies, academia, and health organizations. Their goal was to present a strategy for improving the health of the American people. Their objectives were being used by public and community health organizations to assess current health trends, health programs, and disease prevention programs.

Throughout the 1990s, all states used *Healthy People 2000* objectives to identify emerging public health issues. The success of the program on a national level was accomplished through state and local efforts. Early in the 1990s, surveys from public health departments indicated that 8% of the national objectives had been met, and progress on an additional 40% of the objectives was noted. In the mid-course review published in 1995, it was noted that significant progress had been made toward meeting 50% of the objectives.

In light of the progress made in the past decade, the committee for *Healthy People 2010* proposed two goals. The hope was to reach these goals by such measures as promoting healthy behaviors, increasing access to quality health care, and strengthening community prevention.

The major premise of *Healthy People 2010* was that the health of the individual cannot be entirely separate from the health of the larger community. Therefore the vision for *Healthy People 2010* was "Healthy People in Healthy Communities." The vision for *Healthy People 2020* was "A society in which all people live long, healthy lives." (www.healthypeople.gov/2020) HP 2020 tracked approximately 1300 objectives organized into 42 topic areas, each of which represented an important public health area. In addition, HP2020 contained the Leading Health Indicators, a small, focused set of 12 topics containing 26 objectives identified to communicate and move action on high-priority health issues.

Healthy People 2030 emphasizes a vision of a society in which all people can achieve their full potential for health and well-being across the lifespan with a mission to promote, strengthen, and evaluate the nation's efforts to improve the health and well-being of all people. *HP 2030* highlights leading health indicators and social determinants of health, with five major topic areas and 355 objectives.

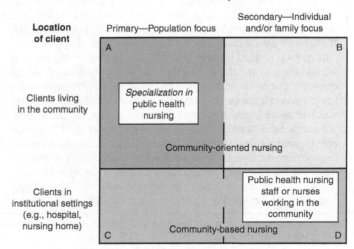

Fig. 1.4 Arenas for Health Care Practice.

public health nurses, historically and at present, focus on providing direct personal care services—including health education—to persons or family units outside of institutional settings (either in the client's home or in a clinic environment), such practice falls into the upper right quadrant (section B) of Fig. 1.4. However, specialization in public health nursing is population-focused and focuses on clients living in the community and is represented by the box in the upper left quadrant (section A).

There are three reasons, in addition to the population focus, that the most important practice arena for public health nursing is represented by section A of Fig. 1.4, the population of free-living clients:

1. Preventive strategies can have the greatest impact on free-living populations, which usually represent the majority of a community.
2. The major interface between health status and the environment (physical, biological, sociocultural, and behavioral) occurs in the free-living population.
3. For philosophical, historical, and economic reasons, prevention-oriented, population-focused practice is most likely to flourish in organizational structures that serve free-living populations (e.g., health departments, health maintenance organizations, health centers, schools, and workplaces).

What roles in the health care system do public health nursing specialists (those in section A of Fig. 1.4) have? Options include director of nursing for a health department, director of the health department, state commissioner for health, director of maternal and child health services for a state or local health department, director of wellness for a business or educational organization, and director of preventive services for an integrated health system. Nurses can occupy all of these roles, but, with the exception of director of nursing for a health department, they are in the minority. Unfortunately, nurses who occupy these roles are often seen as "administrators" and not as public health nursing specialists. However, those who work in such roles have the opportunity to make decisions that affect the health of population groups and the type and quality of health services provided for various populations.

Where does the staff public health nurse or nurse working in the community fit on the diagram in Fig. 1.4? That depends on the focus of the nurse's practice. In many settings, most of the staff nurse's time is spent in community-based direct care activities, where the focus is on dealing with individual clients and individual families, in which case the practice falls into section B of Fig. 1.4. Although a staff public health nurse or a nurse practicing in the community may not be a public health nurse specialist, this nurse may spend some time carrying out core public health functions with a population focus, and thus that part of the role would be represented in section A of Fig. 1.4. In summary, the field of public health nursing can be seen as primarily encompassing two groups of nurses:

- Public health nursing specialists, whose practice is community-oriented and uses population-focused strategies for carrying out the core public health functions (section A of Fig. 1.4)
- Staff public health nurses or clinical nurses working in the community, who are community-based, who may be clinically oriented to the individual client, and who combine

some primary preventive population-focused strategies and direct care clinical strategies in programs serving specified populations (section B of Fig. 1.4)

Sections C and D of Fig. 1.4 represent institutionalized populations. Nurses who provide direct care to these clients in hospital settings fall into section D, and those who have administrative/managerial responsibility for nursing services in institutional settings fall into section C.

Fig. 1.4 also shows that specialization in public health nursing, as it has been defined in this chapter, can be viewed as a specialized field of practice with certain characteristics within the broad arena of community. This view is consistent with recommendations developed at the Consensus Conference on the Essentials of Public Health Nursing Practice and Education (USDHHS, 1985). One of the outcomes of the historical conference was consensus on the use of the terms *community health nurse* and *public health nurse*. It was agreed that the term *community health nurse* could apply to all nurses who practice in the community, whether or not they have had preparation in public health nursing. Thus nurses providing secondary or tertiary care in a home setting, school nurses, and nurses in clinic settings (in fact, any nurse who does not practice in an institutional setting) could fall into the category of community health nurse. Nurses with a master's degree or a doctoral degree who practice in community settings could be referred to as *community health nurse specialists,* regardless of the area of nursing in which the degree was earned. According to the conference statement: "The degree could be in any area of nursing, such as maternal/child health, psychiatric/mental health, or medical-surgical nursing or some subspecialty of any clinical area" (USDHHS, 1985, p. 4). The definitions of the three areas of practice have changed, however, over time.

In 1998 the Quad Council began to develop a statement on the scope of public health nursing practice (Quad Council, 1999 [revised 2005]). The council attempted to clarify the differences between the term *public health nursing* and the term introduced into nursing's vocabulary during health care reform of the 1990s: community-based nursing. The authors recognized that the terms *public health nursing* and *community health nursing* had been used interchangeably since the 1980s to describe population-focused, community-oriented nursing practice and community-based practice. However, the Council decided to make a clearer distinction between community-oriented and community-based nursing practice. In contrast, community-based nursing care was described as the provision or assurance of personal illness care to individuals and families in the community, whereas community-oriented nursing was the provision of disease prevention and health promotion to populations and communities. It was suggested that there be two terms for the two levels of care in the community: *community-oriented care* and *community-based care* (see the list of definitions presented in Box 1.5).

There is a need and a place for a nursing specialty in the community; the nurse in this specialty is more than a clinical specialist with a master's degree who practices in a community-based setting, as was suggested by the Consensus Conference more than 25 years ago. Although in 1984 these nurses were referred to as community health nurses, today they are referred to as

---

BOX 1.5   Definitions of the Key Nursing Areas in the Community

- *Community-oriented nursing practice* is a philosophy of nursing service delivery that involves the generalist or specialist public health and community health nurse. The nurse provides health care through community diagnosis and investigation of major health and environmental problems, health surveillance, and monitoring and evaluation of community and population health status for the purposes of preventing disease and disability and promoting, protecting, and maintaining health to create conditions in which people can be healthy.
- *Community-based nursing practice* is a setting-specific practice whereby care is provided for clients and families where they live, work, and attend school. The emphasis of community-based nursing practice is acute and chronic care and the provision of comprehensive, coordinated, and continuous services. Nurses who deliver community-based care are generalists or specialists in maternal/infant, pediatric, adult, or psychiatric/mental health nursing.

---

nurses in community-based practice (see definitions in the inside cover of this text). Those who provide community-oriented service to specific subpopulations in the community and who provide some clinical services to those populations may be seen as nurse specialists in the community. Although such practitioners may be community-based, they are also community-oriented as public health specialists but are usually focused on only one or two special subpopulations. Preparing for this specialty includes a master's or doctoral degree with emphasis in a direct care clinical area, such as school health or occupational health, and ideally some education in the public health sciences. Examples of roles such specialists might have in direct clinical care areas include case manager, supervisor in a home health agency, school nurse, occupational health nurse, parish nurse, and a nurse practitioner who also manages a nursing clinic.

Table 1.1 illustrates the similarities and differences between Public Health (Community Oriented) Nursing and Community-Based Nursing.

ROLES IN PUBLIC HEALTH NURSING

In community-oriented nursing circles, there has been a tendency to talk about public health nursing from the point of view of a role rather than the functions related to the role. This can be limiting. In discussing such nursing roles, there is a need to have a broader point of view with an emphasis on the functions of the nurse rather than focusing only on the direct care provider orientation. In other words, what do nurses do and how do they relate to a population rather than individual clients? Discussions will be held about how a practice can become more population focused, for an individual practitioner, such as an agency staff nurse, and nurse administrators in public health (one role for public health nursing specialists). This is particularly important because many agencies' nursing administrators, supervisors, or others (sometimes program directors who are not nurses) make the key decisions about how staff nurses will spend their time and what types of clients will be seen and under what circumstances. Public

health nursing administrators who are prepared to practice in a population-focused manner will be more effective than those who are not prepared to do so.

Although their opportunities to make decisions at the population level are limited, staff nurses benefit from having a clear understanding of population-focused practice for three reasons:

- First, it gives them professional satisfaction to see how their individual client care contributes to health at the population level.
- Second, it helps them appreciate the practice of others who are population-focused specialists.
- Third, it gives them a better foundation from which to provide clinical input into decision making at the program or agency level and thus to improve the effectiveness and efficiency of the population-focused practice.

A curriculum was proposed by representatives of key public health nursing organizations and other individuals that would prepare the staff public health nurse or generalist to function as a community-oriented practitioner (Association of State and Territorial Directors of Nursing, 2000). The AACN developed a supplement to the document "The Essentials of Baccalaureate Education for Professional Nursing Practice," which highlights this organization's recommendations for public health nursing (AACN, 2013).

Unfortunately, nursing roles as presently defined are often too limited to include population-focused practice, but it is important not to think too narrowly. Furthermore, roles that entail population-focused decision making may not be defined as nursing roles (e.g., directors of health departments, state or regional programs, and units of health planning and evaluation; directors of programs such as preventive services within a managed care organization). If population-focused public health nursing is to be taken seriously, and if strategies for assessment, policy development, and assurance are to be implemented at the population level, more consideration must be given to organized systems for assessing population needs and managing care.

Redefining nursing roles so that population-focused decision making fits into the present structure of nursing services may be difficult in some circumstances at the present time, but future needs will require that nurses be prepared to make such decisions (IOM, 2010). At this point, it may be more useful to concentrate on identifying the skills and knowledge needed to make decisions in population-focused practice (see Appendix C), to define where in the health care system such decisions are made, and then to equip nurses with the knowledge, skills, and political understanding necessary for success in such positions. Although some of these positions are in nursing settings (e.g., administrator of the nursing service and top-level staff nurse supervisors), others are outside of the traditional nursing roles (e.g., director of a health department).

CHALLENGES FOR THE FUTURE

Barriers to Nurses Specializing in Leadership Roles in Population Health Initiatives

One of the most serious barriers to the development of specialists in public health nursing is the mindset of many nurses that the only role for a nurse is at the bedside or at the client's

TABLE 1.1   Select Examples of Similarities and Differences Between Community-Oriented and Community-Based Nursing

	Community-Oriented Nursing	Community-Based Nursing
Philosophy	Primary focus is on "health care" of individuals, families, groups, and the community or populations within the community	Focus is on "illness care" of individuals and families across the life span
Goal	Preserve, protect, promote, or maintain health and prevent disease	Manage acute or chronic conditions
Service context	Community health care Population health	Family-centered illness care
Community type	Varied; usually local community	Human ecological
Client characteristics	• Individuals at risk • Families at risk • Groups at risk • Communities • Usually healthy • Culturally diverse • Autonomous • Able to define their own problems • Primary decision makers	• Individuals • Families • Usually ill • Culturally diverse • Autonomous • Able to define their own problems • Involved in decision making
Practice setting	• Community agencies • Home • Work • School • Playground • May be organization • May be government	• Community agencies • Home • Work • School
Interaction patterns	• One to one • Groups • May be organizational	• One to one
Type of service	• Direct care of at-risk individuals • Indirect (program management)	• Direct illness care
Emphasis on levels of prevention	• Primary • Secondary (screening) • Tertiary (maintenance and rehabilitation)	• Secondary • Tertiary • May be primary
Roles	**Client and Delivery Oriented: Individual, Family, Group, Population** • Caregiver • Social engineer • Educator • Counselor • Advocate • Case manager	**Client and Delivery Oriented: Individual, Family** • Caregiver
	Group Oriented • Leader (personal health management) • Change agent (screening) • Community advocate/developer • Case finder • Community care agent • Assessment • Policy developer • Assurance • Enforcer of laws/compliance	**Group Oriented** • Leader (disease management) • Change agent (managed-care services)
Priority of nurse's activities	• Case findings • Client education • Community education • Interdisciplinary practice • Case management (direct care) • Program planning and implementation • Individual, family, and population advocacy	• Case management (direct care) • Client education • Individual and family advocacy • Interdisciplinary practice • Continuity of care providers

side (i.e., the direct care role). Indeed, the heart of nursing is the direct care provided in personal contacts with clients. On the other hand, two things should be clear. First, whether a nurse is able to provide direct care services to a particular client depends on decisions made by individuals within and outside of the care system. Second, nurses need to be involved in those fundamental decisions. Perhaps the one-on-one focus of nursing and the historical expectations of the "proper" role of women have influenced nurses to view other ways of contributing, such as administration, consultation, and research, less positively. Fortunately, things are changing. Within and outside of nursing, women have taken on every role imaginable. Further, the number of male nurses is steadily growing; nursing can no longer be viewed as a profession practiced by women exclusively. These two developments have opened doors to new roles that may not have been considered appropriate for nurses in the past.

A second barrier to population-focused public health nursing practice consists of the structures within which nurses work and the process of role socialization within those structures. For example, the absence of a particular role in a nursing unit may suggest that the role is undesirable or inaccessible to nurses. In another example, nurses interested in using political strategy to make changes in health-related policy—an activity clearly within the domain of public health nursing—may run into obstacles if their goals differ from those of other groups. Such groups may subtly but effectively lead nurses to conclude that their involvement in political effort takes their attention away from the client and it is not in their own or in the client's best interest to engage in such activities.

A third barrier is that few nurses receive graduate-level preparation in the concepts and strategies of the disciplines basic to public health (e.g., epidemiology, biostatistics, community development, service administration, and policy formation).

For individuals who want to specialize in public health nursing, these skills are as essential as direct care skills, and they should be given more attention in graduate programs that prepare nurses for careers in public health. There is hope. Fortunately, the curricular expectations for academic programs leading to the doctor of nursing practice (DNP) degree include serious attention to preparing nurses to develop a population perspective as well as the analytical, policy, and leadership skills necessary to be successful as a specialist in public health nursing (AACN, 2006).

Developing Population Health Nurse Leaders

The massive organizational changes occurring in the health delivery system present a unique opportunity to establish new roles for nurse leaders who are prepared to think in population health terms. In a book that is now viewed as a classic, Starr (1982) described the trend toward the use of private capital in financing health care, particularly institution-based care and other health-related businesses. The movement can be thought of as the "industrialization" of health care, which operated very much like a cottage industry or a small business for a very long time. The implications and consequences of this movement are

enormous. First, the goal was to provide investors a return on their investment. Other aspects included more attention to the delivery of primary and community-based care in a variety of settings; less emphasis on specialty care; the development of partnerships, alliances, and other linkages across settings in an effort to build integrated systems, which would provide a broad range of services for the population served; and in some situations adoption of capitation, a payment arrangement in which insurers agree to pay providers a fixed sum for each person per month or per year, independent of the costs actually incurred. Initially with the spread of capitation and now with the development by the Centers for Medicare and Medicaid of value-based reimbursement, health professionals have become more interested in the concept of populations, sometimes referred to by financial officers and others as *covered lives* (i.e., individuals with insurance that pays on a capitated basis). For public health specialists, it is a new experience to see individuals involved in the business aspects of health care, and frequently employed by hospitals, thinking in population terms and taking a population approach to decision making.

This new focus on populations, coupled with the integration of acute, chronic, and primary care that is occurring in some health care systems, is likely to create new roles for individuals, including nurses, who will span inpatient and community-based settings and focus on providing a wide range of services to the population served by the system. Such a role might be director of client care services for a health care system, who would have administrative responsibility for a large program area. There will also be a demand for individuals who can design programs of preventive and clinical services to be offered to targeted subpopulations and those who can implement the services. Who will decide what services will be given to which subpopulation and by which providers? How will nurses be prepared for leadership in the emerging and future structures for health care delivery and health maintenance?

A primary focus of the health care system of the future will be on community-based strategies for health promotion and disease prevention, and on population-focused strategies for primary and secondary care. Directing more attention to developing the specialty of public health nursing as a way to provide nursing leadership may be a good response to the health care system changes. Preparing nurses for population-focused decision making will require greater attention to developing programs at the doctoral level that have a stronger foundation in the public health sciences, while providing better preparation of baccalaureate-level nurses for community-oriented as well as community-based practice.

Some observers of public health have anticipated that if access to health care for all Americans becomes more of a reality, public health practitioners will be in a position to turn over the delivery of personal primary care services to practitioners in accountable care organizations and integrated health plans, and return to the core public health functions. However, assurance (making sure that basic services are available to all) is a core function of public health. Thus even under the condition of improved access to care, there will still be a need to monitor subpopulations in the community to ensure that necessary care is available to all and that its quality is at an acceptable level. When these conditions are not met, public health practitioners are accountable to finding a solution.

Shifting Public Health Practice to Address the Social Determinants of Health and More Vigorous Policy Efforts to Create Conditions for a Healthy Population

The growing concern about the role played by the social determinants of health in contributing to negative health outcomes coupled with the Public Health 3.0 call for public health leaders to be health strategists in their communities suggests that public health leaders need to be more active in assuming community-level leadership in addressing issues like homelessness, food insecurity, and unsafe physical and social environments. This translates into mobilizing various community constituencies to take collaborative action within the constraints of current policies and to mobilize for the policy changes necessary to reduce the barriers to healthy conditions. This also means that public health nurse specialists need to be health strategists in their communities.

In 2012 the Institute of Medicine published a report (IOM, 2012) on shifting public policy from a primary focus of supporting medical care to creating conditions for a healthy population.

A major challenge for the future is the need for public health nursing specialists to be more aggressive in working collaboratively with various groups in the community as well as professional colleagues in institutional settings to deal with barriers to health like the social determinants discussed above. Another challenge is to be more aggressive in their practice of the core public health function of policy development to address (1) the availability of adequate nutrition, (2) the maintenance of a healthy and safe environment in schools, (3) the reduction of secondhand smoke, and (4) assuring access to needed health services.

In the Institute of Medicine's influential report, *The Future of Nursing: Leading Change, Advancing Health* (IOM, 2010), a key message is that "Nurses should be full partners, with physicians and other health professionals, in redesigning health care in the United States" (IOM, 2010, pp. 1–11). In other words, nurses need to be key actors and be prepared for leadership in that area.

As a specialty, public health nursing can have a positive impact on the health status of populations, but to do so it will be necessary to have broad vision; to prepare nurses for roles in community leadership and policy making and in the design, development, management, monitoring, and evaluation of population-focused health care systems and to develop strategies to support nurses in these roles. With the focus on quality and safety education for nurses, public health nursing education will want to reflect this renewed focus and assist nurses who are population focused to develop the competencies noted in the QSEN box.

QSEN FOCUS ON QUALITY AND SAFETY EDUCATION FOR NURSES

QSEN Competency	Competency Definition
Client-centered care	Recognize the client population or designee as the source of control and full partner in providing compassionate and coordinated care based on respect for population preferences, values, and needs
Teamwork and collaboration	Function effectively within nursing and interprofessional teams, fostering open communication, mutual respect, and shared decision making to achieve quality care
Evidence-based practice	Integrate best current evidence with clinical expertise and population preferences and values for delivery of optimal health care
Quality improvement	Use data to monitor the outcomes of the assessment, assurance, and policy development functions and use improvement methods to design and test changes to continuously improve the quality and safety of population health care systems
Safety	Minimize risk for harm to populations and providers through both system effectiveness and nurse performance
Informatics	Use information and technology to communicate, manage knowledge, mitigate error, and support decision making

Prepared by Gail Armstrong, ND, DNP, MS, PhD, professor and assistant dean/DNP program, Oregon Health and Sciences University, and updated by Marcia Stanhope (2020).

⟫ APPLYING CONTENT TO PRACTICE

In this chapter, emphasis is placed on defining and explaining public health nursing practice with populations. The three essential functions of public health and public health nursing are assessment, policy development, and assurance. The Council on Linkages "Core Competencies for Public Health Professionals" revised in 2014 describes the skills of public health professionals, including nurses. In assessment function, one skill is assessment of the health status of populations and their related determinants of health and illness. For policy development, one of the skills is development of a plan to implement policy and programs. For the assurance function, one skill that public health nurses will need is to incorporate ethical standards of practice as the basis of all interactions with organizations, communities, and individuals. These skills can also be linked to the 10 essential services of public health nursing found earlier in this chapter. Assessment of health status is a skill needed for implementing essential service 1, the monitoring of health status to identify community problems. Development of a plan for policy and program implementation is a skill needed for essential service 5, to support individual and community health efforts. Incorporating ethical standards is done in essential service 3 when informing, educating, and empowering people about health issues.

▎ PRACTICE APPLICATION

Population-focused nursing practice is different from clinical nursing care delivered in the community. If one accepts that the specialist in public health nursing is population focused and has a unique body of knowledge, it is useful to debate where and how public health nursing specialists practice. How does their practice compare with that of the nurse specialist in community or community-based nursing?

A. In your public health class, debate with classmates which nurses in the following categories practice population-focused nursing and provide reasons for your choices:
1. School nurse
2. Staff nurse in home care
3. Director of nursing for a home care agency
4. Nurse practitioner in a health maintenance organization
5. Vice president of nursing in a hospital
6. Staff nurse in a public health clinic or community health center
7. Director of nursing in a health department

B. Choose three categories from the preceding list, and interview at least one nurse in each of the categories. Determine the scope of practice for each nurse. Are these nurses carrying out population-focused practice? Could they? How? *Answers can be found on the Evolve site.*

REMEMBER THIS!

- Public health is what we, as a society, do collectively to ensure the conditions in which people can be healthy.
- Assessment, policy development, and assurance are the core public health functions; they are implemented at all levels of government and in communities.
- *Assessment* refers to systematically collecting data on the population, monitoring of the population's health status, and making available information about the health of the community.
- *Policy development* refers to the need to provide leadership in developing policies that support the health of the population; it involves using scientific knowledge in making decisions about policy.
- *Assurance* refers to the role of public health in making sure that essential community-wide health services are available, which may include providing essential personal health services for those who would otherwise not receive them. Assurance also refers to ensuring that a competent public health and personal health care workforce is available.
- The setting is frequently viewed as the feature that distinguishes public health nursing from other specialties. A more useful approach is to use the following characteristics: a focus on populations that are free-living in the community, an emphasis on prevention, a concern for the interface between the health status of the population and the living environment (physical, biological, sociocultural), and the use of political processes to affect public policy as a major intervention strategy for achieving goals.
- According to the 1985 Consensus Conference sponsored by the Nursing Division of the US Department of Health and Human Services, *specialists in public health nursing* are defined as those who are prepared at the graduate level, either master's or doctoral, "with a focus in the public health sciences" (USDHHS, 1985). This is still true today.

- Population-focused practice is the focus of public health nursing. This focus on populations and the emphasis on health protection, health promotion, and disease prevention are the fundamental factors that distinguish public health nursing from other nursing specialties.
- A *population* is defined as a collection of individuals who share one or more personal or environmental characteristics. The term *population* may be used interchangeably with the term *aggregate*.

REFERENCES

American Association of Colleges of Nursing (AACN): AACN Position Statement on the Practice Doctorate in Nursing. Washington, DC, 2004, AACN.

American Association of Colleges of Nursing (AACN): The Essentials of Doctoral Education for Advanced Nursing Practice. Washington, DC, 2006, AACN.

American Association of Colleges of Nursing (AACN): Public Health: Recommended Baccalaureate Competencies and Curricular Guidelines for Public Health Nursing: A Supplement to The Essentials of Baccalaureate education for Professional Nursing Practice" 2013. Accessed at http://www.aacn.nche.edu.

American Nurses Association (ANA): Public Health Nursing: Scope and Standards of Practice. Washington, DC, 2013, ANA.

American Public Health Association (APHA): The Definition and Role of Public Health Nursing in the Delivery of Health Care: A Statement of the Public Health Nursing Section. Washington, DC, 1981, APHA.

American Public Health Association (APHA): The Definition and Practice of Public Health Nursing. 2013. Retrieved on December 28, 2018 at www.apha.org

American Public Health Association (APHA): The Definition and Role of Public Health Nursing: A Statement of the APHA Public Health Nursing Section, *[March 1996 update]*. Washington, DC, 1996, APHA.

Association of Community Health Nursing Educators (ACHNE): Essentials of Master's Level Nursing Education for Advanced Community/Public Health Nursing Practice. Lathrop, NY, 2003, ACHNE.

Association of Community Health Nursing Educators (ACHNE): Essentials of Baccalaureate Nursing Education for Entry Level Community/Public Health Nursing. Wheat Ridge, CO, 2009, ACHNE.

Association of State and Territorial Directors of Nursing (ASTDN): Public Health Nursing: A Partner for Healthy Populations. Washington, DC, 2000, ASTDN.

Blumenthal D, Collins SR. Health care coverage under the Affordable Care Act—a progress report, *N Engl J Med* 371:275–281, 2014.

Bradley EH, Taylor LA. The American Health Care Paradox: Why Spending More is Getting Us Less. Philadelphia, PA, 2013, Public Affairs.

Brooks CJ, Barrett J, Daly J. Lee R, Blanding N, McHugh A, Williams D. A Community-Level Sodium Reduction Intervention, Boston, 2013-2015. Am J Public Health 107, 2017.

Centers for Disease Control and Prevention (CDC). *Ten Great Public Health Achievements in the 20th Century,* 2018. Retrieved November 2020 from: www.cdc.gov.

Centers for Disease Control and Prevention (CDC): *National Public Health Performance Standards Program,* 2018b. Retrieved November 2020 from: www.phf.org.

Centers for Disease Control and Prevention (CDC): *The Community Guide: What Works to Promote Health*, 2014. Retrieved November 2020 from: www.thecommunityguide.org.

Centers for Disease Control (CDC): The public health system and the ten essential services, June 2018c, Atlanta Georgia.

Centers for Medicare and Medicaid Services (CMS), Office of the Actuary, National Health Statistics Group: *The Nation's Health Dollar Calendar Year 2012: Where It Came From, Where It Went*, 2012. Retrieved November 2014 from: http://www.cms.gov.

Centers for Medicare and Medicaid Services (CMS) Office of the Actuary, National Health Statistics Group. *The Nation's Health Dollar Calendar Year 2017* Retrieved December 30, 2018 from www.cms.gov

Chapman DA, Kelley L, Woolf SH: Life Expectancy Maps 2015-2016. VCU Center on Society and Health. Retrieved on December 28, 2018 from http://www.societyhealth.vcu.

Council on Linkages between Academia and Public Health Practice: Core Competencies for Public Health Professionals. Washington, DC, 2010, revised 2014. Retrieved 9/29/2020 from: www.phf.org.

County Health Rankings can be assessed at www.countyhealthrankings.org

DeSalvo KB, Wang YC, Harris A, Auerbach J, Koo D, O'Carroll P. A Call to Action for Public Health to Meet the Challenges of the 21st Century. Perspectives, Discussion Paper, the National Academies. 2017.

Fielding J: Commentary: public health and health care quality assurance—strange bedfellows? *Milbank Q* 87:581–584, 2009.

Koen Füssenich,Wilma J. Nusselder, Stefan K. Lhachimi, Hendriek C. Boshuizen & Talitha F. Feenstra , Potential gains in health expectancy by improving lifestyle: an application for European regions. *Population Health Metrics* 17:1, 2019.

Institute of Medicine (IOM): Improving Health in the Community: A Role for Performance Monitoring. Washington, DC, 1997, National Academies Press.

Institute of Medicine (IOM): Primary Care and Public Health,: Exploring Integration to Improve Population Health. Washington, DC, 2012, National Academies of Sciences Press.

Institute of Medicine: The future of public health. Washington, DC, 1988, National Academy Press.

Institute of Medicine (IOM): The Future of Nursing: Leading Change, Advancing Health. Washington, DC, 2010, National Academies Press.

Institute of Medicine and the National Research Council, The Academies Press, Washington DC, 2018.

Kentucky Center for Smoke-Free Policy: Retrieved December 27, 2018 from www.uky.edu.

Kindig D, Stoddart G: What is Population Health? *Am J Public Health* 93:380-383. 2003.

Murphy SL, Kochanek KD, Xu J, Arias E: Mortality in the United States 2014. National Center Health Statistics Data Brief 229: 1-8. PubMed.

Orszag PR: Health Care and the Budget: Issues and Challenges for Reform *[Statement before the Committee on the Budget, U.S. Senate]*. Washington, DC, June 21, 2007, Congressional Budget Office.

Orszag PR, Emanuel EJ: Health care reform and cost control. *N Engl J Med* 363:601–603, 2010.

Patient Protection and Affordable Care Act & Health Care and Education Affordability Reconciliation Act of 2010, 2010. Retrieved 9/28/ November 2014 from: www.hhs.gov.

Quad Council Coalition Competency Review Task Force: Community/Public Health Nursing Competencies. 2018 Retrieved December 28 from www.quadcouncilphn.org

Quad Council of Public Health Nursing Organizations: Scope and Standards of Public Health Nursing Practice. Washington, DC, 1999 [revised 2005], American Nurses Association.

Quad Council of Public Health Nursing Organizations: Competencies for Public Health Nursing Practice. Washington, DC, 2003 [revised 2009], Association of State and Territorial Directors of Nursing.

Quad Council of Public Health Nursing Organizations: *Quad Council Competencies for Public Health Nurses*, Summer 2011. November 2014 from: www.quadcouncilphn.org.

Quad Council of Public Health Nursing Organizations: Scope and standards of public health nursing practice, Washington, DC, 1999, revised 2003, 2005, 2007, 2013 with the American Nurses Association.

Starr P: The social transformation of American medicine. New York, 1982, Basic Books.

US Department of Health, Education, and Welfare: Healthy People: The Surgeon General's Report on Health Promotion and Disease Prevention, *DHEW (PHS) Publication No. 79-55071*. Washington, DC, 1979, U.S. Government Printing Office.

US Department of Health and Human Services: Promoting Health/Preventing Disease: Objectives for the Nation. Washington, DC, 1980, U.S. Government Printing Office.

US Department of Health and Human Services (USDHHS): Healthy People 2000: National Health Promotion and Disease Prevention Objectives, *DHHS Publication No. 91-50212*. Washington, DC, 1991, U.S. Government Printing Office.

US Department of Health and Human Services, Bureau of Health Professions, Division of Nursing: Consensus Conference on the Essentials of Public Health Nursing Practice and Education [APHA Report Series]. Washington, DC, 1985, American Public Health Association.

US Department of Health and Human Services (USDHHS): Healthy People 2010: Understanding and Improving Health, ed 2. Washington, DC, 2000, U.S. Government Printing Office.

US Department of Health and Human Services (USDHHS): National Center for Health Statistics. Washington, DC, 2010.

US Department of Health and Human Services (USDHHS): Healthy People 2020: The Road Ahead. 2010. Retrieved November 2013 from: www.healthypeople.gov.

US Department of Health and Human Services(USDHHS): Healthy People 2030: Building a healthier future for all, Wash DC, 2020, US Government Printing Office.

US Public Health Service: The Core Functions Project. Washington, DC, 1994 [updated 2008], Office of Disease Prevention and Health Promotion.

Williams CA: Population-focused community health nursing and nursing administration: a new synthesis. In McCloskey JC, Grace HK, editors: *Current Issues in Nursing*, ed 2. Boston, 1985, Blackwell Scientific.

Woolf S, Aron L. Eds. US Health in International Perspective: Shorter Lives, Poorer Health.

2

The History of Public Health and Public and Community Health Nursing

Janna Dieckmann

OBJECTIVES

After reading this chapter, the student should be able to:

1. Discuss historical events that have influenced how current health care is delivered in the community.
2. Trace the ongoing interaction between the practice of public health and that of nursing.
3. Explain significant historical trends that have influenced the development of public health nursing.
4. Examine the contributions of Florence Nightingale, Lillian Wald, and Mary Breckinridge, and the influence

these three nursing leaders had on current public health and nursing.
5. Examine the ways in which nursing has been provided in the community, including settlement houses, visiting nurse associations, official health organizations, and schools.
6. Discuss the status of public health nursing in the 21st century, including the major organizations that have contributed to the current state of public health nursing.

CHAPTER OUTLINE

KEY TERMS

One of the best ways to understand today and plan for tomorrow is to examine the past. This is certainly true for public health and public health nursing. Nurses use historical approaches to examine both the profession's present and its future. Questions are asked: What worked in the past? What did not work? What lessons can be learned about health care, nursing, and the communities in which care is provided? During times of rapid social change, it is important to examine history and try to learn from the events of

the past and build on the events and actions that were effective, and learn from actions and events that were not effective. Current nursing roles in the United States developed from and were influenced by many factors including social, economic, political, and educational. This chapter serves as an introduction to an examination of the past in terms of both public health and nursing.

Historically public health nurses have worked to develop strategies to respond effectively to public health problems. Public health is an interdisciplinary specialty that emphasizes prevention. Nurses have worked in communities to improve the health status of individuals, families, and populations, especially those who belong to vulnerable groups. This work has not been easy for many reasons. One reason is that it is more difficult to measure the effects of prevention than it is to measure the effects of treatment. In recent years, as health care costs have grown, it has become increasingly important to emphasize prevention. There is currently an increased emphasis in public health nursing on population health as was discussed in Chapter 1 and throughout the text. Also the COVID-19 pandemic emphasized the critical role that public health principles and practices play in the health of citizens in the United States and around the world.

Many varied and challenging public health nursing roles originated in the late 1800s, when public health efforts focused on environmental conditions such as sanitation, control of communicable diseases, education for health, prevention of disease and disability, and care of aged and sick persons in their homes. Although the threats to health have changed over time, the foundational principles and goals of public health nursing have remained the same. Many communicable diseases, such as diphtheria, cholera, smallpox, and typhoid fever, have been largely controlled in the United States, but others, such as HIV, tuberculosis, hepatitis, and the emerging virus (flu) strains including the most recent, COVID-19, continue to affect many lives around the world. Certainly with COVID-19, the global nature of the transmission of disease has been evident and frightening. Even though environmental pollution in residential areas has been reduced, communities are now threatened by emissions from the many vehicles on their roads, overcrowded garbage dumps, and pollutants in the air, water, and soil. Natural disasters including hurricanes, tornadoes, floods, and fires continue to challenge public health systems, and bioterrorism and the many human-made disasters threaten to overwhelm existing resources. Research has identified means to avoid or postpone chronic disease, and nurses play an important role in helping implement strategies to modify individual and community risk factors and behaviors. Finally, with the increased numbers of older adults in the United States and their preference to remain at home, additional nursing services are required to sustain the frail, the disabled, and the chronically ill in the community.

Nurses who work in the community have done so to improve the health status of individuals, families, and populations, and they have paid particular attention to high-risk or vulnerable groups. Part of the appeal of public health nursing has been its autonomy of practice, independence in problem solving and decision-making, and the interdisciplinary nature of the specialty. This chapter describes the beginnings of public health, the role of nursing in the community, the contributions made by nurses to public health, and the influence of nurses on community health.

EARLY PUBLIC HEALTH

People in all cultures have been concerned with the events surrounding birth, illness, and death. They have tried to prevent, understand, and control disease. Their ability to preserve health and treat illness has depended on their knowledge of science, the use and availability of technologies, and the degree of social organization. For example, ancient Babylonians understood the need for hygiene and had some medical skills. The Egyptians in approximately 1000 BCE (before the Common Era) developed a variety of pharmaceutical preparations and constructed earth privies and public drainage systems. In England, the Elizabethan Poor Law of 1601 guaranteed assistance for poor, blind, and "lame" individuals. This minimal care was generally provided in almshouses supported by local government. The goal was to regulate the poor and provide a refuge during illness.

The Industrial Revolution in 19th-century Europe led to social changes while making great advances in technology, transportation, and communication. Previous caregiving structures, which relied on families, neighbors, and friends, became inadequate because of migration, urbanization, and increased demand. During this period, small numbers of Roman Catholic and Protestant religious women provided nursing care in institutions and sometimes in the home. Many lay women who performed nursing functions in almshouses and early hospitals in Great Britain were poorly educated and untrained. As the practice of medicine became more complex in the mid-1800s, hospital work required a more skilled caregiver. Physicians and community advocates wanted to improve the quality of nursing services. Early experiments led to some improvement in care, but it was because of the efforts of Florence Nightingale that health care was revolutionized when she founded the profession of nursing.

PUBLIC HEALTH DURING AMERICA'S COLONIAL PERIOD AND THE NEW REPUBLIC

In the early years of America's settlement, as in Europe, the care of the sick was usually informal and was provided by women. The female head of the household typically supervised care during sickness and childbirth and also grew and gathered healing herbs to use throughout the year. This traditional system of care became insufficient as the number of urban residents grew in the early 1800s.

British settlers in the New World influenced the American ideas of social welfare and care of the sick. Just as American law is based on English common law, colonial Americans established systems of care for the sick, poor, aged, mentally ill, and dependents based on England's Elizabethan Poor Law of 1601. Early county or township government was responsible for the care of all dependent residents but provided almshouse charity carefully, economically, and only for local residents. Travelers and people who lived elsewhere were returned to their native counties for care. Few hospitals existed and they were only in larger cities. Pennsylvania Hospital was founded in Philadelphia in 1751 and was the first hospital in what would become the United States.

Early colonial public health efforts included the collection of vital statistics, improvements to sanitation systems, and control of any communicable diseases brought in at the seaports. The colonists did not have a system to ensure that public health efforts were supported or enforced. Epidemics often occurred and strained the limited local organization for health during the 17th, 18th, and 19th centuries (Rosen, 1958).

After the American Revolution, the threat of disease, especially yellow fever, led to public support for establishing government-sponsored, or official, boards of health. By 1800, New York City, with a population of 75,000, had established public health services, which included monitoring water quality, constructing sewers and a waterfront wall, draining marshes, planting trees and vegetables, and burying the dead (Rosen, 1958).

Industrialization attracted increasing numbers of urban residents, leading to inadequate housing and sanitation complicated by epidemics of smallpox, yellow fever, cholera, typhoid, and typhus. Tuberculosis and malaria were always present, and infant mortality was approximately 200 per 1000 live births (Pickett and Hanlon, 1990). American hospitals in the early 1800s were generally unsanitary and staffed by poorly trained workers. Physicians had limited education, and medical care was scarce. Public dispensaries, similar to outpatient clinics, and private charitable efforts tried to provide some care for the poor.

The federal government focused its early public health work on providing health care for merchant seamen and protecting seacoast cities from epidemics. The Public Health Service, still the most important federal public health agency in the 21st century, was established in 1798 as the Marine Hospital Service. The first Marine Hospital opened in Norfolk, Virginia, in 1800. Additional legislation to establish quarantine regulations for seamen and immigrants was passed in 1878.

In the first half of the 1800s, some agencies began to provide lay nursing care in homes, including the Ladies' Benevolent Society of Charleston, South Carolina (Buhler-Wilkerson, 2001); lay nurses in Philadelphia; and visiting nurses in Cincinnati, Ohio (Rodabaugh and Rodabaugh, 1951). Although these programs provided useful services, they were not adopted elsewhere. Table 2.1 presents milestones of public health efforts that occurred during the 17th, 18th, and 19th centuries.

During the mid-19th century national interest increased in addressing public health problems and improving urban living conditions. New responsibilities for urban boards of health reflected changing ideas of public health as the boards began to address communicable diseases and environmental hazards. Soon after it was founded in 1847, the American Medical Association (AMA) formed a hygiene committee to conduct sanitary surveys and develop a system to collect vital statistics. The Shattuck Report, published in 1850 by the Massachusetts Sanitary Commission, was the first attempt to describe a model approach to the organization of public health in the United States. This report called for broad changes to improve the public's health: the establishment of a state health department and local health boards in every town; sanitary surveys and collection of vital statistics; environmental sanitation; food, drug, and communicable disease control; well-child care; health education; tobacco and alcohol control; town planning; and the teaching of preventive medicine in medical schools (Kalisch and Kalisch, 1995). It took 19 years for these recommendations to be implemented in Massachusetts, and they were added in other states much later.

In some areas, charitable organizations addressed the gap between known communicable disease epidemics and the lack of local government resources. For example, the Howard Association of New Orleans, Louisiana, responded to periodic yellow fever epidemics between 1837 and 1878 by providing physicians, lay nurses, and medicine for the sick. The Howard Association established infirmaries and used sophisticated outreach strategies to locate cases (Hanggi-Myers, 1995).

NIGHTINGALE AND THE ORIGINS OF TRAINED NURSING

Even with the growth of technology during this time, cities lacked important public health systems, such as sewage disposal, and also depended on private enterprise for water supply. Previous caregiving structures, which relied on the assistance of family, neighbors, and friends, became inadequate in the early 19th century because of human migration, urbanization, and changing demand. During this period, a few groups of Roman Catholic

TABLE 2.1	Milestones in the History of Community Health and Public Health Nursing: 1600–1865
Year	**Milestone**
1601	Elizabethan Poor Law written
1617	Sisterhood of the Dames de Charité organized in France by St. Vincent de Paul
1789	Baltimore Health Department established
1798	Marine Hospital Service established; later became Public Health Service
1812	Sisters of Mercy established in Dublin, Ireland, where nuns visited the poor
1813	Ladies Benevolent Society of Charleston, South Carolina, founded
1836	Lutheran deaconesses provided home visits in Kaiserswerth, Germany
1851	Florence Nightingale visited Kaiserswerth, Germany, for 3 months of nurse training
1855	Quarantine Board established in New Orleans; beginning of tuberculosis campaign in the United States
1859	District nursing established in Liverpool, England, by William Rathbone
1860	Florence Nightingale Training School for Nurses established at St. Thomas Hospital in London
1864	Beginning of Red Cross

and Protestant women provided nursing care for the sick, poor, and neglected in institutions and sometimes in the home. For example, Mary Aikenhead, also known by her religious name Sister Mary Augustine, organized the Irish Sisters of Charity in Dublin, Ireland, in 1815. These sisters visited the poor at home and established hospitals and schools (Kalisch and Kalisch, 1995).

Florence Nightingale's vision of trained nurses and her model of nursing education influenced the development of professional nursing and, indirectly, public health nursing in the United States. In 1850 and 1851, Nightingale studied the nursing "system and method" during an extended visit to Pastor Theodor Fliedner at his Kaiserswerth, Germany, School for Deaconesses. Her work with Pastor Fliedner and the Kaiserswerth Lutheran deaconesses, with their systems of district nursing, later led her to promote nursing care for the sick in their homes.

During the Crimean War (1854–1856), the British military established hospitals for sick and wounded soldiers in Scutari in Asia Minor. The care of soldiers was poor, with cramped quarters, poor sanitation, lice and rats, not enough food, and inadequate medical supplies (Kalisch and Kalisch, 1995; Palmer, 1983). When the British public demanded improved conditions, Florence Nightingale asked to work in Scutari. Because of her wealth, social and political connections, and knowledge of hospitals, the British government sent her to Asia Minor with 40 women, 117 hired nurses, and 15 paid servants. In Scutari, Nightingale progressively improved the soldiers' health using a population-based approach that improved both environmental conditions and nursing care. Using simple epidemiology measures, she documented a decreased mortality rate from 415 per 1000 at the beginning of the war to 11.5 per 1000 at the end (Cohen, 1984; Palmer, 1983). Like Nightingale and her efforts in Scutari, public health nurses today identify health care needs that affect the entire population. They then mobilize resources and organize themselves and the community to meet these needs.

After the Crimean War, Nightingale returned to England in 1856. Her fame was established. She organized nursing practices and nursing education in hospitals to replace untrained lay nurses with Nightingale nurses. Nightingale thought that nursing should promote health and prevent illness, and she emphasized proper nutrition, rest, sanitation, and hygiene (Nightingale, 1894, 1946). Each of these areas of her early emphasis remains important in the 21st century.

In 1859 British philanthropist William Rathbone founded the first district nursing association in Liverpool, England. His wife had received excellent care from a Nightingale nurse during her terminal illness. He wanted to provide similar care to poor and needy people. Together the work of Nightingale and Rathbone led to the organization of district nursing in England (Nutting and Dock, 1935).

During the last quarter of the 1800s, the number of jobs for women rapidly increased. Educated women became teachers, secretaries, or saleswomen, and less-educated women worked in factories. As it became more acceptable to work outside the home, women were more willing to become nurses. The first nursing schools based on the Nightingale model opened in the United States in the 1870s. The early graduate nurses worked as private duty nurses or were hospital administrators or instructors. The

private duty nurses often lived with the families for whom they cared. Because it was expensive to hire private duty nurses, only the well-to-do could afford their services. Community nursing began in an effort to meet urban health care needs, especially for the disadvantaged, by providing visiting nurses. In 1877 in New York City, trained nurse Francis Root was hired by a New York City mission to visit and care for the sick poor in their homes.

Visiting nurses took care of several families each day (rather than attending to only one client or family as the private duty nurse did), which made their care more economical. The visiting nurse became the key to communicating the prevention campaign, through home visits and well-baby clinics. Visiting nurses worked with physicians, gave selected treatments, and kept temperature and pulse records. Visiting nurses emphasized education of family members in the care of the sick and in personal and environmental prevention measures, such as hygiene and good nutrition (Fig. 2.1). The movement grew, and visiting nurse associations (VNAs) were established in Buffalo (1885), Philadelphia (1886), and Boston (1886). Wealthy people interested in charitable activities funded both settlement houses and VNAs. Wealthy upper-class women who were freed at this time from social restrictions were instrumental in doing charitable work and in supporting the early visiting nurses.

The public wanted to limit disease among all classes of people, partly for religious reasons, partly as a form of charity, but also because the middle and upper classes were afraid of diseases that were prevalent in the large communities of European immigrants. During the 1890s in New York City, about 2,300,000 people were packed into 90,000 tenement houses. The environmental conditions of immigrants in tenement houses and sweatshops were familiar features of urban life across the northeastern United States and upper Midwest. From the beginning, community nursing practice included teaching and prevention. Community interventions led to improved sanitation, economic improvements, and better nutrition. These interventions were credited with reducing the incidence of acute communicable disease by 1901.

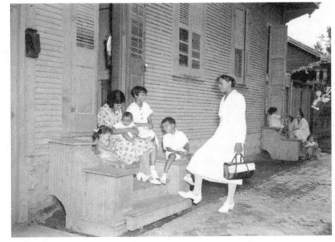

Fig. 2.1 New Orleans Nurse Visiting a Family on the Doorstep. (Courtesy New Orleans Public Library WPA Photograph Collection.)

In 1886 in Boston, two women, to improve their chances of gaining financial support for their cause, coined the term instructive district nursing to emphasize the relationship of nursing to health education. Support for these nurses was also secured from the Women's Education Association, and the Boston Dispensary provided free outpatient medical care. In February 1886, the first district nurse was hired in Boston, and in 1888 the Instructive District Nursing Association was incorporated as an independent voluntary agency (Brainard, 1922).

Other nurses established settlement houses and neighborhood centers, which became hubs for health care and social welfare programs. For example, in 1893 trained nurses Lillian Wald (Fig. 2.2) and Mary Brewster began visiting the poor on New York's Lower East Side. They established a nurses' settlement that became the Henry Street Settlement and later the Visiting Nurse Service of New York City. By 1905, public health nurses had provided almost 48,000 visits to more than 5000 clients (Kalisch and Kalisch, 1995). Lillian Wald emerged as a prominent leader of public health nursing during these decades (Box 2.1). Lillian Wald demonstrated an exceptional ability to develop approaches and programs to solve the health care and social problems of her times. We can learn much from her that can be applied to today's nursing practice.

Jessie Sleet (Scales), a Canadian graduate of Provident Hospital School of Nursing (Chicago), became the first African American public health nurse when the New York Charity Organization

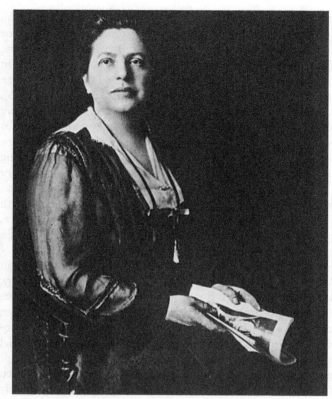

Fig. 2.2 Lillian Wald. (Courtesy Visiting Nurse Service of New York.)

BOX 2.1   Lillian Wald: First Public Health Nurse in the United States

Public health nursing evolved in the United States in the late 19th and early 20th centuries largely because of the pioneering work of Lillian Wald. Born on March 10, 1867, Lillian Wald decided to become a nurse after Vassar College refused to admit her at 16 years of age. She graduated in 1891 from the New York Hospital Training School for Nurses and spent the next year working at the New York Juvenile Asylum. To supplement what she thought had been inadequate training in the sciences, she enrolled in the Woman's Medical College in New York (Frachel, 1988).

Having grown up in a warm, nurturing family in Rochester, New York, her work in New York City introduced her to an entirely different side of life. In 1893, while conducting a class in home nursing for immigrant families on the Lower East Side of New York, Wald was asked by a small child to visit her sick mother. Wald found the mother in bed after childbirth, having hemorrhaged for 2 days. This home visit confirmed for Wald all of the injustices in society and the differences in health care for poor persons versus those persons able to pay (Frachel, 1988).

She believed poor people should have access to health care. With her friend Mary Brewster and the financial support of two wealthy laypeople, Mrs. Solomon Loeb and Joseph H. Schiff, she moved to the Lower East Side and occupied the top floor of a tenement house on Jefferson Street. This move eventually led to the establishment of the Henry Street Settlement. In the beginning, Wald and Brewster helped individual families. Wald believed that the nurse's visit should be friendly, more like a visit from a friend than from someone paid to visit (Dolan, 1978).

Wald used epidemiological methods to campaign for health-promoting social policies to improve environmental and social conditions that affected health. She not only wrote *The House on Henry Street* to describe her own public health

nursing work, but she also led in the development of payment by life insurance companies for nursing services (Frachel, 1988).

In 1909, along with Lee Frankel, Lillian Wald established the first public health nursing program for life insurance policyholders at the Metropolitan Life Insurance Company. She advocated that nurses at agencies such as the Henry Street Settlement provide complex nursing care. Wald convinced the company that it would be more economical to use the services of public health nurses than to employ its own nurses. She also convinced the company that services could be available to anyone desiring them, with fees scaled according to the ability to pay. This nursing service designed by Wald continued for 44 years and contributed several significant accomplishments to public health nursing, including the following (Frachel, 1988):

1. Providing home nursing care on a fee-for-service basis
2. Establishing an effective cost-accounting system for visiting nurses
3. Using advertisements in newspapers and on radio to recruit nurses
4. Reducing mortality from infectious diseases

Lillian Wald also believed that the nursing efforts at the Henry Street Settlement should be aligned with an official health agency. She therefore arranged for nurses to wear an insignia that indicated that they served under the auspices of the Board of Health. Also, she led the establishment of rural health nursing services through the Red Cross. Her other accomplishments included helping to establish the Children's Bureau and fighting in New York City for better tenement living conditions, city recreation centers, parks, pure food laws, graded classes for mentally handicapped children, and assistance to immigrants (Backer, 1993; Dock, 1922; Frachel, 1988; Zerwekh, 1992).

Data from Backer BA: Lillian Wald: connecting caring with action, *Nurs Health Care* 14:122–128, 1993; Dock LL: The history of public health nursing, *Public Health Nurs* 14:522, 1922; Dolan J: *History of nursing*, ed 14, Philadelphia, 1978, Saunders; Frachel RR: A new profession: the evolution of public health nursing, *Public Health Nurs* 5:86–90, 1988; and Zerwekh JV: Public health nursing legacy: historical practical wisdom, *Nurs Health Care* 13:84–91, 1992.

Society hired her in 1900. Although it was hard for her to find an agency willing to hire her as a district nurse, she persevered and was able to provide exceptional care for her clients until she married in 1909. At the Charity Organization Society in 1904 to 1905, she studied health conditions related to tuberculosis among African American people in Manhattan using interviews with families and neighbors, house-to-house canvassing, direct observation, and speeches at neighborhood churches. Sleet reported her research to the Society board, recommending improved employment opportunities for African Americans and better prevention strategies to reduce the excess burden of tuberculosis morbidity and mortality among the African American population (Buhler-Wilkerson, 2001; Hine, 1989; Mosley, 1994; Thoms, 1929). Her work laid the foundation for much of what has characterized public health nursing over the years.

The American Red Cross, through its Rural Nursing Service (later the Town and Country Nursing Service), initiated home nursing care in areas outside larger cities. Lillian Wald secured the initial donations to support this agency, which provided care to the sick, instruction in sanitation and hygiene in rural homes, and improved living conditions in villages and farms. These nurses dealt with diseases such as tuberculosis, pneumonia, and typhoid fever. By 1920, 1800 Red Cross Town and Country Nursing Services were in operation. This number eventually grew to almost 3000 programs in small towns and rural areas.

The emphasis of community nursing has varied and changed over time. In recent years, federal and state financing has influenced the growth or in recent years, the lack of growth. There has rarely been adequate funding to support a comprehensive public health nursing service. In addition to VNAs and settlement houses, a variety of other organizations sponsored visiting nurse work, including boards of education, boards of health, mission boards, clubs, churches, social service agencies, and tuberculosis associations. With tuberculosis then responsible for at least 10% of all mortality, visiting nurses contributed to its control through gaining "the personal cooperation of patients and their families" to modify the environment and individual behavior (Buhler-Wilkerson, 1987, p. 45). Most visiting nurse agencies depended financially on the philanthropy and social networks of metropolitan areas.

Occupational health nursing, originally called industrial nursing, grew out of early home visiting efforts. In 1895 Ada Mayo Stewart began work with employees and families of the Vermont Marble Company in Proctor, Vermont. As a free service for the employees, Stewart provided obstetrical care, sickness care (e.g., for typhoid cases), and some postsurgical care in workers' homes. However, she provided few services for work-related injuries. Although her employer provided a horse and buggy, she often made home visits on a bicycle. Before 1900 a few nurses were hired in industry, such as in department stores in Philadelphia and Brooklyn. Between 1914 and 1943, industrial nursing grew from 60 to 11,220 nurses, reflecting increased governmental and employee concerns for health and safety at work (American Association of Industrial Nurses, 1976; Kalisch and Kalisch, 1995).

School nursing was also an extension of home visiting. In New York City in 1902 more than 20% of children might be absent from school on a single day because of conditions such as pediculosis, ringworm, scabies, inflamed eyes, discharging ears, and infected wounds. Physicians began to make limited inspections of school students in 1897. They focused on excluding infectious children from school rather than on providing or obtaining medical treatment to enable children to return to school. Familiar with this community-wide problem from her work with the Henry Street Settlement, Lillian Wald introduced the English practice of providing nurses for the schools. Lina Rogers, a Henry Street Settlement resident, became the first school nurse. She worked with the children in New York City schools and made home visits to teach parents and to follow up on children absent from school. The school nurses found that many of the children were absent because they did not have shoes or clothing; many were hungry, and others had to take care of the younger children in the family (Hawkins, Hayes, and Corliss, 1994). School nursing was a success; New York City soon added 12 more nurses. School nursing was soon implemented in Los Angeles, Philadelphia, Baltimore, Boston, Chicago, and San Francisco. The scope of school nursing remains highly variable in the United States in the 21st century, and most school nurses are employed directly by a board of education.

CONTINUED GROWTH IN PUBLIC HEALTH NURSING

The *Visiting Nurse Quarterly,* begun in 1909 by the Cleveland Visiting Nurse Association, initiated a professional communication medium for clinical and organizational concerns. In 1911 a joint committee of existing nurse organizations led by Wald and Mary Gardner met to standardize nursing services outside the hospital. They recommended the formation of a new organization to address public health nursing concerns. Their committee invited 800 agencies involved in public health nursing activities to send delegates to an organizational meeting in Chicago in June 1912. After a heated debate on its name and purpose, the delegates established the National Organization for Public Health Nursing (NOPHN) and chose Wald as its first president (Dock, 1922). Unlike other professional nursing organizations, the NOPHN membership included both nurses and their lay supporters. The NOPHN, which worked "to improve the educational and services standards of the public health nurse, and promote public understanding of and respect for her work" (Rosen, 1958, p. 381), soon became the dominant force in public health (Roberts, 1955).

The NOPHN sought to standardize public health nursing education. At that time, newly graduated nurses often were unprepared for home visitation because the diploma schools emphasized care of hospital clients. Thus public health nurses needed education in how to care for the sick at home and to design population-focused programs. In 1914 Mary Adelaide Nutting, working with the Henry Street Settlement, began the first course for postdiploma school training in public health nursing at Teachers College in New York City (Deloughery, 1977). The American Red Cross provided scholarships for graduates of nursing schools to attend the public health nursing course. Its success encouraged the development of other programs, using curricula that might seem familiar to today's nurses. During the 1920s and 1930s, many newly hired public health nurses had to verify completion or promptly enroll in a certificate program in public health nursing. Others took leave for a year to travel to an urban center to obtain this further education. Correspondence courses (distance education) were even acceptable in some areas, for example, for public health nurses in upstate New York.

Public health nurses were active in the American Public Health Association (APHA), which was established in 1872 to facilitate interprofessional efforts and promote the "practical application of public hygiene" (Scutchfield and Keck, 1997, p. 12). The APHA focused on important public health issues, including sewage and garbage disposal, occupational injuries, and sexually transmitted diseases. In 1923 the Public Health Nursing Section (PHNS) was formed within the APHA to provide nurses with a national forum to discuss their concerns and strategies within the larger context of the major public health organization. The PHNS continues to serve as a focus of leadership and policy development for public health nursing.

Public health nursing in voluntary agencies and through the Red Cross grew more quickly than public health nursing supported by local, state, and national government. By 1900, 38 states had established state health departments, following the lead of Massachusetts in 1869; however, these early state boards of health had limited impact because only three states—Massachusetts, Rhode Island, and Florida—annually spent more than 2 cents per capita for public health services (Scutchfield and Keck, 1997).

The federal role in public health gradually expanded. In 1912 the federal government redefined the role of the US Public Health Service, empowering it to "investigate the causes and spread of diseases and the pollution and sanitation of navigable streams and lakes" (Scutchfield and Keck, 1997, p. 15). The NOPHN loaned a nurse to the US Public Health Service during World War I to establish a public health nursing program for military outposts. This led to the first federal government sponsorship of nurses (Shyrock, 1959; Wilner, Walkey, and O'Neill, 1978).

During the 1910s public health organizations began to target infectious and parasitic diseases in rural areas. For example, in 1911 efforts to control typhoid fever in Yakima County, Washington, and to improve health status in Guilford County, North Carolina, led to the establishment of local health units to serve local populations. Public health nurses were the primary staff members of local health departments. These nurses assumed a leadership role on health care issues through collaboration with local residents, nurses, and other health care providers.

The experience of Orange County, California, during the 1920s and 1930s illustrates the growing importance of the nurse in the community. Based on the work of a private physician, social welfare agencies, and a Red Cross nurse, the county board created the public health nurse's position in 1922. Presented with a shining new Model T car sporting the bright orange seal of the county, the nurse began her work by dealing with the serious communicable disease problems of diphtheria and scarlet fever. Typhoid became epidemic when a drainage pipe overflowed into a well, infecting those who drank the water and those who drank raw milk from an infected dairy. Almost 3000 residents were immunized against typhoid. At weekly well-baby conferences, the nurse weighed infants and gave them immunizations and taught mothers how to care for the infants. Also, children with orthopedic disorders and other disabilities were identified and referred for medical care in Los Angeles. The first year of this public health nursing work was so successful that the Rockefeller Foundation and the California Health Department provided funds for more public health professionals.

PUBLIC HEALTH NURSING DURING THE EARLY 20TH CENTURY

The personnel needs of World War I in Europe depleted the ranks of public health nurses, even as the NOPHN identified a need for second and third lines of defense within the United States. Jane Delano in 1909 was appointed both as superintendent of the Army Nurse Corps and chairman of the National Committee on Red Cross Nursing services. She was instrumental in preparing nurses to serve in the military, and she also supported the need for public health nurses to stay at home and serve the needs of those not serving in the military. Over 3 weeks in 1918 the worldwide influenza pandemic swept across the United States. A coalition of the NOPHN and the Red Cross worked to turn houses, churches, and social halls into hospitals for the immense numbers of sick and dying. Some of the nurse volunteers died of influenza. In 2020 we see the same situations occurring with locations for care increasing outside the hospital and with health care workers contracting COVID-19. As the pandemic that began in 2019 spread, public health departments assumed a key role in administering vaccines to groups in priority areas.

Limited funding during the early 20th century was an obstacle to extending nursing services in the community. Most early VNAs relied on contributions from wealthy and middle-class supporters. Consistent with the goal of encouraging economic independence, poor families were asked to pay a small fee for nursing services. In 1909 with encouragement from Lillian Wald in collaboration with Dr. Lee Frankel, the Metropolitan Life Insurance Company began a program using visiting nurse organizations to provide care for sick policyholders. The nurses assessed illness, taught health practices, and collected data from policyholders. By 1912, 589 Metropolitan Life nursing centers provided care through existing agencies or visiting nurses hired directly by the company. In 1918 Metropolitan Life calculated an average decline of 7% in the mortality rate of policyholders and almost a 20% decline in the mortality rate of policyholders' children under the age of 3 years. The insurance company attributed this improvement and its reduced costs to the work of visiting nurses.

Nurses also influenced public policy by advocating for the Children's Bureau and the Sheppard-Towner Program. Wald and other nursing leaders urged that the Children's Bureau be established in 1912 to address national problems of maternal and child welfare. Children's Bureau experts conducted extensive scientific research on the effects of income, housing, employment, and other factors on infant and maternal mortality. Their research led to federal child labor laws and the 1919 White House Conference on Child Health. The Sheppard-Towner Act of 1921, which focused on maternal and infant health, was credited with saving many lives. This act provided federal matching funds to establish maternal and child health divisions in state health departments. Education during home visits by public health nurses emphasized promoting the health of the mother and child and encouraged mothers to seek prompt medical care during pregnancy. Although credited with saving many lives, the program ended in 1929 in response to charges by the AMA and others that the legislation gave too much power to the federal government and too closely resembled socialized medicine (Pickett and Hanlon, 1990). Just as we see today, there has long been an inability to provide public health services because of the lack of funds.

Some nursing innovations were the result of individual commitment and private financial support. In 1925 Mary Breckinridge established the Frontier Nursing Service (FNS). This creative service was based on systems of care in Scotland (Box 2.2 and Fig. 2.3). The pioneering spirit of the FNS influenced the development of public health programs to improve the health care of the rural and often inaccessible populations in the Appalachian region of southeastern Kentucky (Browne, 1966; Tirpak, 1975). Breckinridge introduced the first nurse-midwives into the United States when she deployed FNS nurses trained in nursing, public health, and midwifery. Their efforts

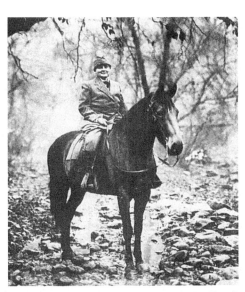

Fig. 2.3 Mary Breckinridge, Founder of the Frontier Nursing Service. (Courtesy Frontier Nursing Service of Wendover, Kentucky.)

led to reduced pregnancy complications and maternal mortality and to one-third fewer stillbirths and infant deaths in an area of 700 square miles (Kalisch and Kalisch, 1995). Today the FNS continues to provide comprehensive health and nursing services to the people of that area and sponsors the Frontier Nursing University.

BOX 2.2 Mary Breckinridge and the Frontier Nursing Service

Born in 1881 into the fifth generation of a well-to-do Kentucky family, Mary Breckinridge devoted her life to the establishment of the Frontier Nursing Service (FNS). Learning from her grandmother, who used a large part of her fortune to improve the education of Southern children, Breckinridge later used money left to her by her grandmother to start the FNS (Browne, 1966).

Tutored in childhood and later attending private schools, Mary Breckinridge did not consider becoming a nurse until her husband died. At that time she wanted to have more adventure in her life and to find opportunities to do something useful for others (Hostutler et al., 2000). In 1907 she enrolled at St. Luke's Hospital School of Nursing in New York. She later married for a second time and had two children. Her second marriage ended after her daughter died at birth and her son died at age 4. From the time of her son's death in 1918, she devoted her energy to promoting the health care of disadvantaged women and children (Browne, 1966).

After World War I and work in postwar France, she returned to the United States, passionate about helping the neglected children of rural America. To prepare herself for what would become her life's work, she studied for a year at Teacher's College, Columbia University, to learn more about public health nursing (Browne, 1966).

Early in 1925 she returned to Kentucky. She decided that the mountains of Kentucky were an excellent place to demonstrate the value of community health nursing to remote, disadvantaged families. She thought that if she could establish a nursing center in rural Kentucky, this effort could then be duplicated anywhere. The first health center was established in a five-room cabin in Hyden, Kentucky. Establishing the center took not only nursing skills but also the construction of the

center and later the hospital and other buildings; it required extensive knowledge about developing a water supply, disposing of sewage, getting electric power, and securing a mountain area in which landslides occurred (Browne, 1966). Despite many obstacles inherent in building in the mountains, six outpost nursing centers were established between 1927 and 1930. The FNS hospital was built in Hyden, Kentucky, and physicians began entering service. Payment of fees ranged from labor and supplies to funds raised through annual family dues, philanthropy, and the fund-raising efforts of Mary Breckinridge (Holloway, 1975).

The FNS established medical, surgical, and dental clinics; provided nursing and midwifery services 24 hours a day; and served nearly 10,000 people spread over 700 square miles. Baseline data were obtained on infant and maternal mortality before beginning services. FNS services are especially remarkable considering the environmental conditions in which rural Kentuckians lived. Many homes had no heat, electricity, or running water. Often physicians were located more than 40 miles from their patients (Tirpak, 1975).

During the 1930s, nurses lived in one of the six outposts, from which they traveled to see clients; they often had to make their visits on horseback. Like her nurses, Mary Breckinridge traveled many miles through the mountains of Kentucky on her horse, Babette, providing food, supplies, and health care to mountain families (Browne, 1966).

Over the years, several hundred nurses have worked for the FNS. Although Mary Breckinridge died in 1965, the FNS has continued to grow and provide needed services to people in the mountains of Kentucky. This service continues today as a vital and creative way to deliver community health services to rural families.

Data from Browne H: A tribute to Mary Breckinridge, *Nurs Outlook* 14:54–55, 1966; Goan MB: *Mary Breckinridge: the frontier nursing service and rural health in Appalachia*, Chapel Hill, NC, 2008, The University of North Carolina Press; Holloway JB: Frontier Nursing Service 1925–1975, *J Ky Med Assoc* 73:491–492, 1975; Hostutler J, Kennedy MS, Mason D, et al: Nurses: then and now and models of practice, *Am J Nurs* 100:82–83, 2000; Tirpak H: The Frontier Nursing Service: fifty years in the mountains, *Nurs Outlook* 33:308–310, 1975.

AFRICAN AMERICAN NURSES IN PUBLIC HEALTH NURSING

African American nurses seeking to work in public health nursing faced many challenges. Nursing education was segregated in the South until the 1960s and elsewhere was also generally segregated or rationed until the mid-20th century. Even public health nursing certificate and graduate education programs were segregated in the South; study outside the South for Southern nurses was difficult to afford, and study leaves from the workplace were rarely granted. The situation improved somewhat in 1936 when collaboration between the US Public Health Service and the Medical College of Virginia (Richmond) established a certificate program in public health nursing for African American nurses, for which the federal government paid nurses' tuition. Discrimination continued during nurses' employment: African American nurses in the South were paid lower salaries than their white counterparts for the same work. In 1925 only 435 African American public health nurses were employed in the United States, and in 1930 only 6 African American nurses held supervisory positions in public health nursing organizations (Buhler-Wilkerson, 2001; Hine, 1989; Thoms, 1929).

African American public health nurses significantly influenced the communities they served (Fig. 2.4). The National Health Circle for Colored People was organized in 1919 to promote public health work in African American communities in the South. One strategy adopted was providing scholarships to assist African American nurses in pursuing university-level public health nursing education. Bessie M. Hawes, the first recipient of the scholarship, completed the program at Columbia University (New York) and was then sent by the Circle to Palatka, Florida. In this small, isolated lumber town, Hawes's first project was to recruit schoolgirls to promote health by dressing as nurses and marching in a parade while singing community

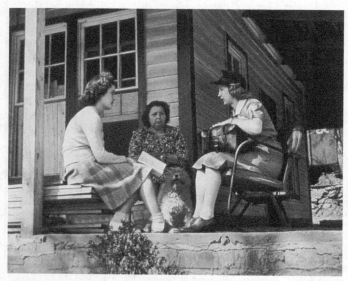

Fig. 2.4 A Public Health Nurse Talks with a Young Woman and her Mother About Childbirth as They Sit on a Porch. (US Public Health Service photo by Perry. Images from the *History of Medicine*, National Library of Medicine, Image ID 157037.)

songs. She conducted mass meetings, led clubs for mothers, provided school health education, and visited the homes of the sick. Eventually she gained the community's trust, overcame opposition, and built a health center for nursing care and treatment (Thoms, 1929).

ECONOMIC DEPRESSION AND THE IMPACT ON PUBLIC HEALTH

The economic depression of the 1930s affected the development of nursing. Not only were agencies and communities unprepared to address the increased needs and numbers of the impoverished, but decreased funding for nursing services reduced the number of employed nurses in hospitals and in community agencies. Federal funding led to a wide variety of programs administered at the state level, including new public health nursing programs; as a result of NOPHN's enormous efforts, public health nursing was included in federal relief programs.

The Federal Emergency Relief Administration (FERA) supported nurse employment through increased grants-in-aid for state programs of home medical care. FERA often purchased nursing care from existing visiting nurse agencies, thus supporting more nurses and preventing agency closures. The FERA program focus varied among states; the state FERA program in New York emphasized bedside nursing care, whereas in North Carolina, the state FERA prioritized maternal and child health and school nursing services. The public health nursing programs of the FERA and its successor, the Works Progress Administration (WPA), were sometimes later incorporated into state health departments.

In another Depression-era initiative, more than 10,000 nurses were employed by the Civil Works Administration (CWA) programs and assigned to official health agencies. "While this facilitated rapid program expansion by recipient agencies and gave the nurses a taste of public health, the nurses' lack of field experience created major problems of training and supervision for the regular staff" (Roberts and Heinrich, 1985, p. 1162).

A 1932 survey of public health agencies found that only 7% of nurses employed in public health were adequately prepared for that role (Roberts and Heinrich, 1985). Basic nursing education emphasized the care of individuals, and students received little information on groups and the community as a unit of service. Thus in the 1930s and early 1940s, new graduates required considerable remedial education when they were hired into public health work (NOPHN, 1944).

During this period, tension persisted between preventive care and care of the sick and the related question of whether nursing interventions should be directed toward groups and communities or toward individuals and their families. Although each nursing agency was unique and services varied from region to region, voluntary VNAs tended to emphasize care of the sick, and official public health agencies provided more preventive services. Not surprisingly, this splintering of services led to a rivalry between "visiting," or community, and "public health" nurses and interfered with the development of comprehensive community nursing services (Roberts and Heinrich, 1985). For example, one household could receive services from several community nurses representing different agencies, with separate visits for a postpartum woman and new baby, for a child sick with scarlet fever, and for an elderly bedridden person. This was confusing and costly, with duplicated services.

One solution was to establish the "combination service," which merged sick-care services and preventive services into one comprehensive agency by combining visiting nurse and official public health agencies. However, in contrast to visiting nurse organizations, public health nurses in official health agencies often had less control of the program because physicians and politicians determined services and the assignment of personnel. The "ideal program" of the combination agency was hard to administer, and many of the combination services implemented between 1930 and 1965 later reverted to their former, divided structures of visiting nurse agencies and official health departments.

Expansion of federal government programs during the 1930s affected the structure of community health resources and led to "the beginning of a new era in public nursing" (Roberts and Heinrich, 1985, p. 1162). In 1933 Pearl McIver became the first nurse employed by the US Public Health Service. In providing consultation services to state health departments, McIver was convinced that the strengths and ability of each state's director of public health nursing would determine the scope and quality of local health services. Together with Naomi Deutsch, director of nursing for the federal Children's Bureau, and with the support of nursing organizations, McIver and her staff of nurse consultants influenced the direction of public health nursing. Between 1931 and 1938 over 40% of the increase in public health nurse employment was in local health agencies. Even so, nationally, more than one-third of all counties still lacked local public health nursing services (Fig. 2.5).

The Social Security Act of 1935 was designed to prevent recurrence of the problems of the Depression. Title VI of this act provided funding for expanded opportunities for health protection and promotion through education and employment of public health nurses. In 1936 more than 1000 nurses completed educational programs in public health. Title VI also provided $8 million to assist states, counties, and medical districts to establish and maintain adequate health services, as well as $2 million for research and investigation of disease (Buhler-Wilkerson, 1985, 1989; Kalisch and Kalisch, 1995).

In the late 1930s and especially in the late 1940s, Congress supported categorical funding to provide federal money for priority diseases or groups rather than for a comprehensive community health program. In response, local health departments designed programs to fit the funding priorities. This included maternal and child health services and crippled children (1935), venereal disease control (1938), tuberculosis (1944), mental health (1947), industrial hygiene (1947), and dental health (1947) (Scutchfield and Keck, 1997). This pattern of funding continues today.

World War II increased the need for nurses both for the war effort and at home. Many nurses joined the US Army and Navy Nurse Corps. US Representative Frances Payne Bolton of Ohio led Congress to pass the Bolton Act of 1943, which established the Cadet Nurses Corps. This legislation funded increased undergraduate and graduate enrollment in schools of nursing, and many of the students studied public health.

Because of the number of nurses involved in the war, civilian hospitals and visiting nurse agencies shifted care to families and nonnursing personnel. "By the end of 1942, over 500,000 women had completed the American Red Cross home nursing course, and nearly 17,000 nurse's aides had been certified" (Roberts and Heinrich, 1985, p. 1165). By the end of 1946, more than 215,000 volunteer nurse's aides had received certificates. During this time, community health nursing expanded its scope of practice. For example, more community health nurses practiced in rural areas, and many official agencies began to provide bedside nursing care (Buhler-Wilkerson, 1985; Kalisch and Kalisch, 1995).

After the war the need increased for services from local health departments to respond to sudden increases in demand for care of emotional problems, accidents, alcoholism, and other responsibilities new to official health agencies. Changes in medical technology improved the ability to screen and treat infectious and communicable diseases. Penicillin, which was developed during the war, became available to treat civilians with rheumatic fever, venereal diseases, and other infections. Job opportunities for public health nurses increased, and nurses comprised a major portion of health department staff. More than 20,000 nurses worked in health departments, VNAs, industry, and schools. Table 2.2 highlights significant milestones in community and public health nursing from the mid-1800s to the mid-1900s.

FROM WORLD WAR II UNTIL THE 1970s

Between 1900 and 1955, the national crude mortality rate decreased by 47%. Many more Americans survived childhood and early adulthood to live into middle and older ages. In 1900 the leading causes of mortality were pneumonia, tuberculosis, diarrhea, and enteritis. By midcentury the leading causes were heart disease, cancer, and cerebrovascular disease. Nurses helped reduce communicable disease mortality through immunization campaigns, nutrition education, and provision of better hygiene and sanitation. Additional factors included improved medications, better housing, and innovative emergency and critical care services.

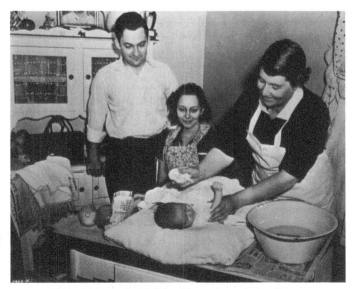

Fig. 2.5 A Nurse from the Visiting Nurse Association Demonstrates Proper Infant Care and Bathing Techniques to the Parents.

TABLE 2.2   Milestones in the History of Community Health and Public Health Nursing: 1866–1944

Year	Milestone
1866	New York Metropolitan Board of Health established
1872	American Public Health Association established
1873	New York Training School opened at Bellevue Hospital, New York City, as first Nightingale-model nursing school in the United States
1877	Women's Board of the New York Mission hired Frances Root to visit the sick poor
1885	Visiting Nurse Association established in Buffalo
1886	Visiting nurse agencies established in Philadelphia and Boston
1893	Lillian Wald and Mary Brewster organized a visiting nursing service for the poor of New York, which later became the Henry Street Settlement; Society of Superintendents of Training Schools of Nurses in the United States and Canada was established (in 1912 it became known as the National League for Nursing Education)
1896	Associated Alumnae of Training Schools for Nurses established (in 1911 it became the American Nurses Association)
1902	School nursing started in New York; Lina Rogers was the first school nurse
1903	First nurse practice acts
1909	Metropolitan Life Insurance Company initiated the first insurance reimbursement for nursing care
1910	Public health nursing program instituted at Teachers College, Columbia University, in New York City
1912	National Organization for Public Health Nursing formed, with Lillian Wald as the first president
1914	First undergraduate nursing education course in public health offered by Adelaide Nutting at Teachers College
1918	Vassar Camp School for Nurses organized; US Public Health Service (USPHS) established division of public health nursing to work in the war effort; worldwide influenza epidemic began
1919	Textbook *Public Health Nursing* written by Mary S. Gardner
1921	Maternity and Infancy Act (Sheppard-Towner Act)
1925	Frontier Nursing Service using nurse-midwives established
1934	Pearl McIver becomes the first nurse employed by USPHS
1935	Passage of the Social Security Act
1941	Beginning of World War II
1943	Passage of the Bolton-Bailey Act for nursing education; Cadet Nurse Program established; Division of Nursing begun at USPHS; Lucille Petry appointed chief of the Cadet Nurse Corps
1944	First basic program in nursing accredited as including sufficient public health content

Increasing numbers of older adults also increased the population at risk for chronic diseases. Nurses now dealt with challenges related to chronic illness care, long-term illness and disability, and chronic disease prevention. In official health agencies, categorical programs focusing on a single chronic disease emphasized narrowly defined services, which might be poorly coordinated with other community programs. Screening for chronic illness was a popular method of both detecting undiagnosed disease and providing individual and community education.

Some VNAs adopted coordinated home-care programs to provide complex, long-term care to the chronically ill, often after long-term hospitalization. These home-care programs established a multidisciplinary approach to complex client care. For example, beginning in 1949, the Visiting Nurse Society of Philadelphia provided care to clients with strokes, arthritis, cancer, and fractures using a wide range of services, including physical and occupational therapy, nutrition consultation, social services, laboratory and radiographic procedures, and transportation. During the 1950s, often in response to family demands and the shortage of nurses, many visiting nurse agencies began experimenting with auxiliary nursing personnel, variously called housekeepers, homemakers, or home health aides. These innovative programs provided a substantial basis

for an approach to bedside nursing care that would be reimbursable by commercial health insurance (such as Blue Cross) and later by Medicare and Medicaid.

During the 1930s and 1940s, more Americans chose to obtain care in hospitals because this was where physicians worked and where technology was readily available to diagnose and treat illness. Health insurance programs now allowed middle-class people to pay for care in hospitals. In 1952 the Metropolitan Life Insurance Company and the John Hancock Life Insurance Company ended their support of visiting nurse services for their policyholders, and the American Red Cross ended its programs of direct nursing service.

Nursing organizations also continued to change. The functions of the NOPHN, the National League for Nursing Education, and the Association of Collegiate Schools of Nursing were distributed to the new National League for Nursing (NLN) in 1952. The American Nurses Association (ANA) continued as the second national nursing organization, after merging with the National Association for Colored Graduate Nurses in 1951.

In 1948 the NLN adopted the recommendations of Esther Lucile Brown's study of nursing education, Nursing for the Future, and this considerably influenced how nurses were prepared. She recommended that basic nursing education take place in colleges and universities. In the 1950s, public health nursing became a required part of most baccalaureate nursing education programs. In 1952 nursing education programs began in junior and community colleges. Louise McManus, a director of the Division of Nursing Education at Teachers College, Columbia University, wanted to see if bedside nurses could be prepared in a 2-year program. The intent was to prepare nurses more quickly than in the past to ease the prevailing nursing shortage (Kalisch and Kalisch, 1995). This would also move more nursing education into American higher education. Mildred Montag, an assistant professor of nursing education at Teacher's College, became the project coordinator. In 1958, when the 5-year study was completed, this experiment was determined to be a success.

EVIDENCE-BASED PRACTICE

Prior to the 20th century, public health nursing emerged from district nursing as described earlier in the chapter. Early in the 20th century the emphasis on preventive care grew. This was a period of growing industrialization and urbanization, considerable immigration, and the growth of infectious diseases. A series of federal programs began that influenced public health nursing. However, despite program expansion, public health nurses still lacked field experience, training, and supervision. The Social Security Act of 1935 strengthened state health organizations and focused on extending services to mothers and children in rural and distressed areas. The next shift was away from direct care to one of education. Following World War II there was an increased need for nurses to meet the needs of families in the community. The health problems of the past took on new forms, and there was a growing body of knowledge that prevention was essential for a healthy nation. The Patient Protection and Affordable Care Act of 2010 was to ensure affordable, accessible, and high-quality health care for the uninsured and those who had inadequate health insurance. This act emphasized preventive care and management of chronic diseases. The relationship between policy, funding, and public health nursing is evident throughout history. The pendulum of what was funded in public health tends to swing from one focus area to another. This article provides detailed information about the changes in public health and public health nursing from 1890 to 1950.

Nurse Use

The influence of nursing should be valued and understood within the context of the time it was being practiced. Students who have an appreciation of nursing's past have a better understanding of nursing and who nurses are. With knowledge of the history of nursing, students can better understand that they are entering a profession with a rich and diverse past and that this can provide a firm platform on which to base their other studies. By studying the history of nursing, they also develop their critical thinking skills, which allows them to question and evaluate information that is presented to them on a daily basis. Students can also learn how policy, economics, and politics influence the direction that public health takes.

From Kub J, Kulbok P, Glick D: Cornerstone documents, milestones, and policies: shaping the direction of Public Health Nursing 1890–1950, *OJIN: Online J Issues Nurs* 20(2):Manuscript 3, 2015.

Currently, associate degree nursing (ADN) programs educate the largest percentage of nurses. Both health care and ADN education have changed; both have moved away from a heavy focus on inpatient care to community-based care. Curricula in ADN programs often include content and clinical experiences in management, community health, home health, and gerontology. These clinical areas have typically been key components of baccalaureate education. The American Association of Colleges of Nursing (AACN) was founded in 1969 to respond to the need for an organization that would further nursing education in American universities and 4-year colleges, including establishing essentials of nursing education for baccalaureate and higher-degree programs.

New personnel also added to the flexibility of the public health nurse to address the needs of communities. Beginning in 1965 at the University of Colorado, the nurse practitioner movement opened a new era for nursing involvement in primary care that affected the delivery of services in community health clinics. Initially, the nurse practitioner was often a public health nurse with additional skills in the diagnosis and treatment of common illnesses. Although some nurse practitioners chose to practice in other clinical areas, those who continued in public health settings made sustained contributions to improving access and providing primary care to people in rural areas, inner cities, and other medically underserved areas (Roberts and Heinrich, 1985). As evidence of the effectiveness of their services grew, nurse practitioners became increasingly accepted as cost-effective providers of a variety of primary care services.

PUBLIC HEALTH NURSING FROM THE 1970s TO THE PRESENT

During the 1970s, nurses made many contributions to improving the health care of communities, including participation in the new hospice movement and through the development of birthing centers, daycare for elderly and disabled persons, drug-abuse treatment programs, and rehabilitation services in long-term care. Adequate funding for population health remained difficult to secure. Growing costs of acute hospital care, medical procedures, and institutional long-term care reduced funding for health promotion and disease prevention programs. The use of ambulatory services, including health maintenance organizations, was encouraged, and utilization of nurse practitioners (advanced-practice nurses) increased. Despite unstable reimbursement, home health care increased its role in the care of the sick at home. By the 1980s, individuals and families assumed more responsibility for their own health, and health education—always a part of community health nursing—became more popular. Consumer and professional advocacy groups urged the passage of laws to prohibit unhealthy practices in public, such as smoking and driving under the influence of alcohol. However, reduced federal and state funds led to decreases in the number of nurses in official public health agencies.

The Division of Nursing of the US Public Health Service conducted and sponsored nursing research beginning in the late 1930s. This expanded in the late 1940s (Uhl, 1965). The National Center for Nursing Research (NCNR) was established in 1985 within the federal National Institutes of Health. The NCNR focused attention on the value of nursing research and promoted the work of nurses. With the effort of many nurses, the NCNR attained institute (rather than center) status in 1993 and became the National Institute of Nursing Research (NINR), reflecting the continued growth in nursing research.

By the late 1980s the public health initiative had declined in its ability to implement its mission and influence the health of the public. The disarray resulting from reduced political support, financing, and effectiveness was clearly described by the Institute of Medicine (IOM) in *The Future of Public Health* (IOM, 1988). Although many people agreed about what the mission of public health should be, there was much less agreement about how to turn the mission of public health into action and effective programs. The IOM report emphasized the core functions of public health as assessment, policy development, and assurance.

The *Healthy People* initiative has influenced goals and priority setting in public health and in public health nursing. In 1979 *Healthy People* proposed a national strategy to improve the health of Americans by preventing or delaying the onset of major chronic illnesses, injuries, and infectious diseases. Specific goals and objectives were established, and the goals were to be evaluated at the end of each decade. Implementation of these strategies has considerably influenced the work of nurses, through their employment in health agencies and through participation in state or local *Healthy People* coalitions (*Healthy People* box). *Healthy People 2020* (US Department of Health and Human Services, 2010) built on the work of *Healthy People 2010* (US Department of Health and Human Services, 2000). Some objectives in *Healthy People 2010* were met; others retained in *Healthy People 2020*, and new ones were added. *Healthy People 2030* built on the work of the previous four editions of *Healthy People*. *Healthy People 2030* objectives are included in each chapter of this text.

Since the 1990s, public concerns about health have focused on cost, quality, and access to services. Despite widespread interest in universal health insurance coverage, neither individuals nor employers are willing to pay for this level of service. The core debate of the economics of health care—who should pay for what—has emphasized the need for reform of medical care rather than comprehensive reform of health care. In 1993 a blue-ribbon group assembled by President Bill Clinton, with First Lady Hillary Rodham Clinton serving as chair, proposed the American Health Security Act. This proposal led to broad discussion of the key issues and concerns in health care, especially the organization and delivery of medical care, with an emphasis on managed care. When Congress failed to pass the American Health Security Act, considerable change followed in health care financing, and the private sector assumed even greater control. As managed care grew, costs were contained, but constraints increased in terms of how to access care and how much and what kind of care would be reimbursed. Throughout these debates, public health was generally ignored. Little attention was given to ensuring that populations and the communities in which they lived were healthy. This omission reflected the large gap between the proposal and actual comprehensive health care reform.

In 1991 the ANA, AACN, NLN, and more than 60 other specialty nursing organizations joined to support health care reform. The coalitions of organizations emphasized the key health care issues of access, quality, and cost. Improved primary care and public health efforts would help build a healthy nation. Professional nursing continues to support revisions in health

care delivery and extension of public health services to prevent illness, promote health, and protect the public (Table 2.3). Chapters 3 (Global and U.S. Public Health Systems) and 5 (Economic Influences) describe the current work to change the way health is provided and who pays for the care.

 ### HEALTHY PEOPLE 2030

History of the Development of Healthy People

In 1979 the groundbreaking *Healthy People: The Surgeon General's Report on Health Promotion and Disease Prevention* stated "the health of the American people has never been better" (US Department of Health, Education and Welfare, 1979, p. 3). But this was only the prologue to deep criticism of the status of American health care delivery. Between 1960 and 1978, health care spending increased 700%—without striking improvements in mortality or morbidity. During the 1950s and 1960s, evidence accumulated about chronic disease risk factors, particularly cigarette smoking, alcohol and drug use, occupational risks, and injuries. But these new research findings were not systematically applied to health planning and to improving population health.

In 1974 the Canadian government published A New Perspective on the Health of Canadians (Lalonde, 1974), which found death and disease to have four contributing factors: inadequacies in the existing health care system, behavioral factors, environmental hazards, and human biological factors. Applying the Canadian approach, in 1976, US experts analyzed the 10 leading causes of US mortality and found that 50% of American deaths were the result of unhealthy behaviors, and only 10% were the result of inadequacies in health care. Rather than just spending more to improve hospital care, clearly, prevention was the key to saving lives, improving the quality of life, and saving health care dollars.

A multidisciplinary group of analysts conducted a comprehensive review of prevention activities. These analysts verified that the health of Americans could be significantly improved through "actions individuals can take for themselves" and through actions that public and private decision makers could take to "promote a safer and healthier environment" (p. 9). Like Canada's New Perspectives, in the United States *Healthy People* (1979) identified priorities and measurable goals. *Healthy People* grouped 15 key priorities into three categories: key preventive services that could be delivered to individuals by health providers, such as timely prenatal care; measures that could be used by governmental agencies, organizations, and industry to protect people from harm, such as reduced exposure to toxic agents; and activities that individuals and communities could use to promote healthy lifestyles, such as improved nutrition.

In the late 1980s, success in addressing these priorities and goals was evaluated, new scientific findings were analyzed, and new goals and objectives were set for the period from 1990 to 2000 through *Healthy People 2000: National Health Promotion and Disease Prevention Objectives* (US Public Health Service, 1991). This process has been repeated every 10 years to develop goals and objectives for the period from 2000 to 2010; 2010 to 2020; and 2020 to 2030. Recognizing the continuing challenge of the use of emerging scientific research to encourage modification of health behaviors and practices, *Healthy People 2030* (US Department of Health and Human Services, USDHHS 2020) was released August 18, 2020. This document builds on the knowledge gained over the past 4 decades and addresses the most current public health priorities and challenges. The ways in which *Healthy People 2030* was developed and how it has been changed since *Healthy People 2020* are discussed in the Preface of the text. In brief, *Healthy People 2030* is more concise and has fewer objectives than were in *Healthy People 2020* in order to make it easier for users to find the objectives relevant to their work.

Like the nurse in the early 20th century who spread the gospel of public health to reduce communicable diseases, today's population-centered nurse uses *Healthy People* to reduce chronic and infectious diseases and injuries through health education, environmental modification, and policy development.

TABLE 2.3 Milestones in the History of Community Health and Public Health Nursing: 1946–2021

Year	Milestone
1946	Nurses classified as professionals by US Civil Service Commission; Hill-Burton Act approved, providing funds for hospital construction in underserved areas and requiring these hospitals to provide care to poor people; passage of National Mental Health Act
1950	25,091 nurses employed in public health
1951	National nursing organizations recommended that college-based nursing education programs include public health content
1952	National Organization for Public Health Nursing merged into the new National League for Nursing; Metropolitan Life Insurance Nursing Program closed
1964	Passage of the Economic Opportunity Act; public health nurse defined by the American Nurses Association (ANA) as a graduate of a bachelor of science in nursing (BSN) program
1965	ANA position paper recommended that nursing education take place in institutions of higher learning; Congress amended the Social Security Act to include Medicare and Medicaid
1977	Passage of the Rural Health Clinic Services Act, which provided indirect reimbursement for nurse practitioners in rural health clinics
1978	Association of Graduate Faculty in Community Health Nursing/Public Health Nursing (later renamed Association of Community Health Nursing Educators)
1980	Medicaid amendment to the Social Security Act to provide direct reimbursement for nurse practitioners in rural health clinics; both ANA and the American Public Health Association (APHA) developed statements on the role and conceptual foundations of community and public health nursing, respectively
1983	Beginning of Medicare prospective payments
1985	National Center for Nursing Research (NCNR) established within the National Institutes of Health (NIH)
1988	Institute of Medicine published *The Future of Public Health*
1990	Association of Community Health Nursing Educators published *Essentials of Baccalaureate Nursing Education*
1991	More than 60 nursing organizations joined forces to support health care reform and published a document entitled *Nursing's Agenda for Health Care Reform*
1993	American Health Security Act of 1993 was published as a blueprint for national health care reform; the national effort, however, failed, leaving states and the private sector to design their own programs
1993	NCNR became the National Institute for Nursing Research, as part of the National Institutes of Health
1993	Public Health Nursing section of the American Public Health Association updated the definition and role of public health nursing
1996	Passage of the Health Insurance Portability and Accountability Act
2001	Significant interest in public health ensues from concerns about biological and other forms of terrorism in the wake of the intentional destruction of buildings in New York City and Washington, DC, on September 11
2002	Office of Homeland Security established to provide leadership to protect against intentional threats to the health of the public
2003–2005	Multiple natural disasters, including earthquakes, tsunamis, and hurricanes, demonstrated the weak infrastructure for managing disasters in the United States and other countries and emphasized the need for strong public health programs that included disaster management
2007	An entirely new Public Health Nursing Scope and Standards of Practice released through the ANA, reflecting the efforts of the Quad Council of Public Health Nursing Organizations
2010	Patient Protection and Affordable Care Act signed by President Barack Obama; *Healthy People 2020* realized by the US Department of Health and Human Services
2011	The Quad Council of Public Health Nursing Organizations published *Competencies for Public Health Nursing*
2013	The American Nurses Association published the second edition of *Public Health Nursing: Scope and Standards of Practice*
2013	The Quad Council of Public Health Nursing Organizations updated *Competencies for Public Health Nursing Practice*
2018	The Quad Council of Community/Public Health Nursing updated *Community/Public Health Nursing Competences;* the USDHHS approved the *Healthy People 2030* framework.
2020	Beginning of the COVID-19 virus in Wuhan, China with subsequent spread around the world; declaration of a pandemic by the World Health Organization on March 11, 2020

During the late 20th and early 21st centuries, challenges continued to trigger growth and change in nursing in the community. Nurse-managed centers now provide a range of nursing services, including health promotion and disease and injury prevention, in areas where existing organizations have been unable to meet community and neighborhood needs. These centers provide valuable services but typically face many challenges in securing adequate funding.

The Affordable Care Act of 2010 has been controversial, and many compromises were made between the House of Representatives and the Senate in the final crafting of this health care act. Much of the Affordable Care Act deals with changes in insurance plans and coverage, and it continues to be controversial with continued debate among congressional members.

Public health nursing, historically and at present, is characterized by reaching out to care for the health of people in need and providing safe and quality care where needed. Currently, many nurses work in the community. Some bring a public health population-based approach and have as their goal preventing illness and protecting health. Other nurses have a community-oriented approach and deal primarily with the health care of individuals, families, and groups in a community. Still other nurses bring a community-based approach that focuses on "illness care" of individuals and families in the community. Each type of nurse is needed in today's communities. It is important that we learn from the past and use time and resources carefully and effectively. Regardless of the level of education of the nurse who provides care in the community, including population-based care, all nurses need to provide care that is safe and of high quality. The accompanying box below describes the history of the Quality and Safety Education for Nurses (QSEN) initiative, which aims to include quality and safety knowledge, skills, and attitudes in all levels of nursing education.

QSEN FOCUS ON QUALITY AND SAFETY EDUCATION FOR NURSES

Although the scope and responsibilities of public health nurses have changed over time, the commitment to quality and safety has remained constant. Since the beginning of population-centered nursing in the United States, the nurses involved in this specialty have been committed to preserving health and preventing disease. They have focused on environmental conditions such as sanitation and control of communicable diseases, education for health, prevention of disease and disability, and, at times, care of the sick and aged in their homes. This long-standing commitment to quality and safety is consistent with the work of the QSEN, a national initiative designed to transform nursing education by including in the curriculum content and experiences related to building knowledge, skills, and attitudes for six quality and safety initiatives (Cronenwett, Sherwood, and Gelmon, 2009). The QSEN work, led by Drs. Linda Cronenwett and Gwen Sherwood at the University of North Carolina, has made great progress in bridging the gap between quality and safety in both practice and academic settings (Brown, Feller, and Benedict, 2010). The six QSEN competencies for nursing are as follows:

1. Patient-centered care: Recognizes the client or designee as the source of control and as a full partner in providing compassionate and coordinated care that is based on the preferences, values, and needs of the client.
2. Teamwork and collaboration: Refers to the ability to function effectively with nursing and interprofessional teams and to foster open communication, mutual respect, and shared decision making to provide quality client care.
3. Evidence-based practice: Integrates the best current clinical evidence with client and family preferences and values to provide optimal client care.
4. Quality improvement: Uses data to monitor the outcomes of the care processes and uses improvement methods to design and test changes to continually improve the quality and safety of health care systems.
5. Safety: Minimizes the risk of harm to clients and providers through both system effectiveness and individual performance.
6. Informatics: Uses information and technology to communicate, manage knowledge, mitigate error, and support decision making (Brown et al., 2010, p. 116).

Of the six QSEN competencies, all but safety were derived from the IOM report *Health Professions Education* (2003). The QSEN team added safety because this competency is central to the work of nurses. Articles have been published to teach educators about QSEN, and national forums have been held. In addition, the AACN has hosted faculty-development institutes for faculty and academic administrators using a train-the-trainer model, and safety and quality objectives have been built in the AACN essentials for nursing education. Similarly, the NLN has incorporated the "NLN Educational Competencies Model" into its educational summits. The six QSEN competencies are integrated throughout the text to emphasize the importance of quality and safety in public health nursing today. Note: The terms *patient* and *care* will be changed to *client* and *intervention* to reflect a public health nursing approach.

Specifically related to the history of nursing, the following targeted competency can be applied:

Targeted Competency: Safety—Minimizes the risk of harm to clients and providers through both system effectiveness and individual performance.

Important aspects of safety include the following:

- Knowledge: Discuss potential and actual impact of national client safety resources initiatives and regulations
- Skills: Participate in analyzing errors and designing system improvements
- Attitudes: Value vigilance and monitoring by clients, families, and other members of the health care team

Safety Question

Updated definitions around client safety include addressing safety at the individual level and at the systems level. The history of public health nursing demonstrates the myriad ways that public health nurses have addressed client safety in their evolving practice. Public health nurses support safety by caring for individuals and providing care for communities and groups. Historically, how have public health nurses addressed safety at the individual client level? How have public health nurses addressed client safety at the systems level? How have public health nurses been involved in system improvements?

Answer: Individual level: A rich part of public health nursing's history has been the development of home visitation, in which clients are cared for in their own environment. Similarly, public health nurses have improved client outcomes by pioneering new models of interventions for maternal–child health and individuals in rural communities.

Systems level: Through their work with communities, public health nurses were an integral part of reducing the incidence of communicable diseases by the mid-20th century. More recently, public health nursing has contributed to health care system improvements through the development of the hospice movement, birthing centers, daycare for elderly and disabled persons, and drug abuse and rehabilitation services. These initiatives have updated the health care system to provide targeted care for previously overlooked populations.

Prepared by Gail Armstrong, PhD, DNP, ACNS-BC, CNE, professor and assistant dean of the DNP Program, Oregon Health and Sciences University.

Today, nurses look to their history for inspiration, explanations, and predictions. Information and advocacy are used to promote a comprehensive approach to addressing the multiple needs of the diverse populations served. Nurses seek to learn from the past and to avoid known pitfalls, even as they seek successful strategies to meet the complex needs of today's vulnerable populations. The How To box describes how to conduct an oral history interview. This is one effective way to learn from the successes and failures of our predecessors.

HOW TO CONDUCT AN ORAL HISTORY INTERVIEW

1. Identify an issue or event of interest.
2. Gather information from written materials.
3. Find a person to interview.
4. Get permission from the person to do the interview, and make an appointment to do so.
5. Gather information about the person's background and the period of interest.
6. Write an outline of your questions. Use open-ended questions because they usually give you more information.
7. Meet with the person being interviewed; use a recording device. Ask for permission to record the interview.
8. Conduct the interview by asking only one question at a time and allowing adequate time for the reply.
9. Clarify points when needed; ask for examples; remember, most people like to talk about themselves.
10. After the interview, write it up as soon as possible, when your recall is best.
11. Compare your written report with the audio recording. There may be times when you can ask the person interviewed to read your report for accuracy.

As plans for the future are made, as the public health challenges that remain unmet are acknowledged, it is the vision of what nursing can accomplish that sustains these nurses. Nurses continue to rely on both nursing and public health standards and competency guides to help chart their practice.

The ANA's (2013) *Scope and Standards of Public Health Nursing Practice*, the Council on Linkages' (2014) *Domains and Core Competencies*, and the Quad Council's (Quad Council Coalition Competency Review Task Force, 2018) *Community/Public Health Nursing(C/PHN) Competencies* provide guidance for the practice of community/public health nursing.

▶ **APPLYING CONTENT TO PRACTICE**

Public Health Nursing, a major journal in the field of public health nursing, publishes articles that broadly reflect contemporary research, practice, education, and public policy for population-based nurses. Begun in 1984, *Public Health Nursing* was published quarterly through 1993 and has been a bimonthly journal since 1994.

More than any other journal, *Public Health Nursing* has assumed responsibility for preserving the history of public health nursing and for publishing new historical research on the field. The contemporary *Public Health Nursing* shares its name with the official journal of the NOPHN in the period 1931 to 1952 (earlier names were used for the official journal from 1913 to 1931, which built on the *Visiting Nurse Quarterly*, published 1909 to 1913).

Public Health Nursing presents a wide variety of articles, including both new historical research and reprints of classic journal articles that deserve to be read and reapplied by modern public health nurses. Original historical research presented in *Public Health Nursing* is varied, from public health nursing education, to public health nurse practice in Alaska's Yukon, to excerpts from the oral histories of public health nurses. Contemporary nurses find inspiration and possibilities for modern innovations in reading the history of public health nursing in the pages of *Public Health Nursing*.

THE ORIGIN AND PROGRESSION OF COVID-19

On December 31, 2019, the government in Wuhan, Hubei Province, China, released the first official report that multiple cases of pneumonia were being treated. On January 12, 2020, it was disclosed that a new virus not seen in humans had been detected. The theory was that the virus originated in a Wuhan market where live fish and animals were sold, and that the virus was transmitted to humans. The first case of the virus in Washington was confirmed January 20, 2020 in a man who had recently traveled there from Wuhan. On March 11, 2020, the World Health Organization declared the virus, which is now known as COVID-19, a pandemic. Since that time, the virus has spread around the world. The countries that have had fewer cases were those that immediately began the three recommended practices to protect a person against the virus: handwashing, social distancing, and wearing a face mask. Some of these countries, despite their best public health practices, have seen up and down surges of the virus. Some countries forced businesses such as restaurants and bars to close; others established distancing rules for these establishments. In the United States, some states imposed a mask rule while others did not do so.

▮ PRACTICE APPLICATION

Mary Lipsky has worked for a VNA in a large urban area for 2 years. She is responsible for a wide variety of services, including caring for older and chronically ill clients recently discharged from hospitals, new mothers and babies, mental health clients, and clients with long-term health problems, such as chronic wounds.

Daily when she leaves the field to go home, she finds that she continues to think about her clients. She keeps going over these and other questions in her mind: Why is it so difficult for mothers and new babies to qualify for and receive Special Supplemental Nutrition Program for Women, Infants, and Children (WIC) services? Why must she limit the number of visits and length of service for clients with chronic wounds? Why are so few services available for clients with behavioral health problems? In particular, she thinks about the burdens and challenges that families and friends face in caring for the sick at home.

A. Why might it be difficult to solve these problems at the individual level, on a case-by-case basis?
B. What information would you need to build an understanding of the policy background for each of these various populations? ***Answers can be found on the Evolve website.***

▮ REMEMBER THIS!

- A historical approach can be used to increase the understanding of public and community health nursing.
- Public health and community health nursing are products of various social, economic, and political forces and incorporate public health science in addition to nursing science and practice.
- Federal responsibility for health care was limited until the 1930s, when the economic challenges of the Depression highlighted the need for and led to the expansion of federal assistance for health care.
- Florence Nightingale designed and implemented the first program of trained nursing, and her contemporary, William Rathbone, founded the first district nursing association in England.

- Urbanization, industrialization, and immigration in the United States increased the need for trained nurses, especially in public and community health nursing.
- The increasing acceptance of public roles for women permitted public and community health nursing employment for nurses and public leadership roles for their wealthy supporters.
- Frances Root was the first trained nurse in the United States who was salaried as a visiting nurse. She was hired in 1887 by the Women's Board of the New York City Mission to provide care to sick persons at home.
- The first VNAs were founded in 1885 and 1886 in Buffalo, Philadelphia, and Boston.
- Lillian Wald established the Henry Street Settlement, which became the Visiting Nurse Service of New York City, in 1893. She played a key role in innovations that shaped public and community health nursing in its first decades, including school nursing, insurance payment for nursing, national organizations for public health nurses, and the US Children's Bureau.
- Founded in 1902, with the vision and support of Lillian Wald, school nursing tried to keep children in school so that they could learn.
- The Metropolitan Life Insurance Company established the first insurance-based program in 1909 to support community health nursing services.
- The NOPHN (founded in 1912) provided essential leadership and coordination of diverse public and community health nursing efforts; the organization merged into the new NLN in 1952.
- Official health agencies slowly grew in numbers between 1900 and 1940, accompanied by a steady increase in public health nursing positions.
- The Sheppard-Towner Act of 1921 expanded community health nursing roles for maternal and child health during the 1920s.
- Mary Breckinridge established the FNS in 1925 to provide rural health care.
- The tension between the nursing roles of caring for the sick and of providing preventive care and the related tension between intervening for individuals and for groups have characterized the specialty since at least the 1910s.
- The challenges of World War II sometimes resulted in extension of community health nursing care and sometimes in retrenchment and decreased public health nursing services.
- By the mid-20th century, the reduced incidence of communicable diseases and the increased prevalence of chronic illness, accompanied by large increases in the population older than 65 years of age, led to a reexamination of the goals and organization of community health nursing services.
- From the 1930s to 1965, organized nursing and community health nursing agencies sought to establish health insurance reimbursement for nursing care at home.
- Implementation of Medicare and Medicaid programs in 1966 established new possibilities for supporting community-based nursing care but encouraged agencies to focus on postacute-care services rather than prevention.
- Efforts to reform health care organization, pushed by increased health care costs during the past 40 years, have focused on reforming acute medical care rather than on designing a comprehensive preventive approach.
- The 1988 *The Future of Public Health* report documented the reduced political support, financing, and impact of increasingly limited public health services at the national, state, and local levels.
- By the late 1990s federal policy changes dangerously reduced financial support for home health care services, threatening the long-term survival of visiting nurse agencies.
- The *Healthy People* program has brought a renewed emphasis on prevention to public and community health nursing.
- In 2011 the Quad Council, an alliance of four national nursing organizations that addresses public health nursing issues, finalized its own set of public health nursing competencies. These competencies were revised in 2013 and again in 2018.
- The five versions of *Healthy People*; recent disasters and acts of terrorism; and the Patient Protection and Affordable Care Act of 2010 have brought a renewed emphasis on the benefits of both public health and nursing.

EVOLVE WEBSITE

http://evolve.elsevier.com/Stanhope/foundations
- NCLEX Review Questions
- Practice Application Answers

REFERENCES

American Association of Industrial Nurses: *The nurse in industry: a history of the American Association of Industrial Nurses, Inc*, New York, 1976, AAIN.

American Nurses Association: *Public health nursing: scope and standards of practice*, Silver Spring, MD, 2013, ANA.

Backer BA: Lillian Wald: connecting caring with action, *Nurs Health Care* 14:122–128, 1993.

Brainard A: *Evolution of public health nursing*, Philadelphia, 1922, Saunders.

Brown R, Feller L, Benedict L: Reframing nursing education: the Quality and Safety Education for Nurses Initiative, *Teach Learn Nurs* 5:115–118, 2010.

Browne H: A tribute to Mary Breckinridge, *Nurs Outlook* 14:54–55, 1966.

Buhler-Wilkerson K: Public health nursing: in sickness or in health? *Am J Pub Health* 75:1155–1161, 1985.

Buhler-Wilkerson K: Left carrying the bag: experiments in visiting nursing. 1977-1909, *Nurs Res* 36:42–45, 1987.

Buhler-Wilkerson K: *False dawn: the rise and decline of public health nursing, 1900-1930*, New York, 1989, Garland Publishing.

Buhler-Wilkerson K: *No place like home: a history of nursing and home care in the United States*, Baltimore, 2001, Johns Hopkins.

Cohen IB: Florence Nightingale, *Sci Am* 3:128–137, 1984.

Council on Linkages between Academic and Public Health Practice: *Core competencies for public health professionals*, Washington DC, 2014, Public Health Foundation, Health Resources and Services Administration.

Cronenwett, L, Sherwood, G, Gelmon, SB: Improving quality and safety education: the QSEN learning collaborative, *Nurs Outlook* 57:304–312, 2009.

Deloughery GL: *History and trends of professional nursing*, ed 8, St. Louis, 1977, Mosby.

Dock LL: The history of public health nursing, *Public Health Nurs*, 1922. (Reprinted by the American Public Health Association).

Dolan J: *History of nursing*, ed 14, Philadelphia, 1978, Saunders.

Frachel RR: A new profession: the evolution of public health nursing, *Public Health Nurs* 5:86–90, 1988.

Goan MB: *Mary Breckinridge: The frontier nursing service and rural health in Appalachia*, Chapel Hill, NC, 2008, The University of North Carolina.

Hanggi-Myers L: The Howard Association of New Orleans: precursor to district nursing, *Public Health Nurs* 12:78, 1995.

Hawkins JW, Hayes ER, Corliss CP: School nursing in America: 1902–1994—a return to public health nursing, *Public Health Nurs* 11:416–425, 1994.

Hine DC: *Black women in white: racial conflict and cooperation in the nursing profession, 1890-1950*, Bloomington, 1989, Indiana University Press.

Holloway JB: Frontier nursing service 1925–1975, *J Ky Med Assoc* 73:491–492, 1975.

Hostutler J, Kennedy MS, Mason D, et al: Nurses: then and now and models of practice, *Am J Nurs* 100:82–83, 2000.

Institute of Medicine: *The future of public health*, Washington, DC, 1988, National Academy of Science.

Institute of Medicine: *Health Professions Education*, Washington, DC, 2003, National Academy of Science.

Kalisch PA, Kalisch BJ: *The advance of American nursing*, ed 3, Philadelphia, 1995, Lippincott.

Lalonde M: *New perspective on the health of Canadians*, Ottawa, ON, 1974, Government of Canada.

Kub, J., Kulbok, P., Glick, D (May 31, 2015) "Cornerstone Documents, Milestones, and Policies: Shaping the Direction of Public Health Nursing 1890-1950" *OJIN: The Online Journal of Issues in Nursing* Vol 20, No 2, Manuscript 3.

Mosley MOP: Jessie Sleet Scales: first black public health nurse, *ABNF J* 5:45, 1994.

National Organization for Public Health Nursing: Approval of Skidmore College of Nursing as preparing students for public health nursing, *Public Health Nurs* 36:371, 1944.

Nightingale F: Sick nursing and health nursing. In Billings JS, Hurd HM, editors: *Hospitals, dispensaries, and nursing*, Baltimore, 1894, Johns Hopkins. (Reprinted New York, 1984, Garland.)

Nightingale F: *Notes on nursing: what it is, and what it is not*, Philadelphia, 1946, Lippincott.

Nutting MA, Dock LL: *A history of nursing*, New York, 1935, GP Putnam's Sons.

Palmer IS: *Florence Nightingale and the first organized delivery of nursing services*, Washington, DC, 1983, American Association of Colleges of Nursing.

Pickett G, Hanlon JJ: *Public health: administration and practice*, St. Louis, 1990, Mosby.

Quad Council Coalition Competency Review Task Force. (2018). *Community/Public Health Nursing Competencies*, Washington DC.

Roberts DE, Heinrich J: Public health nursing comes of age, *Am J Public Health* 75:1162–1172, 1985.

Roberts M: *American nursing: history and interpretation*, New York, 1955, Macmillan.

Rodabaugh JH, Rodabaugh MJ: *Nursing in Ohio: a history*, Columbus, Ohio, 1951, Ohio State Nurses Association.

Rosen G: *A history of public health*, New York, 1958, MD Publications.

Scutchfield FD, Keck CW: *Principles of public health practice*, Albany, NY, 1997, Delmar.

Shyrock H: *The history of nursing*, Philadelphia, 1959, Saunders.

Thoms AB: *Pathfinders: a history of the progress of colored graduate nurses*, New York, 1929, Kay Printing House.

Tirpak H: The Frontier Nursing Service: fifty years in the mountains, *Nurs Outlook* 33:308–310, 1975.

Uhl G: The Division of Nursing: USPHS, *Am J Nurs* 65:82–85, 1965.

US Department of Health, Education and Welfare: *Healthy People: the Surgeon General's report on health promotion and disease prevention*, DHEW Pub no. 79-55071, Washington, DC, 1979, US Government Printing Office.

US Public Health Service: *Healthy People 2000: national health promotion and disease prevention objectives*, Washington, DC, 1991, US Government Printing Office

US Department of Health and Human Services: *Healthy People 2010: understanding and improving health*, Washington, DC, 2000, US Government Printing Office.

US Department of Health and Human Services: *Healthy People 2020: a roadmap to improve America's health*, Washington, DC, 2010, US Government Printing Office.

US Department of Health and Human Services: *Healthy People 2030*, Washington, DC, 2020, USDHHS, Public Health Service.

Wilner DM, Walkey RP, O'Neill EJ: *Introduction to public health*, ed 7, New York, 1978, Macmillan.

Zerwekh JV: Public health nursing legacy: historical practical wisdom, *Nurs Health Care* 13:84–91, 1992.

3

US and Global Health Care

Emma McKim Mitchell and Marcia Stanhope

OBJECTIVES

After reading this chapter, the student should be able to:

1. Describe the events and trends that influence the status of the global and US health care systems.
2. Discuss key aspects of the private health care system.
3. Compare the public health system to primary care.
4. Explain the model of primary health care globally including the United States.
5. Assess the effects of health care and insurance reform on health care delivery.
6. Evaluate the changes needed in public health and primary care to have an integrated health care delivery system.

CHAPTER OUTLINE

KEY TERMS

In September 1978, an international conference was held in the city of Alma-Ata, which at that time was the capital of the Soviet Republic of Kazakhstan. During this conference the Declaration of Alma-Ata and the primary health care model emerged (see https://www.who.int/publications/almaata_declaration_en.pdf). This declaration states that health is a human right and that the health of its people should be the primary goal of every government. One of the main themes of this declaration was the involvement of community health workers and traditional healers in a new health system (World Health Organization [WHO], 1978).

Primary health care (PHC) was introduced, defined, and described. In 2008 the WHO renewed its call for health care improvements and reemphasized the need for public policy makers, public health officials, primary care providers, and leadership within countries to improve health care delivery. The WHO said: "Globalization is putting the social cohesion of many countries under stress, and health systems … are clearly not performing as well as they could and should. People are increasingly impatient with the inability of health services to deliver. … Few would disagree that health systems need to respond better—and faster—to the challenges of a changing world. PHC can do that" (WHO, 2008). (See www.who.int/health. topics/primary health care for more information.)

As defined by the WHO, PHC reflects and evolves from the economic conditions and sociocultural and political characteristics of the country, its populations, and its communities and is based on the application of social, biomedical, and health services research and public health experience. It addresses the main health problems in the community, providing for health promotion, disease prevention, and curative and rehabilitative services (WHO, 1978).

Therefore PHC promotes the integration of all health care systems within a community to come together to improve the health of the community, including primary care and public health.

HEALTH CARE IN THE UNITED STATES

Despite the fact that health care costs in the United States are the highest in the world and make up the greatest percent of the gross domestic product, the indicators of what constitutes good health do not document that Americans are really getting a good return on their investment. In the first decade of the twenty-first century there have been massive and unexpected changes to health, economic, and social conditions as a result of terrorist attacks, hurricanes, fires, floods, infectious diseases, and the 2020 economic recession, often referred to as an economic downturn, due to the COVID-19 outbreak (Smialek, 2020). New systems have been developed to prevent and/or deal with most of the onslaught of these horrendous events. Not all of the systems have worked, including those for containing COVID-19, and many are regularly criticized for their inefficiency and costliness. Simultaneously, new, nearly miraculous advances have been made in treating health-related conditions. Advances in medicine and nursing are keeping people alive who only a few years ago would have suffered and died. These advances save and

prolong lives, and a number of deadly and debilitating diseases have been eliminated through effective immunizations and treatments. There are considerable initiatives to develop vaccines to contain COVID-19, but outcomes cannot yet be predicted. National and global health outcomes have improved through sanitation, clean water supplies, better nutrition, and genetic engineering.

However, attention to all of these advances may overshadow the lack of attention to public health, health promotion, and disease prevention. Several of the most destructive health conditions can be prevented through changes in lifestyle, health screenings, and/or immunizations. The increasing rates of obesity, especially among children; substance use; lack of exercise; violence; and accidents are alarmingly expensive, particularly when they lead to disruptions in health.

This chapter describes a health care system in transition as it struggles to meet evolving global and domestic needs and challenges. The overall health care and public health systems in the United States are described and differentiated, and the changing priorities are discussed. Nurses play a pivotal role in meeting these needs, and the role of the nurse is described. An introduction to global health is provided.

FORCES STIMULATING CHANGE IN THE DEMAND FOR HEALTH CARE

In recent years, enormous changes have occurred in society, in the United States and most other countries of the world. The extent of interaction among countries is stronger than ever, and the economy of each country depends on the stability of other countries. The United States has felt the effects of rising labor costs, and many companies have shifted their production outside the United States to reduce labor costs. It is often less expensive to assemble clothes, automobile parts, and appliances, and to have call distribution centers and call service centers in a less industrialized country and pay the shipping and other charges involved, than to have the items fully assembled in the United States. In recent years the vacillating cost of fuel has affected almost every area of the economy, leading to both higher costs of products and layoffs as some industries have struggled to stay solvent. This has affected the employment rate in the United States. The economic downturn of 2020 left many people unemployed, and many lost their homes because they could not pay their mortgages. When the unemployment rate is high, more people lack comprehensive insurance coverage, since in the United States this has been typically provided by employers. In 2008 the US unemployment rate was 5.8%. In 2012 the unemployment rate had increased to 8.1%, close to double the rate in 2007. In 2016 the rate dropped to 4.9%, and in 2017, 4.4% (Bureau of Labor Statistics [BLS], 2018a). In 2020, with the US shutting down many businesses because of the COVID-19 pandemic, as well as schools and social gatherings, the unemployment rate was 14.7%, the highest since the Great Depression, and it bounced down to 10.2% in July with some businesses opening .

In addition to changes in the labor market, health care services and the ways in which they are financed changed after the implementation of the Patient Protection and Affordable Care Act (ACA, enacted in 2010; Rosenbaum 2011). The ACA continues to be a hot topic for policy debates within the US government. However, with unemployment at record highs, the Affordable Care Act has several options for purchasing health care coverage, and the federal/state partnership to provide Medicaid is an additional option.

Demographic Trends

The population of the world is growing as a result of changing fertility and decreased mortality rates. The greatest growth is occurring in less developed countries, and this is accompanied by decreased growth in the United States and other developed countries. According to historical data of the Centers for Disease Control and Prevention (CDC), the US total fertility rate has been below the replacement level in 43 of the last 45 years (2018). Population replacement level means that for every person who dies, another is born (Hamilton and Kirmeyer, 2017). Both the size and the characteristics of the population contribute to the changing demography.

Seventy-seven million babies were born between the years of 1946 and 1963, giving rise to the often-discussed baby boomer generation (Office for National Statistics, 2014). The oldest of these boomers reached 65 years of age in 2011, and they are expected to live longer than people born previously. The impact on the federal government's insurance program for people 65 years of age and older, Medicare, is expected to be enormous. Medicare spending is projected to grow the fastest among the major health insurance categories between 2021 and 2026, averaging 7.7%. Sustained Medicare growth in both enrollment and per enrollee spending contributes to the spending increase above the 5.7% projected for the national health spending (CMS, 2018).

In 2020 the US population was 331,002,651 people, representing 4.2% of the world's population and the third most populated country in the world, following China and India. From 1960 to 2018 the US foreign-born immigrant population grew from 4.5% of the total population to 13.7%. The future growth rate is likely to be impacted by policy changes implemented at the federal level (US Census Bureau, 2018; Pew, 2020).

According to the Census Bureau (2018), the United States population is made up of 76.3% whites, 18.5% Hispanic or Latino, 13.4% Black or African American, 5.9% Asian, and 2.8% claiming two or more races.

The composition of the US household is also changing. From 1935 to 2016, mortality for both genders in all age groups and races declined (Heron, 2018) as a result of progress in public health initiatives, such as antismoking campaigns, acquired immunodeficiency syndrome (AIDS) prevention programs, and cancer screening programs. Over the last century the leading causes of death have shifted from infectious diseases to chronic and degenerative diseases (NCHS, 2017). The top 10 causes of death in 2016 were diseases of heart; malignant neoplasms; accidents (unintentional injuries); chronic lower respiratory diseases; cerebrovascular diseases; Alzheimer disease; diabetes mellitus; influenza and pneumonia; nephritis, nephrotic syndrome and nephrosis; and intentional self-harm (suicide). These causes accounted for 74% of all deaths in the United States (Heron, 2018).

New infectious diseases are emerging, based on transmission rates throughout the United States and globally. With the exception of COVID-19, new treatments for infectious diseases have resulted in steady declines in mortality among children, as long as parents participate in immunization programs. Recent measles outbreaks throughout the United States and the COVID-19 pandemic demonstrates that continuous focus on control of infectious diseases is essential. The mortality for older Americans has also declined. However, people 50 years of age and older have higher rates of chronic and degenerative illness, and they use a larger portion of health care services than other age groups. The older age groups were also more likely to die from COVID-19 than other age groups in 2020.

Social and Economic Trends

In addition to the size and changing age distribution of the population, other factors also affect the health care system. Several social trends that influence health care include changing lifestyles, a growing appreciation of the quality of life, the changing composition of families and living patterns, changing household incomes, and a revised definition of quality health care.

Americans spend considerable money on health care, nutrition, and fitness (Bureau of Labor Statistics, 2018b), because health is seen as an irreplaceable commodity. To be healthy, people must take care of themselves. Many people combine traditional medical and health care practices with complementary and alternative therapies to achieve the highest level of health. Complementary therapies are those that are used in addition to traditional health care, and alternative therapies are those used instead of traditional care. Examples include acupuncture, herbal medications, and more (National Center for Complementary and Integrative Health, 2017). People often spend a considerable amount of their own money for these types of therapies because few are covered by insurance. In recent years some insurance plans have recognized the value of complementary therapies and have reimbursed for them. State offices of insurance are good sources to determine whether these services are covered and by which health insurance plans.

About 75 years ago income was distributed in such a way that a relatively small portion of households earned high incomes; families in the middle-income range made up a somewhat larger proportion, and households at the lower end of the income scale made up the largest proportion. By the 1970s, household income had risen, and income was more evenly distributed, largely as a result of dual-income families.

Since 1979 and to 2020 two trends in income distribution have emerged. The first is that the average per-person income in the United States has increased. In 2020 there were over 331 million people living in 128 million households in the United States. The second trend is that income was unevenly distributed. Of the households about 12% had incomes below the poverty line. The average income among households in the highest quintile in 2016 was $291,000, more than 10 times the average income of households in the lowest quintile of $21,000 (www.cbo.gov). A quintile is defined as any of five equal groups into which a population can be divided according to the distribution of values of a particular variable, like income. Income within the highest quintile was also significantly skewed toward the very top. The average income among the households in the top 1% of the income distribution was more than 10 times the average income of households in the bottom half of the highest quintile (the 81st to 90th percentiles) (Congressional Budget Office [CBO], 2018). Chapter 5 provides a detailed discussion of the economics of health care and how financial constraints influence decisions about public health services.

Health Workforce Trends

The health care workforce ebbs and flows. The early years of the twenty-first century saw the beginning of what is expected to be a long-term and sizable nursing shortage. Similarly, most other health professionals are documenting current and future shortages. Employment of registered nurses (RNs) is projected to grow 15% from 2016 to 2026, much faster than the average for all occupations. This growth is due to increased focus on preventive care; growing rates of chronic conditions, including heart disease and diabetes; and the aging of America (Bureau of Labor Statistics [BLS], 2018a). Historically, nursing care has been provided in a variety of settings, primarily in the hospital. About 54% of all RNs continue to be employed in hospitals (BLS, 2018b). A few years ago hospitals began reducing their bed capacity as care became more community based. Hospitals have begun to expand their services, including mental health, substance abuse, and long-term care facilities. This growth is due to the factors previously discussed: the ability to treat and perhaps cure more diseases, the complexity of the care and the need for inpatient services, and the growth of the older age group. In 2020, many of the hospital services were diminished by the COVID-19 crisis.

A 2017 Healthcare Survey of Registered Nurses showed that 27% of RNs plan to retire within one year. In addition, 73% of baby boomer RNs plan to retire within three years (Sanborn, 2017). By 2026 there are expected to be at least 438,100 new nursing positions (BLS, 2018c).

There tend to be periodic shortages, especially in the primary care workforce in the United States, as providers choose to be specialists in fields such as medicine and nursing. Primary care providers include generalists who are skilled in preventive health care, diagnostic, and emergency services. The health care personnel trained as primary care providers include family physicians, general internists, general pediatricians, nurse practitioners (NPs), clinical nurse specialists (CNSs), physician assistants, and certified nurse-midwives (CNMs).

NPs, CNSs, and CNMs, considered advanced practice nursing (APN) specialists, are vital members of the primary care teams. Although there is a shortage of primary care physicians, NPs may or may not be able to fill the gap because of state nurse practice acts and medical practice acts, which influence the practice of both groups.

In terms of the nursing workforce, increasing the number of minority nurses remains a priority and a strategy for addressing the current nursing shortage. In 2020 minority nurses represented about 30.1% of the RN population. It is thought that increasing the minority population will help close the health disparity gap for minority populations. (For example, persons from minority groups, especially when language is a barrier, often are more comfortable with and more likely to access care from a provider from their own minority group.)

Technological Trends

The development and refinement of new technologies such as telehealth have opened up new clinical opportunities for nurses and their clients, especially in the areas of managing chronic conditions, assisting persons who live in rural areas, and in providing home health care, rehabilitation, and long-term care. Technological advances promise improved health care services, reduced costs, and more convenience in terms of time and travel for consumers (see Chapter 5). Electronic health records (EHRs) can improve public and population health outcomes by efficiently collecting data in a form that can be shared across multiple health care organizations and leveraged for quality improvement and prevention activities. Reduced costs result from a more efficient means of delivering health care as well as automation (HealthIT, 2018). Advances in health care technology will continue. One example of an effective use of technology is the funding provided by the US Department of Health and Human Services (HHS) and the Health Resources and Services Administration (HRSA) to health centers so they can adopt and implement electronic health records (EHR) and other health information technology (HRSA, 2008). HRSA's Office of Health Information Technology was created in 2005 to promote the effective use of health information technology (HIT) as a mechanism for responding to the needs of the uninsured, underinsured, and special-needs populations (HRSA, 2013).

One innovative use of the EHR in public health is to embed reminders or guidelines into the system. For example, the CDC published health guidelines that contain clinical recommendations for screening, prevention, diagnosis, and treatment. EHRs can improve public health reporting and surveillance and provide additional benefits including the following:

- Three federal programs, Medicaid, the Military Health System within the Department of Defense, and the State Children's Health Insurance Program (SCHIP), have effectively used HIT in several key functions, including outreach and enrollment, service delivery, and care management, as well as communications with families and the broader goals of program planning and improvement.
- Consumers can develop their personalized health record, including an electronic family health history, a tool from the Surgeon General accessed at https://familyhistory.hhs.gov (National Institutes of Health [NIH], 2017). This is an easy-to-use computer application for people to keep a personal record of their family health history.
- Providers can submit electronic data to immunization registries to determine the number of immunized persons within a state. For example, a school health nurse may submit the number of children in a school who have received the necessary immunizations prior to entering school.
- Health and community organizations and providers can submit electronic syndromic surveillance data to public health agencies which will then be submitted to the state

health department to detect disease outbreaks in a locality or the state.

- Laboratories can submit data to the state disease surveillance system to determine numbers of new active cases of a disease or virus such as COVID-19 in a locality or state.

Such information can then be used to direct new or improved public health or population-level health care programs to improve the health of a population, community, or state (www.healthit.gov, 2020).

CURRENT HEALTH CARE SYSTEM IN THE UNITED STATES

Despite the many advances and the sophistication of the US health care system, the system has been plagued with problems related to cost, access, and quality (see more discussion in Chapters 5, 19, and 28). These problems have been affected by the ability of individuals to obtain health insurance. The health care goals of most industrialized countries are similar: they strive for high-quality, affordable care.

Cost

Beginning in 2008 a historic weakening of the national and global economy—the "Great Recession"—led to the loss of 7 million jobs in the United States (Economic Report of the President, 2010). Even as the gross domestic product (GDP), an indicator of the economic health of a country, declined in 2009, health care spending continued to grow and reached $2.5 trillion in the same year (Truffer et al., 2010). In the years between 2017 and 2026, national health spending is expected to grow at an average annual rate of 5.5%, reaching $5.7 trillion by 2026, for a share of about 19.7% of the GDP. This translates into a projected increase in per capita spending (see Chapter 5).

In Chapter 5, additional discussion illustrates how health care dollars are spent. The largest share of health care expenditures goes to pay for acute care, with physician services being the next largest item. The amount of money that has gone to pay for public health services is much lower than for the other categories of expenditures (see Chapter 1). Other significant drivers of the increasingly high cost of health care include prescription drugs, technology, and care for chronic and degenerative diseases.

Following the Great Recession, the economic rebound coincided with the burgeoning Medicare enrollment of the aging baby boomer population. Medicaid recipients were expected to decline as jobs were added to the economy, and the percent of workers covered by employer-sponsored insurance was expected to reflect that growth. Although workers' salaries have not kept pace, the employee's contribution to the employer-sponsored insurance premiums grew to 55% by 2007 (Kaiser Family Foundation, 2018), and the inability of workers to pay this increased cost led to a rise in the percent of working families who were uninsured. It is essential to read about the changes in these facts as the American Affordable Care Act (ACA) was implemented. One change with the ACA is that more individuals have been able to purchase health insurance as employers have shifted more of the cost of health insurance to the employee (KFF, 2018).

Access

Another significant problem has been poor access to health care (Box 3.1). The American health care system is described as a two-class system: private and public. People with insurance or those who can personally pay for health care are viewed as receiving superior care; those who receive lower-quality care are (1) those whose only source of care depends on public funds, or (2) the working poor, who do not qualify for public funds either because they make too much money to qualify or because they are undocumented immigrants.

Employment-provided health care is tied to both the economy and to changes in health insurance premiums. In 2012, before the passing of the ACA, the total number of uninsured persons in the United States was 48 million. In 2016 it was 27.6 million. As discussed, there is a strong relationship between health insurance coverage and access to health care services. Insurance status determines the amount and kind of health care people are able to afford, as well as where they can receive care. Uninsured rates vary by state and region, with individuals living in southern or western states more likely to be uninsured. Eight out of the twelve states with the highest uninsured rates in 2016 were in the South. This is due to different economic conditions, state Medicare expansion status, availability of employer-based coverage, and demographics (Artiga and Damico, 2016). With some small variation the number of uninsured remains about the same in 2020.

The uninsured receive less preventive care, are diagnosed at more advanced disease states, and once diagnosed tend to receive less therapeutic care in terms of surgery and treatment options. As discussed later in this chapter, there are more than 1300 federally funded community health centers throughout the country (HRSA Health Center Program, 2018). Federally funded community health centers provide a broad range of health and social services, using NPs, RNs, physician assistants, physicians, social workers, and dentists. Community health centers serve primarily in medically underserved areas, which can be rural or urban. These centers serve people of all ages, races, and ethnicities, with or without health insurance.

BOX 3.1 CASE STUDY

Public health nurses who worked with local Head Start programs noted that many children had untreated dental caries. Although the children qualified for Medicaid, only two dentists in the area would accept appointments from Medicaid patients. Dentists asserted that Medicaid patients frequently did not show up for their appointments and that reimbursement was too low compared with other third-party payers. They also said the children's behavior made it difficult to work with them, so the waiting list for local dental care was about six years long. Although some nurses found ways to transport clients to dentists in a city 70 miles away, it was very time consuming and was feasible for only a small fraction of the clients. When decayed teeth abscessed, it was possible to get extractions from the local medical center. The health department dentist also saw children, but he, too, was booked for years.

Created by Deborah C. Conway, Assistant Professor, University of Virginia School of Nursing.

Quality

The quality of health care leaped to the forefront of concern following the 1999 release of the Institute of Medicine (IOM) report *To Err Is Human: Building a Safer Health System* (IOM, 2000). As indicated in this ground-breaking report, as many as 98,000 deaths a year could be attributed to preventable medical errors. Some of the untoward events categorized in this report included adverse drug events and improper transfusions, surgical injuries and wrong-site surgery, suicides, restraint-related injuries or death, falls, burns, pressure ulcers, and mistaken client identities. It was further determined that high rates of errors with serious consequences were most likely to occur in intensive care units, operating rooms, and emergency departments. Beyond the cost in human lives, preventable medical errors result in the loss of several billions of dollars annually in hospitals nationwide. Categories of error include diagnostic, treatment, and prevention errors as well as failure of communication, equipment failure, and other system failures. Significant to nurses, the IOM estimated the number of lives lost to preventable errors in medication alone represented more than 7000 deaths annually, with a cost of about $2 billion nationwide.

Although the IOM report made it clear that the majority of medical errors today were not produced by provider negligence, lack of education, or lack of training, questions were raised about the nurse's role and workload and its effect on client safety. In a follow-up report, *Keeping Patients Safe: Transforming the Work Environment of Nurses*, the IOM (2003) stated that nurses' long work hours pose a serious threat to patient safety, because fatigue slows reaction time, saps energy, and diminishes attention to detail. The group called for state regulators to pass laws barring nurses from working more than 12 hours a day and 60 hours a week—even if by choice (IOM, 2003). Although this information is largely related to acute care, many of the patients who survive medical errors are later cared for in the community.

To ensure quality in public health, the accreditation process for public health was developed, through the Public Health Accreditation Board. Outcome analysis demonstrates that public health districts that are accredited have increases in multisector partnerships to promote health in communities, and it strengthens quality improvement and performance management to improve community health. The Public Health Accreditation Board has an interactive US map that identifies health departments that have been accredited and can be accessed at http://www.phaboard.org (PHAB, 2018).

The ability of a public health agency or a community to respond to community disasters is one event that is monitored by the accreditation board. In August 2018, 223 of 416 local, tribal, and state centralized integration systems and multijurisdictional health departments had received accreditation. The accredited health departments served 214 million people. The purpose of the accreditation is to:

- Assist and identify quality health departments to improve performance and quality and to develop leadership
- Improve management
- Improve community relationships (PHAB, 2018)

ORGANIZATION OF THE HEALTH CARE SYSTEM

An enormous number and range of facilities and providers make up the health care system. These include physicians' and dentists' offices, hospitals, long-term care facilities, mental health facilities, ambulatory care centers, freestanding clinics, and clinics housed inside stores and drugstores, as well as free clinics, public health districts, and home health agencies. Providers include nurses, advanced practice nurses, physicians and physician assistants, dentists and dental hygienists, pharmacists, and a wide array of essential allied health providers such as physical, occupational, and recreational therapists; nutritionists; social workers; and a range of technicians. In general, however, the American health care system is divided into the following two, somewhat distinct, components: a private or personal care component and a public health component, with some overlap, as discussed in the following sections. It is important to discuss primary health care (PHC) and examine the interest in developing such a system.

Primary Care System

Primary care, the first level of the private health care system, is delivered in a variety of community settings, such as physicians' offices, urgent care centers, in-store clinics, community health centers, and community nursing centers. Near the end of the past century, in an attempt to contain costs, managed care organizations grew. Managed care is defined as a system in which care is delivered by a specific network of providers who agree to comply with the care approaches established through a case management approach. The key factors are a specified network of providers and the use of a gatekeeper to control access to providers and services. Managed care plans are a type of health insurance that includes contracts with health care providers and medical facilities to provide care for members at reduced costs. These providers make up the plan's network. How much health care is covered is dependent on the network's rules (MedlinePlus, 2017).

The government tried to reap the benefits of cost savings by introducing the managed care model into Medicare and Medicaid, with varying levels of success. The traditional Medicare plan involves Parts A and B. Part C, the Medicare Advantage program, incorporates private insurance plans into the Medicare program, including health maintenance organizations (HMOs) and preferred provider organizations' (PPOs) managed care models and private fee-for-service plans. In addition, Medicare Part D covers prescriptions (see Chapter 5).

Public Health System

The public health system is mandated through laws that are developed at the national, state, or local level. Examples of public health laws instituted to protect the health of the community include a law mandating immunizations for all children entering kindergarten and a law requiring constant monitoring of the local water supply and food service inspections. The public health system is organized into many levels in the federal, state, and local systems. At the local level, health districts provide care that is mandated by state and federal regulations.

The Federal System

The US Department of Health and Human Services (USDHHS, or simply HHS) is the agency most heavily involved with the health and welfare concerns of US citizens. The organizational chart of the HHS (Fig. 3.1; https://www.hhs.gov) shows the office of the secretary, 11 agencies, and an office of support services and operations (USDHHS, 2018a). Ten regional offices are maintained to provide more direct assistance to the states. Their locations are shown in Table 3.1. The HHS is charged with regulating health care and overseeing the health status of Americans. HHS administers more than 100 programs across its operating divisions. HHS goals are to protect the health of all Americans and provide essential human services, especially for those who are least able to help themselves. See Fig. 3.2 and Box 3.2 for the goals and objectives of the

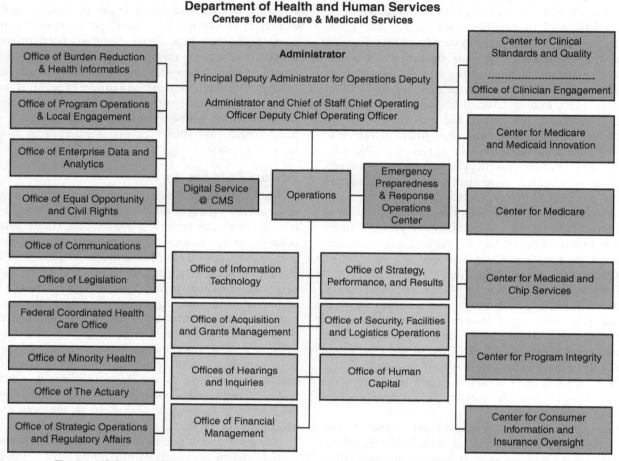

Fig. 3.1 US Department of Health and Human Services Organizational Chart. (From US Department of Health and Human Services. Available at https://www.hhs.gov.)

TABLE 3.1	Regional Offices of the US Department of Health and Human Services	
Region	**Location**	**Territory**
1	Boston	Connecticut, Maine, Massachusetts, New Hampshire, Rhode Island, Vermont
2	New York	New Jersey, New York, Puerto Rico, Virgin Islands
3	Philadelphia	Delaware, District of Columbia, Maryland, Pennsylvania, Virginia, West Virginia
4	Atlanta	Alabama, Florida, Georgia, Kentucky, Mississippi, North Carolina, South Carolina, Tennessee
5	Chicago	Illinois, Indiana, Michigan, Minnesota, Ohio, Wisconsin
6	Dallas	Arkansas, Louisiana, New Mexico, Oklahoma, Texas
7	Kansas City	Iowa, Kansas, Missouri, Nebraska
8	Denver	Colorado, Montana, North Dakota, South Dakota, Utah, Wyoming
9	San Francisco	Arizona, California, Hawaii, Nevada, American Samoa, Commonwealth of the Northern Mariana Islands, Federated States of Micronesia, Guam, Republic of the Marshall Islands, Republic of Palau
10	Seattle	Alaska, Idaho, Oregon, Washington

From US Department of Health and Human Services: *HHS regional offices.* Retrieved from www.hhs.gov.

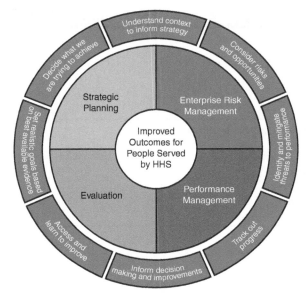

Fig. 3.2 Goals and Objective of the US Department of Health and Human Services. (Retrieved from https://www.hhs.gov.)

HHS strategic plan for fiscal years 2018–22. The Office of Public Health Preparedness was added to assist the nation and states in preparing for bioterrorism after September 11, 2001. The goal of the Office of Global Affairs is to promote global health by coordinating HHS strategies and programs with other governments and international organizations (HHS, 2020). The activities of several key agencies include the US Public Health Service and the US Department of Homeland Security.

The US Public Health Service (USPHS, or simply PHS) is a major component of the HHS. The PHS consists of eight agencies: Agency for Healthcare Research and Quality, Agency for Toxic Substances and Diseases Registry, Centers for Disease Control and Prevention, Food and Drug Administration, Health Resources and Services Administration, Indian Health Service, National Institutes of Health, and Substance Abuse and Mental Health Services Administration. Each has a specific purpose (see Chapter 3 for relevancy of the agencies to policy and providing health care). The PHS also has the Commissioned Corps, which is a uniformed service of more than 6000 health professionals who serve in many HHS and other federal agencies. The surgeon general is head of the Commissioned Corps. The corps fills essential services for public health, such as clinical services, and provides leadership within the federal government departments and agencies to support the care of the underserved and vulnerable populations. The mission of the PHS Commissioned Corps is to protect, promote, and advance the health and safety of the United States. As America's uniformed service of public health professionals, the Commissioned Corps achieves its mission through:

- rapid and effective response to public health needs
- leadership and excellence in public health practices
- advancement of public health science

The core values of the Commissioned Corps are leadership, service, integrity, and excellence (USPHS, 2018). Many nurses have been and are Commissioned Corps members.

Related to public health is the US Department of Homeland Security (USDHS, or simply DHS), which was created in 2003 (USDHS, 2018). The mission of the DHS is to ensure a homeland that is safe, secure, and resilient against terrorism and other hazards. The goals for the department include awareness, prevention, protection, response, and recovery. The DHS works with first responders throughout the United States, and through the development of programs such as the Community Emergency Response Team (CERT) program, trains people to be better prepared to respond to emergency situations in their communities. Nurses working in state and local public health districts, as well as those employed in hospitals and other health facilities, may be called on to respond to acts of terrorism or natural disaster in the course of their careers, and the DHS, along with the Food and Drug Administration (FDA) and CDC, is developing programs to ready nurses and other health care providers for emergency response (USDHS, 2018).

The State System

When the United States faced a pandemic flu outbreak in 2009, the federal government and the public health community quickly prepared to meet the challenge of educating the public and health professionals about the H1N1 flu and making vaccinations available. In 2014 public health within the states was responding to an enterovirus affecting large numbers of children with symptoms of upper respiratory disease and weakness in arms and legs. The virus was considered life threatening (AAP, 2016). In 2020, again the federal government and the public health community quickly responded to the outbreak of COVID-19. This virus had a high rate of infectivity and was deadly.

The rapid spread of the COVID-19 virus challenged federal, state, and local governments to act in ways normally reserved for war, depressions, or natural disasters. The pandemic caused a massive global challenge thought to be likely to last for months to years. All levels of governments using all of the resources available to them were trying to find answers in an attempt to limit economic and human costs. In a crisis that has not been endured by the global community in recent lifetimes, citizens look to their governments for information, guidance, and leadership. They expect to be kept safe and healthy. Public officials are pressured to find solutions to this crisis (Eggers, Flynn et al., 2020).

State and Local Health Departments

As the federal government led the national response to COVID-19, state legislatures and local health departments were on the front lines. All states, territories, and Washington, DC, declared public health emergencies. Federal financial assistance to support public health and the workforce standard was recently issued. This included the Coronavirus Aid, Relief, and Economic Security (CARES) Act that became public law no. 116–136 on March 27, 2020 (Coronavirus Aid, Relief, and Economic Security act or the [CARES act], 2020). This aid package contained $1.5 billion to support state and local public health departments and territories and tribes in their efforts to conduct public health activities, including: the purchase of personal protective equipment, surveillance for COVID-19, laboratory testing to detect positive cases, contact tracing to identify additional cases, infection control and mitigation

BOX 3.2   HHS Strategic Plan, Goals, and Objectives—Fiscal Years 2018–22

Strategic Goal 1: Reform, Strengthen, and Modernize the Nation's Healthcare System
Strategic Goal 2: Protect the Health of Americans Where They Live, Learn, Work, and Play
Strategic Goal 3: Strengthen the Economic and Social Well-Being of Americans Across the Lifespan
Strategic Goal 4: Foster Sound, Sustained Advances in the Sciences
Strategic Goal 5: Promote Effective and Efficient Management and Stewardship

GOAL 1: Strengthen Health Care

Objective A	Make coverage more secure for those who have insurance, and extend affordable coverage to the uninsured.
Objective B	Improve health care quality and patient safety.
Objective C	Emphasize primary and preventive care linked with community prevention services.
Objective D	Reduce the growth of health care costs while promoting high-value, effective care.
Objective E	Ensure access to quality, culturally competent care for vulnerable populations.
Objective F	Promote the adoption and meaningful use of health information technology.

GOAL 2: Advance Scientific Knowledge and Innovation

Objective A	Accelerate the process of scientific discovery to improve patient care.
Objective B	Foster innovation to create shared solutions.
Objective C	Invest in the regulatory sciences to improve food and medical product safety.
Objective D	Increase our understanding of what works in public health and human service practice.

GOAL 3: Advance the Health, Safety, and Well-Being of the American People

Objective A	Promote the safety, well-being, resilience, and healthy development of children and youth.
Objective B	Promote economic and social well-being for individuals, families, and communities.
Objective C	Improve the accessibility and quality of supportive services for people with disabilities and older adults.
Objective D	Promote prevention and wellness.
Objective E	Reduce the occurrence of infectious diseases.
Objective F	Protect Americans' health and safety during emergencies, and foster resilience in response to emergencies.

GOAL 4: Increase Efficiency, Transparency, Accountability, and Effectiveness of HHS Programs

Objective A	Ensure program integrity and responsible stewardship of resources.
Objective B	Fight fraud and work to eliminate improper payments.
Objective C	Use HHS data to improve the health and well-being of the American people.
Objective D	Improve HHS environmental, energy, and economic performance to promote sustainability.

GOAL 5: Strengthen the Nation's Health and Human Service Infrastructure and Workforce

Objective A	Invest in the HHS workforce to meet America's health and human service needs today and tomorrow.
Objective B	Ensure that the nation's health care workforce can meet increased demands.
Objective C	Enhance the ability of the public health workforce to improve public health at home and abroad.
Objective D	Strengthen the nation's human service workforce.
Objective E	Improve national, state, local, and tribal surveillance and epidemiology capacity.

HHS, US Department of Health and Human Services.
From the US Department of Health and Human Services, 2018. Retrieved from https://www.hhs.gov.

at the local level to prevent the spread of the virus, and other public health preparedness and response activities (Centers for Medicare and Medicaid, 2020, March 11).

In addition to this bolus of funding from the CDC, state governments have also issued emergency funding earmarked for state and local public health.

State Health Department Functions

In addition to standing ready for disaster prevention or response, state health departments have other equally important functions, such as health care financing and administration for programs such as Medicaid, providing mental health and professional education, establishing health codes, licensing facilities and personnel, and regulating the insurance industry. State systems also have an important role in direct assistance to local health departments, including ongoing assessment of community health needs.

 LEVELS OF PREVENTION

Related to the Public Health Care System

Primary Prevention
Implement a community-level program such as walking for exercise to assist citizens in improving health behaviors related to lifestyle.

Secondary Prevention
Implement a family-planning program to prevent unintended pregnancies for young couples who attend the local community health center.

Tertiary Prevention
Provide a self-management asthma program for children with chronic asthma to reduce their need for hospitalization.

Nurses serve in many capacities in state health departments; they are consultants, direct service providers, researchers, teachers, and supervisors. They also participate in community assessment, program development, planning, and the evaluation of health programs.

The Local System

The local health system has direct responsibility to the citizens in its community or jurisdiction. Services and programs offered by local health departments vary depending on the state and local health codes that must be followed, the needs of the community, and available funding and other resources. For example, one health department might be more involved with public health education programs and environmental issues, whereas another health department might emphasize direct client care. Local health departments vary in providing sick care or even primary care (see Chapter 28). More often than at other levels of government, public health nurses at the local level provide population-level or direct services. Some of these nurses deliver special or selected services, such as follow-up of contacts in cases of tuberculosis or most recently in cases of COVID-19, or sexually transmitted infections (STIs). They also provide child immunization clinics and in some localities school health nurse services. Others provide more general care, delivering services to families in certain geographic areas. This method of delivery of nursing services involves broader needs and a wider variety of nursing interventions. The local level often provides an opportunity for nurses to take on significant leadership roles, with many nurses serving as directors or managers.

Since the tragedy of September 11, 2001, state and local health departments have increasingly focused on emergency preparedness and response. In case of an event, state and local health departments in the affected area will be expected to collect data and accurately report the situation, to respond appropriately to any type of emergency, and to ensure the safety of the residents of the immediate area, while protecting those just outside the danger zone. This level of knowledge—to enable public health agencies to anticipate, prepare for, recognize, and respond to pandemics, gun violence, terrorist threats, and natural disasters such as hurricanes or floods—has required a level of interstate and federal–local planning and cooperation. Whether participating in disaster simulations or preparing a shelter, nurses play a significant and major role in meeting the challenge of disaster preparedness and response.

FORCES INFLUENCING CHANGES IN THE HEALTH CARE SYSTEM

Although most people are personally satisfied with their own health care provider, at present few people are satisfied with the health care system in general. Costs have been high and have continued to rise while quality and access have been uneven across the country and within communities, depending on the ability to pay. What, then, were some of the factors that might influence health care to change? First, as a nation, citizens must decide what has to be provided for all people, who will be in charge of the system, and who will pay for these services. In recent years, federal and state services have been reduced, and more responsibility for health care delivery has been moved to the private sector. Health care is big business. Health care company stocks are now traded by major stock exchanges, directors receive benefits when profits are high, and the locus of control

has shifted from the provider to the payer. Many competing forces have influenced the changing design of the health care system, some of which are consumers, employers (purchasers), care delivery systems, and state and federal legislation.

First, consumers want lower costs and high-quality health care without limits and with an improved ability to choose providers and services of their choice. Second, employers (purchasers of health care) want to be able to obtain basic health care plans at reasonable costs for their business and employees. Many employers have seen their profits diminish as they put more money into providing adequate health care coverage for employees. Third, health care systems want a better balance between consumer and purchaser demands. Thus they continually watch their own budget and expenses. To maintain a profit while providing quality care, many health care delivery groups have downsized and created alliances, mergers, and other joint ventures. Finally, legislation, especially concerning access and quality, continues to be enacted, thus creating one more force helping shape a health care system. The goal of "evidence-based care" is to ensure high-quality health care.

Many have said that solving the health care crisis requires the institution of a rational health care system that balances equity, cost, and quality. The fact that millions of people have been uninsured, that wide disparities have existed in access, and that a large proportion of deaths each year seem attributable to preventable causes (health care errors as well as tobacco, substance abuse, preventable injuries, and obesity) has indicated that the US health care system is currently not serving the best interests of the population. The WHO has suggested that integrating primary care and public health into a PHC system will be the basis for better health for all world citizens (WHO, 1986a).

Integration of Public Health and the Primary Care Systems

Although primary care and public health share a goal of promoting the health and well-being of all people, these two disciplines historically have operated independently of one another. Problems that stem from this separation have long been recognized, but new opportunities have been emerging for bringing these systems together to promote lasting improvements in the health of individuals, communities, and populations (IOM, 2012).

In recognition of this potential, the CDC and the HRSA, both agencies of the HHS, asked the IOM to convene a committee of experts, including input from nursing, to examine the integration of primary care and public health (IOM, 2012).

To recognize the differences in these two systems, definitions were used to guide the work of the experts. Primary care was defined as "the providing of integrated, accessible health care services by clinicians who are accountable for addressing a large majority of personal health care needs, while developing partnerships with clients and practicing in the context of family and community" (IOM, 1996). Public health was defined as "fulfilling society's interest in assuring conditions in which people can be healthy" (IOM, 1988). The purpose of the integration was to achieve the WHO goal of PHC.

Potential Barriers to Integration

Contrasting the two systems, primary care, which can be either a public or a private entity, is person focused, provides a point of first contact for individuals to address health problems, and is considered comprehensive and provides coordination of individual care. Public health can also be delivered through public and private entities to contribute to the health of society and populations. Local, state, and federal government play a major role in public health. Health departments are legally bound to provide essential public health services and to work with the total community and multiple stakeholders to address community-level health problems. Public health also has specific functions of assurance, assessment, and policy development to address community-level health issues and has a charge to create healthy communities (see Chapter 1).

In addition to differing roles and functions and issues related to funding, different clients and different foci will need to be addressed to form a solid foundation for a partnership. Primary care is largely funded through health insurance, individual client payments, and sometimes through federal grants. Public health is largely funded through tax dollars, federal and state grants, and sometimes health insurance payments through Medicare and Medicaid. Primary care serves the individuals who present to the practice, while public health serves to assess the health problems of the population. Both focus on meeting the most prevalent health needs of the population. Primary care focuses more on the curative aspect of individualized care, while public health focuses more on the prevention of health problems for the population (Levesque et al., 2013).

The common goal of public health and primary care, although these systems operate independently, is to ensure a healthier population. Integration of these two systems has the potential to produce a greater impact on the health of populations than either could have working alone, said the committee of experts convened by the IOM (2012).

The *Healthy People* initiatives, beginning with the US Surgeon General's 1979 report, indicate the long-standing desire to improve population health in the United States.

Primary Health Care

Primary health care (PHC) is the first point of contact people have with the health care system. A combined approach to primary care and public health provides comprehensive, accessible, community-based care that meets the health needs of individuals throughout their life. This includes a variety of services from prevention (vaccinations, family planning, and screenings) to management of chronic health conditions and palliative care (WHO, 2018). This system is composed of public health agencies, community-based agencies and primary care clinics, and health care providers. From a conceptual point of view, PHC is essential care made universally accessible to individuals, families, and the community. Health care is made available to them with their full participation and is provided at a cost that the individual, community, and country can afford. This care is not uniformly available and accessible to all people in many countries, including the United States. Full community participation means that individuals within the community help in defining health problems and in developing approaches to address the problems.

The PHC movement officially began in 1977 when the 30th WHO Health Assembly adopted a resolution accepting the goal of attaining a level of health that permitted all citizens of the world to live socially and economically productive lives. At the international conference in 1978 in Alma-Ata, in Kazakhstan, formerly a Soviet Republic, it was determined that this goal was to be met through PHC. This resolution, the Declaration of Alma-Ata, became known by the slogan "Health for All (HFA) by the Year 2000," which captured the official health target for all the member nations of the WHO. In 1998 the program was adapted to meet the needs of the new century and was deemed "Health for All in the 21st Century" (see discussion of Global Health).

In 1981 the WHO established global indicators for monitoring and evaluating the achievement of HFA. In the *World Health Statistics Annual* (WHO, 1986b), these indicators are grouped into the following four categories:
1. Health policies
2. Social and economic development
3. Provision of health care, and
4. Health status

The indicators suggest that health improvements are a result of efforts in many areas, including agriculture, industry, education, housing, communications, and health care. Because PHC is as much a political statement as a system of care, each United Nations member country interprets PHC according to its own culture, health needs, resources, and system of government. Clearly, the goal of PHC has not been met in most countries, including the United States.

CHECK YOUR PRACTICE

As a senior nursing student, you have been exploring options for future employment. You have developed an interest in working in the community, especially in a primary care clinic setting in a rural community. You wonder why there has not been more emphasis in your nursing program about possible jobs in primary care, and you are aware that in many clinics, a medical assistant is the person who is most accessible to clients. If you are interested in finding a job in primary care, what would you do? How would you present yourself to a potential employer to show how you could benefit the practice and the clients of the practice? How can you, in a primary care position, improve the health of the population in the community? See if you can apply these steps to this scenario. (1) Recognize the cues, look at the literature to see how an RN could be helpful in primary care; (2) analyze the cues; (3) state several and prioritize the hypotheses you have stated; (4) generate solutions for each hypothesis; (5) take action on the number one hypothesis you think best reflects an approach to take to obtain a position in primary care; and (6) evaluate the outcomes you would expect in the population as a result of your employment.

The Changing Role of Registered Nurses in Primary Care

The ACA has brought many changes to health care, with an emphasis on primary care and reducing hospital admissions and length of stay. The role of the nurse in primary care can help achieve both of these goals through an expanded RN role and positions in primary care. RNs are well equipped and trained to coordinate client care; work with all members of the interprofessional team; manage complex comorbidities; promote healthy lifestyles; coordinate medication reconciliation and monitor effects of polypharmacy; bridge the gap between community resources and the people who need them; advocate for clients, families, and community members; and work toward local, state, and federal policy change that improves the health of the community members.

A study by Flinter et al. (2017) identifies the expanding role of the RN in primary care by surveying RNs in 30 different primary care practices. Studies like this demonstrate the expanded role of nurses in primary care and help justify the cost of the care offered by nurses. The 2016 Macy Foundation's conference on Preparing Registered Nurses for Enhanced Roles in Primary Care recommended six domains for improving the involvement of RNs in primary care:

1. Changing the cultures in both nursing schools and practices to place greater value on primary care and the role of nurses in it
2. Redesigning practices to make full use of the expertise of nurses
3. Rebalancing nursing education to elevate primary care content
4. Promoting the career development of nurses in primary care
5. Developing primary care expertise in nursing school faculty
6. Increasing opportunities for interprofessional education and teamwork development in both education and practice (Macy Foundation, 2017)

In 2018 the USDHHS Division of Nursing funded grants to select schools in the United States to develop approaches to include an emphasis on primary care in their nursing curricula.

OVERVIEW OF GLOBAL HEALTH AND NURSING

Many issues make it imperative that nurses know about their effects on global health (Box 3.3). Populations from developing nations may have experienced a lack of access to health care services that could successfully diagnose or treat health issues in their country of origin. Understanding global health and factors that contribute to these health problems better prepares the nurse to develop interventions that are (1) culturally congruent, (2) culturally responsive, and (3) culturally acceptable to the target group.

BOX 3.3 Issues Affecting Global and US Health Care of Populations

- Global warming and the melting of the polar ice caps
- Changing environmental conditions like contaminated water sources
- Worldwide droughts, natural disasters of blizzards, hurricanes, tornadoes, volcanoes, typhoons, and earthquakes
- War, increasing global violence
- Growing populations (impoverished, destitute populations of the world)
- Preventable health care disasters such as malaria, malnutrition, communicable diseases, chronic health problems, and conditions related to environmental pollution
- Lack of access to food, housing, safety, and health care
- The effects of worldwide pandemics (e.g., COVID-19), declining global economy, depletion of food supplies

Data from Alliance of Nurses for Healthy Environments (2018), Bolender et al. (2012, 2013), Fernández-Luqueño et al. (2013), Hunter (2013), World Health Organization (2018c).

The vision of the International Council of Nurses (ICN)'s Leadership for Change program is that nursing is to take a leadership role in helping achieve better health for all (International Council of Nurses, 2018). In June 2018, for example, the ICN Leadership for Change program (sponsored by Johnson & Johnson) trained 36 nurses from 10 provinces in China with a train-the-trainer model. Looking forward, the program aims to cover 12 provinces and support over 500 future nurse leaders (ICN, 2018).

In the document *Health For All 2021*, four goals have been identified to address global and local issues to improve the health of the world:

1. To tackle the determinants of health, taking into account physical, economic, social, cultural, and gender perspectives and ensuring the use of health impact assessment
2. Use health-outcome–driven programs and investments for health development and clinical care
3. Offer integrated family- and community-oriented primary health care, supported by a flexible and responsive hospital system
4. A participatory health development process that involves relevant partners for health at home, school, and work and at local community and country levels, and that promotes joint decision making, implementation, and accountability.

Because of the ease of global travel, contagious and preventable health conditions are not endemic in just an isolated country; they are prevalent around the world. Health professionals and world leaders want to be enlightened about these health issues and want answers on how to address them, which becomes problematic in the countries most afflicted but without the technological infrastructure to help their people.

Many terms are used to describe nations that have achieved a high level of industrial and technological advancement (along with a stable market economy) and those that have not. For the purposes of this chapter, the term developed country refers to those countries with a stable economy and a wide range of industrial and technological development, low child mortality, high gross national income, and a high human asset index (e.g., the United States, Canada.) A country that does not meet these criteria is referred to as a less developed country (e.g., Bangladesh, Somalia, Haiti).

There are more than 6000 rare diseases (Forman et al., 2012), and in developing countries these are often unknown entities in the world of Western medicine (WHO, 2018b). Ongoing health problems needing control in less developed countries include measles, mumps, rubella, and polio; the current health concerns of the more developed countries are problems such as hepatitis, infectious diseases, and new viral strains such as hantavirus, severe acute respiratory syndrome (SARS), H1N1, avian flu, and COVID-19. Chronic health problems such as hypertension and diabetes, and the larger social, yet health-related issues such as terrorism, warfare, violence, and substance abuse are now global issues (Shah, 2014). World travelers may expose themselves to diseases and environmental health hazards that are unknown or rare in their home country and may serve as hosts to various types of disease agents. Examples of diseases that were once fairly isolated and rare but have increased in prevalence are the mosquito-borne viruses of Zika and chikungunya (CMS, 2017, 2018). In 2019 and 2020 world travelers have increased COVID-19 by spreading the virus through travels to countries other than their home country.

In addition to direct health problems, increasing populations, migration between and within countries, political corruption, lack of natural resources, and natural disasters affect the health and well-being of populations.

Nations plagued by civil war and political corruption are faced with chronic poverty, unstable leadership, and lack of economic development. The effects of war and conflict also have devastating effects on a country and the health of its population. These wars have had devastating mental and physical health consequences, leaving each country and its people with few health care services or other resources to sustain life.

As countries promote the goals of HFA21, they realize that they need to improve their economies and infrastructures. They often seek funds and technological expertise from the wealthier and more developed countries. According to the WHO Europe (2013a), HFA21 is not a single, finite goal but a strategic process that can lead to progressive improvement in the health of people. In essence it is a call for social justice and solidarity. Unfortunately, the less developed nations still lack the infrastructure necessary to achieve health promotion and healthy living conditions (Fig. 3.3).

The UN Millennium Development Goals (MDGs), first agreed on by world leaders in 2013, were developed to relieve poor health conditions around the world and to establish positive steps to improve living conditions by the year 2015 (UN, 2013a; see goals in Box 3.4). The Millennium Report (UN, 2015) described the developed nations' responsibility to the betterment of those in less developed nations, as well as areas where progress is still needed. The MDGs highlight the responsibility for action to develop a global partnership.

The MDGs were updated to reflect the Sustainable Development Goals (SDGs) in 2017. These are designed to be a more comprehensive and detailed guide for partners to promote progress into the future (Box 3.4). Strategies for achieving the

---

BOX 3.4   Millennium Development Goals and Sustainable Development Goals

Millennium Development Goals

MDG 1: Eradicate extreme poverty and hunger.
MDG 2: Achieve universal primary education.
MDG 3: Promote gender equality and empower women.
MDG 4: Reduce child mortality.
MDG 5: Improve maternal health.
MDG 6: Combat HIV/AIDS, malaria, and other diseases.
MDG 7: Ensure environmental sustainability.
MDG 8: Develop a global partnership for development.

Sustainable Development Goals

SDG 1: No Poverty
SDG 2: Zero Hunger
SDG 3: Good Health and Well-Being
SDG 4: Quality Education
SDG 5: Gender Equality
SDG 6: Clean Water and Sanitation
SDG 7: Affordable and Clean Energy
SDG 8: Decent Work and Economic Growth
SDG 9: Industry, Innovation, and Infrastructure
SDG 10: Reduced Inequalities
SDG 11: Sustainable Cities and Communities
SDG 12: Responsible Consumption and Production
SDG 13: Climate Action
SDG 14: Life Below Water
SDG 15: Life on Land
SDG 16: Peace, Justice, and Strong Institutions
SDG 17: Partnerships for the Goals

From United Nations: *UN millennium development goals (MDGs)*, 2013. Available at http://www.un.org; United Nations: *UN Sustainable Development Goals (SDGs)*, 2017. Available at https://www.un.org.

---

continuing goals of HFA21 include building on past accomplishments and the identification of global priorities and targets for the first 20 years of the new century.

Nurses need to be informed about global health. Many of the world's health problems directly affect the health of individuals who live in the United States. For example, in 1994 the 103rd US Congress passed the North American Free Trade Agreement (NAFTA), which opened trade borders between the United States, Canada, and Mexico, and allowed increased movement of products and people. Along the United States–Mexico border, an influx of undocumented immigrants in recent years has raised concerns for the health of people who live in this area. NAFTA also provided an impetus and framework for the government of Mexico to modernize its medical system (California Department of Public Health, 2015). The Mexican National Academy of Medicine continues to make health and environmental recommendations to the government, which illustrates the beneficial interactions that have been occurring between Mexico, Canada, and the United States as part of this trade agreement. In July 2020 NAFTA was replaced with a new agreement, titled the United States, Mexico, Canada Agreement, to "modernize" NAFTA. (Office of US Trade Agreements: the United States, Mexico, Canada Agreement to "modernize" NAFTA, Washington, DC, Office of the President of the United States, 2020.)

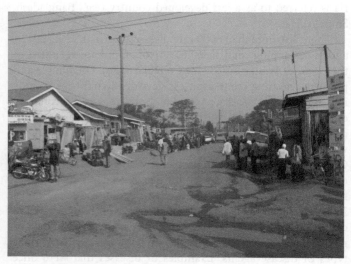

Fig 3.3 The Streets of a Town in Uganda. (Courtesy A. Hunter.)

Nurses play a significant role in obtaining health for the immigrants and undocumented persons who live along the border regions in Texas, New Mexico, Arizona, and California. Nurses supported by private foundations and by local and state public health departments often provide critical and reliable health care in these areas.

The Role of Population Health

According to Williams (2018) population health refers to the health status of a defined population of individuals, including the distribution of the health status within the group, and includes health outcomes, patterns of health determinants, and policies and interventions that link them. Using epidemiologic trends, population health focuses on reducing inequities, improving health in these groups to reduce morbidity and mortality, and assessing emerging diseases and other health risks to a community. A population, often referred to as an aggregate, can be defined by a geographic boundary, by the common personal and environmental characteristics shared by a group of people such as ethnicity or religion, or by the epidemiologic and social conditions of a community.

The factors and conditions that are important considerations in population health are called determinants of health. Population health determinants may include:

- income and social factors,
- social support networks,
- education,
- employment,
- working and living conditions,
- physical environments,
- social environments,
- biology and genetic endowment,
- personal health practices,
- coping skills,
- healthy child development,
- health services,
- sex, and
- culture (WHO, 2014a).

The determinants do not work independently of each other but form a complex system of interactions.

Canada is a leader in promoting the population health approach. Canada has been implementing programs using this framework since the mid-1990s and builds on a tradition of public health and health promotion. Box 3.5 presents the development of the Healthy Cities movement in Toronto. In 2019 Toronto was ranked the number one healthiest city in the world. This successful project was adopted by the WHO and has been implemented in several countries around the world—most specifically Europe, Southeast Asia, Africa, and the Western Pacific (WHO, 2014b). The United States has had several healthy cities designations. A key to the success of this project has been the identification and definition of health issues and of the investment decisions within a population that were guided by evidence about what keeps people healthy.

A Healthy City has four aims: to create a health-supportive environment, achieve a good quality of life, provide basic sanitation and hygiene needs, and supply access to health care.

BOX 3.5 Examples of the Healthy Cities Movement

Toronto, Ontario, Canada, was one of the first cities in North America to become involved in the Healthy Cities movement. Toronto began with a strategic planning committee to develop an overall strategy for health promotion. The committee conducted vision workshops in the community and a comprehensive environmental scan to help identify health needs in Toronto. The outcome was a final report outlining major issues, and it included a strategic mission, priorities, and recommendations for action. The Toronto Healthy City program involved a number of projects. One of them, the Healthiest Babies Possible project, was an intensive antenatal education and nutritional supplement program for pregnant women who were identified by health and social agencies as being at high risk. The program included intensive contact and follow-up of women, along with food supplements. It has been successful in decreasing the incidence of low-birth-weight infants.

Another example is Chengdu, China. Chengdu is located on the upper parts of the Yangtze River. It is surrounded on four sides by the Fu and Nan rivers and was one of the most polluted cities in southwestern China. The pollution created severe environmental problems as a result of industrial waste, raw sewage, and the intensive use of fresh water. The proliferation of slum and squatter settlements exacerbated the social, economic, and environmental problems of the city. The Fu and Nan Rivers Comprehensive Revitalization Plan was started in 1993 as a Healthy Community and City initiative to deal with the growing environmental problems. The principles of participatory planning and partnership were used to raise awareness of the problem among the general public and to mobilize major stakeholders to invest in a sustainable future for Chengdu and its inhabitants. The plan resulted in providing 30,000 households living in the slum and squatter settlements with decent and affordable housing, and with projects to deal with sewage and industrial waste. In addition, the plan was able to improve parks and gardens, turning Chengdu into a clean and green city within the natural flow of its rivers.

From Flynn B, Ivanov L: Health promotion through healthy communities and cities. In *Community and public health nursing*, ed 6, St. Louis, 2004, Mosby, pp 396–411.

The most successful Healthy Cities programs have a commitment of local community members, a clear vision, ownership of policies, a wide array of stakeholders, and a process for institutionalizing the program.

Integration of health determinants into public policies is apparent on the global stage. At the 2009 Nairobi Global Conference on Health Promotion, more than 600 participants representing 100 countries adopted a Call to Action on addressing population health and finding ways to promote health at the global level. Since 1986, with the development of the first Global Conference, until 2009, a large body of evidence and experience has accumulated about the importance of health promotion as an integrative, cost-effective strategy and as an essential component of health systems primed to respond adequately to emerging concerns (WHO, 2010a, 2018b).

As nurses work with immigrants from global arenas or become active participants in health care around the world, understanding such concepts as population health and the determinants of health for a population becomes more important than the most advanced acute care skills. These skills, though important, are intended to help an individual; population health skill sets can help the world.

Global leaders have recognized the need to get nations committed to a common health care agenda. An important effort is needed at the level of recruitment, education, and retention of PHC workers, including public health nurses, primary care nurses, family physicians, and mid-level care workers.

It is well documented that PHC practiced in high-income countries exerts a positive influence on health costs, appropriateness of care, and outcomes for most of the major health indicators. PHC also has more equitable health outcomes than systems oriented toward specialty care.

Nursing and Global Health

Nurses play a leadership role in health care throughout the world. Those with public health experience provide knowledge and skill in countries where nursing is not an organized profession, and they give guidance to the nurses as well as to the auxiliary personnel who are part of the PHC team. In many areas in the developed world, nurses provide direct client care and help meet the education and health promotion needs of the community. They are viewed as strong advocates for PHC, through social commitment to equality of health care and support of the concepts that are contained in the Declaration of Alma-Ata.

In the less developed countries the role and scope of practice of the nurse may be less explicitly defined, and care often depends on and is directed by physicians. Work is needed to support and promote education of nurses, as well as promote professionalization of nursing in countries where this is the case (Fig. 3.4).

Promoting Health/Preventing Disease: Year 2030 Objectives for the Nation

As a WHO member nation, the United States has endorsed PHC as a strategy for achieving the goal of "Health for All in the 21st Century." However, the PHC emphasis on broad strategies, community participation, self-reliance, and a multidisciplinary health care delivery team is not the major strategy for improving the health of the US population. The national health plan for the United States identifies disease prevention and health promotion as the areas of most concern in the nation. Since the 1980s, each decade has been measured and tracked according to health objectives set at the beginning of the decade. The PHS of the HHS publishes the objectives after gathering data from health professionals and organizations throughout the country (see Chapter 1).

Healthy People 2030 was officially launched in 2020 (HHS, 2020). The framework with which measurable health indicators can be tracked builds on the accomplishments of *Healthy People 2020*. This in turn will encourage public health nurses to broaden their scope to all aspects of their clients' lives that may need assessment and intervention, including where they live, the condition of their home, and how the appropriateness of their environment may change as the client ages. The *Healthy People 2030* box presents indicators related to the strengthening of the public health infrastructure. These objectives will assist nurses in having data to show that public health and nurses are changing practice.

 HEALTHY PEOPLE 2030

Selected Objectives That Pertain to Strengthening the Public Health Infrastructure General

- **PHI-01:** Increase the proportion of state public health agencies that are accredited
- **PHI-02:** Increase the proportion of local public health agencies that are accredited community
- **PHI-04:** Increase the proportion of state and territorial jurisdictions that have a health improvement plan
- **PHI-05:** Increase the proportion of local jurisdictions that have a health improvement plan

From US Department of Health and Human Services: *Healthy people 2030*. Available at https://www.healthypeople.gov.

HEALTH CARE DELIVERY REFORM EFFORTS—UNITED STATES

Over the centuries, both health insurance and health care reform have been the focus of numerous discussions and political battles. As can be seen in Chapter 5, the first health insurance plan, established in about 1798 in the United States, was for the Merchant Marines to assist in treating infectious diseases and protecting the ports of entry into the United States. The United States has discussed national health care reform since the 1900s (see Chapter 5). In 1912 Theodore Roosevelt campaigned on a health insurance proposal for industry. Then in 1915 the "progressive reformers" campaigned for a state-based system of compulsory health insurance. In the 1920s the Committee on the Costs of Medical Care suggested group medicine and voluntary insurance, and this movement was labeled as promoting "socialized medicine."

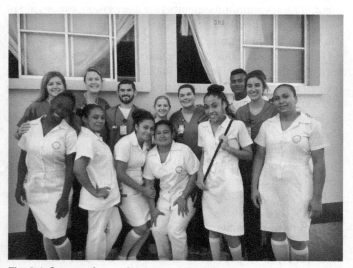

Fig. 3.4 Support for professionalization of nursing in global settings must be in the context of respectful, sustained, cultural engagement. Nursing students from the University of Virginia and the Bluefields Indian and Caribbean University in Bluefields, Nicaragua. (Courtesy E. Mitchell.)

EVIDENCE-BASED PRACTICE

It is often said that the states are the laboratories of democracy. One state, Massachusetts, began an experiment in health reform in 2006. Two years after health reform legislation became effective, only 2.6% of Massachusetts residents were uninsured, the lowest percent ever recorded in any state (Dorn et al., 2009; KFF, 2019). The program became one of the most successful and a model for the ACA. After 5 years, about 98%–99% of all of the commonwealth's citizens were covered by the plan. In 2014, the program was changed to align with the Patient Protection and Affordable Care Act and the program still exists today. In 2019 the uninsured rate was 3% (KFF, 2019).

Although other states have experimented with various programs to decrease the number of uninsured, the Massachusetts plan has had the most success. The health reform plan rests on an individual mandate that requires everyone who can afford insurance to purchase coverage. Those unable to afford insurance receive subsidies that allow low-income individuals and families to purchase coverage. A new state-run program, Commonwealth Care (CommCare), provides benefits to adults who are not eligible for Medicaid but whose incomes fall below 300% of the federal poverty level.

To understand how the state was so successful in this effort toward universal coverage, a group of evaluators met with 15 key informants representing hospitals, community health centers, insurance companies, Medicaid, and CommCare. Several factors, it was found, have contributed to the historic level of coverage seen in the state. Rather than requiring consumers to complete separate applications for programs such as Medicaid, the Children's Health Insurance Program (CHIP), or CommCare, a single-application system provides entry to all the state programs. If an uninsured client was admitted to a hospital or visited a community health center, the client's eligibility was automatically evaluated, and, if eligible, the client would be automatically converted to CommCare coverage, even without completing an application. A "Virtual Gateway" has been developed through which staff of community-based organizations have been trained to complete online applications on behalf of consumers and to provide education and counseling about insurance options to underserved communities. By holding back reimbursement to providers who do not help consumers sign up for one of the available insurance options, hospitals and health centers are motivated to dedicate staff to provide education and counseling to the formerly uninsured. The result is that at least half of the new enrollees in Medicaid and CommCare have been enrolled without filling out any forms on their own. In addition to these efforts, shortly after the reform legislation was enacted, the state financed a massive public education effort to inform consumers about their new options.

Nurse Use

As health reform evolves on the national level, nurses can play a crucial role in driving down the number of uninsured. Nurses should educate themselves so that they can encourage clients to apply and take advantage of all available coverage options. Taking an active role in consumer educational programs is a natural extension of a nurse's role as a client advocate. Nurses can promote legislation to simplify enrollment processes and encourage the development of shared databases for community health care providers, thus preventing consumers from a lack of care or interruption of services in our fragmented health care system.

KFF. Health insurance coverage of the total population. The Henry J. Kaiser Family Foundation; 2019. November 29, 2018. Retrieved August 6, 2019.

Since the 1930s surveys have demonstrated that Americans have shown support of guaranteed access to health care and health insurance and a governmental role in financing of care. Some strides were made in improving access and defining the role of government financing through the passing of Medicare in 1965, with Medicaid as a part of the proposal for Social Security amendments, and the Children's Health Insurance Program (SCHIP) bill passed in 1996. Many proposals have been put forward over the decades for health care reform, as well as health insurance reform. Beginning in the 1970s Senator Ted Kennedy, President Richard Nixon, President Gerald Ford, and President Jimmy Carter all made health-related proposals, all followed by the Health Security Act of President Bill Clinton. None were accepted by Congress (KFF, 2009a). It was not until 2014 the first plan was accepted—the ACA put forth by President Barack Obama and his team.

Nurses and the American Nurses Association (ANA) have been involved in the debates about health care reform over time and developed a healthcare system reform agenda. The ANA (2008) promoted a blueprint for reform that included the following:

- Health care is a basic human right, and so a restructured health care system with universal access to a standard package of essential health care services for all citizens and residents must be assured.
- The development and implementation of health policies that reflect the aims put forth by the Institute of Medicine (safe, effective, patient centered, timely, efficient, equitable) and are based on outcomes research will ultimately save money.
- The overuse of expensive, technology-driven, acute, hospital-based services must give way to a balance between high-tech treatment and community-based and preventive services, with emphasis on the latter.
- A single-payer mechanism is the most desirable option for financing a reformed health care system.

In 2010 the ACA introduced by President Obama was passed after much debate. This act reflects many of the tenets offered by the ANA in its 2008 Health System Reform Agenda and puts into place comprehensive health insurance reforms that began in 2014. The goals of the ACA include improved quality and lower health care costs, provide access to care, and provide for consumer protection. Table 3.2 provides an overview of the key features of the act by year. The ACA has a major focus on prevention. This focus is designed to improve the health of Americans but also help to reduce health care costs and improve quality of care. Through the Prevention and Public Health Fund, the ACA addresses factors that influence health—housing, education, transportation, the availability of quality affordable food, and conditions in the workplace and the environment. By concentrating on the causes of chronic disease, the ACA has begun to move the nation's focus on sickness and disease to one based on wellness and prevention.

In 2016, after the ACA was implemented, ANA's Principles for Health System Transformation outlined an equitable health care system that includes:

- Universal access to a standard package of essential health care services for all citizens and residents
- Optimizing primary, community-based, and preventive services while supporting the cost-effective use of innovative, technology-driven, acute, hospital-based services

TABLE 3.2 Overview of Key Features of the Affordable Care Act by Year

2010

New Consumer Protections
- Putting information for consumers online
- Prohibiting denying coverage of children based on preexisting conditions
- Prohibiting insurance companies from rescinding coverage
- Eliminating lifetime limits on insurance coverage
- Regulating annual limits on insurance coverage
- Establishing consumer assistance programs in the states

Improving Quality and Lowering Costs
- Providing small business health insurance tax credits
- Offering relief for 4 million seniors who hit the Medicare prescription drug "donut hole"
- Providing free preventive care
- Preventing disease and illness
- Cracking down on health care fraud

Increasing Access to Affordable Care
- Providing access to insurance for uninsured Americans with pre existing conditions
- Extending coverage for young adults
- Expanding coverage for early retirees
- Rebuilding the primary care workforce
- Holding insurance companies accountable for unreasonable rate hikes
- Allowing states to cover more people on Medicaid
- Increasing payments for rural health care providers
- Strengthening community health centers

2011

Improving Quality and Lowering Costs
- Offering prescription drug discounts
- Providing free preventive care for seniors
- Improving health care quality and efficiency
- Improving care for seniors after they leave the hospital
- Introducing new innovations to bring down costs

Increasing Access to Affordable Care
- Increasing access to services at home and in the community

Holding Insurance Companies Accountable
- Bringing down health care premiums
- Addressing overpayments to big insurance companies and strengthening Medicare Advantage

2012

Improving Quality and Lowering Costs
- Linking payment to quality outcomes
- Encouraging integrated health systems
- Reducing paperwork and administrative costs
- Understanding and fighting health disparities

Increasing Access to Affordable Care
- Providing new, voluntary options for long-term care insurance

2013

Improving Quality and Lowering Costs
- Improving preventive health coverage
- Expanding authority to bundle payments

Increasing Access to Affordable Care
- Increasing Medicaid payments for primary care doctors
- Open enrollment in the health insurance marketplace begins

2014

New Consumer Protections
- Prohibiting discrimination due to pre-existing conditions or gender
- Eliminating annual limits on insurance coverage
- Ensuring coverage for individuals participating in clinical trials

Improving Quality and Lowering Costs
- Making care more affordable
- Establishing the health insurance marketplace
- Increasing the small business tax credit

Increasing Access to Affordable Care
- Increasing access to Medicaid
- Promoting individual responsibility

2015

Improving Quality and Lowering Costs
- Paying physicians based on value, not volume

For more detail about each of the bulleted statements, please refer to HHS.gov/HealthCare (*Key features of the Affordable Care Act*, 2014. Available at http://www.hhs.gov).

- Encouraging mechanisms to stimulate economic use of health care services while supporting those who do not have the means to share in costs
- Ensuring a sufficient supply of skilled workforce dedicated to providing high-quality health care services

Many states have opted for an expansion of Medicaid under the ACA. Research has focused on access to care and health outcomes since this expansion has taken place. The large body of evidence has demonstrated that expanded Medicaid, as a whole, has had largely positive impacts on coverage; access to

care, utilization, and affordability; and economic outcomes—including impacts on state budgets, uncompensated care costs for hospitals and clinics, and employment and the labor market (Antonisse et al., 2018). Discussions and debates will continue about the impact of the ACA and the IOM's discussions of integrating public health and primary care, reducing cost, increasing quality, and access for all Americans. It is important to focus on the goal: to protect and improve the health of all populations, as well as the ANA tenets for an equitable health care system.

⟩⟩ APPLYING CONTENT TO PRACTICE

Discussions and debates will continue about the impact of the ACA and the IOM's discussions of integrating public health and primary care, reducing cost, and increasing quality and access for all Americans. It is important not to lose sight of the goal: to protect and improve the health of all populations. After spending 18 months in a public policy fellowship and working with the Ways and Means Committee in Congress, Nancy Ridenour, PhD, RN, and Dean of the College of Nursing at the University of New Mexico, described her opportunity to work with others as the ACA was being developed. At a board of nursing celebration in Kentucky in the summer of 2014, Dr. Ridenour explained to the audience that it would be important for nurses to be involved in the implementation of the ACA to promote the success of the health care changes proposed. It is all about the influence of nurses and the nursing profession (Kentucky Board of Nursing, 2014).

Focus efforts on the implementation of the key features of the ACA (Table 3.2) in work with individual clients and populations in your community. An example of this application would be working with families to encourage enrolling children in the state child health insurance programs to assure that the family's children will receive preventive and primary care as needed. Recent evidence based on a national survey of 1143 public health nurses (PHNs) when asked about the ACA and its impact on their perceptions and practice, noted that they are making substantial contributions to the implementation of the ACA. These nurses have been involved in public–private partnerships, access to primary care and care coordination, client navigation, integration of primary care and public health, population health data analysis and health strategies, and community health assessments (Edmonds et al., 2017).

QSEN FOCUS ON QUALITY AND SAFETY EDUCATION IN NURSES

Targeted Competency: Informatics

Use information and technology to communicate, manage knowledge, mitigate error, and support decision making.

Important aspects of informatics include the following:

- **Knowledge:** Identify essential information that must be available in a common database to support interventions in the health care system.
- **Skills:** Use information management tools to monitor outcomes of intervention processes.
- **Attitudes:** Value technologies that support decision making, error prevention, and case coordination.

Informatics Question

Updated informatics definitions focus on having access to the necessary client and system information at the right time to make the best clinical decision. In the US Department of Health and Human Services (HHS) Strategic Plan for 2018–2022, there are five overarching goals. Specifically, Goal 1: Strengthen Health Care, Objective F, focuses on promoting the adoption and meaningful use of health information technology.

Which community data would a public health nurse assess to determine the work that needs to be done in a community related to this HHS strategic goal?

Answer

To assess future work that could be done to effectively address Goal 1, Objective F, public health nurses might gather data and answer questions in the following areas:

- What are the children and adult immunization rates in the community?
- What strategies are used by the health districts and primary care providers to increase vaccine rates?
- Are there characteristics within the unvaccinated population that can be addressed on a system and community level?
- What is the best method to reach this population?
- What strategies would be implemented to educate the unvaccinated?
- Have there been infectious disease outbreaks in the community over the last three years?
- What are the rates of the most common chronic diseases in the community?
- Where are the people living who have these diseases? Is there a cluster of individuals with the chronic disease?
- What resources are available in the community for these chronic diseases?
- How are these resources shared with the population?
- How are these services financed?
- Are communicable and noncommunicable diseases disproportionately affecting a particular group within the population?
- What impact does the environment have on the development of chronic diseases in the community?

Prepared by Gail Armstrong, ND, DNP, MS, PhD, Professor and Assistant Dean/DNP program, Oregon Health and Sciences University, and updated by Marcia Stanhope (2020).

▮ PRACTICE APPLICATION

During a well-child clinic visit, Jenna Wells, RN, met Sandra Farr and her 24-month-old daughter, Jessica. The Farrs had recently moved to the community. Mrs. Farr stated that she knew that Jessica needed the last in a series of immunizations and because they did not have health insurance, she brought her daughter to the public health clinic. On initial assessment, Mrs. Farr told the nurse that her husband would soon be employed, but the family had no health care coverage for the next 30 days. The Farrs also needed to decide which health care package they wanted. Mr. Farr's company offers a preferred provider organization (PPO), a health maintenance organization (HMO), and a community nursing clinic plan to all employees. Neither Mr. nor Mrs. Farr had ever used an HMO or a

community nursing clinic, and they are not sure what services are provided.

Mrs. Farr asks Nurse Wells what she should do.

Nurse Wells should do which of the following?

A. Encourage Mrs. Farr to choose the HMO because it will pay more attention to the family's preventive needs, and direct Mrs. Farr to other sources of health care should the family need to see a provider while they are uninsured.

B. Encourage Mrs. Farr to choose the PPO because it will have a greater number of qualified providers from which to choose, and direct Mrs. Farr to other sources of health care should the family need to see a provider while they are uninsured.

C. Encourage Mrs. Farr to choose the local community nursing center because it is staffed with nurse practitioners who are well qualified to provide comprehensive health care with an emphasis on health education, and direct Mrs. Farr to other sources of health care should the family need to see a provider while they are uninsured.

D. Explain the differences between a PPO, HMO, and community nursing clinic and encourage Mrs. Farr to discuss the options with her husband about signing up for a health insurance plan under the ACA plans, and direct Mrs. Farr to other sources of health care should the family need to see a provider while they are uninsured.
Answers can be found on the Evolve website.

▌ REMEMBER THIS!

- Health care in the United States is made up of a personal care system and a public health system, with overlap between the two systems.
- Primary care is a personal health care system that provides for first contact and continuous, comprehensive, and coordinated care.
- Primary health care is essential care made universally accessible to individuals and families in a community. Health care is made available to them through their full participation and is provided at a cost that the community and country can afford.
- Primary care and the public health systems are part of primary health care.
- Public health refers to organized community efforts designed to prevent disease and promote health of the population.
- Important trends that affect the health care system include political, demographic, social, economic, and technological trends.
- More than 48 million people in the United States were uninsured in 2012, and this was reduced to 27 million by the end of 2019.
- With the implementation of the Affordable Care Act (ACA), by 2016 the numbers of uninsured dropped by 6.3%.
- Many federal agencies are involved in government health care functions. The agency most directly involved with the health and welfare of Americans is the US Department of Health and Human Services (HHS).
- Most state and local jurisdictions have government activities that affect the health care field.
- Health care and insurance reform measures seek to make changes in the cost and quality of and access to the present system, such as the ACA passed in 2010.
- To achieve the specific health goals of programs such as *Healthy People 2030*, primary care and public health must work within the community for community-based care.
- The most sustainable individual and system health changes come when people who live in the community actively participate.
- Nurses are more than able to bridge the gap between individualized care and public health because they have skills in assessment, health promotion, disease and injury prevention, and disease management; knowledge of community resources; and the ability to develop relationships with community members and leaders.

EVOLVE WEBSITE

http://evolve.elsevier.com/Stanhope/foundations/
- Practice Application Answers
- Case Study, with Questions and Answers
- Review Questions

REFERENCES

American Academy of Pediatrics (AAP): *Children and Disasters, Enterovirus D68*, 2016. Retrieved from https://www.aap.org.

American Nurses Association (ANA): *Health System Reform*, Silver Spring, MD, 2008, ANA. Retrieved from https://www.nursingworld.org.

Antonisse L, Garfield R, Rudowitz R, Artiga S. *The effects of Medicaid expansion under the ACA: Updated findings from a literature review*, 2018, Kaiser Family Foundation. Retrieved from https://www.kff.org.

Artiga S, and Damico A. *Health and Health Coverage in the South: A Data Update*, 2016, Kaiser Family Foundation. Retrieved from https://kaiserfamilyfoundation.com.

Bureau of Labor Statistics (BLS), US Department of Labor: *Databases, Tables, and Calculators*, 2018a. Retrieved from https://data.bls.gov.

Bureau of Labor Statistics, US Department of Labor: *Consumer Price Index—2018*, 2018b. Retrieved from https://www.bls.gov.

Bureau of Labor Statistics (BLS), US Department of Labor: *Occupational Outlook Handbook: Registered Nurses*, 2018c. Retrieved from https://www.bls.gov.

Centers for Disease Control and Prevention: *Public Health Genomics: Family History Public Health Initiative*. Atlanta, GA, 2017, CDC, US Department of Health & Human Services.

Centers for Medicare and Medicaid Services: *National Health Expenditure Data*, 2018. Retrieved from https://www.cms.gov.

Congressional Budget Office (CBO): *Trends in the Distribution of Household Income between 1979 and 2018*, 2018, p. 9. Retrieved from https://www.cbo.gov.

Dorn S, Hill I, Hogan S: *The secrets of Massachusetts' success: why 97 % of state residents have health coverage: state health access reform evaluation, Rommneycare-The truth about Massachusetts health care*, 2009. Accessed at mittromneycentral.com, Robert Wood Johnson Foundation. Retrieved from http://www.urban.org.

Economic Report of the President, Washington, DC, 2010, U.S. Government Printing Office. Retrieved from http://www.whitehouse.gov.

Edmonds JK, Campbell LA, Gilder RE: Public health nursing practice in the Affordable Care Act era: A national survey, *Public Health Nurs* 34(1):50–58, 2017. Retrieved from https://onlinelibrary.wiley.com.

Eggers, W. D., Flynn, M., O'Leary, J., & Chew, B. (2020). *Governments Respond to COVID-19*. Retrieved from https://www.ncbi.nlm.nih.gov.

Flinter M, Hsu C, Cromp D, Ladden MD, Wagner EH: Registered nurses in primary care: Emerging new roles and contributions to team-based care in high-performing practices, *J Ambul Care Manage* 40(4):287–296, 2017. Retrieved from https://www.ncbi.nlm.nih.gov.

Hamilton BE, Kirmeyer SE, Division of Vital Statistics: Trends and variations in reproduction and intrinsic rates: United States, 1990–2014, *Natl Vital Stat Rep* 66(2), 2017. Retrieved from https://www.cdc.gov.

Health Information Technology (HealthIT): Rockville, MD, 2018, USDHHS. Retrieved from https://www.healthit.gov.

Health Resources and Services Administration (HRSA): *2017 National Health Center Data*, Washington, DC, 2018, HRSA, US Department of Health and Human Services. Retrieved from https://bphc.hrsa.gov.

Health Resources and Services Administration (HRSA): *HRSA Awards $18.9 Million to Expand Use of Health Information Technology at Health Centers.* Washington, DC, 2018, HRSA, US Department of Health and Human Services. Retrieved from http://archive.hrsa.gov.

Heron M: Deaths: Leading causes for 2016, *Natl Vital Stat Rep* 67(6). Hyattsville, MD, 2018, National Center for Health Statistics.

Institute of Medicine (IOM): *The Future of Public Health*, Washington, DC, 1988, National Academies Press.

Institute of Medicine (IOM): *Primary Care: America's Health in a New Era*, Washington, DC, 1996, National Academies Press. Retrieved from http://www.nap.edu.

Institute of Medicine (IOM): *To Err is Human: Building a Safer Health System*, Washington, DC, 2000, National Academies Press. Retrieved from http://www.iom.edu.

Institute of Medicine (IOM): *Keeping Patients Safe: Transforming the Work Environment of Nurses*, Washington, DC, 2003, National Academies Press. Retrieved from http://www.iom.edu.

Institute of Medicine (IOM): *Primary Care and Public Health: Exploring Integration to Improve Population Health*, Washington, DC, 2012, National Academies Press.

International Council of Nurses, 2018; The ICN Leadership For Change(™) Programme—20 years of growing influence February 2016, International Nursing Review 63(1):15-25

Kaiser Family Foundation: *Focus on Health Reform Massachusetts Health Care Reform: 6 years later*, Washington DC, 2012. Retrieved from https://kaiserfamilyfoundation.com.

Kaiser Family Foundation: *Key Facts about the Uninsured Population*, 2019. Retrieved from https://www.kff.org.

Kaiser Family Foundation: *National Health Insurance—a Brief History of Reform Efforts in the U.S.* 2009a, Kaiser Family Foundation. Retrieved from https://kaiserfamilyfoundation.com.

Kentucky Board of Nursing: 100th anniversary celebration keynote by N. Ridenour, Louisville, KY, 2014.

Levesque JF, Breton M, Senn N, et al.: The interaction of public health and primary care: Functional roles and organizational models that bridge individual and population perspectives, *Public Health Rev* 35:1–27, 2013.

Macy Foundation: *Registered Nurses: Partners in Transforming Primary Care: Proceedings of a conference on Preparing Registered Nurses for Enhanced Roles in Primary Care*, 2017. Retrieved from http://macyfoundation.org.

MedlinePlus. *Managed Care*, Rockville, MD, 2017, US National Library of Medicine. Retrieved from https://medlineplus.gov.

National Center for Complementary and Integrative Health, National Institutes of Health: 2017. Retrieved from https://nccih.nih.gov.

National Center for Health Statistics (NCHS). *Health, United States, 2016: With Chartbook on Long-term Trends in Health*, Hyattsville, MD, 2017, NCHS. Retrieved from https://www.cdc.gov.

National Institutes of Health (NIH): My family health portrait: a tool from the surgeon general, *NIH MedlinePlus* 5(1):4, 2010. Retrieved from http://www.nlm.nih.gov.

Office for National Statistics (ONS): *Vital statistics: population and health reference tables, annual time series data*, 2014.

Pew Research Center: *Tabulations of the 2012 American Community Surveys*, 2020. Retrieved from www.pewresearch.org.

Public Health Accreditation Board: *Accreditation Standards*, 2018. Retrieved from http://www.phaboard.org.

Rosenbaum S, JD. The Patient Protection and Affordable Care Act: Implications for Public Health Policy and Practice, *Public Health Rep.* 2011 Jan-Feb;

Sanborn BJ. As baby boomer nurses retire, concern grows about national shortage. *Healthcare Finance*, 2017. Retrieved from https://www.healthcarefinancenews.com.

Truffer CJ, Keehan S, Smith S, et al.: Health spending projections through 2019: the recession's impact continues, *Health Aff (Millwood)* 29: 522–529, 2010. Retrieved from http://content.healthaffairs.org.

United Nations: *UN millennium development goals (MDGs)*, 2013. Available at http://www.un.org.

United Nations: *UN Sustainable Development Goals (SDGs)*, 2017. Available at https://www.un.org.

US Census Bureau: *Population*, 2018. Retrieved from https://www.census.gov.

US Department of Health and Human Services (HHS): *Strategic Plan: Fiscal Years 2018-2022*, 2018. Retrieved from https://www.hhs.gov.

US Department of Homeland Security (USDHS): *Homeland Security*, 2014. Retrieved from http://www.dhs.gov.

US Public Health Service (USPHS): *The Commissioned Corps of the PHS*, 2018. Retrieved from https://www.usphs.gov.

World Health Organization (WHO): *Primary Health Care*, 2018. Retrieved from http://www.who.int

World Health Organization (WHO): *Primary Health Care: Report of the International Conference on Primary Health Care, Alma-Ata, USSR, September 6-12*, 1978. [Health for All Series No. 1]. Geneva, 1978, WHO.

World Health Organization (WHO): *Basic Documents*, ed 36. Geneva, 1986a, WHO.

World Health Organization (WHO): *World Health Statistics Annual.* Geneva, 1986b, WHO.

World Health Organization (WHO): *The World Health Report 2008: Primary Health Care (Now More Than Ever)*. Geneva, 2008, WHO. Retrieved from http://www.who.int.

World Health Organization (WHO): *The World Health Report 2008: Primary Health Care (Now More Than Ever)*, Geneva, 2008, WHO. Retrieved December 2014 from http://www.who.int.

WHO Europe (2013a); Health 2020. *A European policy framework and strategy for the 21st century (2013)*. Retrieved from WHO Europe Geneva Switzerland

4

Government, the Law, and Policy Activism

Marcia Stanhope

OBJECTIVES

After reading this chapter, the student should be able to:

1. Discuss the structure of the US government and health care roles.
2. Identify the functions of key governmental and quasi-governmental agencies that affect public health systems and nursing
3. Differentiate between the primary bodies of law that affect nursing and health care.
4. Define key terms related to policy and politics.
5. State the relationships between nursing practice, health policy, and politics.
6. Develop and implement a plan to communicate with policy makers on a chosen public health issue.

CHAPTER OUTLINE

KEY TERMS

Nurses are an important part of the health care system and are greatly affected by governmental and legal systems. Nurses who select the community as their area of practice must be especially aware of the impact of government, law, and health policy on nursing, health, and the communities in which they practice. Insight into how government, law, and political action have changed over time is necessary to understand how the health care system has been shaped by these factors. Also, understanding how these factors have influenced the current and future roles for nurses and the public health system is critical for better health policy for the nation.

Nurses have historically viewed themselves as advocates for the health of the population. It is this heritage that has moved the discipline into the policy and political arenas. To secure a more positive health care system, nurse professionals must develop a working knowledge of government, key governmental and quasi-governmental organizations and agencies, health care law, the policy process, and the political forces that are shaping the future of health care. This knowledge and the motivation to be an agent of change in the discipline and in the community are necessary ingredients for success as a population-centered nurse.

DEFINITIONS

To understand the relationship between health policy, politics, and law, one must first understand the definitions of the terms.

1. Policy is a settled course of action, which could be a law, a regulation, or a voluntary practice to be followed by a government or institution to obtain a desired end (CDC, 2015).
2. Public policy is described as all governmental activities, direct or indirect, that influence the lives of all citizens (Birkland, 2016).
3. Health policy, in contrast, is a set course of action to obtain a desired health outcome for an individual, family, group, community, or society (WHO, 2018). Policies are made not only by governments, but also by such institutions as a health department or other health care agency, a family, a community, or a professional organization.

Politics plays a role in the development of such policies. Politics is found in families, professional and employing agencies, and governments. Politics determines who gets what and when and how they get it (Birkland, 2016). Politics is the art of influencing others to accept a specific course of action. Therefore, political activities are used to arrive at a course of action (the policy). Law is a system of privileges and processes by which people solve problems based on a set of established rules; it is intended to minimize the use of force (Hill & Hill, 2018). Laws govern the relationships of individuals and organizations with other individuals and with government. Through political action, a policy may become a law, a regulation, a judicial ruling, a decision, or an order.

After a law is established, regulations further define the course of action (policy) to be taken by organizations or individuals in reaching an outcome. Government is the ultimate authority in society and is designated to enforce the policy whether it is related to health, education, economics, social welfare, or any other society issue. The following discussion explains the role of government in health policy.

GOVERNMENTAL ROLE IN US HEALTH CARE

In the United States, the federal and most state and local governments are composed of three branches, each of which has separate and important functions (USA.gov, 2018). The *executive branch* is composed of the president (or state governor or local mayor) along with the staff and cabinet appointed by this executive, various administrative and regulatory departments, and agencies such as the US Department of Health and Human Services (USDHHS). The *legislative branch* (i.e., Congress at the federal level) is made up of two bodies: the Senate and the House of Representatives, whose members are elected by the citizens of particular geographic areas.

The *judicial branch* is composed of a system of federal, state, and local courts guided by the opinions of the Supreme Court. Each of these branches is established by the Constitution, and each plays an important role in the development and implementation of health law and public policy.

The *executive branch* suggests, administers, and regulates policy. The role of the *legislative branch* is to identify problems and to propose, debate, pass, and modify laws to address those problems. The judicial branch interprets laws and their meaning, as in its ongoing interpretation of states' rights to define access to reproductive health services to citizens of the states.

One of the first constitutional challenges to a federal law passed by Congress was in the area of health and welfare in 1937, after the 74th Congress had established unemployment compensation and old age benefits for US citizens (US Law, 1937a). Although Congress had created other health programs previously, its legal basis for doing so had never been challenged. In *Stewart Machine Co.* v. *Davis* (US Law, 1937b), the Supreme Court (judicial branch) reviewed this legislation and determined, through interpretation of the Constitution, that such federal governmental action was within the powers of Congress to promote the general welfare. It was obvious in 2008 and beyond that unemployment benefits are important to the economy and to individuals who lose jobs during a national economic crisis, including the shutdowns during the COVID-19 crisis (Chikhale, 2017; Rothstein & Valletta, 2017; USAFacts, 2020).

Most legal bases for the actions of Congress in health care are found in Article I, Section 8 of the US Constitution, including the following:

1. Provide for the general welfare.
2. Regulate commerce among the states.
3. Raise funds to support the military.
4. Provide spending power.

Through a continuing number and variety of cases and controversies, these Section 8 provisions have been interpreted by the courts to appropriately include a wide variety of federal powers and activities. State power concerning health care is called police power (Hill & Hill, 2018). This power allows states to act to protect the health, safety, and welfare of their citizens. Such police power must be used fairly, and the state must show that it has a compelling interest in taking actions, especially actions that might infringe on individual rights. Examples of a state using its police powers include requiring immunization of children before being admitted to school and requiring case finding, reporting, treating, and follow-up care of persons with COVID-19. These activities protect the health, safety, and welfare of state citizens.

TRENDS AND SHIFTS IN GOVERNMENTAL ROLES

The government's role in health care at both the state and federal levels began gradually. Wars, economic instability, and political differences between parties all shaped the government's role. The first major federal governmental action relating to health was the creation in 1798 of the Public Health Service (PHS). Then in 1890, federal laws were passed to promote the public health of merchant seamen and Native Americans. In 1934, Senator Wagner of New York initiated the first national health insurance bill. The Social Security Act of 1935 was passed to provide assistance to older adults and the unemployed, and it offered survivors' insurance for widows and children. It also provided for child welfare, health department grants, and maternal and child health projects. In 1948, Congress created the National Institutes of Health (NIH), and in 1965 it passed very important health legislations, creating Medicare and Medicaid to provide health care service payments for older adults, the disabled, and the categorically poor. These legislative acts by Congress created programs that were implemented by the executive branch. In March 2010, legislation was passed and signed by President Obama to improve the health of the nation and access to care, the health reform law, the Patient Protection and Affordable Care Act (US Law, PL 111-148). Changes were made to the implementation of this law by the President and Congress in 2017 (Kaiser Family Foundation, 2017).

The US Department of Health and Human Services (USDHHS) (known previously as the Department of Health, Education, and Welfare [DHEW]) was created in 1953. The Health Care Financing Administration (HCFA) was created in 1977 as the key agency within the USDHHS to provide direction for Medicare and Medicaid. In 2002, HCFA was renamed the Center for Medicare and Medicaid Services (CMS). During the 1980s, a major effort of the Reagan administration was to shift federal government activities to the states, including federal programs for health care. The process of shifting the responsibility for planning, delivering, and financing programs from the federal level to the states is called devolution. Throughout the 1980s and 1990s, Congress increasingly funded health programs by giving block grants to the states. Devolution processes including block granting should alert professional nurses that state and local policies have grown in importance to the health care arena. With the health reform law of 2010, stimulus grants were provided to state and local areas to improve health care access (Congressional Research Service, 2017).

The Health Insurance Portability and Accountability Act (HIPAA) allows working persons to keep their employee group health insurance for up to 16 months after they leave a job (US Law 107-105, 1996). The State Child Health Improvement Act (SCHIP) of 1997 provides insurance for children and families who cannot otherwise afford health insurance (US Law, Title Ten SSA, BBA, 1997).

With the latest health care reform, numerous debates occurred in the House of Representatives and the Senate until there was agreement that the Senate version of the bill would be passed. On March 30, 2010, President Obama signed into law the Health Care and Education Reconciliation Act of 2010, which made some changes to the comprehensive health reform law and included House amendments to the new law (Kaiser Family Foundation, 2017). In 2017, the current congress and president made many changes to the ACA of 2010. These changes can be found at www.kff.org/health-reform.

This discussion has focused primarily on trends and shifts between different levels of government. An additional aspect of governmental action is the relationship between government and individuals. Freedom of individuals must be balanced with governmental powers. After the terrorist attacks on the United States in September 11, 2001 (World Trade Center attack) and October 2001 (anthrax outbreak), much government activity was being conducted in the name of national security.

It is interesting to note that before 2001, Congress and the president, recognizing that the public health system infrastructure needed help, passed The Public Health Threats and Emergencies Act (PL 106-505) in 2000 (US Law, 2000). This law "addresses emerging threats to the public's health and authorizes the secretary of HHS to take appropriate response actions during a public health emergency, including investigations, treatment, and prevention" (Katz et al., 2014, p. 133). This legislation is said to have signaled the beginning of renewed interest in public health as the protector for entire communities. In June 2002, the Public Health Security and Bioterrorism Preparedness and Response Act was signed into law (US Law, 2002, PL 107-188), with $3 billion appropriated by Congress to implement the following antibioterrorism activities:

- Improving public health capacity
- Upgrading of health professionals' ability to recognize and treat diseases caused by bioterrorism
- Speeding the development of new vaccines and other countermeasures
- Improving water and food supply protection
- Tracking and regulating the use of dangerous pathogens within the United States (Katz et al., 2014)

Yet there is considerable debate on just how much governmental intervention is necessary and effective and how much will be tolerated by citizens. For example, in 2010, approximately 49% of citizens were against the new health care reform acts, and political parties would not reach an agreement. In 2016, 52% of citizens were for government intervention in ensuring all Americans have health care coverage and 45% against (Gallup, Inc, 2016).

GOVERNMENT HEALTH CARE FUNCTIONS

Federal, state, and local governments carry out five health care functions, which fall into the general categories of direct services, financing, information, policy setting, and public protection.

Direct Services

Federal, state, and local governments provide direct health services to certain individuals and groups. For example, the federal government provides health care to members and dependents of the military, certain veterans, and federal prisoners. State and local governments employ nurses to deliver a variety of services to individuals and families, frequently on the basis of factors such as financial need or the need for a particular service, such as hypertension, tuberculosis or COVID-19 screening, immunizations for children and older adults, and primary care for inmates in local jails or state prisons. The Evidence-Based Practice box presents a study that examined the use of a state health insurance program.

EVIDENCE-BASED PRACTICE

The purpose of this study was to determine the effects of a public health policy on meeting the primary and preventive care needs of children. A survey was used to collect data from both insured and uninsured children.

"Parents of 4,142 recent enrollees and 5,518 established enrollees in the CHIP (Child Health Insurance program, (referred to as SCHIP at state level) responded to the survey (response rates were 46 percent for recent enrollees and 51 percent for established enrollees)." Comparing uninsured children to CHIP-enrolled children, the results of the survey indicated CHIP enrollees were more likely to have a well-child visit, receive a range of preventive care services, and have client-centered care experiences. They were also more likely than uninsured children to have a regular source of care or provider, and shorter wait times for appointments. CHIP enrollees received preventive care services at similar rates to privately insured children and were more likely to receive effective care coordination services. "However, CHIP enrollees were less likely than privately insured children to have a regular source of care or provider and nighttime and weekend access to a usual source of care." In addition to this study, other outcomes are indicating that CHIP enrollees are benefiting by improved school attendance and graduations.

Nurse Use

This study supports the value of health policy and the need to evaluate the effectiveness of a policy in accomplishing its purposes. The study can be used by nurses to encourage parents to enroll their children in this program and to encourage legislators to continue to support the funding of the program.

Data from Smith KV, Dye C: How Well Is CHIP Addressing Primary and Preventive Care Needs and Access for Children? *Acad Pediatr* May 2015, Vol. 15, No. 3.

Financing

In 2018, the largest shares of total health spending were sponsored by the federal government (28.3%) and the households (28.4%). The private business share of health spending accounted for 19.9% of total health care spending, state and local governments accounted for 16.5%, while other private revenues accounted for 6.9%. These data are very similar from year to year with the governments at all levels and individuals sharing most of the cost burden (CMS, 2020).

The government pays for training some health personnel and for biomedical and health care research (NIH, 2017). Support in these areas has greatly affected both consumers and health care providers. Federal governments finance the direct care of clients through the Medicare, Medicaid, Social Security, and CHIP programs. State governments contribute to the costs of Medicaid and SCHIP (State Child Health Programs). Many nurses have been educated with government funds through grants and loans, and schools of nursing in the past have been built and equipped using federal funds. Governments also have financially supported other health care providers, such as physicians, most significantly through the program of Graduate Medical Education funds.

The federal government invests in research and new program demonstration projects, with NIH receiving a large portion of the monies. The National Institute of Nursing Research (NINR) is a part of the NIH and, as such, provides a substantial sum of money to the discipline of nursing for the purpose of developing the knowledge base of nursing and promoting nursing services in health care (NINR, 2018a).

Useful Information

All branches and levels of government collect, analyze, and disseminate data about health care and health status of the citizens. An example is the annual report, *Health: United States*, compiled each year by the USDHHS (NCHS, 2018). Collecting vital statistics, including mortality and morbidity data, gathering of census data, and conducting health care status surveys are all government activities. Table 4.1 lists examples of available federal and international data sources on the health status of populations in the United States and around the world. These sources are available on the Internet and in the

TABLE 4.1 International and National Sources of Data on the Health Status of the US Population

Organization	Data Sources
International	
United Nations	http://www.un.org/
	Demographic Yearbook
	Population and Vital Statistics Report
World Health Organization	http://www.who.int.
	World Health Statistics Annual
Federal	
Department of Health and Human Services	http://www.hhs.gov
	Health, United States
	Healthy People
	National Health Statistics Reports
	National Vital Statistics System
	National Survey of Family Growth
	National Health Interview Survey
	National Health and Nutrition Examination Survey
	National Hospital Care Survey
	National Nursing Home Survey
	National Ambulatory Medical Care Survey
	National Morbidity Reporting System
	National Immunization Survey
	National Mental Health Services Survey
	Estimates of National Health Expenditures
	AIDS Surveillance
	Nurse Supply Estimates
Department of Commerce	http://www.commerce.gov
	US Census of Population
	Current Population Survey
	Population Estimates and Projections
Department of Labor	http://www.dol.gov
	Consumer Price Index
	Employment and Earnings

governmental documents' section of most large libraries. This information is especially important because it can help nurses understand the major health problems in the United States and those in their own states and local communities.

Policy Setting

Policy setting is a chief governmental function. Governments at all levels and within all branches make policy decisions about health care. These health policy decisions have broad implications for financial expenses, resource use, delivery system change, and innovation in the health care field. One law that has played a very important role in the development of public health policy, public health nursing, and social welfare policy in the United States is the Sheppard-Towner Act of 1921 (US Law, 1921) (Box 4.1).

Public Protection

The US Constitution gives the federal government the authority to provide for the protection of the public's health. This function is carried out in numerous venues, such as by regulating air and water quality and protecting the borders from the influx of diseases by controlling food, drugs, and animal transportation, to name a few. The Supreme Court interprets and makes decisions related to public health, such as affirming a woman's rights to reproductive privacy *(Roe* v. *Wade)*, requiring vaccinations, and setting conditions for states to receive public funds for highway construction/repair by requiring a minimum drinking age.

HEALTHY PEOPLE 2030: AN EXAMPLE OF NATIONAL HEALTH POLICY GUIDANCE

In 1979, the surgeon general issued a report that began a 30-year focus on promoting health and preventing disease

BOX 4.1   The Sheppard-Towner Act

The Sheppard-Towner Act did the following:
- Made nurses available to provide health services for women and children, including well-child and child-development services
- Provided adequate hospital services and facilities for women and children
- Provided grants-in-aid for establishing maternal and child welfare programs
- Set precedents and patterns for the growth of modern-day public health policy
- Defined the role of the federal government in creating standards to be followed by states in conducting categorical programs, such as today's Special Supplemental Nutrition Program for Women, Infants and Children (WIC) and Early Periodic Screening and Developmental Testing (EPSDT) programs
- Defined how the consumer could influence, formulate, and shape public policy
- Defined the government's role in research
- Developed a system for collecting national health statistics
- Explained how health and social services could be integrated
- Established the importance of prenatal care, anticipatory guidance, client education, and nurse–client conferences, all of which are viewed today as essential nursing responsibilities

for all Americans (DHEW, 1979). In 1989, *Healthy People 2000* became a national effort with many stakeholders representing the perspectives of government, state, and local agencies; advocacy groups; academia; and health organizations (USDHHS, 1991).

Throughout the 1990s, states used *Healthy People 2000* objectives to identify emerging public health issues. The success of this national program was accomplished and measured through state and local efforts. The *Healthy People 2010* document focused on a vision of healthy people living in healthy communities (USDHHS, 2000). *Healthy People 2020* had four overarching goals, which can be found in the Healthy People 2020 box; this box compares the goals of *Healthy People* documents from 2000 to 2030.

♥ *HEALTHY PEOPLE 2030*

A Comparison of the Goals of *Healthy People 2000, Healthy People 2010, Healthy People 2020, Healthy People 2030*

Healthy People 2000	Healthy People 2010	Healthy People 2020	Healthy People 2030
• Increase the years of healthy life for Americans • Reduce health disparities among Americans • Achieve access to preventive services for all Americans	• Increase quality and years of healthy life • Eliminate health disparities	• Attain high quality, longer lives free of preventable disease, disability, injury, and premature death • Achieve health equity, eliminate disparities, and improve the health of all groups • Create social and physical environments that promote good health for all • Promote quality of life, healthy development, and healthy behaviors across all life stages	• Attain healthy, thriving lives and well-being, free of preventable disease, disability, injury, and premature death. • Eliminate health disparities, achieve health equity, and attain health literacy to improve the health and well-being of all. • Create social, physical, and economic environments that promote attaining full potential for health and well-being for all. • Promote healthy development, healthy behaviors, and well-being across all life stages. • Engage leadership, key constituents, and the public across multiple sectors to take action and design policies that improve the health and well-being of all.

From US Department of Health and Human Services: *Healthy People 2000, 2010, 2020, 2030,* Washington, DC, Available at http://health.gov/healthypeople.

ORGANIZATIONS AND AGENCIES THAT INFLUENCE HEALTH

International Organizations

In June 1945, following World War II, many national governments joined together to create the United Nations (UN). By charter, the aims and goals of the UN deal with human rights, world peace, international security, and the promotion of economic and social advancement of all the world's peoples. The UN, headquartered in New York City, is made up of six principal divisions: the General Assembly, Security Council, Economic and Social Council, Secretariat, International Court of Justice and the Trusteeship Council. In addition, it is comprised of several subgroups, and many specialized agencies and autonomous organizations. The work of the UN and world conferences continues with agendas to include the development of human beings, eradication of poverty, protection of human rights, investment in health, education, training, trade, economic growth, reduction of disaster risk, and an emphasis on women (United Nations, 2020).

One of the special autonomous organizations growing out of the UN is the World Health Organization (WHO). Established in 1946, WHO relates to the UN through the Economic and Social Council to achieve its goal to attain the highest possible level of health for all persons. "Health for All" is the creed of the WHO. Headquartered in Geneva, Switzerland, the WHO has six regional offices. The office for the Americas is located in Washington, DC, and is known as the Pan American Health Organization (PAHO). The author of this chapter received a grant from PAHO to study the health care delivery system of the United Kingdom and traveled through England, Scotland, and Wales with nurse leaders of the United Kingdom. This could be *you*!

The WHO provides services worldwide to promote health, it cooperates with member countries in promoting their health efforts, and it coordinates the collaborating efforts between countries and the disseminating of biomedical research. Its services, which benefit all countries, include

- a day-to-day information service on the occurrence of internationally important diseases;
- the publishing of the international list of causes of disease, injury, and death;
- monitoring of adverse reactions to drugs; and
- establishing of world standards for antibiotics and vaccines. Assistance available to individual countries includes
- support for national programs to fight disease,
- to train health workers, and
- to strengthen the delivery of health services.

The World Health Assembly (WHA) is the WHO's policy-making body, and it meets annually. The WHA's health policy work provides policy options for many countries of the world in their development of in-country initiatives and priorities; however, although WHA policy statements are important everywhere, they are guides and not laws. The WHA's most recent policy statement on nursing and midwifery was released in 2013 (WHO, 2013a) followed by two global meetings in 2015 (WHA, 2011; WHO 2016). The current worldwide shortage of professional nurses is now on the WHO agenda and is being addressed by many countries (WHA, 2011; WHO, 2010; WHO, 2013a). The WHO recently released a publication on the history of nursing and midwifery (WHO, 2016) and a document discussing global and strategic directions for strengthening nursing and midwifery (WHO, 2016; WHO, 2017). Currently, the WHO publishes information about COVID-19, providing advice for the public, technical guidance for countries, travel advice, situational reports about the status of COVID-19 throughout the world to name a few (WHO, 2020)

The World Health Report, first published in 1995, is WHO's leading publication. Each year the report combines an expert assessment of global health, including statistics relating to all countries, with a focus on a specific subject. The main purpose of the report is to provide countries, donor agencies, international organizations, and others with the information they need to help them make policy and funding decisions.

The presence of nursing in international health is increasing. Besides offering direct health services in every country in the world, nurses serve as consultants, educators, and program planners and evaluators. Nurses focus their work on a variety of public health issues, including the health care workforce and education, environment, sanitation, infectious diseases, wellness promotion, maternal and child health, and primary care.

Many nurse leaders in the United States have served the WHO. Marla Salmon, former dean of nursing at the University of Washington, chaired a global advisory group on nursing and midwifery, and Linda Tarr Whelan served as the US ambassador to the UN Commission on the Status of Women. Virginia Trotter Betts, past president of the American Nurses Association (ANA), served as a US delegate to both the WHA and the Fourth World Conference on Women in Beijing in 1995, where she participated on the negotiating team of the conference to develop a platform on the health of women during their life span. Many US nurse leaders, such as Dr. Carolyn Williams, current author in this book, have been WHO consultants. *This could be you!*

FEDERAL HEALTH AGENCIES

Laws passed by Congress may be assigned to any administrative agency within the executive branch of government for implementing, supervising, regulating, and enforcing. Congress decides which agency will monitor specific laws. For example, most health care legislation is delegated to the USDHHS. However, legislation concerning the environment would most likely be implemented and monitored by the Environmental Protection Agency (EPA), and that concerning occupational health by the Occupational Safety and Health Administration (OSHA) in the US Department of Labor.

US Department of Health and Human Services

The USDHHS is the agency most heavily involved with the health and welfare of US citizens. It touches more lives than any other federal agency. The following agencies of the USDHHS have been selected for their relevance to this chapter.

Health Resources and Services Administration

The Health Resources and Services Administration (HRSA) has been a long-standing contributor to the improved health status of Americans through the programs of services and health professions education that it funds. The HRSA contains the Bureau of Health Workforce, which includes the Divisions of Nursing and Public Health as well as the Departments of Medicine and Dentistry. The Division of Nursing is the key federal focus for nursing education and practice, and it provides national leadership to ensure an adequate supply and distribution of qualified nursing personnel to meet the health needs of the nation.

At the 122nd meeting of the Division of Nursing's National Advisory Council for Nursing Education and Practice (NACNEP), the participants discussed the role of public health nurses in participating in primary care in their communities. The speakers indicated several factors that need to be in place to support the public health nurse role:

- Baccalaureate standard for entry into practice
- Ongoing stable funding for health departments
- Competitive salaries commensurate with responsibilities
- Interventions grounded in and responsive to community needs
- Consideration of health determinants
- Experience in health promotion and prevention
- Long-term trusting relationships in the community (i.e., with clients)
- Established network of community partners
- Commitment to social justice and eliminating health disparities

In the Council's 12th report to Congress (USDHHS, 2014) the Council recommended further investment by the government in public health nursing, arguing the need based on system changes and the Affordable Care Act implementation, greater need to connect public health and care delivery with front-line public health nurses, plus the economic benefits of supporting this investment. The 13th report focused on incorporating interprofessional education and practice into nursing (USDHHS, 2015), and the 14th report provides recommendations for preparing nurses for new roles in population health management (USDHHS, 2016a). The 2018 and 15th report focused on diversity of nurses in the workforce and nurse-led community clinics (2018), while the 2019 and 16th report focused on integrating the social determinants of health into nursing (USDHHS, 2018 and 2019). Through the input of the NACNEP, the Division of Nursing sets policy for nursing nationally.

Centers for Disease Control and Prevention

The Centers for Disease Control and Prevention (CDC) serve as the national focus for developing and applying disease prevention and control, environmental health, and health promotion and education activities designed to improve the health of the people of the United States. The mission of the CDC is to protect America from health, safety, and security threats, both foreign and in the United States. As such, CDC has been on the front line of attempted control of the coronavirus outbreak. Whether diseases start at home or abroad, are chronic or acute, curable or preventable, due to human error or deliberate attack, CDC fights disease and supports communities and citizens to do the same. As such, CDC works to increases the health security of our nation (CDC, 2014a). The CDC seeks to accomplish

its mission by working with partners throughout the nation and the world in the following ways:

- To provide health security
- To detect and investigate health threats
- To tackle the biggest health problems causing death and disability
- To conduct research that will enhance prevention
- To promote healthy and safe behaviors, communities, and environments
- To develop leaders and train the public health workforce, including disease detectives
- To develop and advocate sound public health policies
- To implement prevention strategies
- To promote healthy behaviors
- To foster safe and healthful environments
- To provide leadership and training

The USPHS, since 1798, and the CDC, since 1941, have worked to protect the public from harm. While the Zika virus and COVID-19 are examples of how this is done, there have been numerous examples throughout US history of dangerous epidemics and pandemics and the responses to these epidemics to keep the public healthy. Beginning in 1633 and through 2017, the most dangerous epidemics in the US, in chronological order, were smallpox, yellow fever, cholera, scarlet fever, typhoid fever, influenza (pandemic), diptheria, polio, measles, water contamination, pertussis, and HIV/AIDS. Now, in 2020, the extremely deadly COVID-19 pandemic seemed to have overwhelmed all systems (CDC, 2018; USA Facts, 2020).

The Zika virus outbreak of 2016 is but one example of how the CDC fulfills its mission. Zika virus disease is an arboviral disease usually causing mild illness; however, congenital infection is associated with microcephaly and other birth defects. Although most cases in residents of US states were travel associated, local transmission was reported.

In 2016, a total of 5168 confirmed or probable cases of noncongenital Zika virus disease with symptom onset during January 1 to December 31, 2016, were reported to ArboNET (see Chapter 11) from US states and the District of Columbia. Most (95%) cases were travel-associated. Locally acquired disease accounted for 4% of cases, with transmission occurring in Florida (218) and Texas (6). Forty-seven cases (1%) were acquired through other routes, including sexual transmission (45), laboratory transmission (1), and person-to-person through an unknown route (1).

Because of the recognized numbers of cases, states were asked to report aggregate numbers of cases twice a week along with Zika-related hospitalizations and complications. The CDC implemented an investigation to track the cases and worked with state and local health departments to perform the following:

- Detect the possible outbreak
- Define and find cases
- Generate hypotheses about the likely source
- Test the hypothesis
- Find the point of contamination
- Control the outbreak from further spread
- Decide when the outbreak is over

By 2017, the numbers of cases related to the Zika virus were decreasing. Although the risk for travel-associated Zika virus disease appears to have been decreasing, it is important that persons traveling to areas with a risk for Zika virus transmission be cautioned to continue to take precautions, including using strategies to prevent mosquito bites and sexual transmission.

Sometime in 2019 and in 2020, another landmark event occurred with the arrival of COVID-19. The CDC began case reporting in January 2020. CDC established a case surveillance system database for the nation (see Chapter 17. By April 2020, COVID-19 was added to the National Notifiable Condition list and was classified as "immediately notifiable, and urgent notice within 24 hours." The data to be reported included personal deidentified demographic characteristics, exposure history, disease severity and outcomes, clinical data, laboratory diagnostic test results, and any comorbidities.

Fig. 4.1 presents a CDC map indicating cases per state (USA Facts, 2020). All states were involved. By August 28, 2020, the CDC reported 5,909,997 cases and 181,326 deaths among the US population. By February 25, there were only 18 known cases and 2 deaths. The figure is a map showing the number of confirmed COVID-19 disease cases since January 21, 2020, by state of residence, in 50 US states and territories.

National Institutes of Health

Founded in 1887, NIH today is one of the world's foremost biomedical research centers, and the federal focus point for biomedical research in the United States. The NIH is composed of 27 separate institutes and centers. The goal of NIH research is to acquire new knowledge to help prevent, detect, diagnose, and treat disease and disability, from the rarest genetic disorder to the common cold. The NIH mission is to uncover new knowledge that will lead to better health for everyone. The NIH works toward that mission by conducting research in its own laboratories; supporting the research of nonfederal scientists in universities, medical schools, hospitals, and research institutions throughout the country and abroad; helping in the training of research investigators; and fostering communication of medical and health sciences' information (NIH, 2017).

In late 1985, Congress overrode a presidential veto, allowing the creation of the National Center for Nursing Research within the NIH. In 1993, the Center became one of the divisions of the NIH and was renamed the National Institute of Nursing Research (NINR). The research and research-related training activities previously supported by the Division of Nursing were transferred to the new institute. The NINR is the focal point of the nation's nursing research activities. It promotes the growth and quality of research in nursing and client care, provides important leadership, expands the pool of experienced nurse researchers, and serves as a point of interaction with other bases of health care research. The mission of NINR is to promote and

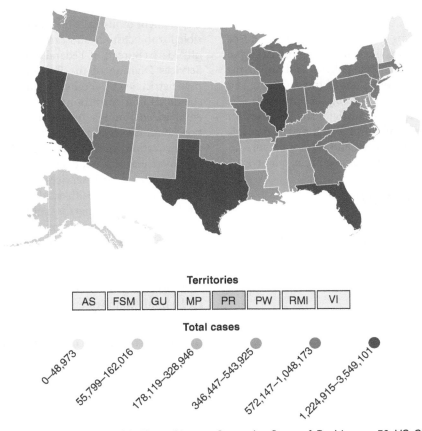

Total number of COVID-19 cases in the US reported to the CDC, by state/territory

Territories

| AS | FSM | GU | MP | PR | PW | RMI | VI |

Total cases

0–48,973   55,799–162,016   178,119–328,946   346,447–543,925   572,147–1,048,173   1,224,915–3,549,101

Fig. 4.1 Number of Confirmed COVID-19 Disease Cases, by State of Residence—50 US States and Territories. (Available at https://covid.cdc.gov/covid-data-tracker/#cases_totalcases, Retrieved March 24, 2021.)

improve the health of individuals, families, communities, and populations.

NINR supports and conducts clinical and basic research and research training on health and illness across the life span. The research focus encompasses health promotion and disease prevention, quality of life, health disparities, and end of life. NINR seeks to extend nursing science by integrating the biological and behavioral sciences, using new technologies to research questions, improving research methods, and developing the scientists of the future (NINR, 2018b).

Agency for Healthcare Research and Quality

The Agency for Healthcare Research and Quality (AHRQ) is the lead federal agency charged with improving the quality, safety, efficiency, and effectiveness of health care for all Americans. As one of 12 agencies within the USDHHS, AHRQ supports health services research that will improve the quality of health care and promote evidence-based decision making. AHRQ is committed to improving care safety and quality by developing successful partnerships and generating the knowledge and tools required for long-term improvement. The goal of AHRQ research is to promote measurable improvements in health care in America. The outcomes are gauged in terms of improved quality of life and client outcomes, lives saved, and value gained for what we spend (AHRQ, 2018).

Centers for Medicare and Medicaid Services

One of the most powerful agencies within the USDHHS is the CMS, which administered Medicare and Medicaid accounts, guided payment policy, and delivery rules for services for millions Americans (CMS, 2018). In addition to providing health insurance, CMS also performs a number of quality-focused health care or health-related activities, including regulating of laboratory testing, developing coverage policies, and improving quality of care. CMS maintains oversight of the surveying and certifying of nursing homes and continuing care providers (including home health agencies, intermediate care facilities for the developmentally disabled, and hospitals). It makes available to beneficiaries, providers, researchers, and state surveyors information about these activities and nursing home quality.

FEDERAL NONHEALTH AGENCIES

Although the USDHHS has primary responsibility for federal health functions, several other departments of the executive branch carry out important health functions for the nation. Among these are the Defense, Labor, Agriculture, and Justice departments.

Department of Defense

The Department of Defense delivers health care to members of the military, to their dependents and survivors, to National Guard and reserve members, and to retired members and their families. The assistant secretary of defense for health affairs administers a variety of health care plans for service personnel: TriCare Prime (a managed care arrangement) and an option for fee-for-service plans called TriCare Standard, as well as TriCare Extra with many other options available. In each branch of the uniformed services, nurses of high military rank are part of the administration of these health services (US Department of Defense, 2018).

Department of Labor

The Department of Labor houses the Occupational Health and Safety Agency, which imposes workplace requirements on industries. These requirements shape the functions of nurses and the types of health services provided to workers in the workplace. A record keeping system required by OSHA greatly affects health records in the workplace. Each state has an agency similar to OSHA that also monitors and inspects industries, as well as the health services delivered to them by nurses (OSHA, 2011).

Department of Agriculture

The Department of Agriculture houses the Food and Nutrition Service, which oversees a variety of food assistance activities. This service collaborates with state and local government welfare agencies to provide food stamps to needy persons to increase their food purchasing power. Other programs include school breakfast and lunch programs, WIC, and grants to states for nutrition education and training. In 2017, 7.3 million women, infants, and children received WIC benefits, with the majority of that being infants and children (USDA, 2018). Although these programs have been successful, the increasing use of the process of giving federal block grants to states (rather than implementing national programs) may threaten the effectiveness of these programs because of differences in how decisions are made at the state level on how to spend money on nutrition (USDA, 2018).

Department of Justice

Health services to federal prisoners are administered within the Department of Justice. The Federal Bureau of Prisons is responsible for the custody and care of approximately 156,083 federal offenders (Bureau of Federal Prisons, 2020). The Medical and Services Division of the Bureau of Prisons includes medical, psychiatric, dental, and health support services with community standards in a correctional environment. Health promotion is emphasized through counseling during examinations, education about effects of medications, infectious disease prevention and education, and chronic care clinics for conditions such as cardiovascular disease, diabetes, and hypertension. The Bureau also provides forensic services to the courts, including a range of evaluative mental health studies outlined in federal statutes. Health care for prisoners is highly regulated because of a series of court decisions on inmates' rights. Bureau also offers community-based facilities that provide work and opportunities to assist offenders. COVID-19 has been an issue. About 1600 inmates and 920 staff were positive for COVID-19 in August of 2020. To reduce the potential for further cases, the bureau initiated a home confinement program for select inmates.

STATE AND LOCAL HEALTH DEPARTMENTS

Depending on funding, public commitment and interest, and access to other resources, programs offered by state and local health departments vary greatly. Many state and local health officials report that employees in public health agencies lack skills in the core sciences of public health, and that this has hindered their effectiveness. The lack of specialized education and skill is a significant barrier to population-based preventive care and the delivery of quality health care to the public. Public health workforce specialists report that the number of retirees expected by 2021 will result in a major shortage of public health workers, including nurses. The state health departments provide health care finances to the local health departments, administration of programs like Medicaid, provide mental health and professional education, establish health codes, license facilities, and regulate the insurance industry. They also provide direct assistance to the local health departments. More often than at other levels of government, nurses at the local level provide direct services. Some nurses deliver special or selected services, such as follow-up of contacts in cases of COVID-19, tuberculosis, or venereal disease, or providing child immunization clinics. Other nurses have a more generalized practice, delivering services to families or populations in certain geographic areas (Beck & Boulton, 2016).

At the local and state levels, coordinating health efforts between health departments and other county or city departments is essential. Gaps in community coordination are showing up in glaring ways as states and communities scramble to address bioterrorism preparedness since September 11, 2001, and since the pandemic of 2020. Health departments are on the front line in such occurrences (see Chapter 28).

IMPACT OF GOVERNMENT HEALTH FUNCTIONS AND STRUCTURES ON NURSING

The variety and range of functions of governmental agencies have had a major impact on the practice of nursing. Funding, in particular, has shaped roles and tasks of population-centered nurses. The designation of money for specific needs, or categorical funding, has led to special and more narrowly focused nursing roles. Examples are in emergency preparedness, school nursing, and family planning. Funds assigned to antibioterrorism cannot be used to support unrelated communicable disease programs like COVID-19 or family planning.

The events of September 11, 2001 have had the public and the profession of nursing concerned about the ability of the present public health system and its workforce to deal with bioterrorism, especially outbreaks of deadly and serious communicable diseases. For example, smallpox vaccinations were stopped in 1972, but immunity lasts for only 10 years; although there have been no reported cases since the early 1970s, almost no one in the United States retains their immunity. Thus, the population is vulnerable to a smallpox outbreak, and smallpox could be used as a weapon of bioterrorism. Two laboratories in the world retain a small amount of the smallpox virus. Because of these potential threats, the US government began to increase production of the vaccine and currently has stockpiled enough vaccine to vaccinate the population in the event of a terrorist attack (NIH, 2014). Few public health professionals are knowledgeable of the symptoms, treatment, or mode of transmission of this disease. Most health professionals, including registered nurses (RNs) who currently work in the United States, have never seen a case of anthrax, smallpox, or plague—the three major biological weapons of concern in the world today. A few have now seen the effects of the Ebola virus and many have experienced the effects of a pandemic. The USDHHS and the federal Office of Homeland Security have provided funds to address serious threats to the people of the United States.

One of the first things to be done is the rebuilding of the crumbling public health infrastructures of each state to provide surveillance, intervention, and communication in the face of future bioterrorism events and natural disasters. On December 19, 2006, President George W. Bush signed the Pandemic and All-Hazards Preparedness Act (PAHPA), which was intended to improve the organization, direction, and utility of preparedness efforts (US Law, 2006). PAHPA centralizes federal responsibilities, requires state-based accountability, proposes new national surveillance methods, addresses surge capacity, and facilitates the development of vaccines and other scarce resources (Morhard and Franco, 2013; USDHHS, 2014). On March 13, 2013, President Barack Obama signed the Pandemic and All-Hazards Preparedness Reauthorization Act into law (US Law, 2013). The 2013 law reauthorizes funding for public health and medical preparedness programs that enable communities to build systems to support people in need during and after disasters (USDHHS, 2016b).

In 2016, the Obama administration developed a guidebook titled the National Security Council guidebook. It was designed to provide direction in the event of something like the COVID-19 pandemic. The guidebook was not used to assist in limiting the effects of the pandemic (Knight, 2020).

THE LAW AND HEALTH CARE

The United States is a nation of laws, which are subject to the US Constitution. The law is a system of privileges and processes by which people solve problems on the basis of a set of established rules. It is intended to minimize the use of force. Laws govern the relationships of individuals and organizations with other individuals and with government. After a law is established, regulations further define the course of actions to be taken by the government, organizations, or individuals in reaching an agreed-on outcome. Government and its laws are the ultimate authority in society and are designed to enforce official policy whether it is related to health, education, economics, social welfare, or any other society issue. The number and types of laws influencing health care are ever increasing. Definitions of law (Hill & Hill, 2018) include the following:

- A rule established by authority, society, or custom
- The body of rules governing the affairs of people, communities, states, corporations, and nations
- A set of rules or customs governing a discrete field or activity (e.g., criminal law, contract law)

These definitions reflect the close relationship of law to the community and to society's customs and beliefs.

The law has had a major impact on nursing practice. Although nursing emerged from individual voluntary activities, society passed laws to give formality to public health and, through legal mandates (i.e., laws), positions and functions for nurses in community settings were created. These functions in many instances carry the force of law. For example, if the nurse discovers a person with smallpox, the law directs the nurse and others in the public health community to take specific actions. In another example, in a mumps outbreak, a nurse and other health professionals are required to report mumps cases. This reporting requirement helps with locating and treating cases so they can be treated or isolated as they occur to prevent further spreading of disease. Three types of laws in the United States have particular importance.

CONSTITUTIONAL LAW

Constitutional law derives from federal and state constitutions. It provides overall guidance for selected practice situations. For example, on what basis can the state *require* quarantine or isolation of individuals with tuberculosis? The US Constitution specifies the explicit and limited functions of the federal government. All other powers and functions are left to the individual states. The major constitutional power of the states relating to population-centered nursing practice is the state's right to intervene in a reasonable manner to protect the health, safety, and welfare of its citizens. The state has *police power* to act through its public health system, but it has limits. First, it must be a "reasonable" exercise of power. Second, if the power interferes or infringes on individual rights, the state must demonstrate that there is a "compelling state interest" in exercising its power. Isolating an individual or separating someone from a community because that person has a communicable disease has been deemed an appropriate exercise of state powers. The state can isolate an individual even though it infringes on individual rights (such as freedom and autonomy), under the following conditions (Gostin & Wiley, 2016):

- There is a compelling state interest in preventing an epidemic (pandemic).
- The isolation is necessary to protect the health, safety, and welfare of individuals in the community or the public as a whole.
- The isolation is done in a reasonable manner.

In such circumstances, the community's rights are more important than the individual rights when there is a threat to the health of the public.

In 2020 there were few legal mandates regarding limiting the spread of COVID-19. However, some restrictions were placed on travel and entry into the US after international travel, and quarantining required for 14 days after receiving a positive test for COVID-19 or exposure to someone who was diagnosed with the disease, although the exposed person may have received a negative test. Follow-up testing was needed at the end of the quarantine. Some states required wearing a mask when with other persons, but it was difficult to monitor and to penalize those who did not comply and the community's health interest were violated by those persons (CDC, 2020).

LEGISLATION AND REGULATION

Legislation is law that comes from the legislative branches of federal, state, or local government. This is referred to as statute law because it becomes coded in the statutes of a government

(Birkland, 2016). Much legislation has an effect on nursing. Regulations are specific statements of law related to defining or implanting individual pieces of legislation or statute law. For example, state legislatures enact laws (statutes) establishing boards of nursing and defining terms such as *registered nurse* and *nursing practice*. Every state has a board of nursing. The board may be found either in the department of licensing boards of the health department or in an administrative agency of the governor's office. Created by legislation known as a state nurse practice act, the board of nursing is made up of nurses and consumers. The functions of this board are described in the nurse practice act of each state and generally include licensing and examination of RNs and licensed practical nurses; licensing and/or certification of advanced practice nurses; approval of schools of nursing in the state; revocation, suspension, or denying of licenses; and writing of regulations about nursing practice and education.

The state boards of nursing operationalize, implement, and enforce the statutory law by writing explicit statements (rules) on what it means to be an RN, and on the nurse's rights and responsibilities in delegating work to others and in meeting continuing education requirements.

All nurses employed in community settings are subject to legislation and regulations. For example, home health care nurses employed by private agencies must deliver care according to federal Medicare or state Medicaid legislation and regulations, so the agency can be reimbursed for those services. Private and public health care services rendered by nurses are subject to many governmental regulations for quality of care, standards of documentation, and confidentiality of client records and communications. All state health departments have a public health practice reference that governs the practice of nurses and others, and state public health laws that define the essential public health services that must be offered in the state as well as the optional services that may also be offered.

JUDICIAL AND COMMON LAW

Both judicial law and common law have great impact on nursing. Judicial law is based on court or jury decisions. The opinions of the courts are referred to as *case law* (Birkland, 2016). The court uses other types of laws to make its decisions, including previous court decisions or cases. Precedent is one principle of common law. This means that judges are bound by previous decisions unless they are convinced that the older law is no longer relevant or valid. This process is called *distinguishing*, and it usually involves a demonstration of how the current situation in dispute differs from the previously decided situation. Other principles of common law such as justice, fairness, respect for individual's autonomy, and self-determination are part of a court's rationale and the basis upon which to make a decision.

LAWS SPECIFIC TO NURSING PRACTICE

Despite the broad nature and varied roles of nurses in practice, two legal arenas are most applicable to nurse practice situations.

The first is the statutory authority for the profession and its scope of practice, and the second is professional negligence or malpractice.

Scope of Practice

The issue of scope of practice involves defining nursing, setting its credentials, and then distinguishing between the practices of nurses, physicians, and other health care providers. The issue is especially important to nurses in community settings who have traditionally practiced with much autonomy.

Health care practitioners are subject to the laws of the state in which they practice, and they can practice only with a license. The states' nurse practice acts differ somewhat, but they are the most important statutory laws affecting nurses. The nurse practice act of each state accomplishes at least four functions: defining the practice of professional nursing, identifying the scope of nursing practice, setting educational qualifications and other requirements for licensure, and determining the legal titles nurses may use to identify themselves. The usual and customary practice of nursing can be determined through a variety of sources, including the following:

- Content of nursing educational programs, both general and special
- Experience of other practicing nurses (peers)
- Statements and standards of nursing professional organizations
- Policies and procedures of agencies employing nurses
- Needs and interests of the community
- Updated literature, including research, books, texts, and journals
- Internet sites if it can be determined that the site is a professional source of information

All of these sources can describe, determine, and refine the scope of practice of a professional nurse. Every nurse should know and follow closely any proposed changes in the practice acts of nursing, medicine, pharmacy, and other related professions. The nurse should always examine all legislation, rules, and regulations related to nursing practice. For example, a review of the pharmacy act will let the nurse know whether to question the right to dispense medications in a family planning clinic in a local health department. Defining the scope of practice forces one to clarify independent, interdependent, and dependent nursing functions.

Just as practice acts vary by state, so do the evolving issues and tensions of scopes of practice among the health professions. In past years, several state legislatures (working closely with the National Council of State Boards of Nursing) embarked on a legislative effort to develop the Interstate Nurse Licensure Compact (NLC). The compact allowed mutual recognition of generalist nursing licensure across state lines in the compact states. In 2017, the Enhanced Nurse Licensure Compact (eNLC) was implemented, replacing the original NLC. Under the eNLC, nurses in participating states are able to have one multistate license, thus able to practice in person or by telehealth within their home state and other eNLC states. As of January 2020, 34 states had adopted the eNLC (NCSBN, 2020).

CHECK YOUR PRACTICE

As a student, you are working as a school health nurse along with an employee of the health department in your community. The state law requires that upon entry into the school system, all children must be vaccinated for childhood communicable diseases. The nurses in the schools may administer the vaccines if a child needs any or all of the required immunizations. A family has recently moved into your school district, and the parents cannot find the immunization record from the prior school system or from the physician in the previous community. The mother insists that the vaccinations are not up to date and wants the child to be able to enter school immediately. You are aware that it only takes one sick child for a major outbreak. To reduce the risk and protect the school population from communicable disease outbreaks, what should you do? See if you can apply these steps to this scenario. (1) Recognize the cues; look at the literature to see how an RN could be helpful in counseling the parent about the significance of her decision; (2) analyze the cues; (3) state several and prioritize the hypotheses you have stated; (4) generate solutions for each hypothesis; (5) take action on the number one hypothesis you think best reflects an approach to take to obtain the cooperation of the mother; and (6) evaluate the outcomes you would expect from your efforts.

Professional Negligence

Professional negligence, or malpractice, is defined as an act (or a failure to act) that leads to injury of a client. To recover money damages in a malpractice action, the client must prove all of the following:

1. The nurse owed a duty to the client or was responsible for the client's care.
2. The duty to act the way a reasonable, prudent nurse would act in the same circumstances was not fulfilled.
3. The failure to act reasonably under the circumstances led to the alleged injuries.
4. The injuries provided the basis for a monetary claim from the nurse as compensation for the injury.

Reported cases involving negligence and population-centered nurses are rare.

An integral part of all negligence actions is the question of who should be sued. When a nurse is employed and functioning within the scope of employment, the employer is responsible for the nurse's negligent actions. This is referred to as the doctrine of *respondeat superior*. By directing a nurse to carry out a particular function, the employer becomes responsible for negligence, along with the individual nurse. Because employers are usually better able to pay for the injuries suffered by clients, they are sued more often than the nurses themselves, although an increasing number of judgments include the professional nurse by name as a codefendant. In some instances, if the agency is found liable, the agency may in turn sue the nurse for negligence. At least, the nurse often loses his or her job.

Thus, it is imperative that all nurses engaged in clinical practice carry their own professional liability insurance. Nurses may have personal immunity for particular practice areas, such as giving immunizations. In some states, the legislature has granted personal immunity to nurses employed by public agencies to cover all aspects of their practice under the legal theory of *sovereign immunity* (Cherry and Jacobs, 2017).

Nursing students need to be aware that the same laws and rules that govern the professional nurse govern them. Students are expected to meet the same standard of care as that met by any licensed nurse practicing under the same or similar circumstances. Students are expected to be able to perform all tasks and make clinical decisions on the basis of the knowledge they have gained or been offered, according to their progress in their educational programs and along with adequate educational supervision.

LEGAL ISSUES AFFECTING HEALTH CARE PRACTICES

Specific legal issues of nursing vary depending on the setting where care is delivered, the clinical arena, and the nurse's functional role. The law, including legislation and judicial opinions, significantly affects each of the following areas of nursing practice. Nurses responsible for setting and implementing program priorities need to identify and monitor laws related to each special area of practice.

School and Family Health

Nurses employed by health departments or boards of education may deliver school and family health nursing. School health legislation establishes a minimum of services that must be provided to children in public and private schools. For example, most states require that children be immunized against certain communicable diseases before entering school. Children must have had a physical examination by that time, and most states require at least one physical at a later time in their schooling. Legislation also specifies when and what type of health screening will be conducted in schools (e.g., vision and hearing testing). These requirements are found in statutory laws of states. Some states are now requiring a simple dental examination in schools for the purpose of referring children to a dental health professional if needed.

Statutes addressing child abuse and neglect make a large impact on nursing practice within schools and families. Most states require nurses to notify police and/or a social service agency of any situation in which they suspect a child is being abused or neglected. This is one instance in which the law mandates that a health professional breach client confidentiality to protect someone who may be in a helpless or vulnerable position. There is *civil immunity* for such reporting, and the nurse may be called as a witness in a court hearing of the case.

Occupational Health

Occupational health is another special area of practice that has specific legal requirements as a result of state and federal statutes. Of special concern are the state workers' compensation statutes, which provide the legal foundation for claims of workers injured on the job. Access to records, confidentiality, and the use of standing orders are legal issues that have great practice significance to nurses employed in industries.

Home Care and Hospice

Home care and hospice services rendered by nurses are shaped through state statutes and have specific nursing requirements for licensure and certification. Compliance with these laws is directly linked to the method of payment for the services. For example, a service must be licensed and certified to obtain payment for services through Medicare. Federal regulations implementing Medicare/Medicaid have an enormous effect on much of nursing practice, including how nurses record details of their visits, record time spent in care activities, and document client care and the client's status and progress.

In addition, many states have passed laws requiring nurses to report elder abuse to the proper authorities, as is done with children and youth. Laws affecting home care and hospice services have focused on such issues as the right to death with dignity, rights of residents of long-term facilities and home health clients, definitions of death, and the use of living wills and advance directives. The legal and ethical dimensions of nursing practice are particularly important. Individual rights, such as the right to refuse treatment, and nursing responsibilities, such as the legal duty to render reasonable and prudent care, may appear to be in conflict in delivering home and hospice services. Much case discussion (sometimes including outside ethics consultation) may be needed to resolve such conflicts.

Correctional Health

Correctional health nursing practice is significantly shaped by federal and state laws and regulations and by recent Supreme Court decisions. The laws and decisions primarily relate to the type and amount of services that must be provided for incarcerated individuals. For example, physical examinations are required for all prisoners after they are sentenced. Regulations specify basic levels of care that must be provided for prisoners, and access to care during illness is a particular focus. Court decisions requiring adequate health services are based on constitutional law. If minimal services are not provided, it is a violation of a prisoner's right to freedom from cruel and unusual punishment. Such decisions provide a framework that strongly influences the setting of nursing priorities. For example, providing care to the sick would take priority over wellness or health education classes.

THE NURSE'S ROLE IN THE POLICY PROCESS

The number and types of laws influencing health care are increasing. Because of this, nurses need to be involved in the policy process and understand the importance of involvement of nursing to the clients they serve.

For nurses to effectively care for their client populations and their communities in the complex US health care system, professional advocacy for logical health policy that considers equality is essential. Professional nurses working in the community know all too well about the health care problems they and their clients encounter daily, and it is through policy and political activism that both big-picture and long-term solutions can be developed.

Although the term *policy* may sound rather lofty, health policy is quite simply the process of turning health problems into workable action solutions. Health policy is developed on the three-legged stool of *access, cost,* and *quality.* The policy process, which is very familiar to professional nurses, includes the following:

- Statement of a health care problem
- Statement of policy options to address the health problem

- Adoption of a particular policy option
- Implementation of the policy product (e.g., a service)
- Evaluation of the policy's intended and unintended consequences in solving the original health problem

Thus, the policy process is very similar to the nursing process, but the focus is on the level of the larger society and the adoption strategies require political action. For most professional nurses, action in the policy arena comes most easily and naturally through participation in nursing organizations such as the State Nurses Association (ANA) at the state level, the Association of Community Health Nursing Educators (ACHNE) or the Association of Public Health Nurses (APHN) at the national or state level, and in certain specialty organizations like the American Public Health Association.

Legislative Action

It is often helpful to review the legislative and political processes that may have been a part of high school education. It becomes important material to remember as a professional career is embarked upon.

The people within geographic jurisdictions elect their legislative representatives and senators. An important part of the legislative process is the work of the legislative staff. These individuals do the legwork, research, paperwork, and other activities that move policy ideas into bills and then into law. In addition to the individual legislator's office, the congressional committee staffs are also important. They are usually experts in the content of the work of a committee, such as a health and welfare committee. Frequently, developing a working relationship with key legislative staffers can be as important to achieving a policy objective as the relationship with the policy maker (i.e., the legislator).

The legislative process begins with ideas (policy options) that are developed into bills. After a bill is drafted, it is introduced to the legislature, given a number, read, and assigned to a committee. Hearings, testimony, lobbying, education, research, and informal discussions follow. If the bill is passed from the legislative committee, the entire House of Representatives hears the bill, amends it as necessary, and votes on it. A majority vote moves the bill to Senate where it is read and amended, and then a vote is taken.

Nurses can be involved in the legislative process at any point. Many professional nursing associations have legislative committees made up of volunteers, governmental relations staff professionals, and sometimes political action committees (PACs), all engaged in efforts to monitor, analyze, and shape health policy.

Common methods of influencing health policy outcomes include face-to-face encounters, personal letters, mailgrams, electronic mail, telephone calls, testimony, petitions, reports, position papers, fact sheets, letters to the editor, news releases, speeches, coalition building, demonstrations, and lawsuits. Depending on the issue, any of these can be effective. Although most businesses, including politics and the policy agendas, are dependent upon the Internet today for instant communication and quick response, all of these methods continue to be of great importance in influencing policy agendas. For example, if a face-to-face encounter is used with a legislator or a staffer, these persons can put a "face on the policy" agenda, and the reality that the policy affects real persons is an important consideration when the legislator or staff pushes the policy agenda forward. Guidelines on communication are provided in the How To box. Tips on communication and visiting legislators and their staffs, as well as general tips on political action, are presented in Boxes 4.2 to 4.4. Political activities in which nurses can and should be involved include a wide variety of activities such as being informed voters (a must!), participating in a political party, registering others to vote, getting out the vote, fundraising for candidates, building networks or communication links for issues (e.g., a phone tree or Internet distribution list), and participating in organizations to ensure their effective involvement in health policy and politics.

HOW TO BE AN EFFECTIVE COMMUNICATOR

- Use simple communications that will be readily understood.
- Choose language that clearly conveys information to individuals of diverse cultures, different ages, and different educational backgrounds.
- Target oral or written communication to the issue and omit jargon unique to medicine and nursing.
- State your expertise on the issue first.
- Briefly describe your education and experience.
- Identify the relevance of the issue beyond nursing.
- Provide information regarding the impact of the issue on the legislator's constituents.
- Present accurate, credible data.
- Do not oversell or give inaccurate information about the problem.
- Present information in an organized, thorough, concise form that is based on factual data (when available).
- Give examples.

BOX 4.2 Tips for Visits with Legislators

- Face-to-face visits are viewed as the most effective.
- Call ahead and ask how much time the staff or legislator is able to give you.
- When you arrive, ask if the appointment time is the same or if a scheduled vote on the House/Senate floor is going to need the legislator's attention.
- Engage in small talk at the beginning of the conversation only if the staff or legislator has time.
- Structure time so that the issue can be briefly presented. The visit will probably be 15 minutes or less.
- Allow an opportunity for the staff or Congress member to seek clarity or ask questions.
- Offer to provide additional information or find answers to questions asked.
- Do not assume that the legislator or the legislator's staff is well informed on the issue.
- Leave a one- or two-page fact sheet on the issue.
- Numbers count. If the views you express are shared by a local nurses' organization or by nurses employed at a health care facility, let the legislator know.
- Invite Congress members and their staffs to conferences or meetings of nurses' organizations or to tour nursing facilities to meet others interested in the same policy issues.
- If appropriate, invite the media and let the legislator know.
- Follow up with a letter of thanks to both the legislator and the staffer.

Modified from previous works of Mason D, Gardner D, Outlaw FH, O'Grady E. *Policy and politics in government*, ed 7, St. Louis, 2016, Elsevier.

BOX 4.3 Tips for Written Communication with Legislators

- Communicate in writing to express opinions, letters or email.
- Identify yourself as a nurse.
- Acknowledge the Congress member's work as positive or negative, but be courteous.
- Follow up on meetings or phone calls with a letter or e-mail.
- Share knowledge about a particular problem.
- Recommend policy solutions so the legislator or staff will know why you are writing.
- The letter should be typed, a maximum of two pages, and focused on one or two issues at most.
- The purpose of the letter should be stated at the beginning.
- Present clear and compelling rationales for your concern or position on an issue.
- If the purpose of the letter is to express disappointment regarding a stance on an issue or a vote that has been cast, the letter should be as positive as possible.
- Write letters thanking a Congress member for taking a particular position on an issue.
- A letter to the editor of the local newspaper or a nursing newsletter praising a legislator's position (with a copy forwarded to the legislator) is welcome publicity, especially during an election year.
- If you visited with the legislator or a staffer, review the major points covered in person and answer any questions that were raised during conversation.
- Have personal business cards and include them with letters.
- Address written correspondence as follows (the same general format applies to state and local officials):

US Senator	US Representative
Honorable Jane Doe	Honorable Jane Doe
United States Senate	House of Representatives
Washington, DC 20510	Washington, DC 20515
Dear Senator Doe:	Dear Representative Doe:

Modified from previous works of Mason D, Gardner D, Outlaw FH, O'Grady E. *Policy and politics in government*, ed 7, St. Louis, 2016, Elsevier.

BOX 4.4 Tips for Action

- Become informed.
- Become acquainted with elected officials.
- Become involved in the state nurses' association.
- Build communication and leadership skills.
- Increase your knowledge about a range of professional issues.
- Expand and strengthen your professional network.
- Build relationships within the profession and with representatives of public and private sector organizations with an interest in health care.
- Be aware of what is taking place in health care beyond the environment and the practice in which you work.
- Communicate with legislators regularly and share expertise and perspective on issues related to health care and nursing.
- Offer your expertise to assist in developing new legislation, modifying existing legislation or regulations.
- Identify yourself as a nurse with associated education and expertise.
- Let people know that nurses are capable of functioning in many different roles and making substantial contributions.
- Be confident.
- Do not burn bridges.
- Be friendly.
- Lend a hand to other nurses. It benefits all of us.
- Find an experienced mentor to work with you if you are new to the policy arena.
- Volunteer, seek appointments, or participate in elections in campaigns.
- Explore opportunities for involvement through internships, fellowships, and volunteer work at all levels (local, state, and national).

Modified from previous works of Mason D, Gardner D, Outlaw FH, O'Grady E. *Policy and politics in government*, ed 7, St. Louis, 2016, Elsevier.

The direct reimbursement of advanced practice nurses (APNs) in the Medicare program is one example of how nurses can use their influence. The inclusion of amendments to Medicare that authorized APN reimbursement regardless of specialty or client location in the Balanced Budget Act of 1997 (US Law, 1997) required the sustained efforts of the ANA and other national nursing organizations over a long period (Phillips, 2018; USDHHS, CMS, 2018). During that time, individual nurses provided testimony to Congress and to MEDPAC (the physicians' political action committee) on the importance of direct reimbursement to APNs. Many APNs worked closely and vigorously with their congressional representatives to lobby for this Medicare amendment. Even more wrote letters and provided position papers and fact sheets to help legislators understand the value of APNs. Although the process took more than 10 years to achieve fully, APN reimbursement in Medicare became a reality. Both the nursing profession and Medicare beneficiaries will benefit from the enhanced access of Medicare clients to APNs.

The ANA was likewise a strong supporter for the Patient Safety Act of 1997 (ANA, 1997) and the Safe Staffing for Nurse and Patient Safety Act (ANA Capitol Beat.Org, 2018) These laws required health care agencies to make public some information on nurse staff levels, staff mix, and outcomes, and it required the USDHHS to review and approve all health care acquisitions and mergers. All of these requirements are to determine any long-term effect on the health and safety of clients, communities, and staff.

On the state legislative level, all 50 states have passed title protection for APNs; this was achieved by individual nurses, state nurses associations, and various nursing specialty groups participating in the legislative process with the 50 state legislators. Title protection means that only certain nurses who meet state criteria can call themselves *advanced practice nurses*.

Regulatory Action

The regulatory process, although it may not be as visible a process as legislation, can also be used to shape laws and dramatically affect health policy. This process should be on the radar screen of professional nurses who wish to successfully participate in policy activity.

At each level of government, the executive branch can and, in most cases, must prepare regulations for implementing policy for new laws and new programs. These regulations are detailed, and they establish, fix, and control standards and criteria for carrying out certain laws. Fig. 4.2 shows the steps in the typical process of writing regulations. When the

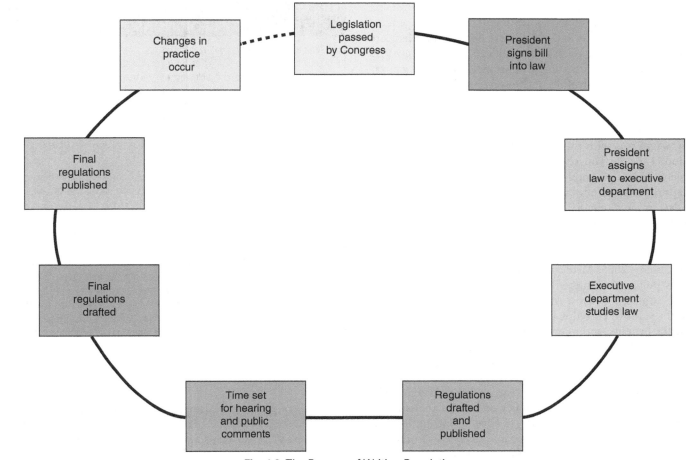

Fig. 4.2 The Process of Writing Regulations.

legislature passes a law and delegates its oversight to an agency, it gives that agency the power to make regulations. Because regulations flow from legislation, they have the force of law.

The Process of Regulation

After a law is passed, the appropriate executive department begins the process of regulation by studying the topic or issue. Advisory groups or special task forces are sometimes formed to provide the content for the regulations. Nurses can influence these regulations by writing letters to the regulatory agency in charge or by speaking at open public hearings. Many letters are now accepted by Internet.

After rewriting, the proposed regulations are put into final draft form and printed in the legally required publication (e.g., at the federal level, the *Federal Register*). Similar registers exist in most states, where regulations from state executive departments, including state health departments, are published. Public comment is called for in written form or oral presentation within a given period.

Revisions made to proposed regulations are based on public comment and public hearing. Depending on the amount and content of the public reaction, final regulations are prepared or more study of the area and issues is conducted. Final published regulations carry the force of law. When regulations become effective, health care practice is changed to conform to the new regulations. Monitoring administrative regulations is essential for the professional nurse, who can influence regulations by attending the hearings, providing comments, testifying, and engaging in lobbying aimed at individuals involved in the writing of the regulations. Concrete written suggestions for revision submitted to these individuals are frequently persuasive and must be acknowledged by government in publishing the final rules. An excellent example of how nurses must continue to influence health policy outcomes, even after positive legislation has passed, occurred after the passage of the Balanced Budget Act of 1997 (US Law, 1997). The HCFA began to implement the BBA '97 through the publication of draft regulations seeking to define APN practice and Medicare reimbursement. The nursing community responded vigorously with negative opinions about the initial restrictive definitions and requirement. Their reactions were effective and reshaped the final regulations to recognize the state definitions for APN practice autonomy.

Final regulations, published in a *Code of Regulations* (both federal and state), usually lead to changes in practice. For example, Medicare regulations setting standards for nursing homes and home health are incorporated into these agencies' manuals. In the case of APN reimbursement, some Medicare fiscal intermediaries have had difficulty in recognizing APNs as appropriate providers, but professional nursing organization advocates have forcefully addressed these implementation barriers.

Nursing Advocacy

Advocacy begins with the art of influencing others (politics) to adopt a specific course of action (policy) to solve a societal problem. This is accomplished by building relationships with the appropriate policy makers—the individuals or groups that determine a specific course of action to be followed by a government or institution to achieve a desired end (policy outcome). Relationships for effective advocacy can be built in a number of ways.

In January 2006, Medicare Part D—the prescription drug benefits policy—became effective. Public health professionals need to continue to assist many vulnerable persons to understand the value of enrolling in Part D, to educate them on how to use the benefits, and to ensure that the populations who are "dually" enrolled in both Medicare and Medicaid are registered. Coordinating efforts among civic, religious, and health care agencies to provide health education is a necessity.

A letter or visit to the district, state, or national office of a legislator to discuss a particular policy or health care issue can be interesting, educational, and effective. Contributions of money, labor, expertise, or influence may also be welcomed by the policy makers involved in setting a course of action to obtain a desired health outcome for an individual, a family, a group, a community, or society (health policy). In addition, one may develop a grassroots network of community and professional friends with a mutual interest in health policy advocacy. The network may be able to promote health policy initiatives for the community. During the Obama presidential campaign, many advocacy networks were established via the Internet and monies were solicited using this process.

Many special-interest groups in health care have the potential, desire, and resources to influence the health policy process. A tremendous advantage that nursing has in advocating for issues and in influencing policy makers is the force of its numbers, since nursing is the largest of the health professions. However, nursing must organize its numbers in such a way that each nurse joins with others to speak with one voice. The greatest effect will be had when all nurses make similar demands for policy outcomes.

Advocacy by expert and committed health professionals can bring about positive change for the profession, the community, and the clients that nurses serve. Keeping up to date on issues within government, professional organizations, law, and public policy is vitally important. Informed activism directed toward a professional role, image, and value for professional nurses, and toward a health care system in the United States that provides high quality and affordable universal access to health care, should be a lifelong commitment for all professional nurses.

QSEN   FOCUS ON QUALITY AND SAFETY EDUCATION FOR NURSES

- Targeted competency: Healthy Public Policy
- Knowledge: Describe strategies for learning about the effects of healthy public policy on program development in the public setting
- Skills: Seek information about outcomes of public health policy applications in populations served in care settings
- Attitudes: Appreciate that following policy is an essential part of the daily work of all professionals

QI Question

The Quad Council competency of policy development and program planning skills indicates that the beginning PHN collects information that will inform policy decisions. Also, the PHN describes the legislative policy development process and identifies outcomes of current health policy relevant to PHN practice. The 2020 outbreak of the coronavirus in the United States brought quick recognition that there was a need for improvement in policies related to infectious disease control. What were the indicators that the infection control policies in place were not sufficient to prevent the spread of disease? Describe the CQI data collection processes that determined the need for policy change. What role did nurses and organized nursing play in improving the infection control policy and guidelines nationally? What has been the outcome of the new policy and how were populations affected both locally and nationally? Did this work have any influence on the outbreak of COVID-19. Why? Why not?

⟫   APPLYING CONTENT TO PRACTICE

An example of how the policy process works follows, involving a nursing organization and individual members. Whether you are a member of a group as described below or working on your own to influence health policy, the steps described here apply.

Over a 15-month time frame, the American Nurses Association was involved in advocating for health care reform. During the presidential campaign, candidates were educated about the nursing profession and ANA's *Agenda for Health System Reform*. ANA and its members participated in national media interviews and local media events. The message was that the association and its members believed that health care is a basic right. ANA collaborated with the nursing community to outline the profession's priorities as proposals were developed in Congress. Testimony was given before three key congressional committees. ANA representatives met with White House and congressional health care reform staff, and took part in two presidential press conferences at the White House.

As reported by ANA, thousands of nurses joined ANA's health care reform team, sending letters to representatives of Congress, sharing their stories, and meeting with members of Congress. They also participated in rallies and events.

For more information on ANA's health care reform work, visit http://www.rnaction.org.

▮   PRACTICE APPLICATION

Larry was in his final rotation in the bachelor of Science in nursing program at State University. He was anxious to complete his final nursing course, because upon graduation he would begin a position as a staff nurse specializing in school health at the local health department. His wife was expecting their first child, and she had been receiving prenatal care at the health department.

Larry was aware that a few years ago the federal government had, by law, provided block grants to states for primary care, maternal–child health programs, and other health care needs of states. He had read the *Federal Register* and knew that the regulations for these grants had been written through USDHHS departments. He was aware that these regulations did not require states to fund specific programs.

Larry read in the local newspaper that the health department was closing its prenatal clinic at the end of the month. When his state had received its block grant, it decided to spend the money for programs other than prenatal care. Larry found that a 3-year study in his own state showed improved pregnancy outcomes as a result of prenatal care. The results were further improved when the care was delivered by population-centered nurses. After Larry's daughter was born, he read in the *Federal Register* that states could apply for federal stimulus funds and receive a grant for home visiting services to support mothers and new babies.

Larry was concerned that, as a student, he would have little influence on how such grant dollars would be spent. However, he decided to call his classmates together to plan a course of action.

What would such an action plan include?

Answers can be found on the Evolve website.

REMEMBER THIS!

- The legal basis for most congressional action in health care can be found in Article I, Section 8, of the US Constitution.
- The five major health care functions of the federal government are direct service, financing, information, policy setting, and public protection.
- The goal of the World Health Organization is the attainment by all people of the highest possible level of health.
- Many federal agencies are involved in government health care functions. The agency most directly involved with the health and welfare of Americans is the US Department of Health and Human Services (USDHHS).
- Most state and local governments have activities that affect nursing practice.
- The variety and range of functions of governmental agencies have had a major impact on nursing. Funding, in particular, has shaped the role and tasks of nurses.
- The private sector (of which nurses are a part) can influence legislation in many ways, especially through the process of writing regulations.
- The number and types of laws influencing health care are increasing. Because of this, involvement in the political process is important to nurses.
- Professional negligence and the scope of practice are two legal aspects particularly relevant to nursing practice.
- Nurses must consider the legal implications of their own practice in each clinical encounter.
- The federal and most state governments are composed of three branches: the executive, the legislative, and the judicial.

- Each branch of government plays a significant role in health policy.
- The US Public Health Service was created in 1798.
- The first national health insurance legislation was challenged in the Supreme Court in 1937.
- *Health: United States* (NCHS, 2018) is an important source of data about the nation's health care problems.
- In 1921 the Sheppard-Towner Act was passed, and it had an important influence on child health programs and population-centered nursing practice.
- The Division of Nursing, the National Institute of Nursing Research, and the Agency for Healthcare Policy and Research are governmental agencies important to nursing.
- Nurses, through state and local health departments, function as consultants, policy advocates, population level and direct care providers, researchers, teachers, supervisors, and program managers.
- The state governments are responsible for regulating nursing practice within the state.
- Federal and state social welfare programs have been developed to provide monetary benefits to the poor, older adults, the disabled, and the unemployed.
- Social welfare programs affect nursing practice. These programs improve the quality of life for special populations, thus making the nurse's job easier in assisting the client with health needs.
- The nurse's scope of practice is defined by legislation and by standards of practice within a specialty.

EVOLVE WEBSITE

http://evolve.elsevier.com/Stanhope/community/
- Answers to Practice Application
- Case Study
- Glossary
- Review Questions

REFERENCES

Agency for Healthcare Research and Quality: *Profile*. Bethesda, 2018, USDHHS. Available at https://www.ahrq. Accessed June 18, 2018.

American Nurses Association: Press Release, ANA Applauds Introduction of Patient Safety Act of 1997. March 1997. Available at: http://www.nursingworld.org. Accessed December 10, 2019.

American Nurses Association Capitol Beat: Introducing the Safe Staffing for Nursing and Patient Safety Act ACT. 3-1-2018. Retrieved from https:anacapitolbeat.org.

Beck AJ, Boulton ML: The public health nurse workforce in US state and local health departments—2012, *Public Health Rep* 131(1): 145-152, 2016.

Birkland TA: *An Introduction to the Policy Process: Theories, Concepts and Models of Public Policy Making*, 4th ed. New York, 2016, Routledge, Taylor & Francis Group.

Bureau of Federal Prisons: *Population Statistics, 2020*. Available at https://www.bop.gov. Accessed June 18, 2020.

Centers for Disease Control and Prevention: *Mission, role and pledge*, 2014a, USDHHS. Available at https://www.cdc.gov. Accessed June 18, 2018.

Centers for Disease Control and Prevention: Zika Cases in the US. Atlanta, 2018a. Available at: www.cdc.gov. Accessed June 1, 2018.

Centers for Disease Control and Prevention: *Definition of Policy*, 2015, USDHHS, Office of the Associate Director for Policy. Available at https://www.cdc.gov. Accessed on May 21, 2018.

Centers for Medicare and Medicaid Services. Washington, DC, 2018. Available at https://www.cms.gov/. Accessed June 18, 2018.

Centers for Medicare and Medicaid Services. National Health Expenditures Fact Sheets. Baltimore, Accessed March 4, 2020.

Cherry B, Jacobs SR: *Contemporary Nursing Issues, Trends and Management*, ed 7. St Louis, 2017, Elsevier.

Chikhale N: The importance of unemployment benefits for protecting against income drops, *Washington Center for Equitable Growth* [online], April 25, 2017.

Congressional Research Service: *Appropriations and fund transfers in the Affordable Care Act, R41301*, February 2017: Redhead CS. Available at https://fas.org. Accessed May 28, 2018.

Department of Health, Education and Welfare: *Improving Health.* Healthy People: The Surgeon General's Report on Health Promotion and Disease Prevention, DHEW Publication No. 79-55071. Washington, DC, 1979, US Government Printing Office. https://profiles.nlm.nih.gov. Accessed June 18, 2018.

Gallup, Inc: *Americans still split on government healthcare role*, December 8, 2016: McCarthy J. Available at http://news.gallup.com. Accessed May 28, 2018.

Gostin LO, Wiley LF: *Public health law: power, duty, restraint*, ed 3, Oakland, 2016, University of California Press.

Hill, G, Hill K: *The People's Law Dictionary*, New York, 2018, ALM media properties. Available at https://dictionary.law.com. Accessed May 21, 2018.

Kaiser Family Foundation: *The uninsured: A primer—key facts about health insurance the uninsured under the Affordable Care Act*, December 2017: Foutz J, Squires E, Garfield R, & Damico, A. Available at http://files.kff.org. Accessed May 28, 2018.

Katz R, Macintyre A, Barbera J: Emergency public health. In Pines JM, Abualenain J, Scott J, et al., eds.: *Emergency care and the public's health.* Hoboken, 2014, John Wiley and Sons, Ltd.

Knight, V: Evidence Shows Obama Team Left a Pandemic Game Plan for Trump Administration, Kaiser Family Foundation, 2020

Mason DJ, Gardner DB, Hopkins Outlaw F, O'Grady ET: *Policy and politics in nursing and health care*, ed 7. St Louis, 2016, Elsevier.

Morhard R, Franco C: The Pandemic and All-Hazards Preparedness Act: Its contributions and new potential to increase public health preparedness. *Biosecur Bioterror* 11(2):145–152, 2013. Available at: http://online.liebertpub.com. Accessed June 18, 2018.

National Center for Health Statistics: *Health: United States, 2017.* Hyattsville, 2018, US Government Printing Office.

National Council of State Boards of Nursing: *Enhanced Nurse Licensure Compact (eNLC) Implementation*. 2020. Available at https://www.ncsbn.org. Accessed June 18, 2020.

National Institutes of Health: *Smallpox : vaccine supply and strength.* Bethesda, 2014, USDHHS. Available at https://www.nih.gov. Accessed June 18, 2018.

National Institutes of Health: *Structure and Goals.* Bethesda, 2017, USDHHS. Available at https://www.nih.gov. Accessed June 18, 2018.

National Institute of Nursing Research: National Institutes of Health: *Funding Opportunities*. Bethesda, 2018a, USDHHS. Available at https://www.ninr.nih.gov. Accessed June 15, 2018.

National Institute of Nursing Research: National Institutes of Health: *Mission and Strategic Plan*. Bethesda, 2018b, USDHHS. Available at https://www.ninr.nih.gov. Accessed June 15, 2018.

Occupational Safety and Health Administration: *OSHA fact sheet: OSHA's bloodborne pathogen standard.* 2011. Available at: https://www.osha.gov. Accessed June 18, 2018.

Phillips SJ: 30th Annual APRN legislative update: improving access to healthcare one state at a time, *The Nurse Practitioner, 43*(1): 27-54, 2018.

Rothstein J, Valletta RG: Scraping by: Income and program participation after the loss of extended unemployment benefits, Washington DC, 2017, *Washington Center for Equitable Growth Working Paper Series.* Available at http://equitablegrowth.org. Accessed May 21, 2018.

Smith, Kimberly V., Dye, Claire. **How well is CHIP addressing primary and preventive care needs and access for children?** *Acad Pediatr*, May 2015, Vol. 15, No. 3.

United Nations: The United Nations System in the Department of Global Communications. New York, 2020, UN.

USA Facts: COVID-19, Impact and Recovery. 2020, USAFacts.org.

USA.gov: *Branches of government*, 2018. Available at https://www.usa.gov. Accessed May 21, 2018.

US Department of Agriculture: *About WIC: WIC at a glance.* Washington, DC, 2018, USDA. Available at https://www.fns.usda.gov. Accessed June 18, 2018.

US Department of Defense: *TRICARE: About Us*, Falls Church, 2018, DOD. Available at https://www.tricare.mil. Accessed June 18, 2018.

US Department of Health and Human Services: *Healthy People 2000: National Health Promotion and Disease Prevention Objectives.* Rockville, 1991, US Government Printing Office. https://www.healthypeople.gov/.

US Department of Health and Human Services: *Healthy People 2010: Understanding and Improving Health*, ed 2. Washington, DC, 2000, US Government Printing Office. https://www.healthypeople.gov/.

US Department of Health and Human Services: *Healthy People 2020.* Washington, DC, 2010. Available at: https://www.healthypeople.gov/. Accessed June 18, 2020.

US Department of Health and Human Services: *Healthy People 2030.* Washington, DC, 2020. Available at: https://www.healthypeople.gov/. Accessed July 18, 2020.

US Department of Health and Human Services, The Division of Nursing's National Advisory Committee on Nursing Education and Practice: *Public Health Nursing: key to our nation's health.* Rockville, 2014, Division of Nursing. Available at https://www.hrsa.gov. Accessed June 18, 2018.

US Department of Health and Human Services, Public Health Emergency, *Pandemic and All Hazards Preparedness Act*, Washington, DC, 2014. Available at https://www.phe.gov. Accessed June 18, 2018.

US Department of Health and Human Services, The Division of Nursing's National Advisory Committee on Nursing Education and Practice: *Incorporating interprofessional education and practice into nursing*. Rockville, 2015, Division of Nursing. Available at https://www.hrsa.gov. Accessed June 18, 2018.

US Department of Health and Human Services, The Division of Nursing's National Advisory Committee on Nursing Education and Practice: *Preparing nurses for new roles in population health management*. Rockville, 2016a, Division of Nursing. Available at https://www.hrsa.gov. Accessed June 18, 2018.

US Department of Health and Human Services, The Division of Nursing's National Advisory Committee on Nursing Education and Practice: *Diversity of the Nursing Workforce*. Rockville, 2018a, Division of Nursing. Available at https://www.hrsa.gov. Accessed June 18, 2020.

US Department of Health and Human Services, The Division of Nursing's National Advisory Committee on Nursing Education and Practice: *Integrating Social Determinants of Health*. Rockville, 2019, Division of Nursing. Available at https://www.hrsa.gov. Accessed June 18, 2020.

US Department of Health and Human Services, Public Health Emergency, *Pandemic and All Hazards Preparedness Reauthorization Act*, Washington, DC, 2016b. Available at https://www.phe.gov. Accessed June 18, 2018.

US Law: 42 USC. Section 161-175, Sheppard-Towner Maternity and Infant Protection Act. 1921.

US Law: 49 Stat 622, Title II. 1937a.

US Law: 42 SC 301, *Stewart Machine Co.* v. *Davis*. 1937b.

US Law: Public Law 107-105, Health Insurance Portability and Accountability Act (HIPAA). 1996.

US Law: Title X of the Social Security Act, BBA '97, State Child Health Improvement Act (SCHIP). 1997.

US Law: Public Law 105-33: Balanced Budget Act, 1997.

US Law: Public Law 106-505: The Public Health Threats and Emergencies Act. 2000.

US Law: 107-188, Public Health Security and Bioterrorism and Response Act. 2002.

US Law: Public Law 109-417: Pandemic and All Hazards Preparedness Act. 2006.

US Law: Public Law 111-148 Patient Protection and Affordable Care Act (PPACA). 2010.

US Law: Public Law 113-5: Pandemic and All-Hazards Preparedness Reauthorization Act, 2013.

World Health Organization: *Health systems financing: the path to universal coverage*. The World Health Report, 2010. Available at http://www.who.int. Accessed June 18, 2018.

World Health Assembly: *Strengthening nursing and midwifery*, 64th session WHA. May 24, 2011. Available at http://apps.who.int. Accessed June 18, 2018.

World Health Organization: *WHO nursing and midwifery progress report: 2008-2012*. 2013a. Available at: http://www.who.int. Accessed June 18, 2018.

World Health Organization: *The global strategic directions for strengthening nursing and midwifery 2016-2020*, Geneva, Switzerland, 2016, WHO. Available at http://www.who.int. Accessed June 18, 2018.

World Health Organization: Coronavirus Disease Pandemic. Geneva, Switzerland, 2020, WHO.

World Health Organization: *Health topics: Health policy,* 2018: WHO. Available at http://www.who.int. Accessed May 21, 2018.

5

Economics of US Health Care Delivery

Whitney Rogers Bischoff

OBJECTIVES

After reading this chapter, the student should be able to:

1. Identify major factors influencing national health care spending.
2. Relate public health and economic principles to nursing and health care.
3. Describe the role of government and other third-party payers in public health care financing.
4. Discuss the implications of health care rationing from an economic perspective.
5. Evaluate levels of prevention as they relate to public health economics.

CHAPTER OUTLINE

KEY TERMS

Health care disparities are differences among population groups in the availability, accessibility, and quality of health care services aimed at prevention, treatment, and management of diseases and their complications, including screening, diagnostic, treatment, management, and rehabilitation services (Ubri and Artiga, 2016).

In the United States, health and health care disparities are routinely seen in individuals who are marginalized because of their socioeconomic status, race, culture, primary language, sexual identity, and, in some cases, gender. How health care is financed and delivered has a direct effect on the ability of all US residents to obtain timely, appropriate care that is affordable. In addition, there is an emerging recognition that social determinants of health (SODH) along with health behavior play a major role in the health of individuals and families (Artiga and Hinton, 2018).

There is strong evidence to suggest that poverty can be directly related to poorer health outcomes. Poorer health outcomes lead to reduced educational outcomes for children, poor nutrition, low productivity in the adult workforce, and unstable economic growth in a population, community, or nation. However, improving health status and economic health is dependent on the "degree of equality" in policies that improve living standards for all members of a population, including the poor.

To address health care disparities, two significant events occurred. In 2010, a significant health reform law, the Patient Protection and Affordable Care Act (PL 111-148) (ACA) was passed by Congress and signed into law on March 23, 2010, resulting in a greater emphasis on access to care, leading to improvements in prevention of illness, patient outcomes, and population health.

To move toward improving a population's health, it was determined that there must be an "investment in public health" by all levels of government. The Prevention and Public Health Fund (PPHF), which was part of the Consolidated Appropriations Act of 2016, was specifically designed to invest in public health in communities (US Department of Health and Human Services [USDHHS], 2016b).

Estimates indicate that public spending on health care makes a difference, although this funding is highly variable from state to state. A baseline of prevention services should be provided to all, regardless of where they live. Several facts are known and based on the literature (Box 5.1) (Barnett and Berchick, 2017; USDHHS, 2016):

The demonstrated consequences of lack of health insurance shown in Box 5.1 continue to hold even as more people come under insurance coverage through the ACA (Kaiser Family Foundation, 2017a):

- Individuals without health insurance are less likely to receive preventive care and treatment for chronic diseases than those with insurance coverage (Kaiser Family Foundation, 2017a).
- Those without health insurance are more likely to be hospitalized for preventable problems and, when hospitalized, receive fewer diagnostic and therapeutic services; they also have higher mortality rates than those with insurance (Kaiser Family Foundation, 2017a).
- Adults without insurance are nearly twice as likely to report being in fair or poor health than those with private insurance (Kaiser Family Foundation, 2017a).

> **BOX 5.1 Facts About the Effects of Public Spending and Health Insurance on Population Health**
>
> - In 2016, approximately 28.1 million (8.8%) of the estimated 320.3 million people in the United States were without health insurance (Barnett and Berchick, 2017). Since many provisions of the Patient Protection Affordable Care Act (PPACA or ACA) went into effect in 2014 and some states expanded Medicaid coverage, the number of uninsured individuals has decreased from levels around 44 million people in 2013 (Kaiser Family Foundation, 2017a).
> - Although the number of uninsured has decreased under the ACA, 45% of uninsured adults cited the high cost of coverage as the reason they were not insured (Kaiser Family Foundation, 2017a).
> - Lack of workplace insurance and failure of some states to expand Medicaid under the ACA are some of the reasons given for remaining uninsured.
> - For households with less than $25,000 annual income, 13.7% did not have health insurance coverage in 2016 (Barnett and Berchick, 2017).
> - Adults younger than 65 years are more likely to be uninsured than children (Barnett and Berchick, 2017).
> - Young adults (ages 19–25 years) were beneficiaries of the ACA provision allowing them to remain on their parent's insurance policy until age 26. This resulted in falling uninsured rates among this group from 2013–2016 of about 11.5% or more for each age between 21 and 28. Even with this change in policy, 17.5% of adults aged 26 were uninsured 2016 (Barnett and Berchick, 2017).
> - The uninsured rate for all children younger than age 19 was 5.4% in 2016. For children living in poverty, the uninsured rate was 7.0%, which was higher than the rate of children not in poverty (5.0%) (Barnett and Berchick, 2017).
> - Minorities are more likely to be uninsured than Whites. Approximately 16% of Hispanics, 10.5% of Black Americans, and 7.6% of Asians were uninsured in 2016, compared with 6.3% of non-Hispanic Whites (Barnett and Berchick, 2017). These uninsured rates are approximately half the uninsured rates reported in 2013 (Kaiser Family Foundation, 2017a). States that expanded Medicaid coverage to more people showed greater gains in insured populations than those that did not (Kaiser Family Foundation, 2017a).
> - More than 8 in 10 (80%) of the uninsured were in working families with income less than 400% of poverty in 2016 (Kaiser Family Foundation, 2017a).
>   - Approximately 75% were from families with one or more full-time workers.
>   - Approximately 11% were from families with part-time workers.
> - Higher level of education, higher household income, and living in a family arrangement is associated with a greater rate of health insurance coverage (Barnett and Berchick, 2017).

- Studies indicate that gaining health insurance restores access to health care considerably and reduces the adverse effects of having been uninsured (Kaiser Family Foundation, 2017a).
- The poor are more likely to receive health care through publicly funded agencies.
- An emphasis on individual health care will not guarantee improvement of a population or a community's health.

Approximately 97% of all health care dollars are spent for individual care, whereas only 2.5% are spent on population-level health care. The 2.5% includes monies spent by the government on public health as well as the preventive health care dollars spent by private sources. These numbers indicate that there has not been a large investment in the public's health or population health in the United States (National Center for Health Statistics [NCHS], 2017). The PPHF increased total state funding for FY17 over FY16 overall, yet it does not reflect the increased need related to the opioid epidemic, growth in population, aging of the population, or emerging infectious diseases or pandemics, such as Zika; flea-, tick-, and mosquito-borne illnesses; and coronavirus (Trust for America's Health, 2018 and USA Facts, 2020).

The United States spends more on health care than any other nation. The cost of health care has been rising more than the rate of inflation since the mid-1960s, yet the US population does not enjoy greater longevity as compared with nations that spend far less than the United States. The current health care system has been reaching the point where it is not affordable and is expected to consume 19.7% of the economy by 2026 (Turnock, 2015; Cuckler, et al., 2018).

An estimated $10 per person invested in community-based prevention programs can lead to improved health status of the population and reduced health care costs (Trust for America's Health, 2016).

Nurses are challenged to implement changes in practice and participate in research, evidence-based practice, and policy activities designed to provide the best return on investment of health care dollars (i.e., to design models of care, at a reasonable price, that improve access or quality of care). Meeting this challenge requires a basic understanding of the economics of the US health care system. Nurses should be aware of the effects of nursing practice on the delivery of cost-effective care.

Although the ACA and the PPHF were showing health care improvements, gains for prevention and access were short lived when in 2017 the 115th US Congress repeatedly attempted to repeal aspects of the ACA. Thus the American Health Care Act of 2017 (CBO, 2017: H.R.1628), often shortened to the AHCA, a US Congress bill introduced to partially repeal the Patient Protection and Affordable Care Act (ACA), was passed into law.

A survey by the Commonwealth Fund found that gains achieved under the ACA were reversing as early as spring 2018 (Collins, et al., 2018). For individuals living in states that did not expand Medicaid under the ACA, the uninsured rate rose to 21%.

PUBLIC HEALTH AND ECONOMICS

Economics is the science concerned with the use of resources, including the production, distribution, and consumption of goods and services. Health economics is concerned with how scarce resources affect the health care industry (McPake et al., 2018). Public health economics, then, focuses on the producing, distributing, and consuming of goods and services as related to public health and where limited public resources might best be spent to save lives or increase the quality of life for the population (USDHHS, 2016a).

Economics provides the means to evaluate the attaining of society wants and needs in relation to limited resources. In addition to the day-to-day decision making about the use of resources, there is a focus on evaluating economics in health care (McPake et al., 2018). Although in the past there has been limited focus on evaluating public health economics, it is becoming more obvious what evaluating public health and preventive care expenditures can do in terms of evaluating cost savings and, more importantly, quality of life (Trust for

America's Health, 2017; Schulte et al., 2016). This type of evaluation will help to present funding proposals to public policymakers (legislators).

Public health financing often causes conflict because of the views and priorities of individuals and groups in society, which may differ from those of the public health care industry. If money is spent on public health care, then money for other public needs, such as education, transportation, recreation, and defense, may be limited. When trying to argue that more money should be spent for population-level health care or prevention, data are becoming available that show the investment is a good one. Public health finance is a growing field of science and practice that involves the acquiring, managing, and using of monies to improve the health of populations through disease prevention and health promotion strategies. This field of study also focuses on evaluating the use of the money and its effect on the public health system (Meit et al., 2013).

Although the public health system had been considered for many years as involving only government public health agencies such as health departments, currently the public health system is known to be much broader and includes schools, industry, media, environmental protection agencies, voluntary organizations, civic groups, local police and fire departments, religious organizations, industry/business, and private sector health care systems, including the insurance industry. All can play a key role in improving population health (Institute of Medicine, 2012; Trust for America's Health, 2017).

The goal of public health finance is to support population focused preventive health services (Meit et al., 2013). Four principles are suggested that explain how public health financing may occur (Sturchio and Goel, 2012):

- The source and use of monies are controlled solely by the government.
- The government controls the money, but the private sector controls how the money is used.
- The private sector controls the money, but the government controls how the money is used.
- The private sector controls the money and how it is used.

When the government provides the funding and controls the use, the monies come from taxes, user fees (e.g., license fees and purchase of alcohol/cigarettes), and charges to consumers of the services.

Services offered at the federal government level include the following:

- Policymaking
- Public health protection
- Collecting and sharing information about US health care and delivery systems
- Building capacity for population health
- Direct care services

Select examples of services offered at the state and local levels include the following:

- Environmental health monitoring
- Population health planning
- Disaster management
- Preventing communicable and infectious diseases
- Direct care services

When the government provides the money but the private sector decides how it is used, the money comes from business and individual tax savings related to private spending for illness prevention care. When a business provides disease prevention and health promotion services to its employees and sometimes families, such as immunizations, health screenings, and counseling, the business taxes owed to the government are reduced. This is considered a means by which the government provides money through tax savings to businesses to use for population health care.

When the private sector provides the money but the government decides how it is used, either voluntarily or involuntarily, the money is used for preventive care services for specific populations. A voluntary example is the private contributions made to reaching *Healthy People 2030* goals. An involuntary example is the Occupational Safety and Health Administration requiring industry to provide the financing to adhere to certain safety standards for use of machinery, air quality, ventilation, and eyewear protection to reduce disease and injury. For example, this has the effect of reducing occupation-related injuries in the population as a whole.

When the private sector is responsible for both the money and its use of resources, the benefits incurred are many. For example, an industry may offer influenza vaccine clinics for workers and families that may lead to "herd immunity" in the community. A business or community may institute a "no-smoking" policy that reduces the risk of smoking-related illnesses to workers, family, and the consumers of the businesses' services. A voluntary philanthropic organization may give a local community money to provide services for assisting low-income communities to improve their environment (Sessions, Fortunato, Johnson, and Panek, 2016).

These are but a few examples of how public health services and the ensuring of a healthy population are not only government related. The partnerships between government and the private sector are necessary to improve the overall health status of populations. This partnership was emphasized in the ACA enacted in 2010. A main feature of the public health ACA coverage included the "individual mandate" that all citizens acquire coverage. Because all individuals were required to purchase coverage, persons previously excluded from insurance coverage were able to get coverage regardless of preexisting conditions. However, the partnership began to unravel after the 2016 presidential election with the president and Congress vowing to "repeal and replace" the ACA.

Toward the end of 2017, Congress's efforts to repeal and replace the ACA were not immediately successful. During December 2017, Congress passed a tax bill which included a provision to repeal the "individual mandate" by removing the penalty on individuals who do not purchase health insurance. Without the individual mandate, costs of coverage for health insurance were expected to increase due to the pool of covered individuals being in poorer health (Jost, 2017, 2018b). This bill disproportionately affected the working poor who may no longer be eligible for health insurance premium subsidies under the new rules.

FACTORS AFFECTING RESOURCE ALLOCATION IN HEALTH CARE

The distribution of health care services is affected largely by the way in which health care is financed in the United States. Third-party coverage, whether public or private, greatly affects the distribution of health care. In addition, socioeconomic status affects health care consumption because it determines the ability to purchase insurance or to pay directly out of pocket for care. A description of the effects of barriers to health care access and the effects of health care rationing on the distribution of health care follows.

Early results after passage of the ACA in 2010 demonstrated that by 2016, when the major components of expanded coverage went into effect, the number of individuals with health insurance had increased (Barnett and Berchick, 2017). These increases were a result of several provisions of the ACA: (a) coverage regardless of preexisting condition, (b) young adults could retain coverage under parents until age 26, (c) voluntary expansion of Medicaid by states to include a greater percentage of the low-income population, (d) subsidies for qualifying individuals buying coverage on the marketplace, (e) availability of coverage outside of employment or government programs through the insurance marketplace, (f) mandated minimum coverage for certain conditions and prevention services, and (g) no lifetime cap on benefits (PL111-148, 2010).

By early 2018, effects of threatening the repeal of key aspects of the ACA by the president and Congress resulted in a robust enrollment in exchange policies; changes to the enrollment process with less marketing, fewer dollars for navigators, and a shorter window to enroll led many to fail to obtain coverage by the open enrollment deadline; enrollment in 2018 did not surpass that of 2017 (Jost, 2018a).

The Uninsured

In 1996, 68% of the total US population had private health insurance. An additional 15% received insurance through public programs, and 17%, or 37 million, were uninsured. In 2008 the number of uninsured persons had increased to 47 million. By 2012 the number had grown to 48 million citizens (DeNavas-Walt et al., 2013). The uninsured landscape changed dramatically from 2013 to 2016 once the full implementation of the ACA went into effect in 2014. In 2013, 41.7 million individuals were uninsured; by 2016 there had been a steady increase in the number of individuals covered by health insurance, and the uninsured rate had dropped to 28 million individuals. The percentage of uninsured dropped from 13.3% in 2013 to 8.7% in 2016 (Barnett and Berchick, 2017). Historically, the typical uninsured person was a member of the workforce or a dependent of this worker. Uninsured workers were likely to be in low-paying jobs, part-time or temporary jobs, or jobs at small businesses. People of color have been more likely to be uninsured than non-Hispanic Whites (Kaiser Family Foundation, 2017b). Until the ACA, these uninsured workers had not been able to afford to purchase health insurance or their employers may not have offered health insurance as a benefit. Others who were typically uninsured were young adults (especially young men), minorities, persons younger than

65 years of age in good or fair health, and the poor or near poor. These individuals may have been unable to afford insurance, may have lacked access to job-based coverage, or, because of their age or good health status, may not have perceived the need for insurance. Eligibility requirements for Medicaid meant the poor were more likely to be insured than the "near poor" also called the "working poor." As changes have occurred in the federal support of the ACA and other health insurance initiatives, some of these individuals, totaling 500,000, have once again found themselves uninsured (Tolbert et al., 2019).

Poor Americans

Socioeconomic status is inversely related to mortality and morbidity for almost every disease. Poor Americans with an income below the poverty level have a mortality rate several times greater than that of middle-income Americans, even after accounting for age, sex, race, education, and risky health behaviors (e.g., smoking, drinking, obesity, and lack of exercise) (Robert Wood Johnson Foundation, 2013; Buettgens, 2018). Historically, the link between poor health and socioeconomic status resulted from poor housing, malnutrition, inadequate sanitation, and hazardous occupations. In the past and still today, explanations include the cumulative effects of a number of characteristics that explain the concept of poverty. These characteristics include: (a) low educational levels, (b) unemployment or low occupational status (blue-collar or unskilled laborer), (c) low wages, (d) being a child or a person older than the age of 65 years, or (e) being a member of a minority group (NCHS, 2012). In addition, mental illness is a causal factor in morbidities, and early mortality is a recognized mortality risk factor, with the mentally ill dying 15 to 30 years earlier than their counterparts without mental illness (Thornicroft, 2011).

Access to Health Services

Access to health services is a public health issue (Wesson et al., 2018; AHRQ, 2017). Medicaid is intended to improve access to health care for the poor. Although persons with Medicaid have improved access to health care compared with the uninsured, Medicaid recipients have difficulty obtaining mental health services from psychiatrists and dental services when compared with the privately insured. Uninsured individuals have far worse access and outcomes. When Medicaid covers the pregnant women and children, the results are impressive and include reduced teen mortality, reduced disability, improved long-run educational attainment, and fewer emergency room (ER) and hospital visits. It remains to be seen how the proposals put forth in the AHCA to cap Medicaid funding to states as well as imposed lifetime caps on funding for services (Kaiser Family Foundation, 2017c).

The primary reasons for delay, difficulty, or failure to access care included: (a) inability to afford health care and (b) a variety of insurance-related reasons, including the insurer not approving, covering, or paying for care; the client having preexisting conditions; and physicians not participating in some insurance plans. Other barriers include lack of transportation, physical barriers, communication problems, child care needs, lack of time or information, or refusal of services by providers. In addition, lack of after-hours care, long office waits, and long travel distance are cited as access barriers. Community characteristics also contribute to individuals' ability to access care. For example, the limited prevalence of managed care and the limited number of safety net providers, as well as the wealth and size of the community, affect accessibility. There is an increasing awareness that culturally congruent health care providers or at least a guarantee of preferred language services are important for some individuals when accessing health care.

Because reimbursement for services provided to Medicaid recipients has been low, physicians are effectively discouraged from serving this population. Although physicians can respond to monetary incentives in client selection, emergency departments are required by law to stabilize every client regardless of ability to pay. Emergency department copayments are modest and are frequently waived if the client is unable to pay; in addition, the hours of operation are convenient for people who work during business hours. Thus low out-of-pocket costs have provided incentives for Medicaid clients and the uninsured to use emergency departments for primary care services.

Poverty level income is adjusted annually for each state by the federal government to indicate how much money an individual or families may earn to qualify for subsidies such as food stamps, Medicaid, and child health improvement program (CHIP). In 2018 the federal poverty level for an individual was $12,140; for a family of four, the poverty level was $25,100. For example, if an individual's income was 133% of the poverty level, then that individual earned no more than $16,146.20 (Federal Register, 2018).

Rationing Health Care

Rationing health care in any form implies reduced access to care and potential decreases in acceptable quality of services offered. For example, health providers may refuse to accept Medicare or Medicaid clients, restrict the appointments available to individuals with these forms of payment, or limit the percent of their patient panel enrolled in these benefits; all are forms of rationing. As with access to care, rationing health care is a public health issue. Where care is not provided, the public health system and nurses must ensure that essential clinical services are available. Managed care was thought to offer the possibility of more appropriate health care access and better-organized care to meet basic health care needs of the total population. A shift in the general approach to health care from a reactive, acute-care orientation toward a proactive, primary prevention orientation has been necessary for some time to achieve not only a more cost-effective but also a more equitable health care system in the United States.

The ACA, while providing coverage to more people, did not eliminate rationing because the law provided for five plans (bronze, silver, gold, platinum, and catastrophic). Each plan had different amounts and types of out-of-pocket spending such as premiums, copays, deductibles, and coinsurance. The state-based American Health Benefit Exchanges provided persons with differing levels of income subsidies to reduce out-of-pocket expenses based on income up to 400% of the poverty level, and some received tax credits and subsidies to assist with out-of-pocket expenses. Benefits varied by state (National Council of State Legislatures, 2014). New proposals under the AHCA passed by Congress in 2017 offered a variety of health plans with a range of premiums. Copays and out-of-pocket costs will come with restricted health coverage based on individual selection and will result in its own form of rationing based on an individual's ability to pay for covered and uncovered care. This discussion has already resulted in Idaho's offering plans that do not meet ACA guidelines but do meet AHCA guidelines (Jost, 2018b).

The Levels of Prevention Box shows examples of the levels of economic prevention strategies.

🗒 LEVELS OF PREVENTION

Economic Prevention Strategies

Primary Prevention
Work with legislators and insurance companies to support Affordable Care Act coverage for health promotion services to reduce the risk of disease.

Secondary Prevention
Encourage clients who are pregnant to participate in prenatal care and WIC (Women, Infants, and Children) programs to increase the number of healthy babies and reduce the costs related to preterm baby care and pregnancy complications.

Tertiary Prevention
Participate in home visits to mothers who are at risk for neglecting or abusing babies to reduce the costs related to abuse and neglect by providing guidance and education on newborn and postpartum care.

❓ CHECK YOUR PRACTICE

At the local nurse-managed clinic for mothers and new babies, you are assigned to assist a population of mothers in understanding the benefits of primary prevention. You are focusing on the Special Supplemental Nutrition Program for Women, Infants, and Children (WIC) program and are encouraging mothers to participate in this program to help their babies have a good start toward a healthy life. Why do you think such a program is important, and why is primary prevention even a focus in health care delivery? See if you can apply these steps to this scenario. (a) Recognize the cues and look at the literature to see why primary prevention is applicable in public health and what steps can the registered nurse (RN) uses to work with a population of mothers; (b) analyze the cues to those answers; (c) state several and prioritize the hypotheses you have stated; (d) generate solutions for each hypothesis; (e) take action on the number one hypothesis you think best reflects an approach to take to obtain the cooperation of the population; and (f) evaluate the outcomes you would expect from your efforts, such as "Did the mothers choose to participate in the program?"

PRIMARY PREVENTION

Society's investment in the health care system has been based on the premise that more health services will result in better health, but non–health care factors also have an effect. Of the major factors that affect health—personal biology and behavior (or lifestyle), environmental factors and policies (including physical, social, health, cultural, and economic environments),

social networks, living and working conditions, and the health care system—medical services are said to have the least effect. Behavior and lifestyle have been shown to have the greatest effect on longevity, with the environment and biology accounting for the greatest effect on the development of all illnesses (National Prevention Council, 2011; NCHS, 2016; Healthy People 2020 and 2010).

The USDHHS has argued that a higher value should be placed on primary prevention. The goal of this approach is to preserve and maximize human capital by investing in primary prevention and public health efforts that reduce disease and disability (e.g., Alzheimer disease prevention, fall prevention, promotion of breastfeeding, heart disease prevention). An emphasis on primary prevention may reduce dollars spent and increase quality of life and longevity. Funding is provided through the PPHF (USDHHS, 2016b).

The return on investment in primary prevention through gains in human capital has not been acknowledged in the past, unfortunately. As a consequence, large investments in primary prevention and public health care have not been made. Reasons given for this lack of emphasis on prevention in clinical practice and lack of financial investment in prevention include the following:

- Provider uncertainty about which clients should receive services and at what intervals
- Lack of information about preventive services
- Negative attitudes about the importance of preventive care
- Lack of time for delivery of preventive services
- Delayed or absent feedback regarding success of preventive measures
- Less reimbursement for these services than curative services
- Lack of organization to deliver preventive services
- Lack of use of services by the poor and elderly
- More out-of-pocket expenses for the poor and those who lack health insurance

A focus on prevention theoretically means reducing the need for and use of medical, dental, hospital, and health provider services. Under fee-for-service payment arrangements, this would mean that the health care system, the largest employer in the United States, would be reduced in size and would become less profitable. However, with the increasing costs of health care and consumer demand and the changes in financing mechanisms, there is a new trend toward financing more preventive care services, as was reflected in the ACA coverage for these services. This trend is based on decades of research into modifiable risks factors associated with the leading causes of death. On the other hand, the millions of Americans with chronic disease and disability are not going to disappear just because the system is more focused on prevention. It is possible that the chronically ill will benefit from a proactive emphasis on prevention but diseases and disabilities will still have to be treated and managed.

Currently, third-party payers cover preventive services, recognizing that the growth of a disease-focused health care system can no longer be supported. Under capitated health plans, health care providers are incentivized to earn money by keeping clients healthy and reducing unnecessary health care use. Through combining client interests with financial interests of the health care industry, primary prevention and public health can be raised to the status and priority currently held by acute care and chronic care. Despite difficulties, methods for determining prevention effectiveness, such as cost effectiveness analysis (CEAs) and cost benefit analysis (CBAs), are becoming standard and used more widely. Two agendas for preventive services have been published that promote the disease prevention agenda:

- The US Preventive Services Task Force, Recommendations for Primary Care Practice (Agency for Healthcare Research and Quality [AHRQ], 2018) for clinicians in primary care that outlines the regular screening and risk factors to identify at various ages
- *The Community Guide* (Community Preventive Services Task Force, 2018), which emphasizes population-level interventions to promote primary prevention

Regardless of the method, prevention-effectiveness analyses (PEAs) are outcome oriented. This area of research seeks to link interventions with health outcomes and economic outcomes and to reveal the tradeoffs between the two. In theory, support for increasing national investment in primary prevention is sound and long standing. Since the public health movement of the mid-19th century, public health officials, epidemiologists, and nurses have been working to advance the agenda of primary prevention to the forefront of the health care industry. Currently, these efforts continue across several disciplines, in both the public and the private sectors, through the efforts for health care reform (*Healthy People 2030* Box).

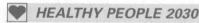

HEALTHY PEOPLE 2030

Objectives Related to Access to Health Services

- **AHS-08:** Increase the proportion of adults who get recommended evidence-based preventive health care
- **ECBP-D07:** Increase the number of community organizations that provide prevention services
- **AHS-R02:** Increase the use of telehealth to improve access to health services
- **AHS-R03:** Reduce the proportion of people younger than 65 years who are underinsured

From US Department of Health and Human Services: *Healthy People 2030*, 2020. Available at http://health.gov/healthypeople.

THE CONTEXT OF THE US HEALTH CARE SYSTEM

The US health care system is a diverse collection of industries that are involved directly or indirectly in providing health care services. The major players in the industry are the health professionals who provide health care services, pharmacy and equipment suppliers, insurers (public/government and private), managed care plans (health maintenance organizations [HMOs], preferred provider organizations), and other groups, such as educational institutions, consulting and research firms, professional associations, and trade unions. Currently, the health care industry is large and its characteristics and operations differ between rural and urban geographic areas.

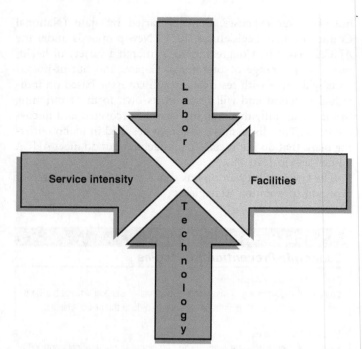

Fig. 5.1 Components of Health Services Development.

In the 21st century, health policy and national politics reflect the importance of health care delivery in the general economy. Conflicts arise between competing special-interest groups that have different goals and objectives when it comes to the producing and consuming of health services. To some degree, this is caused by federal and state policy changes about how health services are financed (public and private).

Fig. 5.1 illustrates the four basic components that make up the framework of health services delivery: service needs and intensity, facilities, technology, and labor. Service intensity is the extent of use of technologies, supplies, and health care services by or for the client. Intensity includes and is a partial measure of the use of technology (NCHS, 2016). Medical technology refers to the set of techniques, drugs, equipment, and procedures used by health care professionals in delivering medical care to individuals. It also includes information technology and the system within which such care is delivered (NCHS, 2016).

Health care systems have developed in four phases from the 1700s through 2019. These developmental stages correspond to different economic conditions. Developmentally, the four components of the health services delivery framework have changed over time, reflecting macrolevel, or societal, changes in morbidity and mortality, national health policy, and economics (Fig. 5.2).

The Preindustrial Era

The first developmental era (1800–1900) was characterized by epidemics of infectious diseases, such as cholera, typhoid, smallpox, influenza, malaria, and yellow fever. Health concerns of the time related to social and public health issues, including contaminated food and water supplies, inadequate sewage disposal, and poor housing conditions. The practice of medicine was unregulated and the quality uneven (Shi and Singh, 2019). Family and friends provided most health care in the home.

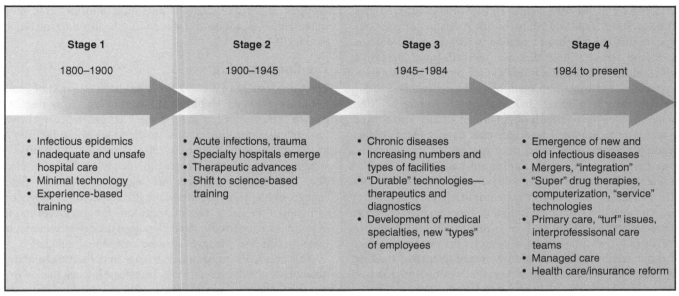

Stage 1	Stage 2	Stage 3	Stage 4
1800–1900	1900–1945	1945–1984	1984 to present
• Infectious epidemics • Inadequate and unsafe hospital care • Minimal technology • Experience-based training	• Acute infections, trauma • Specialty hospitals emerge • Therapeutic advances • Shift to science-based training	• Chronic diseases • Increasing numbers and types of facilities • "Durable" technologies—therapeutics and diagnostics • Development of medical specialties, new "types" of employees	• Emergence of new and old infectious diseases • Mergers, "integration" • "Super" drug therapies, computerization, "service" technologies • Primary care, "turf" issues, interprofessisonal care teams • Managed care • Health care/insurance reform

Fig. 5.2 Developmental Framework for Health Service Needs and Intensity, Facilities, Technology, and Labor.

Hospitals were few in number and suffered from overcrowding, disease, and unsanitary conditions. Sick persons who were cared for in hospitals often died as a result of these conditions. Most people avoided being cared for in a hospital unless there was no alternative. In this first developmental era, health care was paid for by individuals who could afford it, through bartering with physicians, or through charity from individuals or organizations. The first county health departments were established in 1908.

Technology to aid in disease control was very basic and practical but in keeping with the knowledge of the time. The physician's "black bag" contained the few medicines and tools available for treatment. The economics of health care were influenced by the types of health care providers and the number of practitioners, and the labor force then was composed mostly of physicians and nurses who attained their skills through apprenticeships, or on-the-job training. Nurses in the United States were predominantly female, and education was linked to religious orders that expected service, dedication, and charity (Young and Kroth, 2017). The focus of nursing was primarily to support physicians and assist clients with activities of daily living.

The Postindustrial Era

The second developmental era (1900–1980) of US health care delivery was focused on the control of acute infectious diseases. Environmental conditions influencing health began to improve, with major advances in water purity, sanitary sewage disposal, milk and water quality, and urban housing quality. The health problems of this era were no longer mass epidemics but individual acute infections or traumatic episodes (Shi and Singh, 2019).

Hospitals and health departments experienced rapid growth during the late 1800s and early 1900s as technologic advances in science were made (Young and Kroth, 2017). In addition to private and charitable financing of health care, city, county, and state governments were beginning to contribute by providing services for poor persons, state mental institutions, and other specialty hospitals, such as tuberculosis hospitals. Public health departments were emphasizing case finding and quarantine. Although health care was paid for primarily by individuals, the Social Security Act of 1935 signaled the federal government's increasing interest in addressing social welfare problems.

Clinical medicine entered its golden age during this period. Major technologic advances in surgery and childbirth and the identification of disease processes, such as the cause of pernicious anemia, increased the ability to diagnose and treat diseases. The first serologic tests used as a tool for diagnosis and control of infectious diseases were developed in 1910 to detect syphilis and gonorrhea (Shi and Singh, 2019). The first virus isolation techniques were also developed to filter yellow fever virus, for example. The discovery and development of pharmacologic agents, such as insulin in 1922 for control of diabetes, sulfa drugs in 1932 for treatment of infectious diseases, and antibiotics such as penicillin in the 1940s, eradicated certain infectious diseases, increased treatment options, and decreased morbidity and mortality (Shi and Singh, 2019).

Advances in technology and knowledge shifted physician education away from apprenticeships to scientifically based college education, which occurred as a result of the *Flexner Report* in 1910. It was the beginning of medical education as it is today. Nurses were trained primarily in hospital schools of nursing, with an emphasis on following and executing physicians' orders. Nurses in training were required to be unmarried and younger than the age of 30. They provided the bulk of care in hospitals (Young and Kroth, 2017). Public health nurses, who tracked infectious diseases and implemented quarantine procedures, worked more collegially with physicians (Young and Kroth, 2017). In this period the university-based nursing programs were established to accommodate the expanding practice base of nursing. Client education became a nursing function early in the development of the health care delivery system.

The later part of the 20th century (1945–1984) ushered in a shift away from acute infectious health problems of previous stages toward chronic health problems such as heart disease, cancer, and stroke. These illnesses resulted from increasing wealth and lifestyle changes in the United States. To meet society's needs, the number and types of facilities expanded to include, for example, hospital clinics and long-term care facilities. Changes in the overall health of American society also shifted the focus of technology, research, and development. Major technologic advances included developments in the realms of chemotherapeutic agents; immunizations; anesthesia; electrolyte and cardiopulmonary physiology; diagnostic laboratories with complex modalities such as computerized tomography; organ and tissue transplants; radiation therapy; laser surgery; and specialty units for critical care, coronary care, and intensive care. The first "test tube baby" was born via in vitro fertilization, and other fertility advances soon emerged. Negative staining techniques for screening viruses via electronic microscope became available in the 1960s (Shi and Singh, 2019).

Health care providers constituted more than 5% of the total US workforce during this period. The three largest health care employers were hospitals, convalescent institutions, and physicians' offices. Between 1970 and 1984 alone, the number of persons employed in the health care industry grew by 90%. The number of personnel employed in the community also increased. The expansion of care delivery into other sites, such as community-based clinics, increased not only the number but also the types of health care employees.

Technologic advances brought about increased special training for physicians and nurses, and care was organized around these specialties. The ongoing shortage of nurses throughout the century was being seen in the 1970s and early 1980s. Nursing education expanded from hospital-based diploma and university-based baccalaureate education to include associate degree programs at the entry level. As the diploma schools of nursing began closing in the early- to mid-1980s, the number of baccalaureate and associate degree programs began to increase. Graduate nursing education expanded to include the nurse practitioner (NP) and clinical nurse specialist (CNS) to meet increasing demands for the education of nurses in a specialty such as public health. The first doctoral programs in nursing were instituted to build the scientific base for nursing and to increase the number of nurse faculty members.

The role of the commercial health insurance industry increased, and a strong link between employment and the providing of health care benefits emerged. Furthermore, the federal government's role expanded through landmark policymaking that would affect health care delivery well into the 21st century. Specifically, the passage of Titles XVIII and XIX of the Social Security Act in 1965 created the Medicare and Medicaid programs, respectively. The health care system appeared to have access to unlimited resources for growing and expanding.

Throughout the 20th century, many public health advances were achieved. The life expectancy of US citizens increased and has been related to public health activities. The most important achievements were in vaccinations, improved motor vehicle safety, safer workplaces, safer and healthier foods, healthier mothers and babies, family planning, fluoride in drinking water, and recognition of tobacco as a health hazard (Shi and Singh, 2019).

The Corporate Era

The Corporate Era (1980 to 2019) has been a period of limited resources, with an emphasis on containing costs, restricting growth in the health care industry, and reorganizing care delivery. For example, amendments were made to the Social Security Act in 1983 that created diagnostic-related groups and a prospective system of paying for health care provided to Medicare recipients. The 1997 Balanced Budget Act legislated additional federal changes in Medicare and Medicaid. Private-sector employer concerns about the rising costs of health care for employees and fear of profit losses spurred a major change in the delivery and financing of health care. Managed care systems were developed.

This period included drastic change in the settings and organization of health care delivery. Transforming health care organizations became commonplace and buzzwords of the period were reorganization, reengineering, restructuring, and downsizing. Organization mergers occurred at an increased rate to consolidate care, to save money, and to coordinate care across the continuum (i.e., from "cradle to grave"). Merger discussions focused on *horizontal integration,* which indicated the union of similar agencies (e.g., a merger of hospitals), and *vertical integration* between different types of organizations (e.g., an acute care hospital, long-term care institution, and a home health facility).

Initially these pressures brought about hospital closings and a shifting of care to other settings, such as ambulatory and community-based clinics and specialty diagnostic centers that offer technologies such as magnetic resonance imaging (MRI) and sonography. Rehabilitative, restorative, and palliative care, once delivered in the hospitals, was shifted to other settings, such as subacute care hospitals, specialty rehabilitation hospitals, long-term care institutions, and even individual homes. Although the location of care delivery was no longer the traditional acute care hospital, the nature of the care delivered in hospitals changed remarkably, as evidenced by the following:

- Patients admitted to hospitals were more acutely ill.
- Length of stay for patients admitted to hospitals became shorter.
- Care delivery became more intense as a result of these first two changes.
- Management of chronic illness increasingly took place in a home or community setting.

The widespread use of computers and the Internet enabled society to become increasingly sophisticated about health. The public's increasing knowledge about health care and awareness of health care advances influenced the demand for health care, such as diagnostic and therapeutic services for treatment. Furthermore, pharmaceutical companies and other technologic suppliers actively marketed their products to the public through television, printed advertisements, the Internet, and other sources, so clients rapidly became aware of the new technologies.

Health professionals were increasingly dependent on technology to care for clients. Distance, as a barrier to the diagnosis and treatment of disease, was overcome through the use of telemedicine. The insurance industry became the principal buyer of technology for the client. They often made decisions about when and if a certain technology would be used for a client problem. Nurses became dependent on technologies to monitor client progress, make decisions about care, and deliver care in innovative ways.

The shift away from traditional hospital-based care to the community, together with the need to consider new models of care, brought about an increased emphasis on providing primary care, on developing care delivery teams, and on collaborating in practice and education. The substitution of one type of health personnel for another occurred to control care delivery costs. As examples, NPs were replacing physicians as primary care providers, and unlicensed personnel were replacing staff nurses in hospitals and long-term care facilities. These replacements caused much debate, with territorial, or "turf," battles, for example, between physicians and nurses.

The increase in specialization by health professionals led to changes in certification, qualifications, education, and standards of care in health professions. These factors, in turn, caused an increase in the number and kinds of providers to meet the demands of the health care system. In the last part of the 20th century, molecular tools were developed that provided a means of detecting and characterizing infectious disease pathogens and a new capacity to track the transmission of new threats, such as bioterrorism, and determine new ways to treat them.

The Bureau of Labor Statistics predicts that health care support and health care practitioners as well as technical occupations are projected to be the two fastest-growing occupational groups through 2024 (Hogan and Roberts, 2015).

Challenges for the 21st Century

In the 21st century (2020 and the future), the emergence of new and the reemergence of old communicable and infectious diseases are occurring, as well as larger foodborne disease outbreaks and acts of terrorism. Seven out of 10 of all deaths in the United States are related to chronic disease (NCHS, 2017). One in every two Americans has one or more chronic diseases. There is some concern that certain chronic diseases may be caused or intensified by infectious disease processes. Often there are complications that occur as a result of infectious disease, such as human immunodeficiency virus (HIV)/acquired immunodeficiency syndrome (AIDS) and tuberculosis, which can result in chronic lung disease and certain types of cancers because of the compromised immune system. Health behaviors and economics related to poverty are also continuing to build the path to acute and chronic health problems (e.g., the global obesity epidemic; infectious diseases related to sanitation and environmental pollution) (World Health Organization [WHO], 2018). Those who are poor, malnourished, and live in unsanitary conditions have compromised capacity to withstand the types of bodily insults that wealthier and more robust individuals throw off with proper environment, rest, food, and health care. Although some people choose to ignore behavioral factors related to obesity, such as physical activity and eating, those with insufficient income choose foods high in fat and sugar because those are the cheaper foods to obtain. They may use digital media or television as a babysitter for low-cost entertainment (Weese, 2017). The chronic disease burden is concentrated among the poor. Poor people are more vulnerable for several reasons, including increased exposure to risks and decreased access to health services. Chronic diseases can cause poverty in individuals and families and draw them into a downward spiral of worsening disease and poverty.

Investment in chronic disease prevention programs is going to be essential for many low- and middle-income countries struggling to reduce poverty. For the United States, this issue was a focus of the PPACA in 2010. Health promotion and protection, disease surveillance, emergency preparedness, new laboratory and epidemiologic methods, continued antimicrobial and vaccine development, and environmental health research are continuing challenges for this century. The role of technology has also intensified during this century.

Technology is now defined as the application of science to develop solutions to health problems or issues such as the prevention or delay of onset of diseases or the promotion and monitoring of good health. Examples of technology include medical and surgical procedures (e.g., angioplasty, joint replacements, organ transplants), diagnostic tests (e.g., laboratory tests, biopsies, imaging), drugs (e.g., biologic agents, pharmaceuticals, vaccines), medical devices (e.g., implantable defibrillators, stents), prosthetics (e.g., artificial body parts), and new support systems (e.g., electronic health records [EHRs], e-prescribing, telemedicine, and wearable electronics for monitoring and research).

The labor force has been changing to include greater specialization in both licensed and certified providers such as radiology oncologists, geneticists, interventional radiologists, and surgical subspecialists, as well as allied and support professionals such as medical sonographers, radiation technologists, and laboratory technicians. These have all been created to support the use of specific types of technology for diagnosis and treatment (HITC, 2015).

The infrastructure necessary to support more complex technologies is also considered to be a part of health care technology. EHRs and electronic prescribing are methods for coordinating the increasingly complex array of services provided, as well as allowing for electronic checks of quality to reduce medical errors (e.g., drug interactions; best therapy for treatment based on genetics; and decision support systems). Technology applied to health and treatment is exploding, whether from artificial intelligence to solve medical mysteries or three-dimensional (3D) printing to develop low-cost custom prosthetics, the future of technology solutions in health diagnosis, treatment, and rehabilitation has been exploding (The Medical Futurist, 2017). These innovations will require different skills for the provider workforce, greater involvement of patients in their own care, and new opportunities for industry to develop, produce, and maintain these technologies.

In addition to the labor force changes just described, physicians are increasingly moving away from solo practice to group practices, selling primary care practices to hospitals, or working as hospital or corporation employees. Hospital intensivists are the standard of care in 2019, with hospitals employing physicians to be in-house and available to patients and their community physicians to cover nonurgent, urgent, and emergent care while the patient is hospitalized. More NPs and physician assistants can be found working side by side with the physician in the community and in the hospital as members of the office, clinic team, or hospital staff. (See the following QSEN box about teamwork and collaboration.)

Discussions are increasing regarding the integration of public health and primary care and developing the primary health care system.

Public health nurses are more involved with population-centered care, assessment of community needs, and the development or implementation of programs that meet the needs of certain populations. There is a move to provide more care to clients in the home, such as the programs to provide care to new mothers and babies who are defined as at risk. Public health nurses play key roles in developing and implementing plans for bioterrorism and natural disasters in the community.

Nursing education is seeing a dramatic change in this century. There is a recommendation to move all advanced practice nursing to the level of the Doctor of Nursing Practice program, begun in 2000. This has the potential for closing specialist master's programs in nursing or transitioning them to postdoctorate certificate programs. This means the new BSN graduate, for example,

can go into a doctoral program at graduation and become an advanced public health nurse or an NP working in the community. The health care industry is one of the largest employers in the United States and, despite the economic downturn in 2008, has continued to grow. In addition, the largest number of employees in the health care industry are RNs (American Association of Colleges of Nursing, 2017; US Department of Labor, 2017).

Along with other changes in health care delivery and health insurance plans, the ACA (2010) provided an emphasis on prevention and wellness by establishing the National Prevention, Health Promotion, and Public Health Council to coordinate health promotion and public health activities as well as the creation of a PPHF to expand and sustain these activities. It was planned that these activities will assist in the development of a national strategy to improve health, reduce chronic disease rates, and address health disparities. However, cuts to this fund through the Tax Cuts and Jobs Act on December 22, 2017 reduced $750 million from the PPHF, representing 12% of the Centers for Disease Control and Prevention (CDC) budget targeted for state and local programs (Yeager, 2018). Several states have skirted the rules of the PPACA and are now marketing plans with variable coverage that do not comply with the requirements for coverage or premium parity (Jost, 2018b). As an example, a lawsuit seeking to invalidate the ACA (e.g., *Texas et al.* v. *United States et al.,* 2018) was brought before US District Court, Northern District of Texas, Fort Worth Division Court.

TRENDS IN HEALTH CARE SPENDING

Much has been written in the popular and scientific literature about the costs of US health care and how society makes decisions about using available and scarce resources. Given that economics in general and health care economics in particular are concerned with resource use and decision making, any discussion of the economics of health care must consider past and current health care spending. The trends shown here reflect public and private decisions about health care and health care delivery in the past. Past spending reflects past decision making; likewise, past decisions reflect the values and beliefs held by society and policymakers that undergirded policymaking at the time.

According to the Centers for Medicare and Medicaid Services (CMS), national health expenditures reached $3.3 trillion in 2016. This is compared with the $600 billion in health care dollars that were spent in 1990 (CMS, 2016). The CMS predicted total US health spending in 2019 will be $3.8 trillion and $5.7 trillion in 2026 (CMS, 2018a and 2018b). Health spending outpaced increases in the gross domestic product (GDP), accounting for 17.3% of the GDP by 2009 and rising to 17.9% in 2016 and projected to increase to 18.6% of the GDP in 2021. The percentage GDP can be translated into dollars per 100 spent out of pocket. In 2009, $17.30 of every $100 was spent for health care. It also means that in 2009 approximately $8100 was spent on health care for every person in the US population. In 2017, US health spending reached $10,739 per person and was projected to reach $11,559 per person in 2019. Per capita spending grew at a 10-year average rate of 3.5% per year over the 2007 to 2017 period. In 2019, it is projected that out-of-pocket costs

TABLE 5.1 Health Care Expenditures: 1960–2026*

Calendar Year	Total Health Expenditures (in billions of dollars)	Total Health Expenditures per Capita per Person (in billions of dollars)	Percentage of Gross Domestic Product
1960	27.2	146	5.0
1970	74.6	355	6.9
1980	255.3	1,108	8.9
1990	721.4	2,843	12.1
2000	1,369.1	4,855	13.3
2010†	2,598.8	8,412	17.4
2015†	3200.8	9,994	17.7
2018*	3675.3	11,193	18.2
2019*	3867.6	11,670	18.3
2020*	4090.9	12,230	18.4
2026*	5696.2	16,168	19.7

*Projected expenditures.
From Centers for Medicare and Medicaid Services, Office of the Actuary: *National Health Expenditures Aggregate and Per Capita Amounts: 1960–2016 (Historical Table 01).* US Department of Health and Human Services, 2018. www.cms.gov. Accessed July 5, 2018. †*Centers for Medicare and Medicaid Services, Office of the Actuary: *National Health Expenditures and Selected Economic Indicators: 1960–2026 (Projected Table 01 Summary).* US Department of Health and Human Services, 2017. Retrieved July 5, 2018 from www.cms.gov.

would be approximately $20 for every $100 spent, or one-fifth of every $100 earned. Table 5.1 shows the growth in US health care expenditures between 1960 and 2026 (NCHS, 2018).

Public health funding allows states to proactively implement programs that improve health. An investment of $10 per person per year in evidence-based programs in local communities that are proven to increase physical activity, improve nutrition, and prevent smoking or other tobacco use could save the country more than $16 billion annually within 5 years. This is a potential savings of $5.60 for every $1 invested. During fiscal year 2017, the amount spent for public health activities ranged from the healthiest state, Alaska, $281, to the least-healthy state, Nevada, $46 (Trust for America's Health, 2018).

The PPHF was established by the ACA to expand and sustain national investments in evidence-based strategies to improve health outcomes and health care quality. The Prevention Fund has supported nearly $900 million in prevention grants throughout the United States to implement programs that aim to improve health for all, including efforts to prevent infectious diseases such as measles and influenza, and chronic diseases such as diabetes and heart disease. The PPHF funds 12% of the CDC's annual budget and $3 billion in state grants and programs over the next 5 years.

The largest portions of health care expenses were for hospital care and physician services, respectively, in 2016 and again in 2018. Home health care has been exceeding hospital expenditures since 2012 and is expected to rise dramatically in the coming years; it is projected to exceed physician services in terms of expenditures beginning in 2017 (NCHS, 2018).

FACTORS INFLUENCING HEALTH CARE COSTS

Health economists, providers, payers, and politicians have explored a variety of explanations for the rapid rate of increase in health expenses as compared with population growth. That individuals have, over time, consumed more health care is not an adequate explanation. The following factors are frequently cited as having caused the increases in total and per capita health care spending since 1960: inflation, changes in population demographics, and technology and intensity of services (Shi and Singh, 2019).

Demographics Affecting Health Care

Aging. A major demographic change under way in the United States is the aging of the population. Population changes are also affected by illnesses such as AIDS and by chemical dependency epidemics. These changes have implications for providers' health services, and they affect the overall costs of health care. Because the majority of older adults and other special populations receive services through publicly funded programs, the growing health needs among these populations have an effect on costs, payments, and providers associated with Medicaid and Medicare programs. The growing recognition that US Veterans needed more services than the Veterans Administration (VA) could provide resulted in additional funding for these individuals as well (HR 5674, VA Mission Act of 2018). As the population ages and the Baby Boomer generation ages and retires, federal expenditures on Social Security have increased (Congressional Budget Office [CBO], 2018a). At 78 million strong, the oldest of the Baby Boomers—born between 1946 and 1964—are already making demands on federal entitlement programs such as Medicare and Medicaid that will not be sustainable in their current form. In its 2018 Long-Term Budget Outlook, the CBO reports that spending for those programs accounted for approximately 5% of GDP in 2017 and is projected to be 6% of GDP by 2026 (CBO, 2018b).

By 2035, in the absence of change, spending for Medicare alone (which is more likely to be affected by aging Baby Boomers) will be 4% of GDP, and by 2050 it will have grown to 5% in the absence of any changes to health policy (CBO, 2018b). Projections for combined Medicare, Medicaid, and CHIP plus marketplace subsidies (or their equivalent) will reach 10% of GDP by 2050 (CBO, 2018b).

The aging population is expected to affect health services more than any other demographic factor:

- In 1950, more than 50% of the US population was younger than 30 years of age.
- In 1994, 50% of the population was 34 years of age or older.
- In 1990, individuals 65 and older comprised 12% of the population.
- In 2016, they comprised 15% of the population.
- By 2020, projections are that they will comprise 17% of the population.

By 2060 those older than 65 are estimated to comprise up to 25% of the population. In addition, the number of individuals 85 and older is expected to double by 2035 to 6.4 million and triple by 2060 to 19 million people because the population is living longer, healthier lives (US Census Bureau, 2014; US Census Bureau, 2018).

Although many older adults are independent and active, they are likely to experience multiple chronic and degenerative conditions that may become disabling. They are admitted to hospitals more often than the general population, and their average length of stay is more than 3 days longer than the overall average. They visit physicians more often and make up a larger percentage of nursing home residents than the general population (AARP, n.d.).

Life expectancy, at an average of 78.9 years in 2019, and positive health status have been increasing in the United States (Macrotrends, 2020). However, older adults continue to consume a large portion of financial resources. Health care providers are concerned about the growth in the older adult population because public funding sources, such as Medicare, have not been increasing their reimbursement rates sufficiently to cover inflation, and thus providers have been collecting a smaller amount for visits by older adult clients each year.

The aging of the population also spurs concerns about funding their health care because of changes in the proportion of employed individuals to fully retired individuals. Persons in the workforce pay the majority of income taxes and all Social Security payroll taxes. The funding base for Medicare decreases as the population ages, as retirement rates increase, and as the numbers in the workforce decrease. As a result, some policymakers believe that Medicare and system reforms could ensure adequate financing and delivery of health care services to an aging population (PL 111-148, 2010).

Health policy reform options being considered include increased age limits to become eligible for Medicare, means testing (i.e., determining financial need) for Medicare eligibility, increased coverage for long-term care insurance, increased incentives for prevention, and less expensive and more efficient delivery arrangements and care settings (e.g., managed care arrangements). One example of a policy change to reduce the Medicare program burden was the prescription plan (Medicare Part D) that was passed by Congress in 2005 and became effective in January 2006. This plan, although complicated, required most Medicare recipients to provide a copayment for prescription medications.

Although controversial, the plan is thought to provide positive gains for the elderly who did not have prescription drug coverage and could not afford to pay for their prescriptions, while reducing the cost burden for those without coverage who were paying full price for prescriptions (CMS 2017).

The ACA promised to close the "donut hole" coverage gap of variable prescription deductibles and copays for Medicare Part D participants by 2020, but Congress has accelerated the cost savings in the gap to achieve the reductions to 25% of the price of brand name and generic drugs once the deductible and the maximum out-of-pocket cost is met. Some drug plans may offer more comprehensive pharmaceutical coverage for a higher premium (CMS, 2020).

Ethnicity shows health disparities fuel some of the cost of health care in that persons who are racially, ethnically, linguistically, or gender nonconforming tend to have worse health outcomes than non-Hispanic White members of the US population. The population composed of two or more races is the fastest-growing group, followed by Asians and Hispanics; both populations are projected to double by 2060. Although the multiracial and ethnically diverse groups tend to be younger, many in this category will also be aging (US Census Bureau, 2018).

This rich diversity in population will present a challenge to a health care system largely staffed with White middle-class workers. To the extent that the health professions can attract persons who mirror the population they serve, health care can be provided in a way that is congruent with an individual's cultural and health beliefs (Johnson, 2018).

Technology and Intensity

The introduction of innovative technology enhances the delivery of care, but it also has the potential to increase the costs of care. As new and more complex technology is introduced into the system, the cost is typically high. However, clients often demand access to the technology, and providers want to use it. However, in an effort to keep health care costs down, payers have attempted to restrict the use of certain technologies. For example, the drug Viagra, developed for the treatment of impotence by Pfizer Pharmaceuticals, was a controversial technologic advance that, as soon as it was available to the public, was in high demand and prescribed by providers. Initially, use was restricted by payers because of cost. The adoption of new technology demands investment in personnel, equipment, and facilities. Furthermore, new technology adds to administrative costs, especially if the federal government provides financial coverage for the service or is involved in regulating the technology. Table 5.2 outlines federal policy that has affected technology adoption and the cost of health care over time.

Chronic Illness

Chronic illness is a factor that is driving health care spending. Chronic disease accounted for 70% of deaths in the United States (CDC, 2019) and accounted for the majority of the $3.6 trillion spent on health care in 2018. Using Medical Expenditure Panel Survey (MEPS) 2018 data, chronic medical conditions are identified by those costing the most, the number of bed days, work-loss days, and activity impairments (AHRQ, 2019).

TABLE 5.2 Federal Regulations Contributing to Health Care Technology/Cost Controls

Year	Federal Regulation
1906	Prescription drug regulation: Food, Drug, and Cosmetic Act, now the US Food and Drug Administration (FDA)
1935	Social Security Act (PL 74-271): Provides grants-in-aid to states for maternal and child care, aid to crippled children, and aid to the blind and aged
1938	Food, Drug, and Cosmetic Act (PL 75-540): Establishes federal FDA protection for drug safety and protection for misbranded goods, drugs, cosmetics
1946	Hill-Burton Act (PL 79-725): Enacts Hospital Survey and Construction Act providing national direct support for community hospitals; establishes rudimentary standards for construction and planning; establishes community service obligation
1954	Hill-Burton Act amended (PL 83-482): Expands scope of program for nursing homes, rehabilitation facilities, chronic disease hospitals, and diagnostic or treatment centers
1963	Community Mental Health and Mental Retardation Center Construction Act (PL 88-164)
1965	Medicare Title 18; Medicaid Title 19 (PL 89-97): Amendments to Social Security Act provide Medicare and Medicaid to support health care services for certain groups
1966	Comprehensive Health Planning Act (PL 89-749): For health services, personnel, and facilities in federal/state/local partnerships
1971	President Nixon introduces concept of health maintenance organizations (HMOs) as the cornerstone of his administration's national health insurance proposal
1972	Social Security Act Amendments (PL 92-603): Extend coverage to include new treatment technologies for end-stage renal disease; provide for professional standards review organizations to review appropriateness of hospital care for Medicare/Medicaid recipients
1973	HMO Act (PL 93-222): Provides assistance and expansion for HMOs
1975	National Health Planning and Resources Development Act (PL 93-641): Designates local health system areas and establishes a national certificate-of-need (CON) program to limit major health care expansion at local and state levels
1978	Medicare End-Stage Renal Disease Amendment PL 95-292: Provides payment for home dialysis and kidney transplantation Health Services Research, Health Statistics, and Health Care Technology Act PL 95-623 establishes national council on health care technology to develop standards for use
1981	Omnibus Budget Reconciliation Act of 1981 (PL 97-351): Consolidates 26 health programs into 4 block grants (preventives, health services, primary care, and maternal and child health)
1982	Tax Equity and Fiscal Responsibilities Act (PL 97-248): Seeks to control costs by limiting hospital costs per discharge adjusted to hospital case mix
1983	Amended Social Security Act (PL 98-21): Establishes new Medicare hospital prospective payment system based on diagnosis-related groups (DRGs)
1986	1974 Health Planning and Resource Development Act (PL 93-641): was amended and moves certificate of need program to states
1989	Omnibus Reconciliation Act of 1989 (PL 101-239): Creates physician resource–based fee schedule to be implemented by 1992, with emphasis on high-tech specialties of surgery; creates Agency for Healthcare Policy and Research to research effectiveness of medical and nursing services, interventions, and technologies
1990	Ryan White CARE Act (PL 101-381): Authorizes formula-based and competitive supplemental grants to cities and states for human immunodeficiency virus (HIV)-related outpatient medical services Safe Medical Devices Act (PL 101-629): Gives FDA authority to regulate medical devices and diagnostic products
1993	Omnibus Budget Reconciliation Act (OBRA 93) (PL 103-66): Cuts Medicare funding and ends ROE payments to skilled nursing facilities; provides support for immunizations for Medicaid children
1996	Health Insurance Portability and Accountability Act: Protects health insurance coverage for laid-off or displaced workers
1997	Balanced Budget Act of 1997: Creates a new program for states to offer health insurance to children in low-income and uninsured families
1998	Balanced Budget Act of 1997 (PL 105-33): Authorizes third-party reimbursement for Medicare Part B services for nurse practitioners (NPs) and clinical nurse specialists (CNSs)
2003	Medicaid Nursing Incentive Act (HR 2295): Expands direct reimbursement to all NPs and CNSs and recognizes specialized services offered by advanced practice registered nurses such as primary care case management, pain management, and mental health services
2006	Medicare Part D: Provides a plan for prescription payments
2010	Patient Protection and Affordable Care Act (PPACA) passed and signed into law on March 23, 2010
2012	The Affordable Care Act (ACA) provides for $18 million to expand health information technology to 37 health center networks; contraceptive mandate implemented; new insurance policies must cover certain preventive services.
2013	ACA: Health insurance exchanges opened to enrollment
2014	ACA: Insurers may not deny coverage based on preexisting conditions; some states expanded Medicaid eligibility; premium subsidies for qualified individuals; Congress and staff offered ACA Exchange plans exclusively;
2015	Physician reimbursement based on performance
2016	Veterans' health care and benefits improved Access to clinical trials
2017	HR 1628 American Health Care Act (AHCA) passed House and went to Senate for approval May 2017 sought to repeal major provisions of ACA to lower insurance coverage costs. PL 115-97 Tax Cuts and Jobs Act repeals the individual mandate and turns it into a health insurance penalty fee for person who do not obtain coverage prior to 2019.
2018	Proposed legislation related to opioid addiction and treatment: patient access to treatment, eliminating opioid related infections diseases, substance use disorder workforce loan repayment, opioid crisis response

ROE, Return on investment.

FINANCING OF HEALTH CARE

Against the backdrop of today's chronic conditions, it must be appreciated that health care financing has evolved through the 20th and into the 21st century from a system supported primarily by consumers to a system financed by third-party payers (public and private). By 2018 of national health expenditures, the percentage of third-party public insurance payments (Medicaid, CHIP, and Medicare) increased while the percentage of out-of-pocket payments had declined and private health insurance accounted for 34% of payments. Combined state and federal governments paid the greatest percentage of the health care bill (CMS, 2018).

Public Support

The US federal government became involved in health care financing for population groups early in its history. In 1798 the federal government created the Marine Hospital Service to provide medical care for sick and disabled sailors and to protect the nation's borders against the importing of disease through seaports. The Marine Hospital Service is considered the first national health insurance plan in the United States. The National Health Board was established in 1879 and was later renamed the US Public Health Service (PHS). Within the PHS, the federal government developed a public health liaison with state and local health departments to control communicable diseases and improve sanitation. Additional health programs were also developed to meet obligations to federal workers and their families within the PHS, the Department of Defense, and the VA.

Medicare and Medicaid, two federal programs administered by the CMS, account for the majority of public health

care spending. Table 5.3 compares these programs. The CMS is the federal regulatory agency within the USDHHS that is responsible for overseeing and monitoring Medicare and Medicaid spending. This agency routinely collects and reports actual health care use and spending and projects future spending trends. Through these programs, the federal government purchases health care services for population groups through independent health care systems, such as managed care organizations, private practice physicians, and hospitals.

Representing the shift to population health in recent years, there is a new type of provider incentivized by Medicare to be reimbursed based on achieving prevention goals and treatment targets. This shared risk group is called an accountable care organization (ACO). The members of the group agree to care for a specified panel of patients and receive reimbursement on a scale based on number of specific metrics achieved (e.g., diabetic blood glucose checking and eye exams, flu shots, and counseling about smoking or obesity).

Medicare

The Medicare program, established in Title XVIII of the Social Security Act of 1965, provides hospital insurance and medical insurance to persons aged 65 and older, to permanently disabled persons, individuals with amyotrophic lateral sclerosis (ALS), and to persons with end-stage renal disease (ESRD)—altogether approximately 67 million people in 2020. Medicare has two parts: Part A (hospital insurance) covers inpatient hospital care, home health care, hospice care, and skilled nursing care (limited); Part B (noninstitutional care insurance) covers "medically necessary" services such as health care provider services, outpatient care, home health, and other medical services such as diagnostic services, and physiotherapy. In 1999, Medicare Advantage plans

TABLE 5.3	Comparison of Medicare and Medicaid Program Features	
Feature	**Medicare**	**Medicaid**
Where to obtain information	Local Social Security Administration office or website	State Medicaid office or website
Recipients	Client is 65 years or older, is disabled, or has amyotrophic lateral sclerosis (ALS) or permanent kidney failure	Specified low income and needy, children, aged, blind, and/or disabled; those eligible to receive federally assisted income
Type of program	Insurance	Social insurance
Government affiliation	Federal	Joint federal/state
Availability	All states	All states
Financing of hospital insurance	Medicare Trust Fund, dedicated payroll tax, trust fund interest	Federal and state governments
Financing of medical insurance	Beneficiary premium payments, general revenue, interest	Federal and state governments
Types of coverage	Part A. Inpatient, skilled nursing facilities (SNFs), home health services and hospice care Part B. Doctor's services, outpatient care, home health services, durable medical equipment, mental health services, prevention and screening services Part D. Prescription drugs from a formulary (based on plan selected)	Inpatient and outpatient hospital services; nursing facility services: home health, physician services, rural health clinic services, community health center services; laboratory and x-rays; medications as prescribed; family planning; advanced practice nurse services, free-standing birth center services; medical care transportation; tobacco cessation counseling for pregnant women; vaccines for children; many optional services are available by state's choice

From US Department of Health and Human Services, Centers for Medicare and Medicaid Services: *Medicare and You, and Medicaid Benefits*, Baltimore, 2017, USDHHS.

were added to the program (Part C). This is an option that can be chosen for additional coverage. This option includes both Part A and B services. The Part C plans are coordinated care plans that offer HMOs, private fee-for-service plans, and medical savings accounts (MSAs). Part C provides for all health care coverage costs after meeting deductibles, with a uniform level of premium and cost sharing resulting in lower out-of-pocket costs for beneficiaries who opt for a Medicare Advantage plan. An estimated 36% of Medicare beneficiaries elected Part C. New legislation in 2018 allows Part C plans to offer a wider array of services to prevent costly and avoidable procedures (e.g., allowing payment for grab bars to be installed as a way to prevent falls and broken bones), thus reducing overall health spending.

Medicare Part A is primarily financed by a federal payroll tax that is paid by employers and employees. The proceeds from this tax go to the Hospital Insurance Trust Fund, which is managed by the CMS. Part A coverage is available to all persons who are eligible to receive Medicare, with older adults comprising most of these individuals. If a person did not contribute by federal payroll deductions when working, Part A can be obtained by paying a monthly premium upon reaching Medicare eligibility. There is concern about the future of the Medicare Trust Fund because projected expenses may be more than the trust fund resources. Payments to hospitals for covered services have been and continue to be higher than fund growth. Thus Medicare reimbursement policy has been changing in an attempt to control increasing hospital costs. For those with traditional Medicare, Part A requires a deductible from recipients for the first 60 days of services with a reduced deductible for 61 to 90 days of service. The deductible has increased as daily hospital costs have increased. For skilled nursing facility (SNF) care, persons pay nothing for the first 20 days and a cost per day for days 21 through 100 for an episode of care. After 100 days of care, the entire cost is borne by the individual (Medicare.gov, n.d.). Each year the deductibles must be met. The person pays zero for hospice and home health care.

The medical insurance package, Part B, is a supplemental (voluntary) program that is available to all Medicare-eligible persons for a monthly premium. The vast majority of Medicare-covered persons elect this coverage. Part B provides coverage for services other than hospital (physician care, outpatient hospital care, outpatient physical therapy, mental health, and home health care) that are not covered by Part A, such as laboratory services, ambulance transportation, prostheses, equipment, and some supplies. After a deductible, up to 80% of allowable charges are paid for necessary medical and other services. For mental health services, 55% of the costs are paid. Part B resembles the major medical insurance coverage of private insurance carriers.

Since the passing of the Medicare amendments to the Social Security Act in 1965, the cost of Medicare has increased dramatically. Hospital care continues to be the major factor contributing to Medicare costs. However, because of shorter hospital stays, home health and SNF costs have increased dramatically. As a result of rising health costs, Congress passed a law in 1983 that radically changed Medicare's method of payment for hospital services. In 1983 federal legislation (PL 98-21) mandated an end

to cost-plus reimbursement by Medicare and instituted a 3-year transition to a prospective payment system (PPS) for inpatient hospital services (HCFA, 1999). The purpose of the new hospital payment scheme was to shift the cost incentives away from paying for each procedure or service toward reimbursement for an episode of care. The basis for prospective reimbursement is the 468 diagnosis-related groups (DRGs) (see Evidence-Based Practice Box). In addition, the Balanced Budget Act of 1997 determined that payments to Medicare SNFs would be made on the basis of the PPS, effective July 1, 1998 (HCFA 1999). The PPS payment rates cover SNF services, including routine, ancillary, and capital-related costs, and are based on the case mix and geographic location of the SNF (CMS, 2020). In 2001, CMS developed a PPS for DRGs for home health with Health Insurance Prospective Payment System (HIPPS) codes. These changes in payment for services resulted in a closer attention to the cost of care provided, highlighted effective but less expensive alternatives to the usual method of care and noted areas where higher intensity of intervention resulted in better outcomes in terms of patient function or reduced length of stay. In other words, interventions and treatment plans came under scrutiny from a cost and outcome perspective, leading to a focus on evidence-based practice.

EVIDENCE-BASED PRACTICE

This longitudinal cohort study followed a nationally representative sample of patients 65 years and older with and without dementia through their transitions of care from the home to the hospital and from the hospital to the nursing home. Providing effective and efficient care for this population is a priority for the United States because the disease process can be lengthy and their care needs complex because the dementia population may have comorbidities as well as functional limitations. Transitions in care can be fraught with errors, discontinuity of care, and disorientation of the patient that result in multiple costly admissions. The study found that the dementia population experienced frequent transitions between home and hospital and home and nursing home. Often (59.2%), when the dementia clients were discharged from the hospital, there were no home care services.

Nurse Use

Public health nursing initiatives, such as health education, case finding, care management, respite, and other support services, could significantly reduce the amount of hospital admissions in this population. Such interventions could greatly reduce the negative health effects and poor quality of life for this population. The high costs of care for this population could be reduced with services tailored to the needs of this population and its health goals.

Data from Callahan CM, Tu W, Unroe KT, et al: Transitions in care in a nationally representative sample of older Americans with dementia. *J Am Geriatr Soc* 63:1495–1502, 2015.

In 2019 the average amount spent for services for Medicare beneficiaries was reported as $14,151 in the *2019 Annual Report of the Boards of Trustees of the Federal Hospital Insurance and Federal Supplementary Medical Insurance Trust Funds* (2019). The average out-of-pocket spending is greater for those beneficiaries who are 85+ or have declining health. In 2016 Medicare beneficiaries spent 12% of their Social Security income on out-of-pocket health expenses and this is expected to rise by 2030 (Kaiser Family Foundation, 2019). This is because of the limits in Medicare coverage, including certain preventive care, and the limited number of physicians and agencies who accept Medicare and Medicaid payment. Older adults who do not have supplemental insurance must cover the difference between the Medicare payment and the additional costs for services.

Medicaid

The Medicaid program, Title XIX of the Social Security Act of 1965, provides financial assistance to states and counties to pay for medical services for poor older adults, the blind, the disabled, and families with dependent children. The Medicaid program is jointly sponsored and financed with matching funds from the federal and state governments. In 2018, preliminary estimates were that approximately 66 million people were enrolled in Medicaid due in part to Medicaid expansion through the ACA (Medicaid.gov, 2020). Since the expansion of Medicaid under the ACA, Medicaid expansion states show a decrease in the uninsured which is greater than the nonexpansion states. Expansion resulted in a reduction in or elimination of waiting lists for home- and community-based services (Kaiser Family Foundation, 2018a).

Mandatory service benefits include: (Medicaid.gov, n.d.):
- Early Periodic Screening, Diagnosis, and Treatment (EPSDT) services
- Inpatient and outpatient hospital care
- Laboratory and radiology services
- Physician, nurse-midwife, pediatric nurse practitioner (PNP), and family nurse practitioner (FNP) service
- Skilled nursing care at home or in a nursing home
Other services that may be offered are:
- Rural and federally qualified health services
- Freestanding birth center services in licensed facilities
- Tobacco cessation counseling for pregnant women
- Transportation to medical care

The 1972 Social Security amendments added family planning to the list of full-pay services. States can choose to add prescriptions, dental services, eyeglasses, intermediate care facilities, and coverage for the medically indigent as program options. By law, the medically indigent are required to pay a monthly premium.

Any state participating in the Medicaid program is required to provide the mandated services to persons who are below state poverty income levels. Optional programs are provided at the discretion of each state. In 1989, changes in Medicaid required states to provide care for children younger than 6 years of age and to pregnant women less than 133% of the poverty level. For example, if the poverty level were $12,140 (Federal Register, 2018), a pregnant woman could have a household income as high as $16,146.20 and still be eligible to receive care under Medicaid. These changes also provided for pediatric and FNP reimbursement. States that expanded Medicaid offer premium support for individuals to purchase health coverage through American Health Benefit Exchanges.

In the 1990s, states could petition the federal government for a waiver. If the waiver was approved, the states could use their Medicaid monies for programs other than the required basic services. The first waiver to be approved was given to Oregon for their health care reform plan. Other states have received waivers to develop Medicaid managed care programs for special populations. The 2010 health care reform plan provides for new approaches to offering Medicaid services and incentives for states to offer Medicaid services rather than through the waiver option as described previously (PL 111-148, 2010).

Medicaid accounts for more than half of all dollars spent on long-term care services which have historically been SNF based but are increasingly home and community based and include housing supports (Gifford et al., 2017).

Public Health

Most public government agencies operate on an annual budget, and they plan for costs by estimating salaries, expenses, and costs of services for a year. The Prevention for Public Health Fund was also established through the ACA to assist public health agencies, such as health departments, with monies for emergencies such as COVID-19 and WIC (Women, Infants, and Children) programs. Public health agencies receive primary funding from taxes, with additional money for select goods and services through private third-party payers. Selected public health programs receive reimbursement for services as follows: through grants given by the federal government to states for prenatal and child health; through Medicare and Medicaid for home health, nursing homes, and WIC and EPSDT programs; and through collecting of fees on a sliding scale for select client services, such as immunizations (Trust for America's Health, 2018).

In 2011 only 3% of all health care–related federal funds was expended for federal health programs such as WIC, versus 97% for other types of health and illness care (e.g., hospital and physician services). In addition to this 3% allotment, public health funds also came through states and territorial health agencies. State and local governments contributed 16% to public and general assistance, maternal and child health, public health activities, and other related services in 2010. In 2019 the funding had dropped to 2.5% or $274 per person of federal funding (Trust For America's Health 2020).

Other Public Support

The federal government finances health services for retired military persons and dependents through TRICARE, the VA, and the Indian Health Service (IHS). These programs are very important in providing needed health care services to these populations.

The Affordable Care Act: Public Health Support

The ACA provides for PPHFs with emphasis on chronic disease. Funds are allocated to states to implement these provisions. See Table 5.4 for more detail. Also check the state of interest to see what that state is doing to implement this provision in ACA.

Private Support

Private health care payer sources include insurance, employers, managed care, and individuals. Although insurance and consumers have been prominent health care payment sources for some time, the role of employers, managed care, and consumers became increasingly prominent and powerful during the first

TABLE 5.4 **The Affordable Care Act's Prevention and Public Health Fund in Your State**	

• Prevention and Public Health Fund
  • The fund is an unprecedented investment in promoting wellness, preventing disease, and protecting against public health emergencies
	• Much of this work is done in partnership with states and communities to:
	  • Help control the obesity epidemic
	  • Fight health disparities
	  • Detect and quickly respond to health threats
	  • Reduce tobacco use
	  • Train the nation's public health workforce
	  • Modernize vaccine systems
	  • Prevent the spread of HIV/AIDS
	  • Increase public health programs' effectiveness and efficiency
	  • Improve access to behavioral health services

• Preventing Chronic Disease: A Smart Investment	• Chronic diseases: The Prevention Fund helps states:
	  • Tackle the leading causes of death and root causes of costly, preventable chronic disease:
	    1. Detect and respond rapidly to health security threats
	    2. Prevent accidents and injuries

AIDS, Acquired immunodeficiency syndrome; *HIV*, human immunodeficiency virus.
Since the Affordable Care Act was passed in 2010, the US Department of Health and Human Services has awarded $1.25 billion in Prevention Fund grants. In 2016, PPHF funding to all states totaled $624,726,012. Check your state to see what is being done to promote the public's health.

decade of the 21st century, particularly as concerns grew about the use and changing nature of health insurance.

Evolution of Health Insurance

Insurance for health care was first offered for the private sector in 1847 by a commercial insurance company. The purpose of the insurance was to provide security and protection when health care services were needed by individuals. The idea behind insurance was that it provided security, guaranteeing (within certain limits) monies to pay for health care services to offset potential financial losses from unexpected illness or injury related to accidents, catastrophic communicable diseases (e.g., smallpox and scarlet fever), and recurring (but unexpected) chronic illnesses.

A comprehensive study in the 1920s by the Committee on the Costs of Medical Care showed that a small portion of the population was paying most of the costs of medical care for the majority of the people. The Depression of the 1930s, rising medical costs, and the need to spread financial risk across communities spurred the development of the third-party payment system. The system began as a major industry in the 1930s with the Blue Cross system, which initially provided prepayment for hospital care. In 1939 Blue Shield created plans to provide physician payment. The Blue Cross plans began as tax-free, nonprofit organizations established under special enabling legislation in various states.

In the 1940s and 1950s, hospital and medical-surgical coverage increased. Employee group coverage appeared, and profit-making commercial insurance underwriters began offering health insurance packages with competitive premiums. The commercial insurance companies could offer lower premium rates because of the methods used to set rates. Insurance and premium setting, in general, are based on the notion of risk pooling (i.e., insurance companies were willing to risk the unlikely event that all or even a large portion of individuals covered under a plan would need payment for health services at any given time). Blue Cross used a *community rate*, establishing a similar premium rate for all subscribers regardless of illness

potential. In contrast, the commercial companies used an *experience rate*, in which the premium was based on an estimate of the illness *risk* or the number of claims to be made by the subscriber (Shi and Singh, 2019).

Premium competition, the offering of health insurance as a fringe benefit, and the use of health insurance as a negotiable collective bargaining item led to an increase in covered benefits, first-dollar coverage for medical care expenses, and increased employer-paid premiums. In turn, these factors pushed up insurance premium costs and health care costs and enabled insurance plans to cover high-cost segments of the population (the aged, poor, or disabled) because of the number of low-risk enrollees.

The health needs of high-risk populations led to the passage of Medicare and Medicaid legislation. These and other national health programs targeted health care coverage for specific population groups. Because these programs directed additional money into the health care system to subsidize care, there were financial incentives to encourage the providing of services (i.e., the more services that were ordered, the greater the amount of money that would be received). Other incentives were related to the use of services by clients (i.e., the more available the payment was for services that might otherwise have gone unused, the more services that were requested).

Greater increases in health insurance premium cost as well as increasingly high deductibles have resulted in the lowest rate of coverage by workers at large employers to only 61% of those offered coverage. Cost is the often-cited factor in declining health insurance coverage. Driving forces behind rising costs for care include: a) increase in the elderly population; b) waste and duplication of services; c) growth of technology; d) the "health system" focus on illness treatment (more expensive) rather than health promotion (less expensive); e) "defensive medicine," in which additional (usually unnecessary) tests may be ordered to cover all possible causes of a patient's complaints; f) lack of price transparency; and g) fragmentation of plan administration and billing (Shi and Singh, 2019).

Employers

Since the beginning of Blue Cross and Blue Shield, health insurance has been tied to employment and the business sector. This tie was strengthened during World War II to compensate, attract, and retain employees. Since that time, employers have played the major role in determining health insurance benefits. However, with the economic downturn in 2008, employers began to reduce their health insurance benefits or shift the cost of insurance to the employee.

After the economic downturn in 2008, employers shifted more of the cost of health care to the employees. By 2018, premiums had increased 55% since 2007 and 19% since 2012. Premiums in 2018 were projected to be an average of $6,690 for single coverage and $18,764 for family coverage, 4% and 3% increases over the previous year, respectively. These increases exceed inflation, and employee wage rises are lagging behind the rise in health insurance costs (Kaiser Family Foundation, 2017b).

Before the growth of insurance (i.e., before 1930 and the beginning of Blue Cross), the health care consumer had more influence over health care costs because payment was out of pocket. Consumers made decisions about how they would spend their money, making certain tradeoffs (e.g., about the type of health care they were willing to buy and how much they would pay). Entering the system was restricted in large part to those who could afford to pay for care or to those few who could find care financed through charitable and philanthropic organizations. With the beginning of the insurance (or **third-party payer**) system, health care costs were set by payers, and they determined the type of care or service that would be offered and its price. This began to change somewhat in the 1980s with the increased use of managed care.

As the cost of health insurance has increased, some employers, in an effort to bypass the costs established by insurers, have found it more cost effective to self-insure. The employer does this by contracting directly with providers to obtain health care services for employees rather than going through health insurance companies. Some large businesses directly employ on-site providers for care delivery or offer on-site wellness programs. These programs within the private sector offer opportunities for nurses to provide wellness programs and health assessments to screen and monitor employees and their families. This move to self-insure resulted in savings to companies and reduced overall sick-care costs (Shi and Singh, 2019).

From an economic point of view, the shift in responsibility for the cost of health insurance is not bad. In theory, this shift makes consumers more knowledgeable about (sensitive to) the price of health services. This means that they have more information for health care decision making and may consider price in making the decision to access types of health care services. As with employers, employees may choose health insurance voluntarily. Therefore three factors—the shifting of responsibility for health insurance premiums to employees, the changing demographics of the workforce in general, and the loss of employment due to the economic downturn—have resulted in a decline in employee enrollment in health insurance plans. Employees are choosing to use their resources to meet basic needs and are assuming the risks of having an illness for which they may have to pay. Employers will be required to offer coverage also, except for employers with fewer than 50 employees. These two requirements were to be in effect by 2014 unless repealed by Congress.

Given that access to health insurance is tied to employment, there was growing concern in the late 1980s and early 1990s about the employment layoffs and downsizing occurring in private business. Those who lost their jobs lost their ability to pay for health insurance and to qualify to purchase insurance privately. The Health Insurance Portability and Accountability Act of 1996 (HIPAA) was enacted to protect health insurance coverage for workers and families after a job change or loss (Health Care Financing Administration [HCFA], 1999; Nichols and Blumberg, 1998). Although this has increased the number of people who have access to health insurance and health care, there are claims that individual premiums are high, that insurance companies have lost their ability to pool risks, and that HIPAA is just one more federal control mechanism undermining competitive market influences.

Individuals

In 2018, individuals paid approximately 28.4% of total health expenditures out of pocket (CMS, 2020). However, these figures do not reflect the amount of money the consumer pays in taxes to finance government-supported programs such as Medicare and Medicaid, insurance premiums, and money paid for supplemental insurance to cover the gaps in a primary health insurance policy or Medicare.

Managed care is the term used for a variety of health care arrangements that integrate the financing and the delivery of health care. Managed care offers an array of services to purchasers, such as employers, Medicaid, or Medicare, for a set fee. These are called *risk-based plans*. This fee, in turn, is used to pay providers through preset arrangements for services delivered to individuals who are covered (NCHS, 2017). The concept of managed care is based on the notion that the use of costly care could be reduced if consumers had access to care and services that would prevent illness through consumer education and health maintenance. Therefore managed care uses disease prevention, health promotion, wellness, and consumer education strategies to achieve an individual's health goals (Shi and Singh, 2019).

Although they seem relatively new to many clients of care, HMOs have actually been around since the 1940s. The Health Maintenance Organization Act was enacted in 1972, and since that time, the number of individuals receiving care through HMOs and other types of managed care organizations has increased considerably. Managed care is based, in part, on the principles of managed competition. Managed competition was introduced in health care in the late 1980s and early 1990s to address the increasing costs of health care and to introduce quality into the forefront of discussions. **Managed competition** simply means that clients make decisions and choose the health care services they want on the basis of the quality or reputation of the service. Health care is a complex market and not one in which information about health care, health problems, and the costs of care are easy to get. With the passing of the ACA (2010), ACOs have been introduced as a new approach to managing care.

Health-specific savings accounts. The Internal Revenue Service (IRS) provides a number of ways for individuals to save or spend personal funds specifically for health care costs. The four programs are health savings accounts (HSAs), MSAs (Archer MSAs and Medicare Advantage MSAs), health flexible spending arrangements (FSAs), and health reimbursement arrangements (HRAs). These programs are designed to provide tax-advantaged monies for eligible health care costs for individuals who have specific health insurance coverage and meet certain qualifications (IRS, 2017). Money is contributed to an MSA by the employer, and the initial money put into an MSA does not come out of taxable income. In addition, interest earned in MSAs is tax free, and unused MSA money can be held in the account from year to year until the money is used. MSAs, in theory, would allow individuals to make cost/quality tradeoffs and would require that individuals become knowledgeable about health care, become involved in health care decision making, and take responsibility for the decisions made. Providers, in turn, must be willing to provide and disclose information to individuals and give up control of health care decision making. The HIPAA and MSAs are examples of health insurance reform efforts, and these efforts will very likely remain in the forefront of political discussions for some time to come, especially with the health care reform discussions.

HEALTH CARE PAYMENT SYSTEMS

Several methods have been used by public and private sources to pay health care providers for health care services. These include retrospective and prospective reimbursement for paying health care organizations, and fee-for-service and capitation for paying health care practitioners (Shi and Singh, 2019).

Paying Health Care Organizations

Retrospective reimbursement is the traditional reimbursement method, whereby fees for the delivery of health care services in an organization are set after services are delivered (Shi and Singh, 2019). In this scenario, reimbursement is based on either organization costs or charges. The cost method reimburses organizations based on cost per unit of service (e.g., home health visit, patient-day) for treatment and care. Costs include all or a percentage of added, allowable costs. Allowable costs are negotiated between the payer and provider and include items such as depreciation of building, equipment, and administrative costs (e.g., administrative salaries, utilities, and office supplies) (Shi and Singh, 2019). For example, the unit of service in home health is the visit, and the agreed-on price is a set amount of money that the home health agency will be paid for a home visit in the region of the United States in which the home care agency is located.

The *charge method* reimburses organizations on the basis of the price set by the organization for delivering a service (Shi and Singh, 2019). In this case, the organization determines a charge for providing a particular service, provides the service to a client, and submits a bill to the payer; the payer in turn provides payment for the bill. With this method, the charge may be greater than the actual cost to the agency to deliver the service. When the charge method is used, the client often has to pay the difference between what is paid and what is charged.

Prospective reimbursement, or payment, is a more recent method of paying an organization, whereby the third-party payer establishes the amount of money that will be paid for the delivery of a particular service before offering the services to the client (Shi and Singh, 2019). Since the establishment of prospective payment in Medicare in 1983, private insurance has followed by requiring preapprovals before clients can receive certain services, such as hospital admission or mammograms more than once a year. Under this payment scheme, the third-party payer reimburses an organization on the basis of the payer's prediction of the cost to deliver a particular service; these predictions vary by case mix (i.e., different types of clients, with different types, levels, and intensities of health problems), the client's diagnosis, and geographic location. This process is used in the DRG system of the hospital (Shi and Singh, 2019).

Similarly, ambulatory care services received by Medicare recipients are classified into ambulatory payment classes (APCs), which reflect the type of ambulatory clinical services received and resources required (CMS, 2018). Prospective payment to skilled nursing facilities is also adjusted for case mix and geographic variations (CMS, 2017a).

Positive and negative incentives are built into these reimbursement schemes. The retrospective method of payment encourages organizations to inflate prices in one area to offset agency losses in another (Shi and Singh, 2019). The major disadvantage of this system is that little regard is given to the costs involved. This practice of charging a payer at a higher rate to cover losses in providing care is referred to as *cost shifting.*

Prospective cost reimbursement encourages agencies to stay within budget limits and adds an incentive for providing less service to contain or reduce costs. The major disadvantage of this method is that organizations tend to overemphasize controlling costs and sometimes compromise quality of care.

A growth in contracting, or competitive bidding, for health care services, intended to create incentives for providers to compete on price, has occurred as managed care has increased in health care markets. For example, contracting has been used by states to provide Medicaid services to eligible persons. Hospitals and other health care providers that do not have a contract with the state to provide services are not eligible to receive Medicaid payments for client care. Managed care organizations also use this approach to negotiate with health care organizations, such as hospitals, for coverage of services to be provided to covered enrollees, often called *covered lives.*

Paying Health Care Practitioners

The traditional method of paying health care practitioners is known as "fee for service" (Shi and Singh, 2019) and is like the retrospective method just described. The practitioner determines the costs of providing a service, delivers the service to a client, and submits a bill for the delivered service to a third-party payer; the payer then pays the bill. This method is based on usual, customary, and reasonable (UCR) charges for specific services in a given geographic region, determined by periodic regional evaluations of physician charges across specialties (Shi and Singh, 2019). Historically, Medicare, Medicaid, and private insurance companies have used this method of reimbursing physicians.

A major effort to regulate and control the costs of physician fees was introduced in 1990 in the Omnibus Reconciliation Act. After a study by the Physician Payment Review Commission established by Congress, the *resource-based relative value scale* (RBRVS) was established. The RBRVS method reimburses physicians for specific services provided and the amount of resources required to deliver the service. The RBRVS method of reimbursement, adopted by Medicare in 1991, acknowledges the breadth and depth of knowledge required by primary care physicians in the community to provide services aimed at prevention, health promotion, teaching, and counseling.

Preferred provider is similar to prospective reimbursement for health care organizations. Specifically, third-party payers negotiate the amount that practitioners will be paid for a unit of care, such as a client visit, before the delivery of the service, thereby placing a limit on the amount of reimbursement received per patient (Shi and Singh, 2019). In contrast to a fee-for-service arrangement, where the practitioner determines both the services that will be provided to clients and the charges for those services, practitioners being paid through preferred provider are given the rate they will be paid for a client's care, regardless of specific services provided (Shi and Singh, 2019).

Capitation arrangements pay physicians and other practitioners a set amount to provide care to a given client or group of clients for a set period of time and amount of money (sometimes called per member per month rate). This arrangement, typically used by managed care organizations, is one whereby the practitioner contracts with the managed care organization to provide health care services to plan members for a preset and negotiated fee per member. The agreed-on fee is negotiated between the practitioner and the managed care organization before the delivery of services and is set at a discounted rate, and the practitioner and managed care organization come to a legal agreement or contract for the delivery and payment of services. The managed care organization pays the predetermined fee to the practitioner, often before the delivery of services, to provide care to plan members for a set period (Shi and Singh, 2019). Here the provider incentive is to treat adequately on the first patient visit to keep patients healthy and costs low.

Reimbursement for Nursing Services

Historically, practitioners eligible to receive reimbursement for health care services included physicians only. However, nurses who function in certain capacities, such as NPs, CNSs, and midwives, also provide primary care to clients and receive reimbursement for their services. Being recognized as primary care providers and eligible to receive reimbursement has not been an easy achievement. Reportedly, as a result of the passing of the ACA, there are currently more than 200 nurse-managed clinics in the United States providing population-based preventive services, primary care, or specific wellness programs to 46 million Americans (AAN, 2020). Most are receiving financial support through Medicare, Medicaid, contracts, gifts, grants, and private donations.

Hospital nursing care costs have traditionally been included as part of the overall patient room charge and reimbursed as such. Other agencies, such as home health care agencies, include nursing care costs with administrative costs, supplies, and equipment costs. Nursing organizations, such as the American Nurses Association (ANA), have long advocated that nursing care should become a separate budget item in all organizations so that cost studies can show the efficiency and effectiveness of the nursing profession.

Spurred by efforts to control the costs of medical care, effective January 1, 1998, NPs and CNSs were granted third-party reimbursement for Medicare Part B services only, under Public Law 105-33 (ANA, 1999). This new law set reimbursement for NPs and CNSs at 85% of physician rates for the same service, an extension of previous legislation that allowed the same reimbursement rate to NPs and CNSs practicing in rural areas (Buppert, 1999). This law was passed after years of work in this area, including research documenting NP and CNS contributions to health care delivery and client outcomes and after active lobbying efforts by professional nursing organizations.

Data about the cost-to-benefit ratio, efficiency, and effectiveness of nursing care in general have been collected. In 2018, Medicaid began to reimburse for nurse-midwife, PNP, and FNP care (Medicaid.gov). All of these events have moved the discipline toward more autonomy in nursing practice and are serving as a means for providing care in rural and urban areas, serving our most vulnerable populations.

ECONOMICS AND THE FUTURE OF NURSING PRACTICE

Nurses must plan for future changes in health care financing by becoming aware of the costs of nursing services, identifying aspects of care in which cost savings can be safely achieved, and developing knowledge on how nursing practice affects and is affected by the principles of economics. Nursing must continue to focus on improving the overall health of the nation, defining its contribution to the health of the nation, deriving the value of nursing care, and ensuring its economic viability within the health care marketplace. Nurses must effect changes in the health care system by providing leadership in developing new models of care delivery that provide effective, high-quality care, and by assuming a greater role in evaluating client care and nurse performance. It is through their leadership that nurses will contribute to improved decision making about allocating scarce health care resources and will promote primary prevention as an answer to improve many of the current population-level health outcomes.

APPLYING CONTENT TO PRACTICE

The balance of interest within society and health care will continue to shift toward a focus on quality, safety, and elimination of health disparities through public and private sector partnerships. Health care system concerns of the 21st century are expected to focus on examining the quality of health care relative to the costs of care delivered, reduction in disparities, access to care, and health care reform. These changes will result from continued efforts of both the public and private sectors to reform the US health care system. The current era of health care delivery will be noted as a time of vast changes in all sectors of health care delivery. There will be an increased emphasis on SDOH as noted in *Healthy People 2030* with the knowledge that 50% of health outcomes can be attributed to SDOH and health behaviors. Improving SDOH will require nurses to be involved at all levels of policymaking to advocate for education for all ages and abilities; employment; quality of the environment, including public transportation, parks, walkability, and affordable quality housing; types and quality of health services; and social support systems including social integration and community engagement (Artiga and Hinton, 2018).

Nurses will want to plan for future changes in health care financing by becoming aware of the costs of nursing services, identifying aspects of care where cost savings can be safely achieved, and developing knowledge on how nursing practice affects and is affected by the principles of economics. Nursing must continue to focus on improving the overall health of the nation, defining its contribution to the health of the nation, deriving the value of nursing care, and ensuring its economic viability within the health care marketplace. Nurses must effect changes in the health care system by providing leadership in developing new models of care delivery that provide effective, high-quality care and by assuming a greater role in evaluating client care and nurse performance. It is through their leadership that nurses will contribute to improved decision making about allocating scarce health care resources and promoting primary prevention as an answer to improve many of the current population level health outcomes.

PRACTICE APPLICATION

Connie, a nursing student, has identified a population of families in a chronic disease program offered by the local public health department. She is interested in assessing the costs of care to this population and to the agency. Connie approaches the public health nurse administrator and asks the following questions:

A. How is the agency reimbursed for chronic disease management? Has the Affordable Care Act resulted in a greater number of people who can afford these services?
B. Does this population of clients have a responsibility for paying for services?
C. Are nursing care costs known?
D. Are services rationed to the population? On what basis?
E. What effect will the chronic disease management program have on the community population?
Answers can be found on the Evolve website.

REMEMBER THIS!

- From 1800 to 2019, the US health care delivery system experienced four developmental eras, with different emphases on health care economics.
- Four basic components provide the framework for the development of delivery of health care services: service needs and intensity, facilities, technology, and labor (workforce).
- Four major factors have been associated with the growth and development of the health care delivery system: labor and associated costs, technology, service intensity, and available facilities.
- Chronic disease is becoming a major health factor affecting health care spending, with 45% of Americans experiencing at least one chronic disease.
- Health care financing evolved through the 20th century from a system financed primarily by the consumer to a system financed primarily by third-party payers. In the 21st century, the consumer is being asked to pay more.
- To solve the problems of rising health care costs, the Affordable Care Act was passed; this act also included some form of rationing.
- Excessive and inefficient use of goods and services in health care delivery has been viewed as the major cause of rising health care costs.
- Economics is concerned with use of resources, including money, to fulfill society's needs and wants.
- Health economics is concerned with the problems of producing services and programs and distributing them to clients.
- The goal of public health economics is maximum benefits from services of public health providers, leading to health and wellness of the population.
- The goal of public health is to provide the most good for the most people.
- Nurses need to understand basic economic principles to avoid contributing to rising health care costs.
- The gross national product (GNP) reflects the market value of goods and services produced by the United States.
- The GDP reflects the market value of the output of labor and property located in the United States.
- Social issues, economic issues, and communicable disease epidemics and pandemics mark the problems of the 21st century.
- Medicare and Medicaid are two government-funded programs that help to meet the needs of high-risk populations in the United States.
- A majority of the US population has had health insurance. As of 2020 it is not mandated by law, but persons seeking insurance who have not previously been covered will pay a higher premium for their health insurance.
- The uninsured segment represents millions of people, mostly the working poor, older adults, children, and those who lost jobs in the economic downturn of 2008 and the pandemic of 2020. Passage of the ACA in 2010 resulted in a greater number of individuals covered by health insurance.
- Efforts to repeal aspects of the ACA are under way; the impact on number of individuals with adequate insurance is unknown.
- Poverty has a detrimental effect on health.
- Health care rationing has always been a part of the US health care system and will continue to be with health care reform.
- Nurses are cost-effective providers and must be an integral part of health care delivery.

- *Healthy People 2030* is a document that has established US health objectives.
- Human life is valued in health economics, as is money. An emphasis on changing lifestyles and preventive care will reduce the unnecessary years of life lost to early and preventable death.

EVOLVE WEBSITE

http://evolve.elsevier.com/Stanhope/community/
- Answers to Practice Application
- Review Questions

REFERENCES

American Academy of Nursing. Nurse Managed Health Centers: Meeting the Needs of Underserved Populations: 2020, Washington DC.

AARP. Chronic diseases among older adults. n.d., Accessed Sept 2020 at assets.aarp.org.

Agency for Healthcare Research and Quality (AHRQ): *2016 National Healthcare Quality and Disparities Report*, AHRQ Publication No. 17-0001. 2017, 2017. Available at www.ahrq.gov. Accessed July 3, 2018.

Agency for Healthcare Research and Quality: *Guide to clinical preventive services, 2018*, Rockville, 2018, AHRQ. Available at http://www.ahrq.gov.

Agency for Healthcare Research and Quality (AHRQ):Medical Expenditure Panel Survey 2018, Rockville, 2019, AHRQ.

American Association of Colleges of Nursing (AACN): *Nursing Shortage Fact Sheet.* author, 2017. Available at www.aacnnursing. org. Accessed July 5, 2018.

American Nurses Association (ANA): *Medicare reimbursement for NPs and CNSs,* author: 1999.

Artiga S, Hinton E: Beyond health care: the role of social determinants in promoting health and health equity, Kaiser Family Foundation, 2018. Available at https://www.kff.org. Accessed July 23, 2018.

Barnett JC, Berchick, ER: *Current population reports, P60-260, health insurance coverage in the United States: 2016*, US Government Printing Office, 2017.

Buettgens M: The implications of Medicaid expansion in the remaining states, Robert Wood Johnson Foundation, 2018. Available at www.rwjf.org. Accessed July 8, 2018.

Buppert C: HEDIS for the primary care provider: getting an "A" on the managed care report card, *Nurse Pract 24*:84–94, 1999.

Callahan CM, Tu W, Unroe KT, et al: Transitions in care in a nationally representative sample of older Americans with dementia. *J Am Geriatr Soc* 63:1495-1502, 2015.

Centers for Disease Control and Prevention (CDC): Chronic Disease Overview, Atlanta, 2019, CDC.

Centers for Medicare and Medicaid Services (CMS), *Your Medicare coverage: skilled nursing facility (SNF) care,* n.d. Available at https://www.medicare.gov. Accessed July 1, 2018.

Centers for Medicare and Medicaid Services (CMS), *Your Medicare coverage: Part B costs,* n.d. Available at CMS, https://www. medicare.gov. Accessed July 4, 2018.

Centers for Medicaid and Medicare Services (CMS): *Skilled nursing facility PPS.* Baltimore, 2017, US Department of Health and Human Services. Available at http://www.cms.gov. Accessed July 5, 2018.

Centers for Medicare and Medicaid Services (CMS): *MDCR enroll AB 1: total Medicare enrollment,* author, 2016. Available at www.cms.gov. Accessed July 4, 2018.

Centers for Medicare and Medicaid Services. National Health Expenditures Fact Sheets. Baltimore, Accessed March 4, 2020.

Centers for Medicare and Medicaid Services: *Closing the coverage gap—Medicare prescription drugs are becoming more affordable, CMS Product No. 11493,* author, 2017. Available at (https://www.medicare.gov. Accessed June 2018.

Centers for Medicare and Medicaid Services: *Table 01 National Health Expenditures: aggregate and per capita amounts,* author, 2018a. Available at www.cms.gov. Accessed June 2018.

Centers for Medicare and Medicaid Services: *Table 01 National Health Expenditures; aggregate and per capita amounts,* author, 2018b. Available at https://www.cms.gov. Accessed July 5, 2018.

Collins SR, Gunja MZ, Doty MM, et al: First look at health insurance coverage in 2018 finds ACA gains beginning to reverse: *To the Point: Commonwealth Fund,* 2018, Available at: www.commonwealthfund.org. Accessed: July 1, 2018.

Community Preventive Services Task Force: What is the community guide?, Atlanta, 2018,CPSTF.

Congressional Budget Office(CBO): American Health Care Act, 2017. Washington, DC, publication number 52486.

Congressional Budget Office (CBO): *The budget and economic outlook,* US Government Printing Office, 2018a. Available at https://www.cbo.gov. Accessed July 4, 2018.

Congressional Budget Office (CBO): *The 2018 long-term budget outlook,* US Government Printing Office, 2018b. Available at https://www.cbo.gov. Accessed July 1, 2018.

Cuckler GA, Sisko AM, Poisal JA, et al.: National Health Expenditure projections, 2017-26: Despite uncertainty, fundamentals primarily drive spending growth. *Health Affairs* 37(3): 483-493, 2018.

DeNavas-Walt C, Proctor BD, Smith JC: *US Census Bureau, Current Population Reports Income, poverty, and health insurance coverage in the United States 2012,* US Government Printing Office, 2013. Available at www.census.gov. Accessed July 5, 2018.

Federal Register. *Poverty Level Income, 2018.* US Government Printing Office.

Gifford K, Ellis E, Edwards BC, et al.: *Medicaid moving ahead in uncertain times: results from a 50-state Medicaid budget survey for state fiscal years 2017 and 2018,* Kaiser Family Foundation, 2017. Available at https://www.kff.org. Accessed July 4, 2018.

Health Care Financing Administration (HCFA): *HIPAA: The Health Insurance Portability and Accountability Act of 1996.* USDHHS, 1999.

Health IT Consultant Staff [HITC]: *The top 9 most in-demand medical jobs:* author, 2015. Available at https://hitconsultant.net. Accessed July 8, 2018.

Hogan A, Roberts B: *MLR: Monthly Labor Review,* Bureau of Labor Statistics, December 2015. Available at www.bls.gov. Accessed June 2018.

Institute of Medicine: *For the public's health: investing in a healthier future, 2012:* The National Academies Press. Available at www.nap.edu. Accessed June 30, 2018.

Internal Revenue Service (IRS): *Health savings accounts and other tax-favored health plans, Publication No. 969,* author, 2017. Available at www.irs.gov. Accessed July 4, 2018.

Johnson, S. Can we create a fair shot at health? *Culture of health* (blog): Robert Wood Johnson Foundation. 2018. Available at www.rwjf.org. Accessed June 2018.

Jost TS: ACA open enrollment starts amidst tumult: *Health Affairs* 36(12): 2044-2045, 2017.

Jost TS: Mandate repeal provision ends health care calm: *Health Affairs* 37(1): 13-14, 2018a.

Jost TS: Idaho's actions continue challenges for ACA, *Health Affairs* 37(3): 523-524, 2018b.

Kaiser Family Foundation: *Medicare chart book*, ed x., author, 2019.

Kaiser Family Foundation: *The uninsured: a primer: key facts about Americans without health insurance.* Kaiser Commission on Medicaid and the Uninsured 2017a. Available at kaiserfamilyfoundation.files. Accessed July 5, 2018.

Kaiser Family Foundation: *2017 Employer Health Benefits survey,* author, 2017b. Available at www.kff.org. Accessed July 1, 2018.

Kaiser Family Foundation: *Key facts about the uninsured population*: author, 2017c. Available at www.kff.org. Accessed July 1, 2018.

Kaiser Family Foundation: *Implications of the ACA Medicaid Expansion: a look at the data and the evidence,* author, 2018a. Available at www.kff.org. Accessed July 4, 2018.

Kaiser Family Foundation: *Beyond health care: the role of social determinants in promoting health and health equity,* author, 2018b. Available at www.kff.org. Accessed July 4, 2018.

Macrotrends. *US Life Expectancy 1950-2020.* Accessed Sept 2020 at Info@Macrotrends.net.

Medicare.gov: *Part B costs: Centers for Medicare and Medicaid Services,* n.d. Available at www.medicare.gov. Accessed June30, 2018a.

Medicaid.gov: *Medicaid and CHIP total enrollment chart—April 2018*, CMS, 2020, Washington, DC. Available from www.medicaid.gov. Accessed July 4, 2018.

McPake B, Normand C, Smith S, et al.: *Health economics: an international perspective,* 4th ed., Routledge, 2018, New York.

Meit M, Knudson A, Dickman I, et al.: *An Examination of Public Health Financing in the United States.* (Prepared by NORC at the University of Chicago.) Washington, DC: The Office of the Assistant Secretary for Planning and Evaluation. March 2013.

National Center for Health Statistics (NCHS): *Health: United States, 2011 with Special Feature on Socioeconomic Status and Health.* Hyattsville, 2012, US Government Printing Office.

National Center for Health Statistics (NCHS): *Health: United States, 2016 with chartbook on long term trends in health care.* Hyattsville, 2017, US Government Printing Office.

National Center for Health Statistics (NCHS): *US Health care expenditures,* Hyattsville, 2018, US Government Printing Office.

National Conference of State Legislators. American Health Benefits Exchanges, Washington, DC, 2014.

National Prevention Council, *National Prevention Strategy, 2011,* Washington, DC, 2011, USDHHS, Office of the Surgeon General. Available at www.surgeongeneral.gov. Accessed July 3, 2018.

Nichols LM, Blumberg LJ: A different kind of "new federalism"? The Health Insurance Portability and Accountability Act of 1996. *Health Aff* 17:25–42, 1998.

PL: 111-148-The Patient Protection and Affordable Care Act, 2010.

Quad Council Coalition of PHN Organizations: *Competencies for Public Health Nurses, 2018.* Available at www.quadcouncil.phn.org. Accessed Sept 2020.

Robert Wood Johnson Foundation: *Return on investments in public health: saving lives and money,* author, 2013. Available at www. rwjf.org. Accessed July 8, 2018.

Sessions K, Fortunato K, Johnson PRS, et al.: Philanthropy at the intersection of health and the environment. *Health Aff* 35:2142-2147, 2016.

Schulte T, Keating B, and Zaveri H: *Evaluation Technical Assistance Brief: for OAH and ACYF teenage pregnancy prevention grantees,* 2016: CDC. Available at: www.hhs.gov. Accessed July 1, 2018.

Shi L, Singh DA: *Delivering health care in America: a systems approach,* 11th ed. Sudbury, 2019, Jones & Bartlett.

Sturchio JL, Goel A: *The private-sector role in public health: reflections on the new global architecture in health*: Center for Strategic and International Studies, 2012. Available at csis.org. Accessed July 5, 2018.

The Medical Futurist: *The ultimate list of what we can 3D print in medicine and healthcare!* author, 2017. Available at medicalfuturist. com. Accessed July 8, 2018.

Tolbert J. et al: *Key Facts about the uninsured population. Kaiser Family Foundation,* 2019, Available at www.KFF.org.

Thornicroft G: Editorial: Physical health disparities and mental illness: the scandal of premature mortality. *The British Journal of Psychiatry 199*: 441-442, 2011.

Trust for America's Health: *Key health data (by State): public health funding indicator,* 2017: Robert Wood Johnson Foundation. Available at healthyamericans.org. Accessed July 5, 2018.

Trust for America's Health: *Investing in America's Health: A state by state look at Public Health Funding and Key Health Facts:* RWJF, 2020. Accessed Sept, 2020. Available at healthyamericans.org.

Trust for America's Health: *A state-by-state look at public health funding and key health facts:* Robert Wood Johnson Foundation, 2016. Accessed July 8, 2018. Available at healthyamericans.org.

Trust for America's Health: *A funding crisis for public health and safety: state by state public health funding and key health facts 2018,* 2018: Robert Wood Johnson Foundation. Available at healthyamericans.org.

Turnock BJ: *Public health: what it is and how it works,* 6th ed. Boston, 2015, Jones & Bartlett.

Ubri P, Artiga S: *Disparities in health and health care: Five key questions and answers.* Kaiser Family Foundation, 2016. Available at files.kff.org. Accessed July 1, 2018.

USA Facts: COVID-19, Impact and Recovery, 2020. USAFacts.org.

US Census Bureau: *Fueled by aging Baby Boomers, nation's older population to nearly double in next 20 years,* author, 2014, Washington, DC. Available at www.census. Accessed July 1, 2018.

US Census Bureau: *Demographic turning points for the United States: population projections for 2020 to 2060 P25-1144,* author, 2018. Washington, DC. Available at www.census.gov. Accessed July 5, 2018.

US Department of Health and Human Services (USDHHS): *The ACA Prevention and Public Health Fund.* 2016a. Available at www.hhs. gov. Accessed July 5, 2018.

US Department of Health and Human Services: *Prevention and public health fund:* 2016b, author. Available at https://www.hhs.gov. Accessed July 3, 2018.

US Department of Health and Human Services: *Healthy People 2020,* Washington, DC, 2010, Public Health Service.

US Department of Health and Human Services: *Healthy People 2030,* Washington, DC, 2020, Public Health Service.

US Department of Labor: *News release: Bureau of Labor Statistics employment projections—2016-2026,* 2017, author.

US District Court, Northern District of Texas. Texas et al. v. United States et al., 2018. Fort Worth Division Court, Fort Worth, Texas.

VA: Maintaining Internal Systems and Strengthening Integrated Outside Networks Act of 2018 (MISSION). H. R. 5674 [Report No. 115–671, Part I].

Weese, K. 6 things Paul Ryan doesn't understand about poverty (but I didn't, either): 2017. Alternet. Available at www.alternet.org. Accessed July 3, 2018.

Wesson D, Kitaman H, Halloran KH, Tecson K: Innovative population health model associated with reduced emergency department use and inpatient hospitalizations, *Health Affairs* 37(4): 2018. Available at www.healthaffairs.org. Accessed July 3, 2018.

World Health Organization (WHO): *Global health estimates 2016: deaths by cause, age, sex, by country and region, 2000-2016.*

Geneva, 2018, World Health Organization [WHO]. Available at www.who.int. Accessed June 2018.

Yeager A: Cuts to Prevention and Public Health Fund puts CDC programs at risk: *The Scientist*, 2018. Available at www.the-scientist.com. Accessed July 3, 2018.

Young KM, Kroth, PJ: *Sultz & Young's health care USA: understanding its organization and delivery*, 9th ed. Jones & Bartlett Learning, 2017.

6

Ethics in Public and Community Health Nursing Practice

Connie M. Ulrich[a]

OBJECTIVES

After reading this chapter, the student should be able to:

1. Describe a brief history of the ethics of nursing in public and community health.
2. Discuss ethical decision-making processes.
3. Compare and contrast ethical theories and principles, virtue ethics, caring ethics, and feminist ethics.
4. Describe how ethics is part of the core functions of nursing in public health.
5. Analyze codes of ethics for nursing and for public health.
6. Apply the ethics of advocacy to nursing in public health.

CHAPTER OUTLINE

KEY TERMS

[a]We acknowledge Mary Cipriano Silva, Jeanne Merkle Sorrell, and James J. Fletcher for their previous work on this chapter. We have kept their original thoughts in the majority of this chapter and added additional information pertinent to thinking about ethics in public health nursing practice.

INTRODUCTION

Public health and community health nurses focus on prevention, protecting, promoting, preserving, and maintaining health. Working within public health settings, however, can challenge nurses in many ways. First, public health nurses may be the first point of contact for patients and their families within the local community. Therefore these nurses are in a unique position as they work to establish trusting relationships not only with their patients and families but also with a broad array of community groups that represent local interests. As health care providers, nurses navigate personal beliefs, patient and/or family wishes, and community values. They must do so within the parameters of community resources and organizational policy and within the guidelines of their professional codes of conduct. This complex and challenging process has tangible ramifications. Often public health and community health nurses have to weigh or balance the possible risks and benefits to the clients they serve, themselves, their families, and the larger community. In recent years an outbreak of the Zika virus (a mosquito-borne virus) presented a public health threat to communities around the world. The excessive lead levels found in the water in Flint, Michigan, represented a public health threat in that state. Both the Zika virus and the contaminated drinking water presented many ethical issues rooted in social justice, respect of person, and acting in the best interest of a community (Bellinger, 2016). More recently an enormous public health crisis was the onset of COVID-19. As discussed in Chapter 2, this virus began in January 2020 in Wuhan, China, and in weeks spread to most continents around the world. The sudden and massive onslaught of this virus put nurses on the front line for the health care responses and in positions to make high-stakes decisions for patients and for themselves and their families (Pearce, 2020). Nurses during this crisis worked in all areas of health care from screenings to attending the dying. As will be discussed later in the chapter, Provision 2 of the American Nurse's Association Code of Ethics says, "The nurse's primary commitment is to the patient" (ANA, 2015, p v). Provision 5 of the Code states that nurses owe the same duty to self and others. Caring for the patient and oneself and family when there was a threat of COVID-19 exposure created decision-making dilemmas for many nurses. This is especially critical if persons over 60 are part of that family. "Professional nurses historically bring compassionate competent care to disaster response but are challenged to provide care when the nature of their work puts them at increased risk" (ANA, 2020, p 1).

Nurses may struggle about responding during a pandemic; they may choose not to respond if:
- They are in a vulnerable group.
- The nurse feels physically unsafe in the situation due to lack of personal protective equipment (PPE) or inadequate testing.
- There is inadequate support for meeting the nurse's personal or family needs
- The nurse is concerned about professional, ethical, and legal protection for providing nursing care in the COVID-19 pandemic (ANA, 2020, p 2).

- If the nurse lives with family members who are in a high-risk group due to their age or health condition (Maguire B, Shearer K, McKeown J et al., 2020).

Employers have an obligation to provide PPE and not put their employees and their families at risk. In the early days of the COVID-19 pandemic, it was often difficult for organizations to obtain adequate PPE.

A crisis like that caused by COVID-19 can lead to moral distress, that is, knowing (or thinking one knows) the morally right course of action but not being able to act accordingly (Hamric, 2014).

This chapter applies core knowledge of ethics to public health nursing to help nurses develop effective coping strategies for ethical issues, including moral distress and other issues of import. Further, characteristics unique to community health practice are explored.

BRIEF HISTORY OF ETHICS AND BIOETHICS: RELATIONSHIP TO NURSING AND PUBLIC HEALTH

Ethics is both a process for reflection and a body of knowledge that focuses on the study of morality or the moral life (Beauchamp and Childress, 2013). Stated differently, Chadwick and Gallagher (2016) explain that ethics concerns the "oughts" and "shoulds" of practice. Epstein and Turner (2015, p 2) say, "The field of ethics addresses how we ought to treat each other, how we ought to act, what we ought to do, and why." Some useful ethics-related questions are: How should I behave? What actions should I perform? What kind of person should I be? What are my obligations to myself and to others? Ethics is important in all aspects of life and is inherent in nursing; basing actions on ethical principles supports clinical decision making and the practice of nursing. For example, the ethical principles of beneficence (doing good) and nonmaleficence (do no harm) can be traced back to the Hippocratic Oath for health care professionals and provides a framework for patient–clinician relationships (Racher, 2007).

Bioethics, a multidisciplinary subfield of ethics, is the systematic study of ethical issues in research, clinical care, or other areas in the life sciences, using both normative and empirical methodological approaches (Jonsen, 1998; Reich, 1995). Several sentinel historical events have shaped the field of bioethics, including the well-known Nuremberg Tribunals that followed World War II. The Nuremberg Tribunals reviewed the egregious human rights abuses performed under the guise of scientific experimentation by Nazi leaders, including physicians (Grodin et al., 2018). These abuses and the prosecution of their perpetrators led to the development of the Nuremberg Code of 1947, "which provides the foundation for the protection of human subjects in research" (Easley and Allen, 2007, p 367). One of the most important requirements of the Nuremberg Code is the voluntary nature of research (Annas, 2018). Major social movements of the 1960s and 1970s in the United States facilitated further development of the field of bioethics. Examples include the campaign for nuclear disarmament, the civil rights and peace movements, the protests against the war in Vietnam, and new medical technologies that raised challenging ethical questions about life and death (Easley and Allen, 2007). In addition, the first institution in the United States devoted to the study of bioethics was the Hastings Center, founded by Daniel Callahan, PhD, and Willard Gaylin, MD, in 1970. The Hastings Center (2019) addresses core ethical issues that arise in all areas of the life sciences and that affect the health and well-being of individuals, communities, and societies. It remains an excellent resource for nurses and other health care practitioners in the rapidly changing health care landscape.

Despite the atrocities of Nuremberg, violation of human rights in the name of research continued, including the Tuskegee syphilis study sanctioned by the US Public Health Service. From this, the 1974 National Research Act established the National Commission for the Protection of Human Subjects of Biomedical and Behavioral Research; this commission created the seminal Belmont Report (1979). A set of guidelines differentiating clinical practice from research, the Belmont Report also outlines the ethical principles of respect for persons (informed consent and respecting autonomous decisions), beneficence (maximizing the benefits and minimizing the harms), and justice (fair subject selection in research) in the protection of human subjects who participate in research (Belmont Report, 1979).

The field of bioethics continues to evolve as ethical issues remain prevalent in clinical practice and research and as new questions arise in the care of the most vulnerable in our communities. For example, questions abound on how to allocate scarce resources in a just manner both at the micro and macro levels and the benefits and harms of health technologies and research, including renal dialysis, organs for transplants, precision science, genetics and genomics, and emerging and reemerging infectious diseases, among others.

Nurses often encounter three types of ethical issues in the area of biomedical ethics: Policy or social issues such as whether health care is a right or privilege; organizational dilemmas such as multiple loyalties or hierarchies of power; or clinical issues such as breaches of confidentiality (Epstein and Turner, 2015).

FOUNDATIONS OF NURSING AND PUBLIC HEALTH'S CODES OF ETHICS

Modern nursing also has a rich heritage of ethics and morality. Florence Nightingale (1820–1910) is often seen as nursing's first moral leader and nurse in community health. Nightingale saw nursing as a call to service and thought nurses should be people of good moral character. She was a champion of primary prevention, passionate about the need to provide care to the disenfranchised, and committed to the importance of a sanitary environment, as seen in her work with soldiers in the Crimean War (1854–56). The ethical foundations of clinical practice that Nightingale contributed to nursing have endured. Chapter 2 provides details about the many contributions of Nightingale to the development of the nursing profession.

In the 1960s, two seminal events that changed the course of nursing practice occurred. First, the American Nurses Association (ANA) recommended all nursing education occur in institutions of higher education. Before this time, many of the schools of nursing were offered by religious institutions and had ethics included in their curricula. As the process of moving nursing into higher education took place, ethics as a course was removed from many schools of nursing. Often the decision to omit ethics courses was influenced by the need to include more general education courses in the nursing curriculum. Second, because of major advances in science and technology, the field of bioethics began to emerge and was also developing in nursing curricula. It is likely that with the pandemic of 2020, schools of nursing will include more content related to ethics in the curricula.

Nurses' codes of ethics are important in the history of nursing practice in the community. The Nightingale Pledge is generally considered to be nursing's first code of ethics (ANA, 2001). After the Nightingale Pledge, a "suggested" code and a "tentative" code were published in the *American Journal of Nursing* but were not formally adopted. The ANA House of Delegates formally adopted the *Code for Professional Nurses* in 1950. It was amended and revised five more times, until in 2001 the ANA House of Delegates adopted *the Code of Ethics for Nurses with Interpretive Statements.* Most recently, the *Code of Ethics for Nurses* was revised and approved in 2014. As stated by Marsha Fowler (2015), "the *Code of Ethics for Nurses with Interpretive Statements* is remarkable in its breadth and compass. It retains nursing's historical and ethical values, obligations, ideals, and commitments while extending them into the ever-growing art, science, and practice of nursing in 2015" (pp viii–ix).

The International Council of Nurses (ICN) adopted the first known international code of ethics in 1953. Like the *Code of Ethics for Nurses with Interpretive Statements,* it has undergone various revisions and adoptions. The most recent revision of the *ICN Code of Ethics for Nurses* was adopted in 2005, copyrighted in 2006, and revised in 2012 (International Council of Nurses, 2012).

As mentioned earlier in the chapter, the bioethics movement of the late 1960s influenced both nursing ethics and public health ethics. The relationship between public health and ethics has also been made explicit through the development of a code of ethics (Public Health Leadership Society, 2002). After input from many public health professionals and associations, the Code of Ethics for Public Health was approved in 2002 (Olick, 2005). This code, entitled *Principles of the Ethical Practice of Public Health,* defines public health in the following way: "public health not only seeks to assure the health of whole communities but also recognizes that the health of individuals is tied to their life in the community" (Public Health Leadership Society, 2002, p. 1). It also identifies 12 guiding principles, including but not limited to respect for individuals within their communities, community engagement in policies and procedures that affect the community's overall health and well-being, community consent, collaborative practices that support trust within diverse communities, and upholding ethical principles of confidentiality and justice. (For clarity in this chapter, this document is referred to as the Code of Ethics for Public Health unless the official title is used.)

Professional codes provide a foundation from which nurses and other public health advocates can meet their professional and moral obligations to their patients and communities.

Nurses in public health have to honor their professional duties in ways that extend beyond one-on-one care, and this can present unique ethical challenges. Indeed, in public health nursing, the role of prevention is increasingly being informed by genomics as well as other factors. Here, nurses must become more skilled in learning how to reduce the potential influence of genetic risk factors by teaching clients how to live healthier lives, or address the individual health effects of environmental risks within communities, such as drinking water, lead levels, air pollutants, or radiation exposure. Questions that arise in regard to genomics and how this and other factors may affect public health nursing include the following: Should people be held accountable for making unhealthy life choices? To whom should you give information about a genetic predisposition to an environmental health problem? Should society's resources be used for people who knowingly engage in risky behavior? As will be discussed in the Evidence-Based Practice box, what do public health nurses think about the ethics of mandated vaccine education (Navin, Kozak and Deem, 2020)?

ETHICAL DECISION MAKING

Ethical issues are moral challenges facing all health care practitioners and are particularly common in community or public health nursing. Ulrich et al. state that "ethical issues can occur in any situation where profound moral questions of 'rightness' or 'wrongness' underlie professional decision making and the beneficent care of patients" (2010b, p 2511). A timely example of an ethical issue in community or public health nursing at both the individual and community level is the COVID-19 pandemic. Communities struggled with convincing residents to practice social distancing; to self-isolate; to get tested if they had any symptoms or reasons to think they might have contracted the virus; and to see a health care provider if they had difficulty breathing. One of the central ethical issues surrounding the pandemic was informed consent of health care providers as well as the community regarding the risks of contracting the virus and its implications for individual and community health and well-being. From a public health perspective, other ethical issues included concerns about surveillance and tracking measures, availability of personal protective equipment, and quarantine and isolation procedures for hospitalized patients as well as American and foreign citizens who entered or reentered the country. In contrast, ethical dilemmas are human dilemmas and puzzling moral problems in which a person, group, or community can envision morally justified reasons for both taking and not taking a certain course of action (Purtilo and Doherty, 2016; Barrett, 2012).

Making ethical decisions on allocation priorities of a scarce and untested resource such as drugs for COVID-19 that had been used for other diseases such as malaria but had not been scientifically tested for this virus were challenging endeavors. Thus ethical decision making is the part of ethics that focuses on the process of how ethical decisions are made. Ethical theories, principles, and decision-making frameworks help nurses and others think through these issues and dilemmas. Often, ethical content is abstract, which makes decision making more difficult.

Ethical decision-making frameworks use problem-solving processes. They provide guides for making sound ethical decisions that can be morally justified. Some of these frameworks are discussed in this chapter. It is important to remember that when all is said and done, we each make our own decisions. Because we make our own decisions, the following generic ethical decision-making framework may be useful:

1. Identify the ethical issues and dilemmas.
2. Place the ethical issues and dilemmas within a meaningful context.
3. Obtain all relevant facts.
4. Reformulate ethical issues and dilemmas, if needed.
5. Consider appropriate approaches to actions or options (i.e., utilitarianism, deontology, principlism, virtue ethics, care ethics, feminist ethics).
6. Make the decision and take action.
7. Evaluate the decision and the action.

The steps of a generic ethics framework are often nonlinear, and with the exception of the ethical approach, they do not change substantially. Their rationales are presented in Table 6.1. Step 5 (the one exception) lists six approaches to the ethical

TABLE 6.1 Rationale for Steps of an Ethical Decision-Making Framework

Steps	Rationale
1. Identify the ethical issues and dilemmas.	Persons cannot make sound ethical decisions if they cannot identify ethical issues and dilemmas.
2. Place them within a meaningful context.	The historical, sociological, cultural, psychological, economic, political, communal, environmental, and demographic contexts affect the way ethical issues and dilemmas are formulated and justified.
3. Obtain all relevant facts.	Facts affect the way ethical issues and dilemmas are formulated and justified.
4. Reformulate ethical issues or dilemmas if needed.	The initial ethical issues and dilemmas may need to be modified or changed on the basis of context and facts.
5. Consider appropriate approaches to actions or options.	The nature of the ethical issues and dilemmas determines the specific ethical approaches used.
6. Make decisions and take action.	Professional persons cannot avoid choice and action in applied ethics.
7. Evaluate decisions and action.	Evaluation determines whether the ethical decision-making framework used resulted in morally justified actions related to the ethical issues and dilemmas.

decision-making process; these approaches are outlined throughout the chapter in the How To boxes.

Several factors can affect the ethical decision-making process. First, we live in a multicultural society in which nurses face ethical issues and dilemmas related to the diverse cultures, values, and beliefs of their patients, families, and communities. This at times can create conflict. Callahan (2000), cofounder of the Hastings Center, helps explain these conflicts and describes the following four situations for reflection and consideration when working with diverse individuals and communities:

1. Situations that place persons at direct risk for harm, whether psychological or physical
2. Situations in which cultural standards conflict with professional standards
3. Situations in which the greater community's values are jeopardized by values of a smaller culture within that community.
4. Situations in which community customs may cause mild offense or annoyance to other communities, but no major problems

Chapter 7 discusses cultural influences on public health nursing. Applying Callahan's four standards to content in that chapter will be helpful. Callahan (2000) discusses how to consider diversity in the four situations. In situation 1, he says, "we in America imposed some standards on ourselves for important moral reasons; and there is no good reason to exempt subgroups from those standards" (p 43). Regarding situations 2 and 3, Callahan recognizes a challenge between cultural standards of individuals and communities and health care providers' professional standards. Within this scenario, health care providers have to recognize that some groups hold values different from those generally accepted as normative in society. Callahan says, "in the absence of grievous harm, there is no clear moral mandate to interfere with those values" (p 43). However, sometimes there is some degree of moral pressure (not coercion) to intervene with differing values for the sake of community consensus. This often requires compromise and negotiation between differing parties. Finally, regarding situation 4, he notes there is no moral mandate to intervene in non-threatening cultural traditions and values even if they create some degree of burden on others. Intervention only becomes necessary when the imposed burdens cause harm or undue hardship to other groups.

Because decision making is central to the practice of nursing and many decisions are difficult to make, it is useful to consider the experience of moral distress. As noted earlier, moral distress occurs when one is unable to act in a way that he or she thinks is right (consistent with their own personal or professional values, cultural expectations, and/or religious beliefs) due to internal or external constraints. Moral distress is different from what we may consider emotional distress because there is not only an ethical component associated with this phenomenon but also the threat to an individual's moral integrity (Epstein and Delgado, 2010; Hamric, 2014; Ulrich, Hamric, and Grady, 2010a; Campbell et al., 2016). Nurses, as well as other types of health care providers, have experienced moral distress (Epstein and Delgado, 2010; Austin et al., 2008; Chen, 2009; Forde and Aasland, 2008; Hamric and

Blackhall, 2007; Lomis, Carpenter, and Miller, 2009). In a national survey, Ulrich et al. (2007) reported that nurses identified feeling powerless, overwhelmed, frustrated, and fatigued when they cannot resolve ethical issues experienced while working. These reported feelings are psychosocial consequences of moral distress. When this conflict occurs, it can lead to a sense of personal failure in the kind of care nurses give and to subsequent performance issues and may lead to work or career dissatisfaction. However, moral distress may be addressed in some of the following ways:

1. Identifying the type(s) of situation that leads to distress
2. Communicating that concern to your manager and examining ways to work toward addressing the stressor
3. Seeking support from colleagues
4. Seeking support from ethics committees, social workers, and pastoral care, among others
5. Being proactive and expressing one's voice on matters that are ethically concerning

It is often useful to talk with colleagues who may have similar concerns. Additionally, open dialogue with those in leadership positions such as nurse managers can be helpful. Collaboration like this can lead nurses to connect with other services such as ethics committees and social work, both of which have important roles in ethical practice.

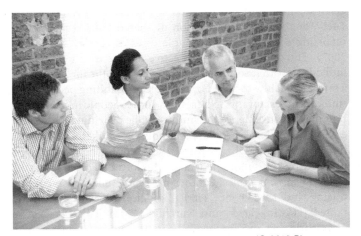

Colleagues Participate in Ethical Decision Making. (© 2012 Photos.com, a division of Getty Images. All rights reserved. Image #92202428.)

Three cases are presented in the chapter. Examine each one using the ethical decision-making processes outlined in the How To boxes and the different codes of ethics provided in the chapter. These cases provide an excellent opportunity to debate your personal beliefs about the application of ethical processes with classmates and to assess your own thoughts, feelings, and possible actions. The cases deal with what the nursing response should be (1) when clients will not assume responsibility for their health, (2) when the question arises about whether parents can adequately care for young children, and (3) when clients are not able or willing to take personal responsibility and do not want the nurse to report the situation.

In each of the three cases, evaluate the National Council of State Boards of Nursing's steps for developing clinical judgment in nursing. This new set of decision-making steps is described in the Preface of the text. They are: recognize cues; analyze cues; prioritize hypotheses; generate solution; take action; and evaluate outcomes. Compare these six steps with the ethical decision-making process you use. Are they complementary or do they suggest different plans of action?

ETHICAL PRINCIPLES AND THEORIES AS GUIDES TO ETHICAL DECISION MAKING

The remainder of this section of the chapter summarizes content about ethical theories and principles. As you read these sections, remember that the ways ethical theories and principles are applied in the community may differ from how they are applied with individuals. As Racher (2007, p 68) aptly says, "Community practice is traditionally based on utilitarianism, adheres to the axiom 'the greatest good for the greatest number,' and supports the position that maximizing benefits to socially disadvantaged groups ultimately benefits society as a whole." Community practitioners work to increase participation in health promotion and manage chronic diseases; they see these actions as benefiting the individual and the community. Public health is concerned with collective action that benefits the greatest number of people, such as having clean water, public safety, or the societal regulation of shared risks, for example, reporting of some communicable diseases (Easley and Allen, 2007). The public health perspective of care may require that individuals forfeit some of their self-interests for the benefits of a safe and healthy society. For example, prohibiting people from smoking in restaurants to benefit the other people in the restaurant may inconvenience the smoker, while providing a healthier environment for all people, including the smoker. Similarly, at times a person's right to privacy and confidentiality may be usurped by the public benefit of disclosure. This might take place during epidemics or other national events when contact tracing and surveillance epidemiological measures are warranted (Gostin, Bayer, and Fairchild, 2003). This perspective was clearly seen during the COVID-19 pandemic when people were required to wear masks to enter most types of buildings ranging from grocery stores to health care provider's offices as well as forms of transportation. Some people wished to resist, but the principle of "caring for the greater good" prevailed, and masks were required.

Utilitarianism and Deontology

At times, decisions are based on outcomes or consequences. In this approach, referred to as consequentialism, the right action is the one that produces the greatest amount of good or the least amount of harm in a given situation. Utilitarianism is a well-known consequentialist ethical theory associated with outcomes or consequences in determining which choice to make. In utilitarianism, the priority is to maximize benefit and minimize harm and to consider what is the greatest good—that is, the end justifies the means.

HOW TO APPLY THE UTILITARIAN ETHICS DECISION PROCESS

1. Determine moral rules that are important to society and that are derived from the principle of utility.[a]
2. Identify the communities or populations that are affected or most affected by the moral rules.
3. Analyze viable alternatives for each proposed action based on the moral rules.
4. Determine the consequences or outcomes of each viable alternative on the communities or populations most affected by the decision.
5. Select the actions on the basis of the rules that produce the greatest amount of good or the least amount of harm for the communities or populations that are affected by the action.

NOTE: Remember that the utilitarian ethics decision process is one of the approaches in step 5 of the generic ethical decision-making framework.

[a]Moral rules of action that produce the greatest good for the greatest number of communities or populations affected by or most affected by the rules.

In other situations, nurses may conclude that the action is right or wrong in itself, regardless of the amount of good that might come from it. This is the ethical theory known as deontology, which is a "theory of duty holding that some features of actions other than or in addition to consequences make actions right or wrong" (Beauchamp & Childress, 2013, p 361). This view is based on the premise that persons should always be treated as ends in themselves and never as mere means to the ends of others (Munson, 2014).

Each theory maintains that there is a universal first principle, the principle of utility for utilitarianism and the categorical imperative for deontology, which serves as a rational norm for behavior and allows us to calculate the rightness or wrongness of each individual action. According to both utilitarianism and deontology, the individual is the special center of moral concern (Steinbock, Arras, and London, 2008). Deontology comes from the Greek roots deon, meaning "duty," and logos, meaning "study of." Giving priority to individual rights and needs refers to the concept that a person's rights and dignity should never (or rarely) be sacrificed to the interests of society (Steinbock, Arras, and London, 2008).

Health professionals have specific obligations that exist because of the practices and goals of the profession. These health care obligations can be interpreted in terms of a set of principles in bioethics as outlined by Beauchamp and Childress (2013): respect for autonomy, nonmaleficence, beneficence, and justice (as shown in Box 6.1). Principlism relies on these ethical principles to guide decision making. As such, the principle of autonomy refers to self-governance. Respecting autonomy requires health care providers to understand a client's ability to decide and act with his or her own plan (Beauchamp and Childress, 2013). Nonmaleficence is the noninfliction of harm and is often closely linked to the principle of beneficence or the duty to act in ways that will benefit others. Distributive justice or social justice refers to the allocation of benefits and burdens to members of society. Benefits refer to basic needs, including material and social goods, liberties, rights, and entitlements. Some benefits of society

BOX 6.1 Ethical Principles

Respect for autonomy: Based on human dignity and respect for individuals, autonomy requires that individuals be permitted to choose those actions and goals that fulfill their life plans unless those choices result in harm to another.

Nonmaleficence: According to Hippocrates, nonmaleficence requires that we do no harm. It is impossible to avoid harm entirely, but this principle requires that health care professionals act according to the standards of due care, always seeking to produce the least amount of harm possible.

Beneficence: This principle is complementary to nonmaleficence and requires that we do good. We are limited by time, place, and talents in the amount of good we can do. We have general obligations to perform those actions that maintain or enhance the dignity of other persons whenever those actions do not place an undue burden on health care providers.

Distributive justice: Distributive justice requires that there be a fair distribution of the benefits and burdens in society based on the needs and contributions of its members. This principle requires that consistent with the dignity and worth of its members and within the limits imposed by its resources, a society must determine a minimal level of goods and services to be available to its members.

are wealth, education, and public services. Among the burdens to be shared are items such as taxes, military service, and the location of incinerators and power plants. Justice requires that the distribution of benefits and burdens in a society be fair. Although it is recognized that distribution should be based on what one needs and deserves, considerable disagreement exists when considering what these terms mean in the context of fairness.

The three primary theories of distributive justice are egalitarian, libertarian, and liberal democratic (Box 6.2).

Although principlism has been used effectively to analyze ethics-related situations in bioethics, it also has its critics (Callahan, 2000, 2003; Walker, 2009). First, some argue that the principles are too abstract and narrow to serve as guides for action. Second, the principles themselves can conflict in a given situation, and there is no independent basis for prioritizing them (Walker, 2009). Third, Walker (2009) contends that there are more than four principles that reflect the "common morality." And, fourth, ethical judgments may depend more on the judgment of sensitive persons than on the application of abstract principles.

HOW TO APPLY THE DEONTOLOGICAL ETHICS DECISION PROCESS

1. Determine the moral rules (e.g., tell the truth) that serve as standards by which individuals can perform their moral obligations.
2. Examine personal motives for proposed actions to ensure that they are based on good intentions in accord with moral rules.
3. Determine whether the proposed actions can be generalized so that all persons in similar situations are treated similarly.
4. Select the action that treats persons as ends in themselves and never as mere means to the ends of others.

NOTE: Remember that the deontological ethics decision process is one of the approaches in step 5 of the generic ethical decision-making framework.

CASE STUDY 1

Applying the Principlism Ethics Decision Process

Jeff Williams, team leader in Home Health Care Services at the county health department, was preparing to visit Mr. Chisholm, a 59-year-old client recently diagnosed as having emphysema. Mr. Chisholm, who was unemployed because of a farming accident several years earlier, was well known to the health department. Hypertensive and overweight, he was also a heavy, long-term cigarette smoker despite his decreased lung function. Mr. Williams visited Mr. Chisholm to find out why the client had missed his latest chest clinic appointment. He also wanted to determine whether the client was continuing his medications as ordered.

As Mr. Williams parked his car in front of his client's house, he could see Mr. Chisholm sitting on the front porch smoking a cigarette. A flash of anger made him wonder why he continued trying to encourage Mr. Chisholm to stop smoking and why he took the time from his busy home-care schedule to follow up on Mr. Chisholm's missed clinic appointments. This client certainly did not seem to care enough about his own health to give up smoking.

During the home visit, Mr. Williams determined that Mr. Chisholm had discontinued the use of his prophylactic antibiotic and was not taking his expectorant and bronchodilator medication on a regular basis. Mr. Chisholm's blood pressure was 210/114 mm Hg, and he coughed almost continuously. Although he listened politely to Mr. Williams's concerns about his respiratory function and the continued use of his medications, Mr. Chisholm simply made no effort to take responsibility for his health care. Even so, another clinic appointment was made, and Mr. Williams encouraged the client to attend.

As he drove to his next home visit, Mr. Williams wondered to what extent he was obligated as a nurse to spend time on clients who took no personal

responsibility for their health. He also wondered if there was a limit to the amount of nursing care a noncooperative client could expect from a service provided in the community.

Consider this case using the principlism ethics decision process:

1. If the nurse wants to respect Mr. Chisholm's right to autonomy, should he try to explain the need for compliance with the treatment plan and urge the client to comply? Or should the nurse tell Mr. Chisholm that he will be given a clinic appointment when he begins to follow the treatment plan? Or should the nurse schedule the next appointment and hope Mr. Chisholm will soon understand why he should follow the care plan? Or is there an action you would choose that is not listed here?
2. What are Mr. Williams's professional responsibilities for Mr. Chisholm's rights to health care?
3. Is there a limit to the amount of care nurses should be expected to give to clients?
4. What authority defines the moral requirements and moral limits of nursing care to clients?
5. Using content in at least one of the How To boxes, apply one of the ethical processes to this case. For example, debate with a classmate whether the deontological ethics decision process is useful in determining the nursing action with Mr. Chisholm. Specifically, examine your motives for being reluctant to continue providing care to this client who seemingly has no desire to promote his own health.
6. What ethical principles are causing distress for the nurse?

Modified from Fry ST, Veatch RM, Taylor C: *Case studies in nursing ethics*, Boston, 2011, Jones and Bartlett Learning, pp 28–29.

BOX 6.2 Three Primary Theories of Distributive Justice

Distributive Justice Theory	Principles
Egalitarian	This view advocates that everyone is entitled to equal rights and equal treatment in society. Ideally, each person has an equal share of the goods of society, and it is the role of government to ensure that this happens. The government has the authority to redistribute wealth if necessary to ensure equal treatment. Thus egalitarians support welfare rights—that is, the right to receive certain social goods necessary to satisfy basic needs. These include adequate food, housing, education, and police and fire protection. Both practical and theoretical weaknesses are inherent in egalitarianism (Beauchamp and Childress, 2013).
Libertarian	The libertarian view of justice advocates for social and economic liberty. Whereas egalitarianism lacks incentives for individuals, libertarianism emphasizes the contribution and merit of the individual (Beauchamp and Childress, 2013). Government has a limited role.
Liberal Democratic	This view values both liberty and equality.
	It is based on Rawls's theory of justice and the "veil of ignorance." Behind this veil, people (or their representatives) are unaware of social position, race, culture, doctrine, sex, endowments, or any other distinguishing circumstances (Rawls, 2001). This is known as the original position and is an exercise to address the inequalities and bargaining advantages that result from birth, natural endowments, and historical circumstances. Without these inequalities, all people are free and equal and can work together as citizens to decide what is fair and therefore just. Once impartiality is guaranteed, Rawls suggests all rational people will choose a system of justice containing the following two basic principles.
	Each person has the same claim to a fully adequate scheme of equal basic liberties, and this scheme is compatible with the same scheme of liberties for all.
	Social and economic inequalities are to satisfy two conditions: first, they are to be attached to offices and positions open to all under conditions of fair equality of opportunity; and second, they are to be to the greatest benefit to the least-advantaged members of society (the difference principle).

HOW TO APPLY THE PRINCIPLISM ETHICS DECISION PROCESS

1. Determine the ethical principles (i.e., respect for autonomy, nonmaleficence, beneficence, justice) that are relevant to an ethical issue or dilemma.
2. Analyze the relevant principles within a meaningful context of accurate facts and other pertinent circumstances.
3. Act on the principle that provides, within the meaningful context, the strongest guide to action that can be morally justified by the tenets foundational to the principle.

NOTE: Remember that using principlism in the ethics decision process is one of the approaches in step 5 of the general ethical decision-making framework.

EVIDENCE-BASED PRACTICE

Since 2015, Michigan has required parents who request nonmedical exemptions (NMEs) from school or daycare immunization mandates to participate in an educational program. These programs are led by public health staff, and generally the staff members are public health nurses. The researchers conducted focus group interviews with 39 of Michigan's waiver educators. In the year after implementing this program, Michigan's nonmedical exemption rates decreased by 35%. This article focused on the educator's ethical reflections and value judgments about immunization, vaccine refusers, the Michigan vaccine education waiver program, and the role of primary care clinicians in promoting childhood immunizations.

The responses of the educators ranged from thinking parents were selfish when they only considered their child and did not value the concept of "for the greater good" to thinking that parents did have the best intentions of their children in determining their actions.

Nurse Use

This study provides information about public health nurses' views on the ethical values and social impact of a state-implemented vaccine education program for families seeking nonmedical exemptions from mandated childhood vaccines. It is difficult to respect the rights of family members if you, the nurse, hold a different view. As a public health nurse, it is essential to always keep in mind what is in the best interests of the community of clients.

Navin MC, Kozak AT, Deem MJ: Perspectives of public health nurses on the ethics of mandated vaccine education, *Nursing Outlook* 68:62–72, 2020.

With the development of a vaccine for COVID-19, the issues discussed above became apparent as people decided if they would take the vaccine.

Virtue, Feminist, and Care Ethic Theories

Several other ethical theories are important to consider in relationship to public health. For example, virtue ethics, one of the oldest ethical theories, dates back to the ancient Greek philosophers Plato and Aristotle. Rather than being concerned with actions as seen in utilitarianism and deontology, virtue ethics asks: What kind of person should I be? Virtue ethics seeks to enable persons to flourish as human beings. Not to be confused with principles, Aristotle defines virtues as acquired, excellent traits of character that dispose humans to act in accord with their natural good. Examples of virtues include benevolence, compassion, discernment, trustworthiness, integrity, and conscientiousness (Beauchamp and Childress, 2013). Virtue ethics emphasizes practical reasoning applied to character development rather than focusing on moral justification by relying on theories and principles. In practice, virtues in nursing shape job responsibilities and patient care. For example, the virtues listed previously contribute to a nurse's role as one of the most trusted health professions.

HOW TO APPLY THE VIRTUE ETHICS DECISION PROCESS

1. Identify communities that are relevant to the ethical dilemmas or issues.
2. Identify moral considerations that arise from a communal perspective and apply the consideration to specific communities.
3. Identify and apply virtues that facilitate a communal perspective.
4. Modify moral considerations as needed to apply to the specific ethical dilemmas or issues.
5. Seek ethical community support to enhance character development.
6. Evaluate and modify the individuals or community character traits that impede communal living.
   NOTE: Remember that the virtue ethics decision process is one of the approaches in step 5 of the generic ethical decision-making framework.

Modified from Volbrecht RM: *Nursing ethics: communities in dialogue,* Upper Saddle River, NJ, 2002, Prentice Hall, p 138.

Care Ethics

Caring in nursing, the ethic of care, and **feminist ethics** are interrelated and converged between the mid-1980s and early 1990s. Nurses have written about caring as the essence of, or the moral ideal, of nursing for many years (Leininger, 1984; Watson, 2007). Caring and the ethic of care are core values of public health nursing and address the importance of the fiduciary relationship between the patient and the care provider.

Carol Gilligan (1982) and Nel Noddings (1984) are often associated with the ethic of care. Gilligan studied the psychological and moral development of women. She conducted her work at a time when the ability to make autonomous and effective decisions was considered masculine. This perpetuated a devaluing of the stereotypical feminine characteristics. Through her work, Gilligan was able to accentuate the feminine experience as distinctive rather than less valuable. She set forth basic premises of responsibility, care, and relationships. In doing so, the link between caring and relationships continued to grow more explicit. From this, it was posited that women not only judge themselves within the context of their relationships, but they also accept and are defined by the responsibility to care for others. Noddings echoed this sentiment and stated an obligation to enhance caring. The commitment that is inherent with caring facilitates ethical ideals. Gilligan and Noddings share a feminine ethic; they believe in the morality of responsibility in relationships that emphasize connection and caring. To them, caring is a moral imperative.

Feminist Ethics

Like virtue ethics and other communitarian views (i.e., the relationship and responsibility between the individual and the community), feminist ethics rejects abstract rules and principles. According to Rogers (2006), feminist ethics is pertinent to public health because it recognizes the role of political and social structures in health. Issues of equity present major challenges in public health. Inequalities in gender, historically affecting females, gave rise to the feminist stance that devaluing and systematic oppression of women are morally wrong. Today, feminism encompasses more than just issues unique to women. Rogers said that the feminist perspective leads people to think critically about the connections among gender, disadvantage,

and health, as well as the distribution of power in public health processes. Feminists advocate economic, social, and political equity. They pay attention to power relations that constitute a community, the rules that regulate it, and who pays and who benefits from membership in the community (Rogers, 2006).

HOW TO APPLY THE CARE ETHICS DECISION PROCESS

1. Recognize that caring is a moral imperative.
2. Identify personally lived caring experiences as a basis for relating to self and others.
3. Assume responsibility and obligation to promote and enhance caring in relationships.
   NOTE: Remember that the care ethics decision process is one of the approaches in step 5 of the generic ethical decision-making framework.

HOW TO APPLY THE FEMINIST ETHICS DECISION PROCESS

1. Identify the social, cultural, political, economic, environmental, and professional contexts that contribute to the identified problem (e.g., underrepresentation of women in clinical trials).
2. Evaluate how the preceding contexts contribute to the oppression of women.
3. Consider how women's lives are defined by their status in subordinate social groups.
4. Analyze how social practices marginalize women.
5. Plan ways to restructure those social practices that oppress women.
6. Implement the plan.
7. Evaluate the plan, and restructure it as needed.
   NOTE: Remember that the feminist ethics decision process is one of the approaches in step 5 of the generic ethical decision-making framework.

Modified from Volbrecht RM: *Nursing ethics: communities in dialogue,* Upper Saddle River, NJ, 2002, Prentice Hall, p 219.

ETHICS AND THE CORE FUNCTIONS OF PUBLIC HEALTH NURSING

In Chapter 1, the three core functions of public health nursing (i.e., assessment, policy development, and assurance) were discussed. The following discussion links these three core functions to ethics.

Assessment

"*Assessment* refers to systematically collecting data on the population, monitoring the population's health status, and making information available about the health of the community" (see Chapter 1). Two ethical tenets support these core functions: beneficence and nonmaleficence. Beneficence refers to "doing good" or maximizing the benefits and minimizing the harms, and this requires clinicians' competency related to knowledge development, analysis, and dissemination. Here one can ask the following: Are the persons assigned to develop community knowledge adequately prepared to collect data on groups and populations? This question is important because the research, measurement, and analysis techniques used to gather information about groups and populations usually differ from the techniques used to assess individuals. Wrong research techniques can lead to wrong assessments, which in turn may hurt rather than help the intended group or population.

QSEN FOCUS ON QUALITY AND SAFETY EDUCATION FOR NURSES

One of the six tenets of Quality and Safety Education for Nurses (QSEN) is patient-centered care (Barton et al., 2009). This chapter has discussed many ways in which an understanding of basic principles of ethics can guide safe and effective nursing practice. Some key aspects of patient-centered care in public health nursing include being certain that the information provided to individuals, families, and communities is accurate and reflects the most current evidence, and that it is presented in a timely fashion. Community health education should take into account the age, gender, and cultural and religious backgrounds of those who receive the information. Giving health information that does not meet these criteria can be unsafe and does not reflect attention to quality nursing care. One of the QSEN competencies related to patient-centered care is as follows: Recognize the patient or designee as the source of control and full partner in providing compassionate and coordinated care based on respect for patient's preferences, values, and needs. Specific aspects of patient-centered care related to communication are as follows:

- **Knowledge:** Integrate understanding of multiple dimensions of patient-centered care: information, communication, and education.
- **Skills:** Communicate patient values, preferences, and expressed needs to other members of the health care team.
- **Attitudes:** Respect and encourage individual expression of patient values, preferences, and expressed needs (Barton et al., 2009, p 315).

- Specific aspects of patient-centered care related to the public health dilemma of serving the good of the population versus serving the good of the individual are as follows:
- **Knowledge:** Explore ethical and legal implications of patient-centered care.
- **Skills:** Recognize the boundaries of therapeutic relationships (Barton et al., 2009, p 315).
- **Attitudes:** Acknowledge the tension that may exist between patient rights and the organizational responsibility for professional ethical care.

Patient-centered ethical activity: Public health is more concerned about the good of the collective group than of the individual. In order to think more closely about quality and safety, debate with a classmate about whether children should be required to have all of the Centers for Disease Control and Prevention vaccines before they can enter school. In this scenario, pretend a parent does not want to give their children all the recommended immunizations because of fear of side effects of the vaccines. To support your argument see http://www.cdc.gov/vaccines/schedules/index.html for what is required. See web articles such as www.responsibility-project.libertymutual.com for the parents' point of view.

Park EJ: The development and implications of a case-based computer program to train ethical decision-making, *Nurs Ethics* 20:943–956, 2013.

Additionally, do the persons selected to develop, assess, and disseminate community knowledge possess integrity? Beauchamp and Childress (2013) define integrity as the holistic integration of moral character. It requires conscientious thought during which people reflect on the rightness or wrongness of actions. The previous discussion of virtue ethics is helpful in exploring this tenet. The importance of integrity is clear: without integrity, the core function of assessment is endangered. Providers lacking integrity pose a risk for misconduct and are a threat to public health. The role of assessment is to provide information to the benefit of public health; any action that deters from this mission is troubling. The second ethical tenet relates to "do no harm." In any public health situation, balancing the benefits and risks is essential. As discussed in regard to the latest pandemic, minimizing harm to both individuals and communities required thoughtful dialogue on personal protective equipment as well as community surveillance and monitoring measures.

Policy Development

Public health nurses are critical to the development of policies that reflect the preferences and goals of their constituents. They are in key positions to provide leadership on the ethical issues that might arise within their communities and can use their unique training and skills to make policy decisions (see Chapter 1). In fact, an important goal of both policy and ethics is to achieve the public good (Silva, 2002), which is a part of the concept of citizenship (Denhardt and Denhardt, 2000; Rogers, 2006; Ruger, 2008). To be effective citizens, people must be both informed about policy and able and willing to do what is in the best interests of the community (Denhardt and Denhardt, 2000). Here, the voice of the community is the foundation on which policy is developed. Silva (2002) also argues that service to others over self is a necessary condition

of what is "good" or "right" policy (Silva, 2002). Denhardt and Denhardt (2000) provide three perspectives on this belief:

1. **Serve rather than steer.** An increasingly important role of the public servant (e.g., nurses and administrators) is to help citizens articulate and meet their shared interests rather than to attempt to control or steer society in new directions (p 553).
2. **Serve citizens, not customers.** The public interest results from a dialogue about shared values rather than the aggregation of individual self-interests. Therefore public servants do not merely respond to the demands of "customers" but focus on building relationships of trust and collaboration with and among citizens (p 555).
3. **Value citizenship and public service above entrepreneurship.** The public interest is better advanced by public servants and citizens committed to making meaningful contributions to society rather than by entrepreneurial managers acting as if public money were their own (p 556).

Service, an enduring nursing value, is at the core of these three perspectives. Service requires ethical action and what is ethical is also good policy (Silva, 2002). Therefore moral leadership from nurses is critical to the development of ethical health care policies.

Assurance

"*Assurance* refers to the role of public health in making sure that essential community health services are available including essential personal health services for those who would otherwise not receive them, and that there is a competent public health and personal health care workforce" (see Chapter 1). The ethical principle of justice can apply to this core function as follows:

1. All persons should receive essential personal health services. Put in terms of justice, "to each person a fair share" or, "to all groups or populations a fair share." This does not necessarily mean that all persons in a society should share all of society's

benefits equally, but that they should share at least essential benefits. Many people think that basic health care for all is essential for social justice.

2. Providers of public health services should be competent and available. Although the Code of Ethics for Public

Health does not speak directly to workforce availability, it does speak directly to ensuring professional competency of public health employees. *Healthy People 2030* discusses both competencies and workforce, as seen in the *Healthy People 2030* box.

CASE STUDY 2

Autonomy and Distributive Justice

Amelia Lewis, a 31-year-old African American woman with multiple diagnoses, has been followed by the local mental health system for over 10 years. Four years ago, while a client at the local day hospital, she met and married another client, James Wood. She became pregnant and now has Tyesha, who is 3 years old. Multiple agencies have followed Ms. Lewis and her little girl, who live in a sparsely furnished apartment in subsidized housing. Mr. Wood lives separately, and he and his family welcome contact with Tyesha, but the relationship between Ms. Lewis and Mr. Wood has deteriorated. A guardian handles all of Ms. Lewis's financial affairs.

Ms. Lewis has issues of trust, and she is often suspicious of the care providers who come to her home. She does rely on some of the professionals with whom she interacts on a weekly or biweekly basis. Her developmental level places her at a stage at which her own needs are her primary focus, and this is not expected to change; her interaction with Tyesha is perfunctory, involving little outward affection. She is unable to understand that Tyesha is not capable of self-care and that her 3-year-old child will not always obey when Ms. Lewis instructs her to do something. Tyesha's needs, level of functioning, and cognitive development are quickly surpassing her mother's ability to cope. Frustration and misunderstanding ensue when Ms. Lewis thinks that Tyesha does not listen to her, and encouragement and parent education have done little to improve the situation as Tyesha gets older and more assertive. This has made toilet training, provision of an appropriate diet, and other aspects of normal child care problematic.

Many services besides those for mental health are involved to help this family of two cope. There is concern about abuse or neglect because of Ms. Lewis's lack of understanding of how to be a parent. Supplemental Security Income provides monetary support because of her mental disability, and they have Medicaid coverage for their health care needs, as well as food stamps and modest financial assistance through Temporary Assistance for Needy Families (TANF). Ms. Lewis cannot currently work and take care of her child because of her mental disability. Before Tyesha's birth, Ms. Lewis held a job and maintained self-care, but the care of Tyesha has precluded her managing employment at this time. Child Protective Services are also monitoring Ms. Lewis's

situation. Ms. Lewis attends a local program to complete her General Education Development (GED), which provides child care during the day. Although Ms. Lewis is not expected to complete her GED, this program provides structured time for Tyesha three times per week. The child is considered developmentally normal at this time. Tyesha is being followed by an infant development program that monitors her progress on developmental issues. The Child Health Partnership, an agency that addresses the needs of challenged families, provides regular visits, family support, and parenting education, and the GED teachers make regular home visits to check on Ms. Lewis and Tyesha. Ms. Lewis thinks things are going just fine.

The Child Health Partnership nurse is concerned about this family and thinks that some permanent resolution of the situation is inevitable. There is minimal coordination of services and no "lead agency" in the family's care. Choose one of the ethical decision processes or one set of code of ethics discussed in the chapter and discuss and debate these questions:

1. Should the nurse involved in the Child Health Partnership program initiate any action to try to coordinate the work of the many agencies involved with this family?
2. Who has a professional responsibility to determine when the mother can no longer cope with the developing child?
3. Whose needs, Ms. Lewis's or Tyesha's, should take precedence?
4. Using one of the ethics decision processes, analyze the role of the nurse in this situation. For example, considering the utilitarian ethics decision process, decide if it is morally right for you to take the child away from the mother. If you do this, what are the implications for the mother, the child, and the community? What would be the possible consequences of removing the child? Of not removing the child? What principles can best guide your decision making? What possible moral dilemmas will you experience?
5. Safety is a core concept of public health nursing. Using two of the six quality and safety competencies (client-centered care and safety) for nurses identified in the Quality and Safety Education for Nurses (QSEN) work, develop a plan of action for the nurse who is caring for this family.

 HEALTHY PEOPLE 2030

Objectives Related to Access to Health Services

- **AHS-04:** Reduce the proportion of people who can't get medical care when they need it.
- **HC/HIT-02:** Decrease the proportion of adults who report poor communication with their health care provider.
- **HC/HIT-03:** Increase the proportion of adults whose health care providers involved them in decisions as much as they wanted.

  Each of these objectives related to access to care reflect important ethical considerations for nurses.

From US Department of Health and Human Services: *Healthy People 2030*, 2020. Retrieved September 3, 2020 at http://www.healthypeople.gov.

NURSING CODE OF ETHICS

As noted in the discussion of history earlier in this chapter, the *Code of Ethics for Nurses with Interpretive Statements* was adopted by the ANA House of Delegates in 2001 and most recently revised in 2015. This code serves three broad purposes, as follows (ANA, 2015):

1. "It is a succinct statement of the ethical values, obligations, duties, and professional ideals of nurses individually and collectively" (p viii).
2. "It is the profession's nonnegotiable ethical standard" (p viii).
3. "It is an expression of nursing's own understanding of its commitment to society" (p viii).

These purposes are reflected in nine provisional statements of the code. The *Code of Ethics for Nurses* and its interpretive statements apply to nurses in community health, although the emphasis for each type of nursing sometimes varies. For example, provision 1 and its interpretive statement primarily address the individual when discussing how the nurse practices with compassion and respect for the person being cared for regardless of the person's status, the person's attributes, or the nature of the health problem. However, it is also recognized under provision 1 that there are times when individual rights may be limited because of public health concerns. The interpretive statements of provisions 2 and 8 are pertinent to public

health nurses, including those who identify as community health nurses. Provision 2 states "the nurse's primary commitment is to the recipients of nursing and health care services—patient or client—whether individuals, families, groups, communities, or populations" (p 5). Provision 8 highlights the need for collaborative practice with other disciplines as well as the public to mitigate health disparities and promote human rights. All nurses have a responsibility to meet the obligations highlighting professional standards, active involvement in nursing, and the integrity of the profession as outlined in the Code (see the *Code of Ethics for Nurses with Interpretative Statements* for all provisions at http://www.nursingworld.org).

CASE STUDY 3

Using the Deontological Decision-Making Process

Because finding affordable housing was difficult, 26-year-old Terry White lived with her 6-month-old son, Tommy, and his father, Billy Smith, in one room of the landlord's house. Ms. White was morbidly obese and was diagnosed with bipolar disease. Mr. Smith had served time for drug dealing and was out on parole and staying straight. Neither had finished high school. Mr. Smith's past drug use had rendered him unable to do much manual labor because of heart damage, but on occasion, he would work in construction to support the family.

Public health nurse Jim Lewis had received a referral on Tommy when he was diagnosed with failure to thrive (FTT) 2 months earlier. Ms. White (who had had two children removed from her custody by Child Protective Services [CPS] in the past) and Mr. Smith seemed to adore their baby, so much so that Ms. White would hold the baby all day long. In the past 2 months, the nurse had taught Ms. White about infant nutrition and gotten her enrolled in the Women, Infants, and Children (WIC) nutrition program; as a result, Tommy had increased his rate of physical growth and was above the 5% level of his growth percentile. Yet he was not meeting his gross motor milestones per Denver Developmental Screening Test II (DDST II) testing. Mr. Lewis thought that Tommy was not allowed to play on the floor enough to progress in sitting, pushing his shoulders up, or crawling. Most of their small room was taken up with the bed and the boxes that stored their belongings. There wasn't really space for "tummy time" or play. When not in the room, the family would take the bus to a discount store and spend the day walking around to get a change of scene.

One week Ms. White told the nurse she was not taking her medications for bipolar disease anymore because they caused her to gain weight. The next week she confided that Mr. Smith had had a "dirty" urine specimen check and would

have to return to prison in the near future. The following week, Mr. Lewis found the family living in a run-down motel because they were evicted after a disagreement with the landlord. Ms. White was agitated, and she told the nurse that they had only $100, Mr. Smith was going to have to return to prison that week, and the motel bill was already $240. Ms. White knew she would be homeless soon without Mr. Smith's support but refused to talk with her social worker about her needs. She asked the nurse not to tell anyone about her situation because she was afraid CPS would take Tommy from her. It was clear to Mr. Lewis that he might not know where Tommy was after they left this motel.

1. Considering the principle of telling the truth, what are Mr. Lewis's professional responsibilities to Ms. White, to Tommy, and to the social worker assigned to this family?

2. Using the generic ethical decision-making framework discussed earlier in the chapter and considering the deontological ethical decision-making process, how should Mr. Lewis respond to Ms. White's request to not tell anyone about their situation? What communication, if any, should the nurse initiate with the social worker? With others?

3. Using virtue ethics, what actions would you take to resolve any moral dilemmas you have about the safety of Tommy in this family situation? If you do not tell anyone about the possible dangers to the child, what moral principles come into play? If you do tell the social worker about the situation and the child is removed from the mother, what moral principles come into play for you?

4. What ethical dilemmas may you experience if you are the nurse in this case? How can you deal effectively with these potential dilemmas?

Created by Deborah C. Conway, assistant professor of nursing (retired), School of Nursing, University of Virginia.

PUBLIC HEALTH CODE OF ETHICS

The *Code of Ethics for Public Health* (Public Health Leadership Society, 2002) was created with the assumption that all humans have the right to adequate health resources. This code consists of 12 principles related to the ethical practice of public health (Box 6.3); this includes those values and beliefs that focus on health, community, and action and a commentary on each of the 12 principles. The preamble describes the collective and societal nature of public health to keep people healthy. In doing so, it reaffirms the World Health Organization's (WHO) definition of health as "a state of complete physical, mental, and social well-being, and not merely the absence of disease"

(WHO, 2014). Similar to other codes of ethics, the 12 value statements incorporate the ethical tenets of preventing harm; doing no harm; promoting good; respecting both individual and community rights; respecting autonomy, diversity, and confidentiality when possible; ensuring professional competency; trustworthiness; and promoting **advocacy** for disenfranchised persons within a community. The Code also lists values and beliefs regarding community and public health. These include the belief that collaboration is a key element of public health, that each person should have opportunities to contribute to public discourse, and that identifying and promoting requirements for health is a primary public health concern.

BOX 6.3 Principles of the Ethical Practice of Public Health

1. Public health should principally address the fundamental causes of disease and requirements for health, aiming to prevent adverse health outcomes.
2. Public health should achieve community health in a way that respects the rights of individuals in the community.
3. Public health policies, programs, and priorities should be developed and evaluated through processes that ensure an opportunity for input from community members.
4. Public health should advocate and work for the empowerment of disenfranchised community members, aiming to ensure that the basic resources and conditions necessary for health are accessible to all.
5. Public health should seek the information needed to implement effective policies and programs that protect and promote health.
6. Public health institutions should provide communities with the information they have that is needed for decisions on policies or programs and should obtain the community's consent for their implementation.
7. Public health institutions should act in a timely manner on the information they have within the resources and the mandate given to them by the public.
8. Public health programs and policies should incorporate a variety of approaches that anticipate and respect diverse values, beliefs, and cultures in the community.
9. Public health programs and policies should be implemented in a manner that most enhances the physical and social environment.
10. Public health institutions should protect the confidentiality of information that can bring harm to an individual or community if made public. Exceptions must be justified on the basis of the high likelihood of significant harm to the individual or others.
11. Public health institutions should ensure the professional competencies of their employees.
12. Public health institutions and their employees should engage in collaborations and affiliations in ways that build the public's trust and the institution's effectiveness.

From the Public Health Leadership Society (PHLS): *Code of ethics for public health,*[a] New Orleans, LA, 2002, Louisiana Public Health Institute. The ethics project was funded in part by the Centers for Disease Control and Prevention.
[a]Officially titled *Principles of the Ethical Practice of Public Health,* as noted by Thomas (2002).

LEVELS OF PREVENTION

Related to Ethics

Primary Prevention
Use the *Code of Ethics for Nurses* to guide your nursing practice.

Secondary Prevention
If you are unable to behave in accordance with the *Code of Ethics for Nurses* (e.g., you speak in a way that does not communicate respect for a client), take steps to correct your behavior. You could explain to the client your error and apologize.

Tertiary Prevention
If you have treated a client or staff member in a way that is inconsistent with ethics practices, seek guidance on other choices you could have made.

Commonalities exist between the *Code of Ethics for Nurses with Interpretative Statements* and the *Code of Ethics for Public Health*. Both codes provide general ethical principles and approaches that are enduring and dynamic. They require nurses to think and act in accordance with the underlying ethics of their profession. They each encourage evidence-based and collaborative approaches for the betterment of health. Although the two codes do not specify (nor should they specify) details for every ethical issue, other mechanisms such as standards of practice, ethical decision-making frameworks, and ethics committees provide further guidance. Nevertheless, these two codes address most approaches to ethical justification, including traditional and emerging ethical theories and principles, humanist and feminist ethics, virtue ethics, professional–individual or community relationships, and advocacy.

ADVOCACY AND ETHICS

Advocacy is a powerful ethical concept in nursing. But what does *advocacy* mean? "Advocacy is the application of information and resources (including finances, effort, and votes) to effect systemic changes that shape the way people in a community live" (Christoffel, 2000, p 722). Bateman (2000) suggests that advocacy includes acting in the client's best interest, maintaining confidentiality, addressing informational needs, acting impartially, and carrying out the preferences and goals of the patient with diligence and competence. *Public health advocacy* is intended "to reduce death or disability in groups of people and that is not confined to clinical settings" (Christoffel, 2000, p 722). Public health includes aggregates or populations and encompasses both preventative and reactionary measures. Thus the problems addressed with public health advocacy affect, or have the potential to affect, a sizeable portion of a community. This form of advocacy was seen in 2020 with the initiation and enforcement of social distancing during the COVID-19 pandemic. Several codes and standards of practice address advocacy and the various roles of nursing. Three are noted here. Advocacy is addressed in the ANA and the Public Health Leadership Society's codes of ethics, as well as the ANA's *Public Health Nursing: Scope and Standards of Practice* (ANA, 2013).

According to the ANA's *Code of Ethics for Nurses with Interpretive Statements,* "The nurse promotes, advocates for, and protects the rights, health, and safety of the patient" (ANA, 2015, p 9). This Code describes advocacy as the nurse's responsibility to take action when the client's best interests are jeopardized by questionable practice on the part of any member of the health team, the health care system, or others. However, Shannon argues that nursing does not bear the "advocacy" label alone. Working with communities as a public health nurse requires collaborative leadership and a team-based approach to address the needs of vulnerable patients (Shannon, 2016).

According to the Public Health Leadership Society's *Code of Ethics for Public Health,* "Public health should advocate and work for the empowerment of disenfranchised community members, aiming to ensure that the basic resources and conditions necessary for health are accessible to all" (Public Health

Leadership Society, 2002, p 1). The Public Health Leadership Society's code elaborates on the preceding principle with two issues: that the voice of the community should be heard and that the marginalized or underserved in a community should receive "a decent minimum" (p 4) of health resources.

According to the ANA's *Public Health Nursing: Scope and Standards of Practice* (ANA, 2013), public health nurses have a moral mandate to establish ethical standards when advocating for health care policy. The preceding standards extend the prior two concepts of advocacy by moving advocacy into the policy arena, particularly health and social policy as applied to populations. Nurses can advocate for access to consistent, effective, efficient health care for all people.

How does ethics fit into dealing with a pandemic? According to Webster and Wocial (2020), "Disasters, including global pandemics such as COVID-19 disrupt standard care and present ethical challenges" (p 18). They state that planning helps prepare for disasters, but in the case of COVID-19, it does not eliminate ethical dilemmas and moral distress. Nurses experience moral distress when they are unable to do what they believe is right for their patients. They say that in caring for people during a pandemic, it is often necessary to move away from Provision 2 of the ANA *Code of Ethics for Nurses with Interpretive Statements* (2015), which advocates for relationship-centered care, and adopt an outcome-based framework (Provision 8), which refers to Promotion of Community and World Health. They note that COVID-19 "puts two ethical frameworks in direct tension with each other" (p 22). That is, nurses try to embrace a principle- or virtue-based framework focusing on respect of the recipient's autonomy and to help them minimize pain and suffering. However, when resources are severely limited, nurses often must adopt a utilitarian framework that asks the nurses to work to achieve the greatest good for the greatest number of people in their care. A fair process during a disaster may not feel fair.

APPLYING CONTENT TO PRACTICE

Throughout this chapter, there has been application of the content related to ethics in public health nursing and the many documents that influence the role of public health nurses. These include the ANA's *Scope and Standards of Public Health Nursing*, the ANA's *Code of Ethics*, the core functions of public health as outlined by the Institute of Medicine, and the *Healthy People 2030* objectives. Ethics is also an integral part of the Core Competencies for Public Health Professionals. The section on analytic and assessment skills states that a public health professional uses "ethical principles in the collection, maintenance, use, and dissemination of data and information," and under leadership and systems thinking, says a professional "incorporates ethical standards of practice as the basis of all interactions with organization, communities, and individuals."

Council on Linkages Between Academia and Public Health Practice: *Core competencies for public health professionals*, Washington, DC, 2014, Public Health Foundation, Health Resources and Services Administration.

PRACTICE APPLICATION

The retiring director of the division of primary care in a state health department had recently hired Ann Jones, a 34-year-old nurse with a master's degree in public health, to be director of the division. Ms. Jones was responsible for monitoring millions of dollars of state and federal money and supervising the funded programs within her division.

She received many requests for funding from a particular state agency that served a large, poor district. The poor people of the district consisted primarily of young families with children and homebound older adults with chronic illnesses. Over the past 3 years, the federal government had allocated considerable money to the state agency to subsidize pediatric primary-care programs, but no formal evaluation of these programs had occurred.

The director of the state agency was a physician who had been in this position for more than 20 years. He was good at obtaining funding for primary-care needs in his district, but the statistics related to the pediatric primary-care program seemed implausible—that is, few physical examinations were performed on the children, which had resulted in extra money in the budget. This unspent federal money was being used to supplement home health care services for the indigent homebound older adults in his district. The thinking of the physician was that he was doing good by providing some needed services to both indigent groups in his district. Ms. Jones experienced moral discomfort because she did not have either the money or the personnel to provide both services.

What should she do?

A. What facts are the most relevant in this scenario?

B. What are the ethical issues?

C. How can Ms. Jones resolve the issues?

NOTE: The preceding case and answers are adapted and paraphrased from a real practice application shared by J. L. Chapin on the inappropriate distribution of primary health care funds {in Silva, M, editor: *Ethical decision-making in nursing administration*, Norwalk, CT, 1990, Appleton & Lange}.)

Answers can be found on the Evolve website.

■ REMEMBER THIS!

- Nursing has a rich heritage of ethics and morality.
- The field of bioethics began to emerge and influence nursing in the late 1960s.
- Ethical decision making is the component of ethics that focuses on the process of how ethical decisions are made.
- Many different ethical decision-making frameworks exist; however, the problem-solving process underlies each of them.
- Ethical decision making applies to all approaches to ethics—utilitarianism, deontology, principlism, virtue ethics, the ethic of care, and feminist ethics.
- Cultural diversity and moral distress make ethical decision making more challenging.
- Classic ethical theories are utilitarianism and deontology.
- Principlism consists of respect for autonomy, nonmaleficence, beneficence, and justice.
- The core functions of nursing in public health (i.e., assessment, policy development, assurance) are all grounded in ethics.
- *Healthy People 2030* discusses access to care.
- The 2015 *Code of Ethics for Nurses* contains nine statements that address the moral standards that delineate nursing's values, goals, and obligations.

- The 2002 *Code of Ethics for Public Health* contains 12 statements that address the moral standards that delineate public health's values, goals, and obligations.
- Advocacy is the act of pleading for or supporting a course of action on behalf of a person, group, or community.
- The *Code of Ethics for Nurses With Interpretive Statements,* the *Principles of the Ethical Practice of Public Health,* and *Public Health Nursing: Scope and Standards of Practice* all address advocacy.
- The processes of public health advocacy include but are not limited to identifying problems, collecting data, developing and endorsing regulations and legislation, enforcing policies, and assessing the policy process.
- The 2020 COVID-19 pandemic raised many ethical questions related to the rights of the individual versus the rights of the greater good; the duty to serve patients when nurses and their families might be put into a difficult risk situation; and the right to enforce such new behaviors as social distancing.

EVOLVE WEBSITE

http://evolve.elsevier.com/Stanhope/foundations
- Case Study, with Questions and Answers
- NCLEX® Review Questions
- Practice Application Answers

REFERENCES

American Nurses Association: *Code of ethics for nurses with interpretive statements*, Washington, DC, 2001, ANA.

American Nurses Association: *Public health nursing: the scope and standards of practice*, Silver Spring, MD, 2013, ANA.

American Nurses Association: *Code of ethics for nurses with interpretive statements*, Washington, DC, 2015, ANA.

American Nurses Association: *Nurses, ethics and the response to the COVID-19 pandemic*, www.nursingworld.org. Posted April 3, 2020. Accessed April 6, 2020.

Annas GJ: Beyond Nazi war crimes experiments: The voluntary consent requirement of the Nuremberg Code at 70, *Am J Public Health*, 108(1):42-46, 2018.

Austin W, Kagan L, Rankel M, Bergum V: The balancing act: psychiatrists' experience of moral distress, *Medicine, Health Care and Philosophy* 11(1):89–97, 2008.

Barrett MS: Ethical decision-making: a framework for understanding and resolving mental health dilemmas. In Ulrich C, editor: *Nursing ethics in everyday practice*, Indianapolis, 2012, Sigma Theta Tau International.

Barton AJ, Armstrong G, Preheim G, Gelmon SB, Andrus LC: A national Delphi to determine developmental progression of quality and safety competences in nursing education, *Nurs Outlook* 57:313-322, 2009.

Bateman N: *Advocacy skills for health and social care professionals*, Philadelphia, PA, 2000, Jessica Kingsley.

Beauchamp TL, Childress JF: *Principles of biomedical ethics*, ed 7, New York, 2013, Oxford.

Bellinger DC: Lead contamination in Flint—an abject failure to protect public health, *N Engl J Med* 374(12):1101-1103, 2016.

Belmont Report: *Ethical principles and guidelines for the protection of human subjects of research*, Washington DC, 1979, Government Printing Office.

Callahan D: Universalism and particularism fighting to a draw, *Hastings Center Report* 30(1): 37–44, 2000.

Callahan D: Principlism and communitarianism, *Journal of Medical Ethics* 29:287–291, 2003.

Campbell SM, Ulrich CM, Grady CA: A broader understanding of moral distress, *Am J Bioeth* 16(12):2-9, 2016.

Chadwick B and Gallagher A: *Ethics and nursing practice,* London, UK, Palgrave, the UK imprint of Macmillan Publishers Limited.

Chapin JL: The inappropriate distribution of primary health care funds. In Silva M, editor: *Ethical decision making in nursing administration*, Norwalk, Conn, 1990, Appleton and Lange.

Chen P: *When nurses and doctors can't do the right thing*, February 5, 2009. Retrieved October 14, 2016 from http://www.nytimes.com/2009/02/06/health/05chen.html.

Christoffel KK: Public health advocacy: process and product, *American Journal of Public Health* 90:722–726, 2000.

Council on Linkages Between Academia and Public Health Practice: *Core competencies for public health professionals*, Washington DC, 2014, Public Health Foundation, Health Resource and Services Administration.

Denhardt RB, Denhardt JV: The new public service: serving rather than steering, *Public Administrative Review* 60:549–552, 2000.

Easley CE, Allen CE: A critical intersection: human rights, public health nursing, and nursing ethics, *Advances in Nursing Science* 30:367–382, 2007.

Epstein B, Delgado S: Understanding and addressing moral distress, *The Online Journal of Issues in Nursing*, 2010. September 30, 2010, 15(3):1-12. 3, Manuscript 1, l.

Epstein B, Turner M: The nursing code of ethics: its value, its history, *The Online Journal of Issues in Nursing*, 20(2), Manuscript 4, May 31, 2015.

Forde R, Aasland OG: Moral distress among Norwegian doctors, *J Medical Ethics* 34(7):521–525, 2008.

Fowler MDM: *Guide to the Code of Ethics for nurses with interpretive statements: Development, interpretation, and application*, ed 2, Silver Spring, MD, 2015, ANA.

Fry ST, Veatch RM, Taylor C: *Case studies in nursing ethics*, ed 4, Sudbury Mass, 2011, Jones and Bartlett Learning.

Gilligan C: *In a different voice: psychological theory and women's development*, Cambridge, MA, 1982, Harvard University.

Gostin LO, Bayer R, Fairchild AL: Ethical and legal challenges posed by severe acute respiratory syndrome: implications for the control of severe infectious disease threats, *JAMA* 290(24):3229–3237, 2003.

Grodin MA, Miller EL, Keely JI: The Nazi physicians as leaders in eugenics and "euthanasia": Lessons for today, *Am Journal of Public Health* 108(1):53-57, 2018.

Hamric AB: A case study of moral distress, *Journal of Hospice and Palliative Nursing* 16(8):457–463, 2014.

Hamric AB, Blackhall J: Nurse-physician perspectives on the care of dying patients in intensive care units: collaboration, moral distress, and ethical climate, *Critical Care Medicine* 35(2):422–429, 2007.

Hastings Center: *Our Mission, 2019*. Retrieved from http://www.the-hastingscenter.org/who-we-are/our-mission/.

International Council of Nurses: *ICN code of ethics for nurses*, Geneva, 2012, ICN.

Jonsen A: *The birth of bioethics*, New York, NY, 1998, Oxford.

Leininger M: *Care: the essence of nursing and health*, Thorofare, NJ, 1984, Slack.

Lomis KD, Carpenter RO, Miller BM: Moral distress in the third year of medical school; a descriptive review of student case reflections, *American Journal of Surgery* 197(1):107–112, 2009.

Maguire BJ, Shearer K, McKeown J, Phelps S, Gerard DR, Handal KA, Maniscalco P, O'Neill BJ: The ethics of PPE and EMS in he COVID-10 Era, *Journal of Emergency Medical Services* April 10, 2020, www.jems.com, accessed April 14, 202

Munson R: *Intervention and reflection: basic issues in medical ethics*, ed 8, Belmont CA, 2014, Thomson Wadsworth.

Noddings N: *Caring: a feminine approach to ethics and moral education*, Berkeley CA, 1984, Berkeley CA, University of California Press.

Olick RS: From the column editor: ethics in public health, *Journal of Public Health Management Practice* 11:258–259, 2005.

Park EJ: The development and implications of a case-based computer program to train ethical decision-making, *Nurs Ethics 20: 943-956, 2013*.

Pearce K: In fight against COVID-19, nurses face high-stakes decisions, moral distress. Discussed by nursing ethics expert Cynda Rushton, www.hub.jhu.edu, Posted April 6, 2020; accessed April 8, 2020.

Public Health Leadership Society: *Public Health Code of Ethics*, Washington DC, 2002, American Public Health Association.

Purtilo R, Doherty RF: *Ethical dimensions in the health professions*, ed 6, St. Louis MO, 2016, Elsevier.

Racher FE: The evolution of ethics for community practice, *J Community Health Nursing* 24:65–76, 2007.

Rawls J, Kelly E, editors: *Justice as fairness: A restatement*, Cambridge MA, 2001, Harvard University Press.

Reich WT: *Encyclopedia of bioethics*, New York, 1995, Macmillan.

Rogers WA: Feminism and public health ethics, *J Med Ethics* 32: 351–354, 2006.

Ruger JP: Ethics in American health 2: an ethical framework for health system reform, *Am J of Public Health* 98:1756–1763, 2008.

Shannon SE: The nurse as the patient's advocate: A contrarian view. In Ulrich CM, Grady C, Hamric AB, Berlinger N, editors: *Nurses at the table: nursing, ethics, and health policy*, New York, 2016, Hastings Center, pp S43–S47.

Silva MC: Ethical issues in health care, public policy, and politics. In Mason D, Leavitt J, Chaffee M, editors: *Policy and politics in nursing and health care*, ed 4, Philadelphia, 2002, Saunders.

Steinbock B, Arras JD, London AJ: *Ethical issues in modern medicine*, ed 7, New York, 2008, McGraw-Hill.

Ulrich C, O'Donnell P, Taylor C, Farrar A, David M, Grady: Ethical climate, ethical stress, and the job satisfaction of nurses and social workers in the United States, *Soc Sci Med* 65:1708-1719, 2007.

Ulrich CM, Hamric A, Grady C: Moral distress: a growing problem in the health professions? *Hastings Center Report* 40(1):20–22, 2010.

Ulrich CM, Taylor C, Soeken K, O'Donnell P, Farrar A, Danis M, Grady C: Everyday ethics: ethical issues and stress in nursing practice, *J of Advanced Nursing* 66(11):2510–2519, 2010.

US Department of Health and Human Services: *Healthy People 2020: a roadmap to improve America's health*, Washington, DC, 2010, US Government Printing Office.

US Department of Health and Human Services: *Healthy People 2030*, Washington DC, 2020, US Government Printing Office.

Volbrecht RM: *Nursing ethics: communities in dialogue*, Upper Saddle River, NJ, 2002, Prentice Hall.

Walker T: What principlism misses, *J of Medical Ethics* 35:229–231, 2009.

Watson J: *Nursing: human science and human care—a theory of nursing*, Burlington, MA, 2007, Jones and Bartlett.

Webster L, Wocial LD: Ethics in a pandemic, *American Nurse Jl*, 15(9):18-23, 2020.

World Health Organization: *Constitution of the World Health Organization, in Basic Documents,* ed. 48, 2014, www.who.int. Accessed April 14, 2020.

7

Culture of Populations in Communities

Cynthia E. Degazon and Bobbie J. Perdue

OBJECTIVES

After reading this chapter, the student should be able to:

1. Discuss ways in which culture can affect nursing practice.
2. Describe methods of developing cultural competence to meet the health needs of culturally diverse individuals, communities, and organizations.
3. Describe major facilitators and barriers to providing culturally competent care for diverse populations.
4. Conduct a cultural assessment of a person from a cultural group other than yours.
5. Develop culturally competent nursing interventions to promote positive health outcomes for clients.
6. Discuss the disparity in the number of minority groups who contracted COVID-19 compared to the majority population.

CHAPTER OUTLINE

KEY TERMS

Nurses have cared for culturally diverse groups since the beginning of this discipline. As early as 1893, nurses in New York City started public health nursing under the leadership of Lillian Wald and provided home care to people who lived in the inner city, particularly immigrants who recently arrived (Anderson and McFarlane, 2015). When nurses were not from the same cultural background as the immigrants, they had to deal with the cultural differences and the persons in their care. Often the same situation still exists; that is, the nurse and client come from different cultural groups and may not recognize or understand their differences.

These first migrants were largely English-speaking White Protestants who thought of themselves as founders and settlers in a new country rather than as immigrants. The first Blacks to arrive in America were free men who brought their own slaves with them. Another early group of people who came to America were Africans brought on slave ships. These Africans were instrumental in developing much of early America with their skills, including farming. They also brought their unique culture with them, and much of that culture has lasted.

Between 1860 and 1910, immigrants to the United States accounted for between 13% and 15% of the overall population largely due to high levels of immigration from Europe. The implementation of restrictive immigration laws between 1921 and 1924 coupled with the Great Depression and World War II led to a sharp drop in immigration in the United States (Batalova, Blizzard, and Bolter, 2020). At present, there is considerable discussion and controversy regarding immigration to the United States. The immigrant population is growing more slowly than in recent years. Also, the makeup of the foreign-born population is changing. Individuals who have immigrated to the United States from Mexico have declined, and in 2018, Canada surpassed the United States as the world's top country for resettling refugees (Batalova, Blizzard, and Bolter, 2020). A more extensive discussion on immigrants can be found later in the chapter.

WHY CULTURAL COMPETENCE MATTERS

Cultural competence is one of the core competences in public health nursing (Quad Council Coalition of Public Health Nursing Organizations, 2018). Likewise, the American Nurses Association, *Scope and Standards of Practice*, 3rd edition (ANA, 2015a) and the *Code of Ethics for Nurses with Interpretive Statements* (ANA, 2015b) specifically address the mandate that nurses treat all patients with respect and with equity. The 4th edition of the ANA *Scope and Standards of Practice* released in 2021 includes content related to respect, equity, inclusion, and social justice. In *The Future of Nursing 2020-2030: Charting a Path to Achieve Health Equity*, released May 2021 by the National Academy of Medicine, considerable attention is given to addressing the social determinants of health and achieving health equity. These standards and recommendations imply that nurses understand cultural competence and try to learn much of the culture from which their clients come as they can. Also, both accreditation agencies for nursing education

programs: the Accreditation Commission for Education in Nursing (ACEN) and the Commission on Collegiate Nursing Education (CCNE), as well as the Joint Commission for the Accreditation of Healthcare Organizations, address the need for cultural competence through their standards and guidelines. Cultural competence entails a combination of culturally congruent behaviors, practice attitudes, and policies that allow nurses to use interpersonal communication, relationship skills, and behavioral flexibility to work effectively in cross-cultural situations (Campinha-Bacote, 2011). In a discussion on the need for cultural competence in home health care, Narayan says "Patients in need of culturally competent care include those characterized by diversity related to race, ethnicity, language, religion, socioeconomic status, sexual orientation, gender identification, mental and physical disabilities, and stigmatized diagnoses (e.g., obesity and substance abuse)" (2020, p. 76).

Cultural competence is an ongoing life process that includes acknowledging the fundamental differences in the ways clients and families respond to illness and treatment, from which might be your response or a more typical Western health care response. It is important for nurses to continuously engage in critical reflection to examine their own values, beliefs, and cultural heritage in order to increase their awareness of how these qualities can influence their care (Douglas et al., 2014). This can include paying attention to dietary practices, pain, death and dying, modesty, eye contact, closeness, and touch.

Ten guidelines, formerly called standards, have been developed by a collaborative task force of members of the American Academy of Nursing (AAN) Expert Panel on Global Nursing and Health and the Transcultural Nursing Society. These standards were developed to serve as a guide for providing culturally competent care. The authors of the standards say that due to the migration of both nurses and clients, it is important to have a set of universally applicable guidelines for providing culturally competent care. The recipient of the nursing care can be an individual, a family, a community, or a population. The standards are based on the principles of social justice and human rights. The 10 standards are (1) knowledge of cultures, (2) education and training in culturally competent care, (3) critical reflection, (4) cross-cultural communication, (5) culturally competent practice, (6) cultural competence in health care systems and organizations, (7) patient advocacy and empowerment, (8) multicultural workforce, (9) cross-cultural leadership, and (10) evidence-based practice and research (Douglas et al., 2014). These guidelines are important because both health care professionals and organizations are responsible for providing the infrastructure needed to deliver safe, culturally congruent, and compassionate care (Douglas et al., 2014).

Purnell (2019, p. 98) developed the Purnell Theory and Model for Culturally Competent Health Care. He developed 11 major assumptions on which he based the model. They are paraphrased, combined and summarized below:

- All health care professions need similar information about cultural diversity, and they share concepts related to global society, family, person and health (1 to 2).

- No culture is better than any others, they are just different, and there are core similarities among cultures with differences within, between, and among cultures, and cultures change slowly (3 to 6).
- The variant cultural characteristics determine the degree to which one varies from the dominant culture, and individuals and families belong to several subcultures (7, 10).
- Persons who participate in their choice of health-related goals, plans and interventions are more likely to comply (8) and culture has a major influence on a person's understanding and response to health care (9).
- Each person has the right to be respected for his or her uniqueness and cultural heritage (11).

CULTURE, RACE, AND ETHNICITY

The concepts of culture, race, and ethnicity influence our understanding of human behavior. These three terms are often used incorrectly. Nurses need to understand the meaning of each when providing culturally competent health care to clients of diverse cultures.

Culture is a set of beliefs, values, and assumptions about life that is widely held among a group of people and that is transmitted across generations (Leininger, 2002a). Culture is an individual concept, a group phenomenon, and an organizational reality. It takes many years for individuals to become familiar enough with a new value and for it to become part of their culture. In response to the needs of its members and their environment, culture provides tested solutions to life's problems.

Culture is transmitted across generations during the processes of learning language and becoming socialized, usually as children. There are three ways in which culture is transferred: (1) vertical transmission, where parents are the primary sources; (2) horizontal, when people within the same generation pass on information; and (3) oblique, between generations of people who are not related, such as religious, social, and educational institutions, and among peers. Parents and family, the most important sources for the transfer of traditions, teach both explicit and implicit behaviors of the culture. The explicit behaviors, such as language, interpersonal distance, and kissing in public, can be observed and allow the individual to identify with other persons of the culture. In this way, people share traditions, customs, and lifestyles with others. The implicit behaviors are less visible and include the way individuals perceive health and illness, body language, difference in language expressions, and the use of titles. These behaviors are subtle and may be difficult for persons to describe, yet they are a part of the culture. For example, deferring to older adults, standing when they enter the room, or offering them a seat suggests a cultural value related to older adults.

Another example of an implicit aspect of culture is the use of language to communicate. For instance, in one culture a sign might read "No smoking is permitted." In another culture the sign might read "Thank you for not smoking." The former statement represents a culture that values directness, whereas the latter values indirectness. Each culture has an organizational

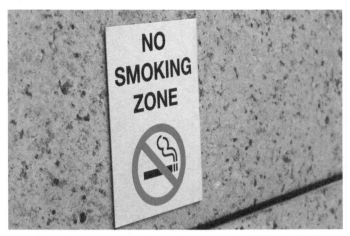

Fig. 7.1 This Sign Is from a Culture that Values Directness in Communication. (© 2012 Photos.com, a division of Getty Images. All rights reserved. Image #122153579.)

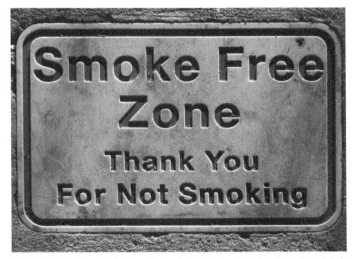

Fig. 7.2 This Sign Is from a Culture that Values an Indirect Approach to Communication. (© 2012 Photos.com, a division of Getty Images. All rights reserved. Image #91883504.)

structure that distinguishes it from others and provides the structure for what members of the cultural group determine to be appropriate or inappropriate behavior (Figs. 7.1 and 7.2).

All cultures are not alike and all individuals within a culture differ. Within a culture, people may speak different dialects, have different religions and religious practices, divergent ages, and different socioeconomic and educational status. Also, in many countries, people who live there may be native to that country or may have immigrated there. If an immigrant, the person may continue to adhere to customs, language, and religion from the native country. Each person should be viewed as a unique human being with differences that are respected.

Race is a biological variation within population groups based on physical markers derived from genetic ancestry such as skin color, physical features, and hair texture. Individuals may be of the same race but of different cultures. For example, African Americans, who may have been born in or trace their heritage to Africa, the Caribbean, North America, or elsewhere,

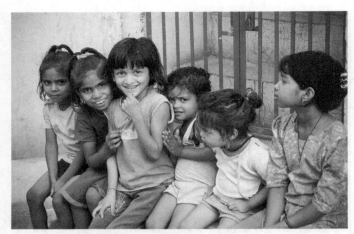

Fig. 7.3 In Countries Around the World, There are Distinct Differences in People Who Represent the Same Cultural Group. (Copyright © 2013 Thinkstock. All rights reserved. Image # 117003112).

are a heterogeneous group, and they should not be viewed as culturally and racially homogeneous. This perception can cause providers to be unaware of cultural differences among individuals who come from different countries but who share similar racial characteristics. This often blurs an understanding of this culturally diverse group.

It is important to understand the growing numbers of interracial families. Before 1989, biracial babies who had one White parent were assigned the race of the non-White parent. Currently the US Census Bureau allows people to choose more than one race (Fig. 7.3).

Ethnicity is the shared feeling of peoplehood among a group of individuals and relates to cultural factors such as nationality, geographical region, culture, ancestry, language, beliefs, and traditions (Giger, 2017). It reflects cultural membership and is based on individuals sharing similar cultural patterns (e.g., beliefs, values, customs, behaviors, traditions) that over time, create a common history that is resistant to change. Ethnicity represents the identifying characteristics of culture (e.g., race, religion, national origin) and is influenced by education, income level, geographical location, and association with people from other ethnic groups. Therefore, a reciprocal relationship exists between the individual and society. Members of an ethnic group give up aspects of their identity and society when they adopt characteristics of the group's identity. However, when the ethnic identity is strong, the group maintains its values, beliefs, behaviors, practices, and ways of thinking.

CULTURAL DIVERSITY

Cultural diversity refers to the degree of variation that is represented among populations based on lifestyle, ethnicity, race, across place of origin and across time. It also includes the social class, gender identity, sexual orientation, and physical abilities/disabilities as well as the changing populations of the world. Although all cultures are not the same, all cultures have the same basic organizing factors (Giger, 2017).

These factors should be explored in a cultural assessment because of the potential for differences among groups. See the Levels of Prevention box for preventions related to cultural differences. Cultural diversity also includes the awareness of the presence of differences among the members of a social group or unit (Darnell and Hickson, 2015). As of July 1, 2019, 60.4% of the population considered themselves to be White alone, not Hispanic or Latino; 13.4% were Black or African American, 1.3% were American Indian and Alaska Native; 5.9% Asian alone; 0.2% were Native Hawaiian and other Pacific Islanders alone (Quick Facts, 2019, United States Census Bureau).

Communication

Effective cross-cultural communication is a core competency for public health professionals and is the fourth domain of the Community/Public Health Nursing (C/PHN) Competencies of the Quad Council Coalition of Public Health Nursing Organizations (2018). Competent communication with the client or family is required for a cultural assessment. It is important to understand variations in patterns of verbal communication and nonverbal communication and to use words that a layperson can understand. Verbal communication entails words used to express ideas and feelings; cultural variations are found, for example, in pronunciation, word meaning, voice quality, use of humor, and speed of talking. For example, many people from the United States and the United Kingdom have English as their first language. However, the word *boot* has different meanings for them. In the United States "a boot" typically refers to something one puts on one's feet; in the United Kingdom the "boot" may refer to what Americans call the trunk of the car. Just as understanding verbal communication is important, so is the understanding of nonverbal communication. Nonverbal communication is the use of body language or gestures to convey a message. Aspects of nonverbal language include eye contact, gestures, body posture, facial expressions, touch, and silence. In some cultures, people might say yes or remain silent when you give an instruction and you interpret that to mean assent. In reality, the person may actually not intend to follow through with the plan of care you just discussed but did not want to appear rude by disagreeing with you. Other areas to consider are how close people in different cultures are comfortable standing when talking with someone, the use of their hands in conversation, or how comfortable the person is with being touched.

An example of misunderstood nonverbal communication occurred when a nurse gave instructions to Asian American clients about taking antituberculin drugs. The clients smilingly responded with "yes, yes." The nurse interpreted this response to mean that the clients understood the instructions and accepted the treatment protocol. A week later, when the clients returned for a follow-up visit, the nurse discovered that the medications had not been taken. The nurse understood that acceptance by and avoidance of confrontation or disagreement with those in authority are important behaviors in the Asian American culture; interventions were therefore adjusted accordingly. The nurse

Related to Cultural Differences (Hypertension, Stroke, and Heart Disease)

Primary Prevention
Provide health teaching about a balanced diet and exercise.

Secondary Prevention
Teach clients and/or family to monitor blood pressure. Teach about diet, keeping in mind the client's cultural preferences. Talk about health beliefs and cultural implications, such as the use of alternative therapies; make sure alternative therapies are compatible with any medications that may be prescribed.

Tertiary Prevention
If blood pressure cannot be controlled by diet, refer the client to a physician or nurse practitioner for medication; advise the client to engage in a cardiac program that will oversee diet and exercise.

repeated the medication instructions and gave the clients an opportunity to raise questions and concerns, and to repeat the instructions that were given. The nurse also discussed the cultural meaning and treatment of tuberculosis. It is important to respect all information that a client shares with you, even when the information is in conflict with your own value system.

Space

Personal space is the physical area individuals need between themselves and others to feel comfortable. When this space is violated, the client may become uncomfortable. Nurses should take cues from clients to place themselves in the appropriate spatial zone and avoid misinterpretation of clients' behavior as they handle their spatial needs. Most cultural groups have spatial preferences. Some groups typically stand close to one another. However, one community may be comfortable with only a 9-inch distance between faces, whereas another group might find that small distance threatening and overly aggressive. It is important to understand the space preferences of the groups with whom you work because you may offend the client by placing yourself at a distance when his or her culture values close proximity to those with whom they speak and vice versa. The issue of space was emphasized during the COVID-19 pandemic when people were urged to practice social distancing and stand at least 6 feet away when around another person.

Social Organization

Social organization refers to the way in which a cultural group structures itself around the family to carry out role functions. In some cultures, family may include people who are not actually related to one another. Find out who is considered to be in the family, who the key decision makers are, and if the needs of the family supersede those of an individual in the family. Nurses should be aware that some Hispanic and Asian cultures place the needs of the family above those of the individual. In the American Indian/Alaskan Native family, members honor and respect their elders. Nurses should advocate for the individual, so that when families make decisions, the individual's needs are also considered. However, members of the family may need to be included in the decision making.

Time Perception

Regarding time, cultures are considered to be future, past, or present oriented. Historically, the American middle-class culture has tended to be future oriented, and individuals were willing to delay immediate gratification until future goals are accomplished. This has begun to change, with some people choosing a more present orientation. In contrast, some cultures may place greater value on quality of life and view present time as being more important than future time. The future is unknown, but the present is known. When nurses discuss health promotion and disease prevention strategies with persons from a present orientation, they should focus on the immediate benefits these clients would gain rather than emphasizing future outcomes.

In cultures that focus on a past orientation (e.g., the Vietnamese culture), individuals may focus on wishes and memories of their ancestors and look to them to provide direction for current situations (Giger, 2017). In a past-oriented culture, time is viewed as being more flexible than in a present-oriented culture. Nurses socialized in the Western culture may view time as money and equate punctuality with goodness and being responsible. Working with clients who have a different perception of time than the nurse can be problematic. Nurses should clarify the clients' perceptions to avoid misunderstanding. It is not realistic to expect clients to change their behavior and adopt the nurse's schedule.

Environmental Control

Environmental control refers to the relationships between humans and nature. Cultural groups might perceive humans as having mastery over nature, being dominated by nature, or having a harmonious relationship with nature. Those who view nature as dominant (e.g., African Americans and Hispanics or Latinos) believe they have little or no control over what happens to them. They may not adhere to a cancer treatment protocol because of the belief that nothing will change the outcome because it is their destiny. These individuals are less likely to engage in illness prevention activities than those who have other worldviews.

Persons who view a human harmony with nature (e.g., African Americans, Asian Americans, and Native Americans/Alaskan Natives) may perceive that illness such as cancer is disharmony with other forces and that medicine can relieve the symptoms but cannot cure the disease. They would seek treatment for the malignancy from the mind, body, and spirit connection because they believe that healing comes from within. These groups are likely to look to naturalistic solutions, such as herbs, acupuncture, and hot and cold treatments, to resolve or cure a cancerous condition. Some clients may view their illness as punishment for misdeeds and may have difficulty accepting care from nurses who do not share their belief. Individuals from cultures that view the environment as being dominant over nature may believe that they have little or no control over a serious illness for which they have been diagnosed. These individuals are less likely to engage in illness management interventions that are harsh and that they cannot trust to lead to a positive health outcome.

Biological Variations

Biological variations are the physical, biological, and physiological differences that distinguish one racial group from another. They occur in areas of growth and development, skin color, enzymatic differences, and susceptibility to disease (Andrews and Boyle, 2016; Giger, 2017). Other common and obvious variations include eye shape, hair texture, adipose tissue deposits, shape of earlobes, thickness of lips, and body configuration. There are also genetic differences that differentially affect some groups. Lactose intolerance is much more common in African Blacks and African Americans than in the general population. Also, Western-born neonates are slightly heavier at birth than those born in non-Western cultures. Mongolian spots are bluish discolorations that are sometimes present on the skin of African American, Asian American, Hispanic or Latino, and Native American/Alaskan Native babies. These discolorations may be mistaken for bruises. When nurses are exposed to situations involving biological variations of which they are unfamiliar, they may create embarrassing situations. Consider the following scenario: The school nurse observes a bluish discoloration on the thigh of a child with brown skin, which she mistook for a bruise. The nurse reported her observation to the child protective agency in her state. When the child's mother arrived to pick her child up at the end of the school day, she was accused of child abuse. The mother had to disprove the allegation before her child could be released into her care.

Nutrition

Nutritional practices are an integral part of the assessment process for all families, especially because they play a prominent role in the health problems of some groups. For many cultures, the preparation and eating of food are social activities, and members of the group come together to celebrate life events and family rituals with food as a focus of the event. Efforts to understand dietary patterns of clients should go beyond relying on membership in a defined group. Knowing clients' nutrition practices makes it possible to develop treatment regimens that will not conflict with their cultural food practices. Box 7.1

BOX 7.1   Assessment of Dietary Practices and Food Consumption Patterns

- What is the social significance of food in the family?
- What foods are most often bought for family consumption?
- What foods are prohibited for the family?
- Does religion play a significant role in food selection?
- Who prepared the food? How is it prepared?
- How much food is eaten? When is it eaten? With whom?
- What kind of restaurants does the family frequent?
- Has the family adopted foods of other cultures?
- What are the family's favorite recipes?

identifies several questions that nurses should ask when conducting a nutritional assessment. In working with clients of different cultures, the nurse might need to consult culturally oriented magazines. For example, some popular magazines such as *Essence, Ebony,* and *Latina* have altered old family recipes using healthier ingredients. These dishes taste good and allow those who use them to continue their old traditions related to food. As another example, many people who subscribe to the Buddhist religion are vegetarian. Their faith teaches self-control as a means to search for happiness. The Buddhist code of morality is in their Five Moral Precepts, and eating meat would conflict with both the first and the fifth (i.e., meat is seen as an intoxicant). These precepts are as follows: harming living things, stealing, engaging in sexual misconduct, lying, or consuming intoxicants, such as alcohol, tobacco, or mind-altering drugs (ElGindy, 2013). Also, Muslims avoid pork and foods cooked with alcohol.

SOCIAL DETERMINANTS OF HEALTH

Social determinants of health are the circumstances in which all people are born, grow, live, work, and age that shape health (Artiga and Hinton, 2018). Social determinants can disproportionally affect ethnically or culturally diverse groups; these determinants are shaped by money, power, education, and other resources. Specifically, according to *Healthy People 2030,* the five areas of social determinants are (1) economic instability, (2) education, (3) social environment, (4) health and health care, and (5) physical environment. Each of these five areas is complex and important in how it affects the health of individuals, families, and communities (USDHHS, 2020).

According to Narayan, "Patients in need of culturally competent care include those characterized by diversity related to race, ethnicity, language, religion, socioeconomic status, sexual orientation, gender identification, mental and physical disabilities, and stigmatized diagnoses (e.g. obesity and substance abuse)" (2019, p. 76.) In addition, COVID-19 often led to a higher propensity for death in African Americans (Strickland et al., 2020) and other minority groups (*Los Angeles Times,* 2020).

A danger also exists in believing that certain cultural behaviors, such as folk practices, are restricted to lower socioeconomic classes. For example, health professionals, such as nurses and physicians, may also use folk systems and complementary and alternative therapies in conjunction with the biomedical system to promote their health and prevent disease. Therefore nurses must conduct a cultural assessment for all individuals when they first come in contact with them. Nurses should be able to distinguish between issues of culture and socioeconomic class and not misinterpret behavior as having a cultural origin when in fact, it should be attributed to the socioeconomic class. It is essential that nurses recognize their own biases as well as try to understand the biases of their clients.

IMMIGRANT ISSUES

As of 2018 there were 44.7 million immigrants living in the United States. This means that 1 in 7 US residents is foreign born. The foreign-born population saw a less than 0.5% growth between 2017 and 2018, which is the lowest annual increase since 2010 (Batalova, Blizzard, and Bolter, 2020). In 2018, Mexicans made up 25% of immigrants to the United States, followed by Indians, Chinese, Filipinos (each about 5%). The remainder of the top ten sources of immigrants were El Salvador, Vietnam, Cuba, and the Dominican Republic (each 3%), and Korea and Guatemala (each 2%).

Immigration has become increasingly controversial in recent years, with increased ambivalence among people in the United States about immigrants and the laws and policies pertaining to them. Since the events of September 11, 2001, and particularly since the inauguration of President Trump in 2017, the national debate about immigration policy has intensified and many laws enacted reflect more difficulty for people seeking visas and more scrutiny of both visa and entry documents (Zong, Batalova, and Hallock, 2018). The complex issues involved with the foreign-born population and health care accessibility restrict the opportunity for public health nurses to provide culturally competent care to this population. These policies may change over time and be less restrictive to foreign-born people and more culturally inclusive.

The median age of the US immigrant population in 2018 was 45.2 years. In contrast the native-born population has a median age of 36.3 years. Note that many children of immigrants are born in the United States, which contributes to the younger age of native-born people (Batalova, Blizzard, and Bolter, 2020).

Place of origin for the immigrant is distinguished from nationality, which refers to the place where the individual has or had citizenship. Foreign-born refers to all residents who were not US citizens at birth, regardless of their current legal or citizen status, or those whose parents were not US citizens. They carry the nationality of their home country.

In 2018 approximately 78% of the US population ages 5 and older regardless of nativity reported speaking English only at home. Spanish is the most common language spoken after English, followed by Chinese (Mandarin and Cantonese), Tagalog and Vietnamese, Arabic, French (including Cajun), and Korean (Batalova, Blizzard, and Bolter, 2020). In 2018, approximately 47% of immigrants ages 5 and older were Limited English Proficient (LEP). At the same time, 32% ages 25 or older had a bachelor's or higher degree, and 80% of Indian immigrant adults had a bachelor's or higher degree. In terms of having a bachelor's degree, "other top countries are: United Arab Emirates (74%), Taiwan (73%); Singapore (70%), and Saudi Arabia (69%)" (Batalova, Blizzard, and Bolter, 2020, p. 9). States with the largest number of immigrants are, in order: California, Texas, Florida, New York, and New Jersey.

In 2018, of the 27.2 million foreign-born workers 16 and older in the United States, over 33% worked in management, professional, and related occupations, including business, science and the arts; 23% in service; 16% in transportation; 15% in sales; and 13% in natural resources, construction, and maintenance. During this year 15% of the immigrants had incomes below the official poverty line compared to 13% of the US-born population (Batalova, Blizzard, and Bolter, 2020).

Approximately one-third of immigrants are insured. Noncitizens are more likely to be uninsured than citizens. "Noncitizens, including lawfully present and undocumented immigrants, were significantly more likely to be uninsured than citizens. Among the nonelderly population, 23% of lawfully present immigrants and more than four in ten (45%) undocumented immigrants were uninsured compared to less than one in ten (9%) citizens" (Artiga, Garfied, and Damico, 2020). Citizen children, including those with at least one noncitizen parent, were significantly more likely to be uninsured compared to children with citizen parents. Immigrants to the United States often bring with them unique cultural, health care, and religious practices that must be respected (Fig. 7.4). A more detailed description of the immigrant populations and what benefits they are eligible to receive can be found at migrationpolicy.org. See "Health Coverage of Immigrants" by the Kaiser Family Foundation, March 18, 2020, for a comprehensive description of what health care benefits are available to specific types of immigrants.

The fear of immigration reinforcement often prevents many immigrants from seeking health care in a timely manner, contributing to poor health outcomes when they do seek health care services. Other factors like living in low-income and segregated neighborhoods (ethnic enclaves) and working in low-wage occupations with exposure to toxic chemicals, poor or other unsafe working situations contribute to poor health outcomes when immigrants seek health care services (United States Department of Health and Human Services, 2018).

? CHECK YOUR PRACTICE

Jorge and his mother, Cecelia, immigrated from El Salvador to the United States seeking refugee status. Before their case could be adjudicated, Cecelia was deported back to El Salvador. Cecelia left Jorge with her sister, Maria, who lives in a small rural town in Texas. As Maria was about to enroll the 5-year-old Jorge in kindergarten, she discovered that she had no record of his immunizations. Maria met with the school's secretary regarding the immunization issue who in turn consulted with the school health nurse as to the appropriate action to be taken.

What is the school health nurse's role in helping to initiate the child's immunization program? What action(s) should the school nurse recommend to the secretary?

Using the clinical judgment and essential cognitive skills developed by the National Council of States Boards of Nursing, how should the school nurse use the six essential skills of: recognize cues; analyze cues; prioritize hypotheses; generate solutions; take action; and evaluate outcomes? What could potentially be the outcome of her nursing care if she omits some of these steps?

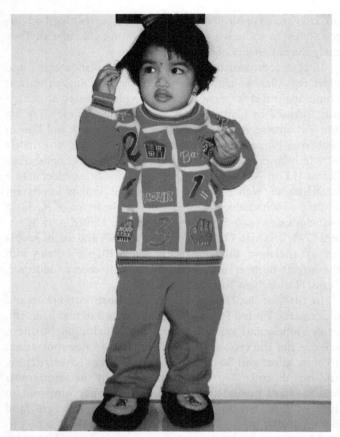

Fig. 7.4 A Child from Nepal Living in the United States. The child has a black dot on her forehead to protect her from the "evil eye."

Types of Foreign-Born

There are four categories of foreign-born. The first category is documented immigrants, also known as lawful permanent residents. In 2016, 49% of this group was naturalized and had become US citizens (Zong, Batalova, and Hallock, 2018). Documented immigrants are not citizens but are legally allowed to live and work in the United States, usually because they fulfill labor demands or have family ties. These individuals usually have a 5-year waiting period living in the United States after receiving "qualified" immigration status before they are eligible to receive entitlements such as Medicaid and Children's Health Insurance Program (CHIP).

The second category of foreign-born consists of refugees and persons seeking asylum. The Refugee Act of 1980 provided a uniform procedure for refugees (based on the United Nations definition) to be admitted to the United States (United States Department of Health and Human Services, 2012). The United States based on international law defines "refugee" as a "person outside the country of his or her nationality who is unable or unwilling to return to that country because of persecution or a well-founded fear of persecution based on his or her race, religion, nationality, membership in a particular social group, or political opinion" (Immigration Forum, January 25, 2019). The president sets the quota for refugees. There were 30,000

admitted in 2019. Refugees are referred primarily by the United Nations High Commissioner for Refugees (Immigration Forum, January 25, 2019). This group of immigrants experience a host of difficulties, and this is particularly true for the younger children, who are at risk for long-term physical, mental, and emotional challenges. Refugees are immediately eligible to receive benefits described for legal immigrants, such as Temporary Assistance for Needy Families, Supplemental Security Income, and Medicaid. The Centers for Disease Control and Prevention (CDC) provides "Refugee's Health Guidelines" designed to promote and improve the health of the refugee, prevent disease, and familiarize refugees with the US health system (Centers for Disease Control, 2016). See also "Guidelines for the US Domestic Medical Examination for Newly Arriving Refugees" which is a screening guideline for state public health departments and health care providers in the United States (CDC, 2020).

The third category of foreign-born is the non-immigrants; these are people admitted to the United States for a limited duration and for a specified purpose. They have a permanent residence outside the United States and include students, tourists, temporary workers, business executives, career diplomats, their spouses and children, artists, entertainers, reporters, and those wishing to receive medical treatment. The fourth category of foreign-born is the undocumented immigrants, or undocumented or illegal aliens. These persons may have crossed a border into the United States illegally, or their legal permission to stay in the United States may have expired. They account for about 11% of the immigrant population. They are mainly from Mexico and Central America (71%), mostly men (54%) between 25 and 44 years of age (53%), homeowners (approximately 33%), majority employed (64%) but uninsured (61%), and slightly more than 50% of them live below the poverty level (Gelatt and Zong, 2018; Migration Policy Institute, 2018). Undocumented immigrants are eligible to receive emergency medical services, immunizations, treatment for the symptoms of communicable diseases, and access to school lunches. They are not eligible to enroll in Medicaid, the CHIP, or the Affordable Care Act (Obamacare), or purchase coverage through the health insurance marketplace. This significantly reduces opportunities to have affordable health insurance and quality health care services (Artiga, Damico, and Young et al., 2016).

Several misperceptions exist about the economic value of allowing immigrants to enter or to stay in the United States. Immigrants who are authorized to work in the United States pay federal, state, and local taxes. Undocumented immigrants also pay taxes but are not entitled to benefits like Medicare and social security. Both documented and undocumented immigrants contribute a large amount of money to the gross domestic product due to their presence in the labor force and the taxes they pay. The dilemma for communities, however, is that immigrants typically pay federal taxes, yet the services they receive are paid for by the states and localities and they are not entitled to tax credits. Even though noncitizens are as likely as citizens to work, they may be in jobs that do not provide health coverage for employees.

In addition to financial constraints on providing health care for immigrants, they often come to the United States with diverse health risks combined with language barriers; social, religious, and cultural backgrounds different from those of their health care providers. The use of traditional healing or complementary health care practices may be unfamiliar to United States health care providers who may lack knowledge about high-risk diseases specific to particular immigrant groups for whom they care. For example, some groups are more at risk for hepatitis B (with its attendant effects on the liver), tuberculosis, intestinal parasites, and visual, hearing, and dental problems. Many of these conditions are either preventable or treatable if managed correctly. Nurses should know the major health problems and risk factors that are specific to the immigrant populations for whom they provide care and to treat them in the context of the culture from which they come.

Often children and adolescents adjust to the new culture more easily than adults. This can lead to a shift in the balance of power between adults and children, contributing to family conflict and at times violence. Inability of elders to acculturate may play a large part in their lack of adherence to health care guidelines. Nurses should be alert for warning signs of family stress and tension, remembering that older family members can help translate their culture, beliefs, religious practices, dietary habits, support systems, and risk factors for the health care provider. They can also assist with decision making and provide support to enable the individual or group seeking care to change behaviors and increase their health promotion practices.

Similarly, understanding the role of the community in the care of immigrants is important. Communities can help clients (and thus providers) with communication, crisis intervention, housing, and emotional and other forms of support. Nurses carefully assess the community and learn what strengths, resources, and talents are available; this includes the traditional practices immigrants use. Many of these practices have therapeutic value and can be blended with traditional Western medicine (Fig. 7.5). The key is to know what practices are being used so the blending can be done knowledgeably. Community members are excellent sources of this information, and nurses working with immigrant populations should use the community assessment, group work, and family techniques described in other chapters to partner with immigrant clients.

The following skills are necessary for the nurse to increase authenticity, accuracy, and approachability when working with immigrant populations:

1. Self-awareness: Recognize the values, beliefs, and practices that comprise your own culture. Nurses, like clients, are influenced by their culture, values, and language.
2. Identify the client's preferred or native language. When nurses do not speak or understand the client's language, they must obtain assistance from an interpreter to ensure that full and effective communication occurs. Health care institutions must provide clients with an interpreter. The interpreter should have knowledge of the client's culture and medical terminology. Interpreters should be trained, qualified, and hired to ensure that they have met minimum standards to provide accurate and safe interpretation. Using family members, friends, and staff who

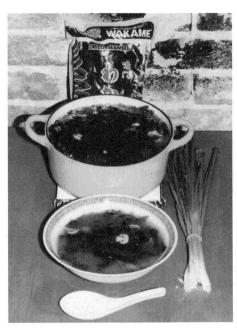

Fig. 7.5 Mi-Yuk Kook (Seaweed Soup) is a Korean Dish Eaten by Postpartum Women to Stop Bleeding and to Cleanse Body Fluids. It is also eaten every birthday.

are not trained as health/medical interpreters can create errors in understanding and communicating, posing grave risks for the client and liability to the health care institution.

While both an interpreter and a translator interpret and translate information from one language to another, there are significant differences between the two. A translator is usually associated with translating written documents such as medical records and legal documents; in contrast, the interpreter is associated with verbal communication that focuses on accurate expression of equivalent meanings rather than on word-to-word equivalence. Experiences of success that nurses report when working with an interpreter include proper use of interpreters to assure that clients understand health care instructions; provision of linguistically appropriate educational material; ability to communicate in the client's language to provide health care instructions; and ensuring proper use of instructions. Experiences of difficulty include language barriers preventing appropriate communications; lack of available interpreters overall and for specific languages; and lack of appropriate translation by interpreters. Nurses can minimize some of these difficulties by learning basic words and sentences of the most commonly spoken languages in the community and observing client reactions when asking them questions. Also, nurses should provide written material in the client's primary language, so that family members can reinforce information when at home with the client. The How To box provides guidelines for using an interpreter.

3. Learn the health-seeking behaviors of your immigrant client and their family members. In asking the client about family members, you might try using a simple genogram, which places family members on a diagram. Ask who the family members are, where they live, and who is missing or deceased.

You might also ask them to talk about holiday celebrations: who comes, who is missing, what do they do?

4. Get to know the community where the immigrant client lives. Read about the culture of your clients. Take a course. Volunteer to participate in the acculturation process of the community (e.g., to give talks, hold forums with free-flowing and two-way communication), and learn who the formal and informal resources are.

5. Get to know some of the traditional practices and remedies used by families and communities. Coordinate health education seminars with traditional healing courses for the community so you can work with, not against them.

6. Learn how cultural subgroups explain common illnesses or events. In cultures where the body and mind are seen as one entity or in cultures in which there is a high degree of stigma associated with mental illness, people or individuals somaticize their feelings of psychological distress. In somatization, psychological distress is experienced as a physical illness.

7. Try to see things from the viewpoint of the client, family, and community and accommodate rather than squash the client's view.

8. Conduct a cultural assessment focusing on what is working, what is not working, and changes that need to be made to accommodate cultural norms and promote positive health behaviors.

HOW TO GUIDELINES FOR SELECTING AND USING AN INTERPRETER

1. The educational level and the socioeconomic status of the interpreter are important. The nurse should know that the interpreter understands the community's interpretation of the disease and understand the community's health care practices around the disease.

2. The gender and/or age of the interpreter may be of concern; in some cultures, women may prefer a female interpreter, men may prefer a male interpreter, and older clients may want a more mature interpreter. Avoid using children as interpreters, particularly when the client is an adult.

   The nurse identifies the client's country of origin and language or dialect spoken before selecting the interpreter. For example, Chinese clients speak different dialects depending on the region in which they were born.

3. The nurse evaluates the interpreter's style, approach to clients, and ability to develop a relationship of trust and respect.

4. The interpreter interprets everything that is said by all the people in the interaction and informs the public health nurse if the content might be perceived as insensitive or harmful to the dignity of the client.

5. The interpreter conveys the content, the spirit of what is said, without omitting or adding.

6. The nurse makes phrase charts and picture cards available.

7. The nurse observes the client for nonverbal messages such as facial expressions, gestures, and other forms of body language. If the client's responses do not fit the question, the nurse should check to be sure that the interpreter understood the question.

8. Increase accuracy in transmission of information by asking the interpreter to translate the client's own words and ask the client to repeat the information that was communicated.

9. The interpreter must maintain confidentiality of all information and interactions.

10. At the end of the interview, the nurse reviews the material with the client and the interpreter to ensure that nothing has been missed or misunderstood.

DEVELOPING CULTURAL COMPETENCE

Many people are taught by and have knowledge of a dominant culture. As long as the person operates within that culture, responses occur without thought to a variety of situations and do not require examination of the cultural context. However, as multiculturalism grows, it becomes increasingly important for health care providers, including nurses and organizations, to provide quality and effective care. For example, consider the situation of a recent immigrant who speaks little English and goes to a community health center because of a urinary tract infection. The nurse understands that she must use strategies that will allow her to effectively communicate with the client; the client has the right to receive effective care, to judge whether she received the care she wanted, and to follow up with appropriate action if she did not receive the expected care. Culturally competent care is provided not only to individuals of racial or ethnic minority groups but also to individuals belonging to groups held together by factors such as age, religion, sexual orientation, and socioeconomic status. Nurses must be culturally competent to provide nursing care that meets the needs of these persons.

Cultural competence in nurses is a combination of culturally congruent behaviors, practice attitudes, and policies that allow nurses to work effectively in cross-cultural situations. The term *competence* refers to performance that is sufficient and adequate. Culturally competent nurses function effectively when caring for clients of other cultures. Culturally competent nurses learn about the cultures of the clients whom they serve and they respect people from other cultures and value diversity; this helps them provide more responsive care.

 HEALTHY PEOPLE 2030

Objectives Related to Cultural Issues

- **AHS-07:** Increase the proportion of persons with a usual primary-care provider.
- **HC/HIT-01:** Increase the proportion of adults whose health care provider checked their understanding
- **HC/HIT-011:** Increase the proportion of adults with limited English proficiency who say their providers explain things to them.

From US Department of Health and Human Services: *Healthy People 2030*, 2020. Available at http://health.gov/healthypeoples.

Nurses must be culturally competent for several key reasons, including the following:

- First, the nurse's culture often differs from that of the client, leading to different understandings of communication, behaviors, and plans for care.
- Second, care that is not culturally competent may increase the cost of health care and decrease the opportunity for positive client outcomes. Clients who do not feel understood may delay seeking care or may withhold key information. For example, if a person is afraid of disapproval, he may not tell the nurse that he is using both folk medicine and Western medicine. The two medicines may have cumulative or contradictory effects that could be dangerous to the client.

TABLE 7.1 The Cultural Competence Framework: Stages of Competence Development

	Culturally Incompetent	Culturally Sensitive	Culturally Competent
Cognitive dimension	Oblivious	Aware	Knowledgeable
Affective dimension	Apathetic	Sympathetic	Committed to change
Skills dimension	Unskilled	Lacking some skills	Highly skilled

From Orlandi MA: Defining cultural competence: an organizing framework. In Orlandi MA, editor: *Cultural competence for evaluators*, Washington, DC, 1992, US Department of Health and Human Services.

- Third, to meet some of the objectives for persons of different cultures as outlined in *Healthy People 2030* (see the *Healthy People 2030* box) (US Department of Health and Human Services, 2020), lifestyle, background, traditions, values, practices, and personal choices must be considered.
- Fourth, legal regulations and accreditation mandates specify that culturally competent health care must be provided so that health disparities can be reduced and ultimately eliminated.

As has been discussed, developing cultural competence is one of the core competencies for public health nurses. It is challenging and at times painful as nurses struggle to adopt new ways of thinking and performing.

Nurses develop cultural competence in different ways, but the key elements are experience with clients of other cultures, an awareness of this experience, and the promotion of mutual respect for differences. Because degrees of cultural competence vary, not all nurses may reach the same level of development. Also, developing cultural competence is a life long process.

Orlandi (1992) suggests that there are three stages in the development of cultural competence: culturally incompetent, culturally sensitive, and culturally competent (Table 7.1). Each stage has three dimensions—cognitive (thinking), affective (feeling), and psychomotor (doing)—that together have an overall effect on nursing care.

A widely used model to explain the process of cultural competence is that of Campinha-Bacote (2011). This model has the following five elements of cultural competence: (1) cultural awareness, (2) cultural knowledge, (3) cultural skill, (4) cultural encounter, and (5) cultural desire.

Cultural awareness is the self-examination and in-depth exploration of one's own biases, stereotypes, and prejudices that influence behavior (Campinha-Bacote, 2011). Nurses who have developed cultural awareness are able to do the following:

- Learn about the cultural dimensions of clients.
- Understand their own behavior and how it helps or hinders the delivery of competent care to persons from cultures other than their own.
- Recognize that health is expressed differently across cultures and that culture influences an individual's responses to health, illness, disease, and death.

For example, at a community outreach program, a nurse was teaching a racially mixed group the screening protocol for the detection of breast and cervical cancer. An African American woman in the group refused to give the return demonstration for breast self-examination. When encouraged to do so, she said, "My breasts are much larger than those on the model. Besides, the models are not like me. They are all White." After hearing the client's comments, the nurse realized that she had made no reference in her talk to the influence of culture or race on screening for breast and cervical cancer.

The nurse talked with the client, asked for her recommendations, and encouraged her to return to the demonstration. The nurse coached the client through the self-examination process while pointing out that regardless of breast size, shape, and color, the technique is the same for feeling the tissue and squeezing the nipple to make certain that there is no discharge. Because this nurse was culturally aware, she neither became angry with herself or the client, nor imposed her own values on the client. Rather, the client talked about her beliefs, attitudes, and feelings about screening for cancer that may be influenced by her culture. Subsequently, the nurse purchased a model of an African American woman's breast to use in future health education programs with African American women. A nurse who was not culturally aware may have misunderstood the client's concerns and acted in a defensive manner. This might have led to lack of information being provided or a confrontation between the nurse and client. See Box 7.2 for questions to ask yourself about your development of cultural awareness.

Cultural knowledge is information about organizational elements of diverse cultures and ethnic groups. Emphasis is on learning about the client's worldview from an ethnic (native) perspective. An understanding of the client's culture decreases misinterpretations and misapplication of scientific knowledge and facilitates the client's cooperation with the health care

BOX 7.2 Early Cultural Awareness

- Think about the first time you had contact with someone you realized was culturally different from you.
- Briefly describe the situation or event. How old were you? What were your feelings? What were your thoughts?
- What did your parents and other significant adults say about those who were culturally different from your family? What adjectives were used? What attitudes were conveyed?
- As you got older, what messages did you get about minority groups from the larger community or culture?
- As an adult, how do you see others in the community talk about culturally different people? What adjectives are used? What attitudes are conveyed? How does this reinforce or contradict your earlier experience?
- What parts of this cultural baggage make it difficult to work with clients from different cultural groups?
- What parts of this cultural baggage facilitate your work with clients?

From Randall-David E: *Culturally competent HIV counseling and education*, McLean, 1994, Maternal and Child Health Clearinghouse.

regimen (Campinha-Bacote, 2011). For example, cultural knowledge informs us that Middle Eastern women may not attend prenatal classes without encouragement and support from the nurse (Meleis, 2005). The reason for this is that attending the classes is about the future of the baby, whereas the mother's main concern may be on the present and what is happening now. If nurses understand the cultural difference in this example, they can select strategies to help the mother understand the value of the classes. In contrast, knowledge about Nigerian culture would allow the nurse to understand that the mother might begin prenatal classes but not continue because Nigerian women view birth as a natural process and not one that they need to attend a class to understand (Ogbu, 2005). Nurses who lack cultural knowledge may develop feelings of inadequacy and helplessness when they cannot effectively help their clients. Although it is unrealistic to expect that nurses will have knowledge of all cultures, they should be aware of and know how to obtain knowledge of cultural influences that affect groups with whom they most frequently interact.

EVIDENCE-BASED PRACTICE

The purpose of this intervention study was to determine if a culturally adapted telephone-delivered smoking cessation program would be feasible and acceptable to Korean Americans. The protocol was implemented over 8 weeks. It consisted of five questionnaires, counseling sessions that included explanation on the harmful effects of smoking, nicotine addiction, and the high mortality rate among Koreans; nicotine replacement patches; family participation; and counseling for relapse. Recruitment of the 31 participants (29 men and 2 women) was facilitated through advertisements on a Korean-speaking radio station. The station reported on smoking related issues and smoking cessation websites. Measures were taken at 1, 2, and 3 months post interventions. The primary outcome was for a 3-month prolonged abstinence as measured by self-report of not smoking a cigarette and corroboration by a family member. The secondary outcome was 7-day point prevalence abstinence. Results were compared with the California Quitline study that used the same interventions, but the cultural adaption was deeper for this study. At 1-month post intervention, 55% (17) participants reported abstinence, and at 3-months, 42% (13) participants achieved prolonged abstinence. Results showed that participants with stronger family ties were less dependent on the nicotine patches. The limitations for the study were that the sample size was small and consisted mostly of men.

Nurse Use

Results of the study emphasize the importance of family in Korean culture. Nurses need to be aware that there is great respect for family and that to accomplish positive health outcomes, it is important to involve the family, using culturally appropriate communications.

Data from Kim SS: A culturally adapted smoking cessation intervention for Korean Americans: preliminary findings. *J Transcult Nurs* 28:24–31, 2017.

The Evidence-Based Practice box provides an example of learning how to meet the needs of a cultural group that is different from that of the nurse.

Cultural skill refers to the effective integration of cultural awareness and cultural knowledge to obtain relevant cultural data and meet the needs of culturally diverse clients. Culturally skillful nurses use appropriate touch during conversation, modify the physical distance between themselves and others, and use

strategies to avoid cultural misunderstandings while meeting mutually agreed-upon goals.

A cultural encounter is the fourth construct essential to becoming culturally competent. Cultural encounter is the process that permits nurses to seek opportunities to engage in cross-cultural interactions with clients of diverse cultures to modify existing beliefs about a specific cultural group and possibly avoid stereotyping (Campinha-Bacote, 2011). Cultural encounters are part of the interpersonal nurse–patient relationship and focus on caring, compassion, presence, caring consciousness, and empathy. There are both direct (face-to-face) and indirect types of cultural encounters. These cultures can be across geographic communities, gender, religion, social class, ethnicities, sexual orientation, or educational level.

An example of a direct cultural encounter is when nurses learn directly from their Puerto Rican American clients about spicy food they avoid when breastfeeding. Indirect cultural encounters occur when nurses share this information about the effect of spicy food on breastfeeding with other nurses. Nurses can develop cultural competence by reading about, taking courses on, and discussing different cultures within multicultural settings.

Cultural desire is the fifth construct in the development of cultural competence. It refers to the nurse's intrinsic motivation to provide culturally competent care (Campinha-Bacote, 2012). Nurses who desire to become culturally competent do so because they want to rather than because they are directed to do so. They are energetic, enthusiastic, and goal directed in providing culturally competent care. Unlike the other constructs, cultural desire cannot be directly taught in the classroom or other educational settings. However, nurses are more likely to demonstrate cultural desire when their work environment reflects a philosophy that values cultural competence at all levels of the organization and for all its clients. Campinha-Bacote (2011) encourages nurses not to be afraid of making mistakes but to enthusiastically try to learn about other people. Box 7.3 lists several important points to remember when trying to increase your cultural competence.

BOX 7.3 Developing Cultural Competency: Points to Remember

- Culture is applicable to groups of Whites, such as Italians or Irish Americans, as well as to racial and ethnic minorities.
- During each interaction with clients, be sensitive to the cultural implications of the encounter.
- Ask questions to stimulate learning about how clients identify and express their cultural background.
- Much diversity exists within groups, and not all persons of the same racial or ethnic group may share the same culture. Assess both cultural group patterns and individual variations within a cultural group to avoid stereotyping.
- When misunderstandings arise, acknowledge the problem and take responsibility for your own errors.
- Be knowledgeable about your own cultural heritage, biases, beliefs, values, and practices when providing care.
- Avoid making assumptions about nonverbal cues when interacting with clients from unfamiliar cultures.
- Use a variety of sources, including clients, to develop cultural knowledge.
- Understand that developing cultural competence is an ongoing journey and an evolving process.

CULTURALLY COMPETENT NURSING INTERVENTIONS

Nurses integrate their professional knowledge with the client's knowledge and practices to negotiate and promote culturally relevant care. Leininger (2002a) suggests that the following three modes of action, based on negotiation between the client and nurse, can guide the nurse in providing culturally competent care: cultural preservation, cultural accommodation, and cultural repatterning. When these decisions and actions are used with cultural brokering, the nurse is able to fulfill the various roles vital to providing holistic care for culturally diverse clients.

Cultural preservation means that the nurse supports and facilitates the use of scientifically supported cultural practices from a person's culture along with those from the biomedical health care system. Examples are acupressure and acupuncture. Acupuncture is an ancient Chinese practice of inserting needles at specific points in the skin to cure disease or relieve pain. These practices are being accepted by increasing numbers of Western practitioners as a legitimate method of health care. It is important to know when clients are blending traditional health practices with those prescribed by the health care provider to make certain they support rather than interfere with one another.

Cultural accommodation means that the nurse supports and facilitates clients in their use of cultural practices when such cultural practices are not harmful to clients. For example, consider the practice of home burial of the placenta. In this example, the delivery room nurse was helpful when Ms. Sanchez asked her not to discard a piece of the amniotic sac that was present on her grandbaby's face immediately after birth. Ms. Sanchez asked the nurse to give it to her instead. The grandmother believed that being born with a piece of the amniotic sac on the face was a visible sign that something special was going to happen in the person's life. The grandmother explained that after she dried the piece of the amniotic sac, she would keep it in a safe place. She would also spend extra time protecting the baby to prevent her from being harmed. Although the delivery room nurse did not know about this practice, she gave the grandmother the piece of the sac as she requested. As another example, using cultural accommodation, a nurse can assist older Chinese American clients to manage more effectively their hypertension by modifying their use of high-sodium soy sauce and substituting low-sodium soy sauce in their cooking. Similarly, African Americans can be guided to use more broiled and boiled foods and eat fewer fried foods.

In providing care to clients who practice the Islamic faith, it is important to understand some of the key tenets of their faith. The Five Pillars of Islam define the duties that each Muslim should practice being consistent with their faith. The second pillar, Salat, can have implications for nurses caring for these patients. Salat says that a Muslim must pray five times a day while facing Mecca, which is in an easterly direction in the United States (Charles and Daroszewski, 2012). The prayers are given in a kneeling position on a prayer mat or carpet. It is important for the agency and the health care professionals to make it possible for these clients to pray at the appointed times. The Qur'an also dictates various health care choices related to contraception and birth, sanitary practices, dietary practices, and medical care concerns, to name a few (Charles and Darowszewski, 2012). In providing culturally appropriate care to Muslim clients, it is important to take into account the tenets of their religion.

Cultural repatterning means that the nurse works with clients to help them reorder, change, or modify their cultural practices when these practices are harmful to them. For example, a culturally competent nurse knows of the high incidence of obesity among Hispanic or Latina women 20 years of age and older. A school nurse was invited to develop a health education program for Hispanic or Latina teenagers in the local high school. While respecting their cultural traditions, the nurse discussed weight management strategies with the teenagers. The nurse understood the teenagers' cultural issues pertaining to food and knew how to negotiate with them. She discouraged the use of fried foods (such as tortillas), sour cream, and regular cheese, and encouraged and demonstrated the use of baked tortillas and of salsa as dip and topping.

In another example, a nurse who was giving prenatal instructions to pregnant Haitian women discovered that many of them were visiting an herbalist to obtain teas that would help them have a "strong baby." The nurse asked for the names of the herbs in the teas they were drinking and scheduled a conference with the pharmacist to discuss the specific ingredients in the herbs and ways they might help the client meet her cultural needs. The nurse found that one of the herbs contributed to high blood pressure, a problem that many of the women were experiencing. She explained to the women why they should not drink the tea with the specific herb. The nurse enlisted the aid of the herbalist because she understood the importance of supernatural causes of illness in the Haitian culture.

Cultural brokering is advocating, mediating, negotiating, and intervening between the client's culture and the biomedical health care culture on behalf of clients. It is important to understand both your culture and that of the client and to resolve or decrease problems that result from individuals in either culture not understanding the other person's values. To illustrate, migrant workers tend to have high occupational mobility; many are poor and have limited formal education. They may seek health care only when they are ill and cannot work. Whenever a nurse interacts with them, it is important to teach them about prevention, health maintenance, environmental sanitation and pesticides, and nutrition because it may be the only opportunity that the nurse will have to treat a particular migrant worker. Nurses also should advocate for the rights of the migrant worker to receive quality health care. For example, the nurse may contact the migrant health services for follow-up or referral care for the migrant worker.

INHIBITORS TO DEVELOPING CULTURAL COMPETENCE

Nurses may fail to provide culturally competent nursing care if they do not understand transcultural nursing, their supervisors are pressuring them to increase productivity by increasing their caseloads, or they are pressured by colleagues who are not knowledgeable about other cultures and who are critical or offended when others use these concepts. These and similar issues can inhibit delivery of culturally competent care and may result in nurse behaviors such as stereotyping, prejudice and racism, ethnocentrism, cultural imposition, cultural conflict, and cultural shock.

- **Stereotyping** means attributing certain beliefs and behaviors about a group to an individual without giving adequate attention to individual differences. Examples of stereotypes are "All Asian people are hardworking" and "All Chinese people are good at math."
- **Prejudice** refers to having a deeply held reaction, often negative, about another group or person. For example, a person may be viewed negatively because of skin color, race, religion, or social standing, with no regard for the worth of the person as an individual.
- **Racism** is a form of prejudice and refers to the belief that persons who are born into a particular group are inferior, for example, in intelligence, morals, beauty, or self-worth. Because of their race, individuals may be denied opportunities that are available to people of other races. Racism can be one of three forms: individual, because of the characteristics of the group of which the person is a member, such as skin color, hair texture, or facial features; institutional, such as discriminatory policies, priorities, and resource allocation pertaining to certain groups; or cultural, in which a culture is viewed in derogatory or stereotypical ways because of, for example, how a group dresses or the language the group uses.
- **Ethnocentrism**, a type of cultural prejudice at the population level, is the belief that one's own group determines the standards for behavior by which all other groups are to be judged. Ethnocentric nurses are unfamiliar and uncomfortable with anything that is different from their culture. Their inability to accept different worldviews often leads them to devalue the experiences of others, judge them to be inferior, and treat people who are different with suspicion or hostility (Andrews and Boyle, 2016). Ethnocentrism contrasts with **cultural blindness**, which is the tendency to ignore all differences among cultures, to act as though these differences do not exist, and as a result, to treat all people the same (when in truth, each person is an individual with unique needs). Nurses who say that they treat all clients the same, regardless of cultural orientation, are demonstrating cultural blindness.
- **Cultural imposition** involves the belief in one's own superiority, or ethnocentrism, and the act of imposing one's values on others. Nurses impose their values on clients when they forcefully promote Western medical traditions while ignoring the clients' value of non-Western treatments such as acupuncture, herbal therapy, or spiritual remedies. A goal for nurses is to develop the approach of **cultural relativism**, in which they recognize that clients have different approaches to their health, and that each culture should be judged on its own merit and not on the nurse's personal beliefs.
- **Cultural conflict** is a perceived threat that may arise from a misunderstanding of expectations between clients and nurses when either group is not aware of cultural differences (Andrews and Boyle, 2016). Although cultural conflict is unavoidable, it is important to know how to manage it while delivering culturally competent care.
- **Cultural shock** is the feeling of helplessness, discomfort, and disorientation experienced by an individual attempting to understand or effectively adapt to another cultural group that differs in practices, values, and beliefs. It results from the anxiety caused by losing familiar sights, sounds, and behaviors.

Being aware of clients' cultural beliefs and knowing about other cultures may help nurses be less judgmental, more accepting of cultural differences, and less likely to engage in the behaviors just listed that inhibit cultural competence.

CULTURAL NURSING ASSESSMENT

A **cultural nursing assessment** is a systematic way to identify the beliefs, values, meanings, and behaviors of people while considering their history, life experiences, and the social and physical environments in which they live.

Skills such as listening, explaining, acknowledging, recommending, understanding, and negotiating help the nurse to be nonjudgmental. It is vital that nurses listen to clients' perceptions of their problems and, in turn, that nurses explain to clients the nurses' perceptions of the problems. Nurses and clients should acknowledge and discuss similarities and differences between the two perceptions to develop suggestions and recommendations for managing problems. Nurses also negotiate with clients on nursing care actions to meet the needs of the clients.

Numerous tools are available to assist nurses in conducting cultural assessments (Andrews and Boyle, 2019, 2016; Leininger, 2002b). The focus of such tools varies, and selection is determined by the dimensions of culture to be assessed.

During an initial contact with clients, nurses should perform a general cultural assessment to obtain an overview of the clients' characteristics. Nurses ask clients about their ethnic background, language, education, religious affiliation, dietary practices, family relationships, hospital experiences, occupation and socioeconomic status, cultural beliefs, and language. Nurses also want to know about clients' distinctive features, perceptions of the health issue, causation, treatment, anticipated results, and the impact the issue might have on the client. This basic data can help nurses understand the clients from the clients' points of view and recognize their uniqueness, thus avoiding stereotyping. Data for an in-depth cultural assessment should be gathered over a period of time and not restricted to the first encounter with the client. This gives both the client and the nurse time to get to know each other, and it helps the client see the nurse in a helping relationship. An in-depth cultural assessment should be conducted in two phases: a data-collection phase and an organization phase.

The data-collection phase consists of three steps:

1. The nurse collects self-identifying data similar to those collected in the brief assessment.
2. The nurse raises a variety of questions that seek information on the clients' perception of what brings them to the health care system, the illness, and previous and anticipated treatments.

QSEN FOCUS ON QUALITY AND SAFETY EDUCATION FOR NURSES

The six quality and safety competencies for nurses that were identified in the Quality and Safety Education for Nurses (QSEN) project are client-centered care, teamwork and collaboration, evidence-based practice, quality improvement, safety, and informatics. Although each of these is important and pertinent to the nursing actions taken with people from cultural groups other than that of the nurse, perhaps the most significant is client-centered care. The chapter presents many guidelines and principles for aiding nurses in providing culturally competent care. Client-centered care is more effective when the nurse and client communicate effectively with one another. Lack of communication may occur when they speak different languages, when they have different cultural practices and expectations that lead them to hear messages differently, or when clients simply do not understand what the nurse is saying and are reluctant to acknowledge it. Nurses must observe for both verbal and nonverbal cues that a message is either understood or not understood. When the latter occurs, the nurse should take action to clarify the message, and this may include asking someone from that cultural group to assist or to enlist the aid of an interpreter (Issel and Bekemeier, 2010).

The following targeted competency applies the QSEN competency of client-centered interventions that reflect cultural competence:

Targeted Competency: Client-Centered Intervention—Recognize the client or designee as the source of control and full partner in providing compassionate and coordinated interventions based on respect for client's preferences, values, and needs.

Important aspects of client-centered intervention include:

Knowledge: Describe strategies to empower clients or families in all aspects of the health care process.

Skills: Communicate client values, preferences, and expressed needs to other members of health care team.

Attitudes: Willingly support client-centered care for individuals and groups whose values differ from own.

Client-centered care question: Competence in providing client-centered interventions involves both effective interviewing of individual clients and developing an awareness of their context. As a community-based clinician, it is helpful to familiarize yourself with the cultural context of your clients. Learning about community resources can sometimes be helpful in learning about the cultural context. You have just been hired as a visiting nurse in a Hispanic community. What community resources could you explore to assist you in providing effective client-centered care?

Answer:

• You might explore community centers. Where are they? How well frequented are the community centers? Which programs are most popular? Which community center programs are health oriented?

• Are community members involved with one or more churches? You might familiarize yourself with elements of this faith tradition.

• Are there community elders who are publicly recognized as leaders in the community? Can you meet with them to understand how the community has changed and evolved over time?

Prepared by Gail Armstrong, ND, DNP, MS, PhD, Professor and Assistant Dean of the DNP Program, Oregon Health and Sciences University.

3. After the nursing diagnosis is made, the nurse identifies cultural factors that may influence the effectiveness of nursing care actions.

In the organization phase, data related to the client's and family's views on optimal treatment choices are examined, and areas of difference between the client's cultural needs and the goals of Western medicine are identified.

A useful site related to cultural assessment is the National Center for Cultural Competence (NCCC) at Georgetown University, which has many links to other useful sites. See https://nccc.georgetown.edu.

The key to a successful cultural assessment lies in nurses being aware of their own culture. The nurse should consider the following suggestions when eliciting cultural information:

• Be sensitive to the cues in the environment and be in tune with the verbal and nonverbal communications before taking action.

• Know about the resources in the community such as schools, churches, clubs and other groups, hospitals, tribal councils, restaurants, taverns, and bars.

• Know the specific areas to focus on before beginning the cultural assessment.

• Select a strategy for gathering cultural data. Possible strategies include in-depth interviews, informal conversations, observations of the client's everyday activities or specific events, survey research, and a case-method approach to study certain aspects of a client.

• Identify a confidante who will help "bridge the gap" between cultures. Be aware that in some cultures the woman's husband

or a close male family friend may be the person from whom the nurse may need to obtain the cultural information.

• Know the appropriate questions to ask without offending the client.

• Interview other nurses or health care professionals who have worked with the specific individual, family, or community to get their input.

• Use a trained interpreter if the client has limited proficiency with English.

• Talk with formal and informal community leaders to gain a comprehensive understanding about significant aspects of community life.

• Be aware that all information has both subjective and objective aspects, and verify and cross-check the information that is collected before acting on it.

• Avoid the pitfalls that may occur when making premature generalizations.

• Be sincere, open, and honest with yourself and the client.

BUILDING CULTURALLY COMPETENT ORGANIZATIONS

Although many of the same guidelines that apply to providing culturally competent care also apply to building culturally competent organizations, there are some areas that should be emphasized at the organizational level. In considering how to build a more culturally competent organization, it is useful to ask these questions:

1. Who lives in the community right now?
2. What kinds of diversity exists?

3. What kinds of relationships are established between cultural groups?
4. Are the different cultural groups well organized?
5. What struggles exist between cultures?
6. What struggles exist within cultural groups?
7. Are these struggles openly recognized and talked about?
8. Are there efforts to build alliances and coalitions between groups?
9. What issues do different cultural groups have in common (Axner, 2015)?

Organizations have a culture that includes policies, procedures, programs, and processes and that incorporates certain values, beliefs, assumptions, and customs (Brownlee and Lee, 2015). Researchers at the University of Kansas have developed a toolbox to help organizations become culturally competent. They note that a culturally competent organizational model has five essential principles: (1) valuing diversity, (2) conducting cultural assessment, (3) understanding the dynamics of difference, (4) institutionalizing cultural knowledge, and (5) adapting to diversity (Brownlee and Lee, 2015). These researchers posit that diversity is reality and that changes in one part of the world affect people everywhere. They cite the following steps as key to building a multicultural organization that recognizes diversity and aims to enable cultural differences to strengthen rather than weaken the organization (Brownlee and Lee, 2015):

- Form a cultural competence committee.
- Write a mission statement.
- Find out what similar organizations have done and develop partnerships.
- Use free resources.
- Complete a comprehensive cultural competence assessment of your organization.
- Find out which cultural groups exist in your community and whether they access community services.
- Have a brown-bag lunch to get staff involved in discussion and activities about cultural competence.
- Ask your personnel about their staff development needs.
- Assign part of your budget to staff development programming in cultural competence.
- Include a cultural competency requirement in job descriptions.

▶▶ APPLYING CONTENT TO PRACTICE

As has been discussed throughout the chapter, culturally competent nursing care uses many of the standards, guidelines, and competencies from key nursing and public health documents. For example, the Council on Linkages (2016) has a set of skills related to cultural competency and a set related to communication that is consistent with the information in this chapter. Likewise, the Quad Council Coalition of Community/Public Health Nursing Organizations (2018) further develops and applies the skills of the Council on Linkages related to both cultural competency and communication to public health nursing practice. As an example, the Council on Linkages states that a necessary skill in public health is to consider "the role of cultural, social, and behavioral factors in the accessibility, availability, acceptability and delivery of public health services." The Quad Council Coalition says that "public health nurses should consider the role of cultural, social, and behavioral factors in the accessibility, availability, acceptability, and delivery of public health nursing services."

- Be sure your facility's location is accessible and respectful of difference.
- Collect resource materials on culturally diverse groups for your staff to use.
- Build a network of natural helpers, community "informants" and other "experts."

Another useful tool is the Andrews/Boyle Transcultural Interprofessional Practice (TIP) Model (2019). This model provides a comprehensive approach for health care teams as they seek to provide culturally congruent care.

▌ PRACTICE APPLICATION

Shu Ping was concerned about her father's deteriorating health and contacted her church friend, Ms. Johnson, a registered nurse, for advice. A public health nurse had been visiting the father since his recent discharge from the hospital, but the father had asked this nurse not to discuss his diagnosis with his family. After several weeks with the family, Ms. Johnson was able to establish a close enough relationship with the father so that she could talk with him privately about his health. He told Ms. Johnson that he was diagnosed with cancer of the small intestine, and he feared he was dying. He did not want the family to know the "bad news." He refused treatment because his view was that people never got better after they were diagnosed with cancer; they always died.

Which of the following actions by the public health nurse would best demonstrate culturally competent care to the family?

A. Discussing the medical treatment and surgical intervention for cancer of the small intestine
B. Discussing with Shu Ping's father the prognosis for a person diagnosed with cancer of the small intestine in the United States
C. With the father's consent, requesting a conference involving the primary physician, the father, and the family to discuss the diagnosis and treatment options
D. Contacting the public health agency and discussing the problem with them

Answers can be found on the Evolve website.

▌ REMEMBER THIS!

- The US population is increasingly diverse which increases the need to understand the culture from which clients come.
- Immigrants often present unique health problems.
- Nurses who do not speak or understand the client's language should use an interpreter. In selecting an interpreter, nurses should consider the clients' cultural needs and respect their right to privacy. If no interpreter is present, translation apps on smart phones can be used.
- Culture is a learned set of behaviors that is widely shared among a group of people; the culture of people helps guide individuals in problem solving and decision making.
- Members of minority groups are overrepresented on the lower tiers of the socioeconomic ladder. Poor economic achievement is also a common characteristic among populations at risk, such as those in poverty, the homeless, migrant

workers, and refugees. Nurses should be able to distinguish between cultural issues and socioeconomic class issues and not interpret behavior as having a cultural origin when, in fact, it is based on the socioeconomic class.

- Culturally competent nursing care is designed for a specific client, reflects the individual's beliefs and values, and is provided with sensitivity. Such nursing care helps improve health outcomes and reduce health care costs.
- Nurses who are culturally competent use cultural knowledge and specific skills, such as intracultural communication and cultural assessment, in selecting interventions to care for clients.
- Four modes of action that nurses may use to negotiate with clients and give culturally competent care are cultural preservation, cultural accommodation, cultural repatterning, and cultural brokering.
- Barriers to providing culturally competent care are stereotyping, prejudice and racism, ethnocentrism, cultural imposition, cultural conflict, and cultural shock.
- Nurses should perform a cultural assessment on every client with whom they interact. Cultural assessments help nurses understand clients' perspectives of health and illness and thereby guide them in discussing culturally appropriate interventions. The needs of clients vary with their age, education, religion, and socioeconomic status.
- Dietary practices are an integral part of the assessment data. Efforts to understand dietary practices should go beyond relying on membership in a defined group and should include individual nutritional practices and religious requirements.
- A variety of steps can be taken to develop culturally competent organizations, and nurses can play a leading role in doing so.

EVOLVE WEBSITE

http://evolve.elsevier.com/Stanhope/foundations
- NCLEX® Review Questions
- Practice Application Answers

REFERENCES

American Nurses Association: Scope and standards of practice, 2015a, www.nursingworld.org. Accessed April 21, 2020 and edition 4, 2021.

American Nurses Association: Code of ethics for nurses with interpretive statements, 2015b, www.nursingworld.org. Accessed April 21, 2020.

Anderson ET, McFarlane J: *Community as partner: theory in practice in nursing*, 7th ed. Philadelphia, 2015, Lippincott Williams and Wilkins.

Andrews MM, Boyle JS: *Transcultural concepts in nursing care*, 7th ed. Philadelphia, 2016, Lippincott Williams and Wilkins.

Andrews MM, Boyle JS: The Andrews//Boyles Transcultural Interprofessional Practice (TIP) Model, *J Transcult Nurs* 30(4):323-330, 2019.

Artiga S, Damico A, Young K et al.: *Health coverage and care for immigrants,* issue brief, Menlo Park, January 2016, The Henry J. Kaiser Family Foundation. http://www.kff.org. Accessed January 20, 2016.

Artiga S, Garfield R, Damico A: *Health coverage and care for immigrants,* Menlo Park, CA, March 2020, The Henry J. Kaiser Family Foundation. http://www.kff.org. Accessed April 25, 2020.

Artiga S, Hinton E: Beyond health care: the role of social determinants in promoting health and health equity, Issue Brief, May 2018, The Henry J. Kaiser Family Foundation, http://www.kff.org. Accessed April 21, 2020.

Axner M: *Understanding culture and diversity in building communities*, Lawrence, 2015, Community Tool Box. University of Kansas. See http://ctb.ku.edu. Accessed October 25, 2020.

Batalova J, Blizzard B, Bolter J: Frequently requested statistics on immigrants and immigration in the United States, Migration Policy Institute, February 14, 2020, https://www.migration policy.org. Accessed April 21, 2020.

Brownlee T, Lee K: *Building culturally competent organizations*, Lawrence, 2015, Community Tool Box. University of Kansas. See http://ctb.ku.edu. Accessed October 25, 2020.

Campinha-Bacote J: Coming to know cultural competence in evolutionary process, *Int J Hum Caring* 15:42–48, 2011.

Campinha-Bacote J: People of African heritage. In Purnell L, Paulanka BJ, editors. *Transcultural health care: a culturally competent approach*, ed 4, Philadelphia, 2012, F.A. Davis, pp. 91-114.

Centers for Disease Control and Prevention. *Refugee health guidelines*, 2016. http://www.cdc.gov/immigrantrefugeehealth/guidelines/refugee-guidelines.html. Accessed April 24, 2020.

Centers for Disease Control and Prevention. *Immigrant and Refugee Health: Guidelines for the US domestic medical examination for newly arriving refugees,* http://www.cdc.gov/immigrantandrefugeehealth, February 7, 2020. Accessed October 2020.

Charles CE, Daroszewski EB: Culturally competent nursing care of the Muslim patient, *Issues Ment Health Nurs* 33:61–63, 2012.

Council on Linkages between Academia and Public Health Practice: *Core competencies for public health professionals*, Washington DC, 2016, Public Health Foundation, Health Resource and Services Administration.

Darnell LK, Hickson SV: Cultural competent patient-centered nursing care, *Nurs Clin N Am* 50:99–108, 2015.

Douglas MK, Rosenkoetter M, Pacquiao DF et al.: Guidelines for implementing culturally competent nursing care, *J Transcult Nurse* 25:109–121, 2014.

ElGindy G: www.minoritynurse.com. Accessed March 30, 2013.

Gelatt J and Zong J: *Settling in: A profile of the unauthorized immigrant population in the United States,* Washington DC, Migration Policy Institute, 2018.

Giger JN: *Transcultural nursing: assessment and intervention*, 7th ed. St Louis, 2017, Elsevier.

Heiman HJ, Artiga S: *Beyond health care: the role of social determinants in promoting health and health equity*, issue brief, Menlo Park, November 2015, The Henry J. Kaiser Family Foundation. http://www.kff.org. Accessed January 20, 2016.

Immigration Forum: Fact sheet: US refugee resettlement, January 26, 2019, author, accessed April 23, 2020.

Issel LM, Bekemeier B: Safe practice of population-focused nursing care: development of a public health nursing concept, *Nurs Outlook* 58:226–232, 2010.

Kim SS: A culturally adapted smoking cessation intervention for Korean Americans: preliminary findings, *J Transcult Nurs* 28:24-31, 2017.

Leininger M: Essential transcultural nursing care concepts, principles, examples, and policy statements. In Leininger MM, McFarland M, editors: *Transcultural nursing: concepts, theories, research, and practices*, 3rd ed. New York, 2002a, McGraw-Hill, pp. 45-69.

Leininger M: The theory of culture care and the ethnonursing research method. In Leininger MM, McFarland M, editors: *Transcultural nursing: concepts, theories, research, and practices*, 3rd ed. New York, 2002b, McGraw-Hill, pp. 71-98.

Los Angeles Times: Editorial: COVID-19 is disproportionately killing minorities. That's not a coincidence, April 8, 2020.

Meleis AI: Arabs. In Lipson JG, Dibble SL, editors: *Providing culturally appropriate care in culture and clinical care*, San Francisco, 2005, UCSF Nursing Press, pp. 42-57.

Migration Policy Institute: Profile of the unauthorized population: United States, 2018, httpss://migrationpolicy.org. Accessed April 23, 2020.

Narayan MC: Cultural competence in home healthcare nursing: Disparity, cost, regulatory, accreditation, ethical and practice issues, *Home Health Care Manag Pract* 33(2):76-80, 2019.

Ogbu M: Nigerians. In Lipson JG, Dibble SL, editors: *Providing culturally appropriate care in culture and critical care*, San Francisco, 2005, UCSF Nursing Press, pp. 243-259.

Orlandi MA, editor: *Cultural competence for evaluators*, Washington, DC, 1992, US Department of Health and Human Services.

Purnell L: Update: The Purnell theory and model for culturally competent health care, *J Transcult Nurs*, 30(2): 98-105, 2019.

Strickland OL, Powell Young, Y, Rees-Miranda C et al.: African-Americans have a high propensity for death from COVID-19: Rationale and causation, *J Natl Black Nurses Assoc*, 31(1):1-12, July 2020.

Quad Council Coalition of Public Health Nursing Organizations: Community/Public Health Nursing (C/PHN) competences, 2018, www.quadcouncilphn.org. Accessed April 20, 2020.

Randall-David E: *Culturally competent HIV counseling and education*, McLean, 1994, Maternal and Child Health Clearinghouse.

US Department of Health and Human Services, Office of Refugee Resettlement: *The Refugee Act*, 2012, Retrieved from https://www/acf/hhs.gov.

US Department of Health and Human Services: *Healthy People 2020*, Washington, DC, 2018, US Government Printing Office.

US Department of Health and Human Services: *Healthy People 2030*, Washington, DC, 2020, US Government Printing Office.

United States Census Bureau: Quick facts, 2019, www.census.gov. Accessed April 18, 2020.

Zong J, Batalova J, and Hallock J. (2018). Frequently requested statistics on immigrants and immigration in the United States. *Migration Policy Institute.* Retrieved from https://www.migrationpolicy.org/article/frequently-requested-statistics-immigrants-and-immigration-united-states, April 21, 2020.

8

Environmental Health

Barbara Sattler

OBJECTIVES

After reading this chapter, the student should be able to:

1. Explain how the environment influences human health and disease.
2. Know which disciplines work most closely with nurses in environmental health.
3. Describe legislative and regulatory policies that have influenced the effect of the environment on health and disease patterns.
4. Describe the skills needed by nurses practicing in environmental health and apply the nursing process to the practice of environmental health.

CHAPTER OUTLINE

KEY TERMS

"Globally 23% of all deaths could be prevented though healthier environments" (World Health Organization, 2019), and an estimated 24% of the global burden of disease can be attributed to environmental factors (Pruss-Ustun et al., 2016). Nurses can define environment in a variety of ways, including homes, schools, workplaces, churches, social organizations, and communities. The environment is everything around us. Each location holds potential health risks. It is both important for and a responsibility of nurses to understand as much as possible about these risks—how to assess them, how to eliminate or reduce them, how to communicate and educate about them, and how to advocate for policies that support healthy environments. We often take the environment for granted and may fail to see the hazards in front of us. For example, how many of us know for certain that our drinking water is safe, or that the air we breathe is free from pollutants that aggravate our individual respiratory functions? Environmental health risks come in the form of poor air and water quality, the use of pesticides, and paint containing lead. Environmental hazards come in the forms of biological, chemical, and radiological hazards. The Clean Air Act signed into law in 1970 and with major revisions in 1977 and 1990 requires the Environmental Protection Agency (EPA) to set National Ambient Air Quality Standards (NAAQS) for six common air pollutants also known as "criteria pollutants." They are ground-level ozone, particulate matter, carbon monoxide, nitrogen dioxide, sulfur dioxide, and lead (EPA, 2018). As will be discussed later, the EPA also provides information about safe drinking water and many of the other environmental hazards.

Factors including genetics, socioeconomic status, and environmental exposure affect environmental health. In evaluating environmental exposures in a home, nurses' assessments can begin with a set of questions: What exposures can you identify in your own home? Do you use pesticides? Does your home have lead-based paint? (The age of a home is a good proxy for identifying the presence of lead-based paint because lead is most likely found in homes built before 1978, when the use of lead was banned in household paint.) Is the paint chipping or peeling? Are any of your appliances or heat sources producing unhealthy levels of carbon monoxide? Have you checked your home for radon, the second largest cause of lung cancer in the United States? How about your workplace? Do you eat fish on a regular basis? (Some fish can have unhealthy levels of mercury.) If so, what kinds of fish?

The American Nurses Association (ANA) calls for all nurses to understand basic environmental health concepts, including knowledge about environmental health and its effect on nursing practice, the Precautionary Principle, nurses' rights to work in a safe workplace and use materials, products, technology, and practices that reflect an evidence-based approach. Other principles relate to quality assessment of the environment, interdisciplinary work in environmental health, involvement in research, and support of nurses who advocate for a safe environment (ANA, 2007).

If children are in the home, are all the toxic cleaning materials and insecticides out of reach? Does the home or apartment have lead in its paint? Beginning in April 2010, any contractor performing renovation or painting in a home, child-care facility, or school built before 1978 and disturbing more than 6 square feet

must be trained and certified in how to prevent lead contamination (EPA, 2019). As long as lead is in good condition and the surface is not broken, it does not pose a health risk. The risk comes when lead flakes or dust falls on surfaces or in the soil near the home. This is a specific risk for young children who tend to put things in their mouths. Exposure to lead can cause premature birth, low birth weight, and brain and nerve damage in a fetus. Lead can cause damage in children to the brain, nervous system, and kidney, as well as behavior, hearing, learning, and bone marrow problems (Fig. 8.1). In adults, it lead can lead to anemia, fertility problems, hearing and vision loss, high blood pressure, kidney damage, nerve disorders, memory and concentration problems, and muscle and joint pain (WebMD, 2018).

Environmental exposures are rarely limited to one location or to one source. For example, the broad category of pesticides includes the insecticides used in homes, the herbicides used in gardens, the pesticide residues on fruits and vegetables, and antimicrobial soaps. Each of these forms of pesticides comes with a potential health risk. Pesticides have been linked to adult liver and prostate cancer (Silva et al., 2016; VoPham et al., 2017). If you have children and regularly use pesticides in your home, you increase their risk of contracting leukemia. The more you use pesticides, the greater the risk of leukemia and this is especially true if they are used inside (Chen et al., 2015). The childhood risk for leukemia increases if the mother was exposed to pesticides, including occupational exposures (Bailey et al., 2014). Many playing fields where children compete in sports are regularly sprayed with pesticides (Gilden et al., 2012). There are other chemicals like the plasticizer bisphenol A (BPA) and phthalates (commonly found in personal care products) that have noncancer endpoints such as endocrine disruption in children (Watkins et al., 2017).

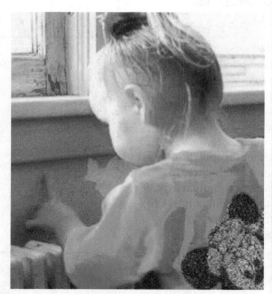

Fig. 8.1 Child in Home With Lead-Based Paint. (From State of Hawaii Department of Public Health. Retrieved September 2012 from http://hawaii.gov/health/environmental/noise/asbestoslead/images2/child.jpg.)

BOX 8.1 General Environmental Health Competencies for Nurses

Basic Knowledge and Concepts

All nurses should understand the scientific principles and underpinnings of the relationship between individuals or populations and the environment (including the work environment). This understanding includes the basic mechanisms and pathways of exposure to environmental health hazards, basic prevention and control strategies, the interdisciplinary nature of effective interventions, and the role of research.

Assessment and Referral

All nurses should be able to successfully complete an environmental health history, recognize potential environmental hazards and sentinel illnesses, and make appropriate referrals for conditions with probable environmental causes. An essential

component is the ability to locate referral sources, access them, and provide information to clients and communities.

Advocacy, Ethics, and Risk Communication

All nurses should be able to demonstrate knowledge of the role of advocacy (case and class), ethics, and risk communication in client care and community intervention with respect to potential adverse effects of the environment on health.

Legislation and Regulation

All nurses should understand the policy framework and major pieces of legislation and regulations related to environmental health.

From Pope AM, Snyder MA, Mood LH, eds: *Nursing, health, and environment,* Washington, DC, 1995, Institute of Medicine, National Academies Press.

Chemical, biological, and radiological exposures that affect our health come from the air we breathe, the water we drink, the food we eat, and the products we use. Nurses need to know how to assess for environmental health risks and develop educational and other preventive interventions to help individuals, families, and communities understand and, where possible, decrease the risks. The National Academy of Science's Institute of Medicine (IOM) recommends that all nurses have a basic understanding of environmental health principles and that these principles be integrated into all aspects of practice, education, advocacy, policies, and research (Pope, Snyder, and Mood, 1995). This chapter explores the basic competencies recommended by the IOM (Box 8.1) and integrates them with the ANA (2007) Principles of Environmental Health. Although developed many years ago, the IOM principles remain useful for today's integration of environmental health into the Standards for Environmental Health Nursing practice. Since 2008 the development of the first environmental health nursing organization, the Alliance of Nurses for Healthy Environments (ANHE), in collaboration with other nursing organizations, has been able to advance the recommendations of the 1995 IOM report (Leffers et al., 2014). The federal government, like important nursing and public health associations, has long recognized the importance of the relationship between environmental risks and diseases. Consistent with this recognition, environmental health is one of the priority areas of the *Healthy People 2030* objectives (see the *Healthy People 2030* box).

♥ HEALTHY PEOPLE 2030

Selected Objectives Related to Environmental Health

EH-03: Increase the proportion of people whose water supply meets Safe Drinking Water Act regulations.

EH-D01: Increase the proportion of schools with policies and practices that promote health and safety.

EH-01: Reduce the number of days people are exposed to unhealthy air.

From US Department of Health and Human Services: *Healthy People 2030,* Washington, DC, 2020, US Government Printing Office.

ENVIRONMENTAL HEALTH SCIENCES

Toxicology

Toxicology is the basic science that studies the health effects associated with chemical exposures. Its corollary in health care is pharmacology, which studies the human health effects, both desirable and undesirable, associated with drugs. In toxicology, only the negative effects of chemical exposures are studied. However, the key principles of pharmacology and toxicology are the same. Just as the dose of a drug influences its effectiveness and its toxicity, the quantity of an air or water pollutant to which we may be exposed will determine the risk for experiencing a negative health effect. Also, the timing of exposure affects the risk for an untoward health effect. For example, during embryonic and fetal development, exposure to toxic chemicals can create immediate harm or create a critical pathway for future disease. Very young children are especially susceptible to exposures because of the immature development of their systems (Wright, 2017).

Both drugs and pollutants can enter the body by a variety of routes. Most drugs are given orally and are absorbed via the gastrointestinal tract. Water- and food-associated pollutants, including pesticides and heavy metals, enter the body via the digestive tract. Some drugs are administered as inhalants, and some pollutants in the air (including indoor air) enter the body via the lungs. Some drugs are applied topically. In work settings, employees can receive dermal exposures from toxic chemicals when they immerse unprotected hands in chemical solutions. Pollution can enter the body via the lungs (inhalation), gastrointestinal tract (ingestion), and skin and mucous membranes (dermal absorption). Some chemicals can cross the placental barrier and affect the fetus. In addition to direct damage to cells, tissues, organs, and organ systems, changes to the DNA can occur from chemical exposures that can change gene expression, which in turn can predict disease. This latter effect is the focus of a relatively new field of biological study—epigenetics. Scientists now understand that many variables predict disease outcomes, including environmental exposures. The onslaught of COVID-19 in early 2020 was an example of a virus that appeared to be transmitted in a variety of ways and was most likely airborne.

When we administer medications to patients, we consider age, weight, other drugs taken, and the underlying health status of the person. We should also make it clear to clients that taking the prescription or over-the-counter drug in greater amounts or more often than recommended can have a toxic effect. Also, combining herbal medicines with others can have harmful interaction effects. In addition, it is important to consider how environmental exposures affect community members. For example, children are more vulnerable to almost all pollutants. Immunocompromised people are more vulnerable to food-borne and waterborne pathogens as they are to the COVID-19 virus. Examples of immunocompromised people are those: (1) infected with the human immunodeficiency virus (HIV), (2) who have acquired immunodeficiency syndrome (AIDS), (3) who are taking chemotherapeutic drugs, or (4) who are organ recipients. When assessing a community's environmental health status, be sure to review the general health status of the community to identify members who may have higher risk factors as well as to assess the environmental exposures. It is also important to teach community residents how to effectively dispose of medications they no longer need.

☐ CHECK YOUR PRACTICE

Many cities and counties sponsor medicine take-back programs during which residents can drop off unused medicines. These community events may be sponsored by the US Drug Enforcement Administration (DEA) or by local law enforcement agencies. You can contact a city or county government's trash and recycling service to learn what is available in the local area. Poison control centers and pharmacists are also a good source of information about disposing of unused medicines. If no take-back program is available, follow these steps:

- Mix medicines (do not crush tablets or capsules) with an unpalatable substance such as used kitty litter, dirt, or used coffee grounds.
- Place the mixture in a container, such as a sealed bag.
- Throw the container in your household trash.
- Scratch out all personal information on the prescription label of your empty container or packaging, then dispose of the container.
- In 2010, the US Drug Enforcement Agency (DEA) began hosting a National Prescription Drug Take-Back event twice a year. Not every drug is taken, so call the local collector to learn about their policies. In 2020, due to the COVID-19 health crisis, the April 25, 2020, event was postponed (www.NationalTakeBackDay 2020).
- There are a small number of drugs that are especially harmful, and possibly fatal, even if only one dose is used by someone other than the person for whom the medication was prescribed.
- The DEA provides a list of medications that can be disposed of by flushing down the sink or toilet.

Knowing about chemicals and using that information in practice can seem like a huge task. Fortunately, chemicals can be grouped into families so that it is possible to understand the actions and risks associated with these groups. The following are examples:

1. Metals and metallic compounds, such as arsenic, cadmium, chromium, lead, and mercury
2. Hydrocarbons, such as benzene, toluene, ketones, formaldehyde, and trichloroethylene

3. Irritant gases, such as ammonia, hydrochloric acid, sulfur dioxide, and chlorine
4. Chemical asphyxiants, including carbon monoxide, hydrogen sulfide, and cyanides
5. Pesticides, such as organophosphates, carbamates, and chlorinated hydrocarbons

EPIDEMIOLOGY

Whereas toxicology is the science that studies the poisonous effects of chemicals, epidemiology is the science that helps us understand the strength of the association between exposures and health effects in human populations. Chapter 10 discusses epidemiology in detail. However, a few points are relevant here because epidemiology is an applied science used in environmental health. Epidemiological studies have helped explain the association between learning disabilities and exposure to lead-based paint dust, as well as asthma exacerbation and air pollution (Smargiasssi et al., 2014; Habre et al., 2014) and gastrointestinal disease and exposure to *Cryptosporidium* in contaminated water (Yoder et al, 2012). Epidemiology also helps in the examination of occupation-related illnesses. Environmental surveillance efforts, such as childhood lead registries, use epidemiological methods to track and analyze incidence, prevalence, and health outcomes.

As discussed in Chapter 10, three major concepts—agent, host, and environment—form the classic epidemiological triangle. This simple model helps explain the often-complex relationships among agent, which may include chemical mixtures (i.e., more than one agent); host, which may refer to a community spanning different ages, both sexes, ethnicities, cultures, and disease states; and environment, which may include dynamic factors such as air, water, soil, and food, as well as temperature, humidity, and wind. Limitations of environmental epidemiology include a reliance on occupational health studies to characterize certain toxic exposures. Studies are usually performed on healthy adults whose biological systems are different from those of neonates, pregnant women, children, the immunosuppressed, and older adults. Geographic information systems (GIS) are used in environmental health studies to code data so that they can be related spatially to a place on Earth. For example, a nurse could combine geographically related data to develop maps to note where the data can be related. Specifically, by taking a data set that geographically notes where children under 10 years of age live and overlaying another data set that notes geographic areas designated by the age of housing stock, a public health nurse could determine locations with the largest number of children who live in areas with older housing stock. Using this information, the nurse could target a lead surveillance and educational program.

MULTIDISCIPLINARY APPROACHES

In addition to toxicology and epidemiology, some earth sciences help explain how pollutants travel in air, water, and soil. Geologists, meteorologists, and chemists all contribute information to help understand how and when humans may be exposed to hazardous chemicals, radiation (such as radon), and biological contaminants. The public health field also depends on food safety specialists, sanitarians, radiation specialists, and industrial hygienists.

The nature of environmental health requires a multidisciplinary approach to assess and decrease environmental health risks. For instance, to assess and address a case of lead-based paint poisoning, the team might include a housing inspector with expertise in lead-based paint or a sanitarian to assess the lead-associated health risks in the home; clinical specialists to manage the clients' health needs; laboratory workers to assess lead levels in the clients' blood as well as in the paint, house dust, and drinking water; and lead-based paint remediation specialists to reduce the lead-based paint risk in the home. This approach could potentially involve the local health department, the state department of environmental protection, the housing department, a tertiary care

setting, and public or private sector laboratories. It is important that nurses understand the roles of each respective agency and organization, know the public health laws (particularly as they pertain to lead-based paint poisoning), and work with the community to coordinate services to address the community's needs. The nurse also might set up a blood-lead screening program through the local health department, educate local health providers to encourage them to systematically test children for lead poisoning, or work with local landlords to improve the condition of their housing stock. Factors contributing to the reduction of lead levels in the United States include elimination of lead in paint, reduction of lead in gasoline, reduction in the number of manufactured food and drink cans and household plumbing components containing lead solder, lead screening laws, and lead paint abatement programs in communities.

QSEN FOCUS ON QUALITY AND SAFETY EDUCATION FOR NURSES

Targeted Competency

Function effectively within nursing and interprofessional teams, fostering open communication, mutual respect, and shared decision making to achieve quality client care.

Important aspects of safety include the following:

- **Knowledge:** Describe scopes of practice and roles of health care team members.
- **Skills:** Assume role of team member or leader based on the situation.
- **Attitudes:** Value the perspectives and expertise of all health team members.

Safety Question

Five of the objectives in *Healthy People 2030* related to environmental health are: Reduce exposure to lead (arsenic, mercury, bisphenol A, and perchlorate): EH-07, EH-08, EH-09, Eh-10, and EH-11." The public health nurse who is working on a project to help mothers develop parenting skills visits a new mother who lives and works on a large farm surrounded by manufacturing plants.

When the nurse drives into the farm on her way to the housing where workers live, she sees that the fields are being sprayed with pesticides from a truck, and

that white smoke is being emitted from two of the plants. She observes that two young children are riding in the back of the truck. What action should she take?

Answer

At the individual level, she should talk with the owner or manager of the farm and remind him or her of the toxicity of pesticides and the danger to those who are in the vicinity of the spraying. She should recommend that he or she not allow anyone to ride in the open portion of the vehicle and that the driver should leave the window closed and wear a mask to protect his or her nose and mouth. She should also advise the mother to limit the time that the children play outside or ride in an open truck when the farmer is spraying the fields or smoke is being emitted from the plants.

At the systems level, she should identify areas where the workers on the area farms congregate, such as churches, social halls, and so forth. Then she should ask if she could provide an educational program on the dangers of coming into contact with pesticides. She could distribute pamphlets about this hazard in local venues where both farm managers and workers will be able to access them. What else might the nurse do?

CLIMATE CHANGE

Climate change is the result of the Earth's warming because of the blanketing effect that is occurring from gases that are primarily man-made and collectively referred to as "greenhouse gases." For a glimpse into this blanketing effect, consider how quickly the interior of a car warms up when we leave the windows closed. On a day that is 80 degrees outside, a car in full sun can heat up to 99 degrees within just 10 minutes. The ever-increasing man-made gases that are now blanketing the Earth's outer atmosphere are deterring the heat that is being created by the sun from being released, thus creating a "greenhouse effect." As a result, the Earth is slowly warming in the same way a car warms, and this is causing our ice caps to melt, our seas to rise, and our climate to change.

Consider also what a difference a couple of degrees means to a human's health—from a body temperature of 98.6°F (37°C) to 100.4°F (38°C). At 98.6°F we feel fine and our body's systems are fine, not so much starting at 100.4. This is a very narrow temperature range. Almost all living things require air, water, food, and a

particular range of temperature. As the Earth's temperature rises, it is placing a wide range of living organisms—from fish to the California redwoods—at risk. Historically, evolution would allow for plant and animal adaptations, but climate change is occurring so quickly that some life forms will not have time to adapt and therefore not survive the impacts of the temperature changes.

In the United States we have seen some of the earlier climate change predictions materialize: long-term warming trends, extreme weather conditions leading to hurricanes, tornadoes, and other fierce storms, fires, as well as disruption in water supplies, agriculture, ecosystems, coastal communities, and vector distribution (Leffers and Butterfield, 2018). These environmental changes due to climate change have brought about enormous eco-consequences. Disasters related to climate change disproportionately affect the poor and most vulnerable including children; the elderly; the sick, especially those with chronic health conditions; and some minority communities, especially those with language barriers, mental health issues, and lack of access to comprehensive health care (Allen, 2015).

Climate changes around the world lead to global warming. The greenhouse effect is influencing the prevalence of global warming. The greenhouse effect refers to the rise in temperature that occurs when the Earth experiences certain gases in the atmosphere, such as water vapor, carbon dioxide, nitrous oxide, and methane, which trap incoming solar radiation from the sun (Afzal, 2007). A certain amount of the greenhouse effect is essential for human life; however, an excess is dangerous. The goal is to reduce the amount of heat in the environment because high temperatures in the presence of sunlight and certain air pollutants can lead to the formation of ground-level ozone. Increased exposure to ozone is associated with increased risk of premature mortality. This risk supports the growing trend toward actions such as walking rather than driving, recycling, and purchasing energy-efficient cars, appliances, and light bulbs. Remember, electricity is wasted each day when lights are left on, so teach clients to turn off lights when not using them to decrease the amount of carbon dioxide (CO_2) greenhouse gas emissions (Fig. 8.2).

There are two concurrent categories of roles for nurses: mitigation and response. There is still much we can do to mitigate the steep upward slope that we are now observing for temperatures, CO_2 levels, desertification, and seawater levels. Working at the individual, community, institutional (school, hospital, etc.), and governmental levels, there is much work to be done to ensure energy-conserving policies and practices, rational transportation practices, and changes in our consumption patterns.

Regarding response preparation, public health nurses must lead the development of contingencies for long-term, high-heat weather conditions, as well as increased storm activities (that include more severe storm patterns), more extensive fires in areas prone to fires, and the associated disaster preparedness. Often, the recovery from extreme climate change is long and complicated when people lose homes and their possessions and when the community infrastructure, including schools and hospitals, is damaged (Allen, 2015). Standing water and warm temperatures are breeding grounds for mosquitoes, and this can increase the disease burden for humans. Other climate-change events that affect health are extreme heat events, air pollution, airborne allergens, and the mental health risks associated with changes in climate that lead to significant community and health disruption (Allen, 2015). For more on disaster preparedness, see Chapter 16 on nurses' roles in disaster management.

EVIDENCE-BASED PRACTICE

As discussed above, climate change endangers the stability of the planet's ecological systems and poses many risks to human survival. In a policy statement for the American Academy of Nursing, Leffers and Butterfield discuss the impact of climate change and identify ways in which nurses can intervene. The consequences of climate change increase the global burden of disease through the various health conditions described above as well as asthma, sudden cardiac death, premature birth, gastrointestinal illness, depression, malnutrition domestic violence, and vector-borne diseases.

Nurse Use

Nurses play significant roles in both reducing and responding to the health consequences of climate change. In addition to clinical care, nurses are involved in research and in influencing policy decisions about climate change. There are both upstream and downstream opportunities for nurses. Upstream opportunities seek to reduce pollution that would affect future generations. Downstream opportunities focus on climate adaptation and response, helping people in the United States to address the health consequences of climate change.

Leffers J and Butterfield P: Nurses play essential roles in reducing health problems due to climate change, *Nursing Outlook* 66:210–213, 2018.

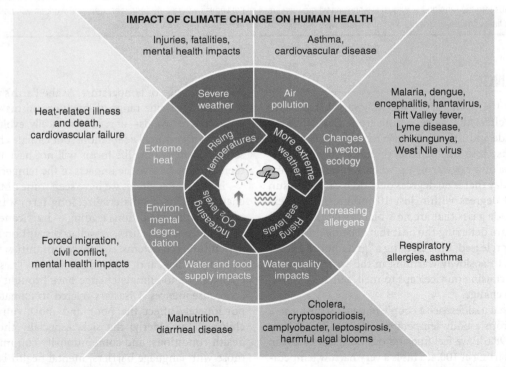

Fig. 8.2 Climate Effects on Health. (From CDC, *Climate and Health*, 2015, www.cdc.gov/climateandhealth/effects/default.htm. Retrieved February 2016.)

The National Environmental Public Health Tracking Network, known as the Tracking Network, is a surveillance system coordinated by the Centers for Disease Control and Prevention (CDC) that collects, integrates, analyzes, interprets, and disseminates data from environmental hazard monitoring and from human exposure and health effects surveillance. At present the CDC is funding 25 states and New York City to build local tracking networks. It is a well-organized and informative source of data on environments and hazards, health effects, and population health (CDC, 2019).

ENVIRONMENTAL HEALTH ASSESSMENT

Environmental health risks can be assessed in various ways. You might assess by environmental factors such as air, water, soil, or food. Or you could assess by setting, such as urban, rural, or suburban. You can also divide the environment into functional locations, such as home, school, workplace, and community. Each of these locations may provide unique environmental exposures and overlapping exposures. For instance, ethylene oxide, the toxic gas used to sterilize equipment in hospitals, is typically found only in a workplace. However, pesticides might be found in all four areas. When assessing environments, determine whether an exposure is in the air, water, soil, or food (or a combination) and whether it is a chemical, biological, or radiological exposure. In any form of assessment, be sure to cover past and present conditions in work, home, and community environments. The How To box demonstrates how to apply the nursing process to environmental health.

HOW TO APPLY THE NURSING PROCESS TO ENVIRONMENTAL HEALTH

If you suspect that a client's health problem is influenced by environmental factors, use the nursing process, noting the environmental aspects of the problem in every step of the process as follows:

1. **Assessment:** Include inventories and history questions that cover environmental issues as a part of the general assessment.
2. **Diagnosis:** Relate the disease and the environmental factors in the diagnosis.
3. **Goal setting:** Include outcome measures that mitigate and eliminate the environmental factors.
4. **Planning:** Look at community policy and laws as methods to facilitate the care needs for the client; include environmental health personnel in the planning.
5. **Intervention:** Coordinate medical, nursing, and public health actions to meet the client's needs.
6. **Evaluation:** Examine criteria that include the immediate and long-term responses of the client, as well as the recidivism of the problem for the client.

When working with individuals, it is important to conduct an environmental health assessment and include questions to assess exposure. One site to use to search for assessments is the Environmental Protection Agency (EPA). For example, see "Guidelines for human exposure assessment" at www.epa.gov.

This assessment was updated in October 2019. A useful nursing exposure was originally prepared by Grace Paranzino, RN, MPH, for the Agency for Toxic Substances and Disease Registry and was updated by Paranzino, Butterfield, Nastoff, and Ranger (2005). A mnemonic was developed to help health professionals remember the questions to ask when taking an environmental history and determine the environmental exposure history. Exposures may occur in any setting in which people spend time; be sure to assess them all. The "I PREPARE" mnemonic can be used when assessing an individual, family, or community. This tool suggests that you do an exposure history to (1) identify current or past exposures; (2) reduce or eliminate current exposures; and (3) reduce adverse health effects. Here is what the letters in "I PREPARE" refer to:

1. I-Investigate potential exposures
2. P-Present work
3. R-Residence
4. E-Environmental concerns
5. P-Past work
6. A-Activities
7. R-Referrals and resources
8. E-Educate (Box 8.2)

A windshield survey is a helpful first step to understanding the potential environmental health risks in a community. If the community is urban, the age and condition of the housing and potential trash problems (and the associated pest problems) can be easily determined by driving around the neighborhood. Note also the proximity to factories, dumpsites, major transportation routes, and other sources of pollution.

In rural communities, pay attention to the use of aerial and other types of pesticide and herbicide spraying. Do people use wood-burning stoves? Do you see or suspect contaminated waterways, and are there industrial-type, large-scale animal feeding facilities that might contribute to pollution?

In addition to the tools used for a general community assessment, some specific tools are available to detect the environmental health risks within a community. The Right to Know section of the chapter describes the types of information available to the public about air and water emissions, drinking water quality, and other environmental sources. Observe also for positive environmental factors such as green spaces in parks and gardens, bike and walking paths, and water features. Two useful web sites that help identify environmental health risks are EnviroFACTs and ToxTown. Using a zip code at EnviroFACTS on the EPA website, you can identify air, land, water, waste, toxic radiation, facilities, compliance, and soil pollution in your area. This site is regularly updated (www.enviro.epa.gov). A second useful site is ToxTown, which is hosted by the National Library of Medicine (NLM). This site provides "information on everyday locations and situations, where you might be exposed to toxic chemicals." It helps consumers understand the risks of exposure, potential health effects, and how to protect themselves. In 2020, the site began adding timely information about COVID-19 (ToxTown.nlm.nih,gov).

BOX 8.2 The "I PREPARE" Mnemonic

An exposure history should identify current and past exposures, have a preliminary goal of reducing or eliminating current exposures, and have a long-term goal of reducing adverse health effects. The "I PREPARE" mnemonic consigns the important questions to categories that can be easily remembered.

I Investigate Potential Exposures
Investigate potential exposures by asking,
- Have you ever felt sick after coming in contact with a chemical, pesticide, or other substance?
- Do you have any symptoms that improve when you are away from your home or work?

P Present Work
At your present work,
- Are you exposed to solvents, dust, fumes, radiation, loud noise, pesticides, or other chemicals?
- Do you know where to find material data safety sheets on the chemicals with which you work?
- Do you wear personal protective equipment?
- Are work clothes worn home?
- Do coworkers have similar health problems?

R Residence
At your place of residence,
- When was your residence built?
- What type of heating do you have?
- Have you recently remodeled your home?
- What chemicals are stored on your property?
- Where does your drinking water come from?

E Environmental Concerns
In your living environment,
- Are there environmental concerns in your neighborhood (i.e., air, water, soil)?

- What types of industries or farms are near your home?
- Do you live near a hazardous waste site or landfill?

P Past Work
About your past work,
- What are your past work experiences?
- What is the longest job you held?
- Have you ever been in the military, worked on a farm, or done volunteer or seasonal work?

A Activities
About your activities,
- What activities and hobbies do you and your family engage in?
- Do you burn, solder, or melt any products?
- Do you garden, fish, or hunt?
- Do you eat what you catch or grow?
- Do you use pesticides?
- Do you engage in any alternative healing or cultural practices?

R Referrals and Resources
Use these key referrals and resources:
- Environmental Protection Agency (http://www.epa.gov)
- National Library of Medicine, TOXNET programs (http://www.nlm.nih.gov)
- Agency for Toxic Substances and Disease Registry (http://www.atsdr.cdc.gov)
- Association of Occupational and Environmental Clinics (http://www.aoec.org)
- Occupational Safety and Health Administration (http://www.osha.gov)
- Local health department, environmental agency, poison control center

E Educate
Use this checklist of educational materials:
- Are materials available to educate the client?
- Are alternatives available to minimize the risk for exposure?
- Have prevention strategies been discussed?
- What is the plan for follow-up?

Prepared by Grace Paranzino, RN, MPH, for the Agency for Toxic Substances and Disease Registry (ATSDR). For more information, contact ATSDR at 1-888-42-ATSDR, or visit the ATSDR's website at http://www.atsdr.cdc.gov.

AIR

Air pollution is a significant contributor to health problems. Air pollution is divided into two major categories: point sources, often called fixed sites, which are individual, identifiable sites, such as smokestacks, and nonpoint sources, which include vehicles, such as cars, trucks, and buses and come from more diffuse exposures. The Clean Air Act regulates air pollution from both point sources and nonpoint sources. Motor vehicles are the greatest single source of air pollution in the United States. The burning of fossil fuels (diesel, industrial boilers, and coal-fired power plants) and waste incineration are two other major contributors. The single greatest source of mercury in our air is coal-fired power plants. Health effects associated with air pollution include asthma and other respiratory diseases, cardiovascular diseases (including heart disease and hypertension), cancer, immunological effects, reproductive health problems (including birth defects), infant deaths, and neurological problems (Smargiassi et al, 2014). According to WHO (2019), approximately 235 million people suffer from asthma; it is common among children, and the strongest risk

factors are genetic factors and inhaled substances and particles that provoke an allergic response or irritate the airways. In the United States, over 26 million people have asthma including 6.1 million children. There is no cure for asthma, but according to the American Lung Association (April 2020), it can be managed (www.lung.org).

Also, many people do not know that a pea-sized amount of mercury is sufficient to contaminate a 25-acre lake and make its fish unfit to eat. Mercury, like lead, is an element, and it persists in the fresh waterways and oceans from which we continue to get our fish. We cannot readily take these elements out once they have been released into the environment; our job is to focus on policies that prevent them from being released. The greatest single source of mercury in our air comes from coal-fired power plants.

Indoor air quality in the workplace, schools, and homes is a growing concern because of the alarming rise in the incidence of asthma in the United States, particularly among children. Both the EPA and the American Lung Association provide excellent materials on indoor air quality. The EPA has a free kit called Indoor Air Quality: Tools for Schools, which includes a video and materials to help people improve the air quality in a

Air Quality Index Levels of Health Concern	Numerical Value	Meaning
Good	0 to 50	Air quality is considered satisfactory, and air pollution poses little or no risk.
Moderate	51 to 100	Air quality is acceptable; however, for some pollutants there may be a moderate health concern for a very small number of people who are unusually sensitive to air pollution.
Unhealthy for Sensitive Groups	101 to 150	Members of sensitive groups may experience health effects. The general public is not likely to be affected.
Unhealthy	151 to 200	Everyone may begin to experience health effects; members of sensitive groups may experience more serious health effects.
Very Unhealthy	201 to 300	Health alert: everyone may experience more serious health effects.
Hazardous	301 to 500	Health warnings of emergency conditions. The entire population is more likely to be affected.

Fig. 8.3 **Air Pollution Can Be Categorized by Health Risks for the Public.** This color coding is used by schools, during weather reports, and other public information sources. (From US Environmental Protection Agency. Available at: https://airnow.gov/index.cfm?action=aqibasics.aqi.)

school building. The major culprits contributing to poor indoor air are carbon monoxide, dust, molds, dust mites, cockroaches, pests and pets, cleaning and personal care products (particularly aerosols), lead, and, of course, environmental tobacco smoke. It is important to assess both the environmental exposures and the human health status in a community. Fig. 8.3 provides a useful way to determine the air quality in a locality and the implications for health. Health status is assessed using local, state, and national health data; by collecting our own data; or by a combination of the two.

Carbon monoxide is a particularly dangerous gas that can be emitted into the air. It is an odorless, colorless, tasteless gas that is produced when carbon-containing fuels, such as oil, kerosene, coal, or wood, are not completely combusted; it can also build up as a result of inadequate natural gas ventilation. Poisoning by carbon monoxide occurs most often in the fall and winter when buildings are being heated. When teaching clients how to avoid exposure to carbon monoxide, be sure to advise them to be aware of the possibility of faulty furnaces, motor vehicles, stoves and gas ranges, and vented gas heaters, which are common sources of carbon monoxide poisoning (Rosenthal, 2006). Because carbon monoxide is so difficult to detect, it is the leading cause of death attributable to poisoning in industrialized nations.

Fracking or hydraulic fracturing is a "process of extracting oil and gas from the Earth by drilling deep wells and injecting a mixture of liquids and chemicals at high pressure (Environmental Health News, 2019). Some of the chemicals used are carcinogenic and toxic and are linked to cancer, gastrointestinal, circulatory, developmental, and neurological disorders (Alliance of Nurses for Healthy Environments {ANHE}, 2017). Fracking chemicals have polluted drinking water and air. Drinking water is most likely to be affected by fracking if it is from private drinking water wells, and the persons most affected by the hazardous air emissions are those with preexisting pulmonary conditions, children, and pregnant women (ANHE, 2017).

WATER

Water is necessary for all forms of life. Human bodies are 70% water. Only 2.5% of the water on this planet is fresh water; saltwater comprises the rest. Much of the freshwater is in the ice of the polar icecaps; groundwater makes up most of what remains, leaving only 0.01% in lakes, creeks, streams, rivers, and rainfall. People's lives are tied to a safe and adequate water supply. Water is necessary for the production of food. In the United States, all public water supplies must test their water in accordance with the EPA's safe drinking water standards and summarize their findings in a *Consumer Confidence Report* (CCR) that is provided to customers annually by July 1st.

Discharges into water bodies from industries, pharmaceuticals for people and animals, and from wastewater treatment systems can contribute to the degradation of water quality. Water quality is also affected by nonpoint sources of pollution, such as storm water runoff from paved roads and parking lots, erosion from clear-cut tracts of land (after timbering and mining), and runoff from chemicals added to soil, such as fertilizers.

LAND

Past and present use of land can affect a community's health. Local governments determine land use through their zoning laws. For example, a zoning law would prevent a housing development from being built on top of a previously used landfill that is now filled in and may look attractive. There are two designations for land that may be contaminated: Superfund sites (highly contaminated sites with associated health risks that are designated by the EPA) and brownfield sites (land that has been used previously that may have contaminated soil and is now slated for redevelopment). Funds are available through both the Superfund and brownfield laws to engage the community and do health assessments.

There seems to be a correlation between the way in which communities are configured and obesity. That is, does the community encourage and support walking or bike riding? Can people shop without needing to do so via a motor vehicle? How long is the average commute time or can people walk to school or work? Is the environment totally built up, and concrete, not grass, covers much of the area?

FOOD

Food and food production are a source of concern. In recent years, foodborne illnesses have been associated with *Salmonella* and *Escherichia coli* O157:H7 in foods such as chicken, eggs, and meats. Good food preparation practices, such as washing and adequate cooking temperature and time, can prevent foodborne illnesses associated with most pathogens. Local health departments are responsible for monitoring food establishments (restaurants, food trucks, etc.) in the community, and the US Department of Agriculture is responsible for oversight of meat, poultry, fish, and produce production. Food safety was highlighted in the news during 2020 when more than one meat packaging plant had a large number of workers who tested positive for COVID-19. A major factor was the close proximity in which workers stood to one another while cutting and handling the meat. Also, when restaurants were allowed to open, rules about cleanliness, mask wearing, and proximity in which customers were allowed to sit were developed.

However, there are also environmental health risks posed by the presence of pesticide residues in our food; the use of recombinant bovine growth hormone (rBGH), which is given to many dairy cows; the administration of antibiotics to beef cattle, pigs, and chickens at nontherapeutic doses that are given to promote growth; and the use of genetically modified organisms (GMOs) for genetically engineered crops.

It is important that nurses understand the term "organic" regarding food labeling. If a food is labeled "Certified Organic," this is a meaningful term that has a legal US Department of Agriculture (USDA) definition. For foods to carry the Certified Organic label, they must have been produced without the use of pesticides, GMOs, or unnecessary (nontherapeutic) antibiotics. If a food is merely labeled "organic," the consumer does not have the same guarantee regarding what chemicals or farming practices have been used. When purchasing foods directly from farmers through farm stands or farmers' markets, consumers can directly ask about the chemicals and farm practices.

THE RIGHT TO KNOW

Several environmental statutes give the public the right to know about hazardous chemicals in the environment. One of the right-to-know laws allows health professionals and community members to access, by zip code, information regarding major sources of pollution being emitted into the air or water in their community. As previously discussed, the EPA "Envirofacts" section on its website provides data on sources of exposure by typing in a zip code. Also, consumer confidence reports (CCR) evaluate water supplies. Nurses should review CCRs, sometimes referred to as *right-to-know reports*, to learn what pollutants have been found in the drinking water. If the drinking water poses an immediate health threat, the water provider must send emergency warnings to the community via the local newspapers, radio, and television. The Freedom of Information Act is a federal law that allows citizens to request public documents.

Employees have the right to know, through the federal Hazard Communication Standard, about the hazardous chemicals with which they work. This standard requires employers (including hospitals) to maintain a list of all hazardous chemicals used on site. Each of these chemicals should have an associated chemical information sheet, known as a *material safety data sheet* (MSDS), written by the chemical manufacturer. These safety sheets, available to any employee or his or her representative, should provide information about the chemical makeup, the health risks, and any special guidance on safe use and handling (e.g., requirements for protective gloves or respiratory protection). For more information on workplace health and safety, see http://www.osha.gov.

RISK ASSESSMENT

Currently, the EPA uses the process of risk assessment when it develops health-based standards. The term risk assessment refers to a process to determine the probability of a health threat associated with an exposure. The following discussion describes the four phases of a risk assessment related to chemical exposures.

First, by accessing toxicological or epidemiological data, determine whether a chemical is known to be associated with negative health effects (in animals or humans). Remember, the available toxicological data will probably be based on animal studies (from which the potential effects on humans are estimated), whereas the results of the epidemiological studies will be for human health effects.

Second, determine whether the chemical has been released into the environment via the air, water, soil, or food. Environmental professionals, such as sanitarians, food inspectors, air and water pollution scientists, meteorologists, environmental engineers, and others, can test for the presence of the suspected chemical in the various media (air, water, soil, food). In performing a risk assessment, determine whether multiple sources of the questionable chemical are present. For example, is lead found in the drinking water, in the ambient air, and in the paint in houses in a given community? If so, the lead will have a cumulative effect and be more of a danger.

In the third phase, estimate how much of the chemical might enter the human body and by which route. This estimate can be based on a one-time exposure, a short-term exposure, or a projected lifetime exposure. Federal standards created for air, water, and other pollutants are based on an estimation of a lifetime exposure. However, in workplace settings, the chemical exposure standards are based on an average exposure during a typical work shift or are set for a maximum exposure at any given time.

The final stage of the risk assessment process takes into account all three of the previous steps and asks the following questions:

• Is the chemical toxic?
• What are the source and amount of the exposure?
• What are the route and duration of the exposure for humans?

The goal is to try to predict the potential for harm on the basis of the estimated exposure. Like all science, risk assessment is subject to interpretation, and there may be more than one interpretation for each step, which could lead to different recommendations. Also, environmental laws are often contentious not only because of public or ecological health concerns but also because economic interests are at stake. Remember that for persons to be harmed by something in the environment, the following factors must be in place and connected:

1. A source of harm that has chemical and/or physical properties
2. An environmental medium for transport—air, water (i.e., surface water or groundwater), or soil
3. A receptor population within the exposure pathway for harm to human health
4. A route of exposure (for humans, these are inhalation, ingestion, and skin absorption)
5. An adequate amount (dose) of the chemical to result in human harm

ASSESSING ENVIRONMENTAL HEALTH RISKS IN CHILDREN

Toxic chemicals can have different effects depending on the timing of exposure. During fetal development, there are periods of heightened sensitivity to the effects of toxic chemicals. During such times, even extraordinarily small exposures can prevent or change a process that may permanently affect normal development. The brain undergoes rapid structural and functional changes during late pregnancy and in the neonatal period. Therefore it is extremely important to safeguard women's environments when they are pregnant.

Fish are a lean, low-calorie, high-quality source of protein. They contain essential nutrients, omega-3 fatty acids, and are low in saturated fats. However, some fish and shellfish (e.g., clams and oysters) may contain chemicals or illness-causing microorganisms like bacteria and viruses that could pose health risks. When the level of contaminants is unsafe, people may be advised to reduce or avoid eating certain fish caught in specific locations. All 50 states and some US territories and tribes issue advisories to tell which fish they can safely eat (EPA, January 3, 2020).

Nurses need to understand the implications that the fish advisories have for their clients and communities while at the same time counseling on the positive contribution of fish to a nutritionally balanced diet. Because more than 100,000 chemicals are used in the world, it is important to understand the possible effects on health.

Companies are not required to divulge all of the results of their private testing. A full battery of neurotoxicity tests is not required even for pesticides that may be sprayed in nurseries and labor and delivery areas, not to mention in homes. To make things even more complicated, risks from multiple chemical exposures are rarely considered when regulations are drafted. Such an omission ignores the reality that both children and adults are exposed to many toxic chemicals, often concurrently. The only exception to this rule is in the case of regulations regarding pesticides that are used on food (Fig. 8.4). This exception was created by the 1996 Food Quality Protection Act, in which Congress acknowledged that children eat foods that may be contaminated by more than one pesticide residue.

Children are especially at risk for environmental hazards because of factors such as poverty, lack of access to health care, and the dangerous environmental situations in which they may live. Children are also at risk because of their size and the immaturity of their systems, such as the respiratory system. Infants and young children breathe more rapidly than adults, and this increase in respiratory rate leads to a proportionately greater exposure to air pollutants. While infants' lungs are developing, they are particularly susceptible to environmental toxicants. Although full function of the lungs is attained at approximately age 6, changes continue to occur in the lungs through adolescence (Fudvoye, et al., 2014; Hsu et al., 2015). Children are short, and thus their breathing zones are lower than those of adults, causing them to have closer contact with the chemical and biological agents on floors, carpeting, and the ground. Children are also at risk during disasters. For example, after Hurricane Katrina, a risk for children was inhaling the

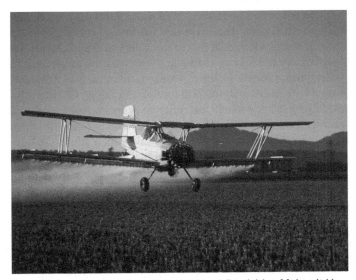

Fig. 8.4 Aerial Application of Agricultural Pesticides Makes It Very Difficult to Control Exposures. The chemicals get tracked into homes of farming communities. (Copyright 2011 Photos.com, a division of Getty Images. All rights reserved. Photo #87531230.)

dangerous toxins from tar balls. Because children are shorter than adults, they were thus closer to the ground and subsequently closer to tar balls than were adults, with greater risk of inhalation. Brief exposure to the crude oil in tar balls can lead to contact dermatitis and skin rashes; longer exposure can lead to erythema, edema, and burning. Gastrointestinal and respiratory effects of this exposure also can occur (Murray, 2011). Children of color and poor children in America are disproportionately affected by a range of environmental health threats, including lead exposure, air pollution, pesticides, incinerator emissions, industrial and agricultural chemicals, and exposures from hazardous waste sites (Suk and Davis, 2008).

Some of the health conditions in children that are associated with environmental factors include autism spectrum disorder; cancer; respiratory diseases, including asthma; obesity; and problems in neurodevelopment (American Cancer Society [ACS], 2016; CDC, 2016). In regard to cancer, only a small percentage of childhood cancers are associated with heredity. However, exposure to ionizing radiation increases the risk of childhood leukemia and possibly other cancers. All of the causes of autism spectrum disorder are not currently known. Environmental factors are thought to be a possible cause, as are biologic and genetic factors. Clearly, the environment plays an important role in children's health. Think about this question: When building a school, should the government require the same environmental assessment of the land as it would if a commercial enterprise, like a hotel, was being placed on the same site? Currently, it requires less stringent environmental assessments.

Children's bodies also operate differently. Some of the protective mechanisms that are well developed in adults, like the blood-brain barrier, are immature in young children, thereby increasing their vulnerability to the effects of toxic chemicals. Finally, the kidneys of young children are less effective at filtering out undesirable toxic chemicals, and these chemicals then continue to circulate and accumulate.

Infants and young children drink more fluids per body weight than adults do, and this increases the dose of contaminants in their drinking water, milk (hormones and antibiotics), and juices (particularly pesticides). If an adult were to drink an amount of water proportionate to the amount an infant drinks, the adult would have to drink about 50 glasses of water a day. Children also eat more per body weight, eat different proportions of food, and absorb food differently from adults. Children consume much greater quantities of fruits and fruit juices than adults do, once again adding exposure to doses of pesticide residues.

REDUCING ENVIRONMENTAL HEALTH RISKS

Preventing problems is less costly, whether the cost is measured in resources consumed or health effects. Education is a primary preventive strategy. When examining the sources of environmental health risks in communities and planning intervention strategies, it is important to apply the basic principles of disease prevention. For a home with lead-based paint, apply the primary prevention strategy of removing that specific source of lead. Good surveillance, a secondary prevention strategy, will not prevent lead exposure, but it may help with early identification of rising blood lead levels. For a symptomatic child brought to a health care provider, a system should be in place for specialists familiar with lead poisoning to provide immediate care; swift medical interventions to reduce blood levels of lead can reduce the risk of further harm. This might be a tertiary prevention response.

For workplace exposures, industrial hygienists have developed a list of precautions for avoiding or minimizing employee exposures to potentially hazardous chemicals. Industrial hygienists are public health professionals who specialize in workplace exposures to hazards—physical, chemical, and biological—that create conditions of health risk (Box 8.3). Once it is established that a human health threat exists, develop a plan of action to eliminate or manage (reduce) the risk. Risk management, which should be informed by the risk assessment process, involves the selection and implementation of a strategy to reduce risks, which can take many forms. For example, the "Three R's for Reducing Environmental Pollution" are as follows:

1. **Reduce:** Reducing consumption reduces waste and unnecessary packaging and nonessentials.
2. **Reuse:** Choosing reusable rather than disposable products creates less waste (e.g., using glass dishes and plastic or metal straws rather than paper ones).
3. **Recycle:** Recycling paper, glass, cans, and plastic decreases pollution.

Risk assessment includes considering ways to dispose of materials. Once waste products are generated, they must be disposed of in one of the following three ways:

1. **Incineration:** Burning can change the chemical composition through heat, but the products of burning, such as ash and air emissions, must be controlled and disposed of using one of the following two options.
2. **Water discharge:** When products are disposed of in water, the water must be treated to ensure that the dose in the water is not great enough to do harm.
3. **Landfilling or burying in soil:** When using landfills or burying products, protections must be put in place, such as liners and leachate pumps and monitors, to avoid seepage of harmful doses into the groundwater or air.

Each of the options for waste disposal is intended to provide a way either to alter the waste product to a less toxic form through chemical intervention (biodegradation) or to store the product in a biounavailable form or place. Because all of the options for disposal can be a problem, prevention is desirable.

BOX 8.3   Industrial Hygiene Controls

- Substitute less hazardous or nonhazardous substances for hazardous ones (e.g., use water-based instead of solvent-based products).
- Isolate the hazardous chemicals from human exposure (closed systems).
- Apply engineering controls (e.g., ventilation systems, including exhausts).
- Reduce the exposures through administrative controls (rotating employees).
- Use personal protective equipment (gloves, respirators, protective clothing).
- Educate employees about controls.

From Levy B, Wegman D, Baron S, Sokas RK: *Occupational and environmental health*, ed 7, New York, NY, 2017, Oxford University Press.

Remember that human effects are intensified in the most sensitive, vulnerable environments, such as estuaries, the nurseries for much of sea and coastal plant and animal life. Some of the most valued food sources are also the most sensitive to pollution. Shellfish are efficient filters of contaminants in the water in which they live. For example, oysters filter and retain almost all contaminants from the water in which they grow. It is impossible to rid them of contaminants after harvesting. The only protection for humans is to grow oysters in environments free from harmful contamination. Safe seafood depends on clean water.

Another form of risk reduction is to reduce the risk from exposure to ultraviolet rays. People need to avoid being outside during peak sun hours and need to wear protective clothing and/or sunblock. To reduce exposure to dangerous heavy metals, special processes can be used at the water filtration plant that supplies the public water. In the home, running the cold water tap for 1 or 2 minutes each morning before collecting water for coffee or drinking will reduce the presence of lead that may have leached from old pipes (or the solder used on them) overnight. In communities that report to the media the local pollution levels, it is important to encourage residents to not exercise or walk excessively outside when the air pollution index is high. Individuals, communities, and nations can reduce risks. In recent years, there have been global agreements to reduce persistent pollutants and decrease global warming. However, not all nations are subscribing to this goal. The national and international news provide many examples of extreme pollution around the world. See WHO, 2020 for ways to intervene in unhealthy environments.

LEVELS OF PREVENTION

Related to the Environment: Lead Exposure

Primary Prevention
Use only non–lead-based paint.

Secondary Prevention
If lead is found in paint, remove this paint and replace with nonlead paint.

Tertiary Prevention
At the first sign of symptoms of lead exposure, take steps to reduce blood lead levels.

Nursing interventions to reduce environmental health risks can also take many forms. Education is a key nursing action. By working with a variety of community members, nurses can explain the relationship between harmful environmental exposures and human health and guide the community toward risk reduction based on both changes in individual behavior and community-wide approaches. For example, a nurse could help clients know how important it is to purchase a carbon monoxide detector. The detectors are designed to measure carbon monoxide levels over time and sound an alarm when the levels reach a specific point. These devices are sold in many stores in the United States.

RISK COMMUNICATION

Risk is a familiar term in nursing practice. We counsel people about risks of pregnancy, communicable disease (especially sexually transmitted disease), intentional and unintentional injury, and personal health-related choices (e.g., smoking, alcohol consumption, diet). Risk assessment in environmental health has focused on characterizing the hazard (i.e., the source), its physical and chemical properties, its toxicity, and the presence of (or potential for) other elements in the exposure pathway—mode of transmission, route of exposure, receptor population, and dose. Risk is typically viewed as the process of estimating the likelihood of an unwanted adverse effect and the probable magnitude and intensity of that effect. For example, an environmental risk assessment of a contaminated site includes a calculation of the dose that might be received through all routes of exposure, the toxicity of the chemical, the size and vulnerability (e.g., age, health) of the population potentially exposed (e.g., resident, future resident, transient), and the likelihood of exposure.

Communication of risk is both an area of practice and a skill. It involves understanding the outrage factors relevant to the risk being addressed so that both can be incorporated in the message, with the result that either action is taken to ensure safety or unnecessary fear is reduced. Outrage factors are those things that cause people to feel a sense of outrage toward a behavior. An example of raising outrage to produce action can be seen in the way people respond to smokers who smoke in public. Because of the fear of secondhand or involuntary, passive smoking, people have advocated to stimulate public policy that limits or bans smoking in public places. When the emphasis on risk went from a voluntary choice of smokers to an involuntary exposure of nonsmokers, the outrage level of the nonsmoking public became high enough to result in legislation guaranteeing smoke-free public spaces (e.g., public buildings, airplanes, restaurants). On the other hand, outrage diminishes when people obtain information about a situation from a trusted source, and nurses are often cited in surveys as trusted sources of information on environmental risks. During the COVID-19 pandemic, there were at least two types of outrage factors: those when people did not wear masks and gloves when they were asked to do so or when they did not practice social distancing in public places. In contrast, some people demonstrated when they were asked to social distance and when their jobs were curtailed due to the virus.

Risk communication includes general principles of good communication. It is a combination of the following:
- *The right information:* Accurate, relevant, and in a language that audiences can understand. It is important to keep the information as concise as possible to ensure that people will read or listen to it.
- *To the right people:* Those affected and those who may not be affected but are worried. Information about the community is essential and includes geographic boundaries, who lives there (demographics), how they get information (i.e., flyers, newspapers, radio, television, the Internet, text messages, word of mouth), where they get together (i.e., school, church,

community center), and who within the community can help plan the communication.

- *At the right time:* For timely action or to allay fear. Risk communication is not a one-time event; it is an ongoing process.

There is also a component of ethics involved in risk communication. The public health goal would likely ask individuals to sacrifice some of their self-interests to benefit the greater good of more people. This could be seen when companies are asked to reduce air or water pollution, even though it might be expensive for them to do so, to protect the health of the people who might be affected. This was clearly seen during the COVID-19 epidemic when businesses were required to close to prevent the spread of the disease. As discussed in Chapter 6, understanding ethics is essential for nurses making their own choices, in describing issues and options within groups, and in advocating for ethical choices. When the sticking points are around competing commodities (e.g., jobs versus environmental protection, production versus conservation, economic development versus the health of the environment), the skillful nurse can change the discussion from "either/or" to "both" by opening new possibilities for ethical and mutually satisfactory outcomes. The following ethical issues may arise in environmental health decisions:

- Who has access to information and when and in what format?
- How complete and accurate is the available information?
- Who is included in decision making and when?
- What and whose values and priorities are given weight in decisions?
- How are short-term and long-term consequences considered?

A review of ethical issues in Chapter 6 may help nurses decide what actions they could and should take in regard to environmental health issues.

GOVERNMENT ENVIRONMENTAL PROTECTION

The federal government is involved with many major pieces of environmental legislation (Box 8.4). The government manages environmental exposures through the development and enforcement of standards and regulations that limit a polluter's ability to put hazardous chemicals into our food, water, air, or soil. The government may also be involved in educating the public about risks and risk reduction. Several federal agencies are involved in environmental health regulation, including the EPA, the Food and Drug Administration, and the Department of Agriculture. In every state, an equivalent state agency exists as well. The local health department may manage environmental health issues at the city or county level. However, environmental protection issues are typically directed by the state using both federal and state laws. The organization and approach to environmental protection vary somewhat among states, but the common essential strategies of prevention and control via the permitting process, establishment of environmental standards, and monitoring, as well as compliance and enforcement, are found in every state.

Potentially harmful pollution that cannot be prevented must be controlled. The first step in the process of controlling pollution is permitting, a process by which the government places limits on the amount of pollution emitted into the air or water.

Industries and businesses whose processes will result in releases (i.e., discharges, emissions) that have the potential for harm are required to obtain environmental permits to construct and operate. A permit is a legally binding document. A range of permits may be required (e.g., stormwater control, construction, operations for air and wastewater discharges, waste management). It is in the permitting process that maximum opportunities to incorporate prevention strategies can be exercised. For example, waste minimization can be included as a permit condition with the agreement of the industry, even if it is not required by law or through regulation.

The permitting process includes submission of an application, which requires details on the proposed operation. During the process, plans are studied, engineering processes are modeled and validated, and technical requirements are reviewed by appropriate regulatory experts. Usually some form of public participation is required or included voluntarily. The public involvement can include public notice, public comment, and public meetings and hearings initiated by the regulatory agency. Public involvement also can take the form of voluntary agreements and dispute resolution between the industry and the community, which may or may not involve a government entity. Limits on what an industry or business can release or emit lawfully are based on environmental standards.

Environmental standards may be expressed as a permitted level of emissions, a maximum contaminant level allowed, an action level for environmental cleanup, or a risk-based calculation. A standard often reflects the level of pollution that will limit a number of excess deaths at a given level of exposure over a specified period. It is the responsibility of the polluters to operate within the standards. Compliance and enforcement are the next steps for controlling pollutions. Compliance refers to the processes for ensuring that permit and standard requirements are met. Cleanup or remediation of environmental damage is another control step. Public information and involvement processes, such as citizen advisory panels or community forums, are integral to the development of standards, ongoing monitoring, and remediation. Monitoring procedures, which must use methods approved by the EPA or scientific consensus, must follow accepted protocols (e.g., maintaining a documented chain of custody of samples to ensure accuracy and protection from contamination at the laboratory after sampling).

ADVOCACY

The more than 3 million nurses in the United States today can and should be a strong voice for their clients. As informed citizens, nurses can work to protect the environmental health of clients, families, and communities. Nurses are seen as trusted sources of information, and they need to serve as reliable sources of environmental health information. They can act in the best interest of public health and use their abilities as educators, advocates, and communicators to affect public policy, laws, and regulations that protect public health. Nurses can serve as a resource for state and federal legislators and their staff. Often, legislators are asked to vote on environmental legislation without a sound understanding of how the legislation may affect

BOX 8.4 Environmental Laws

National Environmental Policy Act (NEPA)

The NEPA established the Environmental Protection Agency (EPA) and a national policy for the environment and provides for the establishment of a Council on Environmental Policy. All policies, regulations, and public laws shall be interpreted and administered in accordance with the policies set forth in this act.

Federal Insecticide, Fungicide, and Rodenticide Act (FIFRA)

FIFRA provides federal control of pesticide distribution, sale, and use. The EPA was given the authority to study the consequences of pesticide usage and requires users such as farmers and utility companies to register when using pesticides. Later amendments to the law required applicators to take certification examinations, registration of all pesticides used in the United States, and proper labeling of pesticides that, if in accordance with specifications, will cause no harm to the environment (summary from FIFRA, 1972).

Clean Water Act (CWA)

The CWA sets basic structure for regulating pollutants to US waters. The law gave the EPA the authority to set effluent standards on an industry basis and continued the requirements to set water quality standards for all contaminants in surface water. The 1977 amendments focused on toxic pollutants. In 1987 the CWA was reauthorized and again focused on toxic pollutants, authorized citizen suit provisions, and funded sewage treatment plants.

Clean Air Act

The Clean Air Act regulates air emissions from area, stationary, and mobile sources. The EPA was authorized to establish National Ambient Air Quality Standards (NAAQSs) to protect public health and the environment. The goal was to set and achieve the NAAQSs by 1975. The law was amended in 1977 when many areas of the country failed to meet the standards. The 1990 amendments to the Clean Air Act intended to meet unaddressed or insufficiently addressed problems, such as acid rain, ground-level ozone, stratospheric ozone depletion, and air toxins. Also in the 1990 reauthorization, a mandate for Chemical Risk Management Plans was included. This mandate requires industry to identify "worst-case scenarios" regarding the hazardous chemicals that they transport, use, or discard (summary from Clean Air Act, 1970).

Occupational Safety and Health Act (OSHA)

The OSHA was passed to ensure worker and workplace safety. The goal was to make sure employers provide an employment place free of hazards to health and safety, such as chemicals, excessive noise, mechanical dangers, heat or cold extremes, or unsanitary conditions. To establish standards for the workplace, the act also created the National Institute for Occupational Safety and Health (NIOSH) as the research institution for OSHA.

Safe Drinking Water Act (SDWA)

The SDWA was established to protect the quality of drinking water in the United States. The SDWA authorized the EPA to establish safe standards of purity and required all owners or operators of public water systems to comply with primary (health-related) standards.

Resource Conservation and Recovery Act (RCRA)

The RCRA gave the EPA the authority to control the generation, transportation, treatment, storage, and disposal of hazardous waste. The RCRA also proposed a framework to manage nonhazardous waste. The 1984 Federal Hazardous and Solid Waste Amendments to this act required phasing out land disposal of hazardous waste. The 1986 amendments enabled the EPA to address problems from underground tanks storing petroleum and other hazardous substances.

Toxic Substances Control Act (TSCA)

The TSCA gives the EPA the ability to track the 75,000 industrial chemicals currently produced or imported into the United States. The EPA can require reporting or testing of chemicals that may pose environmental health risks and can ban the manufacture and import of those chemicals that pose an unreasonable risk. TSCA supplements the Clean Air Act and the Toxic Release Inventory.

Comprehensive Environmental Response, Compensation, and Liability Act (CERCLA or Superfund)

This law created a tax on the chemical and petroleum industries and provided broad federal authority to respond directly to releases or threatened releases of hazardous substances that may endanger public health or the environment.

Superfund Amendments and Reauthorization Act (SARA)

SARA amended the CERCLA with several changes and additions. These changes included increased size of the trust fund, encouragement of greater citizen participation in decision making on how sites should be cleaned up, increased state involvement in every phase of the Superfund program, increased focus on human health problems related to hazardous waste sites, new enforcement authorities and settlement tools, emphasis on the importance of permanent remedies and innovative treatment technologies in cleanup of hazardous waste sites, and superfund actions to consider standards in other federal and state regulations. (Under Superfund legislation, the Federal Agency for Toxic Substances and Disease Registry was established.)

Emergency Planning and Community Right to Know Act (EPCRA)

The EPCRA, also known as Title III of SARA, was enacted to help local communities protect public health safety and the environment from chemical hazards. Each state was required to appoint a State Emergency Response Commission that was required to divide the state into Emergency Planning Districts and establish a Local Emergency Planning Committee (LEPC) for each district.

National Environmental Education Act

The National Environmental Education Act created a new and better coordinated environmental education emphasis at the EPA. It created the National Environmental Education and Training Foundation.

Pollution Prevention Act (PPA)

The PPA focused industry, government, and public attention on reduction of the amount of pollution through cost-effective changes in production, operation, and use of raw materials. Pollution prevention also includes other practices that increase efficient use of energy, water, and other water resources, such as recycling, source reduction, and sustainable agriculture.

Food Quality Protection Act (FQPA)

The FQPA amended the Federal Insecticide, Fungicide, and Rodenticide Act and the Federal Food, Drug, and Cosmetic Act. FQPA changed the way the EPA regulates pesticides. The requirements included a new safety standard of reasonable certainty of no harm to be applied to all pesticides used on foods.

Chemical Safety Information, Site Security, and Fuels Regulatory Act (Amendment to Section 112 of the Clean Air Act)

This act removed from coverage by the Risk Management Plan (RMP) any flammable fuel when used as fuel or held for sale as fuel by a retail facility (flammable fuels used as a feedstock or held for sale as a fuel at a wholesale facility are still covered). The law also limits access to off-site consequence analyses, which are reported in RMPs by covered facilities.

public health. Although not every nurse can be an expert in all aspects of environmental health, every nurse has a basic education in human health and can identify people who may be most vulnerable to environmental insult. Nurses' thoughts about the potential effects of new laws on the health of individuals and communities are valuable to legislators. As communicators and educators, nurses can do the following:

- Write letters to local newspapers responding to environmental health issues affecting the community.
- Participate in blogs or other media that capture the attention of people about the environment and threats to it.
- Serve as a credible source of information at community gatherings, formal governmental hearings, and professional nursing forums.
- Volunteer to serve on local, state, or federal commissions; know the zoning and permit laws that regulate the effects of industry and land use on the community.
- Read, listen, and ask questions. As informed citizens, nurses can lead in fostering community action to address threats to environmental health.

ENVIRONMENTAL JUSTICE AND ENVIRONMENTAL HEALTH DISPARITIES

Some diseases differentially affect different populations. Certain environmental health risks disproportionately affect poor people and people of color in the United States. A poor person of color is more likely to (1) live near a hazardous waste site or an incinerator, (2) have children who are exposed to lead, and (3) have children with asthma, which has a strong association with environmental exposures. Campaigns in communities of color and poor communities to improve the unequal burden of environmental risks strive to achieve environmental justice or environmental equity.

In 1993 the Environmental Justice Act was passed, and in 1994 Executive Order 12898, Federal Actions to Address Environmental Justice in Minority Populations, was signed. These created policies to more comprehensively reduce the incidence of environmental inequity by mandating that every federal agency act in a manner to address and prevent illnesses and injuries. Nursing interventions and involvement in environmental health policies can have a significant effect on the health disparities experienced by our most challenged communities.

UNIQUE ENVIRONMENTAL HEALTH THREATS IN THE HEALTH CARE INDUSTRY: NEW OPPORTUNITIES FOR ADVOCACY

We rarely think of health care facilities as sources of environmental harm. Nurses often lead in reducing the use of mercury-containing products in hospitals. The use of mercury-containing thermometers and sphygmomanometers leads to a risk of breakage, which releases a highly toxic substance into the workplace. Further, when a hospital uses incineration to dispose of its waste, the mercury-containing products will create significant releases of mercury into the air, thus contaminating communities. This

airborne mercury will be present in raindrops. When airborne mercury lands on bodies of water (e.g., lakes, rivers, or oceans), microorganisms in the water convert the mercury into methylmercury, which is highly toxic to humans. The methylmercury is then bioaccumulated in fish: As larger fish eat smaller fish, the body burden of methylmercury increases significantly.

Many synthetic chemicals that contaminate the environment are referred to as persistent bioaccumulative toxins (PBTs) or persistent organic pollutants (POPs). These are chemicals that do not break down in air, water, or soil, or in the plant, animal, and human bodies to which they may be passed. Ultimately, because humans are at the top of the food chain, these chemicals may come to reside in our bodies. For instance, lead, which should not be found in the human body, can be found in the long bones of almost any human in the world because of its ubiquitous use and presence in our environment.

Dioxin, another pollutant that contaminates communities, is created in part by the health care industry. Dioxins are created when we manufacture or burn (incinerate) products that contain chlorine, such as bleached white paper or polyvinyl chloride (PVC) plastics. When dioxins are released into the environment, they are consumed by agricultural animals and by fish. The dioxins are stored in fat cells as they work their way up the food chain. This phenomenon has resulted in dioxin deposition in breast tissue, and dioxin has been found in both cow and human milk. Virtually all women now have dioxin in their breast tissue. Dioxin, an endocrine-disrupting chemical and a strong carcinogen, is associated with several neurodevelopmental problems, including learning disabilities, and is now in every human's body. The solution to this problem is to stop releasing dioxins into the environment. In the health care setting, one way to eliminate the creation and release of dioxins is to stop using products like PVC plastics and select safer alternatives by employing environmentally preferable purchasing policies and practices.

An international campaign called Health Care Without Harm is working to reduce and eliminate the use of mercury and PVC plastic in the health care industry and to eliminate incineration of medical waste. The ANA was a founding member of the Health Care Without Harm campaign, and nurses have taken many leadership roles in the activities in the United States and around the world. The Health Care Without Harm website (http://www.noharm.org) provides outstanding information on greening hospitals and resources about pollution prevention in the health care sector. The face page on their website in 2020 was "Leading the global movement for environmentally responsive health care." On the website you can select the area of the world of interest and see what the latest concern is. For example, in April 2020, concern was expressed about the US withdrawal of support for the World Health Organization during a worldwide health crisis.

REFERRAL RESOURCES

No single source of information about environmental health is available, nor is there a single resource to which individuals or a community can be referred if they suspect an environmental problem. Information is widely accessible on the Internet, but finding an actual person to assist you or the communities you serve may not be as easy. One starting point may be the environmental epidemiology unit or toxicology unit of your state health department or environmental agency. Another local or state resource may be environmental health experts in nursing or medical schools or schools of public health. The Association of Occupational and Environmental Clinics (http://www.aoec.org) is a national network of specialty clinics and individual practitioners available for consultation and sometimes for the provision of educational programs for health professionals.

Local resources include local health and environmental protection agencies, poison control centers, agricultural extension offices, and occupational and environmental departments in schools of medicine, nursing, and public health. Some local and state agencies have developed topical directories to assist in accessing the appropriate staff for specific questions. Many resources have websites that allow ready access through the Internet and can be located by using any of the popular search methods. See Box 8.5 for a list of resources for nurses.

ROLES FOR NURSES IN ENVIRONMENTAL HEALTH

Nurses are involved in many ways in environmental health, whether in full-time work, as an adjunct to existing roles, or as informed and involved citizens. Two of these nursing roles are assessment and referral. Assessment and referral are familiar parts of nursing practice, but they have specific meaning in environmental health. Assessment activities of nurses can range from individual health assessments to being full participants in community assessment or partners in a specific environmental site assessment. Referral resources may vary in communities. One starting point may be the environmental epidemiology or toxicology unit of the state health department or environmental agency. Some of the key nursing functions that are discussed throughout the chapter include the following:

- **Community involvement and public participation:** Organizing, facilitating, and moderating. Making public notices effective, making public forums accessible, and welcoming input. Making information exchange understandable and problem solving acceptable to culturally diverse communities are valuable contributions made by nurses. Skills in community organizing and mobilizing can help communities have a meaningful voice in decisions that affect it.
- **Individual and population risk assessment:** Using nursing assessment skills to detect potential and actual exposure pathways and outcomes for clients cared for in the acute, chronic, and healthy communities of practice.
- **Risk communication:** Interpreting and applying principles to practice. Nurses may serve as skilled risk communicators within agencies, working for industries, or working as independent practitioners. Amendments to the Clean Air Act require major industrial sources of air emissions to have risk management plans and to inform their neighbors of specifics of the risks and plans (Clean Air Act, 1996).
- **Epidemiological investigations:** Having the skills to respond in scientifically sound and humanly sensitive ways to community concerns about cancer, birth defects, and stillbirths that citizens fear may have environmental causes.
- **Policy development:** Proposing, informing, and monitoring action from agencies, communities, and organization perspectives.

BOX 8.5 Environmental Health Resources

Federal Agencies
Agency for Toxic Substances and Disease Registry
Centers for Disease Control and Prevention
Consumer Product Safety Commission
Environmental Protection Agency (EPA)
Office of Children's Environmental Health, EPA
Food and Drug Administration
National Institute for Occupational Safety and Health
National Institute of Environmental Health Sciences
National Institutes of Health
National Cancer Institute
National Institute of Nursing Research
Occupational Safety and Health Administration
National Library of Medicine—TOXNET

State Agencies
State health departments
State environmental protection agencies

Nursing Organizations Focusing on Occupational and Environmental Health
Alliance of Nurses for Healthy Environments
American Association of Occupational Health Nurses

Associations and Organizations
American Association of Poison Control Centers
Association of Occupational and Environmental Clinics
Beyond Pesticides
Center for Health and Environmental Justice
Children's Environmental Health Network
Environmental Defense Fund
Environmental Working Group
Food and Water Watch
Health Care Without Harm
National Academies Press
National Environmental Education Foundation
Natural Resources Defense Council
Pediatric Environmental Health Specialty Units
Pesticide Educational Resources Collaborative
Society for Occupational and Environmental Health
University of California San Francisco Program on Reproductive Health and the Environment

The assimilation of the concepts of environmental health into a nurse's daily practice gives new life to the traditional public health values of prevention, building community, and social justice. There is great congruence with many personal, religious, and spiritual values of stewardship of creation, preserving the gifts of nature, and decision making that provides for quality of life for present and future generations. It is a context for practice in which nurses are welcomed and valued for their contribution.

As nurses learn more about the environment, opportunities for integration into their practice, educational programs, research, advocacy, and policy work will become evident. Opportunities abound for those pioneering spirits within the nursing profession who are dedicated to creating healthier environments for their clients and communities.

▶▶ APPLYING CONTENT TO PRACTICE

Key documents that guide practice in both nursing and public health help practitioners learn how to apply environmental health principles at home and work. Specifically, the core competencies of the Council on Linkages (2014) have, within the domain of public health science skills, a competency that says practitioners will apply "the basic public health sciences (e.g., biostatistics, epidemiology, environmental health sciences, health services administration, and social and behavioral health sciences, and public health informatics) in the delivery of the 10 Essential Public Health Services." The most explicit set of principles were developed by the ANA (2007) in its Principles of Environmental Health for Nursing Practice.

The ANA (2007) lists 10 principles of environmental health. Although all 10 are essential, 4 are mentioned here: Nurses should know about environmental health concepts; participate in assessing the quality of the environment in which they practice; live and use the Precautionary Principle, which refers to using products and practices that do not harm human health or the environment; and take preventive action when uncertain. Another principle points out that healthy environments are sustained through multidisciplinary collaboration, which is a key concept discussed throughout the chapter.

▮ PRACTICE APPLICATION

Two case scenarios related to exposure pathways are presented here. The first involves lead poisoning, and the second involves gasoline contamination of groundwater.

A 3-year-old boy is brought to the county health department with gastric upset and behavior changes that have persisted for several weeks. Billy's parents report that they have been renovating their home to remove lead paint. They had been discouraged from routinely testing their child because their insurance does not cover testing, and they could not find information on where to have the tests done. Their concern has heightened with Billy's persistent symptoms.

You test the level of lead in Billy's blood and find it to be 45 μg/dL. You research lead poisoning and discover that children are at great risk because they absorb lead into the central nervous system. You also find that chronic lead poisoning may have long-term effects, such as developmental delays and impaired learning ability. You refer Billy to his primary-care physician. On further investigation, you find that Billy's home

was built before 1950 and is still under renovation. The sanitarian tests the interior paint and finds a high lead content. Ample amounts of sawdust from sanding are noted in various rooms of the home.

You determine that a completed exposure pathway exists.
A. What would you include in an assessment of this situation?
B. What prevention strategies would you use to resolve this issue?
1. At the individual level?
2. At the population level?

A citizen calls the local health department to report that his drinking water, from a private well, "smells like gasoline." A water sample is collected, and analysis reveals the presence of petroleum products. A nearby rural store with a service station has removed its old underground gasoline storage tanks and replaced them, as required by law. Contaminated soil from the old leaking tank has been removed, and a well to monitor groundwater contamination is scheduled for installation. However, sandy soil has allowed rapid movement of the contamination through the groundwater, and the plume has reached the neighbor's drinking-water well at levels that exceed the drinking-water standard.

What are some possible responses?
Answers can be found on the Evolve website.

▮ REMEMBER THIS!

- Nurses have responsibilities to be informed consumers and to be advocates for citizens in their community regarding environmental health issues.
- Models describing the determinants of health acknowledge the role of the environment in health and disease.
- For many chemical compounds, whether new or familiar, scientific evidence of possible health effects is lacking.
- Prevention activities include education, waste minimizing, and land-use planning. Control activities include environmental permitting, environmental standards, monitoring, compliance and enforcement, and cleanup and remediation.
- Each nursing assessment should include questions and observations about intended and unintended environmental exposures.
- Environmental databases facilitate the easy and immediate access to environmental data useful in assessment, diagnosis, intervention, and evaluation.
- Risk communication is an important skill and must acknowledge the outrage factor experienced by communities with environmental hazards.
- Federal, state, and local laws and regulations exist to protect citizens from environmental hazards.
- Environmental health practice engages multiple disciplines, and nurses are important members of the environmental health team.
- Environmental health practice includes principles of health promotion, disease prevention, and health protection.
- The objectives *of Healthy People 2020* address targets for the reduction of risk factors and diseases related to environmental causes.

EVOLVE WEBSITE

http://evolve.elsevier.com/Stanhope/foundations
- NCLEX® Review Questions
- Practice Application Answers

REFERENCES

Afzal, BM: Global warming: a public health concern, *Online J Issues Nurs* 12:5, 2007.

Allen, PJ: Climate change: it's our problem, *Pediatric Nursing* 41(1):42–46, 2015.

Alliance of Nurses for Healthy Environments: *Public health and fracking*, 2017. Available at Retrieved April 2020..

American Cancer Society: *Cancer facts and figures,* Atlanta GA, 2016, American Cancer Society.

American Lung Association: What is asthma? March 2020, https://www.lung.org,

American Nurses Association: *Principles of environmental health for nursing practice*, Silver Spring, MD, 2007, ANA.

Bailey HD, Fritschi L, Infante-Rivard C, et al: Parental occupational pesticide exposure and the risk of childhood leukemia in the offspring international consortium, *Int J Cancer* 135(9):2157-2172, 2014.

Centers for Disease Control and Prevention: *Facts about ASD*, 2016. Retrieved February 2016 from http://www.cdc.gov.autism/facts.

Centers for Disease Control and Prevention: *National environmental public health tracking network*, 2019. Retrieved April 2020 from http://www.ephtracking.cdc.gov .

Clean Air Act: Risk Management Programs, Section 112(7), Fed Reg Part III EPA, 40 CFR, Part 68, June 20, 1996.

Chen M, Chang CH, Tao L, Lu C: Residential exposure to pesticide during childhood and childhood cancers: a meta-analysis, *Pediatrics* 136(4):719-729, 2015.

Council on Linkages between Academic and Public Health Practice: *Core competencies for public health professionals*, Washington DC, 2014, Public Health Foundation, Health Resources and Services Administration.

Environmental Health News: *After a decade of research, here's what scientists know about the health impacts of fracking*, enh.org/health-impacts-of-fracking-2634432607/html, April 15, 2019. Accessed April 2020.

Environmental Protection Agency: *Lead poisoning is 100% preventable*, 2019. Retrieved April, 2020 from www.cdc/gov.

Environmental Protection Agency: *What are the six common air pollutants?* 2018. Retrieved April 2020 from www.epa.gov/criteria-air-pollutants.

Environmental Protection Agency: *Fish and shellfish advisories and safe eating guidelines*, 2020. http://www.epa.gov/choose-fish-and-shellfish-wisely.

Fudvoye J, Bourguignon JP, Parent AS: Endocrine-disrupting chemicals and human growth and maturation. A focus on early critical windows of exposure, *Vitam Horm* 94:1-25, 2014.

Gilden RC, Friedmann E, Sattler B, Squibb K, McPhaul K: Potential health effects related to pesticide use on athletic fields, *Public Health Nurs* 29(3):198-207, 2012.

Habre R, Moshier E, Castro W, et al: The effect of PM 2.5 and its components from indoor and outdoor sources on cough and wheeze symptoms in asthmatic children, *J Expo Sci Environ Epidemiol*, 24(4):380-387, 2014.

How to safely dispose of your old medications, National prescription drug take back day, 2020, www.nationaltakebackdrug, accessed April 2020. Drugs.com

Hsu HH, Chiu YH, Coull BA, et al: Prenatal particulate air pollution and asthma onset in urban children: identifying sensitive windows and sex differences, *Am J Respir Crit Care Med* 192(9):1052-1059, 2015.

Leffers J and Butterfield P: Nurses play essential roles in reducing health problems due to climate change, *Nurs Outlook,* 66: 210-213, 2018.

Leffers JM, McDermott-Levy R, Smith CM, et al: Nursing education's response to the 1995 Institute of Medicine Report: Nursing, Health and the Environment, *Nurs Forum* 40(4):214–224, 2014.

Levy B, Wegman D, Baron SL, Sokas RK: *Occupational and environmetnal health,* ed 7, New York, 2017, Oxford University Press.

Murray JS: The effects of the Gulf oil spill on children, *J Spec Pediatr Nurs* 16:70–74, 2011.

Paranzino GK, Butterfield P, Nastoff T and Ranger C: I PREPARE: Development and clinical utility of an environmental exposure history mnemonic, *American Association of Occupational Health Nurses,*53(1): 37-42, 2005.

Pope AM, Snyder MA, Mood LH, editors: *Nursing, health, and the environment*, Washington, DC, 1995, Institute of Medicine, National Academies Press.

Pruss-Ustun A, Wolf J, Corvalan C, Bos R, Neira M: World Health Organization: *Preventing disease through healthy environments: a global assessment of the burden of disease from environmental risk, 2016.* Retrieved from http://www.who.int; April 2020.

Rosenthal LD: Carbon monoxide poisoning, *Am J Nurs* 106:40–46, 2006.

Silva JF, Mattos IE, Luz LL, Carmo CN, Aydos RD: Exposure to pesticides and prostate cancer: systematic review of the literature, *Rev Environmen Health*31(3):31—327, 2016.

Smargiassi A, Goldberg MS, Wheeler AJ, et al: Associations between personal exposure to air pollutants and lung function tests and cardiovascular indicates among children with asthma living near an industrial complex and petroleum refineries, *Environ Res* 132C:38–45, 2014.

Suk WA, Davis EA: Strategies for addressing global environmental health concerns, *Ann N Y Acad Sci* 1140:40–44, 2008..

VoPham T, Bertrand KA, Hart JE, et al: Pesticide exposure and liver cancer: a review, *Cancer Causes Conrol* 28(3):211-27, 2017.

Watkins DJ, Sanchez BN, Tellez-Rojo MM, et al: Impact of phthalate and BPA exposure during in utero windows of susceptibility on reproductive hormones and sexual maturation in peripubertal males, *Environ Health* 16(1):69, 2017.

WebMD: *Testing for and removing lead paint*, 2018.

World Health Organization: *Asthma*, 2019. Retrieved April 2020 from www.asthma.who.int.

World Health Organization, *Healthy environments for healthier populations: why do they matter, and what can we do?* 2020, Climate Change, www.who.int. Retrieved April 2020.

Wright RO: Environment, susceptibility windows, development and child health, *Curr Opin Pediatr,* 29(2): 211-217, 2017.

Yoder JS, Wallace RM, Collier SA, et al. Cryptosporidiosis surveillance—United States, 2009-2010, Centers for Disease Control and Prevention (CDC), *MMWR Surveill Summ* 61(5):1–12, 2012.

9

Evidence-Based Practice

Marcia Stanhope and Lisa M. Turner

OBJECTIVES

After reading this chapter, the student should be able to:

1. Define evidence-based practice.
2. Understand the history of evidence-based practice in health care.
3. Analyze the relationship between evidence-based practice and the practice of nursing in the community.
4. Provide examples of evidence-based practice in the community.
5. Identify barriers to evidence-based practice.
6. Apply evidence-based resources in practice.

CHAPTER OUTLINE

KEY TERMS

Emphasis on evidence-based practice (EBP) is a standard to be met in health care delivery in the United States. It is a relevant approach to providing the highest quality of health care in all settings, which will result in improved health outcomes. EBP is important for all professionals who work in social and health care environments, regardless of the client or the setting with which professionals are dealing, including public health nurses who work with populations. Emphasis on EBP has resulted from increased expectations of consumers, changes in health care economics, increased expectations of accountability, advancements in technology, the knowledge explosion fueled by the Internet, and the growing number of lawsuits occurring when there is injury or harm as a result of practice decisions that are not based on the best available evidence (Brower and

Nemec, 2017; Grove and Gray, 2019). Nurses at all levels have an opportunity to improve the practice of nursing and client outcomes.

The Institute of Medicine has set a goal that by 2020 the best available evidence will be used to make 90% of all health care decisions, yet most nurses continue to be inconsistent in implementing EBP. An even greater concern in public health is that the field is lagging behind in developing evidence-based guidelines for the community setting. It is important to recognize that regardless of the level of education, undergraduate or graduate, nurses can be involved in the development, implementation, and evaluation of the effects of EBP (Brooke and Mallion, 2016; Häggman-Laitila et al., 2016; Mathieson, Grande, and Luker, 2019).

Comprehensive databases are available through various Internet sites to assist nurses in applying the most recent best evidence to their clinical practice, like the Cochrane Library database, the Centers for Disease Control and Prevention: Guide to Community Preventive Services, and others.

DEFINITION OF EVIDENCE-BASED PRACTICE

The definition of evidence-based medicine by Sackett et al. (1996) became the first industry standard: "the conscientious, explicit, and judicious use of current best evidence in making decisions about the care of individual clients" (p. 71). Adapting the definition by Sackett et al. (1996), Rychetnik et al. (2004) defined evidence-based public health as "a public health endeavor in which there is an informed, explicit, and judicious use of evidence that has been derived from any of a variety of science and social science research and evaluation methods" (p. 538). Brownson et al. (2009) expanded the definition of evidence-based public health to include "making decisions on the basis of the best available evidence, using data and information systems, applying program planning frameworks, engaging the community in decision making, conducting evaluations, and disseminating what has been learned" (p. 175).

In a position statement on EBP, the Honor Society of Nursing, Sigma Theta Tau International, defined evidence-based nursing as "an integration of the best evidence available, nursing expertise, and the values and preferences of the individuals, families, and communities who are served" (Honor Society of Nursing, Sigma Theta Tau International, 2005). The definition of EBP continues to be broadened in scope and now includes a lifelong problem-solving approach to clinical practice, integrating both external and internal evidence to answer clinical questions and to achieve desired client outcomes (Melnyk and Fineout-Overholt, 2019; Melnyk et al., 2017). *External evidence* includes research and other evidence such as reports and professional guidelines, for example, whereas *internal evidence* includes the nurse's clinical experiences and the client's preferences.

Applied to nursing, evidence-based practice includes the best available evidence from a variety of sources, including research studies, nursing experience and expertise, and community leaders. Culturally and financially appropriate interventions need to be identified when working with communities. The use of evidence to determine the appropriate use of interventions that are culturally sensitive and cost effective is essential.

HISTORY OF EVIDENCE-BASED PRACTICE

During the mid- to late 1970s there was growing consensus among nursing leaders that scientific knowledge should be used as a basis for nursing practice. During that time the Division of Nursing in the US Public Health Service began funding research utilization projects. Research utilization has been defined as "the process of transforming research knowledge into practice" (Stetler, 2001, p. 273) and "the use of research to guide clinical practice" (Estabrooks et al., 2004, p. 293).

Three projects funded by the Division of Nursing received the most attention and were the most influential in shaping nursing's view of using research to guide practice:
- The Nursing Child Assessment Satellite Training Project (NCAST) (Barnard and Hoehn, 1978; King et al., 1981).
- The Western Interstate Commission for Higher Education (WICHE) Regional Program for Nursing Research Development (WICHEN) (Krueger, 1977; Krueger et al., 1978; Lindeman and Krueger, 1977).
- The Conduct and Utilization of Research in Nursing Project (CURN) (Horsley et al., 1978; Horsley et al., 1983).

Using very different approaches and methods, each project tested interventions to facilitate research use in practice.

Although nursing continued to focus on research utilization projects, medicine also began to call for physicians to increase their use of scientific evidence to make clinical decisions. In the late 1970s, David Sackett, a medical doctor and clinical epidemiologist at McMaster University, published a series of articles in the *Canadian Medical Association Journal* describing how to read research articles in clinical journals. The term *critical appraisal* was used to describe the process of evaluating the validity and applicability of research studies (Guyatt and Rennie, 2002). Later, Sackett proposed the phrase "bringing critical appraisal to the

---

EVIDENCE-BASED PRACTICE

The Community Guide is a resource to public health professionals to quickly assess the evidence-based findings of public health interventions. *The Community Guide* consists of a collection of systematic reviews conducted by the Community Preventive Services Task Force (CPSTF). Vaidya et al. (2017) sought to assess the quality of practice-based evidence (PBE) and research-based evidence (RBE) within *The Community Guide*. The researchers developed operational definitions for PBE and RBE, distinguishing RBE studies as those in which there was allocation to intervention and control conditions, whereas PBE studies were studies that assessed an intervention in practice to improve health or other outcomes without allocating individuals or groups to the intervention. The investigators categorized 3656 studies in 202 reviews completed since *The Community Guide* first began. Results showed that 54% of the studies were PBE and 46% RBE.

Furthermore, the researchers noted that community-based and policy reviews used more PBE, whereas health care system and programmatic reviews had more RBE. The researchers concluded that the inclusion of PBE studies in *The Community Guide* reviews indicates that adequate rigor to inform practice is being produced, thus increasing stakeholders' confidence that *The Community Guide* provides recommendations with real-world relevance.

Nurse Use
Public health nurses can be assured that the systematic reviews in *The Community Guide* provide high-quality recommendations with real-world practice relevance. Nurses can continue to add to the literature through conducting evaluative population-focused intervention studies.

Data from Vaidya N, Thota AB, Proia KK, et al: Practice-based evidence in Community Guide systematic reviews, *Am J Public Health* 107(3): 413–420, 2017.

bedside" to describe the application of evidence from medical literature to client care. This concept was used to train resident physicians at McMaster University and evolved into a "philosophy of medical practice based on knowledge and understanding of the medical literature supporting each clinical decision" (Guyatt and Rennie, 2002, p. xiv).

With Gordon Guyatt as Residency Director of Internal Medicine at McMaster, the decision was made to change the program to focus on "this new brand of medicine" that Guyatt eventually called *evidence-based medicine* (Guyatt and Rennie, 2002). Guyatt and Rennie described the goal of evidence-based medicine as being "aware of the evidence on which one's practice is based, the soundness of the evidence, and the strength of inference the evidence permits" (2002, p. xiv).

PARADIGM SHIFT IN USE OF EVIDENCE-BASED PRACTICE

In 1992 the Evidence-Based Medicine Working Group published an article in the *Journal of the American Medical Association* expanding the concept of evidence-based medicine and calling it a *paradigm shift*. A paradigm shift simply means a change from old ways of knowing to new ways of knowing and practicing. Ways of knowing in nursing have included the following:

- The empirical knowledge, or the science of nursing
- The aesthetic knowledge, or the art of nursing
- The personal knowledge, or interpersonal relationships and caring
- Ethical knowledge, or moral and ethical codes of conduct usually established by professional organizations (Carper, 1978)

Nursing practice in the past often focused less on science and more on the other four ways of knowing described here.

According to the Working Group (Evidence-Based Medicine Working Group, 1992), the old paradigm viewed unsystematic clinical observations as a valid way for "building and maintaining" knowledge for clinical decision making". In addition, principles of pathophysiology were seen as a "sufficient guide for clinical practice". Training, common sense, and clinical experience were considered sufficient for evaluating clinical data and developing guidelines for clinical practice. The Working Group cited developments in research over the past 30 years as providing the foundation for the paradigm shift and a "new philosophy of medical practice".

The new paradigm, evidence-based medicine, acknowledged clinical experience as a crucial but insufficient part of clinical decision making. Systematic and unbiased recording of clinical observations in the form of research will increase confidence in the knowledge gained from clinical experience. Principles of pathophysiology were seen as necessary but not sufficient knowledge for making clinical decisions. The Working Group emphasized that physicians needed to be able to critically appraise the research literature to appropriately apply research findings in practice. Knowledge gained from authoritative figures was also deemphasized in the new paradigm (Evidence-Based Medicine Working Group, 1992).

In the years since the Working Group began, the term *evidence-based practice* has been proposed as a term to integrate all health professions. The underlying principle was that high-quality care is based on evidence rather than on tradition or intuition (Chapman, 2018).

Nurses have always used various resources for problem solving. Intuition, trial and error, tradition, authority, institutional standards, prior knowledge, and clinical experience have often been used as the basis for decision making in clinical settings. However, not all of these resources are reliable, and all have not consistently produced desired outcomes (Bower and Nemec, 2017; Weiss et al., 2018). A procedure performed based on intuition or trial and error might be performed successfully sometimes and not at other times. For example, tradition and authority, which comes from texts and policy and procedure manuals, can lead to faulty clinical decision making.

Institutional standards are developed by accrediting agencies (e.g., The Joint Commission), by licensing agencies, and by professional organizations. These standards have been developed in the past primarily by expert opinion and past experiences. The standards may not reflect the best practices in the current environment or from the literature.

Although prior knowledge gained in educational programs, through continuing education, or through experience can be a good teacher, it can also contain bias and quickly become outdated unless a nurse participates in constantly refreshing knowledge. For example, just because a nurse has experience in successfully performing an intervention a certain way today does not mean it is the best way or that it will be successful every time and in the future unless practices are changed based on the most current data.

When EBP was first emphasized in medicine, the focus was on the answer to clinical questions concerning an individual client problem to provide the best diagnosis to implement the best treatment. When nursing became involved in EBP, the focus seemed to shift to answering a clinical question about a health problem experienced by a group of clients (Levin et al., 2010).

The current nursing literature on EBP is primarily associated with applications in the acute and primary care settings, and little is reported about its use in community settings. However, the basic principles of EBP can be applied at the individual level or at the community level. Although definitions of EBP vary widely in the literature, the common thread across disciplines is the application of the best available evidence to improve practice (Brower and Nemec, 2017; Grove and Gray, 2019; Zimmerman, 2017).

EBP has been described as both a process and a product (Dang and Dearholt, 2018; Scott and McSherry, 2009; Zimmerman, 2017). The product is the use of evidence to make practice changes, whereas the process is a systematic approach to locating, critiquing, synthesizing, translating, and evaluating evidence upon which to base practice changes. Systematic reviews of research evidence can potentially assist nurses in putting evidence into practice. Systematic reviews, also known as evidence summaries, provide reliable evidence-based summaries of past research, making it easier for health care professionals to stay current on best practices without having to read a lot of research papers (Holly et al., 2016).

Scott and McSherry (2009) engaged in a process using an extensive literature review to arrive at a definition of evidence-based nursing and to differentiate the definition from evidence-based practice. Based on their review, they arrived at the following definition: Evidence-based nursing is a process whereby evidence, nursing theory, and the nurse's clinical expertise are evaluated and used, in conjunction with the client's involvement, to make critical decisions about the best care for the client. Continuous evaluation of the implementation of care is essential to making clinical decisions about client care for the best possible outcomes. In each chapter there is extensive discussion of an example of how public health nurses have developed and used evidence on which to base population-centered nursing.

TYPES OF EVIDENCE

No matter which definition of EBP is supported, what counts as evidence has been the issue most hotly debated. A hierarchy of evidence, ranked in order of decreasing importance and use, has been accepted by many health professionals. The double-blind randomized controlled trial (RCT) generally ranks as the highest level of evidence followed by:
- Other RCTs
- Nonrandomized clinical trials
- Quasi experimental studies
- Case-controlled reports
- Qualitative studies
- Expert opinion (Grove and Gray, 2019).

Some nurses would argue that this hierarchy ignores evidence gained from clinical experience. However, the definition of evidence-based nursing presented previously indicates that clinical expertise as evidence, when used with other types of evidence, is used to make clinical decisions. Also in the hierarchy of evidence, expert opinion can be gained from the following:
- Non research–based published articles
- Professional guidelines
- National guidelines
- Organizational opinions
- Panels of experts
- The nurse's clinical expertise

Because it is difficult to find or perform RCTs in the community, other types of evidence have been highlighted as the best evidence in public health literature on which to base evidence-based public health practice:
- Scientific literature found in systematic reviews
- Scientific literature used or quoted in one or more journal articles
- Public health surveillance data
- Program evaluations
- Qualitative data obtained from community members and other stakeholders
- Media/marketing data, such as the results of a media campaign to reduce smoking, word of mouth, and personal/professional experience (Brownson et al., 2018)

Within public health practice, guidelines for finding and using evidence include the following:
- Engaging the community in assessment and decision making
- Using data and information systems systematically
- Making decisions on the basis of the best available peer-reviewed evidence (both quantitative and qualitative)
- Applying program planning frameworks (often based in health behavior theory)

- Conducting sound evaluation
- Disseminating what is learned (Brownson et al., 2018)

FACTORS LEADING TO CHANGE

EBP represents a cultural change in practice. It provides an environment to improve both nursing practice and client outcomes. Nursing is known for providing care based on the following:
- Environmental and client assessments
- Critical observations
- Development of questions or hypotheses to be explored
- Collecting data from the environment through community or organizational assessments
- Client history
- Physical assessment
- Review of past heath records
- Analyzing the data to develop plans of care, whether for the individual client, family, group, or community
- Drawing conclusions upon which to base care for the purpose of improving client outcomes (Bowers, 2018; Melnyk et al., 2017)

However, several factors have been identified in the literature that support implementation of EBP or that will need to be overcome for nursing and other disciplines to successfully implement EBP. These factors include the following:
- Knowledge of research and current evidence
- Ability to interpret the meaning of the evidence
- Individual professional's characteristics, such as a willingness to change, or personal viewpoints about the quality and credibility of evidence
- Commitment of the time needed to implement EBP and to engage in education and directed practice
- The hierarchy of the practice environment and the level of support of managers and the ability to engage in autonomous practice
- The philosophy of the practice environment and the willingness to embrace EBP
- The resources available to engage in EBP, such as amount of work, proper equipment, computer-based EBP programs, and information systems
- The practice characteristics, such as leadership and colleague attitudes
- Links to outside supports such as teaching facilities like a teaching health department or a university
- Political constraints and the lack of relevant and timely public health practice research (Bowers, 2018; Duncombe, 2018; Kristensen et al., 2016; Melnyk et al., 2017; Pereira et al., 2018; Schaefer & Welton, 2018)

BARRIERS TO EVIDENCE-BASED PRACTICE

Although a community agency may subscribe in theory to the use of EBP, actual implementation may be affected by the realities of the practice setting. Community-focused nursing agencies may lack the resources needed for its implementation in the clinical setting, such as time, funding, computer resources, and knowledge. Nurses may be reluctant to accept findings and feel threatened when long-established practices are questioned. Cost can also be a barrier if the clinical decision or change will require more funds than the agency has available. Compliance can be a barrier if the client will not follow the recommended intervention. Public health departments are moving toward EBP and are seeking accreditation through the national public health accreditation board. The accreditation process began in 2011 (Public Health Accreditation Board, 2020).

STEPS IN THE EVIDENCE-BASED PRACTICE PROCESS

EBP is a philosophy of practice that respects client values (Melnyk et al., 2010). The seven-step EBP process was described as follows:

0. Cultivating a spirit of inquiry
1. Asking clinical questions
2. Searching for the best evidence
3. Critically appraising the evidence
4. Integrating the evidence with clinical expertise and client preferences and values
5. Evaluating the outcomes of the practice decisions or changes based on evidence
6. Disseminating EBP results (Melnyk and Fineout-Overholt, 2019)

Yes, their first step is step 0. This process was initially described as a five-step process by others (Dawes et al., 2004; Dicenso et al., 2005). The unique features of the Melnyk et al. (2010) model are the emphasis on the spirit of inquiry and the sharing of the results of the process (Melnyk and Fineout-Overholt, 2019).

Step Zero involves a curiosity about the interventions that are being applied. Do they work, or is there a better approach? In public health nursing, for example, are there better parenting outcomes if the parents attend classes at the health department? Or are home visits to new mothers and babies more effective for achieving a healthy baby?

Step 1 requires asking questions in a "PICOT" format. Although Melnyk et al. (2010) developed a specific process for the PICOT, the process was first described by Sackett (1996), who discussed the following:

- The need to define the *(P)opulation* of interest
- The *(I)ntervention* or practice strategy in question
- The population or intervention to be used for *(C)omparision*
- The *(O)utcome* desired
- The *(T)ime frame*.

Step 2 involves searching for the best evidence to answer the question. This step involves searching the literature. In the case of the previous example, a literature search would focus on a search of key terms like *public health nursing, parenting of new babies, parenting classes,* and *home visits.*

Step 3 requires a critical appraisal of the evidence found in step 2. To appraise the literature found, Melnyk and Fineout-Overholt (2019) suggest asking three questions about each of the articles found in the literature search: (1) the validity, (2) the importance, and (3) whether or not the results of the article will help you as a nurse provide quality care for your clients.

Step 4 is the step in which the evidence found is integrated with clinical expertise and client values. Institutional standards and practice guidelines, as well as cost of care and support of the health care environment to implement the findings, are all factors considered in this step.

Step 5 requires an evaluation of the outcomes of practice decisions and changes that were based on the answers to the first four steps. The goal in evaluation is a positive change in quality of care and health care outcomes. For example, in a randomized controlled study evaluating the effects of a home visit program on asthma outcomes and costs for children with uncontrolled asthma, researchers noted the program improved health outcomes and reduced urgent care use and costs (Campbell et al., 2015).

Step 6 is disseminating outcomes of the results to others, to colleagues, to the employing agency's administration, to faculty and other students, and through a poster or podium presentation of student nurse organizations or professional organizations. Professional organizations often sponsor student presentations for undergraduates as well as graduate students. Sharing of information is most important because it prevents each individual nurse from trying to find the best answer to the same question answered by someone else, and it gives us the basis for asking new questions. Sharing makes practice more efficient and improves quality and health care outcomes.

In a busy community practice setting, it is often difficult for nurses to access evidence-based resources. Using evidence-based clinical practice guidelines is one way for nurses to provide evidence-based nursing care in an efficient manner. Clinical practice guidelines are usually developed by a group of experts in the field who have reviewed the evidence and made recommendations based on the best available evidence. The recommendations are usually graded according to the quality and quantity of the evidence.

APPROACHES TO FINDING EVIDENCE

Returning to the previous example, the clinical question has been stated, and the population has been defined as new mothers and babies. Two interventions will be compared. The outcome is stated as healthy babies, and the time frame may be 6 months or 1 year or another time at which the outcomes of the interventions will be evaluated.

Four approaches are described that allow the nurse to read research/non-research evidence in a condensed format. The first, a systematic review, is "a method of identifying, appraising, and synthesizing research evidence. The aim is to evaluate and interpret all available research that is relevant to a particular research question" (Cochrane Library, 2019). A systematic review is usually done by more than one person and describes the methods used to search for and evaluate the evidence. Systematic reviews can be accessed from most databases, such as Medline and CINAHL.

The Cochrane Library is an electronic database that contains regularly updated evidence-based health care databases maintained by the Cochrane Collaboration, a not-for-profit organization (http://www.cochrane.org). The Cochrane Library is composed of three main branches: systematic reviews, trials register, and a methodology database. The Cochrane Library publishes systematic reviews on a wide variety of topics. Systematic reviews differ from traditional literature review publications in that systematic reviews require more rigor and contain less opinion of the author. Systematic reviews for public health can be found in the Guide to Community Preventive Services, the Cochrane Public Health Group, the Centre for Reviews and Dissemination, and the Campbell Collaboration (Box 9.1).

BOX 9.1 Resources for Implementing Evidence-Based Practice

The following resources can assist nurses in developing evidence-based nursing practice:

1. *PubMed* (http://www.pubmed.gov/) is a bibliographical database developed and maintained by the National Library of Medicine. Bibliographical information from Medline is covered in PubMed and includes references for nursing, medicine, dentistry, the health care system, and preclinical sciences. Full texts of referenced articles are often included. Searches can be limited to type of evidence (e.g., diagnosis, therapy) and systematic reviews.

2. The *Cochrane Database of Systematic Reviews* is a collection of more than 1000 systematic reviews of effects in health care internationally. These reviews are accessible at a cost via the website (http://www.cochrane.org). Nurses may also have free access from a medical library.

3. The *Evidence-Based Nursing Journal* (http://ebn.bmjjournals.com/) is published quarterly. The purpose of the journal is to select articles reporting studies and reviews from health-related literature that warrant immediate attention by nurses attempting to keep pace with advances in their profession. Using predefined criteria, the best quantitative and qualitative original articles are abstracted in a structured format, commented on by clinical experts, and shared in a timely fashion. The research questions, methods, results, and evidence-based conclusions are reported. The website for the journal is http://www.evidence-basednursing.com.

4. The Honor Society of Nursing, Sigma Theta Tau International, sponsors the online peer-reviewed journal *Worldviews on Evidence-Based Nursing* that publishes systematic reviews and research articles on best evidence that supports nursing practice globally. The journal is available by subscription (https://www.sigmanursing.org/).

5. The Community Preventive Services Task Force is an independent, nonfederal task force appointed by the director of the Centers for Disease Control and Prevention (CDC). Information about the Task Force may be found at the website http://www.thecommunityguide.org. The Task Force is charged with determining the topics to be addressed by *The Community Guide* and the most appropriate means to assess evidence regarding population-based interventions. The Task Force reviews and assesses the quality of available evidence on the effects of essential community preventive services. The multidisciplinary Task Force determines the scope of *The Community Guide,* which will be used by health departments and agencies to determine best practices for preventive health in populations.

6. The US Preventive Services Task Force (USPSTF) is an independent panel of private-sector experts in prevention and primary care. The USPSTF conducts rigorous, impartial assessments of the scientific evidence for the effectiveness of a broad range of clinical preventive services, including screening, counseling, and preventive medications. Its recommendations are considered the "gold standard" for clinical preventive services. The mission of the USPSTF is to evaluate the benefits of individual services based on age, gender, and risk factors for disease; make recommendations about which preventive services should be incorporated routinely into primary medical care and for which populations; and identify a research agenda for clinical preventive care. Recommendations of the USPSTF are published as the *Guide to Clinical Preventive Services.* The guide is available online at https://www.ahrq.gov.

7. The Centers for Disease Control and Prevention (https://www.cdc.gov) publishes guidelines on immunizations and sexually transmitted diseases. Guidelines are developed by experts in the field appointed by the US Department of Health and Human Services and the CDC.

8. Cochrane Public Health Review Group (PHRG), formerly the health promotion and public health field, aims to work with contributors to produce and publish Cochrane reviews of the effects of population-level public health interventions. The PHRG undertakes systematic reviews of the effects of public health interventions to improve health and other outcomes at the population level, not those targeted at individuals. Thus it covers interventions seeking to address macroenvironmental and distal social environmental factors that influence health. In line with the underlying principles of public health, these reviews seek to have a significant focus on equity and aim to build the evidence to address the social determinants of health. (Visit http://www.ph.cochrane.org/.)

9. Centre for Reviews and Dissemination (CRD) is part of the National Institute for Health Research and is a department of the University of York. CRD, which was established in 1994, is one of the largest groups in the world engaged exclusively in evidence synthesis in the health field. CRD undertakes systematic reviews evaluating the research evidence on health and public health questions of national and international importance. (Visit http://www.york.ac.uk/crd.)

10. Campbell Collaboration, named after Donald Campbell, was founded on the principle that systematic reviews on the effects of interventions will inform and help improve policy and services. The collaboration strives to make the best social science research available and accessible. Campbell reviews provide high-quality evidence of what works to meet the needs of service providers, policy makers, educators and their students, professional researchers, and the general public. Areas of interest include crime, justice, education, and social welfare. (Visit http://www.campbellcollaboration.org/.)

11. The Putting Public Health Evidence in Action Training Workshop is an interactive training curriculum created by the Cancer Prevention and Control Research Network to support program planners and health educators in using evidence-based approaches. (Visit http://cpcrn.org.)

The second approach, meta-analysis, is a specific method of statistical synthesis used in some systematic reviews, where the results from several studies are quantitatively combined and summarized (Grove and Gray, 2019). A well-designed systematic review or meta-analysis can provide stronger evidence than a single randomized controlled trial.

The integrative review is a form of a systematic review that does not have the summary statistics found in the meta-analysis because of the limitations of the studies that are reviewed (e.g., small sample size of the population). Narrative review is a review done on published papers that support the reviewer's particular point of view or opinion and is used to provide a general discussion of the topic reviewed. This review does not often include an explicit or systematic review process.

Undergraduate students often perform narrative reviews. However, it is important to learn the process for systematic reviews, especially the use of the results of systematic reviews. Reading systematic reviews that have been completed is helpful in answering the question related to the EBP process (Pierce, 2018).

What counts as evidence has also been argued in the public health literature (Brownson et al., 2018). RCTs, which are the highest level of evidence used to make clinical decisions, are appropriate for evaluating many interventions in medicine but are often inappropriate for evaluating public health interventions. For example, an RCT can be designed ethically to test a new medication for diabetes, but not for a smoking cessation intervention. In a smoking cessation intervention, subjects could not be assigned randomly to smoking or nonsmoking

HOW TO DEVELOP AN EVIDENCE-BASED PRACTICE GUIDE FOR A COMMUNITY PREVENTIVE SERVICE

- Form a coordination team to guide the review process.
- Develop a conceptual framework, called a logic model for the review.
- Identify and select interventions that the review will cover.
- Define and develop a conceptual approach for evaluating the interventions, called an analytic framework.
- Identify criteria for including and excluding studies.
- Use the criteria to search for, retrieve, and screen abstracts.
- Review the full text of every study and code the data from each using *The Community Guide* abstraction form.
- Assess the quality of each study.
- Summarize all of the evidence found, called the body of evidence.
- Identify issues of applicability and barriers to implementation (when available) for recommended interventions.
- Summarize information about other benefits or harms that might result from the interventions.
- Identify and summarize evidence gaps.
- Develop recommendations and findings.
- Conduct an economic evaluation of the interventions found to be effective.

From Community Preventive Services Task Force: *Our methodology: what are the steps in The Community Guide review process,* 2018. Available at https://www.thecommunityguide.org.

groups because a smoking cessation intervention is not appropriate for someone who does not smoke. In this situation, a case-control study would be most appropriate. Today there are many community-based clinical trials assisting in finding answers to the questions of which population-level intervention has the best outcomes. (Visit the CDC website to review these trials.)

HOW TO DEVELOP AN EVIDENCE-BASED PROTOCOL

Evidence-based protocols are a recognized approach to providing quality client care. Such protocols enhance the abilities of providers and can reduce health care errors. The following are steps to developing a protocol:

- Enlist committed leadership support that ensures consistent staff participation in the EBP process.
- Develop a committed team that works together for a set time period (e.g., 1 year) to discuss and evaluate practice protocols.
- Identify a clinical issue.
- Identify current policies, protocols, and resources related to the clinical issue.
- Recognize current practices, identifying gaps and additional resources needed to follow best-practice guidelines.
- Develop a protocol that logically follows the flow of patient care and coincides with the caregivers' thought processes.
- Align patient education materials with the new protocol.
- Develop effective dissemination methods, such as providing education and reminders of new protocol, role-modeling changes, and gathering feedback from clinicians.
- Implement the protocol.
- Establish evaluation and sustainability practices for the new protocol, such as through use of a checklist to monitor adherence and identify additional education needs.

From Dols JD, Muñoz LR, Martinez SS, et al.: Developing policies and protocols in the age of evidence-based practice, *J Contin Educ Nurs* 48(2):87–92, 2017.

APPROACHES TO EVALUATING EVIDENCE

One approach used in evaluating evidence is grading the strength of evidence. When evidence is graded, the evidence is assigned a "grade" based on the number and type of well-designed studies and the presence of similar findings in all of the studies. Grading evidence has been debated so strongly that in 2002 the Agency for Healthcare Research and Quality (AHRQ) commissioned a study to describe existing systems used to evaluate the usefulness of studies and strength of evidence. The report reviewed 40 systems and identified three domains for evaluating systems for the grading of evidence: quality, quantity, and consistency (West et al., 2002). The *quality* of a study refers to the extent to which bias is minimized. *Quantity* refers to the number of studies, the magnitude of the effect, and the sample size. *Consistency* refers to studies that have similar findings, using similar and different study designs (Haine-Schlagel et al., 2014).

As indicated, many frameworks exist for evaluating the strength and the usefulness of the evidence found in the literature and other sources, such as professional standards. A popular framework was developed by AHRQ. Fineout-Overholt et al. (2010) have also developed an approach for evaluating evidence. Although these approaches vary in the factors they evaluate, the best approach to choose is one that evaluates not only the strength but also the usefulness of the evidence. Table 9.1 provides an example of an approach for evaluating evidence.

The strength of the literature is measured by the type of evidence it represents. For example, the RCT is the evidence that has the greatest strength upon which to make a clinical decision. In contrast, opinion articles, descriptive studies, and professional reports of expert committees have less strength. The usefulness of the evidence is measured by whether the evidence is valid, whether it is important, and whether it can be used to assist in making practice decisions or changes in the community environment and with the population of interest to improve outcomes (Melnyk et al., 2017).

The best RCT conducted in a hospital setting on using an intervention to prevent falls may not be applicable at all in a community setting. Therefore, although it may be a strong study with outcomes that improve health, it may not have the usefulness for applicability in the community because of the setting in which it was conducted.

Shaughnessy et al. (1994) proposed criteria for evaluating the usefulness of evidence, calling the process *patient-oriented evidence that matters* (POEM). In general, the reader should ask the following questions: "What are the results? (Are they important?) Are the results valid? How can the results be applied to client care?". POEMs research summaries can be found at https://www. essentialevidenceplus.com (Essential Evidence Plus, 2018). Brownson et al. (2013 proposed that the following questions be asked for EBP (plus suggested application examples):

- What is the size of the public health problem? What is the need for improved health outcomes for new mothers and babies in our community?
- Can interventions be found in the literature to address the problem (e.g., home visits or parenting classes)?

TABLE 9.1 Typology for Classifying Interventions by Level of Scientific Evidence

Type/Category	Strength/How Established	Considerations for the Level of Scientific Evidence—Quality	Quantity/Consistency Data Source Examples
Evidence-based I	Peer review via systematic or narrative review	Based on study design and execution External validity Potential side benefits or harms Costs and cost effectiveness	*Community Guide to Clinical Preventive Services* Cochrane reviews Narrative reviews based on published literature
Effective II	Peer review	Based on study design and execution External validity Potential side benefits or harms Costs and cost effectiveness	Articles in the scientific literature Research-tested intervention programs (123) Technical reports with peer review
Promising III	Written program evaluation without formal peer review	Summative evidence of effectiveness Formative evaluation data Theory consistent, plausible, potentially high reach, low cost, replicable	State or federal government reports (without peer review) Conference presentations
Emerging IV	Ongoing work, practice-based summaries, or evaluation works in progress	Formative evaluation data Theory consistent, plausible, potentially high reaching, low cost, replicable Face validity	Evaluability assessments Pilot studies NIH CRISP database Projects funded by health foundations

CRISP, The Computer Retrieval of Information on Scientific Projects *NIH,* National Institutes of Health.
From Brownson RC, Fielding JE, Maylahn CM: Evidence-based public health: a fundamental concept for public health practice, *Annu Rev Public Health* 30:175–201, 2009.

- Is the intervention useful in this community, with this population, or with populations at risk (e.g., the low income or uninsured)?
- Is the intervention the best one, or are there other ways to address the problem considering cost and potential health outcomes for the population? (Assess cost and health outcomes of both of the interventions before choosing, including the nurses available to make home visits or who have the skills to teach the parenting class.)

Multiple variables are considered important in determining the quality of evidence used to make clinical decisions (Polit and Beck, 2018):

- *Sample selection:* Sample selection should be as unbiased as possible. For example, a sample is randomly selected when each subject has an equal chance of being selected from the population of interest. Random selection offers the least bias of any type of sample selection. Other types of sample selection such as convenience sampling contain researcher or evaluator bias.
- *Randomization:* When testing an intervention, randomly assign participants to either the intervention or control group. This type of assignment is less biased than if participants are allowed to choose the group they want to join.
- *Blinding:* The researcher or evaluator should not know which participants are in the experimental (treatment) group or which are in the control group. The researcher or evaluator is "blinded" as to who is receiving the treatment and who is not receiving the treatment.
- *Sample size:* The sample size should be large enough to show an effect of the intervention. In general, the larger the sample size, the better.
- *Description of intervention:* The intervention should be described in detail and explicitly enough that another person could duplicate the study if desired.

- *Outcomes:* The outcomes should be measured accurately.
- *Length of follow-up:* Depending on the intervention, the participants should be followed for a long enough period of time to determine if the intervention continued to work or if the results just happened by chance.
- *Attrition:* Few subjects should have dropped out of the study.
- *Confounding variables:* Variables that could affect the outcome should be accounted for either by statistical methods or by study measurements.
- *Statistical analysis:* Statistical analysis should be appropriate to determine the desired outcome.

? CHECK YOUR PRACTICE

Exploring the Evidence

You are the chief public health nurse for the local health department in a community with a high rate of sexually transmitted infections (STIs) among the adolescent population.

There is a law in your state requiring abstinence-only education in public schools.

The board of education approaches you, questioning why the rate is high, what is being done to reduce the rate, and how the public school system might help in reducing the rate. WHAT WOULD YOU DO?

- What data would you need to investigate the high STI rate?
- What evidence-based interventions could you recommend to the school board? Is abstinence-only education a recommended evidence-based intervention to reduce STI risk?

See if you can apply these steps to this scenario. (1) Recognize the cues, looking at available data about rates of STI in your community and the state; (2) analyze the cues looking at "why" the rate is so high; 3. state several and prioritize the hypotheses you have stated; (4) generate solutions for each hypothesis; (5) take action on the number one hypothesis you think best reflects what is going on in the community; and (6) evaluate the outcomes you would expect as a result of changing approaches to public health services offered in the community to reduce the rate.

APPROACHES TO IMPLEMENTING EVIDENCE-BASED PRACTICE

The first step toward implementing EBP in nursing is recognizing the current status of one's own practice and believing that care based on the best evidence will lead to improved client outcomes (Melnyk et al., 2010; Melnyk and Fineout-Overholt, 2019; Melnyk et al., 2017). Since EBP is a relatively new concept, many practicing nurses are not familiar with the application of EBP and may lack computer and Internet skills necessary to implement EBP. Also, implementation will be successful only when nurses practice in an environment that supports evidence-based care. Public health nurses consider EBP a process to improve practice and outcomes and use the evidence to influence policies that will improve the health of communities.

CURRENT PERSPECTIVES

Cost Versus Quality

Much of the pressure to use EBP comes from third-party payers and is a response to the need to contain costs and reduce legal liability. Nurses must question whether the current agenda to contain health care costs creates pressure to focus on those research results that favor cost saving at the expense of quality outcomes for clients. Outcomes include client and community satisfaction and the safety of care. Costs can be weighed against outcomes when EBP is used to show the best practices available to reduce possible harm to clients (Grove and Gray, 2019; Melnyk, 2017).

LEVELS OF PREVENTION

Using Evidence-Based Practice

According to evidence collected by the Community Preventive Services Task Force, the following are interventions supported by the literature at each level of prevention:

Primary Prevention

Extended and extensive mass media campaigns reduce youth initiation of tobacco use.

Secondary Prevention

Client reminders and recalls via mail, telephone, e-mail, or a combination of these strategies are effective in increasing compliance with screening activities, such as those for colorectal and breast cancer.

Tertiary Prevention

Diabetes self-management education in community gathering places improves glycemic control.

From Community Preventive Services Task Force: *The Community Guide.* Available at https://www.thecommunityguide.org; https://www.cdc.gov.

Individual Differences

EBP cannot be applied as a universal remedy without attention to client differences. When EBP is applied at the community level, best evidence may point to a solution that is not sensitive to cultural issues and distinctions and thus may not be acceptable to the community. Ethical practice in communities requires attention to community differences.

QSEN   FOCUS ON QUALITY AND SAFETY EDUCATION FOR NURSES

Targeted Competency: Evidence-Based Practice—Integrate best current evidence with clinical expertise and client and family preferences and values for delivery of optimal interventions.

Important aspects of EBP include:

- **Knowledge:** Describe EBP to include the components of research evidence, clinical expertise, and client and family values.
- **Skills:** Locate evidence reports related to clinical practice topics and guidelines.
- **Attitudes:** Value the need for continuous improvement in clinical practice based on new knowledge.

Evidence-Based Practice Question

As a nurse in the community, you are working within an Hispanic community that has a high prevalence of gestational diabetes. You decide to initiate a focus group with clients who attend the obstetrics and gynecology clinic at the health department to explore potential gestational diabetes intervention for this community.

1. Go to *The Community Guide* website at https://www.thecommunityguide.org. This website is a collection of evidence-based findings from the Community Preventive Services Task Force (CPSTF).
2. On the home page, click on the "topics" drop-down menu and select "diabetes."
3. Click on the "Diabetes Prevention: Lifestyle Interventions to Reduce Risk of Gestation Diabetes" 2017 systematic review.

4. Review and summarize the CPSTF findings and considerations for implementation.
5. What baseline data might you gather from your focus group participants to be best informed in how to tailor the evidence-based recommendations for this community?

Answer

- The CPSTF findings indicate strong evidence for lifestyle interventions that provide supervised exercise classes, either alone or in combination with other components, and sufficient evidence for lifestyle interventions that provide education and counseling for diet or physical activity, diet activities, or a combination of these components.
- Understanding the common facilitators and barriers to the recommended lifestyle interventions for this community is a good starting place. How many participants are able to get the recommended about of exercise each week? What helps those who are able to exercise (e.g., childcare, affordable classes, accessible classes)? For those unable to exercise, what stands in their way (e.g., time, money, lack of social support)? What types of food do they eat? How do these lifestyle behaviors compare to the recommendations in *The Community Guide*?
- Developing an intervention with assistance from leaders in the community would be a helpful strategy. It will likely be more accepted and impactful if the EBP guidelines are tailored to the specific needs of the community.

Originally prepared by Gail Armstrong, ND, DNP, MS, PhD, Professor and Assistant Dean/DNP program, Oregon Health and Sciences University. Updated in 2018 by Lisa Turner, PhD, RN, PHCNS-BC, Associate Professor, Berea College.

Appropriate Evidence-Based Practice Methods For Population-Centered Nursing Practice

Gaining a number of perspectives in a situated community is important for nurses using EBP. Nursing has a legitimate role to play in interprofessional community-focused practice and can contribute to its evidence base. Nurses are obliged to ensure that the evidence applied to practice is acceptable to the community. Establishing an EBP culture depends on the use of both qualitative and quantitative research approaches or the best evidence available at the time. For example, a quantitative research study of a community health center could provide information about patterns of client use, the cost of various services, and the use of different health care providers. However, when quantitative research is combined with qualitative research, the nurse can gain an understanding of *why* clients use or do not use the services and help the health center be both clinically effective and cost-effective. Evidence from multiple research methods has the potential to enrich the application of evidence and improve nursing practice (Weiss et al., 2018). The Quality and Safety Education for Nurses (QSEN) box gives an example of how to use evidence for making a change in a community's health.

The rising cost of health care will demand a more critical look at the benefits and costs of EBP. Finding resources to implement EBP will continue to be a challenge requiring creative strategies. An emphasis on quality care, equal distribution of health care resources, and cost control will continue. Implementing EBP can assist nurses in addressing these issues in the clinical setting. However, EBP can save money by providing the best care possible.

As nurses implement EBP in an environment focused on cost savings, the potential for governments, managed care organizations, or other health care agencies to endorse reimbursement of health care options solely on the basis of cost, without allowing for individual variation or considering environmental issues, will continue to be a concern. Nurses must use caution in adopting EBP in a prescriptive manner in different community environments. One aspect of the Affordable Care Act (PL 111-148) addresses the development of task forces on preventive services and community preventive services to develop, update, and disseminate EBP recommendations on the use of community preventive services. In addition, grant programs to support EBP delivery in the community are addressed in the Affordable Care Act of 2010.

Although the Internet is one source of evidence data (see Box 9.1), there may be a lack of quality indicators to evaluate the myriad websites claiming to contain evidence-based information. It is essential to evaluate the quantity of the information on the website, whether it comes from a reputable agency or scholar, and whether the source of the website has a financial interest in the acceptance of the evidence presented.

HEALTHY PEOPLE 2030 OBJECTIVES

Healthy People 2030 objectives offer a systematic approach to health improvement. See the *Healthy People 2030* box for the most recent objectives to improve clients' understanding of EBP and how they can contribute to health care decisions.

 HEALTHY PEOPLE 2030

Information access is important to assure clients and communities have the correct information to make EBP health care decisions. The *Healthy People 2030* objectives related to providing resources are as follows:

- **AHS-R01:** Increase the use of telehealth to improve access to health services.
- **HC/HIT-05:** Increase the proportion of adults with broadband Internet.
- **HC/HIT-06:** Increase the proportion of adults offered online access to their medical record.
- **HC/HIT-D09:** Increase the proportion of patients who can view, download, and send their electronic health information.
- **PHI-D03:** Increase the proportion of vital records/health statistics programs that are nationally accredited.
- **PHI-R06:** Enhance the use and capabilities of informatics in public health.

From US Department of Health and Human Services: *Healthy People 2030*. HHS, 2020. Available at https://health.gov/our-work/healthy-people-2030.

EXAMPLE OF APPLICATION OF EVIDENCE-BASED PRACTICE TO PUBLIC HEALTH NURSING

This example describes the Intervention Wheel, a population-based practice model for public health nursing. The model consists of three levels of practice at the community, systems, and individual/family levels. It also consists of 17 public health interventions for improving population health. The model was originally developed using a qualitative grounded theory process but did not include a systematic review of evidence to support the interventions or their application to practice. Initially, the model was developed from an extensive analysis of the actual work of 200 practicing public health nurses working in a variety of settings. The 17 interventions grew out of this analysis, as did the three levels of practice. The authors indicated that the original intent was to provide a description of the scope and breadth of public health nursing practice.

Because of the positive response to the Intervention Wheel, the decision was made to complete a systematic review of the evidence supporting the use of the Intervention Wheel. The goal was to examine the evidence underlying the interventions and the levels of practice. The systematic review involved answering six questions, a comprehensive search of literature, a survey of 51 bachelor of science in nursing (BSN) programs in 5 states, and a critique (by 5 graduate students) of the 665 pieces of evidence found in the literature review for rigor (strength and usefulness). After limiting the final review to 221 sources of evidence, each source was independently rated by at least 2 members of a 42-member panel of practicing public health nurses and educators. The 42-member panel met to reach consensus on the outcomes of the reviews. The outcomes were field-tested with 150 practicing nurses and then critiqued by a national panel of 20 experts.

The Intervention Wheel presented is the result of this systematic review and critique (Keller et al., 2004). Although this critique may appear overwhelming, the undergraduate or graduate student may be involved in such a systematic critique as one of many participants contributing to the outcome of such a review. Table 9.2 applies some of the interventions to the core functions of public health.

TABLE 9.2   Core Public Health Functions and Related Evidence-Based Nursing Interventions

Core Functions	Related Nursing Interventions
Assessment	Diagnose and investigate health problems and hazards in the community.
	Mobilize community partnerships to identify and solve health problems.
	Link people to needed health services.
	Use evidence-based practice for new insights and innovative solutions to health problems.
Policy development	Inform, educate, and empower communities about health issues.
	Develop policies and plans using evidence-based practice that supports individual and community health efforts.
Assurance	Monitor health status to identify community health problems.
	Enforce laws and regulations that protect health and ensure safety.
	Ensure the provision of health care that is otherwise unavailable.
	Ensure a competent public health and personal health care workforce.
	Use evidence-based practice to evaluate effectiveness, accessibility, and quality of personal and population-based services.

CASE STUDY

Developing an Evidence-Based Health Promotion Program

Jamie Lee is the occupational health nurse at the T-shirt factory in town. Recently the health clinic at the T-shirt factory had budget cuts, resulting in the reduction of services and personnel. The once full-time clinic is now open only 3 days a week, and Ms. Lee no longer has support staff to help her with her paperwork responsibilities.

From her interactions with the workers, Ms. Lee has observed several risky health behaviors (e.g., unhealthy diets, smoking) among them. Although she is very busy in the clinic, Ms. Lee would like to develop a health promotion program to address these risky health behaviors, but she is not sure where to start.

▶ APPLYING CONTENT TO PRACTICE

It is important for nurses to acknowledge and understand EBP. They can participate by applying EBP or they can add to the research base for public health through active programs of research, participating in systematic reviews, or reviewing the best evidence available to them by reading published systematic reviews. Nurses can demonstrate leadership in supporting EBP by becoming change agents, fostering a cultural change in the practice environment, and assisting nurses who do not know how to use EBP to make a difference in practice.

For example, nurses who have recently graduated are knowledgeable about the use of evidence in practice. The new nurses can assist nurses who have been out of school for a while to find sources of evidence upon which to base their practice, such as referring them to *The Community Guide*. Using evidence in practice will demonstrate its value, but implementation can be difficult because of lthe sheer volume of evidence and increasing population needs. Sharing knowledge and engaging in teamwork can help overcome these barriers.

Nurses have an important role to play in developing and using clinical guidelines for community practices. Use of a community development model and engaging in community partnerships will ensure that the community's perspective is included.

Nurses active in EBP can devote attention to understanding how best to incorporate the guidelines into practice demonstrating practice excellence. EBP offers the opportunity for shared decision making because it can help nurses focus their thinking, observe process outcomes, and thus improve care for clients by communicating with leaders and other nurses what they have observed. Participation in EBP offers continuing professional growth and a feeling of value, recognition for contributions, and respect from peers and administrators (Dols et al., 2017; Melnyk et al., 2017).

▮ PRACTICE APPLICATION

A nurse who is the director of a public health clinic is in the process of analyzing how best to expand services to operate as a full-time clinic in the most cost-effective and clinically effective manner. The director gathers evidence from the literature on public health clinics in rural settings to evaluate cost and clinical effectiveness of various models. The nurse also considers evidence from the following sources in the decision-making process: client satisfaction research data, knowledge of clinic staff, expert opinion of community advisory board members, evidence from community partners, and data on service needs in the state. Having examined the evidence, the nurse decides that incremental (step-by-step) growth toward full-time status is warranted. Evidence of needs in the community and analysis of statistical data indicate that the addition of wellness services for children is a priority, and a pediatric nurse practitioner is hired as a first step to assist the public health nurses while planning for full-time status continues.

A. Evaluation of the evidence gathered demonstrates which of the following?
   1. Effectiveness of the intervention in communities
   2. Application of the data to populations and communities
   3. Existence of positive or negative health outcomes
   4. Economic consequences of the intervention
   5. Barriers to implementation of the interventions in communities
B. Explain how this example applies principles of EBP.
   Answers can be found on the Evolve website.

▮ REMEMBER THIS!

- Evidence-based practice (EBP) was developed in other countries before its use in the United States.
- Application of EBP in relation to clinical decision making in population-centered nursing concentrates on interventions and strategies geared to communities and populations rather than to individuals.
- Nurses at all levels have an opportunity to improve the practice of nursing and client outcomes.

- Evaluating the strength and usefulness of evidence is essential to finding the best evidence on which to make practice decisions.
- EBP includes interventions based on theory, expert opinions, provider knowledge, and research.
- Use of a community development model and community partnership model involves community leaders in making decisions about best practices in their community.

EVOLVE WEBSITE

http://evolve.elsevier.com/Stanhope/community/
- Answers to Practice Application
- Case Study
- Review Questions

REFERENCES

Barnard K, Hoehn R: *Nursing Child Assessment Satellite Training: Final Report*, Hyattsville, 1978, DHEW, Division of Nursing.

Bowers B: Evidence-based practice in community nursing, *Br J Community Nurs* 23(7): 336–337, 2018.

Brooke JM, Mallion J: Implementation of evidence-based practice by nurses working in community settings and their strategies to mentor student nurses to develop evidence-based practice: a qualitative study, *Int J Nurs Pract* 22(4):339–347, 2016.

Brower EJ, Nemec R: Origins of evidence-based practices and what it means for nurses, *Int J of Childbirth Educ* 32(2):14–18, 2017.

Brownson RC, Baker EA, Deshpande AD, Gillespie KN: *Evidence-based public health*, ed 3. New York, 2018, Oxford University Press.

Brownson RC, Fielding JE, Maylahn CM: Evidence-based public health: a fundamental concept for public health practice, *Annu Rev Public Health* 30:175–202, 2009.

Campbell JD, Brooks M, Hosokawa P, Robinson J, Song L, Krieger J: Community health worker home visits for Medicaid-enrolled children with asthma: effects on asthma outcomes and costs, *Am J Public Health* 105(11):2366–2372, 2015.

Carper BA: Fundamental patterns of knowing in nursing, *ANS Adv Nurs Sci* 1(1):13–23, 1978.

Chapman A: Evidence based practice and public health, *HLG Nursing Bulletin* 37(3/4):90–93, 2018.

Community Preventive Services Task Force (CPSTF): *The Community Guide*, 2018. Retrieved from http://www.thecommunityguide.org.

Cochrane Library: *Cochrane handbook for systematic reviews of interventions,* version 6, 2019. Retrieved from www.cochrane.org.

Dawes M, Davies P, Gray A, et al: *Evidence-Based Practice: a Primer for Health Care Professionals*, ed 2. London, 2004, Churchill Livingstone Elsevier.

Dicenso A, Guyatt G, Ciliska D, editors: *Evidence-Based Nursing: a Guide to Clinical Practice*, St. Louis, 2005, Elsevier Mosby.

Dols JD, Muñoz LR, Martinez SS, et al.: Developing policies and protocols in the age of evidence-based practice, *J Contin Educ Nurs* 48(2):87-92, 2017

Duncombe DC: A multi-institutional study of the perceived barriers and facilitators to implementing evidence-based practice, *J Clin Nurs* 27(5/6):1216–1226, 2018.

Essential Evidence Plus: *POEMs research summaries*, 2018. Retrieved from https://www.essentialevidenceplus.com.

Estabrooks CA, Winther C, Derksen L: Mapping the field: a bibliometric analysis of the research utilization literature in nursing, *Nurs Res* 53:293–303, 2004.

Evidence-Based Medicine Working Group: Evidence-based medicine: a new approach to teaching the practice of medicine, *JAMA* 268:2420–2425, 1992.

Fineout-Overholt E, Melnyk B, Stillwell SB, Williamson KM: Critical appraisal of the evidence: part 1: an introduction to gathering, evaluating, and recording the evidence, *Am J Nurs* 110(7):47–52, 2010.

Grove SK, Gray J: *Understanding nursing research—building an evidence-based practice*, ed 7, St. Louis, 2019, Elsevier Saunders.

Guyatt G, Rennie D, editors: *Users' guides to the medical literature: a manual for evidence-based clinical practice*, Chicago, 2002, AMA.

Häggman-Laitila A, Mattila LR, Melender HL: A systematic review of journal clubs for nurses, *Worldviews Evid Based Nurs* 13(2): 163–171, 2016.

Haine-Schlagel R, Fettes DL, Garcia AR, Brookman-Frazee L, Garland AF: Consistency with evidence-based treatments and perceived effectiveness of children's community-based care, *Community Ment Health J* 50(2):158–163, 2014.

Honor Society of Nursing, Sigma Theta Tau International: *Evidence-based nursing position statement,* 2005. Retrieved from http://www.nursingsociety.org.

Horsley JA, Crane J, Bingle J: Research utilization as an organizational process, *J Nurs Admin* 8:4–6, 1978.

Horsley JA, Crane J, Crabtree MK, et al: *Using Research to Improve Nursing Practice: A Guide*, San Francisco, 1983, Grune & Stratton.

Keller LO, Strohschein S, Lia-Hoagberg B, Schaffer MA: Population-based public health interventions: practice-based and evidence-supported. Part I, *Public Health Nurs* 21(5):453–468, 2004.

King D, Barnard KE, Hoehn R: Disseminating the results of nursing research, *Nurs Outlook* 29:164–169, 1981.

Kristensen N, Nymann C, Konradsen H: Implementing research results in clinical practice—the experiences of healthcare professional, *BMC Health Serv Res* 16:48, 2016.

Krueger JC: Utilizing clinical nursing research findings in practice: a structured approach, *Commun Nurs Res* 9:381–394, 1977.

Krueger JC, Nelson AH, Wolanin MO: *Nursing Research: Development, Collaboration and Utilization*, Germantown, 1978, Aspen.

Lindeman CA, Krueger JC: Increasing the quality, quantity, and use of nursing research, *Nurs Outlook* 25:450–454, 1977.

Mathieson A, Grande G, Luker L: Strategies, facilitators and barriers to implementation of evidence-based practice in community nursing: a systematic mixed-studies review and qualitative synthesis, *Primary Health Care Research & Development,* 20(E6). doi:10.1017/S1463423618000488

Melnyk BM, Gallager-Ford L, Fineout-Overholt E: *Implementing the evidence-based practice competencies in healthcare—a practical guide for improving quality, safety, & outcomes*, Indianapolis, IN, 2017, Sigma Theta Tau International.

Melnyk BM, Fineout-Overholt E, Stillwell SB, Williamson KM: Evidence-based practice: step by step: the seven steps of evidence-based practice, *Am J Nurs* 110(1):51–53, 2010.

Melnyk BM, Fineout-Overholt E: *Evidence-Based Practice in Nursing and Healthcare: A Guide to Best Practice*, ed 4. Philadelphia, 2019, Wolters Kluwer Health.

Pereira F, Pellaux V, Verloo H: Beliefs and implementation of evidence-based practice among community health nurses: a cross-sectional descriptive study, *J Clin Nurs* 27(9/10): 2052-2061, 2018.

Pierce LL, Reuille KM: Instructor-created activities to engage undergraduate nursing research students, *J Nurs Educ* 57(3): 174–177, 2018.

Polit DF, Beck CT: *Essentials of Nursing Research: Appraising Evidence for Nursing Practice*, ed 9, Philadelphia, 2018, Wolters Kluwer.

Public Health Accreditation Board: *Accredited health departments*, 2020. Retrieved from http://www.phaboard.org.

Rychetnik L, Hawe P, Waters E, Barratt A, Frommer M: A glossary for evidence based public health, *J Epidemiol Community Health* 58(7):538–545, 2004.

Sackett DL, Rosenberg WMC, Gray J, et al: Evidence-based medicine: what it is and what it isn't, *BMJ* 312:71–72, 1996.

Schaefer JD, Welton JM: Evidence based practice readiness: a concept analysis, *J Nurs Manag* 26(6):621–629, 2018.

Stetler CB: Updating the Stetler model of research utilization to facilitate evidence-based practice, *Nurs Outlook* 49:272–279, 2001.

US Department of Health and Human Services: *Healthy People 2030*. HHS, 2020. Available at https://health.gov/our-work/healthy-people-2030.

Vaidya N, Thota AB, Proia KK, et al: Practice-based evidence in Community Guide systematic reviews, *Am J Public Health* 107(3):413–420, 2017.

Weiss ME, Bobay KL, Johantgen M, Shirey MR: Aligning evidence-based practice with translational research: opportunities for clinical practice research, *J Nurs Adm* 48(9):425–431, 2018.

West S, King V, Carey TS, Lohr KN, McKoy N, Sutton SF, Lux L: *Systems to rate the strength of scientific evidence: summary*, Rockville MD, 2002, Agency for Healthcare Research and Quality.

Zimmerman K: Essentials of evidence based practice, *Int J Childbirth Educ* 32(2):37–43, 2017.

10

Epidemiologic Applications

Swan Arp Adams and DeAnne K. Hilfinger Messias

OBJECTIVES

After reading this chapter, the student should be able to:

1. Define epidemiology and describe its basic elements and approach.
2. Identify elements of the epidemiologic triangle and the ecological model and describe the interactions among these elements in both models.
3. Discuss the steps in the epidemiologic process.
4. Explain the basic epidemiologic concepts of population at risk, natural history of disease, levels of prevention,

host-agent-environment relationships, and the web-of-causation model.
5. Differentiate between descriptive and analytic epidemiology.
6. Explain how nurses use epidemiology in public health practice.

CHAPTER OUTLINE

KEY TERMS

The term *epidemiology* comes from the Greek terms *logos* ("study"), *demos* ("people"), and *epi* ("upon"). Literally this would be "the study of what is upon the people." Epidemiology is the basic science of public health; it is study of the distribution and determinants of disease in populations. For example, you would use epidemiology to see if a disease is more common among men or women or if the disease is seen more in older versus younger people. The term originally referred to the spread of infectious epidemics such as cholera or tuberculosis (TB). Now the term is more inclusive and involves infectious diseases and chronic diseases, such as cancer and cardiovascular disease, as well as mental health and other health-related events, such as intentional injuries (accidents), violence, occupational and environmental exposures and their effects, and positive health states. Epidemiology has been an essential science in trying to understand what causes COVID-19, its transmission and incubation, and how to trace those who have been near someone who tested positive for the virus.

DEFINITIONS

Health is the core concept in nursing and epidemiology. A holistic approach to health, including the incorporation of epidemiologic principles, is particularly appropriate for nurses. Epidemiology has been defined as "the study of the occurrence and distribution of health-related states ore events in specified populations, including the study of the determinants influencing such states, and the application of the knowledge to control the health problems" (Porta, 2014). Epidemiology investigates the distribution or the patterns of health events in populations to understand health outcomes in terms of what, who, where, when, how, and why: What is the outcome? Who is affected? Where are they? When do events occur? The focus is on descriptive epidemiology because

it seeks to describe the occurrence of a disease in terms of person, place, and time (Weiss and Koepsell, 2014). The how and why, or determinants of health events, are those factors, exposures, characteristics, behaviors, and contexts that determine (or influence) the patterns: How does it occur? Why are some people affected more than others? Determinants may be individual, relational or social, communal, or environmental. This focus on investigation of causes and associations is called analytic epidemiology.

Epidemiology, like both the research process and nursing process, consists of a set of steps. The first step is to answer the "what" question by defining the outcome. The health outcome can be a disease, or it can refer to injuries, accidents, or even wellness (Weiss and Koepsell, 2014). Epidemiologic methods are used to quantify the frequency of occurrence and characterize both the case group and the population from which they come. Epidemiology played a key role in the refinement of the case definition for acquired immunodeficiency syndrome (AIDS) and will be essential to determining ways to understand COVID-19. The aim in epidemiology is to describe the distribution (i.e., determine how, where, and when the disease occurs) and to look for factors that explain the pattern of the disease or the risk for occurrence (i.e., answer the questions of why and how the disease occurs).

Like nursing, epidemiology builds on and draws from other disciplines and methods, including clinical medicine and laboratory sciences, social sciences, quantitative methods (especially biostatistics), and public health policy and goals. Epidemiology focuses on populations, whereas clinical medicine focuses on the diagnosis and treatment of disease in individuals. Epidemiology studies populations to (1) monitor the health of the population, (2) understand the determinants of health and disease in communities, and (3) investigate and evaluate interventions to prevent disease and maintain health.

Effective nursing interventions bridge the disciplines of clinical medicine and epidemiology, incorporating a focus on both individual and collective strategies. Epidemiologic methods are used extensively to determine to what extent the goals of *Healthy People 2030* (US Department of Health and Human Services, 2020) have been met and to monitor the progress of those objectives not fully met at present.

Epidemiology is true detective work. For example, consider a man who visited a country other than where he lived. Within 3 days, he was experiencing nausea and diarrhea. The epidemiologic process could help to determine what action should be taken. Specifically, what did he eat or drink? Did others eat or drink the same things? Are other people with him experiencing the same symptoms? After a thorough review of the "what, who, where, and when," he realizes that the only thing he did differently from others with him was use water from the bathroom faucet to brush his teeth. Others in his group had used bottled water. Although he knew that people often react negatively to water that is different from their own, he was so accustomed to using tap water to brush his teeth that he did so in this new location without thinking about the effects it might have for him. Similarly, three women shared a meal, and all ate everything, except for one person who did not eat any green peppers. Thirty minutes after eating, the two women who ate the green peppers had painful gastrointestinal symptoms. The only thing different in what they had to eat and drink that day were the peppers. One can conclude that the peppers may not have been washed carefully or had some other way of having bacteria attached to them. Using the epidemiologic process is more complex with COVID-19 because it is spread through the air, and it is difficult when people gather in groups, especially large groups, to know who was the COVID-19-positive person.

♥ HEALTHY PEOPLE 2030

Examples of Epidemiologic Objectives in Healthy People 2030

- **D-09:** Reduce the rate of death in adults with diabetes.
- **FS-07:** Increase the proportion of people who wash their hands and surfaces often when preparing food.
- **DS-10:** Increase the proportion of people who refrigerate food within 2 h after cooking.

From US Department of Health and Human Services: *Healthy People 2030*, Washington, DC, 2020, US Government Printing Office.

HISTORY

Hippocrates, in the 4th century BCE, was one of the first people to use the ideas that are now part of epidemiology (Merrill, 2017). He examined health and disease in a community by looking at geography, climate, the seasons of the year, the food and water consumed, and the habits and behaviors of the people. His approach, like descriptive epidemiology, looked at how health is influenced by personal characteristics, place, and time.

In the 18th and 19th centuries, comparison groups began to be used to measure change or the effects of some action or treatment on an experimental group. Also at this time, quantitative methods (i.e., numeric measurements or counts) were beginning to be used. One of the most famous studies using a comparison group is the mid-19th-century investigation of cholera by John Snow, whom some call the "father of epidemiology" (Merrill, 2017). By mapping cases that clustered around one public water pump during a London cholera outbreak, Snow was able to show how the water supply and cholera were associated. He observed that cholera rates were higher among households supplied by water companies whose water came from downstream than among households whose water came from farther upstream, where it was subject to less contamination. Snow conducted a "natural experiment," as seen in Table 10.1, and documented that foul water was the vehicle for transmission of the agent that caused cholera (Weiss and Koepsell, 2014).

In nursing, Florence Nightingale contributed to the development of epidemiology in her work with British soldiers during the Crimean War (1854 to 1856). At this time, sick soldiers were cared for in cramped quarters that had poor sanitation, were overrun with lice and rats, and had insufficient food and medical supplies. She looked at the relationship between the conditions of the environment and the recovery of the soldiers. Using simple epidemiologic measures of rates of illness per 1000 soldiers, she was able to show that improving environmental conditions and adding nursing care decreased the mortality rates of the soldiers (Cohen, 1984; Palmer, 1983). These same principles can be applied today in the many countries that experience war leading to poor food, water, and sanitary conditions. That is, if the environment is improved and better care provided, the rate of illnesses and death can be reduced.

During the 20th century, several changes in society influenced the further development of epidemiology. Some of these were the Great Depression of the 1920s in the United States;

TABLE 10.1 Household Cholera Death Rates by Source of Water Supply in John Snow's 1853 Investigation			
Company	**Number of Houses**	**Deaths From Cholera**	**Deaths per 10,000 Households**
Southwark and Vauxhall	40,046	1263	315
Lambeth	26,107	98	37

From Snow J: On the mode of communication of cholera. In *Snow on cholera*, New York, 1855, The Commonwealth Fund.

World War II; a rising standard of living for many but poverty for others; improved nutrition; better sanitation; the development of antibiotics, vaccines, and cancer chemotherapies; decreased birth rates in some countries; and decreases in infant and child mortality in many nations. People began to live longer, and these shifts in the age distribution of the population led to increases in the rates of several age-related chronic diseases such as coronary heart disease (CHD), stroke, cancer, and senile dementia. In 1900 the leading causes of death were (1) pneumonia and influenza, followed by (2) TB and (3) gastritis, enteritis, and colitis; then came (4) heart diseases, (5) symptoms of senility, (6) vascular lesions affecting the central nervous system (CNS), (7) chronic nephritis and renal sclerosis, (8) unintentional injuries, (9) malignant neoplasms, and (10) diphtheria. In 2018 heart disease was the leading cause of death. Other leading causes included cancer, accidents, chronic lower respiratory diseases, cerebrovascular disease, Alzheimer disease, diabetes mellitus, influenza and pneumonia, nephritis, nephrotic syndrome and nephrosis, and intentional self-harm. COVID-19 was added to the top 10 leading causes of death in 2020. The leading causes of death worldwide are similar to those in the United States. However, lung disease, road injury, diarrheal diseases, and TB are all major causes of death worldwide but are not among the top 10 in the United States (Elflein, 2020).

During the 20th century a shift occurred from looking for single agents, such as the infectious agent that causes cholera, to determining the multifactorial etiology or the many factors or combinations of factors that contribute to disease. This is referred to as an ecological model. An example of multifactorial etiology can be found in the complex number and type of factors that cause cardiovascular disease. People began to realize that not all of the diseases of older people were the result of the degenerative processes of aging. Rather, it became clear that many behavioral and environmental factors supported or encouraged the development of diseases. This information led to the belief that some diseases could be prevented and other diseases could at least be delayed.

In addition, the development of genetic and molecular techniques increased the ability of the epidemiologist to classify persons in terms of exposures or inherent susceptibility to disease. Examples included the identification of genetic traits that indicated an increased risk for breast cancer and markers that identified exposures to environmental toxins such as lead or pesticides. These developments are of particular interest to nurses who work with people in their living and work environments and understand the interaction of the environment(s) on health and well-being. Furthermore, nurses in the community can assess a broad range of health outcomes as well as factors that contribute to wellness and illness.

Unfortunately, in recent years new infectious diseases (e.g., Ebola, the Zika virus, Lyme disease, methicillin-resistant *Staphylococcus aureus* [MRSA], the H1N1 and H3N2 viruses, and COVID-19) and new forms of old diseases (e.g., drug-resistant strains of TB, new forms of *Escherichia coli*) have emphasized the dangers that can occur with these diseases. In addition, potential threats from terrorist use of infectious agents (e.g., anthrax, smallpox) have once again placed the epidemiology of infectious diseases in the spotlight. Epidemiologic methods also have been applied to a broader spectrum of health-related outcomes, including accidents, injuries and violence, occupational and environmental exposures, psychiatric and sociologic phenomena, health-related behaviors, and health services research.

HOW NURSES USE EPIDEMIOLOGY

Nurses play a key role in the community's interdisciplinary team, looking at health, disease causation, and how to both prevent and treat illness. Nurses use epidemiology in the community to examine factors that affect the individual, family, and population group because it is more difficult to control these factors in the community than in the hospital. Specifically, it is difficult to control the environment, including water and food supplies; air quality conditions, including pollutants; disposal of garbage and trash; insects and animals that carry infectious diseases; quality of paint used to ensure it contains no lead; or what comes in the mail. Therefore community residents are often exposed to many factors affecting their health.

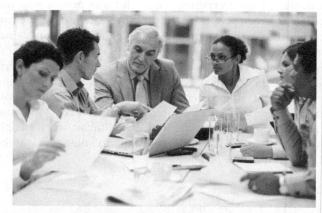

Nurses Work in an Interdisciplinary Team to Solve Epidemiologic Problems. (© 2012 Photos.com, a division of Getty Images. All rights reserved. Image #121198999.)

Nurses are involved in the surveillance and monitoring of disease trends. In settings such as homes, schools, workplaces, clinics, and health care organizations, nurses can identify patterns of disease in a group. For example, if several children in a school become sick with abdominal problems within a short period (e.g., a 24-hour period), the nurse would try to determine what these children had in common. For instance, did they eat the same food, drink from the same source of water, or swim in the same pool? Likewise, if workers in a plant displayed a similar pattern of symptoms, the nurse would look for factors in the workplace to locate the cause. The reason for looking at the workplace first is that it is the setting the individuals have in common. During the pandemic that began in 2020, nurses played a key role in the testing of people around the world for the virus.

Care of clients, families, and population groups in the community uses the following steps of the nursing process: (1) assessment,

(2) diagnosis, (3) planning, (4) implementation, and (5) evaluation. When using the nursing process, epidemiology provides baseline information for assessing needs, identifying problems, designing appropriate strategies to evaluate the problems, setting priorities to develop a plan of care, and evaluating how effective the care was. The information learned from the Human Genome Project completed in 2003 will continue to be the basis of new discoveries about the consequences of genetic variations and the outcomes of the interaction between genes and the environment. Nurses, in their focus on health, can use the information that is now available and will increasingly become available as a result of further research. The "Essential Nursing Competencies and Curricula Guidelines for Genetics" will help nurses to care for individuals, families, communities, and populations by including genetic and genomic information in their practice. For example, this information could assist a nurse to recognize whether a newborn is at risk for morbidity or mortality resulting from errors in genetic metabolism and when there is a history of a genetic mutation in the family (American Nurses Association, 2006).

CHECK YOUR PRACTICE

A 40-year-old woman returns from a cancer center after learning that she has an ATM gene mutation and that this may cause her to have a higher risk of developing certain types of cancers. There is a likely increased risk for breast, ovarian, and pancreatic cancer. One of her options is a prophylactic mastectomy, which has been shown to significantly reduce the risk of breast cancer. That will be a difficult decision for her to make. However, the other difficult decision will be whether she will inform members of her family of this information because they could also be affected. Consider the following questions:

1. Would you do nothing until she decides whether she will have the mastectomy or not and learns more about the ATM gene?
2. Would you suggest that she think carefully about whether she should tell her siblings and other family members who may also be at increased risk?
3. If she decides to tell her family, should she encourage them to have genetic testing?
4. Would you recommend that she meet with a genetic counselor before she tells her family members?
5. How can you be assured that she is aware of the Genetic Information Nondiscrimination Act (GINA), which prohibits health insurers and most employers from discriminating against individuals based on genetic information (including the results of genetic tests and family history information)?
6. You might encourage her to visit http://www.ginahelp.org. What other steps would you take to advise and counsel her effectively?
7. Using the six essential clinical judgment steps developed by the National Council of State Boards of Nursing (NCSBN): recognize cues; analyze cues; prioritize hypotheses; generate solutions; take action, and evaluate outcomes, would you take further actions than those in the first five questions in this clinical scenario? If you take further actions, what specifically would they be? What questions would you ask to determine and analyze the cues in order to develop your hypotheses, plan of action, and steps to take to evaluate the outcome of your nursing care?

The sections that follow discuss the "tools of epidemiology" that are needed by nurses who work in community settings.

CASE STUDY

Church Picnic

Mary Miles is the nurse epidemiologist for the Warren County Health Department. A local church contacted Ms. Miles when several church members became sick after the annual church picnic. Of the 200 people who attended the picnic, 100 were ill with diarrhea, nausea, or vomiting. Ten people required emergency medical treatment or hospitalization. Incubation periods ranged from 1.5 to 30 hours, with a mean of 6 hours and a median of 3.5 hours. Duration of illness ranged from 1 to 80 hours, with a mean of 30 hours and a median of 15 hours.

The annual church picnic is a potluck lunch buffet. The menu included macaroni casserole (brought by the Joneses), turkey with gravy and stuffing (brought by the Smiths), potato salad (brought by the Changs), green bean casserole (brought by the Champs), chili (brought by the Turners), homemade bread (brought by Granny Ivy), chocolate cake (brought by the Bushes), and cookies (brought by the Beckmans). Ms. Miles interviewed the church members who were ill and found that three food items were significantly associated with illness: turkey, gravy, and stuffing.

Ms. Miles interviewed the Smiths, who brought the turkey, gravy, and stuffing to the picnic. Review of food-handling procedures indicated that the turkey had cooled for 4 hours at room temperature after cooking—a time and temperature sufficient for bacterial growth and toxin production. Furthermore, the same utensils were used for both the turkey and other foods before and after cooking.

Ms. Miles talked with the Smiths about proper food-handling practices, emphasizing hand washing, proper cooling and preserving methods, and better equipment and utensil sanitation. Ms. Miles also offered a similar class to the church congregation.

1. For the nurse to evaluate why people at the picnic became sick, what questions should she ask the people who brought the food?
   A. Cooking time and how they cooked the food
   B. Hygiene of their equipment
   C. Sources of the water used in cooking the food
   D. All of the above
2. Identify the agent, host, and environment in this.
3. Is Ms. Miles performing descriptive epidemiology or analytic epidemiology?
4. Which level of prevention is Ms. Miles exemplifying?
   A. Primary prevention
   B. Secondary prevention
   C. Tertiary prevention
   D. Combination of the above
   E. None of the above

Answers can be found on the Evolve website.

Contrast this form of epidemiologic investigation with the onset of the COVID-19 pandemic. It was often difficult to do contact tracing due to the large numbers of people in proximity to the person(s) who tested positive for the virus. Consider the difficulty if the person testing positive was a passenger on a cruise ship; someone who attended a demonstration; or someone who participated in a large social event. Contact tracing has been used for decades by state and local health departments to slow or stop the spread of infectious diseases. Applying the concept of contact tracing to the spread of COVID-19, you would:
- Let people know they may have been exposed to COVID-19 and should monitor their health for signs and symptoms of COVID-19
- Help people who may have been exposed to COVID-19 get tested

- Ask people to self-isolate if they have COVID-19 or self-quarantine if they are a close contact of someone with COVID-19

BASIC CONCEPTS IN EPIDEMIOLOGY

Measures of Morbidity and Mortality

Proportions, Rates, and Risk

Epidemiology looks at the distribution of health states and events. Because people differ in their probability or risk for disease, the primary concern is how they differ. Today epidemiologists use tools such as geographic information systems (GISs) to study health-related events to identify disease distribution patterns, similar to how John Snow mapped cases of cholera in one area of London. However, mapping of cases is limited in what it can reveal. A larger number of cases may simply be the result of a larger population with more potential cases or the result of a longer period of observation. Any description of disease patterns should take into account the size of the population at risk for the disease. That is, we should look not only at the numerator (the number of cases) but also at the denominator (the number of people in the population at risk) and at the amount of time each was observed. For example, 50 cases of influenza might be seen as a serious epidemic in a population of 250 but would be a low rate in a population of 250,000. Using rates and proportions instead of simple counts of cases takes the size of the population at risk into account.

Epidemiologic studies rely on rates and proportions. A proportion is a type of ratio in which the denominator includes the numerator. For example in 2017, there were 2,813,503 deaths recorded in the United States, of which 647,457 were reported to have been caused by heart disease; the proportion of deaths attributed to heart disease at a given time was 647,457/2,813,503 = 0.230, or 23.0%. Because the numerator must be included in the denominator, proportions can range from 0 to 1. Proportions are often multiplied by 100 and expressed as a percentage, literally meaning "per 100." However, in public health statistics, if the proportion is very small, we use a larger multiplier to avoid small fractions, so the proportion may be expressed as a number per 1000 or per 100,000.

A rate is a measure of the frequency of a health event in different populations at certain periods (Porta, 2014). A rate is a ratio, but it is not a proportion because the denominator is a function of both the population size and the dimension of time, whereas the numerator is the number of events. Furthermore, depending on the units of time and the frequency of events, a rate may exceed 1. As its name suggests, a rate is a measure of how quickly something is happening: how rapidly a disease is developing in a population or how rapidly people are dying. Rates deal with change: moving from one state of being to another, from well to ill, from alive to dead, or from ill to cured. Because they deal with events (i.e., moving from one state of being to another), time is involved. We must follow a population over time to observe the changes in state, and we typically exclude from the population being followed those persons who

have already experienced the event. Using the same 2017 data for number of deaths and deaths due to heart disease, you have number of deaths = 2,813,503 divided by 100,000 is 2814. Then calculate the death rate from heart disease by 647, 457 divided by 2814 = 230.1 per 100,000.

Risk refers to the probability that an event will occur within a specified period. A population at risk is the population of persons for whom there is some finite probability (even if small) of that event occurring. For example, although the risk for breast cancer in men is small, a few men do develop breast cancer and therefore are part of the population at risk. There are some outcomes for which certain people would never be at risk (e.g., men cannot be at risk for ovarian cancer, nor can women be at risk for testicular cancer). In contrast, a high-risk population would include those persons who, because of exposure, lifestyle, family history, or other factors, are at greater risk for disease than the population at large. For example, although everyone in the population is at risk for human immunodeficiency virus (HIV) infection and AIDS, persons who have multiple sexual partners without adequate protection or who use intravenous drugs are in the high-risk population for HIV infection. However, others may unknowingly be at high risk, such as women who think they are in monogamous relationships and do not know that their partners have sexual relations with other individuals. Genetic testing is becoming more common, but most tests for disease indicate only susceptibility to disease, not certainty. Similarly, screening tests are never perfect, so there is always some probability of misclassifying a person. Similarly, a person's risk of developing COVID-19 is great if that person has been in contract with a person who has the virus. The person with the virus may be asymptomatic when the infection is transferred to the other person(s). The risk decreased as people were vaccinated for the virus and as people continued to wear masks inside and observe social distancing behaviors.

Epidemiologists and other health professionals examine measures of morbidity, especially incidence proportions, incidence rates, and prevalence proportions, to learn about the risk for disease, the rate of disease development, and the levels of existing disease in a population, respectively.

Measures of Incidence

Measures of incidence reflect the number of new cases or events in a population at risk during a specified time. An incidence rate quantifies the rate of development of new cases in a population at risk, whereas an incidence proportion indicates the proportion of the population at risk that experiences the event over some period of time (Rothman, 2012). The population at risk is considered to be persons without the event or outcome of interest but who are at risk for experiencing it. People who already have the disease or outcome of interest are excluded from the population at risk for this calculation because they already have the condition and are no longer at risk for developing it. The incidence proportion is also referred to as the *cumulative incidence rate* because it reflects the cumulative effect of the incidence rate over the time period. The risk for disease is a function of both the rate of new disease development and the length of time the population is at risk. The interpretation can be for an individual (i.e., the probability that the person will become ill) or for a population (i.e., the proportion of a population expected to become ill over that period). In epidemiology, we often calculate proportions on the basis of population frequencies. These frequencies are then translated into personal risk statements for people representative of the population on which the estimates are based.

For example, suppose a health department and hospital partner want to develop an intensive, broad-based screening program in an area with overcrowded housing, limited access to services, and underuse of preventive health practices. They might include physical examinations; tuberculin skin tests with follow-up chest radiography where indicated; cardiovascular, glaucoma, and diabetes screening; and mammography for women and prostate screening for men older than 45 years of age. Of the 8000 women screened, 35 were previously diagnosed with breast cancer; by screening and follow-up, 20 with no history of breast cancer were found to have cancer of the breast. We could follow the 7945 women in whom no breast cancer was detected and note the number of new cases of breast cancer detected over the following 5 years. Assuming no losses to follow-up (i.e., moved away or died from other causes), if 44 women were diagnosed over the 5-year period, the 5-year incidence proportion of breast cancer in this population would be as follows:

$$\frac{44}{7945} = 0.005538, \text{ or } 553.8 \text{ per } 100,000$$

Note the multiplication by 100,000, so that the number of cases is expressed as per 100,000 women. A cumulative incidence rate estimates the risk for developing the disease in that population during that time. In addition, as a proportion, each event in the numerator must be represented in the denominator, and only those persons at risk for the event counted in the numerator may be included in the denominator.

A ratio can be used as an approximation of a risk. For example, the infant mortality "rate" is the number of infant deaths (infants are defined as being younger than 1 year of age) in a given year divided by the number of live births in that same year. It approximates the risk for death in the first year of life for live-born infants in a specific year. Some of the infants who die that year were born in the previous year, and some of the infants born that year may die in the following year before their first birthday. However, because approximately two-thirds of infant deaths occur within the first 28 days of life, the number of infants in the numerator (i.e., deaths in a given year) but not in the denominator (i.e., live births in that same year) will be small. It can be assumed that current year's deaths from the previous year's cohort approximately equal the deaths from the current year's cohort occurring in the following year. Although technically a ratio, this is an approximation to the true proportion and therefore an estimate of the risk.

The terms endemic, outbreak, epidemic, and pandemic describe how common a condition is at a point in time related to how common it was at an earlier time. An endemic condition is present when the number of cases present is approximately

what one would expect. The health condition occurs at a steady rate among the population. An example would be malaria in Africa. An outbreak refers to a condition that occurs in excess of what would be expected at the endemic level. An example would be the increased rate of measles among unvaccinated US children who visited a theme park in 2015. An epidemic occurs when the rate of disease, injury, or other condition exceeds the usual (i.e., endemic) level of that condition and spreads over a larger geographic area. An example would be the 2014 to 2016 Ebola outbreak in West Africa. No specific threshold of incidence indicates that an epidemic exists. Because of the virtual eradication of smallpox globally, any occurrence of smallpox might be considered an epidemic by this definition. In contrast, given the high rates of ischemic heart disease in the United States, a large increase of cases would be needed before an epidemic was noted, although some might argue that the current high rates in contrast to earlier periods already indicate an epidemic. A pandemic is an epidemic that spreads globally. Before the onset of the COVID-19 pandemic, the best-known pandemic was the 1918 Spanish influenza, which infected more than one-third of the world's population, and a more recent example was the severe acute respiratory syndrome (SARS) virus in 2003 (Grennan, 2019).

In thinking about infectious diseases, it is important to talk about herd immunity. Herd immunity is "the resistance of a group of people to an attack by a disease to which a large proportion of the members of the group are immune. If a large percentage of the members of the group are immune, the entire population may be protected; not just those who are immune" (Celentano and Szklo, 2018, p 27). Herd immunity can be provided when a large percentage of the population have either been vaccinated or have had the disease. Herd immunity will not be protective if a number of people who live, work, or go to school in the same area chose not to be vaccinated or have not had the illness.

Prevalence Proportion

The prevalence proportion is a measure of existing disease in a population at a particular time (i.e., the number of existing cases divided by the current population). It is also possible to calculate the prevalence of a specific risk factor or exposure. In the breast cancer example given earlier, the screening program discovered 35 of the 8000 women screened had previously been diagnosed with breast cancer and 20 women with no history of breast cancer were diagnosed as a result of the screening. The prevalence proportion of current and past breast cancer events in this population of women would be as follows:

$$\frac{55}{8000} = 0.006875, \text{ or } 687.5 \text{ per } 100,000$$

A prevalence proportion is not an estimate of the risk for developing disease because it is a function of both the rate at which new cases of the disease develop and how long those cases remain in the population. In this example, the prevalence of breast cancer in this population of women is a function of how many new cases develop and how long women live after the diagnosis of breast cancer. A fairly constant prevalence might be seen, for example, if improved survival after diagnosis were offset by an increasing incidence rate. The duration of a disease is affected by case fatality and cure. (For simplicity, in this example, women with a history of the disease are counted in the prevalence proportion even though they may have been cured.) A disease with a short duration (e.g., an intestinal virus) may not have a high prevalence proportion even if the rate of new cases is high because cases do not accumulate (see the discussion of point epidemic). A disease with a long course will have a higher prevalence proportion than a rapidly fatal disease that has the same rate of new cases.

Incidence and Prevalence Compared

The prevalence proportion measures existing cases of disease and is affected by factors that influence risk (i.e., incidence) and factors that influence survival or recovery (i.e., duration). Prevalence proportions are useful in planning health care services because they indicate the level of disease existing in the population and therefore the size of the population in need of services. However, prevalence measures are less useful when we are looking for factors related to disease etiology. Because prevalence proportions reflect duration in addition to the risk for getting the disease, it is difficult to sort out what factors are related to risk and what factors are related to survival or recovery. In mathematic notation,

$$p/(1-P) \cong I \times D,$$
$$\text{or, when } P \text{ is small } (<0.1), \text{ the } P \cong I \times D,$$

where P = prevalence, I = incidence rate, and D = average duration.

For example, the 5-year survival rate for breast cancer is approximately 85%, but the 5-year survival rate for lung cancer in women is only approximately 15%. Even if the incidence rates of breast and lung cancer were the same in women (and they are not), the prevalence proportions would differ because, on average, women live longer with breast cancer (i.e., it has a longer duration). In contrast, incidence rates and incidence proportions are the measure of choice to study etiology because incidence is affected only by factors related to the risk for developing disease and not to survival or cure. In the previous example about screening, the health department would want to know both the existing level of TB in the area (the prevalence) to plan services and direct prevention and control measures, and the rate at which new cases are developing (the incidence) to study risk factors and evaluate the effectiveness of prevention and control programs (see the "How To" box).

Attack Rate

One final measure of morbidity often used in infectious disease investigations is the attack rate, or the proportion of persons who are exposed to an agent and develop the disease. Attack rates are often specific to an exposure; for example, food-specific attack rates are the proportion of persons becoming ill after eating a specific food item.

Mortality Rates

Several key mortality rates are shown in Table 10.2. Many commonly used mortality rates are not true rates but are proportions,

---

HOW TO ASSESS HEALTH PROBLEMS IN A COMMUNITY

1. Examine local epidemiologic data (e.g., incidence, morbidity, and mortality rates) to identify major health problems.
2. Examine local health services data to identify major causes of hospitalizations and emergency department visits. Consult with key community leaders (e.g., political, religious, business, educational, health, and cultural leaders) about their perceptions of identified community health problems.
3. Mobilize community groups to elicit discussions and identify perceived health priorities within the community (e.g., focus groups, neighborhood forums, or community-wide forums).
4. Analyze community environmental health hazards and pollutants (e.g., water, sewage, air, toxic waste).
5. Examine indicators of community knowledge and practices of preventive health behaviors (e.g., use of infant car seats, safe playgrounds, lighted streets, seat belt use, designated driver programs).
6. Identify cultural priorities and beliefs about health among different social, cultural, racial, or national origin groups.
7. Assess community members' interpretations of and degrees of trust in federal, state, and local assistance programs.
8. Engage community members in conducting surveys to assess specific health problems.

Think about how the above eight steps would be modified if you were going to assess for the incidence or prevalence of COVID-19 in your community.
Note: This process is similar to the intake/assessment process used by nurses, that includes obtaining medical and family history (analogous to #1 and #2 above), identifying health concerns of the patient (analogous to #3 and #5 above), performing clinical exam (analogous to #4 above), and evaluating patient knowledge, beliefs, and personal risk (analogous to #5–#8).

---

because the population changes throughout the year. Although measures of mortality reflect serious health problems and changing patterns of disease, they have limited usefulness. They provide information only about fatal diseases and do not provide direct information about either the level of existing disease in the population or the risk for getting a particular disease. In addition, a person may have one disease (e.g., prostate cancer) yet die of a different cause (e.g., stroke). This tendency became prominent during COVID-19 when people had a chronic health condition and contracted the virus. What was the actual cause of death?

Note than many commonly used mortality rates listed in Table 10.2 are in fact proportions, not true rates. Because the population changes during the course of a year, we typically take an estimate of the population at midyear as the denominator for annual rates because the midyear populations approximate the amount of person-time contributed by the population during a given year.

The crude annual mortality rate is an estimate of the risk for death for a person in a given population for that year. These rates are multiplied by a scaling factor, usually 100,000, to avoid small fractions. The result is then expressed as the number of deaths per 100,000 persons. Although a crude mortality rate is calculated easily and represents the actual death rate for the total population, it has certain limitations. It does not reveal specific causes of death, which change in relative importance over time. In addition, the mortality rate is affected by the

TABLE 10.2 Common Mortality Rates

Rate/Ratio	Definition and Example
Crude mortality rate	Usually an annual rate that represents the proportion of a population who die from any cause during the period, using the midyear population as the denominator Example: In 2016 there were 2,744,248 deaths in a total population of 323,127,513, or 849.3 per 100,000: $$\frac{2,744,248}{323,127,513} = 849.3 \text{ per } 100,000$$
Age-specific rate	Number of deaths among persons of given age group per midyear population of that age group Example: 2016 age-specific mortality rate for 20- to 24-year-olds: $$\frac{21,763}{22,381,028} = 97.2 \text{ per } 100,000$$
Cause-specific rate	Number of deaths from a specific cause per midyear population Example: 2016 cause-specific rate for accidents: $$\frac{161,374}{323,127,513} = 5.9 \text{ per } 100,000$$
Case fatality rate	Number of deaths from a specific disease in a given period divided by number of persons diagnosed with that disease Example: If 87 of every 100 persons diagnosed with lung cancer die within 5 years, the 5-year case fatality rate is 87%. The 5-year survival rate is 13%.
Proportionate mortality ratio	Number of deaths from a specific disease per total number of deaths in the same period Example: In 2016 there were 635,260 deaths from diseases of the heart, and 2,744,248 deaths from all causes: $$\frac{635,260}{2,744,248} = 0.231 \text{ or } 23\%$$
Infant mortality rate	Number of infant deaths before 1 year of age in a year per number of live births in the same year Example: In 2016 there were 23,161 infant deaths and 3,945,875 live births: $$\frac{23,161}{3,945,875} = 286.97 \text{ per } 100,000 \text{ live birth or } 5.87 \text{ per } 1000 \text{ live births}$$
Neonatal mortality rate	Number of infant deaths under 28 days of age in a year per number of live births in the same year Example: In 2016 there were 15,282 neonatal deaths and 3,945,875 live births: $$\frac{15,282}{3,945,875} = 3.87 \text{ per } 1000 \text{ live births}$$
Postneonatal mortality rate	Number of infant deaths from 28 days to 1 year in a year per number of live births in the same year Example: In 2016 there were 7879 postneonatal deaths and 3,945,875 live births: $$\frac{7,879}{3,945,875} = 2.00 \text{ per } 1000 \text{ live births}$$

From Xu JQ et al.: Deaths: leading causes for 2016, *Natl Vital Stat Rep* 67(5), 2018; Martin JA et al.: Births: final data for 2016, *Natl Vital Stat Rep* 67(1), Hyattsville, MD: National Center for Health Statistics, 2018.

population's age distribution, because older people are at much greater risk for death than younger people.

Mortality rates are also calculated for specific groups (e.g., age-, gender-, or race-specific rates). In these instances, the number of deaths occurring in the specified group is divided by the population at risk, now restricted to the number of persons in that group. This rate is then viewed as the risk for death for persons in the specified group during the period of observation.

The cause-specific mortality rate is an estimate of the risk for death from some specific disease in a population. It is the number of deaths from a specific cause divided by the total population at risk, usually multiplied by 100,000. Two related measures should be distinguished from the cause-specific mortality rate. The case fatality rate (CFR) is the proportion of persons diagnosed with a particular disorder (i.e., cases) who die within a specified period. It is considered an estimate of the risk for death within that

period for a person newly diagnosed with the disease (e.g., the proportion of persons with a disease who die during the natural history of the disease). Because the CFR is the proportion of diagnosed persons who die within the period, 1 minus the CFR yields the survival rate. For example, if the 5-year CFR for lung cancer is 86%, then the 5-year survival rate is only 14% (Remington et al., 2016).

The second measure to be distinguished from the cause-specific mortality rate is the proportionate mortality ratio (PMR), the proportion of all deaths resulting from a specific cause. The denominator is not the population at risk for death, but the total number of deaths in the population; therefore the PMR is not a rate, nor does it estimate the risk for death. The magnitude of the PMR is a function of both the number of deaths from the cause of interest and the number of deaths from other causes. If deaths from certain causes decline over time, the PMR for deaths from other causes that remain relatively constant (in absolute numbers) may increase. For example, unintentional accidents accounted for 4.1 deaths per 100,000 persons 10 to 14 years of age in the United States in 2016, which is 28.1% of all deaths in this age group (the PMR). By comparison, accidents (unintentional injuries) caused 49.1 deaths per 100,000 persons 65 to 74 years of age in 2016, which is less than 2.7% of all deaths in this age group (Heron, 2018). This demonstrates that, although the risk of death from a motor vehicle accident was almost 12 times greater in the older age group (based on the rates), such accidents accounted for a greater proportion of all deaths in the younger group (based on the PMR). The reason is that there is a much greater risk of death from other causes in the older group.

Infant mortality is used around the world as an indicator of overall health and availability of health care services. The most common measure, the infant mortality rate (IMR), is the number of deaths to infants in the first year of life divided by the total number of live births. Because the risk for death declines considerably during the first year of life, neonatal (i.e., newborn) and postneonatal mortality rates are also of interest.

Epidemiologic Triangle: Agent, Host, and Environment

Epidemiologists understand that disease results from complex relationships among causal agents, susceptible persons, and environmental factors. These three elements—agent, host, and environment—are called the epidemiologic triangle (Fig. 10.1A). Changes in one of the elements of the triangle can influence the occurrence of disease by increasing or decreasing a person's risk for disease. Fig. 10.1B shows that agent and host, as well as their interaction, are influenced by the environment in which they exist. They also may influence the environment.

Specifically, these elements or variables are defined as follows:
- Agent: An animate or inanimate factor that must be present or lacking for a disease or condition to develop
- Host: A living species (human or animal) capable of being infected or affected by an agent
- Environment: All that is internal or external to a given host or agent and that is influenced and influences the host and/or agent

Examples of these three components are listed in Box 10.1.

Causal relationships (one thing or event causes another) are often more complex than the epidemiologic triangle conveys. The term web of causality recognizes the complex interrelationships of many factors interacting, sometimes in subtle ways, to increase (or decrease) the risk for disease. In addition, associations are sometimes mutual, with lines of causality going in both directions. Some researchers have advocated for a new paradigm that goes beyond the two-dimensional causal web and considers multiple levels of factors that affect health and disease (Macintyre and Ellaway, 2000). This is consistent with the ecological model for population health supported by the 2002 report of the Institute of Medicine (IOM) that expands epidemiologic studies both upward to broader contexts such as neighborhood characteristics and social context and downward to the genetic and molecular level. The ecological model treats

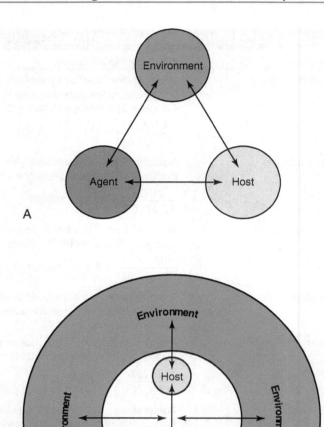

Fig. 10.1 (A and B) Two models of the agent-host-environment interaction (the epidemiologic triangle).

BOX 10.1 Examples of Agent, Host, and Environmental Factors in the Epidemiologic Triangle

Agent
- Infectious agents (bacteria, viruses, fungi, parasites)
- Chemical agents (heavy metals, toxic chemicals, pesticides)
- Physical agents (radiation, heat, cold, machinery)

Host
- Genetic susceptibility
- Immutable characteristics (age, sex)
- Acquired characteristics (immunologic status)
- Lifestyle factors (diet, exercise)

Environment
- Climate (temperature, rainfall)
- Plant and animal life (agents, reservoirs, or habitats for agents)
- Human population distribution (crowding, social support)
- Socioeconomic factors (education, resources, access to care)
- Working conditions (levels of stress, noise, satisfaction)

the multiple determinants of health as interrelated and acting synergistically (or antagonistically), rather than as discrete factors. This model encompasses determinants at many levels: biologic, mental, behavioral, social, and environmental factors, including policy, culture, and economic environments, and includes a life span perspective. The IOM's vision of "healthy people in healthy communities" requires a model that recognizes that healthy communities are more than a collection of healthy individuals and that the characteristics of communities affect the health of people who live in them (IOM, 2002).

Levels of Preventive Interventions

The goal of epidemiology is to identify and understand the causal factors and mechanisms of disease, disability, and injuries so that effective interventions can be implemented to prevent the occurrence of these adverse processes before they begin or before they progress. The natural history of disease is the course of the disease process from onset to resolution (Porta, 2014). The three levels of prevention—primary, secondary, and tertiary—provide a framework often used in public health practice. See the Levels of Prevention box later in the chapter.

Primary prevention refers to interventions that promote health and prevent the occurrence of disease, injury, or disability. Primary prevention is aimed at individuals and groups who are susceptible to disease but have no discernible pathological process (i.e., they are in a state of prepathogenesis). An example of primary prevention is when a nurse provides health education and training for schoolteachers about proper hand hygiene, social distancing, and the importance of wearing a face mask, and for the students to not share food or drinks with one another. These skills became important when schools opened in 2020 and some allowed in-person classes. Immunizations are another example of primary prevention, as are teaching about the importance of wearing seat belts and about taking folic acid supplementation at preconception to prevent neural tube defects, fluoridation of water supplies to prevent dental caries, and actions taken to reduce human exposure to agents that may cause cancer.

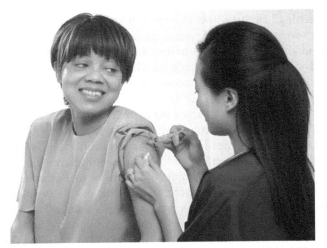

Immunizations are an Integral Part of Primary Prevention. (© 2012 Photos. com, a division of Getty Images. All rights reserved. Image #147673258).

CASE STUDY

Inmates at the Local Jail

An infection preventionist (IP) at a local hospital contacted the nurse epidemiologist at the local health department to report that the hospital had received three laboratory reports of *Acinetobacter baumannii* infection from inmates at the local jail. The IP stated that the jail typically sends all of its laboratory specimens to the hospital for processing. The IP said that the specimens were obtained from wounds and collected within a 2-month period.

1. The nurse epidemiologist suspects an outbreak and launches an investigation for which reason?
   A. This is an unusual problem.
   B. There is a potential risk to the public.
   C. There is a causal pathway.
   D. All of the above
2. The nurse epidemiologist decided to visit the jail. Based on what she knows about the transmission of *A. baumannii,* she should collect which of the following information?
   A. Underlying infections and chronic diseases of inmates
   B. Medical procedures performed in the jail
   C. The number of air exchanges in the jail
   D. All of the above
   E. A and B only
3. The nurse epidemiologist discovers that all of the infected inmates have their wound dressings changed on the same day of the week in the same treatment room. She notices there is no sink or evidence of hand sanitizer in the treatment room. She recommends all of the following strategies *except:*
   A. Installing hand-hygiene stations in convenient locations in treatment rooms
   B. Cleaning and disinfecting examination tables after each inmate is seen
   C. Educating staff on proper wound care and hand hygiene
   D. Antibiotics for all inmates and staff
4. The nurse epidemiologist decides to educate all staff about the organism, including how it is transmitted and prevention strategies. This level of prevention is
   A. Primary
   B. Secondary
   C. Tertiary

Case prepared by Mary Beth White-Comstock, MSN, RN, CIC.
Answers can be found on the Evolve website.

Secondary prevention refers to interventions designed to increase the probability that a person with a disease will have that condition diagnosed early enough that treatment is likely to result in a cure. Health screenings are at the core of secondary prevention. Early and periodic screenings are critical for diseases such as breast cancer, for which there are few specific primary prevention strategies. Screening programs are discussed in the section on screening that follows. Testing for COVID-19 in 2020 emphasized the need for screening if persons had symptoms or had been exposed to someone with the disease.

Interventions at the secondary level of prevention may occur in community settings as well as in primary and secondary levels of health care services. For example, a nurse may teach an asthmatic client to recognize and avoid exposure to asthma triggers and assist the family to implement specific protection strategies such as replacing carpets, keeping air systems clean and free of mold, staying inside when the pollution level is high, and avoiding pets. A nurse also might ask a family about their history of cancer, heart disease, diabetes, and mental illness as part of a client's health history and then follow up with education about appropriate screening procedures. Other secondary prevention interventions include mammography to detect breast cancer, Papanicolaou (Pap) smears to detect cervical cancer, colonoscopy for early detection of colon cancer, and prenatal screening of pregnant women to screen for gestational diabetes. In developing countries, oral rehydrating therapy (ORT) is an excellent example of secondary prevention. If safe water is available, ORT can be used to treat infant diarrheal disease. To do so you would prepare a homemade ORT solution of water, sugar, and salt to give to infants.

Tertiary prevention includes interventions aimed at limiting disability and interventions that enhance rehabilitation from disease, injury, or disability. Interventions for tertiary prevention occur most often at secondary and tertiary levels of care (e.g., specialized clinics, hospitals, rehabilitation centers) but also may occur in community and primary care settings. Examples of tertiary prevention are medical treatment, physical and occupational therapy, and rehabilitation. With the emergence of new drug-resistant strains of TB, nurses now face the challenge of designing and implementing programs to increase long-term compliance and provide aftercare for clients in a variety of community settings. An example of tertiary prevention for persons diagnosed with active TB is directly observed therapy (DOT), discussed in Chapter 12.

SCREENING

Screening, a key component of many secondary prevention interventions, involves the testing of groups of individuals who are at risk for a specific condition but do not have symptoms. The goal is to determine the likelihood that these individuals will develop the disease. From a clinical perspective, the aim of screening is early detection and treatment when these result in a more favorable prognosis. From a public health perspective, the objective is to sort out efficiently and effectively those who probably have the disease from those who probably do not, again to detect early cases for treatment or begin public health prevention and control programs. A screening test is not a diagnostic test. Effective screening programs must include referrals for diagnostic evaluation for those who have positive findings on screening, to determine if they actually have the disease and need treatment.

As public health advocates, nurses are responsible for planning and implementing screening and prevention programs targeted to the at-risk populations. Nurses working in schools, worksites, primary care facilities, and public health agencies may work together to target at-risk populations on the basis of occupational and environmental risks. Successful screening programs have several characteristics related to both the tests and the target population (Box 10.2). In planning screening programs for a specific population (e.g., school, workplace, community), nurses need to take into consideration various factors. These include the characteristics of the health problem, the screening tests available, and the population (Noonan et al., 2017). Screening is recommended for health problems that have a high prevalence, are

---

BOX 10.2 Characteristics of a Successful Screening Program

1. *Valid (accurate):* A high probability of correct classification of persons tested
2. *Reliable (precise):* Results consistent from place to place, time to time, and person to person
3. *Capable of large-group administration:*
   a. Fast in both the administration of the test and the procurement of results
   b. Inexpensive in both personnel required and materials and procedures used
4. *Innocuous:* Few, if any, side effects; minimally invasive test
5. *High yield:* Able to detect enough new cases to warrant the effort and expense (*yield* defined as the amount of previously unrecognized disease that is diagnosed and treated as a result of screening)
6. *Ethical and effective:* Meets the desired public health goal with health benefits that outweigh any moral or ethical infringements

---

relatively serious, and can be detected in early states and for which effective treatment is available. The population should be easily identifiable and accessible, amenable to screening, and willing and able to seek treatment or follow-up procedures. Criteria for evaluating the suitability of screening tests include cost effectiveness, ease and safety of administration, availability of treatment, ethics of administration or widespread implementation, sensitivity, specificity, validity, and reliability (Celetano and Szklo, 2018; McKeown and Learner, 2009).

Nurses must stay current about screening guidelines because these are regularly reviewed and revised on the basis of epidemiologic research results. It is useful for nurses to know how to access information provided by the US Preventive Services Task Force (USPSTF). The USPSTF is an independent, volunteer group of national experts in prevention and evidence-based medicine that makes recommendations about clinical preventive services such as screening tests, counseling services, and preventive medications. They make annual recommendations on a selected group of health risks according to category of health risk, age group, gender, and type of preventive service (i.e., counseling, preventive medication, or screening). Examples of recommendations in 2020 were for "Sexually transmitted infections: behavioral counseling" and "Unhealthy drug use: screening." In 2019, two examples of screening recommendations were published for pancreatic cancer and cognitive impairment in older adults. To understand how the process works, consider the update for "Statin use for the primary prevention of cardiovascular disease in adults: preventive medication." This topic was reviewed in 2016 and was updated in 2020. This is a useful site for nurses to know the current recommendations for a wide range of health conditions and possible illnesses.

As community health advocates and educators, nurses plan and implement screening and prevention programs for high-risk populations. For example, the primary goal of screening younger people is to promote lifestyle changes. As people live longer, there appears to be a greater emphasis among the older population in participating in health-promoting activities such as those recommended by the USPSTF regarding diet, exercise, social interaction, and a variety of other key topics.

See http://www.uspreventiveservicestaskforce.org for details on recommendations, the year the recommendation was published, and analyses still in progress.

Criteria for evaluating the usefulness of a screening test include cost effectiveness, ease and safety of administration, availability of treatment, ethics of administration, or widespread implementation, sensitivity, specificity, validity, and reliability (Celentano and Szklo, 2018).

Reliability, Validity, and Surveillance

Reliability

It is important to pay attention to the precision, or reliability, of the measure (i.e., its consistency or repeatability) and the accuracy of the measure, its validity (i.e., whether it is really measuring what we think it is and how exact the measurement is). Suppose you want to screen for blood pressure in a community. You will take blood pressure readings on a large number of people, perhaps following up with repeated measures for individuals with higher pressures. If the readings of the sphygmomanometer used for the screening vary so that two consecutive readings are not the same for the same person, the sphygmomanometer lacks precision or reliability. The instrument would be unreliable even if the overall mean of repeated measurements were close to the true overall mean for the persons measured. The problem would be that the readings would not be reliable for any individual, which is what a screening program requires.

On the other hand, suppose the readings are reliably reproducible but unknown to you, they tend to be approximately 10 mm Hg too high. This instrument is producing precise readings, but the uncorrected (or uncalibrated) instrument lacks accuracy (or validity). In short, a measure can be consistent without producing valid results.

The following three major sources of error can affect the reliability of tests:

1. Variation inherent in the trait being measured (e.g., blood pressure changes with time of day, activity, level of stress, and other factors)
2. Observer variation, which can be divided into intraobserver reliability (i.e., consistency by the same observer) and interobserver reliability (i.e., level of consistency from one observer to another)
3. Inconsistency in the instrument, which includes the level of internal consistency of the instrument (e.g., whether all items in a questionnaire measure the same thing) and the stability (i.e., for test-retest reliability) of the instrument over time

Validity: Sensitivity and Specificity

Validity in a screening test is typically measured by sensitivity and specificity. Sensitivity quantifies how accurately the test identifies those with the condition or trait. Sensitivity represents the proportion of persons with the disease whom the test correctly identifies as positive (true positives). High sensitivity is needed when early treatment is important and when identification of every case is important. As seen during the testing for determining if a person had COVID-19, the sensitivity of the

test was important. People who tested positive were told to self-isolate for a specified number of days, and later in the process to identify other people with whom they had been in contact so that contract tracing could be carried out.

Specificity indicates how accurately the test identifies those *without* the condition or trait (i.e., the proportion of persons whom the test correctly identifies as negative for the disease [true negatives]). High specificity is needed when rescreening is impractical and when it is important to reduce false-positive results. The sensitivity and specificity of a test are determined by comparing the test results with results from a definitive diagnostic procedure (sometimes called the *gold standard*). For example, the Pap smear is used frequently to screen for cervical dysplasia and carcinoma. The definitive diagnosis of cervical cancer requires a biopsy with histologic confirmation of malignant cells.

The ideal for a screening test is 100% sensitivity and 100% specificity. That is, the test is positive for 100% of those who actually have the disease, and it is negative for all those who do not have the disease. In practice, sensitivity and specificity are often inversely related. That is, if the test results are such that it is possible to choose some point beyond which a person is considered positive (a "cutpoint"), as in a blood pressure reading to screen for hypertension or a serum glucose reading to screen for diabetes, then moving that critical point to improve the sensitivity of the test will result in a decrease in specificity, or an improvement in specificity can be made only at the expense of sensitivity.

A third measure associated with sensitivity and specificity is the predictive value of the test. The positive predictive value (also called *predictive value positive*) is the proportion of persons with a positive test who actually have the disease, interpreted as the probability that an individual with a positive test has the disease. The negative predictive value (or *predictive value negative*) is the proportion of persons with a negative test who are actually disease-free.

Two or more tests can be combined in series or in parallel to enhance sensitivity or specificity. In series testing, the final result is considered positive only if all tests in the series were positive, and it is considered negative if any test was negative. For example, if a blood sample was screened for HIV, a positive enzyme-linked immunosorbent assay (ELISA) might be followed with a Western blot test, and the sample would be considered positive only if both tests were positive. Series testing enhances specificity, producing fewer false-positives, but sensitivity will be lower. In series testing, sequence is important; a very sensitive test is often used first to pick up all cases, including false-positives, and then a second, very specific test is used to eliminate the false-positives. In parallel testing, the final result is considered positive if any test was positive and is considered negative only if *all* tests were negative. To return to the example of a blood sample being tested for HIV, a blood bank might consider a sample positive if a positive result was found on either the ELISA or the Western blot. Parallel testing enhances sensitivity, leaving fewer false-negatives, but specificity will be lower.

Surveillance involves the systematic collection, analysis, and interpretation of data related to the occurrence of disease and the health status of a given population. Surveillance systems are often classified as either active or passive (Lee, Tuetsch, et al., 2010). Passive surveillance is the more common form used by most local and state health departments. Health care providers in the community report cases of notifiable diseases to public health authorities through the use of standardized reports. Passive surveillance is relatively inexpensive but is limited by variability and incompleteness in provider reporting practices. Active surveillance is the purposeful, ongoing search for new cases of disease by public health personnel, through personal or telephone contacts or the review of laboratory reports or hospital or clinic records. Because active surveillance is costly, its use is often limited to brief periods for specific purposes as in the emergence of a newly identified disease, a particularly severe disease, or the reemergence of a previously eradicated disease. The practice of surveillance was of importance during the COVOD-19 pandemic. See Chapter 17, Surveillance and Outbreak Investigation.

BASIC METHODS IN EPIDEMIOLOGY

Sources of Data

It is important to know early in any epidemiologic study how the data will be obtained (Celentano and Szklo, 2018; Weiss and Koepsell, 2014). The following three major categories of data sources are commonly used in epidemiologic investigations:

1. Routinely collected data: census data, vital records (i.e., birth and death certificates), and surveillance data (i.e., systematic collection of data concerning disease occurrence) as carried out by the Centers for Disease Control and Prevention (CDC)
2. Data collected for other purposes but useful for epidemiologic research: medical, health department, and insurance records
3. Original data collected for specific epidemiologic studies

The first two types of data are often referred to as *secondary data*, and the third type is considered *primary data.*

Routinely Collected Data

Vital records are the primary source of birth and mortality statistics. Registration of births and deaths is mandated in most countries and provides one of the most complete sources of health-related data. However, the quality of specific information varies. For example, on birth certificates, sex and date of birth are fairly reliable, whereas reports of gestational age, level of prenatal care, and smoking habits of the mother during pregnancy are less reliable. On death certificates, the quality of the cause-of-death information varies over time and from place to place, depending on diagnostic capabilities and custom. Vital records are readily available in most areas; they are inexpensive and convenient and allow study of long-term trends. However, mortality data are informative only for fatal diseases or events.

The US census is conducted every 10 years and provides population data, including demographic distribution (i.e., age, race, sex), geographic distribution, and additional information about economic status, housing, and education. These data provide denominators for various rates. The American Community Survey is an ongoing survey conducted by the US Census Bureau. Data from these surveys provide information about the status of the population and for public health planning and evaluation.

Data Collected for Other Purposes

Hospital, physician, health department, and insurance records provide information on morbidity, as do surveillance systems, such as cancer registries and health department reporting systems, which solicit reports of all cases of a particular disease within a geographic region. Other information, such as occupational exposures, may be available from employer records. School and employment attendance and absenteeism records are another potential source of data that may be used in epidemiologic investigations.

Epidemiologic Data

The National Center for Health Statistics (NCHS) sponsors periodic health surveys and examinations in carefully drawn samples of the US population. Examples are the National Health and Nutrition Examination Survey (NHANES), the National Health Interview Survey (NHIS), and the National Hospital Discharge Survey (NHDS). The CDC also conducts or contracts for surveys such as the Youth Risk Behavior Surveillance System (YRBSS), Pregnancy Risk Assessment Monitoring System (PRAMS), and the Behavioral Risk Factor Surveillance System (BRFSS). These surveys provide information on the health status and behaviors of the population. However, for many studies, the only way to obtain the needed information is to collect the required data in a study specifically designed to investigate a particular question. The design of such studies is discussed later.

With the National Institutes of Health's recent emphasis on transdisciplinary approaches to science, disciplines that have not traditionally partnered together are beginning to recognize the benefits of combining methodologies to tackle public health problems. An example of this is the increase in collaborative research between public health professionals and geographers, aimed at furthering understanding of the influence of "place on health outcomes." Within the field of geography, a GIS (often termed "ArcGIS" after the software used) allows for mapping data to the exact location of specific occurrences or events (e.g., a family residence, the location where they receive medical care, or the number of fast-food restaurants within a 1-mile radius of the residence).

This type of integrated geographic and public health data mapping allows researchers and public health professionals to conduct more detailed assessments of the environments of individuals, families, and communities. A GIS can be used to examine health issues such as access to prenatal care, mapping the distribution of health exposures or outcomes and linking data with geocoded addresses of individuals to sources of potentially toxic exposures. The Evidence-Based Practice box describes a way in which nursing students conducted a study to examine if environmental factors co-occur in areas with high asthma rates in Head Start (HS) program attendees.

EVIDENCE-BASED PRACTICE

In this study a convenience sample of 56 children with asthma who were enrolled in HS were chosen. They were ages 3 to 5 years. A GIS using ArcGIS 10.4 was used to geocode and map aggregated home addresses through the census track level using vector map analysis. Location, race, economic status, pollution remediation sites, age of housing, and blood lead levels were assessed for areas with high asthma concentration. What they found is most children with asthma resided in one census tract, which was only 1% of the total service area. Fifty-six percent of housing was built before 1960, with only 10% after 1990, suggesting deteriorating conditions. Environmental remediation sites were found in the vicinity of the asthma cases. The research question was: Are there environmental factors to which these HS children are exposed that may contribute to poor asthma outcomes?

Nurse Use

The need for proactive interventions to decrease asthma risk/poor asthma outcomes with HS was clear. A GIS locates children with high susceptibility to asthma. By using this technology, public health nurses can target interventions and education families about environmental exposures and asthma risk factors. However, unless the nurses and others advocate for changes in the environmental conditions, the education of families will not be fully effective.

Quaranta JE, Swaine J, Ryszka S: Preschool asthma: examining environmental influences using geographic information systems, *Public Health Nurs* 37(3):405–411, May/June 2020.

Rate Adjustment

Rates, which are essential in epidemiologic studies, can be misleading when compared across different populations. For example, the risk for death increases considerably after 40 years of age, so a higher crude death rate is expected in a population of older people in contrast to a population of younger people (Celentano and Szklo, 2018; Weiss and Koepsell, 2014; Rothman, 2012). Comparing the overall mortality rate in an area with a large population of older adults with the rate in a younger population would be misleading. Methods that adjust for differences in populations can be used to compare death rates. Age adjustment is based on the assumption that a population's overall mortality rate is a function of the age distribution of the population and the age-specific mortality rates.

Age adjustment can be performed by direct or indirect methods. Both methods require a *standard population,* which can be an external population, such as the US population for a given year, a combined population of the groups under study, or some other standard chosen for relevance or convenience.

A direct adjusted rate applies the age-specific death rates from the study population to the age distribution of the standard population. The result is the (hypothetical) death rate of the study population if it had the same age distribution as the standard population. The indirect method, as the name suggests, is more complicated. The age-specific death rates of the standard population applied to the study population's age distribution result in an index rate that is used with the crude rates of both the study and standard populations to produce the final indirect adjusted rate, which is also hypothetical. The indirect method may be required when the age-specific death rates for the study population are unknown or unstable (e.g., based on relatively small numbers).

Often, instead of an indirect adjusted rate, a standardized mortality ratio (SMR) is calculated. This is the number of observed deaths in the study population divided by the number of deaths expected on the basis of the age-specific rates in the standard population and the age distribution of the study population (Celentano and Szklo, 2018; Szklo and Nieto, 2018).

Comparison Groups

Comparison groups are often used in epidemiology. To decide if the rate of disease is the result of a suspected risk factor, the exposed group should be compared with a group of comparable unexposed persons. For example, you might investigate the effect of smoking during pregnancy on the rate of low-birth-weight infants by calculating the rate of low-birth-weight infants born to women who smoked during their pregnancy. However, the hypothesis that smoking during pregnancy is a risk factor for low birth weight is supported only when the low-birth-weight rate among smoking women is compared with the (lower) rate of low-birth-weight infants born to nonsmoking women.

Ideally you want to compare one group of people who all have a certain characteristic, exposure, or behavior with a group of people exactly like them except they all lack that characteristic, exposure, or behavior. In the absence of that ideal, you can either randomize people to exposure or treatment groups in experimental studies or select comparison groups that are comparable in observational studies. It is especially important in observational studies to control for confounding variables or factors.

DESCRIPTIVE EPIDEMIOLOGY

Descriptive epidemiology describes the distribution of disease, death, and other health outcomes in the population according to person, place, and time. This type of epidemiology provides a picture of how things are or have been and describes the who, where, and when of disease patterns. In contrast, analytic epidemiology looks for the determinants of the patterns observed—the how and why. That is, epidemiologic concepts and methods are used to identify what factors, characteristics, exposures, or behaviors might account for differences in the observed patterns of disease occurrence. Descriptive and analytic studies are observational. In these studies the investigator observes events as they are or have been and does not intervene to change anything or to introduce a new factor. However, experimental or intervention studies include interventions to test preventive or treatment measures, techniques, materials, policies, or drugs.

Person

Personal characteristics of interest in epidemiology include race, ethnicity, sex, age, education, occupation, income (and related socioeconomic status), and marital status. Age is the most important predictor of overall mortality. The mortality curve by age drops sharply during and after the first year of life to a low point in childhood, then begins to increase through adolescence and young adulthood, and after that increases sharply through middle and older ages (Celentano and Szklo, 2018). Mortality and morbidity differ by sex and by race. For example, among males, intentional self-harm accounts for approximately 2.5% of all deaths but intention self-harm is not among the leading causes of death for women. In contrast, septicemia, influenza, and pneumonia account for more deaths among women than men. Assault, or homicide, accounts for approximately 3% of all deaths among the Black population but is not even among the leading causes of death for other races and ethnicities (Elfein, 2020). Disparities were also found in the incidence of COVID-19 among underrepresented racial/ethnic groups. "Persons of color might be more likely to become infected with SARS-Co-V-2, the virus that causes COVID-19, experience more several COVID-19-associated illness, including that requiring hospitalization, and have higher risk for death from COVID-19" (Moore, Ricaldi, Rose et al., 2020).

There are also substantial differences in mortality and morbidity rates by sex. Female infants have a lower mortality rate than comparable male infants, and the survival advantage continues throughout life (Xu, 2018). However, patterns for specific diseases vary. For example, women have lower rates of CHD until menopause, after which the gap narrows. For rheumatoid arthritis, the prevalence among women is greater than among men (Remington et al., 2016).

Although the concept of race as a variable for public health research has come under scrutiny (Fullilove, 1998), there are clear differences in morbidity and mortality rates by race in the United States (Kochanek, 2017). According to the Office of Minority Health (OMH, 2015), racial and ethnic minority groups are among the fastest-growing populations in the United States, yet they have poorer health and remain chronically underserved by the health care system. Data in the OMH report *HHS Action Plan to Reduce Racial and Ethnic Health Disparities Implementation Progress Report* highlighted some of the significant health disparities within the leading categories of death in the United States. For example, in 2016 the overall IMR was 5.87 deaths per 1000 live births, but the IMR among African Americans was 11.76 per 1000 live births (Xu, et al., 2018), and the gap has been widening in recent years. Racial and ethnic health disparities have been observed in a wide range of diseases and health behaviors, from infant mortality to diabetes, heart disease, cancer, and HIV. Although there has been some progress toward meeting the goal of eliminating racial/ethnic disparities, with improvement in rates for most health status indicators across all racial/ethnic groups, the improvements have not been uniform across groups and "substantial differences among racial/ethnic groups persist" (OMH, 2015). Among American Indians and Alaska Natives, several health indicators actually worsened from 1990 to 1998. The IMR declined in all groups, but it remains 2.3 times higher for infants born to non-Hispanic African American mothers than for those born to White non-Hispanic mothers. Similarly, the overall age-adjusted mortality rate was 22% higher in the African American population than in the White population in 2016, and it was higher for 10 of the 15 leading causes of death (Xu et al., 2017). Although individual characteristics such as race, gender, and immigration status are of interest to epidemiologists, there has been increasing focus on social, economic, and cultural contexts and processes underlying racial and ethnic inequalities in health, such as discrimination (Fuller et al., 2005; Matoba et al., 2017).

Place

When looking at the distribution of a disease, examine geographic patterns. Does the rate of disease differ from place to place (e.g., with local environment)? If geography had no effect on disease occurrence, random geographic patterns might be seen, but that is often not the case. For example, at high altitudes, oxygen tension is lower, which might result in smaller babies. Other diseases reflect distinctive geographic patterns. For example, Lyme disease is transmitted from animal reservoirs to humans by a tick vector. Disease is more likely to be found in areas in which there are animals carrying the disease, a large tick population for transmission to humans, and contact between the human population and the tick vectors (Heymann, 2014). Geographic variations can be caused by:

- Differences in the chemical, physical, or biologic environment
- Differences in population densities, customary patterns of behavior and lifestyle, or other personal characteristics

Geographic variations might occur because of high concentrations of a religious, cultural, or ethnic group that practices certain health-related behaviors. The high rates of stroke found in the southeastern United States are likely to be the result of social and personal factors that have little to do with geographic features per se. Other neighborhood-level variables include the unemployment and crime rate, education levels, racial segregation, social cohesion, and access to important services (Fuller et al., 2005; Patel, 2015).

Time

Time is the third component of descriptive epidemiology. In relation to time, epidemiologists ask these questions: Is there an increase or decrease in the frequency of the disease over time? Are other temporal (and spatial) patterns evident? Temporal patterns could include secular trends, point epidemic, cyclical patterns, and event-related clusters.

Secular Changes

Long-term patterns of morbidity or mortality rates (i.e., over years or decades) are called secular trends. Secular trends may reflect changes in social behavior or practices. For example, increased lung cancer mortality rates in recent years reflect a delayed effect of the increased smoking in prior years. In addition, the decline in cervical cancer deaths is primarily the result of widespread screening with the Pap test (Remington et al., 2016).

Some secular trends may result from increased diagnostic ability or changes in survival (or case fatality) rather than in incidence. For example, case fatality from breast cancer has decreased in recent years, although the incidence of breast cancer has increased. Some, although not all, of the increased incidence is the result of improved diagnostic capability. These two trends result in a breast cancer mortality curve that is flatter than the incidence curve (Remington et al., 2016). Relying on mortality data alone does not accurately reflect the true situation. Secular trends also are affected by changes in case definition or revisions in the coding of a disease according to the International Classification of Diseases (ICD).

A point epidemic is a time-and-space–related pattern that is important in infectious disease investigations and as an indicator for toxic exposures. A point epidemic is most clearly seen when the frequency of cases is graphed against time. The sharp peak characteristic of such graphs indicates a concentration of cases over a short interval of time. The peak often indicates the population's response to a common source of infection or contamination to which they were all simultaneously exposed. Knowledge of the incubation or latency period (i.e., the time between exposure and development of signs and symptoms) for the specific disease entity can help to determine the probable time of exposure. A common example of a point epidemic is an outbreak of gastrointestinal illness from a food-borne pathogen. Nurses who are alert to a sudden increase in the number of cases of a disease can chart the outbreak, determine the probable time of exposure, and, by careful investigation, isolate the probable source of the agent.

In addition to secular trends and point epidemics, there are also cyclical time patterns of disease. Seasonal fluctuation is a common type of cyclical variation in some infectious illnesses. Seasonal changes may be influenced by changes in the agent itself, changes in population densities or behaviors of animal reservoirs or vectors, or changes in human behaviors resulting in changing exposures (e.g., being outdoors in warmer weather and indoors in colder months). In addition, calendar events may create artificial seasons, such as holidays and tax-filing deadlines, that are associated with patterns of stress-related illness. Patterns of accidents and injuries also may be seasonal, reflecting differing employment and recreational patterns. Some disease cycles, such as influenza, have patterns of smaller epidemics every few years, depending on the strain, with major pandemics occurring at longer intervals (Heymann, 2014). Public health workers need to pay attention to cyclical patterns so that they are prepared to meet possible increased demands for service.

A third type of temporal pattern is nonsimultaneous, event-related clusters. These are patterns in which time is not measured from fixed dates on the calendar but from the point of some exposure, event, or experience presumably held in common by affected persons, although not occurring at the same time. An example of this pattern would be vaccine reactions during an immunization program. Clearly, if vaccinations are being given on a regular basis, nonspecific symptoms, such as fever, headaches, or rashes, might be seen fairly consistently over time, making identification of a cluster related to the vaccinations difficult. However, if the occurrence of symptoms is plotted against the amount of time since vaccination, the number of vaccine reactions is likely to peak at some period after the immunization. Another example would be natural disasters such as hurricanes and their impact on public health. Often after hurricanes, particularly those causing significant damage to natural resources, an increase in acute infectious diseases will be seen due to lack of safe water, adequate hygiene, and sanitation. After Hurricane Maria passed through Puerto Rico on September 20, 2017, officials reported a significant increase in cases of leptospirosis (bacterial infection that can lead to kidney damage, meningitis, brain damage, liver failure, and even death). By October of 2017, officials had 121 confirmed cases of leptospirosis compared with 60 in a usual year (Henry J. Kaiser Family Foundation, https://www.kff.org, accessed May 31, 2018).

CASE STUDY

The Dean of the School of Nursing held an open house on August 26 to welcome new and returning nursing students. Approximately 50 nursing students and professors attended. Light appetizers and cider were served. On the morning of August 28, two nursing students reported to the student health clinic with nausea and vomiting. Later that day, three other students reported to the clinic with headache, nausea, and vomiting. Two of the five students reported that their symptoms began the evening of August 27, and the other three reported symptom onset the morning of August 28. Two nursing professors called in sick with nausea and diarrhea on August 28. Both attended the dean's open house and a reception earlier in the week.

What would you do?

The student health nurse notified the nurse epidemiologist at the local health department that she has seen five nursing students with gastrointestinal symptoms. She reports their names, dates of birth, and dates and times of onset of symptoms.

1. The nurse epidemiologist at the health department develops a line list to organize the data. The line list includes the information reported by the student health nurse. What is the term used to describe the type of epidemiology associated with time, place, and person?
   A. Descriptive
   B. Analytic
   C. Scientific
   D. Environmental

2. The nurse epidemiologist notes that the infections are clustered in time, place, and person. She interviews all of the ill nursing students and learns that all of them attended the open house at the dean's home. What should the nurse do next?
   A. Close the nursing school
   B. Arrange to collect stool specimens
   C. Contact the dean
   D. Quarantine all of the open house attendees

3. The nurse epidemiologist notifies the student health nurse that all of the stool specimens were positive for norovirus. Based on the incubation period for norovirus (12–48 h) and the dates of onset of symptoms, the nurse epidemiologist suspects the students were exposed to the virus at or around the same time. She hypothesizes that the nurses contracted norovirus from a contaminated item consumed at the open house event. She makes arrangements to meet with the dean to discuss the situation and gather additional information. What information would be useful to the nurse epidemiologist?
   A. A list of items served at the event
   B. A list of persons who prepared and served the refreshments
   C. A list of students, faculty, and staff who attended the event
   D. A list of faculty and student absences
   E. All of the above

4. The nurse epidemiologist decides to interview everyone (ill and well) who attended the open house. This type of study is called a:
   A. Case-control study
   B. Cohort study
   C. Longitudinal study
   D. Case study

5. Based on the data analysis, the nurse epidemiologist determined that the fresh vegetable tray was associated with illness. She also learned that two of the food handlers were not feeling well during the event. What measures should she take at this point to control the outbreak?
   A. Try to obtain stool specimens from the catering staff
   B. Educate catering and serving staff about safe food preparation
   C. Encourage food service staff not to prepare or serve food when they are ill with gastrointestinal symptoms
   D. Call the Better Business Bureau

Case prepared by Mary Beth White-Comstock, MSN, RN, CIC.

ANALYTIC EPIDEMIOLOGY

Descriptive epidemiology deals with the *distribution* of health outcomes. The goal of analytic epidemiology is to discover the *determinants* of outcomes—the how and the why. Analytic epidemiology deals with the factors that influence the observed patterns of health and disease and increase or decrease the risk for adverse outcomes. This section discusses analytic study designs and the related measures of association derived from them. Table 10.3 summarizes the advantages and disadvantages of each design.

Cohort Studies

The cohort study is the standard for observational epidemiologic studies. It comes closest to the idea of a natural experiment

(Rothman, 2012). The term *cohort* is used in epidemiology to describe a group of persons who are born at about the same time. In analytic studies, cohort refers to a group of persons generally sharing some characteristic of interest. They are enrolled in a study and followed over time to observe some health outcome (Porta, 2014). Because of this ability to observe the development of new cases of disease, cohort study designs allow for calculation of incidence rates and therefore estimates of risk for disease. Cohort studies may be prospective or retrospective (Celentano and Szklo, 2018; Szklo and Nieto, 2018; Rothman, 2012).

Prospective Cohort Studies

In a prospective cohort study (also called a *longitudinal* or *follow-up study*), subjects who do not have the outcome under

TABLE 10.3   Comparison of Major Epidemiologic Study Designs

Study Design	Advantages	Disadvantages
Ecological	Quick, easy, inexpensive first study Uses readily available existing data May prompt further investigation or suggest other or new hypotheses May provide information about contextual factors not accounted for by individual characteristics	Ecological fallacy: the associations observed may not hold true for individuals Problems in interpreting temporal sequence (cause and effect) More difficult to control for confounding and "mixed" models (ecological and individual data); more complex statistically
Cross-sectional (correlational)	Gives general description of the scope of problem; provides prevalence estimates Often based on population (or community) sample, not just who sought care Useful in health service evaluation and planning Data obtained at once; less expense and quicker than cohort because of no follow-up Baseline for prospective study or to identify cases and controls for case-control study	No calculation of risk; prevalence, not incidence Temporal sequence unclear Not good for rare disease or rare exposure unless there is a large sample size or stratified sampling Selective survival can be a major source of selection bias; surviving subjects may differ from those who are not included (e.g., death, institutionalization) Selective recall or lack of past exposure information can create bias
Case-control (retrospective, case comparison)	Less expensive than cohort; smaller sample required Quicker than cohort; no follow-up Can investigate more than one exposure Best design for rare diseases If well designed, it can be an important tool for etiologic investigation Best suited to a disease with a relatively clear onset (timing of onset can be established so that incident cases can be included)	Greater susceptibility than cohort studies to various types of bias (selective survival, recall bias, selection bias in choice of both cases and controls) Information on other risk factors may not be available, resulting in confounding Antecedent-consequence (temporal sequence) not as certain as in cohort Not well suited to rare exposures Gives only an indirect estimate of risk Generally limited to a single outcome because of sampling effect on disease status
Prospective cohort (concurrent cohort, longitudinal, follow-up)	Best estimate of disease incidence Best estimate of risk Fewer problems with selective survival and selective recall Temporal sequence more clearly established Broader range of options for exposure assessment	Expensive in terms of time and money More difficult organizationally Not good for rare diseases Attrition of participants can bias the estimate Latency period may be very long; may miss cases May be difficult to examine several exposures
Retrospective cohort (nonconcurrent cohort)	Combines advantages of both prospective cohort and case-control Shorter time (even if follow-up into the future) than prospective cohort Less expensive than prospective cohort because it relies on existing data Temporal sequence may be clearer than case-control	Shares some disadvantages with both prospective cohort and case-control Subject to attrition (loss to follow-up) Relies on existing records that may result in misclassification of both exposure and outcome May have to rely on a surrogate measure of exposure (e.g., job title) and vital records information on cause of death

investigation are classified on the basis of the exposure of interest at the beginning of the follow-up period. The subjects are then followed for some period of time to determine the occurrence of disease in each group. The question is, "Do persons with the factor (or exposure) of interest develop (or avoid) the outcome more frequently than those without the factor (or exposure)?"

For example, a cohort of subjects could be recruited who would be classified as physically active ("exposed") or sedentary ("not exposed"). If you had adequate information, you could quantify the amount of the "exposure." You could then follow these subjects over time to determine the development of CHD. This study design avoids the problem of selective survival seen in other designs. The cohort study also has the advantage of allowing estimation of the risk for acquiring disease for those who are exposed compared with those who are unexposed (or less exposed). This ratio of cumulative incidence rates is called the risk ratio or *relative risk*.

Suppose 1000 physically active and 1000 sedentary middle-aged men and women were enrolled in a prospective cohort study. All were free of CHD at enrollment. Over a 5-year follow-up period, regular examinations detect CHD in 120 of the sedentary men and women and in 48 of the active men and women. Assuming no other deaths or losses to follow-up, the data could be presented as shown in Fig. 10.2.

The incidence of CHD in the active group is $(a/[a + b]) = 48/1000$, and the incidence of CHD in the sedentary group is $(c/[c + d]) = 120/1000$. The relative risk is:

$$(48/100) + (120/1000) = 0.4$$

Because physical activity is protective for CHD, the relative risk is less than 1. In this example, over a 5-year period, the risk for CHD in persons who are physically active compared with the risk among sedentary persons was 0.4. In the cohort study design, subjects are enrolled before disease onset, and this allows the researcher to study more than one outcome, calculate incidence rates and estimate risk, and establish the temporal sequence of exposure and outcome with greater clarity and certainty. The researcher may need a large sample to ensure that enough cases are observed to provide statistical power to detect meaningful differences between groups and may have to wait a long time for some diseases to develop.

Retrospective Cohort Studies

Retrospective cohort studies combine some of the advantages and disadvantages of case-control studies and prospective cohort studies. These studies rely on existing records, such as employment, insurance, or hospital records, to define a cohort that is classified as having been exposed or unexposed at some time in the past. The cohort is followed over time using the records to determine if the outcome occurred. Retrospective cohort (also called *historical cohort*) studies may be conducted entirely using past records or may include current assessment or additional follow-up time after study initiation. This approach saves time; however, its accuracy relies on existing historical records.

Case-Control Studies

In the case-control study, subjects are enrolled *because* they are known to have the outcome of interest (these are the cases) or they are known *not* to have the outcome of interest (these are the controls). Case-control status is verified using a clear case definition and some previously determined method or protocol (e.g., by an examination, laboratory test, or medical chart review). Information is then collected on the exposures or characteristics of interest, frequently from existing sources, subject interview, or questionnaire (Rothman, 2012; Szklo and Nieto, 2018). The question in a case-control study is "Do persons with the outcome of interest (cases) have the exposure characteristic (or a history of the exposure) more frequently than those without the outcome (controls)?"

Because of the method of subject selection in case-control studies, neither incidence nor prevalence can be calculated directly. In a case-control study, an odds ratio tells us how much more (or less) likely the exposure is to be found among cases than among controls. The odds of exposure among cases (*a* and *c* in the table that follows) are compared with the odds of exposure among controls (*b* and *d*). The ratio of these two odds provides us with an estimate of the relative risk.

Suppose a research group wanted to study risk factors for suicide attempts among adolescents. To do so, they would enroll 100 adolescents who had attempted suicide and select 200 adolescents from the same community with no history of a suicide attempt. The research group's goal is to determine if the adolescents had a history of substance abuse. Through a questionnaire and use of medical records, they learned that 68 of the 100 adolescents who had attempted suicide had a history of substance abuse. They also found that 36 of the 200 adolescents with no suicide attempt had a history of substance abuse. The information could be presented as shown in Fig. 10.3.

The odds of a history of substance abuse among suicide attempters are *a/c*, or 68/32, whereas the odds of substance abuse among controls are *b/d*, or 36/164. The odds ratio (equivalent to *ad/bc*) is the following:

$$\frac{68 \times 164}{36 \times 32} = 9.68$$

This would be interpreted to mean that adolescents who attempted suicide are almost 10 times more likely to have a history of substance abuse than are adolescents who have not

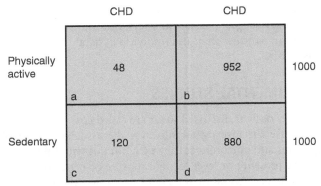

Fig. 10.2 Cohort Study. *CHD*, Coronary heart disease.

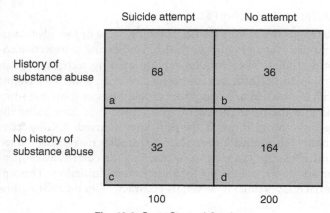

Fig. 10.3 Case-Control Study.

attempted suicide. Note that an odds ratio of 1 is indicative of no association (i.e., the odds of exposure are similar for cases and controls). An odds ratio less than 1 suggests a protective association; that is, cases are less likely to have been exposed than controls. Because case-control studies know the number of cases involved, they do not require a large sample or take a long follow-up time. They may have biases. *Bias* is a systematic deviation from the truth. Because these studies begin with existing diseases, differential survival can produce biased results. The use of recently diagnosed (or "incident") cases may reduce this bias. Because exposure information is obtained from subject recall or past records, there may be errors in exposure assessment or misclassification.

Cross-Sectional Studies

The cross-sectional study provides a snapshot, or cross-section, of a population or group (Celentano and Szklo, 2018). Information is collected on current health status, personal characteristics, and potential risk factors or exposures all at once. In the cross-sectional study there is a simultaneous collection of information necessary for the classification of exposure and outcome status. Historical information can also be collected (e.g., past diet, history of radiation exposures). Surveys are one type of data collection for cross-sectional studies. They may be administered in person, over the telephone, by mail, or via a website or personal electronic device. Surveys have both advantages and disadvantages, and it is important to learn about both before conducting a survey.

One way cross-sectional studies evaluate the association of a factor with a health problem is to compare the prevalence of the disease in those with the factor (or exposure) with the prevalence of the disease in the unexposed. For this reason, they are often called prevalence studies. The ratio of the two prevalence rates is an indication of the association between the factor and the outcome. If the prevalence of CHD in smokers were twice as high as the prevalence among non-smokers, the prevalence ratio would be 2. If a factor is unrelated to the prevalence of a disease, the prevalence ratio will be close to 1. A value less than 1 may suggest a protective association. For example, the prevalence of CHD is lower among physically active people than among sedentary persons. Thus

the prevalence ratio for the association between physical activity and CHD should be less than 1. Use caution in interpreting prevalence ratios because the prevalence measure is affected by cure, survival, and migration and does not estimate the risk for *getting* the disease.

Cross-sectional studies are subject to bias resulting from selective survival. That is, persons with existing cases who have survived to be in the study may be different from those diagnosed at approximately the same time who died and are unavailable for inclusion. Suppose physical activity not only reduced the risk for CHD but also improved survival among those with CHD. Sedentary persons with CHD would then have higher fatality rates than physically active persons who developed CHD. Higher rates of physical activity might be observed in a group of CHD survivors than in a general population without CHD. This might occur because of the survival advantage and also because of the participation of the survivors in cardiac rehabilitation programs. However, it might erroneously appear that physical activity was a risk factor for heart disease.

Ecological Studies

An ecological study is a study that is a bridge between descriptive and analytic epidemiology. The descriptive component looks at variations in disease rates by person, place, or time. The analytic component tries to determine if there is a relationship between disease rates and variations in rates for possible risk (or protective) factors. The identifying characteristic of ecological studies is that only aggregate data, such as population rates, are used, rather than data on individuals' exposures, characteristics, and outcomes. Examples include the following:

1. Information on per capita cigarette consumption in relation to lung cancer mortality rates in several countries, several groups of people, or the same population at different times
2. Comparisons of rates of breastfeeding and of breast cancer
3. Average dietary fat content and rates of CHD
4. Unemployment rates and level of psychiatric disorder

Ecological studies often use existing, readily available rates and are therefore quick and inexpensive to conduct. However, they are subject to ecological fallacy (i.e., associations observed at the group level may not hold true for the individuals who make up the groups, or associations that actually exist may be masked in the grouped data). This can occur when other factors operate in these populations for which the ecological correlations do not account. For that reason, ecological studies may suggest possible answers, but they require confirmation in studies that use individual data (Koepsell and Weiss, 2014).

EXPERIMENTAL STUDIES

The study designs discussed so far are called *observational studies* because the investigator observes the association between exposures and outcomes as they exist but does not intervene to alter the presence or level of any exposure or behavior. In contrast, in experimental or intervention studies, the investigator initiates a treatment or intervention to influence the risk for or course of disease. These studies test whether interventions can prevent disease or improve health. Both observational and experimental studies generally use comparison (or control) groups. In experimental studies, persons can be randomly assigned to a particular group, an intervention (i.e., a treatment or exposure) is applied, and the effects of the intervention are measured. The two types of intervention studies are clinical trials and community trials.

Clinical Trials

The goal of a clinical trial is generally to evaluate the effectiveness of an intervention, such as a medical treatment for disease, a new drug or existing drug used in a new or a different way, a surgical technique, or other treatment. In clinical trials, subjects should be randomly assigned to groups. In randomization, treatments are assigned to patients (subjects) so that all possible treatment assignments have a predetermined probability, but neither subject nor investigator determines the actual assignment of any participant. Randomization avoids the bias that may result if subjects choose to be in one group or the other or if the investigator or clinician chooses subjects for each group.

Masking or "blinding" treatment assignments is a second aspect of treatment allocation. In general, it is best to use a double-blinded study in which neither subject nor investigator knows who is getting which treatment. Clinical trials usually are the best way to show causality because of the objective way in which subjects are assigned and the greater control over other factors that could influence outcome. Like cohort studies, they are prospective and provide the clearest evidence of correct temporal sequence. Clinical trials tend to be conducted in a contrived (versus natural) situation, under controlled conditions, and with patient populations. That means that treatment may not be as effective when applied under more realistic clinical or community conditions in a more diverse patient population. There are also more ethical considerations involved in experimental studies than in observational studies. For example, is it fair to withhold a treatment, if the treatment truly appears to have the potential to alleviate a disease, to evaluate this treatment systematically using both an experimental and a control group? Finally, clinical trials are expensive in terms of time, personnel, facilities, and, in some cases, supplies.

Community Trials

Community trials are similar to clinical trials in that an investigator determines the exposure or intervention. However, community trials often deal with health promotion and disease prevention rather than treatment of existing disease. The intervention is usually undertaken on a large scale, and the unit of treatment is a community, region, or group rather than individuals. Although a pharmaceutical product such as fluoridation of water or mass immunizations may be involved in a community trial, these trials often involve educational, programmatic, or policy interventions. Examples of community interventions would be measuring the rates of diabetes or cardiovascular disease in a community in which the availability of exercise programs and facilities was increased or in which a much larger supply of healthful, fresh foods was made available.

Although community trials provide the best means of testing whether changes in knowledge or behavior, policy, programs, or other mass interventions are effective, they do pre-sent some problems. For many interventions, it may take years for the effectiveness to be evident (e.g., the effect of changing the availability of exercise and healthful food on the rates of either diabetes or heart disease). While the study is being carried out over time, other factors can influence the outcome either positively (i.e., making the intervention look more effective than it really is) or negatively (i.e., making the intervention look less effective than it really is). Comparable community populations without similar interventions for comparative analysis are often difficult to find. Even when comparable comparison communities are available—especially when the intervention is improved knowledge or changed behavior—it is difficult and unethical to prevent the control communities from making use of generally available information, effectively making them less different from the intervention communities. Finally, because community trials are often undertaken on a large scale and over long periods, they can be expensive, require a large staff, have complicated logistics, and need extensive communication about the study.

CAUSALITY

Statistical Associations

One of the first steps in assessing the relationship of a factor with a health outcome is determining whether a statistical association exists. If the probability of disease seems unaffected by the presence or level of the factor, no association is apparent. In contrast, if the probability of disease does vary according to whether the factor is present, there is a statistical association. Sample size, strength of association, and variance of measures can all affect statistical significance. For example, to determine if eating habits affect the onset of hypertension, a statistical association between the factor (diet) and the health outcome (hypertension) would need to be established. If the probability of disease seems unaffected by the presence or level of the factor, no association is apparent. On the other hand, if the probability of disease does vary according to whether the factor is present, there is a statistical association. The earlier discussion of null values is pertinent at this point. When an observed measure of association (e.g., a risk ratio) does not differ from the null value, there is no evidence of an association between the factor and the outcome being studied. To say a result is statistically significant means that the observed result is unlikely to be due to chance. Sample size affects statistical significance.

Bias

A statistically significant result may also be observed because of bias, a systematic error as a result of the study design, the way it is conducted, or a confounding factor. For example, if there were a gumball machine with colors randomly mixed and three red ones in a row came out, that would be due to chance. However, if the person loading the gumball machine had poured in a bag of red ones first, then green ones, then yellow ones, it would not be surprising to get three red ones in a row because of the way the machine was loaded. In epidemiologic studies, results are sometimes biased because of the way the study was "loaded" (i.e., the way the study was designed or the way subjects were selected, information was collected, and subjects were classified). Although the types of bias are numerous, there are three general categories of bias (Rothman, 2012). Bias can be attributed to the following:

1. **Selection or the way subjects enter a study:** Selection bias has to do with selection procedures and the population from which subjects are drawn, and it may involve self-selection factors. *Example:* Are teenagers who agree to complete a questionnaire on alcohol, tobacco, and other drug use representative of the total teenage population?

2. **Misclassification of subjects once they are in the study:** This is information, or classification (or misclassification), bias. It is related to how information is collected, including the information that subjects supply or how subjects are classified.

3. **Confounding or bias resulting from the relationship between the outcome and study factor and some third factor not accounted for.** *Example:* There is a well-known association between maternal smoking during pregnancy and low-birth-weight babies. There is also an association between alcohol consumption and smoking that is not due to chance, nor is it causal (i.e., drinking alcohol does not cause a person to smoke, nor does smoking cause a person to drink alcohol). If we were to investigate the association between alcohol consumption and low birth weight, smoking would be a confounder because it is related to both alcohol consumption and low birth weight. Failure to account for smoking in the analysis would bias the observed association between alcohol use and low birth weight. In practice, we can often identify potentially confounding variables and adjust for them in the analysis.

Assessing for Causality

The existence of a statistical association does not necessarily mean that a causal relationship exists or that causality is present. As just discussed, the observed association may be a random event (due to chance) or may be the result of bias from confounding or from flaws in the study design or execution. Statistical associations, although necessary to an argument for causality, or causal inference, are not adequate proof. Some epidemiologists refer to criteria for causality, a term originally used to evaluate the link between an infectious agent and a disease but revised and elaborated to also apply to other outcomes. Although various lists of guidelines have been proposed, the seven guidelines listed in Box 10.3 are often used (Weiss and Koepsell, 2014).

BOX 10.3 Guidelines for Causal Inference

1. **Strength of association:** A strong association between a potential risk factor and an outcome supports a causal hypothesis (i.e., a relative risk of 7 provides stronger evidence of a causal association than a relative risk of 1.5).

2. **Consistency of findings:** Repeated findings of an association with different study designs and in different populations strengthen a causal inference.

3. **Biologic plausibility:** Demonstration of a physiologic mechanism by which the risk factor acts to cause disease enhances the causal hypothesis. Conversely, an association that does not initially seem biologically defensible may later be discovered to be so.

4. **Demonstration of correct temporal sequence:** For a risk factor to cause an outcome, it must precede the onset of the outcome.

5. **Dose-response relationship:** The risk for developing an outcome should increase with increasing exposure (either in duration or quantity) to the risk factor of interest. For example, studies have shown that the more a woman smokes during pregnancy, the greater is the risk for delivering a low-birth-weight infant.

6. **Specificity of the association:** The presence of a one-to-one relationship between an agent and a disease (i.e., the idea that a disease is caused by only one agent and that agent results in only one disease lends support to a causal hypothesis, but its absence does not rule out causality). This criterion grows out of the infectious disease model in which it is more often though not always satisfied and is less applicable in chronic diseases.

7. **Experimental evidence:** Experimental designs provide the strongest epidemiologic evidence for causal associations, but they are not feasible or ethical to conduct for many risk factor–disease associations.

APPLICATIONS OF EPIDEMIOLOGY IN NURSING

Nurses need to know and be able to use epidemiology. Nurses regularly collect, report, analyze, interpret, and communicate epidemiologic data in many of the areas in which they work. Nurses involved in the care of persons with communicable diseases use epidemiology daily as they identify, report, treat, and provide follow-up on cases and contacts of TB, gonorrhea, gastroenteritis, and viruses such as COVID-19. School nurses also function as epidemiologists, collecting data on the incidence and prevalence of accidents, injuries, and illnesses in the school population. They are also key players in the detection and control of local epidemics, such as outbreaks of lice. As described earlier in this chapter, nurses across practice settings are actively involved in activities related to primary, secondary, and tertiary prevention (see the discussion of levels of prevention and the Levels of Prevention box).

LEVELS OF PREVENTION

Related to Cardiovascular Disease

Primary Prevention
Discuss with clients a low-fat diet and the need for regular physical exercise.

Secondary Prevention
Implement blood pressure and cholesterol screening; give a treadmill stress test.

Tertiary Prevention
Provide cardiac rehabilitation, medication, and surgery.

Some nursing jobs are specifically based in epidemiologic practice. These include nurse epidemiologists and environmental risk communicators employed by local health departments, as well as hospital infection control nurses. Nurses are key members of local fetal and infant mortality review boards, which examine cases of newborn deaths for identifiable risk factors and quality of care measures. Members of these review boards may include public health and maternal and child nurses as well as representatives from hospital labor and delivery and neonatal intensive care units. Nurses play a key role in disaster preparedness in their communities, and this work includes knowledge of epidemiology.

Nursing documentation on patient charts and records is an important source of data for epidemiologic reviews. Patient demographics and health histories are often collected or verified by nurses. As nurses collect and document patient information, they might not be thinking about the epidemiologic connection. However, the reliability and validity of such data can be key factors in the quality of future epidemiologic studies.

QSEN FOCUS ON QUALITY AND SAFETY EDUCATION FOR NURSES

Targeted Competency: Informatics—Use information and technology to communicate, manage knowledge, mitigate error, and support decision making. Important aspects of informatics include:

- **Knowledge:** Identify essential information that must be available in a common database to support client care.
- **Skills:** Use information management tools to monitor outcomes of care processes.
- **Attitudes:** Value nurses' involvement in design, selection, implementation, and evaluation of information technologies to support client care.

Informatics Question

Determine If a Health Problem Exists in the Community

Nurses are involved in the surveillance and monitoring of health phenomena. Planning for resources and personnel often requires quantifying the level of a problem in the community. For example, to know how different districts compare in the rates of infants with very low birth weight, you would calculate the prevalence of infants with very low birth weight in each district:

1. Determine the number of live births in each district from birth certificate data obtained from the vital records division of the health department.
2. Use the birth weight information from the birth certificate data to determine the number of infants born weighing less than 1500 g in each district.
3. Calculate the prevalence of births of infants with very low birth weights by district as the number of infants weighing less than 1500 g at birth divided by the total number of live births.
4. If the number of births of infants with very low birth weights in each district is small, use several years of data to obtain a more stable estimate.

Prepared by Gail Armstrong, ND, DNP, MS, PhD, Professor and Assistant Dean of the DNP Program, Oregon Health and Sciences University.

►► APPLYING CONTENT TO PRACTICE

It is important that nurses understand the relationship between population health concepts and clinical practice. Within the field of epidemiology, the definition of *population* is not necessarily confined to large groups of people, such as a population of the United States. Population health concepts also apply to other types of groups, such as the collective group of clients at one clinical practice site. In this case, the clinical epidemiologic application of population health concepts is evident in questions such as: What are the factors that contribute to the health and illness of issues among clients that I see in my clinic? Why do some of my clients fare better than others with the same disease conditions? What alternative clinical practices might help my clients? All of these clinical questions incorporate epidemiologic concepts of describing the *burden of disease* in a population, identifying and understanding *determinants of health,* and examining possible *root causes* of health outcomes. Two important documents highlight ways in which epidemiologic knowledge and skills are essential in nursing practice. The Council on Linkages between Academia and Public Health Practice (2014) outlined essential analytic/ assessment and public health science skills, and the Quad Council Coalition of Public Health Nursing Competencies (2018) provided details and examples of ways to implement these skill sets in nursing practice.

▮ PRACTICE APPLICATION

You are a nurse at a local health department where Rob Jones, a 46-year-old African American, comes for a routine blood pressure check. He mentions that his father recently died of prostate cancer and that he is worried about himself. Further assessment reveals that his father was diagnosed with prostate cancer when he was 52 years old and that Mr. Jones's uncle, who is 56, was recently diagnosed with prostate cancer. You know from Mr. Jones's health history that he smokes a pack of cigarettes per day and eats fried food frequently.

Which action would be your best choice?

A. Give Mr. Jones a digital rectal examination and prostate-specific antigen (PSA) test immediately to screen for prostate cancer.
B. Do not discuss or provide prostate cancer screening with him, because he is younger than 50 years.
C. Advise Mr. Jones to be tested immediately for the prostate cancer gene, because of his family history.
D. Inform him of the risks and benefits of prostate cancer testing and of his increased personal risk for prostate cancer because of his family history, smoking, and dietary habits. Involve him in the decision-making process about prostate cancer screening.

Answers can be found on the Evolve website.

REMEMBER THIS!

- Epidemiology is the study of the distribution and determinants of health-related events in human populations and the application of this knowledge to improving the health of communities.
- Epidemiology is a multidisciplinary science that recognizes the complex interrelationships of factors that influence disease and health at both the individual and the community level; it provides the basic tools for the study of health and disease in communities.
- Epidemiology is a multidisciplinary practice that recognizes the complex interrelationships of factors that influence disease and health at both the individual and community level.
- Epidemiologic methods are used to describe health and disease and to investigate the factors that promote health or influence the risk for, or distribution of, disease. This knowledge can be useful in planning and evaluating programs, policies, and services and in clinical decision making.
- Basic epidemiologic concepts include the interrelationships among the agent, host, and environment (the epidemiologic triangle); the interactions of multilevel factors, exposures, and characteristics (causal web) affecting the risk for disease; and the levels of prevention corresponding to stages in the natural history of disease.
- Primary prevention involves interventions to reduce the incidence of disease by promoting health and preventing disease processes from developing.
- Secondary prevention includes programs (e.g., screening) designed to detect disease in the early stages, before signs and symptoms are clinically evident, to intervene with early diagnosis and treatment.
- Tertiary prevention provides treatments and other interventions directed toward persons with clinically apparent disease, with the aim of lessening the course of the disease, reducing disability, or rehabilitating the client.
- Epidemiologic methods are also used in the planning and design of screening (secondary prevention) and community health intervention (primary prevention) strategies and in the evaluation of their effectiveness.
- Basic epidemiologic methods include the use of existing data sources to study health outcomes and related factors and the use of comparison groups to assess the association between exposures or characteristics and health outcomes.
- Epidemiologists use rates and proportions to quantify levels of morbidity and mortality.
- Prevalence proportions provide a picture of the level of existing cases in a population at a given time.
- Incidence rates and proportions measure the rate of new case development in a population and provide an estimate of the risk for disease.
- Descriptive epidemiologic studies provide information on the distribution of disease and health states according to personal characteristics, geographic region, and time. This knowledge enables practitioners to target programs and allocate resources more effectively and provides a basis for further study.
- Analytic epidemiologic studies investigate associations between exposures or characteristics and health or disease outcomes, with the goal of understanding the etiology of disease. Analytic studies provide the foundation for understanding disease causality and for developing effective intervention strategies aimed at primary, secondary, and tertiary prevention.

EVOLVE WEBSITE

http://evolve.elsevier.com/Stanhope/foundations

- Case Study, with Questions and Answers
- NCLEX Review Questions
- Practice Application Answers

REFERENCES

American Nurses Association: *Essential nursing competencies and curricula guidelines for genetics and genomics*, Silver Spring, MD, 2006, ANA.

Celentano DO , Szklo M: *Gordis Epidemiology*, 6th ed, Philadelphia. PA, 2018, Elsevier.

Cohen IB: Florence Nightingale, *Sci Am* 250:128–137, 1984.

Council on Linkages between Academic and Public Health Practice: *Core competencies for public health professionals*, Washington DC, 2014, Public Health Foundation/Health Resources and Services Administration.

Elflein J: Leading causes of death in the United States 2018, https:www.statista.com

Fullilove MT: Comment: abandoning "race" as a variable in public health research—an idea whose time has come, *Am J Public Health* 88:1297-1298, 1998.

Fuller CM, Borrell LN, Latkin CA, et al.: Effects of race, neighborhood, and social network on age at initiation of injection drug use, *Am J Public Health* 95:689–695, 2005.

Heymann DL, editor: *Control of communicable diseases manual*, ed 20, Washington, DC, 2014, American Public Health Association.

Institute of Medicine: *The future of the public's health in the 21st century*, Washington, DC, 2002, National Academies Press. Retrieved May 2012 from http://www.iom.edu/Reports.

Kochanek KD, Murphy SL, Xu JQ, Arias, E: *Mortality in the United States, 2016*, NCHS Data Brief, no 293, Hyattsville, MD, 2017, National Center for Health Statistics.

Koepsell TD, Weiss NS: *Epidemiologic methods: studying the occurrence of illness*, New York, 2014, Oxford University Press.

Lee MN, Teutsch SM, Thacker SB, St Louis ME: *Principles and practice of public health surveillance*, New York, 2010, Oxford University Press.

Macintyre S, Ellaway A: Ecological approaches: rediscovering the role of the physical and social environment. In Berkman LF, Kawachi I, eds: *Social epidemiology*, New York, 2000, Oxford University Press, pp 332-348.

Matoba N, Collins JW Jr: Racial disparity in infant mortality, *Semin Perinatol* 41(6):354–359, 2017.

Moore JT, Ricaldi JN, Rose CE et al., Disparities in incidence of COVID-19 among underrepresented racial/ethnic groups in counties identified as hotspots during June 5-18, 2020—22 states, February-June 2020, *MMWR Morb Mortal Wkly Rep*. ePub, August 14, 2020, Vol 69.

Noonan M, Galvin R, Doody O, Jomeen J: A qualitative meta-synthesis: public health nurses, role in the identification and management of perinatal mental health problems, *J Adv Nurs* 73(3): 545–557, 2017.

Office of Minority Health (USDHHS, OMH): *HHS Action Plan to Reduce Racial and Ethnic Health Disparities Implementation Progress Report*, Washington, DC, 2015, Office of the Assistant Secretary for Planning and Evaluation

Palmer IS: *Florence Nightingale and the first organized delivery of nursing services*, Washington, DC, 1983, American Association of Colleges of Nursing.

Patel RC, Baek J, Smith MA, Morgenstern LB, Lisabeth LD: Residential ethnic segregation and stroke risk in Mexican Americans: the Brain Attack Surveillance in Corpus Christi project, *Ethn Dis* 25(1):11–18, 2015.

Porta M: *A dictionary of epidemiology*, ed 6, New York, 2014, Oxford University Press.

Quad Council Coalition Competency Review Task Force: Community/Public Health Nursing Competencies, 2018.

Quaranta JE, Swaine J, Ryszka S: Preschool asthma: examining environmental influences using geographic information systems, *Public Health Nursing*, 37(3): 405-411, May/June 2020.

Remington PL, Brownson RC, Wegman MV: *Chronic disease epidemiology and control*, ed 4, Washington DC, 2016, American Public Health Association.

Rothman KJ: *Epidemiology: an introduction*, ed 2, New York, 2012, Oxford University Press.

Snow J: On the mode of communication of cholera. In *Snow on cholera*, New York, 1855, The Commonwealth Fund.

Szklo M, Nieto FJ: *Epidemiology: beyond the basics*, ed 4, Boston, 2018, Jones & Bartlett.

US Department of Health and Human Services: *Healthy People 2030*, Washington, DC, 2020, US Government Printing Office.

Weiss NS, Koepsell TD: *Epidemiologic methods: studying the occurrence of illness*, New York, NY, 2014, Oxford University Press.

Xu JQ, Murphy SL Kochanek KD, et al.: Deaths: Leading causes for 2015, National Vital Statistics Reports; vol 66 no 6. Hyattsville, MD: 2017, National Center for Health Statistics.

Xu JQ, Murphy SL, Kochanek KD, Bastian BA, Arias C: Deaths: Final data for 2016, *National Vital Statistics Reports* 64(2):1–119, Hyattsville MD, 2018, National Center for Health Statistics.

11

Infectious Disease Prevention and Control

Susan C. Long-Marin and Donna E. Smith

OBJECTIVES

After reading this chapter, the student should be able to:

1. Discuss the current effect and threats of infectious diseases on individuals, families, communities, and society.
2. Explain how the elements of the epidemiologic triangle interact to cause infectious diseases.
3. Provide examples of infectious disease control interventions at the three levels of public health prevention.
4. Explain the multisystem approach to the control of communicable diseases.

5. Discuss the factors contributing to newly emerging or reemerging infectious diseases.
6. Discuss issues related to obtaining and maintaining appropriate levels of immunization against vaccine-preventable diseases.
7. Describe issues and agents associated with foodborne illness and appropriate prevention measures.

CHAPTER OUTLINE

KEY TERMS

As evidenced by the rapid and widespread transmission of COVID, concern about infectious and emerging diseases has grown tremendously beginning in 2020. Migration can increase the spread of infectious diseases when people travel or move from one place to another. This chapter presents an overview of communicable diseases that nurses most often encounter. Diseases are grouped according to descriptive category (by mode of transmission or means of prevention). A detailed discussion of sexually transmitted diseases or infections (STDs or STIs), human immunodeficiency virus (HIV), acquired immunodeficiency syndrome (AIDS), viral hepatitis, and tuberculosis (TB) is provided in Chapter 12. Although not all infectious diseases are directly transferred from person to person, the terms *infectious diseases* and *communicable diseases* are used interchangeably throughout this chapter.

HISTORICAL AND CURRENT PERSPECTIVES

In 1900, communicable diseases were the leading causes of death in the United States. Since that time, improved sanitation and nutrition, the discovery of antibiotics, and the development of vaccines have ended some epidemics such as diphtheria and typhoid fever and greatly reduced the incidence of others such as TB. In ·1900, respiratory and diarrheal diseases were major killers, and TB was the second leading cause of death. Since 1989, the United States has worked toward the goal of eliminating TB. The pace of decline has slowed in recent years; however, provisional 2019 data reported 8920 new cases of TB (Schwartz, Price, Pratt, and Langer, 2020). The World Health Organization (WHO) estimated that in 2018, an estimated 10.0 million people fell ill with TB. The distinction is not equal around the world. The countries reporting the largest number of cases were southeast Asia, Africa, and the western Pacific, with fewer cases in the eastern Mediterranean, the Americas, and Europe (WHO, 2019a). As people live longer, chronic diseases—heart disease, cancer, and stroke—have replaced infectious diseases as the leading causes of death in the United States. However, infectious diseases have not vanished. In 2020, COVID-19 became a major cause of morbidity and mortality around the world, with the United States having some of the highest rates in the world. Infectious diseases remain a cause of concern, and they persist as the leading cause of death for children and adolescents worldwide, especially those in low-income countries, killing an estimated 6 million people a year (WHO 2018). Organisms once susceptible to antibiotics are becoming increasingly drug resistant; this may result in vulnerability to diseases previously thought to no longer be a threat. In addition, in the 21st century, infectious diseases have become a means of terrorism.

New killers emerge, and old familiar diseases take on different, more virulent characteristics. In 1918 the country suffered enormously from the influenza pandemic referred to as the "Spanish Flu." Consider the following developments over the past 45 years. HIV was first recognized in the 1980s, but there is still no vaccine, although new drugs offer prevention and treatment.

In the summer of 1993, in the southwestern United States, healthy young adults were stricken with a mysterious and unknown but often fatal respiratory disease that is now known as hantavirus pulmonary syndrome. In 1994 a severe invasive strain of *Streptococcus pyogenes* group A, called by the press the "flesh-eating" bacteria, was identified. This devastating disease occurs when bacteria enter a wound such as from an insect bite, burn, or cut, and leads to necrotizing fasciitis, which results in death in one of four affected persons (see information on necrotizing fasciitis at http://www.WebMD or on the Centers for Disease Control and Prevention [CDC] website: http://www.cdc.gov). Consumption of improperly cooked hamburgers and unpasteurized apple juice contaminated with a highly toxic strain of *Escherichia coli*, O157:H7, caused illness and death in children across the country. In 1996, 10 states had outbreaks of diarrheal disease traced to imported fresh berries. The implicated organism in these outbreaks is *Cyclospora cayetanensis* (a coccidian parasite). A person becomes infected when consuming food or water contaminated with the parasite, and the symptoms can last from 2 days to 2 weeks. It is important to be cautious about this parasite when traveling to other countries.

Also in 1996, the fear that "mad cow disease" (bovine spongiform encephalopathy [BSE]) could be transferred to humans through beef consumption led to the slaughter of thousands of British cattle and a ban on the international sale of British beef. Although not seen in the United States until 2003, when a BSE case was imported from Canada, BSE was reported in many countries, including several in Europe, as well as in Japan, Canada, and Israel.

Vancomycin-resistant *Staphylococcus aureus* (VRSA) was reported in 1997; previously, vancomycin had been considered the only effective antibiotic against methicillin-resistant *S. aureus* (MRSA). MRSA is increasingly a problem for people who acquire the bacteria in the hospital, and there is a growing incidence of community-acquired MRSA. These latter outbreaks are associated with (but not limited to) places in which people share facilities, such as locker rooms, prisons, and other close bathing areas.

Ebola hemorrhagic fever, a sporadic but highly fatal virus, was unknown to most people nearly 45 years ago. Since its discovery in 1976, the majority of cases and outbreaks of Ebola virus disease have occurred in Africa. The 2014 to 2016 Ebola outbreak in West Africa began in a rural setting of southeastern

Guinea, spread to urban areas and across borders within weeks, and became a global epidemic within months (CDC, 2019a). An air traveler brought a case to the United States, and a small number of nurses and other health care workers who went to help treat Ebola in west Africa contracted the disease. By January 2015, there were 8650 reported deaths due to this epidemic. The majority of cases of Ebola and deaths were in Guinea, Liberia, and Sierra Leone (CDC, 2019a). Ebola virus is spread through direct contact with blood or body fluids and can enter the person's body through broken skin or unprotected mucous membranes. This virus can also be spread through needlesticks by needles that are contaminated with the virus, infected fruit bats or primates, and possibly from contact with semen from a man who has recovered from Ebola (CDC, 2019a).

In 1999 the first Western Hemisphere activity of West Nile virus (WNV), a mosquito-transmitted illness that can affect livestock, birds, and humans, occurred in New York City. By 2002, WNV, believed to be carried by infected birds and possibly mosquitoes in cargo containers, had spread across the United States as far west as California and was reported in Canada and Central America as well. Any person with a febrile or acute neurologic illness who has recently been exposed to mosquitoes, blood transfusion, or organ transplantation should be evaluated for WNV. Most symptomatic persons have an acute febrile illness that can include headache, weakness, myalgia, or arthralgia; gastrointestinal symptoms and a transient maculopapular rash are also often observed. Both Ebola and WNV are discussed in more detail later in the chapter.

In addition, in early 2003, severe acute respiratory syndrome (SARS), a previously unknown disease of undetermined etiology and no definitive treatment, emerged with major outbreaks in China, Hong Kong, Taiwan, Vietnam, Singapore, and Canada, with additional cases reported from 20 locations around the world. This syndrome ended as suddenly as it had begun, with only a few cases being reported since 2003.

In the 21st century, foodborne infections again have made headlines as E. coli–infected spinach sickened and killed individuals across the United States. In 2008 tomatoes were blamed for a nationwide outbreak of salmonellosis but were ruled innocent when the green chilies that accompanied them in salsa were found to be the actual culprits. Salmonella again made the news as contaminated peanut butter forced recalls across the United States, sickened hundreds, and resulted in several deaths. Even chocolate chip cookie dough was not safe; a national recall in 2009 followed the discovery that people had been sickened after eating raw dough contaminated with E. coli. Perhaps the most publicized infectious disease event of 2009 was the advent of a new strain of flu, novel influenza A H1N1. First reported from Mexico and rapidly acquired by travelers to that country, H1N1 spread quickly across the world, causing the WHO to declare a pandemic and stimulate the race for a vaccine. During the 2013 to 2014 flu season in the United States, H1N1 became a predominant strain, primarily affecting young and middle-aged people. In 2012 the Middle Eastern respiratory syndrome coronavirus, or MERS-CoV, similar to SARS, appeared in the Arabian Peninsula and affected people there and those who traveled there. The reservoir for this disease is unknown but appears to be associated with camels. The first cases of MERS-CoV in the United States were reported in 2014 in individuals who had traveled from Saudi Arabia.

Previously seen in other parts of the world, the first case of chikungunya virus was reported in the Americas in 2013. Transmitted by mosquitos, chikungunya most commonly involves fever and sometimes severe joint pain as well as headache, muscle pain, conjunctivitis, and rash. For most people, the disease is mild and self-limiting, although joint pain may persist for some time. There is neither a specific treatment nor vaccine. Primates and humans are thought to be the main reservoirs, and person-to-mosquito-to-person transmission can occur. Cases in the United States typically involved travelers to infected areas outside the country. Another mosquito-borne virus, Zika, made major news in 2015 with an initial widespread outbreak in Brazil. First identified in 1947, Zika virus, seemingly a mild-mannered disease, was reported in only a handful of cases across equatorial Africa and Asia until outbreaks in 2007 and 2013 in the Pacific islands revealed a more aggressive virus causing large outbreaks and resulting in neurologic conditions such as microcephaly and Guillain-Barré syndrome. In Brazil, as in the outbreaks in the Pacific islands with no immunity among the population, Zika virus spread throughout the country and to surrounding countries, leaving in its wake thousands of children with neurologic birth defects, devastated families, and an economic impact that will last for decades as the cost of raising these medically fragile children mounts. At the beginning of 2016, the WHO declared a Public Health Emergency of International Concern (PHEIC), a status previously reserved for diseases such as Ebola and polio, which was not lifted until the end of the year. Women were advised to delay pregnancy, and, in the United States, pregnant women were warned to avoid mosquitos and traveling to infected areas. Some fans and athletes chose not to attend the 2016 Summer Olympics in Rio de Janeiro. Refraining from sexual activity with travelers from infected areas was also added to warnings when it was discovered that Zika virus could be transmitted sexually. As of 2018, there were no mosquito-transmitted cases of Zika in the United States (CDC, 2019b).

In the early years of the 21st century, worldwide, the leading causes of deaths from infectious diseases were respiratory infections, diarrheal diseases, HIV/AIDS, TB, malaria, meningitis, pertussis, measles, hepatitis B, and other infectious diseases (Fauci and Morens, 2012). COVID-19 has joined this list of causes of death from an infectious disease. Infections are unpredictable and can have an explosive global effect as people move around the world. This has been incredibly apparent with the onset of COVID-19. Most infectious diseases are caused by a single agent, and general disease control measures, such as sanitation, chemical disinfection, hand washing, social distancing, mask wearing, vector control, and specific medical measures such as vaccination or antimicrobial treatment, can influence the outcome of the infection. See the How To box in the section of the chapter on prevention and control of communicable diseases for ways to prevent infection transmission at home. In 2012 Fauci and Morens emphasized ways to prevent contracting an infectious disease when they said, "Infectious diseases are acquired specifically and directly as a result of our behaviors and lifestyles" (p. 455). They pointed out that we contract infectious diseases from social gatherings, travel and transportation, sexual activity, occupational exposures, sports and recreational activities, what we eat and drink, our pets, the environment, and even from people in hospitals. These warnings remain pertinent. Infectious diseases are expensive. There are costs due to lost wages, medications, and other forms of health care.

Because of the morbidity (rate of an illness or abnormal quality), mortality (rate of death), and associated cost of infectious diseases, the national health promotion and disease prevention goals outlined in *Healthy People 2030* list objectives for reducing the incidence of these illnesses in the sections on Infectious Disease and in Foodborne Illness (see the *Healthy People 2030* box). The objectives provide information on how to prevent infectious diseases that nurses can use in health education.

HEALTHY PEOPLE 2030

Selected Objectives Related to Infectious Diseases and Foodborne Illness
- **IID-D03:** Increase the proportion of adults age 19 years or older who get recommended vaccines.
- **FS-02:** Reduce infections causes by Shiga toxin–producing *E. coli.*
- **FS-10:** Increase the proportion of people who refrigerate food within 2 hours after cooking.

From US Department of Health and Human Services: *Healthy People 2030,* Washington, DC, 2020a, US Government Printing Office.

TRANSMISSION OF COMMUNICABLE DISEASES

Agent, Host, and Environment

The transmission of communicable diseases depends on the successful interaction of the infectious agent, the host, and the environment. These three factors make up the epidemiologic triangle (Fig. 11.1), as discussed in Chapter 10 (epidemiologic approaches). Changes in the characteristics of any of the factors may result in disease transmission. Consider the following examples. Not only may antibiotic therapy eliminate a specific pathologic agent, but it also may alter the balance of normally occurring organisms in the body. As a result, one of these agents overruns another and disease, such as a yeast infection, occurs. HIV performs its deadly work not by directly poisoning the host but by destroying the host's immune reaction to other disease-producing agents. Individuals living in the temperate climate of the United States do not contract malaria at home, but they may become infected if they change their environment by traveling to a climate in which malaria-carrying mosquitoes thrive. As these examples illustrate, the balance among agent, host, and environment is often precarious and may be unintentionally disrupted.

Agent Factor

Four main categories of infectious agents can cause infection or disease: bacteria, fungi, parasites, and viruses. The individual agent may be described by its ability to cause disease and by the

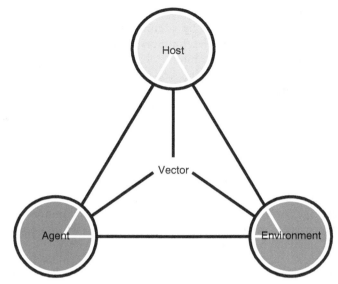

Fig. 11.1 The Epidemiologic Triangle of Disease. (From Gordis L: *Epidemiology,* Philadelphia, 1996, Saunders.)

nature and the severity of the disease. *Infectivity, pathogenicity, virulence, toxicity, invasiveness,* and *antigenicity,* terms commonly used to characterize infectious agents, are defined in Box 11.1.

Host Factor

A human or animal host can harbor an infectious agent. The characteristics of the host that may influence the spread of disease are host resistance, immunity, herd immunity, and infectiousness of the host. Resistance is the ability of the host to withstand infection, and it may involve natural or acquired immunity.

Natural immunity refers to species-determined, innate resistance to an infectious agent. For example, opossums rarely contract rabies. Acquired immunity is the resistance acquired by a host as a result of previous natural exposure to an infectious agent. Having measles once protects against future infection. Acquired immunity may be induced by active or passive immunization. Active immunization refers to the immunization of an individual by administration of an antigen (infectious agent or vaccine) and is usually characterized by the presence of an antibody produced by the individual host. Vaccinating children against childhood diseases is an example of inducing active immunity. Passive immunization refers to immunization through the transfer of a specific antibody from an immunized individual

BOX 11.1 Six Characteristics of an Infectious Agent
- **Infectivity:** The ability to enter and multiply in the host
- **Pathogenicity:** The ability to produce a specific clinical reaction after infection occurs
- **Virulence:** The ability to produce a severe pathologic reaction
- **Toxicity:** The ability to produce a poisonous reaction
- **Invasiveness:** The ability to penetrate and spread throughout a tissue
- **Antigenicity:** The ability to stimulate an immunologic response

to a nonimmunized individual, such as the transfer of antibody from mother to infant or by administration of an antibody-containing preparation (i.e., immunoglobulin or antiserum). Passive immunity from immunoglobulin is almost immediate but short lived. It is often induced as a stopgap measure until active immunity has time to develop after vaccination. Examples of commonly used immunoglobulins include those for hepatitis A, rabies, and tetanus.

Herd immunity refers to the immunity of a group or community. It is the resistance of a group of people to invasion and spread of an infectious agent. Herd immunity is based on the resistance of a high proportion of individual members of a group to infection. It is the basis for increasing immunization coverage for vaccine-preventable diseases. Higher immunization coverage will lead to greater herd immunity, which in turn will block the further spread of the disease.

Infectiousness is a measure of the potential ability of an infected host to transmit the infection to other hosts. It reflects the relative ease with which the infectious agent is transmitted to others. Individuals with measles are extremely infectious; the virus spreads readily on airborne droplets. A person with Lyme disease cannot spread the disease to other people (although the infected tick can). COVID-19 is a highly infectious disease that is primarily airborne. Considerable effort and resources were devoted to finding a vaccine and to achieve herd immunity throughout the world.

Environment Factor

The environment refers to the physical, biologic, social, and cultural factors that are external to the human host. These environmental factors facilitate the transmission of an infectious agent from an infected host to other susceptible hosts. Reduction in communicable disease risk can be achieved by altering these environmental factors. Using mosquito nets and repellents to avoid bug bites, avoiding having even small amounts of standing water that can breed mosquitos, installing sewage systems to prevent fecal contamination of water supplies, and washing utensils after contact with raw meat to reduce bacterial contamination are all examples of altering the environment to prevent disease. *Healthy People 2030* recommends not using the same cutting board for different foods. For example, you would not cut vegetables or fruit on the same board that you used to cut raw chicken without thoroughly cleaning the board.

Modes of Transmission

Infectious diseases can be transmitted horizontally or vertically. Vertical transmission occurs when the infection is passed from parent to offspring via sperm, placenta, milk, or contact in the vaginal canal at birth. Examples of vertical transmission are transplacental transmission of HIV and syphilis. Horizontal transmission is the person-to-person spread of infection through one or more of the following four routes: direct or indirect contact, common vehicle, airborne, or vector-borne. Most STDs are spread by direct sexual contact. Enterobiasis, or pinworm infection, can be acquired

through direct contact or indirect contact with contaminated objects such as toys, clothing, and bedding. A growing problem of horizontal transmission is that of bedbugs, which are often found in bedding and other soft surfaces. Common vehicle refers to transportation of the infectious agent from an infected host to a susceptible host via food, water, milk, blood, serum, saliva, or plasma. Hepatitis A can be transmitted through contaminated food and water; hepatitis B can be transmitted through contaminated blood. Legionellosis and TB are both spread via contaminated droplets in the air. Vectors are arthropods such as ticks and mosquitoes or other invertebrates such as snails that can transmit the infectious agent by biting or depositing the infective material near the host.

Disease Development

Exposure to an infectious agent does not always lead to an infection. Similarly, infection does not always lead to disease. Infection depends on the infective dose, the infectivity of the infectious agent, and the immunocompetence of the host. It is important to differentiate infection and disease, as clearly illustrated by the HIV/AIDS epidemic. Infection refers to the entry, development, and multiplication of the infectious agent in the susceptible host. Disease is one of the possible outcomes of infection, and it may indicate a physiological dysfunction or pathologic reaction. An individual who tests positive for HIV is infected, but if that person shows no clinical signs, the individual is not diseased. Similarly, an individual who tests positive for HIV and also exhibits clinical signs of AIDS is both infected and diseased. This same series of events are present in COVID-19.

Incubation period and *communicable period* are not synonymous. Incubation period is the time interval between invasion by an infectious agent and the first appearance of signs and symptoms of the disease. The incubation periods of infectious diseases vary from between 2 and 4 hours for staphylococcal food poisoning to between 10 and 15 years for AIDS (HIV stage III). Communicable period is the interval during which an infectious agent may be transferred directly or indirectly from an infected person to another person. The period of communicability for influenza is 3 to 5 days after the clinical onset of symptoms. Hepatitis B–infected persons are infectious many weeks before the onset of the first symptoms and remain infective during the acute phase and chronic carrier state, which may persist for life.

Disease Spectrum

Persons with infectious diseases may exhibit a broad spectrum of disease ranging from subclinical infection to severe and fatal disease. Those with subclinical or nonapparent infections are important from the public health point of view because they are a source of infection but may not be receiving the care that those with clinical disease are receiving. They should be targeted for early diagnosis and treatment. Those with clinical disease may exhibit localized or systemic symptoms and mild to severe illness. The final outcome of a disease may be recovery, death, or something in between, including a carrier state, complications requiring an extended hospital stay, or disability requiring rehabilitation.

At the community level, the disease may occur in endemic, epidemic, or pandemic proportion. Endemic refers to the constant presence of a disease within a geographic area or a population. Pertussis is endemic in the United States. Epidemic refers to the occurrence of a disease in a community or region in excess of normal expectancy. Although people tend to associate large numbers with epidemics, even one case can be termed *epidemic* if the disease is considered eliminated from that area. For example, one case of polio, a disease that is considered eliminated from the United States, would be considered epidemic. Pandemic refers to an epidemic that occurs worldwide and affects large populations. This was seen with COVID-19, a virus that rapidly spread worldwide. HIV disease is both epidemic and pandemic because the number of cases is growing rapidly across various regions of the world. Zika virus and novel influenza A H1N1 were both emerging infectious diseases and were responsible for recent pandemics.

SURVEILLANCE OF COMMUNICABLE DISEASES

When conducting surveillance, you gather information about *who, when, where,* and *what;* these elements are then used to answer *why.* A good surveillance system collects, organizes, and analyzes current, accurate, and complete data for a defined disease condition. The resulting information is promptly released to those who need it for effective planning, implementation, and evaluation of disease prevention and control programs. Infectious disease surveillance incorporates and analyzes data from a variety of sources. Box 11.2 lists 10 commonly used data elements.

Surveillance for Agents of Bioterrorism

Since September 11, 2001, greater emphasis has been placed on surveillance for any disease that might be associated with the intentional release of a biologic agent. The concern is that because of the interval between exposure and disease, a covert release may go unrecognized and without response for some time if the resulting outbreak closely resembles a naturally occurring one. Health care providers need to be alert to (1) temporal or geographic clustering of illnesses (e.g., people who attended the same public gathering or visited the same location), especially those with clinical signs that resemble an infectious disease outbreak—previously healthy people with unexplained fever accompanied by sepsis, pneumonia, respiratory failure, rash, or flaccid paralysis; (2) an unusual age distribution for a common disease (e.g., chickenpox-like disease in adults without a child source case); and (3) a large number of cases of acute flaccid paralysis, such as that seen in *Clostridium botulinum* intoxication. Although more active infectious disease surveillance is being encouraged because of the potential for bioterrorism, the positive benefit is increased surveillance for other communicable diseases as well.

Because of the heightened concern about possible bioterrorist attacks, various sorts of syndromic surveillance systems have been developed by public health agencies across the country. These systems are essential for many other outbreaks and activities other than bioterrorism. These systems incorporate factors such as the previously mentioned temporal and geographic clustering and unusual age distributions with groups of disease symptoms or syndromes (e.g., flaccid paralysis, respiratory signs, skin rashes, gastrointestinal symptoms) with the goal of detecting early signs of diseases that could result from a bioterrorism-related attack. Syndromic surveillance systems may include tracking emergency department visits sorted by syndrome symptoms, as well as other indicators of illness, including school absenteeism and sales of selected over-the-counter medications. In recent years, the tracking of cold medicines used to make crystal methamphetamine has received considerable attention. Nurses are frequently involved at different levels of the surveillance system. They collect data, make diagnoses, investigate and report cases, and provide information to the general public. Nurses may investigate sources and contacts in outbreaks of pertussis in school settings or shigellosis in daycare; TB testing and contact tracing; collecting and reporting information about notifiable communicable diseases; and providing morbidity and mortality statistics to those who request them, including the media, the public, service planners, and grant writers. See Chapter 17 for a complete discussion of surveillance and outbreak investigation.

List of Reportable Diseases

Notifiable or reportable diseases are those in which regular, frequent, and timely information about each case is needed for the prevention and control of the disease. The requirements for disease reporting in the United States are mandated by state rather than federal law and may vary slightly from state to state. State health departments, on a voluntary basis, report cases of selected diseases to the CDC through the National Notifiable Diseases Surveillance System (NNNDSS). The list of notifiable diseases may be revised as new diseases emerge or disease incidence declines. In 2019 there were 127 National Notifiable Conditions. The list can be found on the CDC website under the heading of *Nationally notifiable conditions* (CDC, 2019c).

BOX 11.2 10 Basic Elements of Surveillance

1. Mortality registration
2. Morbidity reporting
3. Epidemic reporting
4. Epidemic field investigation
5. Laboratory reporting
6. Individual case investigation
7. Surveys
8. Use of biologic agents and drugs
9. Distribution of animal reservoirs and vectors
10. Demographic and environmental data

EMERGING INFECTIOUS DISEASES

Emergence Factors

Emerging infectious diseases are those in which the incidence has increased in the past several decades or has the potential to increase in the near future. These emerging diseases may include new or known infectious diseases. Consider the following examples. Ebola virus was identified in 1976 when sporadic outbreaks occurred in Sudan and Zaire. Ebola virus is a mysterious killer with a high mortality rate, has no licensed vaccine or known treatment, and has no recognized reservoir in nature. It appears to be transmitted through direct contact with bodily secretions and can be contained once cases are identified. It is not clear why outbreaks occur. The CDC has current information on the Ebola virus and its fellow virus Marburg.

WNV is a mosquito-borne seasonal disease that was first identified in Uganda in 1937 and in the United States in 1999. How WNV first arrived in the United States is not known, but the answer most likely involves infected birds or mosquitoes. Because the virus was new in this country and the outbreak of 2002 caused many deaths, WNV gained media attention. However, for the majority of people, infection with WNV has no clinical signs or only mild flulike symptoms. In a small percentage of individuals, a more severe, potentially fatal neuroinvasive form may develop. After first appearing in New York City in 1999, the virus spent several years quietly spreading up and down the East Coast without remarkable morbidity or mortality. This situation changed abruptly in the summer of 2002, when WNV was reported across the country and was accompanied by significant avian, equine, and human mortality. As of October 6, 2020, a total of 42 states had reported WNV infections in people, birds, or mosquitoes, and 279 cases in people were reported to the CDC, with 212 of these cases being neuroinvasive (CDC, 2020a).

Periodic outbreaks appear to result from a complex interaction of multiple factors, including weather. Extensive rain followed by dry periods support mosquito reproduction and may play a role in WNV. Because there is no human vaccine, only a vaccine for horses, preventing human infection depends on mosquito control and preventing mosquito bites. The CDC website for WNV provides details and maps of recent WNV activity.

Table 11.1 illustrates factors, operating singly or in combination, which can influence the emergence of these diseases (CDC, 1994). Except for microbial adaptation and changes made by the infectious agent, such as those likely in the emergence of E. coli O157:H7, H1N1 and possibly Zika virus, most of the emergence factors are consequences of activities and behavior of the human hosts and environmental changes such as deforestation, urbanization, and industrialization. The rise in households with two working parents has increased the number of children in daycare, and with this shift has come an increase in diarrheal diseases such as shigellosis. Changing sexual behavior and illegal drug use influence the spread of HIV and other STDs. Before the use of large air-conditioning systems with cooling towers, legionellosis was virtually unknown. Modern transportation systems closely and quickly connect regions of the world that for centuries had little contact. Insects and animals, as well as humans, may carry disease between continents on ships and planes. Immigrants, legal and undocumented, as well as travelers bring with them a variety of known and potentially unknown diseases. To prevent and control these emerging diseases, effective ways to educate people and change their behavior and to develop effective drugs and vaccines must be developed. In addition, current surveillance systems must be strengthened and expanded to improve the detection and tracking of these diseases. The list of emerging infectious diseases changes as has been seen in the last few years. Selected emerging infectious diseases, including a brief description of the diseases and symptoms they cause, their modes of transmission, and causes of emergence, are listed in Table 11.2. Progress in addressing emerging infectious disease as well as current findings and topics can be found in the CDC journal *Emerging Infectious Diseases*. The journal is published monthly and is available online at http://wwwnc.cdc.gov.

TABLE 11.1   Factors That Can Influence the Emergence of New Infectious Diseases

Categories	Specific Examples
Societal events	Economic impoverishment, war or civil conflict, population growth and migration, urban decay
Health care	New medical devices, organ or tissue transplantation, drugs causing immunosuppression, widespread use of antibiotics
Food production	Globalization of food supplies, changes in food processing and packaging
Human behavior	Sexual behavior, drug use, travel, diet, outdoor recreation, use of child-care facilities
Environment	Deforestation or reforestation, changes in water ecosystems, flood or drought, famine, global changes (e.g., warming)
Public health	Curtailment or reduction in prevention programs, inadequate communicable disease infrastructure surveillance, lack of trained personnel (epidemiologists, laboratory scientists, vector and rodent control specialists)
Microbial adaptation	Changes in virulence and toxin production, development of drug resistance, microbes as cofactors in chronic diseases

From Centers for Disease Control and Prevention: Addressing emerging infectious disease threats: a prevention strategy for the United States (Executive Summary), *MMWR* 43 (No. RR-5):1-16, 1994.

TABLE 11.2 Examples of Emerging Infectious Diseases

Infectious Agent	Diseases/Symptoms	Mode of Transmission	Causes of Emergence
Borrelia burgdorferi	Lyme disease: rash, fever, arthritis, neurological and cardiac abnormalities	Bite of infective *Ixodes* tick	Increase in deer and human populations in wooded areas
Cryptosporidium	Cryptosporidiosis; infection of epithelial cells in gastrointestinal and respiratory tracts	Fecal-oral, person-to-person, waterborne	Development near watershed areas; immunosuppression
Ebola-Marburg viruses	Fulminant, high mortality, hemorrhagic fever	Direct contact with infected blood, organs, secretions, and semen	Unknown, likely human invasion of virus ecological niche
Escherichia coli O157:H7	Hemorrhagic colitis; thrombocytopenia; hemolytic uremic syndrome	Ingestion of contaminated food, especially undercooked beef and raw milk	Likely caused by a new pathogen
Hantavirus	Hemorrhagic fever with renal syndrome; pulmonary syndrome	Inhalation of aerosolized rodent urine and feces	Human invasion of virus ecologic niche
Human immunodeficiency virus (HIV)-1	HIV infection; acquired immunodeficiency syndrome (AIDS) (HIV stage III); severe immune dysfunction, opportunistic infections	Sexual contact with or exposure to blood or tissues of infected persons; perinatal	Urbanization; lifestyle changes; drug use; international travel; transfusions; transplant
Human papillomavirus (HPV)	Skin and mucous membrane lesions (warts); strongly linked to cancer of the cervix and penis	Direct sexual contact, contact with contaminated surfaces	Newly recognized; changes in sexual lifestyle
Influenza A H1N1 virus (novel, pandemic)	Influenza: fever, cough, headache, myalgia, prostration, possibly gastrointestinal signs	Person-to-person, airborne (droplet), and contact (direct and indirect)	Antigenic shift
Influenza A H5N1 virus (novel, avian)	Influenza: fever, cough, headache, myalgia, prostration	Direct contact with infected poultry or birds; limited person-to-person transmission	Antigenic shift
Legionella pneumophila	Legionnaires' disease: malaise, myalgia, fever, headache, respiratory illness	Air cooling systems, water supplies	Recognition in an epidemic situation
Pneumocystis jiroveci	Acute pneumonia	Unknown; possibly airborne or reactivation of latent infection	Immunosuppression
Severe acute respiratory syndrome (SARS)	Severe and acute pneumonia	Person-to-person, airborne (droplet) and direct and indirect contact with respiratory secretions and other bodily fluid	Unknown; newly recognized coronavirus; possible animal transmission into Chinese population
West Nile virus	No clinical signs to mild flulike symptoms to fatal neuroinvasive disease	Bite of infected mosquitoes; infected birds serve as reservoirs	International travel and commerce

Based on information from Heymann DL, editor: *Control of communicable diseases manual,* ed 20, Washington, DC, 2014, American Public Health Association; Fauci AS, Touchette NA, Folkers GK: Emerging infectious diseases: a 10-year perspective from the National Institute of Allergy and Infectious Diseases, *Emerg Infect Dis* 11(4):519–525, 2005.

CASE STUDY

Li Ming emigrated to America from Tibet with her father and brother after her mother's death. During a trip to the emergency room with a fever, hemoptysis, and cough, she was diagnosed with drug-resistant tuberculosis and placed in directly observed therapy (DOT), which meant a nurse from the local health department had to witness her ingesting her medication daily. Ms. Ming found taking the medication to be a big problem; swallowing the pills caused her to gag. She was embarrassed to have to take them in front of a nurse, and that made the whole situation even harder. Fortunately, all the rest of the family had negative purified protein derivative (PPD) skin tests and needed to be tested only periodically.

Ms. Ming was thin but not emaciated. She spoke English well enough to communicate with the nurse, Rachel Jones, who told her she could take her time swallowing the medication. They chatted each day about Ms. Ming's life in Tibet and her adjustment to America. Ms. Ming worked in a beauty salon washing hair. Although she was 25 years old, her father did not want her to date, and so she never had.

Ms. Jones worked to decrease Ms. Ming's anxiety. She taught Ms. Ming some relaxation exercises that Ms. Ming was able to use. During the first week of visits, it took about an hour for the pills to be ingested. A month later the pill taking was down to 15 min and she no longer gagged. See if you can apply these steps to this clinical situation to get Ms. Ming to take her medication and to reduce her anxiety. (1) Recognize the cues; (2) analyze the cues; (3) state several cues and prioritize the hypotheses you have developed; (4) generate solutions for each hypothesis; (5) take action on your higher priority hypothesis; and (6) evaluate the outcomes you expect.

Were there other actions that Ms. Jones might have taken with this patient? How can you apply this case in the community?

Created by Deborah C. Conway, Assistant Professor (retired), School of Nursing, University of Virginia.

PREVENTION AND CONTROL OF INFECTIOUS DISEASES

In 2011, the CDC published *A CDC Framework for Preventing Infectious Disease: Sustaining the Essentials and Innovating for the Future,* a plan for preventing and controlling infectious threats through a "strengthened, adaptable, and multi-purpose U.S. public health system." The plan was reviewed in 2018 and remains current. See the plan at http://www.cdc.gov. Infectious disease can be prevented and controlled. The goal of prevention and control programs is to reduce the prevalence of a disease to a level at which it no longer poses a major public health problem. In some cases, diseases may even be eliminated or eradicated. The goal of elimination is to remove a disease from a large geographic area such as a country or region of the world. Eradication is removing a disease worldwide by ending all transmission of infection through the complete extermination of the infectious agent. The WHO officially declared the global eradication of smallpox on May 8, 1980 (Evans, 1985). The Americas were certified to be polio free in 1994. Because of the devastating effects of polio, the WHO partnered with national governments, Rotary International, the CDC, and the United Nations Children Fund (UNICEF) in the Global Polio Eradication Initiative. This initiative has worked tirelessly to immunize people against polio. Ways to prevent infectious disease in homes are listed in the How To box. This CDC box provides easy to understand and detailed information on the seven topics in the box.

HOW TO PREVENT INFECTIOUS DISEASE IN YOUR HOME
- Wash your hands (when and how).
- Routinely clean and disinfect surfaces (bathroom and kitchen).
- Handle and prepare food safely (separate and do not cross-contaminate one food with another; cook at proper temperature; refrigerate food promptly).
- Get immunized.
- Use antibiotics appropriately.
- Be careful with pets.
- Avoid contact with wild animals.

From Centers for Disease Control and Prevention: *An ounce of prevention keeps the germs away: seven keys to a safer healthier home,* Atlanta, 2008, CDC. Retrieved October 2020 from http://www.cdc.gov/ounce ofprevention

---

Primary, Secondary, and Tertiary Prevention

As discussed in previous chapters, the three levels of prevention in public health are *primary, secondary,* and *tertiary.* In the prevention and control of infectious disease, the goal of primary prevention is to reduce the incidence of disease by preventing it before it happens, and in this, governments often provide assistance. Many interventions at the primary level, such as federally supplied vaccines and "no shots, no school" immunization laws, are population based because of public health mandate. Nurses deliver many childhood immunizations in public and community health settings, check immunization records in daycare facilities, and monitor immunization records in schools. Nurses often provide the teaching necessary to prevent communicable diseases. Consider the primary prevention efforts that took place during the COVID-19 pandemic.

The goal of secondary prevention is to prevent the spread of disease once it occurs. These activities center on rapid identification of potential contacts of a reported case. Contacts may be (1) identified as new cases and treated or (2) determined to be possibly exposed but not diseased and appropriately treated with prophylaxis. Public health disease control laws assist in secondary prevention because they require investigation and prevention measures for individuals affected by a communicable disease report or outbreak. These laws can extend to the entire community if the exposure potential appears great enough (i.e., an outbreak of smallpox, epidemic influenza, or COVID-19). Nurses perform much of the communicable disease surveillance and control work in this country and are often responsible for reporting cases so that transmission can be reduced. In addition, nurses perform much of the screening, such as for TB, HIV, and STDs (or STIs). Nurses were very much involved with the screening for COVID-19 throughout the country. Education can be both primary and secondary prevention.

Nurses who work in clinics, home health, schools, and other sites provide tertiary prevention care that is designed to reduce complications and disabilities through treatment and rehabilitation. This care may include helping people to recover and return to their previous or a new level of health, as well as aspects of primary and secondary care to prevent the continuation of the infectious disease and its further spread. Include family in all aspects of prevention, including tertiary, to help develop a treatment plan for the affected person and to prevent transmission of the disease.

Effective control of communicable diseases requires a multisystem approach. The primary goals and examples of such an approach include the following:

1. Improving host resistance to infectious agents and other environmental hazards, such as by improved hygiene, practicing social distance, wearing a mask when in a public place or near other people, nutrition, physical fitness, and immunization coverage and providing drugs for prevention and treatment, as well as aids for improved mental health. In some locales, trash accumulates, dead animals are on the sides of roads, and standing water is a breeding ground for mosquitos.
2. Improve safety of the environment, such as by improved sanitation, clean water, and clean air; teaching proper cooking and storage of food; and control of vectors and animal reservoir hosts.
3. Improve public health systems by increasing access to health care and appropriate and timely health education and improving surveillance and reporting.
4. Facilitate social and political change to ensure better health for all people, such as by individual, group, and community action and legislation.

See the Levels of Prevention box.

LEVELS OF PREVENTION
Related to Infectious Disease Interventions

Primary Prevention
Goal: To prevent the occurrence of disease
- Educate about safe food-handling practices in the home.

Secondary Prevention
Goal: To prevent the spread of disease
- Immediately evaluate the possible source of any foodborne outbreak.

Tertiary Prevention
Goal: To reduce complications and disabilities through treatment and rehabilitation
- Immediately treat any foodborne infection.

AGENTS OF BIOTERRORISM

Both the attacks of September 11, 2001, and the subsequent anthrax attacks demonstrated the possibilities for the intentional release of a biologic agent, or bioterrorism. The CDC suggests that the biologic agents most likely to be used in a bioterrorist attack are those that both have the potential for high mortality and can be easily disseminated, with the results of major public panic and social disruption. The diseases and infectious agents of highest concern are anthrax *(Bacillus anthracis)*, plague *(Yersinia pestis)*, smallpox *(Variola major)*, botulism *(C. botulinum)*, tularemia *(Francisella tularensis)*, and selected hemorrhagic viruses (Filoviridae and Arenaviridae). See the CDC Emergency Preparedness and Response website http://emergency.cdc.gov for more information.

Anthrax

Until the fall of 2001, anthrax was more commonly a concern of veterinarians and military strategists than the general public. After September 11, 2001, the news of deaths caused by letters deliberately contaminated with anthrax and sent through the postal service profoundly changed our view of this infectious disease. Anthrax is an acute disease caused by the spore-forming bacterium *B. anthracis.* It is found naturally in soil and often affects domestic and wild animals. It is not spread from human to human but typically from handling products from infected animals or eating undercooked meat from affected animals (CDC, 2015). Anthrax is not contagious.

Anthrax is an organism that perpetuates itself by forming spores. A spore is a cell that is dormant but may come to life under the right conditions. Domestic and wild animals such as cattle, sheep, goats, antelope, and deer can get infected when they breathe in or ingest spores in contaminated soil, plants, or water. People get infected when spores get into the body such as when they breathe in spores, eat food, or drink water contaminated with spores, or get spores in a cut or scrape in the skin. It is uncommon for people in the United States to get infected with anthrax. It is most often found in agricultural regions of Central and South America, sub-Saharan Africa, central and southeastern Asia, southern and eastern Europe, and the Caribbean (CDC, 2015). Symptoms often appear within 7 days of coming in contact with the bacterium. Treatment for a person who is exposed but not yet sick generally includes an antibiotic combined with anthrax vaccine; treatment for a person after infection is usually a 60-day course of antibiotics. Success depends on the type of anthrax and how soon treatment begins.

Smallpox

Formerly a disease found worldwide, smallpox has been considered eradicated since 1979. The last known natural death from smallpox occurred in Somalia in 1977. The United States stopped routinely immunizing for smallpox in 1982. The only documented existing virus sources are located in freezers at the CDC in Atlanta and a research institute in Novosibirsk, Russia. Controversy exists over the destruction of these viral stocks, but scientists and public health officials continue to assert that there is a need to perform research using this virus in the event there is an accidental or intentional exposure. The WHO is responsible for smallpox research.

Smallpox could be a leading candidate as an agent of bioterrorism. Susceptibility is 100% in the unvaccinated (those vaccinated before 1982 are not considered protected, although they may possess some immunity), and the fatality rate is estimated at 20% to 40% or higher. Vaccinia vaccine, the immunizing agent for smallpox, can be protective even after exposure. The WHO does not recommend vaccination for the general public; however, laboratory workers should be vaccinated. Because of the potential for bioterrorism and the fact that many health care providers have never seen this disease, it is important to become familiar with the clinical and epidemiologic features of smallpox and how it is differentiated from chickenpox (see the How To box) (Heymann, 2014).

HOW TO DISTINGUISH CHICKENPOX FROM SMALLPOX

Chickenpox (Varicella)	Smallpox (Historical Variola Major)
Sudden onset with slight fever and mild constitutional symptoms (both may be more severe in adults)	Sudden onset of fever, prostration, severe body aches, and occasional abdominal pain and vomiting, as in influenza
Rash is present at onset	Clear-cut prodromal illness, rash follows two to four days after fever begins decreasing
The classic symptom is a rash that turns into itchy, fluid-filled blisters that eventually turn into scabs.	Progression is macular, papular, vesicular, and pustular, followed by crusted scabs that fall off after three to four weeks if client survives
Rash may first appear on the chest, back, and face and then spread over the entire body including the mouth, eyelids, or genital area	Rash starts as small red spots on the tongue and in the mouth and can spread to all parts of the body in 24 hours
Lesions appear in "crops" and can be at various stages in the same area of the body	Lesions are all at same stage in all areas
Vesicles are superficial and collapse on puncture; mild scarring may occur	Vesicles are deep-seated and do not collapse on puncture; pitting and scarring are common

See these CDC sites: Chickenpox: Signs and symptoms, April 2021; Evaluating patients for symptoms of smallpox, n.d.; Smallpox: signs and symptoms, 2016.

Despite the availability of a vaccine, chickenpox is still a common disease of childhood and may be seen in susceptible adults as well. Although many health care providers are familiar with chickenpox, most have never seen a case of smallpox. Because of the potential for smallpox to be used as a bioweapon, nurses and other practitioners should familiarize themselves with the differences in presentation between the two diseases. The rash pattern for each disease is distinctive, but it has been observed that in the first 2 to 3 days of development, the two may be indistinguishable. Infectious disease texts and posters provide a pictorial description. If a smallpox infection is suspected, the local health department should be notified immediately.

VACCINE-PREVENTABLE DISEASE

Vaccines are one of the most effective methods of preventing and controlling communicable diseases. The smallpox vaccine, which left distinctive scars on so many shoulders, is no longer in general use because the smallpox virus has been declared totally eradicated from the world's population. Despite threats of bioterrorism, there are no plans to reintroduce universal smallpox immunization with the existing vaccine because of potential side effects. Diseases such as polio, diphtheria, pertussis, and measles, which previously occurred in epidemic proportions, are now controlled by routine childhood immunization. However, they have not been eradicated, so children need to be immunized against these diseases. In the United States "no shots, no school" legislation has resulted in the immunization of most children by the time they enter school. However, many infants and toddlers, the group most vulnerable to these potentially severe diseases, do not receive scheduled immunizations despite the availability of free vaccines. Surveys show that inner-city children from minority and ethnic groups are particularly at risk for incomplete immunization. Children from religious communities whose beliefs prohibit immunization and children with parents who have philosophical objections to immunization may receive no protection at all. Studies also show low levels of vaccination against pneumonia in senior citizens and lower levels of influenza coverage in adults from minority and ethnic groups. Research also suggests that adolescents have lower rates of coverage than children or adults, perhaps because they do not as frequently access preventive care. *Healthy People 2030* includes several objectives about obtaining and maintaining appropriate levels of immunization in all age groups. (Additional information on vaccine-preventable diseases may be found at the CDC website: http://www.cdc.gov/vaccines/.)

Because many children receive their immunizations at public health departments, nurses play a major role in increasing immunization coverage of infants and toddlers. Nurses track children known to be at risk for underimmunization and call or send reminders to their parents. They help to avoid missed immunization opportunities by checking the immunization status of every young child encountered, whether the clinic or home visit is related to immunization or not. In addition, they organize immunization outreach activities in the community that deliver immunization services; provide answers to parents' questions and concerns about

EVIDENCE-BASED PRACTICE

Infants younger than 6 months of age are at greatest risk for complications and death from pertussis because they are too young to be fully immunized. Since 2012 the CDC has recommended that pregnant women be vaccinated with Tdap (tetanus, reduced diphtheria, acellular pertussis) between 27 and 36 weeks' gestation to allow for a transfer of maternal antibodies, offering protection to the infant until its first pertussis vaccination at age 2 months. However, despite evidence that this practice does offer protection, uptake of Tdap has been slow, with the CDC reporting 48.8% coverage in 2016. In this study, the University of Kansas Medical Center created a pop-up message for the electronic medical record system in their obstetrics clinic to provide a reminder of the CDC recommendation. The physician could then choose to order the vaccine directly from the message screen or note the reason for not doing so (patient declines, other with comment, not indicated). Although the pop-up could be ignored, unless the physician selected one of the options, it would continue to appear at every visit for the patient between 27 and 36 weeks of pregnancy. Nurses could also view the pop-up when checking clients in, allowing them to introduce the topic of Tdap before it was broached by the physician. A comparison of the same 4-month period preintervention and postintervention showed a statistically significant 15.7% increase in coverage, moving from 44.6% of 531 patients to 60.3% of 574 patients ($P < .0001$). No differences were noted in the characteristics of the women who did and did not receive the vaccine. This simple medical records alert resulted in increasing uptake of Tdap among pregnant women at this clinic by over a third.

Nurse Use

The adult public has been slow to embrace Tdap. One reason may be lack of awareness of the availability of the vaccine and/or of the importance it plays in keeping infants safe. There are a variety of ways to approach this issue, starting with consumer awareness and provider education and advocacy. This study shows how a change in standard practice within an institution had a dramatic effect on Tdap immunization in pregnant mothers. Whether Tdap or other issues that require attention, nurses manage clinics and take leadership roles in hospitals, physicians' offices, health departments, and safety-net health services, which puts them in a position to both assess where there are opportunities for intervention and to change practice in order to address important public health concerns.

American College of Obstetricians and Gynecologists (ACOG): 2018 Annual Meeting, Abstract 8L, Simple alert increases prenatal uptake of Tdap vaccine. *Medscape Medical News*, April 29, 2018. Available at https://www.medscape.com. Accessed August 31, 2018.

immunization; and educate parents about why immunizations are needed, about inappropriate contraindications to immunization, and about the importance of completing the immunization schedule on time.

Routine Childhood Immunization Schedule

The CDC regularly publishes the recommended immunization schedule for children ages birth to 15 months and 18 months to 18 years. Persons 19 years and older should follow the Recommended adult immunization schedule. The CDC also discusses "catch-up" doses and describes actions for special situations (CDC, 2020b). The recommended vaccine schedule is complex and changes, so consult the CDC website for current information. Other useful sites related to immunization schedules and requirements are those of the American Academy of Pediatrics (http://www.aap.org) and the American Academy of Family

Physicians (http://www.aafp.org). These sites are updated regularly and provide consistent information.

Measles

Measles is an acute, highly contagious respiratory disease that, although considered a childhood illness, can occur in adolescents and young adults. Symptoms include fever, runny nose, sneezing, cough, a rash all over the body, small white spots on the inside of the cheek (Koplik spots), and a red, blotchy rash beginning several days after the respiratory signs. Measles is caused by the rubeola virus and is spread through the air by inhalation of infected aerosol droplets; by direct contact with infected nasal or throat secretions or with articles freshly contaminated with the same nasal or throat secretions; breathing; coughing; or sneezing. The contagious nature, combined with the fact that people are most contagious before they know they are infected, makes measles a disease that can spread rapidly. Infection with measles confers lifelong immunity (Heymann, 2014).

Measles was declared eliminated in the United States in 2000, and it is rare in North and South America because of the high level of vaccination. The majority of people who get measles are unvaccinated. This disease is still common in many parts of the world, and travelers can bring measles into the United States. In addition, US citizens should be vaccinated for measles before they travel internationally. In 2012, there were 55 cases reported to the CDC compared with 1282 cases in 2019. More than 73% of the cases in 2019 were linked to outbreaks in New York. Measles is more likely to spread and cause outbreaks in communities where groups of people remain unvaccinated (CDC, 2020c). The WHO collects data from countries around the world based on the reports that they received. There has been a resurgence of measles in many countries. As of November 2019, there were 413,308 confirmed measles cases reported to WHO through official monthly reporting by 187 Member States in 2019 (WHO, 2019b).

Healthy People 2030 has a section under the heading of "health behaviors" that lists a variety of objectives related to vaccinations (US Department of Health and Human Services [USDHHS], 2020b). Nurses receive reports of cases, investigate them, initiate control measures for outbreaks, and use every opportunity to immunize adolescents and young adults who lack documentation of two doses of measles vaccine. Nurses who work in regions in which undocumented residents are common, where groups obtain exemption from immunization on religious grounds, where preschool coverage is low, or where international visitors are frequent need to be especially alert for cases of measles and the need for prompt outbreak control among particularly susceptible populations.

Rubella

The rubella (German measles, 3-day measles) virus causes a mild febrile disease characterized by enlarged lymph nodes and a fine, pink rash that is often difficult to distinguish from those of measles or scarlet fever. In contrast to measles, rubella is only moderately contagious. Transmission is through inhalation of or direct contact with infected droplets from respiratory tract secretions of infected persons. Children may show few or no symptoms, and adults usually experience several days of low-grade fever, headache, malaise, runny nose, and conjunctivitis before the rash appears. Many infections occur without a rash (Heymann, 2014).

Since the introduction of a vaccine in 1969, cases of rubella in the United States have dropped greatly. This decrease has changed the epidemiology of the disease. Although still considered a childhood illness, rubella can occur in adolescents and young adults. Pregnant women are at particular risk in that rubella infection can cause intrauterine death, spontaneous abortion, and congenital anomalies (known as congenital rubella syndrome [CRS]) in the baby, including deafness, cataracts, heart defects, mental retardation, and liver and spleen damage. Unimmunized immigrants do not necessarily import disease, but their unimmunized status leaves them vulnerable to infection once they arrive. Eliminating rubella and CRS will require many of the same efforts discussed for other vaccine-preventable diseases, including achievement and maintenance of high rates of immunization among children; ensuring vaccination among women of childbearing age, especially those who are foreign born; continued aggressive surveillance; and rapid response to outbreaks. The best protection against rubella is the MMR (measles-mumps-rubella) vaccine. Rubella and CRS were considered eliminated from the United States in 2004, although it is still common in other parts of the world (CDC, 2017b).

Pertussis

Pertussis also called whooping cough because of the "whooping" sound that the person makes when gasping for air after a coughing fit. Coughing fits can last up to 10 weeks. Pertussis begins as a mild upper respiratory tract infection that progresses to an irritating cough and in 1 to 2 weeks, may become paroxysmal (a series of repeated violent coughs). Pertussis is caused by the bacterium *Bordetella pertussis* and is transmitted via an airborne route through contact with infected droplets. It is highly contagious and is considered endemic in the United States. Infants who have not been vaccinated yet and the elderly are the most likely to experience serious disease and death. Vaccination against pertussis, delivered in combination with diphtheria and tetanus, is a part of the routine childhood immunization schedule. Treatment of infected individuals with antibiotics such as erythromycin may shorten the period of communicability but does not relieve symptoms unless given early in the course of the infection. Prophylactic treatment with antibiotics is recommended for family members and close contacts of infected individuals, regardless of immunization status and age, if there is a child in the house younger than the age of 1 year, or a woman in the last 3 weeks of pregnancy, or to prevent ongoing transmission within the family (Heymann, 2014).

More than 200,000 children previously got pertussis each year. Two vaccines protect again this disease: DTaP protects young children from diphtheria, tetanus, and pertussis; and Tdap protects preteens, teens, and adults. This virus typically begins like a cold so people may not know they are spreading whooping cough (USDHHS, 2020a).

In the mid-2000s the epidemiology of pertussis changed with incidence increasing in children 7 to 10 years old, many of whom had been fully vaccinated, suggesting that the acellular vaccine DTaP, introduced in 1997 for the entire childhood series in response to concerns over serious side effects in some children after DTP, may not offer the duration of protection seen with the whole-cell vaccine. Tdap (tetanus, reduced strength diphtheria, acellular pertussis) was licensed in 2005 as a booster for adults in place of their next tetanus vaccination and adolescents, with routine recommendation for immunization at 11 to 12 years. The reduction in rates in preteens 11 to 12 years old demonstrated immediate protection from Tdap, but increasing incidence in those 13 to 14 years old suggested waning immunity with no durable protection. Although waning immunity may not be completely protective, evidence indicates that boostered individuals will experience milder disease when infected. The downside of mild disease is that this lack of symptoms may have the unintended consequence of making these people excellent inapparent-carriers (CDC, 2012). Nonetheless, vaccination with DTaP and Tdap continues to be recommended as the single most effective strategy in reducing illness and death from pertussis (Fig. 11.2). Pregnant women and close contacts to their babies are especially encouraged to be vaccinated in an effort to prevent disease in infants, the group most likely to experience severe complications and death. In addition to maintaining high rates of immunization, prevention efforts also included publicizing Tdap, increasing awareness of pertussis in adolescents and adults among providers, and promptly implementing treatment and control in the face of outbreaks (CDC, 2017a).

Because pertussis does have a cyclical pattern with periodic outbreaks, it is important for nurses to work with the community to maintain the highest possible levels of immunization coverage to minimize these occurrences. Because of the contagious nature of pertussis, nurses play a major role in limiting transmission during outbreaks by ensuring appropriate treatment of family members and close contacts (CDC, 2018).

Influenza

Influenza (flu) is a viral respiratory infection often indistinguishable from the common cold or other respiratory diseases. Transmission is airborne and through direct contact with infected droplets. Unlike many viruses that do not survive long in the environment, the flu virus may survive for many hours in dried mucus. Outbreaks are common in the winter and early spring in areas in which people gather indoors, such as in schools and nursing homes. Everyone 6 months and older should get a flu vaccine in the fall. September and October are good times to get the vaccine. It is especially important to get a flu vaccine when COVID-19 is present. People at high risk are those 65 years and older; adults with chronic health conditions; pregnant women; persons with asthma, heart disease, stroke, or diabetes; persons with HIV/AIDS, cancer, or chronic kidney disease; children with neurologic conditions; and racial and ethnic minority groups (CDC, 2020d). The CDC has useful information for these specific high-risk groups.

Gastrointestinal and respiratory symptoms are common. Because symptoms do not always follow a characteristic pattern, many viral diseases that are not influenza are often called *flu*. The most important factors to note about influenza are its epidemic nature and the mortality that may result from pulmonary complications, especially in older adults and children younger than 2 years of age (Heymann, 2014).

People of all ages need
WHOOPING COUGH VACCINES

DTaP for young children	Tdap for preteens	Tdap for pregnant women	Tdap for adults
✓ 2, 4, and 6 months ✓ 15 through 18 months ✓ 4 through 6 years	✓ 11 through 12 years	✓ During the 27–36th week of each pregnancy	✓ Anytime for those who have never received it

www.cdc.gov/whoopingcough

Fig. 11.2 Pertussis Vaccination Schedule. (From www.cdc.gov. Pertussis (Whooping Cough). Last reviewed January 19, 2019.)

QSEN FOCUS ON QUALITY AND SAFETY EDUCATION FOR NURSES

Targeted Competency: Safety—Minimizes risk for harm to clients and providers through both system effectiveness and individual performance. Important aspects of safety include the following:

- **Knowledge:** Discuss potential and actual impact of national client safety resources, initiatives, and regulations
- **Skills:** Use national client safety resources for own professional development and to focus attention on safety in care settings
- **Attitudes:** Value relationship between national safety campaigns and implementation in local practices and practice settings

Safety Question:

Pertussis has become an increasing infectious disease concern.

- Look into local statistics around pertussis occurrence. Has there been an increased occurrence of pertussis over the past 5 years?
- How do your local statistics compare with national statistics for pertussis from the Centers for Disease Control and Prevention?
- What might be some systems approaches to educating your community about the risk for pertussis?
- What might be some systems approaches to providing pertussis vaccinations to the appropriate populations?
- What data points will you want to track to assess whether your interventions have been effective?

Prepared by Gail Armstrong, ND, DNP, MS. PhD, Professor and Assistant Dean of the DNP Program, Oregon Health and Sciences University.

There are four types of influenza viruses: A, B, C, and D. Type A is usually responsible for large epidemics, whereas outbreaks from type B are more regionalized. Type C epidemics are sporadic, less common, and usually result in only mild illness. Type D is seen primarily in cattle and not known to infect people. Influenza viruses often change in the nature of their surface appearance or their antigenic makeup. Types B and C are fairly stable viruses, but type A changes constantly. This means that in some years the flu vaccine that is developed does not have complete accuracy due to the changes in the flu type. Minor antigenic changes are referred to as *antigenic drift,* and they result in yearly epidemics and regional outbreaks. Major changes such as the emergence of new subtypes are called *antigenic shift;* these occur only with type A viruses. Antigenic shift and drift lead to epidemic outbreaks every few years and pandemic outbreaks every 10 to 40 years, as seen with novel influenza A H1N1 in 2009.

The preparation of influenza vaccine each year is based on the best possible prediction of what type and variant of the virus will be most prevalent that year. Because of the changing nature of the virus, yearly immunization is necessary and in the United States is given in early fall before the flu season begins. There is a flu vaccine that is specific for people older than 65 years of age.

The use of influenza antiviral drugs should be considered in the nonimmunized or groups at high risk for complications. Evidence also suggests that antivirals can decrease the number of deaths in hospitalized influenza patients. The neuraminidase inhibitors (oseltamivir, zanamivir) have activity against influenza A and B viruses. The adamantanes (amantadine, rimantadine) have activity only against influenza A viruses and are not recommended for use at this time in the United States because of resistance. There have been incidences, worldwide and in the United States, of H1N1 virus resistance to oseltamivir. Current guidelines indicate antiviral treatment should be guided by surveillance data on circulating viruses and confirmatory testing of viral subgroups. CDC annually publishes *Recommendations for Influenza Antiviral Medications* (CDC, 2020e). Read more about influenza at http://www.cdc.gov.

Healthy People 2030 recommends increasing the proportion of the population vaccinated annually against influenza and pneumococcal disease. See objective IID-09: Increase the proportion of persons who are vaccinated annually against seasonal influenza. Nurses often spearhead influenza immunization campaigns that target older adults. In the past, examples included flu clinics at polling places during elections or at community centers and churches during "senior vaccination Sundays." Many of these sites were put on hold during the COVID-19 pandemic. Persons living in nursing homes, residences for older adults, prisons, and other congregate living arrangements are at risk because influenza can spread rapidly with severe consequences through such living arrangements. As with children, nurses should check immunization history and encourage immunization for every older adult encountered in a clinic or home visit. Nurses should get immunized against influenza to protect themselves as well as the patients whom they serve, and they should be role models for health promotion and disease prevention. Prevention of the flu virus

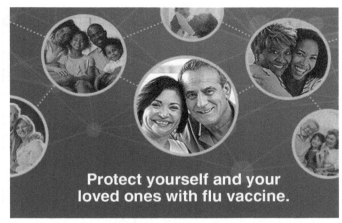

Fig. 11.3 Get Your Flu Vaccine. (From www.cdc.gov.Influenza.)

follows the same precautionary measures as those used to prevent the spread of COVID-19 (Fig. 11.3).

FOODBORNE AND WATERBORNE DISEASES

Protecting a nation's food supply from contamination by all virulent microbes is complex, costly, and time consuming. *Healthy People 2030* in its sections on foodborne illness and safe food handling states that approximately one in six people in the United States get foodborne illnesses each year. Illness is often caused by bacteria, such as *Campylobacter, E. coli, Listeria, and Salmonella.* It is estimated that more than 100,000 people annually are hospitalized due to foodborne illnesses and 3000 die (USDHHS, 2020b). Foodborne illnesses are preventable. According to *Healthy People 2030,* you can prevent these illnesses by safe handling in food production, processing, and storage. WHO has developed *Five Keys to Safer Food,* which remains a current guide for ways to prevent foodborne illness (Box 11.3 and Fig. 11.4).

Foodborne illness, often called "food poisoning," can be categorized as either a food infection or food intoxication. Food infection results from bacterial, viral, or parasitic infection of food and includes salmonellosis, hepatitis A, and trichinosis. Food intoxication results from toxins produced by bacterial growth, chemical contaminants (heavy metals), and a variety of disease-producing substances found naturally in certain foods such as mushrooms and some seafood. Examples of food intoxications are botulism, mercury poisoning, and paralytic shellfish poisoning. Table 11.3 presents some of the most common agents of food intoxication, their incubation period, source, symptoms, and pathology. Although it is not a hard-and-fast rule, food infections are associated with incubation periods of 12 hours to several days after ingestion of the infected food, whereas food intoxications become obvious within minutes to hours after ingestion. Botulism is a clear exception to this rule, with an incubation period up to several days or more in adults.

The spectrum of foodborne illness is constantly changing, and foodborne illnesses affect people of all socioeconomic levels, races, sexes, ages, occupations, educations, and areas of

BOX 11.3   Five Keys to Safer Food

1. Keep clean.
   * Wash your hands before handling food and often during food preparation.
   * Wash your hands after going to the toilet.
   * Wash and sanitize all surfaces and equipment used for food preparation.
   * Protect kitchen areas and food from insects, pests, and other animals.
2. Separate raw and cooked.
   * Separate raw meat, poultry, and seafood from other foods.
   * Use separate equipment and utensils, such as knives and cutting boards, for handling raw foods.
   * Store food in containers to avoid contact between raw and prepared foods.
3. Cook thoroughly.
   * Cook food thoroughly, especially meat, poultry, eggs, and seafood.
   * Bring foods such as soups and stews to boiling to make sure that they reach 70°C (158°F). For meat and poultry, make sure that juices are clear, not pink. Ideally use a thermometer.
4. Keep food at safe temperatures.
   * Do not leave cooked food at room temperature for more than 2 h.
   * Refrigerate promptly all cooked and perishable food (preferably less than 5°C [41°F]).
   * Keep cooked food piping hot (more than 60°C [140°F]) before serving.
   * Do not store food too long even in the refrigerator.
   * Do not thaw frozen food at room temperature.
5. Use safe water and raw materials.
   * Use safe water, or treat it to make it safe.
   * Select fresh and wholesome foods.
   * Choose foods processed for safety, such as pasteurized milk.
   * Wash fruits and vegetables, especially if eaten raw.
   * Do not use food beyond its expiration date.

From World Health Organization: *Five keys to safer food,* Geneva, 2008, WHO. Retrieved October 2020 from www.who.int.

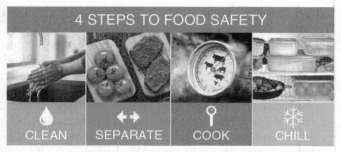

4 STEPS TO FOOD SAFETY

| CLEAN | SEPARATE | COOK | CHILL |

Fig. 11.4 Four Steps to Food Safety. (From http://www.cdc.gov/foodsafety. Last reviewed August 13, 2020.)

residence. The very young, old, and debilitated are the most susceptible and have the highest burden of morbidity and mortality. FoodNet is a CDC sentinel surveillance system targeting 10 sites across the country and collecting information from laboratories on disease caused by nine enteric pathogens transmitted commonly through food. FoodNet is a collaborative effort among the CDC, the US Department of Agriculture (USDA), and the US Food and Drug Administration (FDA). The surveillance includes 15% of the US population. FoodNet collects data on the following pathogens: *Salmonella, Campylobacter, Shigella, Cryptosporidium, Cyclospora, Listeria, E. coli, Vibrio,* and *Yersinia* (CDC, 2020f).

In recent years, headlines have described foodborne illness related to peanut butter, cookie dough, spinach, lettuce, tomatoes, chili peppers, strawberries, raspberries, oysters, uncooked eggs, poultry and hamburger, raw milk, unpasteurized apple cider, and other foods. Recalls of food products have been a

TABLE 11.3   Commonly Encountered Food Intoxications

Causal Agent	Incubation Period	Duration	Clinical Presentation	Associated Food
Staphylococcus aureus	30 min–7 h	1–2 days	Sudden onset of nausea, cramps, vomiting, and prostration, often accompanied by diarrhea; rarely fatal	All foods, especially those likely to come into contact with food-handlers' hands that may be contaminated from infections of the eyes and skin
Clostridium perfringens (strain A)	6–24 h	1 day or less	Sudden onset of colic and diarrhea, maybe nausea; vomiting and fever unusual; rarely fatal	Inadequately heated meats or stews; food contaminated by soil or feces becomes infective when improper storage or reheating allows multiplication of organism
Vibrio parahaemolyticus	4–96 h	1–7 days	Watery diarrhea and abdominal cramps; sometimes nausea, vomiting, fever, and headache; rarely fatal	Raw or inadequately cooked seafood; period of time at room temperature usually required for multiplication of organisms
Clostridium botulinum	12–36 h; sometimes days	Slow recovery; could be months	Central nervous system signs; blurred vision, difficulty in swallowing and dry mouth, followed by descending symmetrical flaccid paralysis of an alert person; "floppy baby" in infant; fatality <15% with antitoxin and respiratory support	Home-canned fruits and vegetables that have not been preserved with adequate heating; infants have become infected from ingesting honey

Data from Heymann DL, ed.: *Control of communicable diseases manual,* ed 20, Washington, DC, 2014, American Public Health Association.

common occurrence. Anyone can acquire foodborne illness; however, the very young, old, and debilitated are likely to be more susceptible.

Salmonellosis

Salmonellosis is a bacterial disease that affects the intestinal tract. This bacterium typically lives in animal and human intestines and is shed through feces. Humans are most often infected through contaminated water or food such as that which is eaten raw or is undercooked, including meat, poultry, eggs, or egg products. Some people have no symptoms; others develop diarrhea, fever, and abdominal cramps within 8 to 72 hours. Symptoms also can include a sudden onset of headache, nausea, vomiting, chills, and blood in the stool (Mayo Clinic, 2019). Onset is typically within 48 hours of ingestion, but the clinical signs are impossible to distinguish from those of other causes of gastrointestinal distress. Diarrhea and lack of appetite may last several days, and dehydration may be severe. Although morbidity can be significant, death is uncommon except among infants, older adults, and the debilitated. The rate of infection is highest among infants and small children. It is estimated that only a small proportion of cases is recognized clinically and that only 1% of clinical cases are reported. The number of *Salmonella* infections yearly may actually number in the millions (Heymann, 2014).

Outbreaks occur commonly in restaurants, hospitals, nursing homes, and institutions for children. The transmission route is eating food that comes from an infected animal or food contaminated by feces of an infected animal or person. Raw or undercooked meat, meat products, and poultry; uncooked eggs; unpasteurized milk and dairy products; and contaminated produce are the foods most often associated with salmonellosis. However, regional and national outbreaks have resulted from vegetables (e.g., lettuce, green onions, tomatoes, chili peppers) and peanut butter. Animals are the common reservoir for the various *Salmonella* serotypes, although infected humans also may fill this role. Animals are more likely to be chronic carriers. Risk factors include increased exposure through international travel or owning a pet bird or reptile; stomach or bowel disorders caused by antacids, inflammatory bowel disease, or recent use of antibiotics and immune problems. Although *Salmonella* infection is usually not life threatening, it can cause dehydration, bacteremia, and reactive arthritis. Prevention is the same as that described in the box that describes keys to safe food.

Escherichia Coli O157:H7

E. coli O157:H7 belongs to the enterohemorrhagic category of *E. coli* serotypes that produce a strong cytotoxin called Shiga toxin and are collectively known as Shiga toxin–producing *E. coli* (STEC). *E. coli* serotypes in this group can cause a potentially fatal hemorrhagic colitis. *E. coli* bacteria normally live in the intestines of healthy people and animals, and most types are harmless or cause brief diarrhea. The *E. coli* O157:H7 can cause severe stomach cramps, bloody diarrhea, and vomiting. It is most often caused by contaminated water or food such as raw vegetables, undercooked ground beef, unpasteurized milk, and

some fresh produce such as spinach or lettuce (Mayo Clinic, 2020). There is often person-to-person transmission in daycare centers, homes, and institutions. Outbreaks also have been associated with petting zoos. Children, persons with a weakened immune system, and older adults are at highest risk for clinical disease and complications. Hemolytic uremic syndrome (HUS) is seen in approximately 15% of cases among children and a smaller number of adults and may result in acute renal failure (Heymann, 2014).

Hamburger is often involved in outbreaks because the grinding process exposes pathogens on the surface of the whole meat to the interior of the ground meat, effectively mixing the once-exterior bacteria thoroughly throughout the hamburger so that searing the surface no longer suffices to kill all bacteria. Tracking the contamination is complicated by the fact that hamburger is often made of meat ground from several sources. The best protection against this pathogen, as with most foodborne agents, is to thoroughly cook food before eating it.

Waterborne Disease Outbreaks and Pathogens

Waterborne pathogens usually enter water supplies through animal or human fecal contamination and often cause enteric disease. They include viruses, bacteria, and protozoans. Hepatitis A virus is probably the best known waterborne viral agent, although other viruses may be transmitted by this route (i.e., enteroviruses, rotaviruses, paramyxoviruses). The most important waterborne bacterial diseases are cholera, typhoid fever, and bacillary dysentery. However, other *Salmonella* types, *Shigella*, *Vibrio*, and *Campylobacter* species and various coliform bacteria, including *E. coli* O157:H7, may be transmitted in the same manner. In the past, the most important waterborne protozoans have been *Entamoeba histolytica* (amebic dysentery) and *Giardia lamblia*, but outbreaks of cryptosporidiosis in municipal water have called attention to the importance of protecting sources of water. Protozoans do not respond to traditional chlorine treatment as do enteric and coliform bacteria, and their small size requires special filtration. *Giardia* is often an issue for US citizens who travel to other countries and have no immunity from the protozoans in those countries. *Giardia* is a microscopic parasite passed via stool and can survive for weeks or months. It can be contracted by swallowing water while swimming, drinking water or ice made from infected sources, eating foods prepared in infected water, or having contact with someone with giardiasis. The symptoms include diarrhea, gas, greasy stools that can float, stomach or abdominal cramps, upset stomach, nausea, and dehydration. It may last 2 to 6 weeks. The treatment is to drink fluids and get medication. The CDC provides the most up-to-date information on these diseases and pathogens.

The CDC defines an outbreak of waterborne disease as an incident in which two or more persons experience similar illness after consuming water that epidemiologic evidence implicates as the source of that illness. Only a single incident is required in cases of chemical contamination. The CDC and the Environmental Protection Agency (EPA) maintain a collaborative surveillance program for collection and periodic reporting of data on the occurrence and causes of waterborne disease outbreaks.

VECTOR-BORNE DISEASE AND ZOONOSES

The infectious agent in vector-borne diseases is transmitted by a carrier, or vector, usually an arthropod (i.e., mosquito, tick, fly), either biologically or mechanically. With *biologic transmission,* the vector is necessary for the infectious agent to develop. Examples include the mosquitos that carry Zika virus and malaria and the fleas that transmit the plague. *Mechanical transmission* occurs when an insect contacts the infectious agent with its legs or mouthparts and carries it to the host. For example, flies and cockroaches may contaminate food or cooking utensils.

Vector-borne diseases typically involve zoonotic cycles and require an animal host or reservoir. Vector-borne diseases commonly found in the United States are those associated with ticks, such as Lyme disease *(Borrelia burgdorferi),* ehrlichiosis *(Ehrlichia),* anaplasmosis *(Anaplasma phagocytophilum),* and Rocky Mountain spotted fever (RMSF) *(Rickettsia rickettsii).* Nurses who work with large immigrant populations or with international travelers may encounter Zika, chikungunya, malaria, and dengue fever, all carried by mosquitoes but rarely transmitted in the United States. WNV is an example of endemic mosquito-borne viral diseases, which include St. Louis, LaCrosse, and Western and Eastern equine encephalitis. Plague *(Y. pestis)* is carried by fleas of wild rodents.

Lyme Disease

Parents in Lyme, Connecticut, concerned about the unusual incidence of juvenile rheumatoid arthritis in their children, were the first to bring attention to this tick-borne infection that now bears their town's name. First described in 1975, Lyme disease became a nationally notifiable disease in 1991 and is now the most commonly reported vector-borne disease in the United States. Lyme disease is transmitted by ixodid ticks that are associated with the white-tailed deer and the white-footed mouse. This disease typically occurs in summer during tick season, and it has been reported throughout the United States, with 95% of cases concentrated in rural and suburban areas of the northeast, mid-Atlantic, and north central states, especially Wisconsin and Minnesota.

Clinically, Lyme disease is divided into three stages. Stage I is characterized by erythema chronicum migrans, a distinctive skin lesion often called a *bull's-eye lesion* because it begins as a red area at the site of the tick attachment that spreads outward in a ring like fashion as the center clears. Approximately 50% to 70% of infected persons develop this lesion 3 to 30 days after a tick bite. The skin lesion may be accompanied or preceded by fever, fatigue, malaise, headache, muscle pains, and a stiff neck, as well as tender and enlarged lymph nodes and migratory joint pain. Most clients diagnosed in this early stage respond well to 10 to 14 days of amoxicillin or doxycycline.

If not treated during the first stage, Lyme disease can progress to stage II, which may include additional skin lesions, headache, and neurologic and cardiac abnormalities. Clients who progress to stage III have recurrent attacks of arthritis and arthralgia, especially in the knees, which may begin months to years after the initial lesion. The clinical diagnosis of classic Lyme disease with the distinctive skin lesion is straightforward. Illness without the lesion is more difficult to diagnose because serologic tests are more accurate in stages II and III than in stage I (Heymann, 2014).

Measures for preventing exposure to ticks include reducing tick populations, avoiding tick-infested areas, wearing protective clothing when outdoors (i.e., long sleeves and long pants tucked into socks), using repellants, and immediately inspecting for and removing ticks when returning indoors. Ticks require a prolonged period of attachment (6 to 48 hours) before they start blood feeding on the host; prompt tick discovery and removal can help prevent transmission of disease. When outdoors, permethrin sprayed on clothing and tick repellents containing 20% to 30% diethyltoluamide (DEET) can offer effective protection. Use of DEET should be avoided in children younger than 2 years, because of reports of significant toxicity, including skin irritation, anaphylaxis, and seizures. Read more about tick-associated diseases at the CDC website: http://www.cdc.gov/ticks/. See Fig. 11.5 for a graphic picture of tick removal.

❓ CHECK YOUR PRACTICE

A client who was bitten by a tick while working in his tree-covered lawn comes to see you. He knew it was important to remove the tick in the correct manner. You know exactly how to correctly remove the tick. You remove the tick while simultaneously teaching the client how to do this if he ever gets another tick bite. The steps that you follow are:

1. Use fine-tipped tweezers to grasp the tick as close to the skin's surface as possible.
2. Pull upward with steady, even pressure. Do not twist or jerk the tick because this could cause the mouthparts to break off and remain in the skin. Should you break the mouthparts, remove them with tweezers. If you cannot remove them, leave them alone, and let the area heal.
3. After removing the tick, thoroughly clean the bite area and your hands with rubbing alcohol, an iodine scrub, or soap and water.
4. Dispose of the live tick by putting it in alcohol, placing in a sealed bag/container, wrapping it tightly with tape, or flushing it down the toilet.
5. Never crush a tick with your fingers.
6. If you develop a rash or fever within several weeks after removing the tick, see a health care professional. (CDC, 2019d)

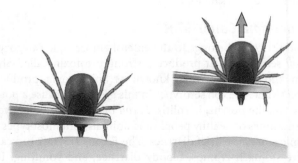

Fig. 11.5 The Progression of Tick Removal. (From Centers for Disease Control and Prevention. Tick Removal. https://www.cdc.gov/ticks, 2019.)

Rocky Mountain Spotted Fever

RMSF is a serious tickborne illness which can be deadly if not treated early. It is spread by several species of ticks in the United States, including the American dog tick *(Dermacentor variabilis),* Rocky Mountain wood tick *(Dermacentor andersoni),* and, in parts of the southwestern United States and Mexico, the brown dog tick *(Rhipicephalus sanguineus).* RMSF cases occur throughout the United States but are most commonly reported from North Carolina, Tennessee, Missouri, Arkansas, and Oklahoma. It is seldom seen in the Rocky Mountains. The infectious agent is *R. rickettsii.* The tick vector varies according to geographic region. RMSF is not transmitted from person to person. It is thought that one attack confers lifelong immunity.

Clinical signs include a sudden onset of moderate to high fever, severe headache, chills, deep muscle pain, and malaise. Approximately 50% of cases experience a rash on the extremities that spreads to most of the body. Many cases of what has been referred to as "spotless" RMSF may actually be caused by recently identified forms of human *ehrlichiosis,* another tickborne infection. RMSF responds readily to treatment with tetracycline. A definitive diagnosis can be made with paired serum titers. Because early treatment is important in decreasing morbidity and mortality, treatment should be started in response to clinical and epidemiologic considerations rather than waiting for laboratory confirmation. Doxycycline is the recommended antibiotic treatment for RMSF in adults and children (Heymann, 2014).

Diseases of Travelers

Individuals traveling outside the United States need to be aware of and take precautions against potential diseases to which they may be exposed. Which diseases and what precautions depend on the individual's health status, the destination, the reason for travel, and the length of travel. Persons who plan to travel in remote regions for an extended period may need to consider rare diseases and take special precautions that would not apply to the average traveler. Consultation with public health officials can provide specific health information and recommendations for a given situation. Nurses often staff public health travel clinics and provide this information based on CDC recommendations. The CDC offers a wide variety of information for both medical professionals and travelers at their Travelers' Health webpage, including the Yellow Book, *CDC Health Information for International Travel,* which in addition to being available online, can be ordered in hard copy or accessed from mobile devices. To read more about travelers' health, consult the CDC website https://www.cdc.gov.

On return from visiting exotic places, travelers may bring back with them an unplanned souvenir in the form of disease. Therefore, in a presenting client, it is important to ask about a history of travel. Even the apparently healthy returned traveler, especially one who was in a tropical country for some time, should undergo routine screening to rule out acquired infections. Likewise, refugees and immigrants may arrive with infectious disease problems ranging from helminthic infections to diseases of major public health significance, such as TB, malaria, Zika virus, cholera, HIV disease, and hepatitis. Nurses may deal with these diseases because refugees and immigrants, especially the undocumented, are often treated through the public health system. Zika virus has not been reported in the United States since 2017. It first emerged in Uganda in 1947. Zika virus is transmitted by Aedes mosquitoes (Fauci and Morens, 2016). This virus emerged in the Bahia region of Brazil and moved to several other countries fairly rapidly. It came to the United States via persons who traveled to or moved from areas with active Zika virus transmission.

Malaria

Malaria is a mosquito-borne disease caused by a parasite. People with malaria often experience fever, chills, and flu like illness. Left untreated, they may develop severe complications and die. In 2018 an estimated 228 million cases of malaria occurred worldwide and 405,000 people died, mostly children in the African region. Approximately 2000 cases of malaria are diagnosed in the United States each year. The vast majority of cases in the United States are in travelers and immigrants returning from countries where malaria transmission occurs, many from sub-Saharan Africa and south Asia. Transmission is through the bite of an infected *Anopheles* mosquito. Currently, there is no vaccine available to prevent malaria, although several are in development. Malaria can be a severe, potentially fatal disease (especially when caused by *Plasmodium falciparum*), and treatment should be initiated as soon as possible. Which drug regimen chosen to treat a patient with malaria depends on the clinical status of the patient, the type (species) of the infecting parasite, the area where the infection was acquired and its drug-resistance status, pregnancy status, and finally, history of drug allergies, or other medications taken by the patient (CDC, 2020g).

Foodborne and Waterborne Diseases

As in the United States, much foodborne disease abroad can be avoided if the traveler eats thoroughly cooked foods prepared with reasonable hygiene; eating foods from street vendors may not be a good idea. Trichinosis, tapeworms, and fluke infections, as well as bacterial infections, result from eating raw or undercooked meats. Raw vegetables may act as a source of bacterial, viral, helminthic, or protozoal infection if they have been grown with or washed in contaminated water. Fruits that can be peeled immediately before eating, such as bananas, are less likely to be a source of infection. Dairy products should be pasteurized and appropriately refrigerated.

Water in many areas of the world is not potable (safe to drink), and drinking this water can lead to infection with a variety of protozoal, viral, and bacterial agents, including amoebae, *Giardia, Cryptosporidium,* hepatitis, cholera, and various coliform bacteria. Unless traveling in an area where the piped water is known to be safe, only boiled water (boiled for 1 minute), bottled water, or water purified with iodine or chlorine compounds should be consumed. Ice should be avoided since freezing does not inactivate these agents. If the water is questionable, choose coffee or tea made with boiled water, carbonated beverages without ice, beer, wine, or canned fruit juices. Chapter 2 in the CDC Yellow Book offers useful information on food and water consumption for travelers and can be found at https://www.cdc.gov.

Diarrheal Diseases

Travelers often suffer from diarrhea, so much so that colorful names, such as Montezuma's revenge, turista, and Colorado quickstep, exist in our vocabulary to describe these bouts of intestinal upset. Some of these diarrheas do not have infectious causes; they result from stress, fatigue, schedule changes, and eating unfamiliar foods. Acute infectious diarrheas are usually of viral or bacterial origin. *E. coli* probably causes more cases of traveler's diarrhea than all other infective agents combined. Protozoan-induced diarrheas such as those resulting from *Entamoeba* and *Giardia* are less likely to be acute, and they more commonly present once the traveler returns home. Travelers need to pay special attention to what they eat and drink. Read more about travelers' health at the CDC website: http://www.cdc.gov. The 2020 CDC Yellow Book is about traveler's health.

Zoonoses

A zoonosis is an infection transmitted from a vertebrate animal to a human under natural conditions. Zoonotic diseases can be caused by viruses, bacteria, parasites, and fungi. They are common diseases. The agents that cause zoonoses do not need humans to maintain their life cycles; infected humans have simply somehow managed to get in their way. Means of transmission include animal bites (bats and rabies), inhalation (rodent excrement and hantavirus), ingestion (milk and listeriosis), direct contact (rabbit carcasses and tularemia), and arthropod intermediates. This last transmission route means that some vector-borne diseases also may be zoonoses. For example, white-tailed deer harbor ticks that can carry Lyme disease, and rats and ground squirrels may be infected with fleas that can transmit plague. Other than vector-borne diseases, some of the more common zoonoses in the United States include toxoplasmosis *(Toxoplasma gondii)*, cat-scratch disease *(Bartonella henselae)*, brucellosis (*Brucella* species), leptospirosis *(Leptospira interrogans)*, listeriosis *(Listeria monocytogenes)*, salmonellosis (*Salmonella* serotypes), and rabies (family Rhabdoviridae, (genus *Lyssavirus*). Many of the emerging infections such as avian influenza A, H5N1, WNV, monkey pox, hantavirus pulmonary syndrome, and variant Creutzfeldt-Jakob disease are zoonoses. In addition, among the diseases considered best candidates for weapons of bioterrorism, anthrax, plague, tularemia, and some of the hemorrhagic fever viruses (e.g., Lassa) are all zoonoses.

Rabies (Hydrophobia)

Rabies, one of the most feared of human diseases, has the highest case fatality rate of any known human infection—essentially 100%. To date, fewer than 10 cases of human survival from clinical rabies have been reported, and only two have not had a history of preexposure or postexposure prophylaxis. In the United States, rabies is mostly found in wild animals like bats, raccoons, skunks, and foxes. However, in many other countries dogs still carry rabies, and most rabies deaths in people around the world are caused by dog bites. Most dogs in the United States are vaccinated for rabies (CDC, 2020h).

Rabies is transmitted to humans by introducing virus-carrying saliva into the body, usually via an animal bite or scratch.

Transmission may also occur if infected saliva comes into contact with a fresh cut or intact mucous membranes. Rabies is found in neural tissue and is not transmitted via blood, urine, or feces. Airborne transmission has been documented in caves with infected bat colonies. Transmission from human to human is theoretically possible but has been documented only in the case of organ transplants harvested from individuals who died of undiagnosed rabies. Guidelines for organ donation exist to minimize this possibility (Heymann, 2014). The best protection against rabies remains vaccinating domestic animals—dogs, cats, cattle, and horses. If a person is bitten, clean the bite wound thoroughly with soap and water and immediately consult a physician. Suspicion of rabies should exist if the bite is from a wild animal or an unprovoked attack from a domestic animal. Even when there is no suspicion of rabies, a physician should be contacted because tetanus or antibiotic prophylaxis may be indicated.

No successful treatment exists for rabies once symptoms appear, but if given promptly and as directed, postexposure prophylaxis with human rabies immunoglobulin and rabies vaccine can prevent development of the disease. Two products are available for use as rabies vaccine in the United States: human diploid cell vaccine (HDCV) and purified chick embryo cell culture vaccine (PCECV). Four 1-mL doses of vaccine are injected into the deltoid muscle (CDC, 2014). Reactions to the vaccine are fewer and less serious than with previously used vaccines. Individuals who deal frequently with animals, such as zookeepers, laboratory workers, and veterinarians, may choose to receive the vaccine as preexposure prophylaxis. The decision to administer the vaccine to a bite victim depends on the circumstances of the bite and is made on an individual basis.

Recommendations for prevention of and vaccination for rabies in animals are found in the Compendium of Animal Rabies Prevention and Control compiled by the National Association of State Public Health Veterinarians, Inc. (Brown et al., 2016). Recommendations for administering post exposure prophylaxis (PEP)are provided by the Advisory Committee for Recommendations on Immunization Practices and are available through local public health officials or the CDC (CDC, 2020i). Decisions on whether an exposure has occurred requiring the use of PEP may not always be straightforward, and public health officials are helpful in making these treatment decisions.

PARASITIC DISEASES

Parasites are organisms that depend on a host to survive. Endoparasites, those that live within the body, are classified into four major groups: nematodes (roundworms), cestodes (tapeworms), trematodes (flukes), and protozoa (single-celled animals). Nematodes, cestodes, and trematodes are all referred to as helminths, along with acanthocephalans or thorny-headed worms, which are not as commonly involved in human infections. Table 11. 4 presents examples of relatively common diseases caused by parasites from these groups. Ectoparasites remain on the surface of a host's body to feed. Examples are ticks, fleas, lice, and mites that attach or burrow into the skin. Many parasitic infections are vector-borne and/or zoonotic.

TABLE 11.4 Examples of Diseases Resulting from Endoparasitic Infection by Category

Category	Parasite	Disease
Cestodes	*Taenia saginata, Taenia solium*	Beef tapeworm, pork tapeworm
Nematodes Intestinal Blood/tissue	*Ancylostoma, Necator* *Ascaris, Toxocara* Enterobius vermicularis Trichuris trichiura Dracunculiasis medinensis Onchocerca volvulus Wuchereria bancrofti	Ancylostomiasis, necatoriasis (hookworm) Ascariasis, toxocariasis (roundworm) Enterobiasis (pinworm) Trichuriasis (whipworm) Guinea worm Onchocerciasis (river blindness) Lymphatic filariasis (elephantiasis)
Trematodes	*Schistosoma* sp.	Schistosomiasis (snail fever)
Protozoans	*Entamoeba histolytica*	Amebiasis
	Giardia lamblia	Giardiasis
	Leishmania spp.	Leishmaniasis
	Plasmodium spp.	Malaria
	Toxoplasma gondii	Toxoplasmosis
	Trichomonas vaginalis	Trichomoniasis
	Trypanosoma spp.	African sleeping sickness, Chagas disease

Based on information from Heymann DL, editor: *Control of communicable diseases manual,* ed 20, Washington, DC, 2014, American Public Health Association.

Parasitic diseases are more prevalent in rural areas of low-income countries than in the United States. Contributing factors are tropical climate and inadequate prevention and control measures. Poor sanitation, a lack of cheap and effective drugs, and a scarcity of funding lead to high reinfection rates even when control programs are attempted. Parasitic organisms result in a wide spectrum of diseases, including leading causes of death and disability in Africa, Asia, Central America, and South America. Examples include malaria, schistosomiasis, guinea worm disease, river blindness (onchocerciasis), leishmaniasis, amoebiasis, African sleeping sickness, Chagas disease, and lymphatic filariasis. These parasitic diseases not only cause major mortality in endemic regions but also tremendous morbidity. Debilitation from infection may result in an inability to attend school or work as well as growth retardation, developmental disabilities, and cognitive impairment in young children, all of which contribute to significant economic burden for the countries affected.

Intestinal Parasitic Infections

Enterobiasis (pinworm) is the most common helminthic infection in the United States. Pinworm infection is seen most often among children and is most prevalent in crowded and institutional settings. Pinworms resemble small pieces of white thread and can be seen with the naked eye. Diagnosis is usually accomplished by pressing cellophane tape to the perianal region early in the morning. Treatment with oral vermicides and concurrent disinfection is highly effective (Heymann, 2014). The opportunities for widespread indigenous transmission of these intestinal parasites are reduced because of improved sanitary conditions in this country. Effective drug treatment is available for these intestinal parasitic infections.

Cryptosporidiosis (crypto) is caused by a microscopic parasite that causes this diarrheal disease. Both the parasite and the disease are called crypto. Although the disease is spread in many ways, the most common is via water, both drinking and recreational water. Crypto may be found in soil, food, water, or surfaces that have been contaminated with the feces from infected humans or animals. Crypto is not spread by contact with blood. The groups most at risk are children in daycare, childcare workers, parents of infected children, international travelers, people who drink unfiltered or untreated water, and older adults. The symptoms include watery diarrhea, stomach cramps or pain, dehydration, nausea, vomiting, fever, and weight loss. The symptoms can last 1 to 2 weeks. Nitazoxanide has been approved by the FDA for the treatment of persons with a healthy immune system (CDC, 2019e).

Parasitic Opportunistic Infections

Opportunistic infections (OIs) are those more frequent or more severe in individuals immunocompromised by HIV infection. Before the introduction of routine prophylactic treatment and potent-combination, highly active antiretroviral therapies (ARTs), OIs were the leading cause of illness and death in this group. Some of the protozoan parasitic OIs seen in clients with HIV disease and others who are immunocompromised include *Pneumocystis jiroveci* pneumonia (PCP), cryptosporidiosis, microsporidiosis, and isosporiasis, all producing diarrheal disease and transmitted by fecal–oral contact, as well as toxoplasmosis. With the advent of ARTs, the incidence of OIs in American clients with HIV disease has dropped dramatically. Isosporiasis was always rare, but the rates for cryptosporidiosis and microsporidiosis also have declined markedly. Although no longer seen with the frequency of the past, toxoplasmosis and PCP have not disappeared. They are more likely to appear in individuals unaware of their HIV disease or without good access to health care. Guidelines for prevention and treatment of OIs are regularly updated by the Panel on Opportunistic Infections in HIV-Infected Adults and Adolescents, representing opinion from the CDC, the National Institutes of Health, and the HIV Medicine Association of the Infectious Diseases Society of America. See http://aidsinfor.nih.gov.

T. gondii is a coccidial organism harbored by cats infected by ingesting other infected animals. Although rodents, ruminants, swine, and poultry and other birds may have infective organisms in their muscle tissue, only cats carry this parasite in their intestinal tract, allowing the excretion of infected eggs. People contract the disease through contact with infected cat feces or eating improperly cooked meat. In most healthy people, toxoplasmosis produces a mild to inapparent infection, but in immunodeficient individuals, the disease may, in addition to rash and skeletal muscle involvement, result in cerebritis, pneumonia, chorioretinitis, myocarditis, or death. CNS infection is common with HIV disease. Because toxoplasmosis is not a nationally reportable disease, it is not possible to get accurate numbers of cases. However, toxoplasmosis is a leading cause of foodborne illness deaths in the United States. Correct diagnosis by nurses and other health care workers leads to appropriate treatment and client education for preventing and controlling parasitic infections. The diagnosis of parasitic diseases is based on history of travel, characteristic clinical signs and symptoms, and the use of appropriate laboratory tests to confirm the clinical diagnosis. It is important to know what specimens to collect, how and when to collect them, and what laboratory techniques to use to establish a correct diagnosis. Effective drug treatment is available for most parasitic diseases. Measures for prevention and control of parasitic diseases include early diagnosis and treatment, improved personal hygiene, safer sex practices, community health education, vector control, and improvements in sanitary control of food, water, and waste disposal.

HEALTH CARE–ACQUIRED INFECTIONS

Previously referred to as nosocomial infections, health care–acquired infections (HAIs) are infections acquired during hospitalization or developed within a hospital or other health care setting. They may involve clients, health care workers, visitors, or anyone who has contact with a hospital, clinic, or medical office. Invasive diagnostic and surgical procedures, broad-spectrum antibiotics, and immunosuppressive drugs, along with the original underlying illness, leave hospitalized clients particularly vulnerable to exposure to virulent infectious agents from other clients and indigenous hospital flora from health care staff. Good hand hygiene is essential in any health care setting. The CDC maintains the National Healthcare Safety Network, a voluntary, Internet-based surveillance system managed by the Division of Healthcare Quality Promotion at the CDC, to provide national data on the epidemiology of HAIs in the United States. See http://ww.cdc.gov/hai for more information about how to prevent HAIs and antibiotic resistance. In 2020 a module on COVID-19 for long-term care facilities was added.

Infection control practitioners play a key role in hospital infection surveillance and control programs. Without a qualified and well-trained person in this position, the infection control program is ineffective. Many infection control practitioners are nurses. Their common job titles are *infection control nurse, infection control coordinator*, and *nurse epidemiologist*.

▶▶ APPLYING CONTENT TO PRACTICE

Public health involves the prevention of disease, promotion of health, and protection against hazards that threaten the health of the community, as reflected in the public health logo and summed up in the mission "assuring conditions in which people can be healthy." The three core functions of public health in achieving this mission as defined in 1988 by the Institute of Medicine in Recommendations for the Future of Public Health are *Assessment, Policy Development*, and *Assurance*. These three have been further divided into the "Ten Essential Services of Public Health" as a means of evaluating the effectiveness of public health efforts.

This chapter presents communicable diseases that commonly challenge the health of a community as well as prevention and control roles for public health nurses. Examples of some of the "Essential Services" under which these roles fall are presented by core function.

Assessment: (1) Monitor health/identify problems, and (2) diagnose and investigate health problems. Examples include surveillance, investigation, and identification of reportable communicable disease cases. **Policy Development:** (3) Inform, educate, and empower, and (4) mobilize community partnerships. Examples include evaluating immunization status, explaining the reason for immunizations and how to comply with the immunization schedule, organizing community partners to provide immunizations and documentation through a registry, and mounting a community campaign to inform the community of the importance of age-appropriate immunization. **Assurance:** (5) Enforce laws and regulations, and (6) link to services and provide care. Examples include assuring compliance with communicable disease control laws through treatment or prophylaxis for exposure to reportable diseases, excluding diseased students from daycare or school, and linking individuals without insurance to follow-up care for communicable disease treatment or exposure.

▍ PRACTICE APPLICATION

The rising numbers of foreign-born residents in communities that did not previously have large immigrant populations provide a challenge to those involved with communicable disease control, especially in outbreak situations. Language barriers, specific cultural practices, travel to and from their home countries, and undocumented status all contribute to opportunities for infection and present obstacles to prevention and control. It is common for diseases such as TB, brucellosis, measles, hepatitis B, COVID-19, and parasitic infections to originate in other countries and be diagnosed only after arrival of the person in the United States. People coming from countries without, with newly established, or with poorly enforced vaccination programs may be unimmunized. These people are particularly susceptible to infection in outbreak situations. For example, many people coming from Latin America have not been immunized against rubella. Differences in cultural practices can lead to outbreaks of foodborne illness. Listeriosis outbreaks often are linked to dairy products (cheese and ice cream) and some produce such as celery, sprouts, and cantaloupe.

In the face of a single infectious disease report or an outbreak situation, when working with communities whose members speak little English, it is vital (1) to have a means of communication, (2) to be able to provide a culturally appropriate message, and (3) to have an established level of trust. Ideally, these requirements are addressed before an outbreak occurs, allowing a prompt and efficient response when immediate action is needed.
A. What would be a useful first step in building trust with a largely non–English-speaking immigrant community?
   1. Hold a health fair in the community.

2. Provide incentives to use health department services.
3. Identify trusted community leaders, such as religious leaders, and ask for their help in developing a plan.
4. Distribute a brochure in the target community's language.

B. What might best encourage undocumented residents to respond to a request to be immunized during an outbreak situation?
   1. Use an already established public health program to provide interpreter services, making it clear that proof of immigration status is not required for services.
   2. Place a request in the newspaper in the language of the targeted individuals.
   3. Involve trusted community leaders in making the request.
   4. Explain the severity of the consequences of lack of immunization.

C. What means of communication would work best when targeting largely non–English-speaking communities of recent immigrants? Select all that apply.
   1. Publish newspaper articles in the target language.
   2. Request radio announcements in the target language.
   3. Post fliers in the target language in the community.
   4. Enlist trusted community leaders to make announcements.

D. How would public health officials best go about developing information to effectively reach a largely non–English-speaking community of recent immigrants?
   1. Use the services of the local university communications department.
   2. Ask community leaders to work with translators and prevention specialists to develop messages using their own words.
   3. Hire a professional to translate an existing well-developed English-language brochure.
   4. Use brochures provided by the state health department.

Answers can be found on the Evolve website.

▌ REMEMBER THIS!

- The burden of infectious diseases is high in both human and economic terms. Preventing these diseases must be given high priority in our present health care system. These enormous costs were seen with COVID-19 transmission.
- The successful interaction of the infectious agent, host, and environment is necessary for disease transmission. Knowledge of the characteristics of each of these three factors is important in understanding the transmission, prevention, and control of these diseases.
- Effective intervention measures at the individual and community levels must be aimed at breaking the chain linking the agent, host, and environment. An integrated approach focused on all three factors simultaneously is an ideal goal to strive for but may not be feasible for all diseases. It was for this reason that during the rapid and extensive spread of COVID-19, mask wearing and social distancing were instituted.
- Health care professionals must constantly be aware of vulnerability to threats posed by emerging infectious diseases. Most of the factors causing the emergence of these diseases are influenced by human activities and behavior.

- Infectious diseases are preventable. Preventing infection through primary prevention activities is the most cost-effective public health strategy.
- Effective control of communicable diseases requires the use of a multisystem approach focusing on improving host resistance, improving the safety of the environment, improving public health systems, and facilitating social and political changes to ensure health for all people.
- Communicable disease prevention and control programs must move beyond providing drug treatment and vaccines. Health promotion and education aimed at changing individual and community behavior must be emphasized.
- Nurses play a key role in all aspects of prevention and control of communicable diseases. Close cooperation with other members of the interdisciplinary health care team must be maintained. Mobilizing community participation is essential to successful implementation of programs.

EVOLVE WEBSITE

http://evolve.elsevier.com/Stanhope/foundations
- Case Study, with Questions and Answers
- NCLEX Review Questions
- Practice Application Answers

REFERENCES

American College of Obstetricians and Gynecologists (ACOG): 2018 Annual Meeting, Abstract 8L, Simple alert increases prenatal uptake of Tdap vaccine, *Medscape Medical News*, April 29, 2018. Available at: https://www.medscape.com. Accessed August 31, 2018.

Brown CM, Slavinski S, Ettestad P, Sidwa TJ, Sorhage FE: Compendium of animal rabies prevention and control, 2016, *J Am Vet Med Assoc* 248(5):505–517, 2016

Centers for Disease Control and Prevention: *An ounce of prevention keeps the germs away: seven keys to a safer healthier home*, Atlanta, 2008, CDC. Retrieved October 2020 from http://www.cdc.gov/ounceofprevention/.

Centers for Disease Control and Prevention: *Addressing emerging infectious disease threats: a prevention strategy for the United States*, Atlanta, 1994, CDC.

Centers for Disease Control and Prevention: Pertussis epidemic–Washington 2012, *MMWR Morb Mortal Wkly Rep* 61(04):61-65, 2012.

Centers for Disease Control and Prevention: *Anthrax: basic information, 2015*, Retrieved October 2020 from https://www.cdc.gov.

Centers for Disease Control and Prevention (CDC): *Pertussis Vaccination*, 2017a. Retrieved July 2018 from https://www.cdc.gov.

Centers for Disease Control and Prevention (CDC): *Rubella (German Measles, Three-Day Measles)*, September 15, 2017b, Retrieved October 2020 from https://www.cdc.gov.

Centers for Disease Control and Prevention (CDC): *2017 Final Pertussis Surveillance Report*, 2018. Retrieved July 2018 from https://www.cdc.gov.

Centers for Disease Control and Prevention (CDC): *Ebola (Ebola virus disease)* September 18, 2019a, Retrieved October 2020 at https://www.cdc.gov.

Centers for Disease Control and Prevention (CDC): *Zika virus: prevention and transmission,* May, 2019b, Retrieved October 2020 from https://www.cdc.gov.

Centers for Disease Control and Prevention: *2019 National Notifiable Conditions,* 2019c, Retrieved October 2020 from https://www.cdc.gov.

Centers for Disease Control and Prevention (CDC): *Tick removal and testing,* April 22, 2019d, Retrieved October 2020 from https://www.cdc.gov

Centers for Disease Control and Prevention (CDC): *Parasites– Cryptosporidum (also known as Crypto),* July 1, 2019e, Retrieved October 2020 from https://www.cdc.gov.

Centers for Disease Control and Prevention (CDC): *West Nile Virus: Preliminary Maps and Data for 2020,* October 6, 2020a, Retrieved October 2020, from https://www.cdc.gov.

Centers for Disease Control and Prevention (CDC): *Immunization schedules. Table 1: Recommended child and adolescent immunization schedule for ages 18 years or younger, United States, 2020.* February 3, 2020b, Retrieved October 2020 from https://www.cdc.gov.

Centers for Disease Control and Prevention: *Measles (Rubeola),* August 19, 2020c, Retrieved October 2020 from https://www.cdc.gov.

Centers for Disease Control and Prevention: *Influenza (Flu):* October 16, 2020d, Retrieved October 2020 from https://www.cdc.gov.

Centers for Disease Control and Prevention: *Flu antiviral,* August 31, 2020e, Retrieved October 2020 from https://www.cdc.gov.

Centers for Disease Control and Prevention: Preliminary incidence and trends of infections with pathogens transmitted commonly though food. Foodborne diseases active surveillance network, 10 US Sites, 2016-2019, *MMWR Morb Mortality,* April 30 2020f, Retrieved October 2020 from https://www.cdc.

Centers for Disease Control and Prevention: *Malaria treatment (United States),* May 7, 2020g, Retrieved October 2020 from https://www.cdc.gov.

Centers for Disease Control and Prevention: *Rabies,* September 25, 2020h, Retrieved October 2020 from https://www.cdc.gov.

Centers for Disease Control and Prevention: *Advisory Committee on immunization practices (ACIP),* September 23, 2020i, Retrieved October 2020 from https://www.cdc.gov.

Centers for Disease Control and Prevention: *Healthy pets and people,* 2014.

Evans AS: The eradication of communicable diseases: myth or reality? *Am J Epidemiol* 122:199–207, 1985.

Fauci AS, Touchette NA, Folkers GK: Emerging infectious diseases: a 10-year perspective from the National Institute of Allergy and Infectious Diseases, *Emerg Infect Dis* 11(4):519-525, 2005.

Fauci, AS, Morens DM: The perpetual challenge of infectious disease, *N Engl J Med* 366:454–461, 2012.

Fauci AS, Morens DM: Zika virus in the Americas–yet another arbovirus threat, *N Engl J Med* January 13, 2016. Published online at http://NEJM.org.

Heymann DL, editor: *Control of communicable diseases manual,* ed 20, Washington, DC, 2014, American Public Health Association.

Mayo Clinic: *Salmonella infection,* October 11, 2019, Retrieved October 2020 from mayoclinic.org.

Mayo Clinic: *E. coli,* October 10, 2020, Retrieved October 2020 from mayoclinic.org.

Schwartz N, Price S, Pratt R, Langer A: Tuberculosis–United States, 2019, *MMWR Morb Mortal Wkly Rep,* 69 (11):286-289, March 20, 2020.

US Department of Health and Human Services: *Vaccines; Whooping cough (Pertussis):* January 2020a, Retrieved October 2020.

US Department of Health and Human Services: *Healthy People 2030b,* Washington, DC, 2020b, US Government Printing Office.

World Health Organization: *Five keys to safer food,* Geneva 2008, WHO. Retrieved October 2020 from http://www.who.int/foodsafety/publications/consumer/en/5keys_en.pdf.

World Health Organization (WHO): *The top 10 causes of death, Fact sheet,* WHO News, 2018a. Available at: http://www.who.int. Accessed July 28, 2018.

World Health Organization (WHO): *Global tuberculosis report 2019: executive summary, 2019a.* Retrieved October 2020 from http://who.int.

World Health Organization: *Measles-global situation,* 2019b, Retrieved October 2020 from http://who.int.

12

Communicable and Infectious Disease Risks

Erika Metzler Sawin and Tammy Kiser

OBJECTIVES

After reading this chapter, the student should be able to:

1. Describe the natural history of human immunodeficiency virus (HIV) infection and plan appropriate client education at each stage.
2. Explain the clinical signs of selected communicable diseases.
3. Describe the scope of the problem with HIV, sexually transmitted diseases (STDs), hepatitis, and tuberculosis (TB), and identify groups that are at greatest risk.
4. Analyze behaviors that place people at risk for contracting selected communicable diseases.
5. Describe nursing actions to prevent these diseases and care for people who experience these diseases.

CHAPTER OUTLINE

KEY TERMS

Knowledge about the risk for communicable diseases changes often as some diseases become resistant to methods of treatment, new diseases emerge, new treatments are developed, and some diseases increase in the number of people affected while others show a decline. Concern about infectious diseases prompted the continuation of objectives for sexually transmitted infections (STI) in *Healthy People 2030* (USDHHS, 2020). The overall goal is to "Reduce sexually transmitted infections and their complications and improve access to STI care." The STI objectives are organized into these categories: STIs-general; adolescents; infectious diseases; lesbian, gay, bisexual, and transgender (LGBT); pregnancy and childbirth; preventive care; and vaccination. The *Healthy People 2030* box lists examples of objectives related to HIV and human papillomavirus (HPV). Because these diseases are often acquired through behaviors that can be avoided or changed or through immunizations, nursing actions focus particularly on disease prevention. Prevention of communicable diseases, including those not transmitted via sexual contact, can take the form of vaccine administration (as for hepatitis A and hepatitis B and HPV), early detection (for TB), or teaching clients about abstinence or safer sex. Individuals who live with these chronic infections can transmit them to others. This chapter describes selected communicable diseases and their nursing management, including primary, secondary, and tertiary prevention. STIs are also called sexually transmitted infections (STDs), because many times the infections are asymptomatic. *Healthy People 2030* uses the term STIs and the Centers for Disease Control and Prevention use the term STDs. In this chapter, the term *STDs* will be used.

 HEALTHY PEOPLE 2030

- **IID-07:** Reduce infections of HPV types prevented by the vaccine in young adults
- **HIV-06:** Reduce the rate of mother-to-child HIV transmission
- **IID-08:** Increase the proportion of adolescents who get recommended doses of the HPV vaccine

From US Department of Health and Human Services: *Healthy People 2030*, Washington, DC, 2020, US Government Printing Office.

HUMAN IMMUNODEFICIENCY VIRUS INFECTION

Human immunodeficiency virus (HIV) infection has had an enormous political and social impact on society. Controversies have arisen over many aspects of HIV. Fears about HIV may lead to attitudes of blaming clients for their infections and to discrimination. These beliefs are magnified by the fact that this disease has commonly afflicted two groups who have been largely stigmatized by society: homosexuals and injection drug users (Hall et al., 2017). Debates have arisen over how to control disease transmission and how to pay for related health services. An ongoing debate involves whether clean needles should be distributed to injection drug users to prevent the spread of HIV.

Overall from 2014 to 2018, the rate of diagnoses of HIV infection decreased in all 50 states, the District of Columbia and the six US dependent areas. However, rates increased in some subgroups and decreased in others (CDC, 2020a). The overall rate was 11.5 per 100,000 population (p. 9). In 2018 the highest rate of HIV infection was in adults aged 25 to 29 (32.6 per 100,000 persons), followed by adults between the ages of 20 and 24 (27.9 per 100,000 persons) (p. 11). At the end of 2018, 1,040,352 adults and adolescents were living with diagnoses of HIV infection (p. 17). For details related to a range of categories of persons diagnosed with HIV see the following section in the CDC: HIV Surveillance Report, 2018. Medicaid and Medicare primarily support the health care delivery costs of those infected. Many people with HIV qualify for Medicaid or Medicare because they are indigent or fall into poverty when paying for health care over the course of the illness. The lifetime cost of HIV care in 2015 for one client infected with HIV at the mean age of 35 was $326,500 (Schackman et al., 2015). The Ryan White HIV/AIDS Program, through the Ryan White HIV/AIDS Treatment Extension Act of 2009, provides care for persons with HIV infection (Health Resources and Service Administration [HRSA, 2019]). This program provides funds for health care in the geographic areas with the largest number of AIDS cases. Health services that are covered include emergency services, services for early intervention and care (sometimes including coverage of health insurance), and drug reimbursement programs for HIV-infected individuals. The AIDS Drug Assistance Programs (ADAPs) are awards that pay for medications on the basis of the estimated number of persons living with AIDS in the individual state (HRSA, 2019).

Natural History of Human Immunodeficiency Virus Infection

HIV is a virus that attacks the body's immune system. If not treated, it can lead to AIDS (acquired immunodeficiency syndrome). There is no cure for HIV, but with proper medical care, the disease can be controlled. The natural history of HIV includes three stages: the primary infection (within a month of contracting the virus), followed by a period when there are no symptoms (clinical latency), and then a final stage of symptomatic disease (Buttaro et al., 2017). When HIV enters the body, it can cause a mononucleosis-like syndrome referred to as a *primary infection* that can last for a few weeks. This may go unrecognized. Initially the body's CD4 white blood cell count drops for a brief time when the virus is most plentiful in the body. The immune system increases antibody production in response to this initial infection, which is a self-limiting illness. Some people have flulike symptoms within 2 to 4 weeks after infection, and these symptoms may last for a few days to several weeks. Possible symptoms are fever, chills, rash, night sweats, muscle aches, sore throat, fatigue, swollen lymph nodes, and mouth ulcers (CDC, 2020b). An antibody test at this stage is usually negative, so it is often not recognized as HIV.

After 6 weeks to 3 months, HIV antibodies appear in the blood. Although most antibodies serve a protective role, HIV antibodies do not. Their presence does help in the detection of HIV infection because tests show their presence in the bloodstream. During this prolonged incubation period, clients experience a gradual deterioration of the immune system and can transmit the virus to others. The use of highly active anti-retroviral therapy (HAART) has greatly increased the survival time of persons with HIV/AIDS.

Acquired immunodeficiency syndrome (AIDS, a.k.a HIV Stage 3) is the last stage on the long continuum of HIV infection and is the most severe phase. People with AIDS have a badly impaired immune system and this makes them susceptible to illnesses, called opportunistic infections (CDC, 2020b). People are diagnosed with AIDS when their CD4 cell count drops below 22 cells/mm, or if they develop opportunistic infections.

QSEN FOCUS ON QUALITY AND SAFETY EDUCATION FOR NURSES

Sexually Transmitted Diseases

Targeted Competency: Evidence-Based Practice (EBP)—Integrate best current evidence with clinical expertise and client/family preferences and values for delivery of optimal care.

- Knowledge: Explain the role of evidence in determining best clinical practice.
- Skills: Locate evidence reports related to clinical practice topics and guidelines.
- Attitudes: Value the concept of EBP as integral to determining best clinical practice.

Client-Centered Care Question

Evidence supports the fact that some medications previously effective in treating sexually transmitted diseases (STDs) no longer are effective. If you learned that a colleague was planning to use a treatment that is no longer considered effective to treat a specific STD, what would you do to ensure that the care the client receives is based on current evidence?

Answer

With your colleague, collect current treatment guidelines information about that specific STD. The first place that you might look would be the Centers for Disease Control guidelines for HIV, especially the section on Living with HIV. The National Institutes of Health is also helpful. For example, you might look at HIV Treatment Guidelines for the use of antiretroviral agents in adults and adolescents living with HIV. See HIV/AIDS Treatment Guidelines/AIDSinfo at aidsinfo.nih.gov.guidelines.

Many of the AIDS-related opportunistic infections are caused by microorganisms that are commonly present in healthy individuals but do not cause disease in persons with an intact immune system. These microorganisms increase in persons with HIV/AIDS as a result of a weakened immune system. Bacteria, fungi, viruses, or protozoa can cause opportunistic infections. The most common opportunistic diseases are *Pneumocystis jiroveci* (formerly *carinii*) pneumonia and oral candidiasis; other diseases are pulmonary TB, invasive cervical cancer, and recurrent pneumonia. TB can spread rapidly among immunosuppressed individuals. Thus HIV-infected individuals must be carefully screened for TB and deemed noninfectious before admission to such settings as long-term care facilities, correctional facilities, and drug treatment facilities.

Transmission

HIV is transmitted through exposure to blood, semen, transplanted organs, vaginal secretions, and breast milk (Heymann, 2014). It is not transmitted through casual contact such as touching or hugging someone who has HIV infection. Also, HIV is not transmitted by insects, coughing, sneezing, touching office equipment, or sitting next to or eating with someone who has HIV infection. The modes of transmission are listed in Box 12.1. Rare transmission methods include accidental needlestick injury, organ transplants, and blood transfusions (Heymann, 2014).

Potential blood and tissue donors are interviewed to screen for a history of high-risk activities, and they are screened with the HIV antibody test. Blood or tissue is not used from individuals who have a history of high-risk behavior or who are HIV infected. In addition to being screened, coagulation factors used to treat hemophilia and other blood disorders are made safe through heat treatments to inactivate the virus. Screening has significantly reduced the risk for transmission of HIV by blood products and organ donations. The presence of an STD infection such as chlamydia or gonorrhea increases the risk for HIV infection, and HIV may also increase the risk for other STDs. This may result from any of the following: open lesions providing a portal of entry for pathogens; STDs decreasing the host's immune status, resulting in a rapid progression of HIV infection; and HIV changing the natural history of STDs or the effectiveness of medications used in treating STDs (Heymann, 2014).

Nurses can educate people about the modes of transmission and can be role models for how to behave toward and provide supportive care for those with HIV infection. An understanding of how transmission occurs will help family and community members feel more comfortable in relating to and caring for persons with HIV.

Epidemiology and Surveillance of Human Immunodeficiency Virus and Acquired Immunodeficiency Syndrome

Nurses must identify the trends of HIV infection in the populations they serve so they can screen clients who may be at risk and adequately plan prevention programs and illness care resources. For example, knowing that AIDS disproportionately

---

BOX 12.1 Modes of Transmission of Human Immunodeficiency Virus

Human immunodeficiency virus can be transmitted in the following ways:
- Sexual contact, involving the exchange of body fluids with an infected person
- Sharing or reusing needles, syringes, or other equipment used to prepare injectable drugs
- Perinatal transmission from an infected mother to her fetus during pregnancy or delivery or to an infant when breastfeeding
- Transfusions or other exposure to human immunodeficiency virus–contaminated blood or blood products, organs, or semen

affects minorities assists the nurse to set priorities and plan services for these groups. Factors such as geographic location, age, and ethnic distribution are tracked to more effectively target programs. Since AIDS was first identified in the United States in 1981, the number of people diagnosed with AIDS in the United States was 1,232,246 in 2018 (CDC, 2020a). Many of the people living with HIV are unaware that they have the infection. People most often contract or transmit HIV through sexual behaviors and needle or syringe use. According to the CDC, "Only certain body fluids—blood, semen, pre-seminal fluid, rectal fluids, vaginal fluids, and breast milk—from a person who has HIV can transmit HIV. These fluids must come in contact with a mucous membrane or damaged tissue or be directly injected into the bloodstream (from a needle or syringe) for transmission to occur" (CDC, 2019a). In the United States, the first common method to spread HIV is via anal or vaginal sex with someone who has HIV and is not using a condom or taking medicines to prevent or treat HIV. The second most common transmission method is via sharing needles or syringes, rinse water or other equipment used to prepare drugs for injection with someone who has HIV. HIV can live in a used needle for up to 42 days (CDC, 2019a).

Nurses need also to know that AIDS disproportionately affects minorities in order to set priorities and plan services. Factors such as geographic location, age, and ethnic distribution are tracked to more effectively target programs. African Americans have the largest HIV disease burden of any racial/ethnic group in the United States; African American rates of new HIV infection are 8 times higher than in whites, the highest prevalence of those living with HIV is in the African American community, and the highest proportion of people diagnosed with HIV stage 3 (AIDS) are African American (CDC, 2017a). This overrepresentation is associated with poverty, since African Americans have a higher poverty rate than do other groups. This reflects decreased access to prevention and treatment and lack of awareness of HIV infection. Stigma, fear, and homophobia play a role as well (CDC, 2017a). Specifically, in 2018, the highest HIV rate in the United States was 39.2 for blacks/African Americans followed by 16.4 for Hispanic/Latinos; 13.3 for persons of multiple races; 11.3 for Native Hawaiians and other Pacific Islanders; 7.7 for American Indians/Alaska Native; 4.8 for whites; and 4.7 for Asians. The diagnosis of HIV infection attributed to male-to-male sexual contact accounted for nearly 94% of diagnoses in the United States in 2018 (CDC, 2020a). Transgender people are also at high risk, particularly transgender women. Because of data collection limitations, it is difficult to estimate HIV prevalence in transgender communities. However, data from countries that collect data for transgender women separately from MSM indicate that HIV prevalence is nearly 50 times higher than for other adults of reproductive age (UNAIDS, 2018).

Youth are a group that need special attention in regard to HIV. In 2018, of the 37,832 new HIV diagnoses in the United States and dependent area, 21% were among youth; of these most were among young gay and bisexual men (CDC, 2020c).

Compared to all people with HIV, youth have the lowest rates of viral suppression. Also, several challenges make it difficult for youth to learn how to reduce their risk or to get care and treatment if they have HIV. Some of these barriers are: Low rates of testing; substance use; low rates of condom use; number of partners; older partners; socioeconomic challenges; low rates of pre-exposure prophylaxis (PrEP) use; feelings of isolation; stigma and misperceptions about HIV; and high rates of STDs (CDC, 2020c). For more information visit www.cdc.gov/hiv.

Human Immunodeficiency Virus Testing

The HIV antibody test is the most commonly used screening test for determining infection. This test does just as its name implies: it does not reveal whether an individual has symptomatic AIDS, nor does it isolate the virus. It does indicate the presence of the antibody to HIV. The most commonly used form of this test is the enzyme-linked immunosorbent assay (EIA). The EIA effectively screens blood and other donor products. To minimize false-positive results, a confirmatory test, the Western blot, is used to verify the results. False-negative results may also occur after infection and before antibodies are produced. Sometimes referred to as the window period, this can last from 6 weeks to 3 months.

Rapid HIV antibody testing using oral fluid samples (e.g., OraQuick, Home Access HIV-1 Test System) is 99.5% accurate and provides results within 20 minutes, allowing immediate results to be given. This is the only FDA-approved rapid self-test. You can buy a rapid self-test kit at a pharmacy or online (CDC, 2020d). In addition to the rapid results, this test may appeal to persons who fear having their blood drawn. If the test is positive, go to a health care provider for follow-up testing. There is also a mail-in test that allows a person to collect dried blood from a fingerstick at home. The sample is then sent to a lab for testing, and a health care worker provides the results.

Routine voluntary HIV testing is recommended for adults ages 13 to 64 at least once. People at high risk for contracting HIV should be tested more often. See the CDC site on HIV: testing for details (CDC, 2020d). Voluntary screening programs for HIV may be either confidential or anonymous; the process for each is unique. Confidential testing involves reporting by identifying the person's name and other identifying information; this information is considered protected by confidentiality. With anonymous testing, the client is given an identification code number that is attached to all records of the test results and is not linked to the person's name and address (CDC, 2020d).

Demographic data such as sex, age, and race may be collected, but there is no record of the client's name and associated identifying information. An advantage of anonymous testing may be that it increases the number of people who are willing to be tested. The anonymity eliminates their concern about the possibility of arrest or discrimination. However, anonymous testing does not allow for follow-up if the test is positive because the client's name and address are not available.

Caring for Clients with Acquired Immunodeficiency Syndrome in the Community

Because AIDS is a chronic disease, affected individuals continue to live and work in the community. They have bouts of illness interspersed with periods of wellness in which they are able to return to school or work. When they are ill, much of their care is provided in the home. The nurse teaches families and significant others about personal care and hygiene, medication administration, standard precautions to ensure infection control, and healthy lifestyle behaviors such as adequate rest, balanced nutrition, and exercise. It is essential that clients adhere to their HAART regimen because administration must be consistent to be effective (Heymann, 2014). Nurses need to educate clients about accurate medication administration.

The Americans with Disabilities Act of 1990 and other laws protect persons with HIV/AIDS against discrimination in housing, at work, and in other public situations (HIV.gov, 2017). Policies regarding school and worksite attendance have been developed by most states and localities on the basis of these laws.

Nurses can rely on these policies to provide direction for the community's response when an individual develops HIV infection. Nursing actions include the following:

- Identifying resources such as social and financial support services
- Implementing school and work policies
- Assisting employers by educating managers about how to deal with ill or infected workers to reduce the risk of breaching confidentiality or wrongful actions such as termination

HIV-infected children should attend school because the benefits of attendance far outweigh the risks for transmitting or acquiring infections. None of the cases of HIV infection in the United States have been transmitted in a school setting. An interdisciplinary team made up of the child's physician, public health personnel, the child's parent or guardian, and the nurse should make decisions about educational and care needs. Individual decisions about risk to the infected child or others should be based on the behavior, neurological development, and physical condition of the child. Children with HIV infection have impaired immunity; therefore; it is important that they have regular recommended immunizations. Attendance may be inadvisable if cases of childhood infections, such as chickenpox or measles, are in the school, because the immunosuppressed child is at greater risk for suffering complications. Alternative arrangements, such as home-bound instruction, might be instituted if a child is unable to control body secretions or displays biting behavior.

A growing number of services are available for persons with HIV/AIDS. Voluntary and faith-based groups, such as community organizations or AIDS support organizations, are available in some localities to address their many needs. Services include counseling, support groups, legal aid, personal care services, housing programs, and community education programs. Nurses collaborate with workers from community organizations in the client's home and may advise these groups in their supportive work. The federal government and many organizations have established toll-free numbers and websites to provide information.

Considerable work has been done and progress is being made in finding effective methods to prevent and treat HIV. Preexposure prophylaxis, or PrEP, is a new HIV prevention method for people who do not have the infection but would like to reduce their risk for becoming infected. PrEP requires taking a pill daily to prevent the HIV virus from getting into the body. It has been shown to be effective for people at very high risk for HIV infection through sex or injection drug use (CDC, 2020e). Studies have shown that PrEP reduces the risk of getting HIV from sex by about 99% when taken daily and about 74% for those who inject drugs. Currently, there are two medications, sold under the brand names of Truvada and Descovy that are approved for daily use as an HIV prevention method (CDC, 2020e). Truvada is recommended for people at risk through sex or injection drug use, and Descovy is recommended to prevent HIV through sexual encounters. In addition to strictly adhering to the medication protocol, the person must first be tested to make sure he or she is HIV negative.

HIV treatment involves taking medicines that slow the progression of the virus in the body. HIV is a retrovirus. The drug combination used for treatment are called antiretroviral therapy (ART). These drugs reduce the amount of virus (viral load) in a person's blood and body fluids. ART also reduces the chance of transmitting HIV to others if the drug is taken correctly. ART is typically a combination of three or more drugs that have the best likelihood of lowering the amount of HIV in the body (CDC, 2019b).

SEXUALLY TRANSMITTED DISEASES

Sexually transmitted diseases (STDs) are a major public health challenge in the United States. The numbers of new cases of gonorrhea, herpes simplex virus (HSV), HPV, and chlamydia continues to increase. Chlamydia is the most commonly reported infectious disease, and gonorrhea is the second most common. The common STDs listed in Table 12.1 are grouped according to their having either a bacterial or viral cause. The bacterial infections include gonorrhea, syphilis, and chlamydia. Most of these infections are cured with antibiotics with the exception of the newly emerging antibiotic-resistant strains of gonorrhea. STDs caused by viruses cannot be cured. These are chronic diseases leading to a lifetime of symptom management and infection control. The viral infections include HSV and HPV, also referred to as genital warts. The hepatitis A and hepatitis B viruses, which may also be transmitted via sexual activity, are discussed in the section of this chapter on hepatitis.

Gonorrhea

Gonorrhea is the second most commonly reported notifiable disease in the United States, and the CDC estimates that about 583,405 Americans had the disease in 2018, and this was a

TABLE 12.1 Summary of Sexually Transmitted Diseases

Disease/Pathogen	Incubation	Signs and Symptoms	Diagnosis	Treatment	Nursing Implications
Bacterial					
Chlamydia: *Chlamydia trachomatis*	Poorly defined—probably 7–14 days or longer	*Man:* None or nongonococcal urethritis (NGU); painful urination and urethral discharge; epididymitis *Woman:* None or mucopurulent cervicitis (MPC), vaginal discharge; if untreated, progresses to symptoms of PID: diffuse abdominal pain, fever, chills	Nucleic acid amplification test (NAAT) of male urine and female endocervix	One of following treatments: Doxycycline 100 mg orally bid ×7 days; Azithromycin 1 g orally ×1 Alternative regimens: Erythromycin base 500 mg orally qid × 7 days; Erythromycin ethylsuccinate 800 mg orally qid ×7 days; Levofloxacin 500 mg orally, daily ×7 days Ofloxacin 300 mg orally bid ×7 days *See CDC for further notes about which medications are good, inexpensive, and dose level.*	Refer partners of past 60 days; counsel client to use condoms and to avoid sex for 7 days after start of therapy and until symptoms are gone in both client and partners; medication teaching Annual screening recommended for all sexually active women under 25, and women over 25 with new or multiple sexual partners
Gonorrhea: *Neisseria gonorrhoeae*	1–14 days, can be longer	Man: Urethritis, purulent discharge, painful urination, urinary frequency; epididymitis Woman: None, or symptoms of PID	Gram stain of discharge, culture on selective media, or NAAT	For uncomplicated gonorrhea: Ceftriaxone 500 mg IM	Refer partners of past 60 days; return for evaluation if symptoms persist; counsel client to use therapy until complete and symptoms are gone in both client and partners; medication teaching
Syphilis: *Treponema pallidum*	10–90 days, usually 3 weeks Stages are generally diagnosed by appearance of hallmark symptoms	Primary: usually single, painless chancre; if untreated, heals in few weeks Secondary: low-grade fever, malaise, sore throat, headache, lymphadenopathy, and rash Early latency: asymptomatic, infectious lesions may recur Late latency: Asymptomatic, noninfectious except to fetus of pregnant women Gummas of skin, bone, mucous membranes, heart, liver CNS involvement: paresis, optic atrophy Cardiovascular involvement: aortic aneurysm, aortic value insufficiency	Nontreponemal serological test such as the rapid plasma reagin. If that is positive, then confirm with a treponemal serological test. Early in the disease, these test results may be negative. Examine smears of lesion exudate using darkfield microscopic examination, PCR, or lesion biopsy. For patients with neurologic abnormalities, consider neurosyphilis, diagnosed by CSF cell testing.	For primary, secondary, or early latent 1 year: benzathine penicillin G 2.4 million units, IM once Latent >1 year or latent of unknown duration: benzathine penicillin G 7.2 million units total in 3 doses of 2.4 million units IM at 1-week intervals See CDC treatment guidelines for treatment of syphilis in children or pregnancy, neurosyphilis, and congenital syphilis or if the person has a penicillin allergy.	Counsel to be tested for HIV and other STIs; screen all partners of past 3 months; reexamine client at 3 and 6 months. Universal precautions should be used with all syphilis patients.

Viral	Incubation	Signs and symptoms	Diagnosis	Treatment	Prevention
Human immunodeficiency virus (HIV)	4–6 weeks *Seroconversion:* 6 weeks to 3 months *AIDS:* month to years (average, 11 years)	*Possible:* Acute mononucleosis-like illness (lymphadenopathy, fever, rash, joint and muscle pain, sore throat) Appearance of HIV antibody *Opportunistic diseases:* Most commonly *Pneumocystis jiroveci* pneumonia, oral candidiasis, Kaposi sarcoma	*HIV antibody test:* EIA or Western blot test; OraSure (SmithKline Beecham) is an oral HIV-1 antibody testing system, test results in about 3 days CD4+ T-lymphocyte count of less than 200/µL with documented HIV infection, or diagnosis with clinical manifestation of AIDS as defined by CDC	Prophylactic administration of zidovudine (ZDV) immediately after exposure may prevent seroconversion Postexposure prophylaxis (PEP) should begin as soon as possible. Choice of antiviral drug therapy is made based on toxicity and drug resistance. Combinations of drugs are considered, such as ZDV and 3TC. Drug selection is complicated and evolving. Preexposure prophylaxis (PrEP) was approved in 2012, consisting of daily tenofovir disoproxil fumarate plus emtricitabine (TDF/FTC) for use among sexually active, at-risk adults.	HIV education and counseling; partner referral for evaluation; medication education; assessment and referral Men who have sex with men should be tested annually for HIV, chlamydia, syphilis, and gonorrhea.
Genital warts: human papillomavirus (HPV)	2–3 months; range is 1–20 months	Often asymptomatic or subclinical infection; painless lesions near vaginal openings, anus, shaft of penis, vagina, cervix, with less common sites being throat, respiratory tract, mouth, or conjunctiva; lesions are textured, cauliflower appearance; may remain unchanged over time	Visual inspection for lesions; Pap smear	Prevention: Gardasil vaccine No cure; one-third of lesions will disappear without topical treatment.	Education about HPV vaccine. Warts and surrounding tissues contain HPV, so removal of warts does not completely eradicate virus; examination of partners not necessary, since treatment is only symptomatic; condom use may reduce transmission; medication application
Genital herpes simplex virus (HSV)	2–12 days	Vesicles, painful ulceration of penis, vagina, labia, perineum, or anus; lesions last 5–6 weeks and recurrence is common; may be asymptomatic	Presence of vesicles; viral culture (obtained only when lesions present and before they have scabbed over). See CDC site for genital herpes for more details.	No cure; Antiviral medications can prevent or shorten outbreaks during the time the person takes the medication. Daily antiviral medication can reduce the likelihood of transmission to partners. See CDC guidelines for recurrent infection, treatment for persons with HIV infection, and daily suppressive therapy.	Refer partners for evaluation; teach client about likelihood of recurrent episodes and ability to transmit to others even if asymptomatic; condom use; annual Pap smear. Health care providers should wear gloves when in direct contact with possible infectious lesions or mucous membranes.

AIDS, Acquired immunodeficiency syndrome; *CDC,* Centers for Disease Control and Prevention; *CNS,* central nervous system; *CSF,* cerebrospinal fluid; *EIA,* enzyme-linked immunosorbent assay; *IM,* intramuscular; *PCR,* polymerase chain reaction; *PID,* pelvic inflammatory disease ; *STI,* sexually transmitted infection.

From Centers for Disease Control and Prevention: Sexually transmitted diseases treatment guidelines, *MMWR Morb Mortal Wkly Rep* 64(3), 2015. Retrieved from https://www.cdc.gov; Heymann D: *Control of communicable diseases manual,* 20th ed. Washington, DC, 2014, American Public Health Association; Sancta St. C, Barbee L, Workowski KA, et al: Update to CDC's treatment guidelines for gonococcal infection, 2020, *Weekly* 69(50):1911-1916, December 18, 2020.

63% increase from 2014 (CDC, 2019c). The South had the highest rate of reported gonorrhea cases, followed by the Midwest, the West, and the Northeast. The rate in 2018 was higher for males than for females. The magnitude of the increase in males (0.6% from 2017 to 2018) is likely due either from increased transmission or increased case ascertainment. The rates of reported gonorrhea cases continued in 2018 to be highest among adolescents and young adults, with persons between 15 and 44 years accounting for 91.6% of the cases (CDC, 2019c). The reported rate is also highest among Blacks, being 7.7 times higher than in Whites. In comparison with the rate among Whites, the rate among American Indians/Alaska Natives was 4.6 times higher; Native Hawaiians/Pacific Islanders was 2.6 times higher; Hispanics 1.6 times higher; and Asians was half the rate of Whites (CDC, 2019c). These numbers are not exact because gonorrhea may be unreported by health care providers and because clients who are asymptomatic do not seek treatment and are therefore not identified. *Neisseria gonorrheae* is a gram-negative intracellular diplococcal bacterium that infects the mucous membranes of the genitourinary tract, rectum, and pharynx. Gonorrhea can be transmitted by having vaginal, anal, or oral sex with a person who has the disease. It can be transmitted via fluids even if a male does not ejaculate. It can also be spread from an untreated mother to the infant during childbirth. Gonorrhea is identified as either uncomplicated or complicated. Uncomplicated gonorrhea refers to limited cervical or urethral infection. Complicated gonorrhea includes salpingitis, epididymitis, systemic gonococcal infection, and gonococcal meningitis. The signs and symptoms of infection in males are purulent and copious urethral discharge and dysuria. Symptoms in males are typically significant enough for the person to seek treatment. These symptoms include a burning sensation when urinating or a white, yellow, or green discharge from the penis. Some men may get swollen or painful testicles. In men, gonorrhea can cause epididymitis, a painful condition of the testicles that if untreated can lead to infertility. In contrast, symptoms in women are often asymptomatic and may be confused with a bladder or vaginal infection (CDC, 2015). Treatment may not be sought, and this could allow the disease to continue to spread and possibly not be detected until pelvic inflammatory disease (PID) occurs. In women, infection with *N. gonorrheae* is a major cause of PID, ectopic pregnancy, and infertility. Untreated gonorrhea can increase a person's risk for acquiring or transmitting HIV (CDC, 2015).

As a result of increasing drug resistance, treatment of gonorrhea is becoming more complex. In 2005 there were five treatments for gonorrhea and at this time, there is only one treatment, which is injected ceftriaxone combined with oral azithromycin, both in single doses, simultaneously and under direct observations (CDC, 2018a). The increase in antibiotic-resistant infections is partially attributed to the indiscriminate or illicit use of antibiotics as a prophylactic measure by persons with multiple sexual partners. To ensure proper treatment and cure, those diagnosed with gonorrheal infection should return for health care if symptoms persist, have all partners evaluated for infection and treated if necessary, and remain sexually abstinent for 77 days (CDC, 2018a).

The development of PID is a risk for women who remain asymptomatic and do not seek treatment. PID is a serious infection involving the fallopian tubes (salpingitis) and is the most common complication of gonorrhea but may also result from chlamydia infection. Its symptoms include fever, abnormal menses, and lower abdominal pain, but PID may not be recognized because the symptoms vary among women. PID can result in ectopic pregnancy and infertility related to fallopian tube scarring and occlusion. It may also cause stillbirths and premature labor (CDC, 2019c).

Syphilis

Syphilis is caused by a member of the treponemal group of spirochetes, *Treponema pallidum*. It infects moist mucous or cutaneous membranes and is spread through direct contact, usually by sexual contact or from mother to fetus. Transmission via blood transfusion may occur if the donor is in the early stages of disease (Heymann, 2014).

Syphilis rates in the United States declined between 1990 and 2001 but have been steadily increasing since then, with last reported rates of primary and secondary syphilis (P & S) rates at 10.8 cases per 100,000 people in 2018. This rate represents a 14.9% increase from 2017. In 2018, the West had the highest rate of reported P & S syphilis cases, followed by the South, the Northeast, and the Midwest. Reported cases of P & S syphilis continue to be characterized by a high rate of HIV coinfection, particularly among men having sex with men (MSM). In 2018, the rate was highest among Blacks, being 4.7 times the rate among Whites (6.0 cases per 100,000 population). The rate among Native Hawaiians/other Pacific Islanders was 2.7 time that of Whites; among American Indian/Alaska Natives 2.6 times; among Hispanics 2.2 times; and among Asians 0.8 times greater than the rate among Whites. In recent years the number of infected women has increased (CDC, 2019d).

The clinical signs of syphilis are divided into primary, secondary, and tertiary infections. Latency, a period when an individual is free of symptoms but has serological evidence, may occur early or late in the infection. All cases of syphilis that are untreated progress to latent infection. During early latency, skin and mucous membrane lesions may be apparent (Heymann, 2014).

Primary Syphilis

When syphilis is acquired sexually, the bacteria produce infection in the form of a chancre at the site of entry. The lesion begins as a macula, progresses to a papule, and later ulcerates. If left untreated, this chancre persists for 3 to 6 weeks and then in most cases disappears (Heymann, 2014).

Secondary Syphilis

Secondary syphilis occurs when the organism enters the lymph system and spreads throughout the body. Signs include rash, lymphadenopathy, and mucosal ulceration. Symptoms of secondary syphilis may include skin rash, lymphadenopathy, and lesions of the mucous membranes (Heymann, 2014).

Tertiary Syphilis

About one-third of untreated syphilis patients will demonstrate signs and symptoms of tertiary syphilis (Heymann, 2014). Tertiary syphilis can lead to blindness, congenital damage, cardiovascular damage, or syphilitic psychoses. A further complication can be the development of lesions of the bones, skin, and mucous membranes, known as gummatous lesions. Tertiary syphilis usually occurs several years after initial infection and is rare in the United States because the disease is usually cured in its early stages with antibiotics. Tertiary syphilis is a major problem in developing countries.

Congenital Syphilis

When primary and secondary syphilis rates increase, so do the rates of congenital syphilis (CS), which has increased each year since 2012 to a 2018 rate of 1306 reported cases leading to a national rate of 33.1 cases per 100,000 births (CDC, 2019d). Syphilis is transmitted transplacentally and, if untreated, can cause premature stillbirth, blindness, deafness, facial abnormalities, crippling, or death. Signs include jaundice, skin rash, hepatosplenomegaly, or pseudoparalysis of an extremity. Preferred treatment is penicillin G administered parenterally (CDC, 2015).

Chlamydia

Chlamydia infection, caused by the bacterium *Chlamydia trachomatis,* infects the genitourinary tract and rectum of adults and causes conjunctivitis and pneumonia in neonates. Transmission occurs when mucopurulent discharge from infected sites, such as the cervix or urethra, comes into contact with the mucous membranes of a non infected person. Because the cervix of teenage girls and young women is not fully matured and may be more susceptive to infection, they are an especially high-risk group if they are sexually active. Like gonorrhea, the infection is asymptomatic in men in as many as 90% of cases and in women in as many as 70% to 95% of cases and is called a "silent" disease (Heymann, 2014). If symptoms do appear, they typically do so within 1 to 3 weeks after exposure. If left untreated, chlamydia can result in PID. When chlamydia infection is present, symptoms in women include dysuria, urinary frequency, and purulent vaginal discharge. If the infection spreads from the cervix to the fallopian tubes, some women may have no symptoms, and others have lower abdominal pain, low back pain, nausea, fever, pain during intercourse, or bleeding between menstrual periods. In men, the urethra is the most common site of infection, resulting in non-gonococcal urethritis (NGU). The symptoms of NGU are dysuria and urethral discharge. Epididymitis is a possible complication.

Chlamydia is the most common reportable infectious disease in the United States. In 2018, there were 1,758,668 cases of chlamydial infections reported to the CDC in 50 states and the District of Columbia. The rates of reported cases were highest in the South, followed by the West, Midwest, and Northeast. Of these reported cases in 2018, 1,145,063 were in females and 610,447 were in males. In terms of age, the rates of reported chlamydia were highest among persons aged 15 to 24 years. In terms of race/ethnicity the highest reported rates were among Black, American Indian/Alaska Native and Native Hawaiian/other Pacific Islander persons (CDC, 2019e). Prevention is important because chlamydia can cause PID, ectopic pregnancy, infertility, and neonatal complications. Women under 25 years of age are the most commonly infected with chlamydial infection because of inconsistent use of barrier contraceptives, multiple sexual partners, and a history of infection with other STDs. The CDC recommends annual chlamydia screening for all sexually active women younger than age 25 years and women over 25 years who are an increased risk for infection such as those with new or multiple sex partners. Chlamydia can be effectively treated with antibiotics (CDC, 2019e).

Herpes Simplex Virus 2 (Genital Herpes)

There are two types of herpes caused by HSV. The first is oral herpes that is usually caused by HSV-1 and results in cold sores or fever blisters in or around the mouth. Two types of herpes simplex viruses (HSV-1 and HSV-2) cause genital herpes. The majority of genital herpes infections are caused by HSV-2, and these herpes infections are more likely to be recurrent (CDC, 2015). However, an increasing number of genital herpes infections are caused by HSV-1; these infections are more common in young women and MSM (CDC, 2015).

As is true for other viral STDs, there is no cure for herpes infection, and it is considered a chronic disease. The virus is transmitted through direct exposure and infects the genitalia and surrounding skin. After the initial infection the virus remains latent in the sacral nerve of the central nervous system and may reactivate periodically with or without visible vesicles.

Signs and symptoms of HSV infection include the presence of painful lesions that begin as vesicles and ulcerate and crust within 1 to 4 days. The first episode is typically longer and is usually characterized by more lesions than seen in subsequent infections. Lesions may occur on the vulva, vagina, upper thighs, buttocks, and penis and have an average duration of 11 days (Fig. 12.1). The vesicles can cause itching and pain and may be accompanied by dysuria or rectal pain. Although the ability to

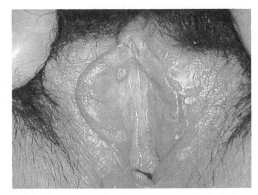

Fig. 12.1 *Herpes genitalis.* (From Habif TP: *Clinical dermatology: a color guide to diagnosis and therapy,* ed 5, St. Louis, 2010, Mosby.)

pass the infection to others is higher with active lesions, some individuals can spread the virus even when they are asymptomatic. There can be a prodromal phase before lesions develop that includes tingling and paresthesia at the site (Heymann, 2014).

HSV-2 seroprevalence is decreasing. However, this prevalence is likely underrated because HSV-1 infections are rising, and a large number of people have no symptoms; thus HSV is difficult to identify and diagnose. Also, HSV is not nationally reportable. The majority of people with HSV-2 have never been told that they have it (CDC, 2017b). The consequences of genital herpes are of particular concern for women and their children. HSV-2 infection is linked with the development of cervical cancer. There is also an increased risk of fatal newborn infection during vaginal delivery with active lesions (Heymann, 2014). A pregnant woman who has active lesions at the time of giving birth should have a cesarean delivery before the rupture of amniotic membranes to avoid fetal contact with the herpetic lesions, whereas those who have no clinical evidence of herpes lesions should be delivered vaginally. A small number of infants are infected in utero. The clinical infection in infants may present as liver disease, encephalitis, or infection limited to the skin, eyes, or mouth (Heymann, 2014).

Human Papillomavirus Infection

Human papillomavirus (HPV) results in genital warts. Two specific types of HPV (HPV 16 and HPV 18) cause cervical cancer, accounting for 70% of cervical cancer cases (Heymann, 2014). HPV is the most common STD in the United States, although it is not reportable (CDC, 2017c). Transmission of HPV occurs through direct contact with warts that result from HPV and can infect the mouth, genitals, and anus. Genital warts are most commonly found on the penis and scrotum in men, and on the vulva, labia, vagina, and cervix in women. They appear as textured surface lesions, with what is sometimes described as a cauliflower appearance. The warts are usually multiple and vary between 1 mm and 1 cm in diameter. They may be difficult to visualize, so careful examination is required (Buttaro et al., 2017).

The CDC recommends a 2-dose schedule for people who get the first dose before their 15th birthday. In a 2-dose series, the second dose should be given 6 to 12 months after the first dose. A 3-dose schedule is recommended for people who get the first dose on or after their 15th birthday. Useful sites to check about current HPV vaccines are the CDC and the American Cancer Institute. As of 2019 the only approved vaccine in the United States is Gardasil 9 (CDC, 2019f). The recommended age for vaccination in both girls and boys is 11 to 12 years old, but it is also recommended for females aged 13 to 26 years old, males 13 to 21, transgender people, bisexual people, and MSM, as well as for people who have certain immunocompromising conditions (CDC, 2018b). The vaccine can be given as early as 9 years of age (CDC, 2018b). However, complete vaccination coverage is an issue. Experts recommend several strategies to increase vaccination rates in adolescent girls and boys, such as a reminder/recall system to increase vaccination rates and consideration of use of schools as a vaccination site. The 2-dose schedule is now recommended for cost saving and efficacy, when initiated before the age of 15 (CDC, 2018b).

Once HPV infection occurs, the goal of therapy is to eliminate the warts. Genital warts spontaneously disappear over time, as do skin warts. However, because the condition is worrisome for the client and HPV may lead to the development of cervical neoplasia, treatment of the warts through surgical removal, laser therapy, or cytotoxic agents is often done (Buttaro et al., 2017).

Complications of HPV infection may be especially serious for women. The link between HPV infection and cervical cancer has been established and is associated with specific types of the virus (CDC, 2018c). Other cancers attributed to HPV include vaginal, penile, anal, and oropharyngeal; the latter are more common in men (CDC, 2018c). Pap smears are vitally important because they allow for microscopic examination of cells to detect HPV, which can be surgically removed if detected early (Heymann, 2014). Infection is exacerbated in both pregnancy and immune-related disorders, which are believed to result from a decrease in cell-mediated immune functioning. HPV may infect the fetus during pregnancy and can result in a laryngeal papilloma that can obstruct the infant's airway. Genital warts may enlarge and become friable during pregnancy, and therefore surgical removal may be recommended. One challenge of HPV prevention is that condoms do not necessarily prevent infection. Warts may grow where barriers, such as condoms, do not cover, and skin-to-skin contact may occur.

HEPATITIS

Viral hepatitis refers to a group of infections that primarily affect the liver. These infections have similar clinical presentations but different causes and characteristics. Brief profiles of the types of hepatitis are presented in Table 12.2.

Hepatitis A Virus

Hepatitis A virus (HAV) is a vaccine-preventable disease of the liver caused by the HAV. It is usually transmitted from person to person through the fecal–oral route or via contaminated food or water (CDC, 2020f). The virus level in the feces appears to peak 1 to 2 weeks before symptoms appear, making individuals highly contagious before they realize they are ill (Heymann, 2014). Since the vaccine was developed in 1995, the cases of HAV have declined with the exception of several cases associated with imported food (CDC, 2018d). The vaccine is recommended for children over 1 year; however, the rate of vaccination remains low (CDC, 2018d). Persons most at risk for HAV infection are travelers to countries with high rates of infection, children living in areas with high rates of infection, injection drug users, MSM, and persons with clotting disorders or chronic liver disease. The incidence of HAV increased 850% from 2014 to 2018, and this was largely due to people who use drugs and those who are homeless. Males are most likely to have HAV; as are people between the ages of 30 and 39; and Whites are the largest group affected. In 2018, there were 12,474 reported cases of HAV (CDC, 2020f).

Hepatitis A is found worldwide. In developing countries where sanitation is inadequate, epidemics are not common because most adults are immune from childhood infection. In countries with

TABLE 12.2 Viral Hepatitis Profiles (Cases Reported in the United States in 2018)

	Hepatitis A	Hepatitis B	Hepatitis C
Incubation period	Average, 28 days; range, 15–50 days	Average, 90 days; range, 60–150 days	Average range: 14-84, range, 14–182 days
Mode of transmission	Fecal–oral, contaminated food/water	Blood-borne, sexual, perinatal	Primarily blood-borne; also sexual and perinatal
Incidence	Reported cases 12,474,–Estimated 24,900	Reported acute cases 3,322; Estimated: 21,600	Reported acute cases 3,621; Estimated 50
Chronic carrier state?	No	Yes, 5% of adult cases; 90% of infants; 25%–50% of children aged 1–5 years	Yes, 75%–85% or more of cases
Diagnosis	Serological test (anti-HAV), viral isolation	Serological tests (e.g., HBsAg), viral isolation	Serological tests (anti-HCV)
Sequelae	No chronic infection	Chronic liver disease; liver cancer	Chronic liver disease; liver cancer
Vaccine availability	Yes, vaccination of all children at 1 year, children in areas of high disease rates recommended; travelers to endemic regions; men who have sex with men; injection and noninjection drug users	Yes, vaccination of infants recommended; all children who have not been already immunized; individuals with exposure risks; men who have sex with men; people with end-stage renal disease, people with HIV infection	No
Control and prevention	Good hygiene (e.g., hand washing); proper sanitation	Preexposure vaccination; reduce exposure risk behaviors	Screening of blood/organ donors; reduce exposure risk behaviors

Updates on any of these sexually transmitted diseases can be found on the Centers for Disease Control and Prevention website by typing in exactly which disease is of interest. See www.cdc.gov.
Examples are *Viral hepatitis surveillance 2016,* Atlanta, 2016, and Centers for Disease Control and Prevention: *Viral hepatitis surveillance-United States 2018.* https://www.cdc.gov/hepatitis/statistics/SurveillanceRpts.htm, July 2020. (Accessed September 2020).
See also St Cyr S, Barbee L, Workowski KA, et al., Gonococcal infection, 2020, *MMWR Morb Mortality Wkly Rep,* 2020: 69)1911-1916

improved sanitation, outbreaks are common in daycare centers whose staff must change diapers, among household and sexual contacts of infected individuals, and among travelers to countries where hepatitis A is endemic. In many outbreaks, one individual is the source of an infection that may become community-wide. In other cases, hepatitis A is spread through food contaminated by an infected food handler, contaminated produce, or contaminated water. The source of infection may never be identified in many outbreaks (Heymann, 2014).

HAV is a self-limited disease that does not lead to chronic infection. Children under 6 years of age often have no symptoms, so the disease goes unrecognized. Most adults and older children typically have symptoms that last about 2 months. Signs and symptoms may include one or more of the following: "fever, fatigue, nausea, vomiting, loss of appetite, abdominal pain, dark urine, and clay-colored stools" (CDC, 2020f, p. 5). Severe cases of HAV may require hospitalization. Vaccination and good sanitation and personal hygiene are the best ways to prevent infection. People who travel often or for long periods in countries in which the disease is endemic should have the HAV vaccine. Candidates for immunoglobulin administration and vaccine after exposure to HAV are listed in Box 12.2 (CDC, 2018d; Heymann, 2014).

Hepatitis B Virus

The number of new cases of hepatitis B virus (HBV) in the United States is decreasing as a result of the use of HBV vaccine. HBV is also a vaccine-preventable liver disease that is transmitted when blood, semen, or another body fluid from a person infected with the virus enters the body of someone who is not

BOX 12.2 Recommendations for Administration of Hepatitis A Vaccine

- Are traveling to countries where hepatitis A is common
- Are a man who has sex with other men
- Use illegal drugs
- Have a chronic liver disease such as hepatitis B or hepatitis C
- Are being treated with clotting-factor concentrates
- Work with hepatitis A–infected animals or in a hepatitis A research laboratory
- Expect to have close personal contact with an international adoptee from a country where hepatitis A is common

Centers for Disease Control and Prevention: *Hepatitis A vaccine: what you need to know,* Atlanta, 2016, CDC. http://www.cdc.gov/vaccines/hcp/vis/visstatements/hep-a.pdf. Accessed August 2016.

infected (CDC, July 2020f). The groups with the highest prevalence are injection drug users, persons with STDs or multiple sex partners, immigrants and refugees and their descendants who came from areas where there is a high endemic rate of HBV, health care workers, clients on hemodialysis, and inmates of long-term correctional institutions (Buttaro et al., 2017).

HBV is spread through blood and body fluids and, like HIV, is referred to as a *blood-borne pathogen.* It has the same transmission properties as HIV and thus, individuals should take the same precautions to prevent the spread of both HIV and HBV. A major difference is that HBV remains alive outside the body for a longer time than HIV and thus has greater infectivity. The virus can survive for at least 1 week dried at room temperature on environmental surfaces, and therefore infection control measures are paramount in preventing transmission from client to client (Heymann, 2014).

Infection with HBV results in either acute or chronic HBV infection. The acute infection is self-limited, and individuals develop an antibody to the virus and successfully eliminate the virus from the body. They subsequently have lifelong immunity against the virus. Symptoms range from mild, flulike symptoms to a more severe response that includes jaundice, extreme lethargy, nausea, fever, and joint pain. Any of these more severe symptoms may result in hospitalization. A second possible outcome from infection is chronic HBV infection, which more likely occurs in persons with immunodeficiency (Heymann, 2014). These individuals cannot rid their bodies of the virus and remain lifelong carriers of the hepatitis B surface antigen (HBsAg). As carriers, they can transmit the HBV to others. They may develop hepatic carcinoma or chronic active hepatitis. The signs and symptoms of chronic hepatitis B include anorexia, fatigue, abdominal discomfort, hepatomegaly, and jaundice (Heymann, 2014).

HBV infection can be prevented by immunization, prevention of nosocomial occupational exposure, and prevention of sexual and injection drug use exposure. Vaccination is recommended for persons with occupational risk, such as health care workers, and for infants. Protection from HBV consists of a series of 3 intramuscular injections, with the second and third doses administered 1 and 6 months after the first (Heymann, 2014). Pregnant women should be tested for HBsAg; if the mother is positive, newborns require hepatitis B immune globulin in addition to the hepatitis B vaccine within 12 hours of birth, and then at 1 and 6 months thereafter (Schillie et al., 2018). If the individual is not protected by vaccination and exposure to HBV occurs, hepatitis B immune globulin is given as soon as possible (within 24 hours is optimal) and the hepatitis B vaccine given (Schillie et al., 2018).

CASE STUDY 12.1

Hepatitis

On Friday afternoon, Jane Brown, the nurse epidemiologist at the Bertrand County Health Department, had just finished her last influenza vaccine clinic for the season. She sat down at her desk to respond to telephone and e-mail messages. She found a voice mail message that Dr. Smith, a local physician, left earlier in the day to report two cases of acute hepatitis B infection. Dr. Smith said both of these patients were elderly and lived in an assisted living facility. He stated that he would fax a copy of the reportable disease form and the laboratory results to the health department that day. He said that he was calling not only to report the infections but to seek direction on what to advise the facility.

Ms. Brown read the form Dr. Smith had faxed and confirmed that both patients are in their 80s, live at the same address, and have laboratory evidence of acute hepatitis B infection. She is puzzled by the report because she has never seen an acute case of hepatitis B in an elderly person. In fact, she has only had three reported cases of acute hepatitis B infection in her 5 years at the health department: one in an infant, another in a health care worker who had a needlestick injury, and the other in a 40-year-old man with a history of intravenous drug use.

Ms. Brown called the physician to discuss the report and gather additional information about the cases. She learned that the physician had left for the day, but she spoke with his nurse, Sally Johnson. Ms. Johnson said that both patients were seen the prior week for complaints of nausea, lethargy, and weight loss, and one had yellowing of the skin. Based on their presenting symptoms, Dr. Smith decided to perform a hepatitis B and C panel and draw blood to evaluate their liver enzymes. The hepatitis C antibody results were negative, but the liver enzymes were elevated and the hepatitis B surface antigen was positive, along with the hepatitis B core immunoglobulin M. The remaining markers were negative. The patients have no known history of exposure to hepatitis B, drug abuse, or multiple sex partners, and both have lived in the facility for over 5 years. Ms. Brown explains to the nurse that this is an unusual event and that she will launch an investigation to try to identify the source of transmission and help the assisted living facility effectively manage the residents. She called the facility immediately to set up a meeting with the administrator that evening.

Check Your Practice

1. Which term describes the system the physician used to collect, organize, and report disease information?
   A. Screening
   B. Surveillance
   C. Distribution
   D. Rate adjustment

2. What data source would *not* be useful to the nurse epidemiologist in this situation?
   A. Medical records
   B. Facility staff (administrator, nurse supervisor, nursing staff, housekeeping)
   C. Policy and procedure manuals
   D. Food history
   E. Medication administration log

In analyzing the data, Ms. Brown identifies commonalities among the two patients. She learns that both patients live in the same unit, eat in the same dining hall, are diabetic, and receive blood glucose monitoring. Ms. Brown knows that the hepatitis B virus can be transmitted by blood, so she decides to observe the nurse performing glucose monitoring. She sees that the nurse used a penlet device to secure the lancets that are used on the residents and that all residents have their own glucometer. The nurse uses a separate lancet for each patient, but the same penlet is used on each resident. Ms. Brown also observes dried blood on the lancet. Based on this observation, she decides to test all of the diabetic residents for hepatitis B infection.

3. What level of prevention is the nurse exercising in this situation?
   A. Primary
   B. Secondary
   C. Tertiary
   D. None

Ms. Brown reviews the hepatitis B testing results and learns that one patient has chronic hepatitis B infection and three other patients have had the infection in the past but are no longer infected. She recommends hepatitis B vaccine for all of the residents and staff who are susceptible to the infection.

4. Immunizations represent what level of prevention?
   A. Primary
   B. Secondary
   C. Tertiary
   D. None

Now apply these steps to this case: (1) Recognize the cues about what might have taken place; (2) analyze the cues to see if your observations are correct, (3) develop your hypotheses or assumptions about what could have occurred and then prioritize them; (4) generate potential solutions to each of the hypotheses you developed; (5) if you were Ms. Brown, what action would you take? (6) evaluate the outcomes you got or expected to get from the action that Ms. Brown took.

Case prepared by Mary Beth White-Comstock, MSN, RN, CIC.

The Occupational Safety and Health Administration (OSHA) mandates specific activities to protect workers from HBV and other blood-borne pathogens. Potential exposures for health care workers are needlestick injuries and mucous membrane splashes. The OSHA standard requires employers to identify the risk for blood exposure to various employees. If employees perform work that involves potential exposure to the body fluids of other people, employers are mandated to offer the HBV vaccine to the employee at the employer's expense and to offer annual educational programs on preventing HBV and HIV exposure in the workplace. Employees have the right to refuse the vaccine.

Hepatitis C Virus

Hepatitis C virus (HCV) is a liver disease caused by the HCV, a blood-borne virus. HCV is transmitted when blood or body fluids of an infected person enter an uninfected person. Today most people are infected with hepatitis C by sharing needles or other equipment to inject drugs. Groups at highest risk include health care workers and emergency personnel who are accidentally exposed, infants of infected mothers, and injection drug users who share needles or other drug use equipment. Risk is greatest for persons exposed to infected blood. Others at risk include hemodialysis patients (from dialysis equipment shared with infected persons) and recipients of donor organs and blood products before 1992 (USPSTF, 2016).

In 2018, 3621 cases of acute hepatitis C were reported to the CDC, and there were an estimated 50,300 infections. Over 65% of acute hepatitis C cases reported to the CDC in 2018 were among personas aged 20 to 39. Males were most likely to contract HCV, and the most likely groups were American Indians/Alaska Natives. The clinical signs of hepatitis C may be so mild that an infected individual does not seek medical attention. The incubation period ranges from 2 weeks to 6 months. Clients may experience fatigue and other nonspecific symptoms. Acute hepatitis C is a short-term illness that occurs about 6 months after exposure; of those with the acute disease, approximately 15% to 25% have the disease clear without treatment, and about 75% to 85% develop chronic or lifelong infection. Chronic hepatitis C can lead to cirrhosis, liver cancer, and death (CDC, July 2020f).

Primary prevention of HCV infection includes screening of blood products and donor organs and tissue; risk reduction counseling and services, including obtaining an injection drug use (IDU) history; and infection control practices. Secondary prevention strategies include testing of high-risk individuals, including those who currently inject drugs or injected drugs in the past, have HIV infection, have abnormal liver tests or liver disease, received blood or an organ transplant before 1992, are on hemodialysis, and have been exposed to blood on the job through a needle or injury with a sharp object (CDC, 2018d).

TUBERCULOSIS

Tuberculosis (TB) is a mycobacterial disease caused by *Mycobacterium tuberculosis*. Transmission usually occurs through exposure to the tubercle bacilli in airborne droplets from persons with pulmonary TB who talk, cough, or sneeze. TB disease in the lungs can cause symptoms such as: a cough that lasts 3 weeks or more; pain in the chest; coughing up blood or sputum (phlegm from deep inside the lungs). Other symptoms are weakness or fatigue; weight loss; lack of appetite; chills; fever; or sweating at night (CDC, 2016). The incubation period is 4 to 12 weeks. The most critical period for development of clinical disease is the first 6 to 12 months after infection. About 5% of those initially infected may develop pulmonary TB or extrapulmonary involvement. The infection in about 95% of those initially infected becomes latent, but in about 10% of otherwise healthy individuals, it may be reactivated later in life. The chance of reactivation of latent infections increases in immunocompromised persons, substance abusers, underweight and undernourished persons, and persons with diabetes, silicosis, or gastrectomies (Heymann, 2014). TB is an especially difficult and typically fatal disease for persons who are positive for HIV disease (WHO, 2020).

The World Health Organization (WHO) reported that 1.5 million people died from TB in 2018. TB is one of the top 10 causes of death worldwide and the leading cause from a single infectious agent. In 2018, it was estimated that 10 million people contracted TB worldwide. Many of these cases are resistant to rifampicin, the most effective first-line drug for treating TB (WHO, 2020). In 2018, the largest number of new TB cases were in the southeast Asia region; followed by the African region; and then the western Pacific region. Specifically, 87% of cases occurred in 30 high-TB–burden countries, with the following eight countries accounting for two thirds of new TB cases: India, China, Indonesia, Philippines, Pakistan, Nigeria, Bangladesh, and South Africa. In 2019, there were 8920 new cases provisionally reported in the United States; that represents a 1.1% decline from 2018. Non-US–born persons had a TB rate of 15.5 times greater than the rate among persons born in the United States. Many of these cases are attributed to reactivation of latent TB infection (Schwartz, Price, Pratt, and Langer, 2020). The WHO estimates that one-fourth of the world's population has latent TB, meaning that individuals are infected with TB bacteria, but they are not yet ill, nor can they transmit the disease (WHO, 2020). Worldwide, TB drug resistance is a significant issue. Resistance can be caused by people not completing the full course of treatment; provider prescription error; poor quality drugs; or lack of TB drug availability. Types of drug-resistant TB include multidrug resistant TB (MDRTB), defined as resistant to rifampin and isoniazid, and extremely drug-resistant TB (XDRTB), which is MDRTB plus added resistance to fluoroquinolones and at least three injectable second-line drugs (e.g., amikacin, kanamycin, and capreomycin) (WHO, 2017). Drug-resistant TB is a significant concern to people with weak immune systems, such as HIV-infected individuals.

To prevent TB, the CDC works with public health agencies in other countries to improve screening and reporting of cases, and to improve treatment strategies (Fig. 12.2). This includes coordination of treatment for infected individuals who migrate to the United States. This coordination is particularly significant between Mexico and the United States.

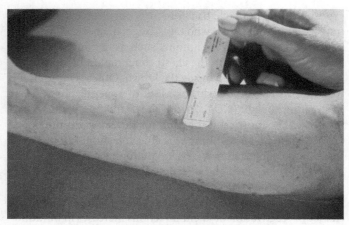

Fig. 12.2 Testing for Tuberculosis Infection. (Courtesy Centers for Disease Control and Prevention, Public Health Image Library [PHIL] ID 3752. http://CDC/Donald Kopanoff.)

The most effective tuberculin skin test (TST) is the Mantoux test. The TST, previously referred to as purified protein derivative (PPD) test, is used for initial screening. It can be followed by chest radiography for persons with a positive skin reaction and pulmonary symptoms. Persons who are immunosuppressed by drugs or who have diseases such as advanced TB, AIDS, or measles may not have the ability to mount an immune response to the TST, so the result may be a false-negative skin test reaction resulting from allergy (nonreaction). A second issue with the TST is that a positive result may come from an earlier TST boosting the person's ability to respond to the infection and not

from a recent infection. Therefore, it is difficult to determine whether the infection is old or recent. A blood test (in vitro gamma release interferon assays [IVGRA]) is available and is increasingly used for providing clinical care (CDC, 2018e). One example is the QuantiFERON-TB blood test to detect *M. tuberculosis* infection. Diagnosis can also be made through stained sputum smears and other body fluids to determine the presence of acid-fast bacilli (for presumptive diagnosis) and culture of the tubercle bacilli for definitive diagnosis. The How To box describes how to read a TST.

Clients with TB should be treated promptly with the appropriate combination of multiple antimicrobial drugs. Effective drug regimens used in the United States include isoniazid and in some instances, rifampin. Treatment regimens for persons with active symptomatic infection may be different from the regimens used for persons with latent TB infection or with HIV (Buttaro et al., 2017). Treatment failure may be due to clients' poor adherence in taking the medication, which can result in drug resistance. Nurses usually administer TSTs and provide education on the importance of compliance to long-term therapy. They also may be involved in directly observed therapy (DOT) and contact investigations of cases in the community.

NURSE'S ROLE IN PROVIDING PREVENTIVE CARE FOR COMMUNICABLE DISEASES

From prevention to treatment, the nurse functions as a counselor, educator, advocate, case manager, and primary care provider. Appropriate interventions for primary, secondary, and tertiary prevention are reviewed. In primary prevention, the

---

HOW TO PERFORM A TUBERCULIN SKIN TEST

Apply and Read the Tuberculin Skin Test

- For the Mantoux test, inject 0.1 ml of purified protein derivative (PPD) with a 26.27 or 30 gauge needle
- Read the reaction 48–72 h after injection. Typically read the results in 48-72 hours.
- Measure only induration.
- Record results in millimeters.

Tuberculin Skin Test Interpretation

The test is positive if the induration is ≥ 5 mm in the following:
- Immunosuppressed clients
- Persons known to have human immunodeficiency virus (HIV) infection
- Persons whose chest radiograph is suggestive of previous tuberculosis (TB) that was untreated
- Close contacts of a person with infectious TB
- Organ transplant recipients

Test is positive if the induration is ≥ 10 mm in the following:
- Persons with certain medical conditions, such as diabetes, alcoholism, or drug abuse
- Persons who inject drugs (if HIV negative)
- Foreign-born persons from areas where TB is common
- Children under 4 years of age
- Residents and staff of long-term care facilities, jails, and prisons

Test is positive if the induration is ≥15 mm in the following:
- All persons more than 4 years of age with no risk factors for TB (Buttaro et al., 2017)

CASE STUDY 12.2

Tuberculosis Screening in a Homeless Population

Jill Miles is the nurse epidemiologist for the Warren County Health Department. Part of Ms. Miles's role at the health department is to administer tuberculosis (TB) screening to at-risk populations and to track TB cases seen in the county. Ms. Miles has identified the homeless population in Warren County as a high-risk population for TB.

Ms. Miles has already implemented a TB education program at the homeless shelter. Every other month, she goes to the shelter and teaches a class about TB—what it is, who is at risk, and why to get a TB screening test. Furthermore, every person who wishes to stay at the shelter must receive a TB screening test.

Yesterday, the homeless shelter contacted Ms. Miles and reported that one of the men staying at the shelter tested positive for active TB, but they now cannot find him. The shelter director suspects the man has left to work at one of the rural farms that offer temporary work, but he does not know which farm.

Ms. Miles talks to the men at the shelter who spoke with the client. She learns that the client, José, is in his 30s and speaks only Spanish. The friends give Ms. Miles some leads of possible farms to which José may have gone. Ms. Miles calls the farms and speaks to the farm managers. Luckily, Ms. Miles discovers one of the farm managers had recently been at the shelter to recruit workers. She visits the farm and, through interviewing the newly hired men, finds José, the missing person with active TB. Because of José's transient lifestyle, Ms. Miles decides to enroll him in directly observed therapy (DOT) for TB treatment. DOT will provide a hotel room and meals for him while he receives TB treatment.

nursing process is used to care for clients with communicable diseases. Nurses are in an ideal position to affect the outcomes of communicable diseases, and their influence begins with primary prevention.

Primary Prevention

Primary prevention aims to keep people healthy and avoid the onset of disease. First, assess for risk behavior and provide relevant intervention through education on how to avoid infection, mostly through healthy behaviors. To assess the risk for acquiring an infection, obtain a history that focuses on potential exposure, which varies with the specific organism being studied and its mode of transmission. The questions to be asked can be especially challenging with clients who have an STD. The nurse should obtain a sexual and injection drug use history for clients and their partners. The sexual history provides information that leads to the need for specific diagnostic tests, treatment approaches, and partner notification. It also facilitates evaluation of risk factors and is necessary for the nurse to be able to provide relevant education for the client's lifestyle. A thorough sexual history requires obtaining personal and sensitive information. Ask about the types of relationships, the number of sexual partners and encounters, and the types of sexual behaviors practiced. The confidential nature of the information and how it will be used should be shared with the client to establish open communication and goal-directed interaction. Most clients feel uneasy disclosing such personal information. The nurse can ease this discomfort by remaining supportive and open during the interview to facilitate honesty about intimate issues. The nurse serves as a model for discussing sensitive information in a candid manner. When discussing precautions, use direct and simple language to describe specific behaviors. This encourages the client to openly discuss sexuality during this interaction and with future partners.

LEVELS OF PREVENTION

Related to Nursing Interventions

Primary Prevention
- Provide community education about prevention of communicable diseases to well populations.
- Vaccinate for hepatitis A virus (HAV) or hepatitis B virus (HBV).
- Provide community outreach for education and needle exchange.

Secondary Prevention
- Administer tuberculin skin test (TST).
- Test and counsel for human immunodeficiency virus (HIV).
- Notify partners and trace contacts.

Tertiary Prevention
- Educate caregivers of persons with HIV about standard precautions.
- Maintain long-term directly observed therapy (DOT) for tuberculosis (TB) treatment.
- Identify community resources for providing supportive care (e.g., funds for purchasing medications).
- Set up support groups for persons with herpes simplex virus 2.

Nurses who are uncomfortable discussing topics such as sexual behavior or sexual orientation are likely to avoid assessing risk behaviors with the client. They will then be ineffective in identifying risks and helping clients modify risky behaviors. Nurses can gain confidence in conducting sexual risk assessments by understanding their own values and feelings about sexuality and realizing that the purpose of the interaction is to improve the client's health. The nurse's comfort in discussing sexual behavior can be improved by using role playing to practice assessments of sexual and intravenous drug use behavior and by contracting with clients to make behavior changes.

Identifying the number of sexual injection drug using partners and the number of contacts with these partners provides information about the client's risk. The chance of exposure decreases as the number of partners decreases, so people in mutually monogamous relationships are at low risk for acquiring STDs. You can obtain this information by asking, "How many sex (or drug) partners have you had over the past 6 months?" Try to avoid basing assumptions about the sexual partner or partners on the client's sex, age, ethnicity, or any other factor. Stereotypes and assumptions about who people are and what they do are common problems that keep interviewers from asking the questions that lead to obtaining useful information. For example, it should not be taken for granted that if a man is homosexual, he always has more than one partner. Be aware also that the long incubation of HIV and the subclinical phase of many STDs lead some monogamous individuals to assume erroneously that they are not at risk.

It is important to determine whether the person has sexual contact with men, women, or both. This information can be obtained simply by asking a direct question. This lets the client know that the nurse is open to hearing about these behaviors, and thus the nurse is more likely to obtain information that is relevant to sexual practices and risk. Women who are exclusively lesbian are at low risk for acquiring STDs, but bisexual women may transmit STDs between male and female partners. In addition, it is possible for men to have sexual contact with other men and not label themselves as homosexual. Therefore, education to reduce risk that is aimed at homosexual men will not be heeded by men who do not see themselves as homosexual. In such situations, the nurse can ask, "When was the last time you had sex with another man?"

Certain sexual practices are more likely to result in exposure to and transmission of STDs. Dangerous sexual activities include unprotected anal or vaginal intercourse, oral–anal contact, and insertion of finger or fist into the rectum. These practices introduce a high risk for transmission of enteric organisms or result in physical trauma during sexual encounters. The nurse can obtain information about sexual encounters by asking, "Can you tell me the kinds of sexual practices in which you engage? This will help determine what risks you may have and the type of tests we should do." Clients who engage in genital–anal, oral–anal, or oral–genital contact will need throat and rectal cultures for some STDs, as well as cervical and urethral cultures.

Drug use is linked to STD transmission in several ways. Drugs such as alcohol put people at risk because these drugs

EVIDENCE-BASED PRACTICE

This descriptive study asked 93 largely low-income HIV-infected Latino men about their sexual practices, substance use history, and HIV disclosure patterns. A complicated picture emerged, indicating that presentation and reporting of sexual preference and behavior did not necessarily match actual orientation and behavior. This is important because the HIV rate in the Latino community is increasing, and careful history taking and question asking can help nurses to better understand the range of sexual practices and communication behaviors of their patients, hopefully leading to a better understanding of HIV disclosure patterns.

In this sample, many of the HIV-infected men also had a high rate of substance use, including 56% of the men reporting alcohol use in the past 3 months, 87.4% using marijuana, 71.9% using crack cocaine, 40.4% using IV drugs, and 35.6% reporting sharing needles. Latino men who identified as straight engaged in risky practices such as sharing needles (56%) or having sex with a partner who uses needles (54.3%) at higher rates than gay or bisexual men in this sample. Additionally, HIV testing (and therefore perceived susceptibility to contracting HIV) was typically associated with sexual orientation in this study, meaning that men who identified as straight or bisexual received testing at lower rates than gay men. HIV disclosure to partners varied among groups as well, with gay men (67.5%) most frequently disclosing their HIV-positive status to a partner than straight (57.6%) or bisexual (50%) men.

Results indicate that public health interventions for Latino straight men in particular should identify and focus on IV drug use, needle sharing, and unprotected sex as high-risk behaviors that lead to contracting HIV. Clinicians should also be aware that there is much diversity in sexual behavior for straight, gay, and bisexual people and to be aware of this when discussing self-care, risk, and protective factors with clients. For instance, gay does not always equal same-sex sexual practices, and straight does not always indicate heterosexual sex.

Nurse Use

This study highlights the importance of a nuanced history taking in terms of sexual history and substance use as an important part of maximizing public health interventions. Nurses can play a large role in open and honest HIV disclosure behavior by carefully addressing a range of risk behaviors and possible barriers to testing, indicated by this sample of HIV-positive ethnic minority men.

Data from Champion JD, Szlachta A: Self-identified sexual orientation and sexual risk behavior among HIV-infected Latino males, *J Assoc Nurses AIDS Care* 27(5):285–294, 2016.

can lower inhibitions and impair judgment about engaging in risky behaviors. Addictions to drugs may cause individuals to acquire the drug or money to purchase the drug through sexual favors. This increases both the frequency of sexual contacts and the chances of contracting STDs. Thus the nurse should obtain information on the type and frequency of drug use and the presence of risk behaviors. The administration of vaccines to prevent infection such as for hepatitis A and B is an example of primary prevention.

Interventions to prevent infection are aimed at preventing specific infections. These interventions can take several forms and include, for example, education on how to prevent infection or the availability of vaccines. For example, on the basis of the information obtained in the sexual history and risk assessment just described, the nurse can identify specific education and counseling needs of the client. The nursing interventions focus on contracting with clients to change behavior and reduce their risk in regard to sexual practice.

Safer Sex

Sexual abstinence is the best way to prevent STDs. However, for many people sexual abstinence is not realistic, and teaching how to make sexual behavior safer is critical. Safer sexual behavior includes masturbation, dry kissing, touching, fantasy, and vaginal and oral sex with a condom.

If used correctly and consistently, condoms can prevent both pregnancy and most STDs because they prevent the exchange of body fluids during sexual activity. Condom failure may occur from incorrect use rather than condom breakage. Thus information about proper use of condoms and how to communicate with a partner is also necessary. The nurse has many opportunities to convey this information during counseling. Condom use may be viewed as inconvenient, messy, or decreasing sensation. Consuming alcohol may accompany sexual activity and decrease condom use. Nurses can use role playing to help clients gain skill in discussing safer sex by role modeling and by practicing communication skills.

Female condoms can also be a barrier to body fluid contact and therefore protect against pregnancy and STDs. The main advantage of the female condom is that the female controls its use. The FC2 female condom is the only one approved in the United States by the FDA. Because it is made of polyurethane, it is also useful if a latex sensitivity develops to male condoms. Symptoms of latex allergy include penile, vaginal, or rectal itching or swelling after use of a male condom or diaphragm. The female condom consists of a sheath over two rings, with one closed end that fits over the cervix. The condoms are often free at public health clinics, or cost ranges from $2.50 to $3.00 per condom.

Clients should understand that it is important to know the risk behavior of their sexual partners, including a history of injection drug use and STDs, bisexuality, and any current symptoms. This is because each sexual partner is potentially exposed to all the STDs of all the persons with whom the other partner has been sexually active.

Drug Use

Injection drug use is risky because the potential for injecting blood-borne pathogens, such as HIV, HBV, and HCV exists when needles and syringes are shared. During IDU, small quantities of drugs are repeatedly injected. Blood is withdrawn into the syringe and is then injected back into the user's vein. Individuals should be advised against using injectable drugs and sharing needles, syringes, or other drug paraphernalia. People who inject drugs are difficult to reach for health care services. Effective outreach programs include using community peers, increasing accessibility of drug treatment programs combined with HIV testing and counseling, and long-term repeat contacts after completion of the program.

Community Outreach, Education, and Evaluation

Because of the illegal nature of injectable drugs and the poverty associated with HIV, many people at risk have neither the inclination nor the resources to seek health care. Nurses may work to establish programs within communities because the opportunities for counseling on the prevention of HIV and other STDs are increased by bringing services into the neighborhoods of those at risk. Before the onset of the COVID-19 pandemic, public health workers went into communities to disseminate information on safer sex, drug treatment programs, and discontinuation of drug use or safer drug use practices (e.g., using new needles and syringes with each injection). Some programs provide sterile needles and syringes, condoms, and literature about anonymous test sites.

Using primary prevention, nurses can educate healthy groups about prevention of communicable diseases. During the COVID-19 pandemic, much of the health teaching was done electronically rather than in person. Prior to the pandemic, information about modes of transmission, testing, availability of vaccines, and early symptoms could be provided to groups in the community to help prevent the spread of STDs and HIV. When talking with groups about HIV infection, be sure to discuss the following:

- The number of people infected with HIV and the number who are living with AIDS
- Modes of transmission of the virus
- How to prevent infection
- Testing services
- Common symptoms of illness
- Providing a compassionate response to those affected
- Available community resources
- Content about other STDs because the mode of transmission (sexual contact) is the same
- Information on these diseases, including the distribution, incidence, and consequences of the infection for individuals and society

Evaluation is based on whether risky behavior has changed to safe behavior and, ultimately, whether illness is prevented. Condom use is evaluated for consistency of use if the client is sexually active. Other behaviors, such as abstinence or monogamy, can be evaluated for their implementation.

Secondary Prevention

Secondary prevention includes screening for diseases to ensure their early identification and treatment and follow-up with contacts to prevent further spread. In general, client teaching and counseling should include education about preventing self-reinfection, managing symptoms, and preventing the infection of others. HIV screening is recommended for all patients in health care settings unless the patient declines testing. Persons at high risk should be tested annually.

Human Immunodeficiency Virus Test Counseling

Universal testing for HIV infection should be routine for all clients aged 13 to 64 years (CDC, 2018f). Younger adolescents and older adults who are at increased risk should be screened as well. As of April 2020, there was no data to support that people with HIV were at greater risk for COVID-19 than were people not considered in the high-risk category. Routine HIV testing should be a part of all annual physicals, laboratory tests for every pregnancy, and all hospital visits, without securing special permission. Clients can decline or "opt out" of HIV testing, but the benefits of testing are considerable. For persons who have engaged in high-risk behavior, the nurse should recommend annual HIV testing. Individuals with the following characteristics are considered at risk and should be offered HIV testing: those with a history of STDs

(which are transmitted through the same behavior and may decrease immune functioning), multiple sex partners, or IDU; those who have unprotected intercourse (i.e., without using a condom or preexposure prophylaxis [PrEP]) (CDC, 2020b); those who have intercourse with someone who has another partner and those who have had sex with a prostitute; men with a history of homosexual or bisexual activity; and those who have been a sexual partner to anyone in one of these groups.

Testing enables clients to benefit from early detection and treatment, as well as risk reduction education. If HIV infection is discovered before the onset of symptoms, early monitoring of the disease process and CD4 lymphocyte counts or viral loads is indicated. In addition, prophylactic therapy with antiretroviral therapy and/or antibiotics may begin in order to delay the onset of symptomatic illness.

There are three types of available tests: nucleic acid tests (NAT); antigen/antibody tests, and antibody tests. Tests are typically performed using blood or oral fluid, but they can also be performed using urine. The NAT looks for actual virus in the blood and involved drawing blood from a vein. This test is expensive and is not used unless a person recently had a high-risk exposure or has early HIV infection symptoms. Results may take several days. The antigen/antibody tests look for both HIV antibodies and antigens. The test is recommended if the testing is done in a lab, and it involves drawing blood or done via a fingerstick. Results from the rapid antigen/antibody test done via a fingerstick can be available in 30 minutes or less. HIV antibody tests look for antibodies to HIV in blood or oral fluids. The rapid antibody test done via fingerstick or with oral fluid can provide results in 30 minutes or less. Most rapid tests and the only currently approved HIV self-test are antibody tests (CDC, 2020g).

A negative test may not reveal infections that were acquired within several weeks before the test. Evidence of HIV antibody takes from 6 to 12 weeks to develop. All clients who are antibody positive should be counseled about the need to reduce their risks and notify partners. If the client is unwilling or hesitant to notify past partners, the nurse will do partner notification (or contact tracing). Clients should seek treatment from their primary health care provider so that physical evaluation can be performed and, if indicated, antiviral or other therapies begun. Box 12.3 describes the responsibilities of individuals who are HIV positive.

Psychosocial counseling is indicated when positive HIV test results precipitate acute anxiety, depression, or suicidal ideation. The client should be informed about available counseling services. The person should be cautioned to consider carefully who should be informed of the test results. Many individuals have told others about their HIV-positive test, only to experience isolation and discrimination. Plans for the future should be explored, and clients should be advised to avoid stress, drugs, and infections to maintain optimal health.

Partner Notification and Contact Tracing

Partner notification, also known as contact tracing, is an example of a population-level intervention aimed at controlling communicable diseases. Partner notification programs usually occur in conjunction with reportable disease requirements and are carried out by most health departments. It involves confidentially

BOX 12.3 Responsibilities of Persons Who Are Human Immunodeficiency Virus Infected

- Have regular medical evaluations and follow-ups.
- Do not donate blood, plasma, body organs, other tissues, or sperm.
- Take precautions against exchanging body fluids during sexual activity.
- Inform sexual or injection drug–using partners of the potential exposure to HIV or arrange for notification through the health department.
- Inform health care providers of the HIV infection.
- Consider the risk of perinatal transmission and follow up with contraceptive use.

HIV, Human immunodeficiency virus.

identifying and notifying exposed individuals of clients who are found to have reportable diseases. This could result in, for example, family members and close contacts of individuals with TB being given a TST, which may be administered in the home. Contract tracing was difficult during the COVID-19 pandemic because on many occasions, and against health care advice, large groups gathered for rallies, demonstrations and so forth. Often, the participants did not wear face masks or maintain an acceptable social distance. When hundreds or thousands of people gather and the virus is detected in some, it is difficult to use contract tracing to notify the exposed individuals. Contract tracing was more effective in venues such as in-person classes where teachers knew the children and youth who were in close proximity to a person who tested positive for the virus.

Individuals diagnosed with a reportable STD are asked to provide the names and locations of all partners so that these individuals can be informed of their exposure, receive counseling, and obtain the necessary referral and/or treatment. The originally diagnosed (index case) clients may be encouraged to notify their partners (can be sexual and/or injection drug partners) and to encourage them to seek treatment. If the client agrees to do so, suggestions on how to inform their partners and how to deal with possible reactions can be discussed. In some instances, clients may feel more comfortable if the nurse notifies those who are exposed. If clients contact their partners about possible infection, the nurse contacts health care providers or clinics to verify positive test results or microscopic findings and treatment of the index case.

If the originally diagnosed client prefers not to participate in notifying partners, the public health nurse contacts the partners by phone, certified delivery letter, or home visit, depending on the circumstances, and counsels them to seek evaluation and treatment.Often, the client is treated for the STI at the health department. At this appointment the client is offered literature regarding the STD for which they need treatment, receives risk-reduction counseling, and is offered testing for the other STDs. The identity of the infected client who names sexual and injection drug–using partners cannot be revealed. Maintaining confidentiality is critical with all STDs.

Tertiary Prevention

Tertiary prevention can apply to many of the chronic viral STDs and TB. For viral STDs, much of this effort focuses on managing symptoms and maintaining psychosocial support. Many clients report feeling contaminated and thus feel lower self-worth. Support groups may be available to help clients cope with chronic STDs, such as genital herpes or genital warts.

Directly Observed Therapy

In DOT programs for TB medication, nurses observe and document individual clients taking their TB drugs. When clients prematurely stop taking TB medications, there is a risk of resistance to medications. This can affect an entire community of people who are susceptible to this airborne disease. Health professionals share in the responsibility of adhering to treatment, and DOT ensures that TB-infected clients have adequate medication. Thus, DOT programs are aimed at the population level to prevent antibiotic resistance in the community and to ensure effective treatment at the individual level. Many health departments have DOT home health programs to ensure adequate treatment. DOT short course (DOTS) is a variation applied in specific countries of the world to combat multidrug-resistant TB (WHO, 2017; CDC, 2018g).

The management of AIDS at home may include monitoring physical status and referring the family to additional care services for maintaining the client at home. Case management is important in all phases of HIV infection. It is especially important to ensure that clients have adequate services to meet their needs. This may include ensuring that medication can be obtained through identifying funding resources, maintaining infection control standards, reducing risk behaviors, identifying sources of respite care for caretakers, or referring clients for home or hospice care. Nursing interventions include teaching families about managing symptomatic illness by preventing deteriorating conditions such as diarrhea, skin breakdown, and inadequate nutrition.

Standard Precautions

It is important to teach caregivers about infection control in the home. This became especially apparent during the COVID-19 pandemic, where people were told repeatedly in all forms of media to wash their hands for 20 seconds, wear face masks when around other people; maintain a social distance of at least 6 feet from other people. It became a time when friends and family no longer hugged one another.

Standard precautions must be taught to caregivers in the home setting. All blood and articles soiled with body fluids must be handled as if they were infectious or contaminated by bloodborne pathogens. Gloves should be worn whenever hands might touch nonintact skin, mucous membranes, blood, or other fluids. A mask, goggles or face shield, and gown should also be worn if there is potential for splashing or contact with infectious material during any care. All protective equipment should be worn only once and then disposed of. If the skin or mucous membranes of the caregiver come in contact with body fluids, the skin should be washed with soap and water, and the mucous membranes should be flushed with water as soon as possible after the exposure. Thorough handwashing with soap and water—a major infection control measure—should be conducted whenever hands become contaminated and whenever gloves or other protective equipment (e.g., mask, gown) is removed. Soiled clothing or linen should be washed in a washing machine filled with hot water, using bleach as an additive, and dried on the hot-air cycle of a dryer. Face masks should be washed often if they are cloth and reusable.

APPLYING CONTENT TO PRACTICE

This chapter emphasizes the epidemiology and prevention of selected communicable diseases, as well as the public health nursing services provided to clients. The Council on Linkages Domains and Core Competencies are addressed through activities in caring for clients with communicable diseases. Examples of how these eight domains are used in providing nursing care to clients with communicable disease are as follows:

Domain 1, Analytic Assessment Skills, is achieved through the review of the incidence and prevalence rates of communicable diseases to determine population health status.

Domain 3, Communication Skills, is applied when public health nurses teach how to prevent and treat infections.

Domain 4, Cultural Competency Skills, is met through understanding the various social and behavioral factors that make health care acceptable to diverse populations.

Council on Linkages between Academic and Public Health Practice: *Core competencies for public health professionals,* Washington, DC, 2014. Public Health Foundation/Health Resources and Services Administration.

PRACTICE APPLICATION

Yvonne Jackson is a 20-year-old woman who visits the Hopetown City Health Department's maternity clinic. Examination reveals she is at 14 weeks of gestation. She is single but has been in a steady relationship for the past 6 months with Phil. She states that she has no other children. The HIV test is routinely performed during the initial prenatal visit. The results are positive.

Yvonne is shocked and emotionally distraught about the positive test results. Understanding that Yvonne will not be able to concentrate on all of the questions and information that need to be covered, the nurse sets priorities regarding essential information to obtain and provide during this visit.

A. List the relevant factors to consider on the basis of this information.

B. What questions do you need to ask with regard to controlling the spread of HIV to others?

C. What information is most important to give to Yvonne at this time?

D. What follow-up does the nurse need to arrange for Yvonne? **Answers can be found on the Evolve website.**

REMEMBER THIS!

- Most communicable diseases discussed in this chapter are preventable because they are transmitted through specific and known behaviors.
- Sexually transmitted diseases (STDs) are among the most serious public health problems in the United States. Not only is there an increased incidence of drug-resistant gonococcal infection, but other STDs, such as HPV (genital warts), human immunodeficiency virus (HIV), and herpes simplex virus (HSV) (genital herpes), are associated with cancer.
- STDs affect certain groups in greater numbers. Factors associated with risk include being younger than 25 years, being a member of a minority group, residing in an urban setting, being impoverished, and using crack cocaine.

- It is important for nurses to educate clients about ways to prevent communicable diseases.
- Many STDs are asymptomatic.
- Aside from death, the most serious complications caused by STDs are pelvic inflammatory disease, infertility, ectopic pregnancy, neonatal morbidity and mortality, and neoplasia.
- Hepatitis A is often silent in children, and children are a significant source of infection to others.
- The use of vaccine in children has led to a reduced incidence of Hepatitis A.
- Hepatitis C is the most common blood-borne pathogen in the United States.
- The emergence of multidrug-resistant TB has prompted the use of directly observed therapy (DOT) in the United States and other countries to ensure adherence to drug treatment regimens.
- Early detection of communicable diseases is important because it results in early treatment and prevention of additional transmission to others. Treatment includes effective medications, stress reduction, and proper nutrition.
- Partner notification, or contact tracing, is done by identifying, contacting, and ensuring evaluation and treatment of persons exposed to sexual and injectable drug–using partners. Contact tracing is also conducted for tuberculosis (TB), hepatitis A virus (HAV), and COVID-19.
- Most of the care (both home and outpatient) that is provided for HIV is done within the community setting, which reduces direct health care costs but increases the need for financial support of home and community health services.

EVOLVE WEBSITE

http://evolve.elsevier.com/Stanhope/foundations
- Case Study, with Questions and Answers
- NCLEX® Review Questions
- Practice Application Answers

REFERENCES

Buttaro T, Trybulski J, Polgar Bailey P, et al.: *Primary care: a collaborative practice,* 5th ed. St Louis, 2017, Elsevier.
Centers for Disease Control and Prevention: Sexually transmitted diseases treatment guidelines, 2015. *MMWR Recomm Rep* 64(3): 1–137
Centers for Disease Control and Prevention: Tuberculosis: Signs and symptoms, Atlanta, 2016, CDC. Retrieved September 2020 from http://www.cdc.gov/TB.
Centers for Disease Control and Prevention: *HIV Surveillance Report: Diagnoses of HIV Infection and AIDS in the United States and Dependent Areas, 2016,* vol 28, 2017a. Retrieved from http://www.cdc.gov/hiv/topics/surveillance/resources/reports/.
Centers for Disease Control and Prevention: *Genital herpes: CDC fact sheet,* Atlanta, August 2017b, CDC. Retrieved October 2020 from http://www.cdc.gov/genitalherpes-CDCfactsheet.
Centers for Disease Control and Prevention: *Sexually Transmitted Disease Surveillance 2016,* Atlanta, 2017c, US Department of Health and Human Services. Retrieved September 2020 from http://www.cdc.gov/std.

Centers for Disease Control and Prevention: *Gonococcal infections—2015 STD treatment guidelines*, 2018a. Retrieved from https://www.cdc.gov/std/tg2015/gonorrhea.htm.

Centers for Disease Control and Prevention: *Clinician factsheets and guidance*, 2018b. Retrieved from https://www.cdc.gov/hpv/hcp/clinician-factsheet.html.

Centers for Disease Control and Prevention: *CDC—human papillomavirus (HPV) and cancer*, 2018c. Retrieved from https://www.cdc.gov/cancer/hpv/index.htm.

Centers for Disease Control and Prevention: *US 2016 surveillance data for viral hepatitis*, 2018d, Atlanta, Retrieved from https://www.cdc.gov/hepatitis/statistics/2016surveillance/index.htm.

Centers for Disease Control and Prevention: *TB incidence in the US 2018*, 2018e, Atlanta, CDC. Available at http://www.cdc.gov/tb/statistics/tbcases.htm. Accessed 2018.

Centers for Disease Control and Prevention: *Prevention: HIV basics*, 2018f, Atlanta, CDC, Retrieved from https://www.cdc.gov/hiv/basics/prevention.html.

Centers for Disease Control and Prevention: *TB incidence in the U.S*, 2018g. Atlanta, CDC, Retrieved from https://www.cdc.gov/tb/statistics/tbcases.htm

Centers for Disease Control and Prevention: Sexually transmitted disease surveillance 2018, Atlanta, 2019a, CDC. Retrieved September 2020 from http://www.cdc.gov/sexuallytransmitteddiseasesurveillance2018.

Centers for Disease Control and Prevention: *HIV transmission*, Atlanta, 2019b, CDC. Retrieved September 2020 from http://www.cdc.gov/hiv/hivtransmission.

Centers for Disease Control and Prevention: *Sexually transmitted disease surveillance, 2018 Gonorrhea*, Atlanta, 2019c, CDC. Retrieved September 2020 from http://www.cdc.gov/std/gonorrhea.

Centers for Disease Control and Prevention: *Sexually transmitted disease surveillance, 2018, Syphilis*, Atlanta, 2019d, CDC. Retrieved September 2020 from http://www.cdc.gov/std/syphilis.

Centers for Disease Control and Prevention: *Sexually transmitted disease surveillance 2018, Chlamydia*, Atlanta, September 2019e, CDC. Retrieved September 2020 from http://www.cdc.gov/sexually transmitted disease surveillance 2018, chlamydia.

Centers for Disease Control and Prevention: *Human Papillomavirus (HPV): HPV vaccine schedule and dosing*, 2019f, Retrieved October 2020 from http://www.cdc.govHumanPapillomavirus.

Centers for Disease Control and Prevention: *HIV Surveillance Report, 2018 updated*, Atlanta, 2020a, CDC, Retrieved September 2020 from http://www.cdc.gov/hiv/library/reports/surveillance.

Centers for Disease Control and Prevention: *About HIV*, Atlanta, 2020b, CDC, Retrieved September 2020 at http://www.cdc.gov/hiv/abouthiv.

Centers for Disease Control and Prevention: *HIV and youth*, Atlanta, 2020c, Retrieved September 2020 at http://www.chc.gov/hivandyouth.

Centers for Disease Control and Prevention: *HIV self-testing (home testing)*, 2020d. CDC. Available at http://www.cdc.gov/hiv/. Accessed September 2020.

Centers for Disease Control and Prevention: *PrEP*, Atlanta, 2020e, CDC. Retrieved Septetember 2020 from http://www.cdc.gov hiv/PrEP.

Centers for Disease Control and Prevention: *Viral hepatitis surveillance-United States 2018*, Atlanta, July 2020f, CDC. Retrieved September 2020 from http://www.cdc.gov/hepatitis/2018surveillance /Rpts.htm.

Centers for Disease Control and Prevention: *HIV: Types of HIV tests*, Atlanta, 2020g, Retrieved September 2020 at http://www.cdc.gov/hiv/testing.

Champion JD, Szlachta A: Self-identified sexual orientation and sexual risk behavior among HIV-infected Latino males. *J Assoc Nurses AIDS Care* 27(5):285–294, 2016.

Council on Linkages Between Academic and Public Health Practice: *Core competencies for public health professionals*, Washington, DC, 2014, Public Health Foundation/Health Resource and Services Administration.

Hall HI, Song R, Tang T, et al.: HIV trends in the United States: Diagnoses and estimated incidence, *JMIR Public Health Surveill* 3(1):e8, 2017.

Health Resources and Service Administration: *About the Ryan White HIV/AIDS program*. Washington, DC, 2019. Retrieved September 2020 from http://hab.hrsa.gov.about-ryan-white-hivaidsprogram.

Heymann D: *Control of communicable diseases manual*, 20th ed. Washington, DC, 2014, American Public Health Association.

HIV.gov: *Workplace rights*, 2017. Retrieved from https://www.hiv.gov/hiv-basics/living-well-with-hiv/your-legal-rights/workplace-rights.

Schackman BR, Fleishman JA, Su AE, et al.: The lifetime medical cost savings from preventing HIV in the United States, *Med Care* 53(4):293–301, 2015.

Schwartz, Price, Pratt and Langer: Tuberculosis-United States, 2019, *MMWR Morb Mortal Wkly Rep* 69(11): 286-289.

Schillie S, Vellozzi C, Reingold A, et al.: Prevention of hepatitis B virus infection in the United States: Recommendations of the advisory committee on immunization practices, *MMWR. Recomm Rep* 67:1–31, 2018.

UNAIDS: Fact sheet-latest statistics on the status of the AIDS epidemic, 2018, Retrieved from http://www.unaids.org/en/resources/fact-sheet.

US Department of Health and Human Services: *Healthy People 2030*, Washington, DC, 2020, US Government Printing Office. Retrieved September 2020 from https://www.healthypeople.gov/2030.

United States Preventive Services Task Force (USPSTF): *Final recommendation statement: Hepatitis C: Screening*, 2016. Retrieved from https://www.uspreventiveservicestaskforce.org/Page/Document/RecommendationStatementFinal/hepatitis-c-screening.

World Health Organization (WHO): Global tuberculosis report 2017, Geneva, 2017, WHO Press. Available at http://www.who.int/tb/publications/global-report/en/. Accessed September 2020.

World Health Organization: *Tuberculosis*, Geneva, 2020, WHO. Retrieved September 2020 from http://www.who.int/tuberculosis.

13

Community Assessment and Evaluation

Mary E. Gibson and Esther J. Thatcher

OBJECTIVES

After reading this chapter, the student should be able to:

1. Understand the importance of community assessment, the community, the community client, community health, and partnership for health.
2. Use the nursing process to create a community assessment for a selected community.
3. Develop a prioritized community problem list and nursing diagnosis, and a care plan for a community.
4. Decide which methods of assessment, planning, implementation, and evaluation are most appropriate for application in the community.

CHAPTER OUTLINE

KEY TERMS

I believe that the community—in the fullest sense: a place and all its creatures—is the smallest unit of health and that to speak of the health of an isolated individual is a contradiction in terms.

Wendell Berry

INTRODUCTION

Communities are the environments where we live and work. Naturally, the community's ability to serve the needs of its members determines key aspects in the health of the community. The public health nurse (PHN) is in an ideal position to view the "community as client," and to begin to identify and harness the strengths present to meet the challenges faced by the community. Health is an interdependent concept. As defined by the World Health Organization (WHO), "Health is a state of complete physical, mental and social well-being and not merely the absence of disease or infirmity" (WHO, 1948). The influences of environment, public services and policies, and economics play a large role in the health of the community.

As PHNs, we use the nursing process from assessment through evaluation to promote a community's health. This process begins with community assessment (sometimes called community needs assessment)—one of the core functions of public health nursing—which involves getting to know the community inside and out. It is a logical, systematic approach to identifying community needs, clarifying problems, and identifying community strengths and resources. In this chapter specific community concepts will be clarified, including community as client, a snapshot of the nurse's role in communities, and the process for undertaking a community assessment using mostly secondary data.

COMMUNITY DEFINED

Throughout history, humans have formed cooperative social groups that enhanced the survival chances of individual group members. Even today, communities that rally together in solidarity tend to recover faster after a disaster or other event (Boyd and Richerson, 2009; Mercy Corps, 2017). Each generation defines and seeks community in different ways; the "millennial" generation of young adults has received much interest in how their definitions of community influence their work, housing, social, and political lives (Feldman et al., 2017). But what do we mean by *community*, and how might being part of a community influence a person's health?

There are many definitions of community. At its simplest, a **community** is a group of people, as in a defined population, who share something in common, such as geographic location, interests, or values (The Community Guide, n.d.; MacQueen et al., 2001). The WHO defines community as "a group of people, often living in a defined geographical area, who may share a common culture, values and norms, and are arranged in a social structure according to relationships which the community has developed over a period of time" (WHO, 2004, p 16). A community is a system, not just the sum of the characteristics of its inhabitants. In most definitions, the community includes

three factors: people, place, and function. *People* are the community members or residents. An aggregate is a population or group of individuals in the community who share common personal or environmental characteristics. *Place* can be a geographic location or other shared spaces such as the Internet. *Function* refers to the aims and activities of the community.

Community is a concept rather than simply a specific place, and individuals living in the same place may describe their community differently. When an organization asks a nurse to perform a community assessment, community usually refers to a specific population, an aggregate with specific characteristics living within the area that an organization serves, such as a school district, or a geographic area such as a county. However, it is important to remember that individuals within this defined area could view the community through a different lens. Understanding the many identities of community is part of the community assessment and is best done through talking with and or collecting data about residents and stakeholders.

COMMUNITY AS CLIENT

Nursing Care of the Community as Client

Population-focused health care is highly relevant in the current health care environment, and the community as client is important to nursing practice for several reasons. The community is the client when the nursing focus is on the collective or common good of the population, instead of only on individual health. When focusing on the community as client, direct primary, secondary, or tertiary preventive interventions can be a part of population-focused community health practice (Sidorov and Romney, 2016). For example, sometimes these interventions are provided to individuals and family members because their health needs are common community-related problems. Changes in individual or population health will ultimately affect the health of the community.

Improved health of the community remains the overall goal of nursing intervention. This is often accomplished through individual interventions. For example, addressing intimate partner violence, child abuse, or elder abuse is intended primarily to impact the effects of abuse on society and ultimately on the population as a whole. Similarly, diagnosing or treating a client for tuberculosis reduces the risk to other community members, thereby reducing the risk of an epidemic in the community. Since 1965, large-scale campaigns to encourage smoking reduction or cessation among groups and individuals and laws that prohibit smoking in specific public spaces have resulted in significantly lower smoking rates in the adult population (42% in 1965 compared with 15.5% in 2016) (Centers for Disease Control and Prevention [CDC], 2018a).

Focusing on the community client highlights the complexity of the change process. Change for the benefit of the community client must often occur at several levels, ranging from the individual to society as a whole. For example, health problems caused by lifestyle, such as lack of exercise, overeating, and speeding, cannot be solved simply by asking individuals to choose health-promoting habits. Society must also provide healthy choices. Most individuals find changing their habits independently extremely difficult—indeed, sometimes impossible. The support of family members, friends, and community health care systems and relevant social policies are necessary for success. Individuals who have lifestyle health problems are often blamed for their illness because of their choices (e.g., to smoke), often referred to as "blaming the victim." In his classic work, Ryan (1976) points out that the "victim" cannot always be blamed and expected to correct the problem without changes also being made in the helping professions and public policy.

Commitment to the health of the community client requires a process of change from the individual, the family, and the community. One nursing role emphasizes individual and direct personal interventions, another nursing role focuses on the family as the unit of service, and a third centers on the community. The most successful change processes often arise from collaborative practice models that involve the community and nurses in joint decision making (Joyce et al., 2015). Nurses must remember that collaboration means shared roles and a cooperative effort in which participants want to work together. Participants must see themselves as part of a group effort and share in the process, beginning with planning and including decision making. This means sharing not only the power but also the responsibility for the outcomes of the intervention. Viewing the community as client and thus as the target of service means a commitment to two key concepts: (1) community health and (2) partnership. These two concepts form not only the *goal* (community health) but also the *means* of population-centered practice (partnership).

Goals and Means of the Community as Client

Population-centered practice seeks healthful change for the whole community's benefit (Fawcett et al., 2015). Although the nurse may work with individuals, families or other groups, aggregates, or institutions, the resulting changes are intended to affect the whole community. For example, an occupational health nurse's target typically includes preventing illness and injury and maintaining or promoting the health of an entire company workforce. Because of this focus, the nurse might help an individual disabled worker to become independent in activities of daily living. The nurse could also take action to make the whole community better able to support persons with disabilities. These actions might include promoting vocational rehabilitation services in the community and advocating for local policies that improve equal opportunities for disabled workers.

PHNs join professionals from many other fields in fulfilling the core functions of assessment, assurance, and policy development for the ten essential public health services (CDC, 2018b) (see Chapter 1). The community assessment process described in this chapter is a key role of PHNs. The findings of the assessment process guide actions of *assurance*, or ensuring that all community members have access to high-quality health services. *Policy development* includes informing and mobilizing community members to advocate for business and government policies that improve health.

The community as client perspective guides decisions about allocation of resources and services to create the greatest benefit for the community. Sometimes this means spreading the benefit

---

BOX 13.1 Ethical Concepts Applied to a Community's Health

- **Utilitarianism** means doing the greatest good for the greatest number of people.
- **Distributive justice** means treating people fairly and distributing resources and burdens equitably among the members of a society.
- **Social justice** means ensuring that vulnerable groups are included in equitable distribution of resources.

---

to as many people as possible in the community. For example, clean air and water are resources needed by everyone in a community. At other times, the community will experience the greatest benefit if resources are prioritized for groups within the community who are in high-risk categories. Three main ethical concepts that guide the community as client perspective are utilitarianism, distributive justice, and social justice (Box 13.1).

The outcomes of these concepts should be a reduction in health disparities between privileged and marginalized social groups. Nurses can use these concepts to carefully consider how to best allocate scarce resources, such as health services and funding, in ways that benefit the whole community. More information on ethics in community practice is found in other chapters of this book.

COMMUNITY HEALTH

Community health is reflected in the health behaviors and subsequent outcomes of its residents and also by the ability of the community as a system to support healthy individuals. Nurses caring for the community as the client identify effects that these complex community parts have on individuals' health; they work with all parts of a community to achieve the goal of a healthy community. Betty Neuman's Health Care Systems Model illustrates this system well (Beckman and Fawcett, 2017).

Neuman's model views systems as greater than the sum of their parts; the strength of each part of a community and the synergy between these parts contribute to the ability of its residents to be healthy. Community systems provide stability and protection from chronic or sudden stressors such as homelessness, health declines, disease outbreaks, or disasters, like the COVID-19 pandemic.

The WHO (2014) describes four aims of healthy communities as:

(1) supporting individual health,
(2) promoting quality of life,
(3) distributing the resources needed for basic sanitation and hygiene, and
(4) creating accessible health care services.

Healthy People 2030

An important guideline available for nurses working to improve the health of the community is *Healthy People 2030,* a publication from the US Department of Health and Human Services (USDHHS, 2020). It offers a vision of the future for public health and specific objectives to help attain that vision.

The *Healthy People 2030* vision recognizes the need to work collectively, in community partnerships, to bring about the changes that will be necessary to fulfill this vision. PHNs can be an integral part of making this happen. *Healthy People 2030* provides the foundation for a national health promotion and disease prevention strategy built on five goals:

- Attain healthy, thriving lives and well-being, free of preventable disease, disability, injury, and premature death.
- Eliminate health disparities, achieve health equity, and attain health literacy to improve the health and well-being of all.
- Create social, physical, and economic environments that promote attaining full potential for health and well-being for all.
- Promote healthy development, healthy behaviors and well-being across all life stages.
- Engage leadership, key constituents, and the public across multiple sectors to take action and design policies that improve the health and well-being of all.

Healthy People helps to access data on changes in the health status of the US population; these data also inform each new decade's goals and objectives. Communities across the United States are encouraged to adopt *Healthy People* goals and objectives. Communities, which may be as small as neighborhoods or large as municipalities, may alter the goals and objectives to meet their own needs, and/or use them to set priorities for their region and population groups. *Healthy People* priorities are those aspects of health that are the most critical to overall health and well-being and can be improved using our available knowledge (USDHHS, 2020).

Community Partnerships

Partnering with community members is a key element of a successful community health program or intervention. Involving community members not only in the data collection process, but in all phases of the assessment, ensures that the data collected are more accurate and more relevant to the concerns of the community. Partnerships also promote community members' investment in the success of the assessment and in the resulting projects to improve community health. Therefore successful strategies for improving community health must include community partnerships as the basic means or key for improvement. Some community assessment models feature community partnerships as a central activity, such as **Mobilizing for Action through Planning and Partnerships (MAPP)** (National Association of County and City Health Officials [NACCHO], 2016).

Nurse-community partnerships can take many forms. A successful democratic partnership requires hard work from all parties and is usually achieved only through a long-term commitment to the process, wherein diverse community members and health care professionals share all resources and work equitably. Coalitions are formal partnerships in which individuals and organizations serve in defined capacities such as steering committees, advisory committees, and work groups. Coalitions are *active partnerships*, in which all participants share leadership and decision making to some degree. Unfortunately, some community health efforts view community residents only as sources of information and receivers of interventions; this limits residents to *passive participation*. Passive participation is a negative nurse-community partnership approach. A positive approach is one in which all partners are actively involved and share power in assessing, planning, and implementing needed community changes (Ocloo and Matthews, 2016).

Community members who are recognized as community leaders (whether professionals, pastors, government officials, or interested citizens) possess credibility and skills that health professionals often lack. The community member–professional partnership approach specifically emphasizes active participation of the community or its representatives in healthy change (Jagosh et al., 2015).

Partnership, as defined here, is an essential concept for nurses to know and use, as are the concepts of community, community as client, and community health. Experienced nurses know that partnership is important because health is not a static reality but is continuously generated through new and increasingly effective means of community member–professional collaboration. Other active professional service providers such as schoolteachers, public safety officers, and agricultural extension agents play a large part in the overall health of the community. A partnership in identifying strengths and problems and in setting goals is especially important because it brings commitment from all persons involved, an essential component of successful change.

Partnerships involving nurses working with community organizations offer one of the most effective means for interventions because they actively involve the community and build on existing community strengths. Nurses working with community groups and organizations can fulfill many different roles including media advocacy, political action, community-based health communication, social marketing, and outreach facilitation. Regardless of what roles nurses fulfill as their contribution to the partnership, they must remember to "start where the people are" (Minkler 2012).

Kaiser and colleagues (2017) looked at the challenges and possible solutions in developing partnerships with communities. Community partnerships involve both influence and power, respecting voices of all community members, nurses doing *with* rather than *to* the partner, while recognizing the partner's role throughout the process as active and empowered, not passive. Mutually determined goals and plans of action, and the assignment of roles and responsibilities, are negotiated. Through the goal is that community partners become more effective at working independently to solve and prioritize their own problems and make their own decisions and being active in the change process.

The PHNs must work hard to include members of a setting, neighborhood, or organization while developing trust and providing the community with a central role throughout the process.

One historical example of a nurse-community partnership remains an inspiring story of this important work (Box 13.2).

The Nurse's Role in the Community

The nurse's ability to establish credibility and trust in the community is important in doing a complete community assessment. The nurse may be considered to be an *insider* if he or she

BOX 13.2 Nurse and Community Partnership for Change

Nancy Milio was a young, White PHN when she began working with an inner-city African American community in Detroit during the 1960s. Together, she and community members identified needs and designed a program to meet them. Milio's painstaking process of working *with* the community to create a Moms and Tots Center, where mothers and children could access primary health care and child care, is a sentinel example of community partnership. The true value of this partnership was demonstrated when the Detroit riots occurred in 1967, and the storefront where the clinic was located remained intact while surrounding structures burned; the local rioters had spared the clinic because it "belonged to the people" (Milio, 2000; DeGuzman and Keeling, 2012).

grew up in the community, has personal ties to the people there, or comes from a similar cultural or ethnic background. This may increase community members' willingness to speak openly and partner with the nurse, unless this status disadvantages or compromises the nurse's impartiality or objectivity. Nurses who are new to the community or have few insider connections can increase their familiarity with the community and its residents through taking part in informal community activities, such as shopping, attending church, or participating in organizations. They can also partner with trusted insiders in the community, such as *gatekeepers* and *community health workers* (CHWs).

Gatekeepers refer to formal or informal community leaders who create opportunities for nurses to meet diverse members of the community (Kaiser et al., 2017). For example, a church pastor may act as a gatekeeper by introducing a nurse to the congregation, thus increasing the likelihood that the church members will trust the nurse enough to provide information or to serve as partners in the assessment and throughout any planning, intervention, and evaluation.

CHWs are not professional or licensed health care providers but are community members from diverse backgrounds who receive training to do health outreach work. CHWs can assist nurses in doing community health assessments in several ways. They extend the reach of the nurse by being able to do many activities that are part of the community assessment process. They can also serve as gatekeepers, using their own insider status to engage community members in the assessment process (Olaniran, 2017).

COMMUNITY AS PARTNER: THE PROCESS FROM ASSESSMENT TO EVALUATION

Community Assessment

Community assessment put quite simply is taking detailed stock of a community both from the outside in and from the inside out for the purpose of identifying and analyzing conditions therein. Community assessment, sometimes called community needs assessment, is one of three core functions of public health. This process requires clinical judgment and critical appraisal of multiple types of data from a variety of sources, and it requires a clear knowledge and understanding of the community as client. People, place, and function are the foundational dimensions of a community and need to be defined as part of the assessment process. These dimensions guide the gathering of data. Data can be primary or secondary. There might be many reasons for conducting a community assessment, but for public health nursing the purpose is usually to identify community health needs and to develop strategies to address them. The purpose of this section is to provide a clear method for completing a comprehensive community assessment, using the tools of the nursing process adapted to communities. The CDC (2015) offers a clear set of common elements that constitute a community assessment (Box 13.3). An example of Santa Cruz, California's very comprehensive and ongoing community assessment (2017) can be accessed at https://www.appliedsurveyresearch.org/scccap/.

Why Community Assessment?

Community assessments may be done for various reasons. For example, a PHN and a community may want to:

- conduct an assessment to learn more about community needs or strengths,
- locate confirmation data to address a recognized community problem,
- focus on setting priorities to address health issues in communities.

Organizations may also be required to complete community assessments for regulatory or accreditation standards. For example, the Affordable Care Act directed nonprofit hospitals to perform community health needs assessments. In some cases, administrators will perform these assessments, but PHNs are ideal choices to lead the community in this required activity. Public health personnel are the recognized experts in this arena.

CHECK YOUR PRACTICE

As a senior nursing student, you have been asked by the local health department to conduct a community assessment of the central district of the city. What would you do? How would you approach this assignment? See if you can apply these steps to this scenario. (1) Recognize the cues, looking at available data from past assessments in your community and the state; (2) analyze the cues looking at issues related to the central district; (3) state several and prioritize the hypotheses you have stated; (4) generate solutions for each hypothesis; (5) take action on the number one hypothesis you think best reflects what is going on in central district and compare with the community at large; and (6) evaluate the outcomes you would expect as a result of this assessment.

BOX 13.3 Common Elements of Assessment and Planning Frameworks

- Organize and plan
- Engage the community
- Develop a goal or vision
- Conduct community health assessment(s)
- Prioritize health issues
- Develop community health improvement plan (in this case, Nursing Diagnosis)
- Implement and monitor community health improvement plan
- Evaluate process and outcomes

Source: CDC *Assessment and Planning Models, Frameworks and Tools* 2014A, www.cdc.gov/stltpublichealth/ch/assessment.html.

The recent formation of the Public Health Department Accreditation Board placed responsibility to implement standards for uniform performance with health departments in the United States. These standards include enhanced surveillance of community health services through regularly conducted community assessments (Swider et al., 2017).

Assessment is one of the three core functions of public health (CDC Core Functions, 2011). Public health nursing places assessment at the forefront of PHN competencies. The Quad Council Coalition of public health nursing (2018) has defined community/public health nursing competencies to include six major domains across three levels of practice. The domain of assessment and analytic skills (Box 13.4) details the competencies specific to community assessment across the first tier of public health nursing practice. This first level is applied to beginning and staff PHNs.

Assessing the health of the community requires a broad definition of health, including consideration of the economic, social, physical, and mental health of the population. Access to resources that provide for these broad needs and services will be part of the assessment process.

The PHN should place the assessment of community strengths as high on the list, while recognizing limitations as problems in the development of an assessment plan. It is important to value both strengths and problems in the assessment, planning, implementation, and evaluation process.

Communities have both resources and needs. A balanced approach to the assessment, highlights community strengths, often referred to as assets, as well as problems to identify the community vehicles already present for positive change. Community strengths can later be called upon in the planning and intervention phases of the process to address the challenges the community faces. This strength-based approach may be better received by communities and funders, and promotes the inclusion of key informants and interested stakeholders; it can make strategic planning a part of the process.

Data Sources—Types

Measures of health status take more than one form. Numeric data put out by a recognized agency (e.g., the US Census Bureau, CDC, or Robert Wood Johnson Foundation) are referred to as secondary data (collected by someone else). Secondary data are obtained through existing reports on the community, including census, vital statistics, and numeric reports (e.g., morbidity and mortality information or information from reference books).

Information that is gleaned from telephone surveys, personal interviews, or focus groups conducted by those who are assessing the community, or derived from personal connections or key informants, is considered primary data. Primary data are collected directly through interaction with community members, which may include community leaders or interested stakeholders.

Community assessment requires both types of data and are included when analyzing the assessment data for a comprehensive view of the community.

Health Indicators—Secondary Sources of Data

Even before setting foot in the community it is possible to learn a great deal about its residents' health status. Health indicators are numeric measures of health outcomes, such as morbidity and mortality, as well as determinants of health and population characteristics. In general, these data are from *secondary* sources such as websites or printed materials. Table 13.1 lists several of these sources.

Creation of a set of health indicator data during a community health assessment serves several purposes. First, it creates a "snapshot" of health conditions that can guide the assessment team during the analysis and problem prioritization phases. Second, it is an important and easily comprehensible means of communicating the results of the assessment to the larger community. Third, it is an effective way to compare the current health status in the community with the same community at different time points, with other communities, or with larger populations such as state or national data.

There are two important considerations for selecting which indicators to include in an assessment: the priorities of the community and comparability with other data. Ideally, diverse community stakeholders should participate in identifying health indicators that address their interests or concerns. Stakeholders include anyone with a personal or occupational interest or concern in a community's life. If the health indicators are to be compared with other assessments, then use similar measures when possible. For example, the total number of deaths in a

---

BOX 13.4   Assessment and Analytic Skills

1A1. Assess the health status and health literacy of individuals and families, including determinants of health, using multiple sources of data.

1A2a. Use an ecological perspective and epidemiologic data to identify health risks for a population.

1A2b. Identify individual and family assets, needs, values, beliefs, resources, and relevant environmental factors.

1A3. Select variables that measure health and public health conditions.

1A4. Use a data collection plan that incorporates valid and reliable methods and instruments for collection of qualitative and quantitative data to inform the service for individuals, families, and a community.

1A5. Interpret valid and reliable data that impacts the health of individuals, families, and communities to make comparisons that are understandable to all who were involved in the assessment process.

1A6. Compare appropriate data sources in a community.

1A7. Contribute to comprehensive community health assessments through the application of quantitative and qualitative public health nursing data.

1A8. Apply ethical, legal, and policy guidelines and principles in the collection, maintenance, use, and dissemination of data and information.

1A9. Use varied approaches in the identification of community needs (i.e., focus groups, multisector collaboration, SWOT analysis).

1A10. Use *information technology* effectively to collect, analyze, store, and retrieve data related to public health nursing services for individuals, families, and groups.

1A11. Use evidence-based strategies or promising practices from across disciplines to promote health in communities and populations.

1A12. Use available data and resources related to the determinants of health when planning services for individuals, families, and groups.

SWOT, Strengths, Weaknesses, Opportunities and Threats Analysis done within the community.

TABLE 13.1	Frequently Used Secondary Sources for Health Indicator Data	
Behavioral Risk Factors Surveillance Survey (BRFSS)	http://www.cdc.gov	Wide variety of data on individuals' health status, health behaviors, and preventive health services
CDC Social Determinants of Health	https://www.cdc.gov	CDC-supported data on income, education level, employment, social vulnerability, and health conditions
CDC Wonder	http://wonder.cdc.gov/	Public health data on births, mortality, infectious diseases, cancer, and environment
County Health Rankings	http://www.countyhealthrankings.org/	Collates county-level data on a wide range of health outcomes and health determinants
Dartmouth Atlas of Health Care	http://www.dartmouthatlas.org	Distribution and outcomes of health care services, in chart and map formats
Local advocacy organizations		Organizations that specialize in social issues such as homelessness, child abuse, or domestic violence
National Center for Health Statistics: FastStats	https://www.cdc.gov	US government website that gathers data from multiple sources and provides an extensive topic index
State Cancer Profile	http://statecancerprofiles.cancer.gov	Incidence of cancer types by race/ethnicity, sex, and geography
State Health Access Data Assistance Center (SHADAC)	http://statehealthcompare.shadac.org/	Provides access to data about health statistics by demographic breakdown. Statistics can be compared state to state.
US Census	http://www.census.gov	Demographic and economic data

CDC, Centers for Disease Control and Prevention.

BOX 13.5 Secondary Source Data Questions

Questions to ask about data from secondary sources:
- How current is the reported information?
- When was the site last updated?
- How credible is the data source?
- Is an author identified?
- Are demographic data reported about the people?
- Are data reported about different community systems?
- Is there any obvious bias in the reporting of data?
- Are community voices represented?

---

community is different from the annual rate of deaths per 100,000 population. Box 13.5 gives additional tips on obtaining high-quality data.

Healthy People 2030 and County Health Rankings are useful resources for health indicators. The County Health Rankings report is updated annually and provides county-level data for a wide variety of health indicators, and also compares county rankings within and across states (www.countyhealthrankings.org).

Health Indicators—Primary Sources of Data

Primary data involve the researcher or community members at the community level. Various methods can be used to collect the data such as participant observation, key informant interviews, surveys, town hall meetings, focus groups, Photovoice, spatial data, or windshield surveys. Participant observation refers to the deliberate sharing in the life of a community, for example, participating in a local fair or festival or attending a political or social event. Visiting or attending an event can be a window through which to view the community. In addition, participant observation can be a fun way to experience community events.

Key informants can be identified through formal or informal channels in the community. Meeting with key informants and identifying local issues, strengths, and concerns from their viewpoint constitutes an important component of the overall assessment. See How To box for more information.

HOW TO IDENTIFY A KEY INFORMANT
- Talking to key informants is a critical part of the community assessment.
- Key informants are not always people who have a formal title or position.
- Key informants often have an informal role within the community.
- County health department nurses and church leaders are often key informants. They also know many community members and can identify other key informants.

Town hall meetings are opportunities for local constituents to come together, usually to discuss a particular issue or proposal that influences all members of the community. Many town hall meetings have been held recently, for example, to address the issue of health care reform.

A focus group is similar to an interview in that it collects data mainly through asking open-ended questions to a small group rather than an individual to prompt discussions or generate ideas that individual interviews might not. Focus groups work well when the topic is not a sensitive one and participants feel comfortable speaking out about the issue with the group.

Some details regarding focus groups include:
- They should be structured to balance a diversity of perspectives with opportunities for in-depth understanding of the chosen topics.
- The question guide should address the goals for the data: for example, a free-flowing discussion of ideas or obtain specific information from each participant.
- Up to 6 to 8 participants who are homogenous in characteristics should be recruited through community channels such

as churches, associations, and other places where people gather (Guest et al., 2017; Vance et al., 2017).

• One moderator leads the discussion, an assistant takes written notes, and the session is often audio recorded, then transcribed and included in the analysis.

Photovoice

Photovoice, also called photo elicitation, is a community assessment technique in which community members take photos to represent a topic or theme about community health (Lennon-Dearing and Price, 2018). Photovoice has been used with many types of community participants but can be especially useful in working with groups that may be marginalized or have little power, such as youths, the elderly, individuals living in poverty, or those involved in substance abuse. Photovoice is a way for participants to communicate powerful messages about their experiences, without the need for words.

The basic process to incorporate Photovoice into a community assessment is in the following How To Box.

HOW TO USE PHOTOVOICE IN COMMUNITY ASSESSMENT

• **Train community participants:** in Photovoice methods, including the topic of interest, basic photography techniques, obtaining written consent and ethical and safety issues.

• **Take photos:** Participants take the cameras into their communities and take photographs that reflect the topic.

• **Display photos:** The photos are collected from the participants and then printed or digitally projected for group participants, and sometimes members of the public, to view them.

• **Discuss photos:** Viewing the photos is meant to spark discussions that provide additional information about the topic of interest to raise awareness and to start conversations among diverse stakeholders.

• **Analyze and report results:** Analyze the information gathered by participants in photovoice activity and through discussions, and with photos, report to the community about the findings of the community assessment (Florian, 2016).

Spatial Data

Most of the information gathered in a community assessment has a spatial component; it is located somewhere in the community like health care services, food stores, schools, bus routes, factories, highways, bodies of water, and parks. Demographic data can also be spatial. These data can be collected in neighborhood or other areas about residents, such as age, racial or ethnic background, health characteristics, income, home value, and crime rates. This defines the population for the community assessment. By assessing the spatial distribution of health resources and disparities, programs can be placed where the impact will be greatest for the population.

Maps are useful in compiling spatial data from primary or secondary sources. Maps can support decision making about community health priorities. Later, maps can be used to plan programs and interventions and communicating the findings to a wide range of stakeholders and encouraging their participation in discussions about the findings.

During a community assessment, spatial data can be collected in several ways. One low-tech approach is to note the address or nearest street intersection of a place and later draw it onto a map. For example, a public health study analyzed geographic data for demographic patterns of poor birth outcomes in an urban area (MacQuillan et al., 2017). They found that children living near a major roadway were much more likely to experience hospital admissions for asthma.

Community Health Assessment Models

There are many existing models of community health assessment, making it possible to conduct an assessment without the need to design the process from scratch. Table 13.2 provides examples of commonly used models that assess for a broad array of community health concerns. The WHO's Healthy Cities initiative offers another approach to population-centered health assessment. An example of the assessment data that support this approach is found at http://www.healthycity.org.

Other assessment models focus on specific topics. For example, the CDC (2018) developed the Community Assessment for Public Health Emergency Response (CASPER) toolkit for rapid needs assessment of communities affected by disasters or other emergencies. Another example is the Built Environment Assessment Tool Manual, a toolkit to assess the human-built features of a community that affect physical activity, nutrition, and other aspects of health (physical and social aspects of a community related to walking and bicycling) (CDC, 2017).

Selecting an assessment model or designing your own can be guided by several criteria. What are your goals for the assessment? What are the resources available for the assessment project, such as time, people, budget, and access to the community? Is there an existing model that aligns with your goals and is feasible in terms of your available resources? (See Chapter 18 for How To develop a Program. This can be applied to the assessment of the community.)

COMMUNITY AS PARTNER

The community-as-partner model is based on nursing processes and theories and emphasizes the dynamic nature of community systems as integral to the health of residents (Anderson and McFarlane, 2015). A key feature of this model is its division of the community structure into subsystems that can serve as an organizational structure for community health assessments. The subsystems of the community structure consist of physical environment, health and social services, economy, transportation and safety, politics and government, communication, education, and recreation. Each of these subsystems represents distinct functions and organizations within the community that can be assessed separately. However, they also interact to create the complex community environment in which people live and function. Each subsystem may protect the health of community members by addressing a particular need. Understanding the relative success of each of these subsystems in promoting health and safety can provide important insights about the community's ability to respond to health problems.

TABLE 13.2 Interprofessional Community Health Assessment Models

Assessment Model	Example
Health Impact Assessment (HIA) is a process to predict the effects on health from projects or policies such as land use, community design, transportation, or industrial facilities. The outcome of an HIA is to provide recommendations to minimize negative health impacts, and monitor results. *Learn more at https://www.naccho.org.*	Community officials in East Aldine District, a suburb of Houston, Texas, worked with health researchers to perform an HIA on a proposed town center development for this previously rural area. The HIA found positive health impacts such as better access to healthy food retailers and health care facilities, and enhanced opportunities for physical activity and active transport. These were predicted to improve health of economically vulnerable residents, such as those without cars and the elderly (Cummings et al., 2016).
Mobilizing for Action through Planning and Partnerships (MAPP) is a strategic planning process to select high-priority public health issues and to match them with resources. Public health agencies lead the MAPP, but participation of community members and agencies is a major focus. *Learn more at https://www.naccho.org.*	A public health department in Virginia assessed the 5 counties and independent city in its district to identify top health issues needing action. Through partnerships with 61 agencies and gathering data from more than 2000 residents, the MAPP process selected top priorities as obesity, mental health and substance abuse, pregnancy outcomes, and tobacco use (Thomas Jefferson Health District, 2016).
Community Health Assessment and Group Evaluation (CHANGE) is a tool to help communities annually gather and organize data about community health, plan programs, and monitor changes over time. Five community sectors are assessed: community at large, community institution/organization, health care, school, and work site. *Learn more at https://www.cdc.gov* (CDC, 2018).	Researchers in a rural Missouri county used the CHANGE tool to assess why rates of chronic disease were high. Through interviews with representatives from each of the five sectors, they identified challenges, assets, and potential partnerships for addressing chronic disease (Stewart, Visker, and Cox, 2013).
Community Health Needs Assessment (CHNA) is a set of guidelines for nonprofit hospitals to assess the communities they serve, and is a requirement under the Patient Protection and Affordable Care Act (ACA). Community input and other sources provide data on priority health problems, barriers to health care access, and vulnerable populations. *Learn more at http://www.cdc.gov* (Rosenbaum 2013).	Nursing students partnered with a hospital in rural Minnesota to complete the CHNA. They gathered data through surveys and interviews with residents and organizational leaders. They identified three priority health problems, and differentiated assets and barriers to addressing these problems in different community institutions serving vulnerable populations (Madelia Community Hospital & Clinic, 2013).

HOW TO CONDUCT A COMMUNITY ASSESSMENT

Getting Started

In the previous section, several models of community assessment are discussed. This section will offer a step-by-step method to complete a community assessment. In beginning the assessment, the nurse should identify one model that will guide the assessment.

The community assessor(s) should plan to visit and interact in the community and collect data about *people, place,* and *function* over a month or more to get a feel for the community and create as full a picture as possible. A "feet on the ground" approach will yield rich data and visiting the community and interacting with its members is essential to the process. Very comprehensive assessments will require community coalitions and inclusion of key stakeholders, such as those included in MAPP assessments; expanding the participant group may extend this stage over many months or years (NACCHO: www.naccho.org).

The first step of the community assessment is to define the community and the geographic boundaries, the population within the boundaries, the purpose of the assessment, and a data collection plan identified.

Windshield Survey

Windshield surveys are a method of simple observation. They provide a quick overview of a community and can be used

along with photographs and interviews to get a general overall sense of the community (Table 13.3). This can be the first step in the process of generating data that help to identify the community, trends, stability, and changes that all serve to define the health of the community. The nurse riding in a vehicle can observe many dimensions of a community's life and environment through the windshield but walking the streets can also provide similar information. Under those circumstances, one can readily observe common characteristics of people in the community, neighborhood gathering places, the rhythm of community life, housing quality, and geographic boundaries (see How To box below and Table 13.3). A windshield survey can be used by itself for a short and simple assessment.

HOW TO OBTAIN A QUICK ASSESSMENT OF A COMMUNITY

One way to get a quick initial sense of the community is to do a windshield assessment, using a format like the one provided in Table 13.3.

Nurses interested in conducting a windshield assessment need to take public transportation, have someone else drive while they take notes, or plan to stop frequently to write down what they see.

The windshield survey example is organized into 15 elements with specific questions related to each element.

Nurses who use this approach will have an initial descriptive assessment of the community when they are finished.

If interventions are planned, a more thorough and more comprehensive process will be necessary.

TABLE 13.3 Windshield Survey Guidelines (Adapted)

Each community has its own characteristics. These characteristics along with demographic data provide valuable information in understanding the population that lives within the community and the health status, strengths/limitations, risks, and vulnerabilities unique to the "population of interest." Once you have defined a "community of interest" to assess, a *windshield survey* is the equivalent of a community head-to-toe assessment. The best way to conduct a windshield survey is with more than one person, allowing for one to observe and take notes. Having one pair of eyes on the road, you can benefit from having other individuals notice the unique characteristics of the community; a shared experience provides additional insight. As you analyze your findings, it may be necessary to make a second tour to fill in any blanks. Many of us take these characteristics for granted in our own community, but they provide a rich context for understanding communities and populations and often have significant impact on the health status of the community in general.

Elements	Description
Boundaries	What defines the boundary? Roads, water, railroads? Does the area have a name? A nickname?
Housing and zoning	What is the age of the houses? What kind of materials are used in the construction? Describe the housing, including space between them, general appearance and condition, and presence of central heating, air conditioning, and modern plumbing.
Open space	Describe the amount, condition, and use of open space. How is the space used? Is it safe? Attractive?
Commons	Where do people in the neighborhood hang out? Who hangs out there and at what hours during the day?
Transportation	How do people get from one place to another? If they use public transportation, what kind and how effective is it? How timely? Personal autos? Bikes, etc.? Are there pedestrians? Does the area appear to be safe?
Social service centers	Do you see evidence of recreation centers, parks, social services, offices of doctors, dentists, pharmacies?
Stores	Where do residents shop? How do they get to the shops? Do they have groceries or sources of fresh produce? Is this a "food desert"?
Street people and animals	Who do you see on the streets during the day? Besides the people, do you see animals? Are they loose or contained?
Condition of the area	Is the area well kept, or is there evidence of trash, abandoned cars or houses? What kind of information is provided on the signs in the area?
Race and ethnicity	What is the racial mix of the people you see? What do you see about indices of ethnicity? Places of worship, food stores, restaurants? Are signs in English or other languages? (If the latter, which ones)?
Religion	What indications do you see about the types of religion residents practice?
Health indicators	Do you see evidence of clinics, hospitals, mental illness, and/or substance abuse?
Politics	What indicators do you see about politics? Posters, headquarters?
Media	Do you see indicators of what people read? If they watch television? Listen to the radio? Can you tell if residents use social media? Availability of Internet?
Business and industry	What type of business climate exists? Manufacturers? Light or heavy industry? Large employers? Small business owners? Retail? Hospitality industry? Military installation? Do people have to seek employment elsewhere?

Adapted and revised by M. Gibson & J. Lancaster from: Mizrahi TM: School of Social Work, Virginia Commonwealth University, Richmond VA, September 2008; Stanhope MS, Knollmueller RN: *Public and Community Health Nurse's Consultant: A Health Promotion Guide*, St. Louis, 1997, Mosby.

Community "Place" and "People" Identified

The first step of the community assessment is to define the community (i.e., geographic boundaries, the population within the boundaries, the purpose of the assessment, and a data collection plan identified).

Morbidity and mortality data should be tabulated identifying the top three causes of morbidity and mortality and also comparing the local data to the state, national, and previous years' local data. Are there conditions in the causes of illness or death that are rising or declining according to past data? Looking at this information and linking with the information derived from primary data will help to focus priorities. Identifying health indicators such as obesity rates, smoking rates, and causes of morbidity and mortality can clarify the needs of the population to be served.

Identification of Health Assets and Challenges

Once you have pulled together your data into an organized format, the community problems and strengths should emerge. Using a targeted approach will help you to summarize these in

QSEN FOCUS ON QUALITY AND SAFETY EDUCATION FOR NURSES

Targeted Competency: Population-Centered Care—Recognizes the clients within the population served as the source of control and as a full partner in providing compassionate and coordinated care that is based on the preferences, values, and needs of the population.

- **Knowledge:** understanding of multiple dimensions of population-centered care
- **Skill:** for the community population elicits values, preferences, and expressed needs as part of interview of population representatives
- **Attitude:** show support for the population members whose values differ from one's own

Question

The Quad Council Coalition core competency of analytic and assessment skills indicates the beginning PHN should collect data, both quantitative and qualitative, to be used in community assessment. The PHN then assesses data collected as part of the community assessment process to make inferences about the populations (values, culture, preferences for health care)

To develop, revise, or even improve the population health care delivery, how would the PHN use the outcomes of the community assessment? What steps would the nurse take to make change based on population level choices?

a clear way. With the resulting "list" of identified problems and assets, you will be ready to prioritize your results (Box 13.6).

Prioritizing

Once the data are collated and clarified on paper, the themes can be placed in the context of the earlier identified community priorities. In this way, community involvement and input in the assessment process will make your assessment and planning relevant to the community and create the opportunity to meet the community's identified needs. Try to identify within your secondary data a rationale for the community's identified need. In other words, you might compromise. Attempting to implement programs that are not recognized as most relevant by the community can result in lack of community buy-in and ultimate program failure.

For example, although secondary data may document that increased mortality due to heart disease should be the community's highest priority as evidenced by higher-than-average mortality from heart disease, the community might see a different need, such as elder care or child care, as the highest priority. There is no clear guide in this prioritizing process but testing ideas about perceived need and actual data-driven information with community stakeholders and key informants helps the PHN come to an optimal way to prioritize problems and identify target areas for improvement. Just as in the hospital setting, make the patient (in this case, the community) the center of your focus. Box 13.6 can assist you in steps to prioritize the community problem list. Identifying the top three community problems or needs should then lead to creating the priority nursing diagnoses (see Use of Secondary Data Sources).

The ethical concepts of utilitarianism and justice can help you navigate the negotiations and advocacy inherent in prioritizing one health problem over another. A priority problem would ideally be one that affects a large proportion of the community. Social justice means advocating for the most vulnerable populations in a community, to ensure that their problems receive higher priority than the problems found throughout the general population. For example, secondary data might find that infant mortality occurs rarely in the community, but if there is a wide disparity among racial groups in infant mortality rates, social justice would call for this problem to be given higher priority in order to address underlying determinants of health that may cause the disparity.

BOX 13.6 Problem Priority Criteria

Criteria that have been helpful in ranking identified problems include the following:
- Community awareness of the problem
- Community motivation to resolve or better manage the problem
- Nurse's ability to influence problem solution
- Availability of expertise to solve the problem
- Severity of the outcomes if the problem is unresolved
- Speed with which the problem can be solved

Community Nursing Diagnosis

The community health nursing diagnosis in this phase of the process helps clarify the prioritized problems and is an important first step to planning. Community diagnoses clarify the target population for care and identify the factors contributing to the identified problem. As the analysis of the data proceeds, the implementation plan can be formed. In the planning phase, the PHN identifies community-focused interventions, along with ways to measure outcomes. At this point in the analysis of data, collaborating with community partners and colleagues will assist in the objectivity of the analysis and uncover potentially diverse data interpretations (Anderson and McFarlane, 2015). Community diagnoses should consider the community's strengths and assets. There are several standardized classification systems to accommodate this diagnosis formation. The Omaha system and the North American Nursing Diagnosis Association (NANDA) are two prominent systems of classification. NANDA includes several community diagnoses and health-seeking behaviors that can apply to communities, although certain diagnoses may require some adaptation to the community (Herdman and Kamitsuru, 2014). The NANDA system provides a useful format for the diagnosis statement but is confining in its strict parameters mostly limited to individual and family systems. It does not include much about community level diagnosis, but the format may be helpful to develop a community diagnosis.

This format includes:
- Identification of the problem:
- Its relation to factors, stressors, or health issues
- The supporting data that document the problem.

It is recommended that the use of this problem layout may be helpful. For example, a diagnosis statement might read: Increased level of infant mortality in Community X **related to** inadequate access to prenatal care, high teen birth rate and few obstetrical providers in city; **as evidenced by** infant mortality rate of 8 infant deaths per 1000 live births, a preterm birth rate of 15%, teen birth rate of 75/1000 females, and 3 obstetrical providers for a population of 30,000.

Community nursing diagnosis language must describe at the aggregate level—in other words, the community level—responses to actual and potential illnesses and life processes. This also means that the defining characteristics for community diagnoses must be observable and measurable at the aggregate level. To do this, community-level data must be used. The community survey data are an example of community-level data. The comparison of local data with state, regional, or national data, as rates and across multiple years, is one key means of identifying community-level problems, as well as patterns and trends.

The community nursing diagnosis drives the plan. The expected outcomes and evaluations derived from the nursing diagnosis systems suggest subsequent evaluation measures for identified needs or problems. Just as problems are recognized and prioritized, so can strengths be identified that may offer avenues through which the PHN can address existing challenges facing the community.

Planning, Implementation, and Evaluation

Once interventions and evaluation measures are identified through the nursing diagnosis framework, the PHN arrives at a new step in the nursing process—the planning phase. This includes analyzing and establishing priorities among community health problems already identified through nursing diagnosis, establishing goals and objectives, and identifying intervention activities for implementation that will accomplish the objectives. These interventions must be clearly supported by the community stakeholders in order for the community to buy in to the identified program plans. Intervention activities, the means by which objectives are met, are the strategies that clarify what must be done to achieve the objectives or the ways change will be effected. The next phase of the nursing process is program implementation. This involves enacting the plan for improved community health using the identified goals and objectives.

Finally, upon implementation of the program and by using the established evaluation measures, the PHN can measure the success of the program and determine community satisfaction with the outcome. These evaluation criteria will already be identified through the nursing diagnosis format chosen.

The planning and implementation strategies should be based on the community's problems AND its strengths, as well as the priorities of the community members. If the identified problem is not resolved to the satisfaction of the community at large following program implementation, the PHN will return to the data-gathering phase and begin the process again using the updated data. This can be an ongoing, circular process, just like the nursing process. After planning for implementation management, the evaluation of outcomes is the next step (see Chapter 18).

Personal Safety in Community Practice

Effective nursing practice starts with personal safety, and this remains important throughout the community assessment process. An awareness of the community and common sense are the two best guidelines for judgment. For example, common sense suggests not leaving anything valuable on a car seat and not leaving your car unlocked. Similar guidelines apply to the use of public transportation. Calling ahead to clients to schedule meetings will help prevent delays or confusion, and it gives the nurse an opportunity to lay the groundwork for the meeting. If there is no telephone and no access to a neighbor's telephone, plan to establish a time for any future meetings during the initial visit. Regardless of whether there has been telephone contact, there are rare situations when a meeting is postponed because the nurse arrives at a location where people are unexpectedly loitering by the entrance and the nurse has concerns about personal safety.

For nurses who either are just beginning their careers in the community or are just starting a new position, three clear sources of information will help answer many questions about personal safety:

1. *Other nurses, social workers, or health care providers who are familiar with the dynamics of a given community:* They can provide valuable insights into when to visit, how to get there, and what to expect, because they function in the community themselves.

2. *Community members:* The best sources of information about the community are the community members themselves, and one benefit of developing an active partnership with community members is their willingness to share their insight about day-to-day community life.

3. *The nurse's own observations:* Knowledge gained during the data collection phase of the process should provide a solid basis for an awareness of day-to-day community activity. Nurses with experience practicing in the community generally agree that if they feel uncomfortable in a situation, they should trust their instincts and leave.

▶▶ APPLYING CONTENT TO PRACTICE

In this chapter, the focus is placed on the partnership between the public health nurse and the community throughout the process of community assessment, problem identification, planning, intervention, and evaluation. One of the Institute of Medicine's (IOM) three core functions of public health is assessment. The process of community assessment outlined and described in this chapter closely follows The Council on Linkages' *Core Competencies for Public Health* (adopted June 26, 2014). This includes the need for public health nurses to "maintain relationships that improve health in a community." Among other identified competencies for public health providers, including public health nurses, is that one "assesses community health status and factors influencing health in a community (e.g., quality, availability, accessibility, and use of health services; access to affordable housing)." This chapter presents the means by which public health nurses can construct a composite database containing assessment data from a wide variety of sources. This initial community assessment phase also directly links with The Quad Council Domains of Public Health Practice: Domain #1: Assessment and Analytic Skills; Domain #5: Community Dimensions of Practice Skills; and Domain #6: Public Health Sciences Skills. The Council on Linkages' *Core Competencies for Public Health* also emphasizes the public health nurse's ability to develop "community health assessments using information about health status, factors influencing health, and assets and resources." Development of goals and objectives along with their problem correlates as part of the community health assessment directly relates to this competency.

■ PRACTICE APPLICATION

Lily, a nurse in a small city, became aware of the increased incidence of respiratory diseases through the windshield survey conducted by a public health team and the data collected. After speaking with the local chapter of the American Lung Association, and during family visits, Lily noticed that many members of the population and parents were smokers. Because most of the families Lily visited had small children, she became concerned about the effects of secondhand smoke on the health of the infants and children in her family population caseload.

Further review of her windshield assessment of this community indicated that the community recognized several problems, including school safety and the risk of water pollution, in addition to the smoking problem that Lily had identified. Talks with different community members revealed that they wanted each of these identified problems "fixed," although these same community members were uncertain about how to start. In deciding which of the three identified problems to address first, which criterion would be most important for Lily to consider?

A. The amount of money available

B. The level of community motivation to "fix" one of the three identified problems

C. The number of people in the community who expressed a concern about each of the three identified problems

D. How much control she would have in the process

Answers can be found on the Evolve website.

REMEMBER THIS!

- Most definitions of community include three dimensions: (1) networks of interpersonal relationships that provide friendship and support to members, (2) residence in a common locality, and (3) shared values, interests, or concerns.
- A community is defined as a locality-based entity, composed of systems of formal organizations reflecting societal institutions, informal groups, and aggregates that are interdependent and whose function or expressed intent is to meet a wide variety of collective needs.
- A community practice setting is insufficient reason for stating that practice is oriented toward the community client. When the location of the practice is in the community but the focus of the practice is the individual or family, the nursing client remains the individual or family, not the whole community.
- Population-centered practice is targeted to the community—the population group in which healthful change is sought.
- Community health as used in this chapter is defined as the meeting of collective needs through identification of problems and management of behaviors within the community itself and between the community and the larger society.
- Most changes aimed at improving community health involve, out of necessity, partnerships among community residents and health workers from a variety of disciplines.
- Assessing community health requires gathering existing data and interpreting the database.
- Five methods of collecting data useful to the nurse are analysis of existing secondary data, conducting windshield surveys, and primary data collection through informant interviews, participant observation, or surveys.
- Nurses should identify and partner with gatekeepers, formal or informal community leaders, to gain entry or acceptance into the community.
- The planning phase includes analyzing and establishing priorities among community health problems already identified, establishing goals and objectives, and identifying intervention activities that will accomplish the objectives.
- Once high-priority problems are identified, broad relevant goals and objectives are developed; the goal is generally a broad statement of the desired outcome, and the objectives are precise statements of the desired outcome.
- Intervention activities, the means by which objectives are met, are the strategies that clarify what must be done to achieve the objectives, the ways change will be effected, and the way the problem will be interpreted.

- Implementation, the next phase of the nursing process, means transforming a plan for improved community health into achieving goals and objectives.
- Simply defined, evaluation is the appraisal of the effects of some organized activity.

EVOLVE WEBSITE

http://evolve.elsevier.com/Stanhope/foundations
- Case Study, with Questions and Answers
- NCLEX® Review Questions
- Practice Application Answers

REFERENCES

Anderson ET, McFarlane J: *Community as Partner: Theory and Practice in Nursing*, ed 6. Philadelphia, 2015, Lippincott Williams & Wilkins.

Applied Survey Research, Santa Cruz County Community Assessment Project, year 23, 2017. Available at https://www.appliedsurveyresearch.org . Accessed June 22, 2018.

Beckman, Sarah and Fawcett, Jacqueline, "Neuman Systems Model: Celebrating Academic-Practice Partnerships" (2017). *IPFW eBooks*. 1. https://opus.ipfw.edu.

Boyd R, Richerson PJ: Culture and the evolution of human cooperation. *Philosophical Transactions of the Royal Society B: Biological Sciences*, 364(1533): 3281-3288, 2009.

CDC: *Preparedness and Response for Public Health Disasters: Community Assessment for Public Health Emergency Response (CASPER)*, 2018. Available at https://www.cdc.gov. Accessed May 22, 2018.

CDC: *Trends in Current Cigarette Smoking among Adults, United States*, 2018a. Available at http://www.cdc.gov. Accessed Sept 1, 2018.

CDC: *Assessment & planning models, frameworks & tools*. 2015. Available at http://www.cdc.gov Accessed April 25, 2018.

CDC. Core Functions of Public Health and How they Relate to the 10 Essential Services https://www.cdc.gov. 2011 Accessed Sept. 1. 2018b

CDC. Ten essential public health services and how they include addressing social determinants of health inequities. Available at https://www.cdc.gov. Accessed June 16, 2018.

CDC. *The Built Environment Assessment Tool Manual*, 2017. Available at https://www.cdc.gov. Available at May 15, 2018.

DeGuzman PB, Keeling AW: Addressing disparities in access to care: lessons from the Kercheval Street Clinic in the 1960's. *Policy Polit Nurs Pract* 12(4):199–207, 2012.

Fawcett J, Ellenbecker CH. A proposed conceptual model of nursing and population health, *Nursing outlook*. 63(3):288-98, 2015.

Feldman D, Thayer A, Wall M, et al: *The 2017 Millennial Impact Report: An Invigorated Generation for Causes and Social Issues. 2017*. Available at http://www.themillennialimpact.com. Accessed June 15, 2018.

Florian J, Roy NM, Quintiliani LM, Truong V, Feng Y, Bloch PP, et al. Using Photovoice and Asset Mapping to Inform a Community-Based Diabetes Intervention, Boston, Massachusetts, 2015. *Prev Chronic Dis* 2016;13:160160.

Guest G, Namey E, McKenna K: How many focus groups are enough? Building an evidence base for nonprobability sample sizes, *Field Methods* Feb;29(1):3-22, 2017.

Herdman TH, Kamitsuru S (eds): *NANDA International Nursing Diagnoses: Definitions & Classification, 2015-2017*. Oxford, 2014, Wiley Blackwell.

Jagosh J, Bush PL, Salsberg J, et al: A realist evaluation of community-based participatory research: partnership synergy, trust building and related ripple effects, *BMC Public Health* 15(1):725, 2015.

Joyce BL, Harmon MJ, Pilling LB, et al: The preparation of community/public health nurses: Amplifying the impact, *Public Health Nursing* 32(6):595-7, 2015.

Kaiser BL, Thomas GR, Bowers BJ: A case study of engaging hard-to-reach participants in the research process: Community Advisors on Research Design and Strategies (CARDS)®, *Research in Nursing & Health*: 40(1):70-9, 2017.

Lennon-Dearing & Price: Women living with HIV tell their stories with photvoice. *Journal of Human Behavior in the Social Environment*, 2018.

MacQueen KM, McLellan E, Metzger DS, et al: What is community? An evidence-based definition for participatory public health, *Am J Public Health: 91(12):1929–1938, 2001.*

MacQuillan EL, Curtis AB, Baker KM, et al: Using GIS mapping to target public health interventions: examining birth outcomes across GIS techniques. *Journal of Community Health*. 42(4):633-8, 2017.

Mercy Corps: Driving resilience: Market approaches to disaster recovery Sept 2017, Portland Oregon

Milio N: 9226 *Kercheval: The Storefront that Did Not Burn*. Ann Arbor, MI, 2000, University of Michigan.

Minkler M: *Community Organizing and Community Building for Health and Welfare*, New Brunswick, NJ, 2012, Rutgers University Press.

National Association of County and City Health Officials NACCHO): *Mobilizing for Action through Planning and Partnerships (MAPP)*, 2016. Available at http://www.naccho.org. Accessed June 22, 2018.

Ocloo J, Matthews R. From tokenism to empowerment: progressing patient and public involvement in healthcare improvement. *BMJ Qual Saf*. Mar 18:bmjqs-2015, 2016.

Olaniran, A, Smith H, Unkels R, Bar-Zeev S, van den Broek N: 2017. *Who is a community health worker? – a systematic review of definitions*. National Center for Biotechnology Information, U.S. National Library of Medicine 8600 Rockville Pike, Bethesda MD, 20894 USA.

Lennon-Dearing R, Price J: Women living with HIV tell their stories with photovoice. *J Human Behavior in the Social Env* Mar 2:1-4, 2018.

Quad Council Coalition Competency Review Task Force. (2018). *Community/Public Health Nursing Competencies*. Available at http://www.quadcouncilphn.org. Accessed June 21, 2018.

Ryan W, editor: *Blaming the victim*. New York, 1976, Free Press.

Sidorov J, Romney M: The Spectrum of Care. In Nash DB, Fabius RJ, Skoufalos A, Clarke JL, Horowitz MR (editors): *Population Health: Creating a Culture of Wellness*, ed. 2, Philadelphia, PA, 2016, Jones & Bartlett Learning.

Swider SM, Berkowitz B, Valentine-Maher S, et al: Engaging communities in creating health: leveraging community benefit. *Nurs Outlook* 65(5):657-60, 2017.

Thomas Jefferson Health District: *Mobilizing for Action Through Planning and Partnerships: MAPP 2 Health. 2016.* Available at http://www.vdh.virginia.gov. Accessed May 22, 2018.

USDHHS: *Healthy People 2030*. Washington DC, 2020, US Government Printing Office.

Vance DE, Gakumo CA, Childs GD, et al: Perceptions of brain health and cognition in older African Americans and Caucasians with HIV: a focus group study, *J Assoc Nurses in AIDS Care* 28(6): 862-76, 2017.

Windshield Survey. Adapted by J. Lancaster from: Mizrahi TM: School of Social Work, Virginia Commonwealth University, Richmond VA, 1992; Stanhope MS, Knollmueller RN: *Public and Community Health Nurse's Consultant: a Health Promotion Guide*, St. Louis, 1997, Mosby.

World Health Organization: *A glossary of terms for community health care and services for older persons.* In Centre for Health Development: Ageing and Health Technical Report, Vol 5. 2004. Available at http://www.who.int. Accessed March 7, 2014.

World Health Organization: *Preamble to the Constitution of the World Health Organization as adopted by the International Health Conference, New York, 19-22 June, 1946; signed on 22 July 1946 by the representatives of 61 States (Official Records of the World Health Organization, no. 2, p. 100) and entered into force on 7 April 1948.* Available at http://www.who.int. Accessed Sept. 1, 2018.

World Health Organization: *Types of healthy settings*, 2014. Available at http://www.who.int. Accessed March 7, 2014.

14

Health Education in the Community

Victoria P. Niederhauser

OBJECTIVES

After reading this chapter, the student should be able to:

1. Discuss ways that people learn.
2. Identify the steps and principles that guide health education.
3. Describe the importance of literacy, especially health literacy, in health promotion and health education.
4. Examine types of health education, including written, spoken, and social media.
5. Describe how nurses can work with groups to promote the health of individuals and communities.
6. Explore potential ethical issues that might arise in the practice of health education.

CHAPTER OUTLINE

KEY TERMS

One of the best ways to manage health care costs is to help people stay healthier. Nurses are ideal health care practitioners to lead in health promotion through health education because (1) they educate clients across all three levels of prevention: primary, secondary, and tertiary; and (2) they work with individuals, families, groups, and communities. The goal is to help clients attain optimal health, prevent health problems, identify and treat health problems early, and minimize disability. Education allows individuals to make knowledgeable health-related decisions, assume personal responsibility for their health, and cope effectively with alterations in their health and lifestyles. Often the goal in health promotion and health education is helping clients change their behaviors; a key part of public health nursing practice is to teach people to promote health, prevent illness, and manage chronic illness.

This chapter discusses ways to develop the educational aspect of health promotion programs for individuals, groups, and the community. Discussion includes information about how people learn, the sequence of actions that a nurse follows when developing an educational program, using selected models of health promotion, and the important topic of literacy, especially health literacy. The role of groups in health promotion is also presented. Many of the objectives of *Healthy People 2030* address the importance of health promotion, and selected objectives are cited in this chapter.

HEALTHY PEOPLE 2030 OBJECTIVES FOR HEALTH EDUCATION

As mentioned in chapters throughout the text, *Healthy People 2030* lists national health needs and outlines goals and objectives designed to improve health. The *Healthy People 2030* educational objectives emphasize the importance of educating various populations. The document says that "effective health communication is critical to health and well-being." Many of the objectives related to specific health conditions or health populations imply that health communication is critical to their success. That is, when objectives under such topics as physical activity and nutrition direct people to exercise and eat healthy foods, the success of attaining the objectives will depend on effective health communication. *Healthy People 2030* points out that health communication is often complex, and it is important for health care providers to communicate clearly and use methods like teach-back and shared decision making to help people make better informed decisions about their health. This attention to clarity also includes electronic health information that should be accurate and easy to access and understand.

♥ HEALTHY PEOPLE 2030

Selected examples related to health education are as follows:
- **HC/HIT-R01:** Increase the health literacy of the population.
- **HC/HIT-06:** Increase the proportion of adults offered online access to their medical record.
- **ECBP-D03:** Increase the proportion of worksites that offer an employee health promotion program.

US Department of Health and Human Services: *Healthy People 2030*, Washington, DC, 2020, US Government Printing Office.

In designing, implementing, and evaluating health education activities, it is important to learn about the primary health problems in the community, as well as education principles related to learning and teaching. The goal of an educational program is to teach what people think they want to learn and in ways that facilitate their learning. In public health, it is important for learners to participate in identifying their learning needs. Then education programs are designed to meet the health need or problem in that population. In general, these programs involve educating individual members of the population about health promotion, illness prevention, and treatment. For example, in a community in which childhood and adolescent asthma is a problem, a community-based asthma education and training program can be developed. If childhood obesity is a major health concern, a program to educate children in their schools and their parents or caregivers about healthy eating, cooking, and exercise may be useful.

To develop a community-based educational program for education about asthma or childhood obesity, the nurse would need to follow a set of steps. The steps are listed here and discussed in detail throughout the chapter. Typical steps to follow in developing a health education program include (1) *identify* a population-specific learning need for the community health client; (2) *select* one or more learning theories to use in the education program; (3) *consider* which educational principles are most likely to increase learning and choose those that are most appropriate and feasible; (4) *examine* educational issues, such as population-specific or cultural concerns, identify barriers to learning, such as limited literacy or limited or lack of health literacy, and choose the most appropriate teaching and learning strategies based on the age, gender, cultural background, education, and learning needs of the learners; (5) *design and implement* the educational program using carefully chosen strategies; (6) *evaluate* the effects of the educational program. The steps used in educational programs parallel those of the nursing process—assessment, planning, implementation, and evaluation.

🧬 HEALTH EDUCATION AND INFLUENCE OF GENOMICS

As has been discussed in many chapters of this text, there is a correlation among weight, health, and exercise. It has recently been determined that even if obesity is in your genes, regular exercise can help keep pounds from accruing to you. Researchers at the University of North Carolina at Chapel Hill found that people who carried the FTO gene variant that increases the risk of obesity could reduce the effects of their DNA by approximately one-third by engaging in regular exercise. One thing that the study shows is that people do not have to be victims to their genes. They have choices. With this gene variant, regular exercise can interrupt to some extent the effects on weight. Overall the research team found that exercise weakened the gene variant's effects by approximately 30%.

Source: Graff M, Scott RA. Justice AE, et al: Genome-wide physical activity interactions in adiposity—A meta-analysis of 200,452 adults, PLOS, *Genetics* 13(8):e1006972. Accessed May 2020.

EDUCATION, LEARNING, AND CHANGE

Education is an activity designed to help people change their knowledge, attitudes, and skills about a specific topic. Knowledge is the least difficult area to change, followed by attitudes, and the most difficult area to change is behavior. Nurses provide people with health information so they can improve their decision-making abilities and thereby decide if they will change their behavior. Education includes providing knowledge and skills. Learning occurs when the recipient receives the knowledge and skills. Remember that learning involves change, and change is difficult for many people.

People learn in a variety of ways. Many people learn best through active involvement in their learning, while other learners are like sponges and prefer to simply soak up the information that is presented. Learners accept information based on many factors, including what they already know, what they believe, the culture in which they have been raised, their generational experiences related to learning, and how well they can understand and relate to the information that they receive. What people hear is filtered through their past experiences; the social groups to which they belong; assumptions, values, level of attention, and knowledge; and the esteem in which they hold the person communicating the information. Effective health education is a competency that is included in many documents that describe the role of public health professionals, including nurses.

A variety of educational principles can be used to guide the selection of health information for individuals, families, communities, and populations. Three of the most useful categories of educational principles are those associated with the nature of learning, the educational process, and the skills of effective educators.

The Nature of Learning

One way to think about the nature of learning is to examine the cognitive (thinking), affective (feeling), and psychomotor (acting) domains of learning. Each domain has specific behavioral components that form a hierarchy of steps, or levels. Each level builds on the previous one. Understanding these three learning domains is crucial in providing effective health education (Bloom et al., 1956). First, consider assumptions about how adults learn. Specifically, adults are motivated to learn when (1) they think they need to know something, (2) the new information is compatible with their prior life experiences, (3) they value the person(s) providing the information, and (4) they believe they can make any necessary changes that are implied by the new information (Knowles et al., 2015).

Cognitive Domain

The cognitive domain includes memory, recognition, understanding, reasoning, application, and problem solving, and is divided into a hierarchical classification of behaviors. Learners master each level of cognition in order of difficulty and move up the learning hierarchy (Bloom et al., 1956). Start by assessing the cognitive abilities of the learners. This is especially important when learners have a limited level of literacy either of the language used in the instruction or of the content presented. A later section will discuss literacy in general and health literacy in particular. Teaching above or below a person's level of understanding can lead to frustration and discouragement. The components of the cognitive domain are as follows (Bloom et al., 1956):

1. **Knowledge:** Requires recall of information
2. **Comprehension:** Combines recall with understanding
3. **Application:** New information is taken in and used in a different way
4. **Analysis:** Breaks communication down into parts to understand both the parts and their relationships to one another
5. **Synthesis:** Builds on the first four levels by assembling them into a new whole
6. Evaluation: Learners judge the value of what has been learned

Affective Domain

The affective domain includes changes in attitudes and the development of values. For affective learning to take place, nurses consider and attempt to influence what learners feel, think, and value. Because the attitudes and values of nurses may differ from those of their clients, it is important to listen carefully to detect clues to feelings that learners have that may influence learning. It is difficult to change deeply rooted attitudes, beliefs, interests, and values. To make such changes, people need support and encouragement from those around them. Affective learning, like cognitive learning, consists of the following series of steps:

1. **Knowledge:** Receives the information
2. **Comprehension:** Responds to the information received
3. **Application:** Values the information
4. **Analysis:** Makes sense of the information
5. **Synthesis:** Organizes the information
6. **Evaluation:** Adopts behaviors consistent with new values

Psychomotor Domain

The psychomotor domain includes the performance of skills that require some degree of neuromuscular coordination and emphasizes motor skills (Bloom et al., 1956). Clients are taught a variety of psychomotor skills, including bathing infants, changing dressings, giving injections, measuring blood glucose levels, taking blood pressures, and walking with crutches, as well as many skills related to health promotion exercises.

When you are teaching a skill, first show clients how to do the skill. You can show the client using pictures, a model, or a device or via a live demonstration, video, CD, or the Internet. There are many helpful teaching materials available on YouTube. Next, have clients practice by repeat demonstration to validate that what was being taught was learned. In addition, if the teaching is being done in a class, participants may learn by observing one another master a task. Psychomotor learning depends on learners meeting the following three conditions (Bloom et al., 1956). The learner must have the following:

- The *necessary ability,* including both cognitive and psychomotor ability. For example, you may find that a person with Alzheimer disease can follow only one-step instructions. Thus you need to tailor your education plan to that person.
- A *sensory image* of how to carry out the skill. For example, when teaching a group of women how to cook heart-healthy meals, ask the women to describe their kitchen and how they would actually go about the shopping and cooking process.
- *Opportunities to practice* the new skills. Provide practice sessions during the program to help the client adapt the skill to the home or work environment where the skill will be performed.

CASE STUDY

Teaching About Diabetes

To apply the three learning domains, consider this clinical situation: In the community being served, the nurse identifies a large number of women who are newly diagnosed as having diabetes. The nurse's goals would include: (1) learning what the women know about their health condition; (2) providing basic information about diabetes and self-care (cognitive domain); and (3) teaching them how to determine the correct amount of insulin and the correct way to do the injection (psychomotor domain). It is important to demonstrate insulin injection and ask each woman to do a repeat demonstration to verify that she has the necessary ability and dexterity to self-inject insulin. During the teaching session, the nurse learns that the women have a limited understanding of the possible long-term complications of diabetes. Teaching at this level will include the affective domain in that the women may be denying the seriousness of their illness. They may think that a disease that causes limited pain and discomfort in its early stages cannot lead to many complications if not properly managed. In this case the nurse would be guided by six principles of effective education. First, the nurse would convey the information clearly, using words that the women understand. A place for the teaching would be chosen that is private and comfortable,

and the nurse would organize the teaching approach to fit the needs of the learner. In diabetes education, it is important to give information and demonstrate self-injection and then ask the learners to practice in the class what they are learning. Evaluation of the effectiveness of the session(s) can be accomplished by asking the learners what they have learned and by watching and listening to them as they discuss and practice their new learning.

Application to other clinical examples: How would you apply the three domains of learning to developing an educational session for a group of women who have young children in the home and need to be better informed about safety practices in terms of water, stoves, poisons, medicines, tools, and so forth? Remember to consider abilities and deficiencies. Now apply the six clinical judgment steps to this second clinical example. What cues would you look for in the home to determine if the home had issues related to safety? Next, analyze the cues you detect.

Then develop and prioritize your hypotheses about what the issues are in this home. You would then develop possible solutions for each of your hypotheses and begin to take action on your highest prior goal. Finally, you would evaluate the outcomes you and the family have achieved.

QSEN FOCUS ON QUALITY AND SAFETY EDUCATION FOR NURSES

Targeted Competency: Client-Centered Care—Key aspects of client-centered care include the following:

- **Knowledge:** Integrate understanding of multiple dimensions of client-centered care: information, communication, and education.
- **Skills:** Communicate client values, preferences, and expressed needs to other members of the health care team.
- **Attitudes:** Respect and encourage individual expression of client values, preferences, and expressed needs.

Client-Centered Care Question

Providing health information in a way that is not understandable or useful to the recipient is a poor form of client-centered communication. If you were teaching a group of four women about wound care after surgery, what steps would you take to ensure that the message the women received was the message that you intended to send?

Answer: Begin by providing the needed information by describing each step; you might include an easy-to-understand handout in the language the four women understand, or you might give them a CD to take home that has the information on it. Next, you would demonstrate how to clean the wound. Then you would ask each woman to repeat the cleaning process that you just demonstrated. Finally, you would ask each woman if she has the facilities and supplies to clean the wound at home; then you would ask each woman if she had any questions or concerns that you might answer. What else would you do?

Data from Cronenwett L, Sherwood G, Barnsteiner J, et al: Quality and safety education for nurses, *Nurs Outlook* 55:122–131, 2007.

THE EDUCATIONAL PROCESS

The educational process builds on an understanding of education, learning, and how people learn. The five steps of the educational process are discussed next.

Identify Educational Needs and Develop Goals and Objectives

To learn about clients' health education needs, conduct a needs assessment. Assessment steps are listed in Box 14.1. Once needs are identified, prioritize them beginning with the most critical educational needs. Factors that can influence a person's learning needs and ability to learn include demographic, physical, geographic, economic, psychological, social, and spiritual characteristics. Also consider the learner's knowledge, skills, and motivation to learn, as well as resources available to support and possibly prevent learning. Resources include printed, audio or visual materials, equipment, agencies, and other individuals. Many useful audio and visual resources can be found electronically. Barriers for the presenter include lack of time, skill, confidence, money, space, energy, and organizational support.

After you identify the learner's needs, develop the goals and objectives for the educational program. Goals are broad, long-term expected outcomes, such as, "Each child in the third-grade class will participate in 30 minutes of daily physical exercise 4 days per week for 2 months." Program goals should deal directly with the clients' overall learning needs, and for the third graders, the learning need is to know the importance of exercise and fitness to their health.

BOX 14.1 Steps of a Needs Assessment

1. Identify what the client wants to know. (Consider *Healthy People 2030* educational objectives.)
2. Collect data systematically to obtain information about learning needs, readiness to learn, and barriers to learning.
3. Analyze assessment data that have been collected and identify cognitive, affective, and psychomotor learning needs.
4. Think about what will increase the client's ability and motivation to learn.
5. Assist the client to prioritize learning needs.

Objectives are specific, short-term criteria that are met as steps toward achieving the long-term goal, such as, "Within 2 weeks, each child will be able to demonstrate at least 2 exercises they have learned." Objectives are written statements of an intended outcome or expected change in behavior and should define the minimum degree of knowledge or ability needed by a client. Objectives must be stated clearly and defined in measurable terms, and they typically imply an action (Knowles et al., 2015).

Select Appropriate Educational Methods

Choose educational methods that will facilitate the efficient and successful accomplishment of program goals and objectives. The methods also should be appropriately matched to the strengths and needs of both the client and the presenter. Choose the simplest, clearest, and most succinct manner of presentation and avoid complex program designs. Try to vary the methods to hold the attention of the learners and to meet the needs of different learners. Some people learn best by being actively involved in the program (Fig. 14.1), such as by brainstorming, role playing, simulation, games, group participation, demonstrations, and field trips. Others learn by a more solitary approach, such as watching a video, listening to a guest speaker, case studies, reading printed materials, or reflecting on how they might apply the content to their health situation.

Educators also need to be able to deliver presentations, lead group discussions, organize role plays, provide feedback to learners, share case studies, use media and materials, and, where indicated, administer examinations. Consider the content to include, how to organize and sequence the information, what your rate of delivery will be, whether you need to include repetition, how much practice time should be included, how you will evaluate the effectiveness of the teaching, and ways that you can provide reinforcement and rewards (Box 14.2).

When choosing educational methods, consider age, gender, culture, developmental disabilities or special learning needs, educational level, knowledge of the subject, and size of the group. For example, clients with a visual impairment need more verbal

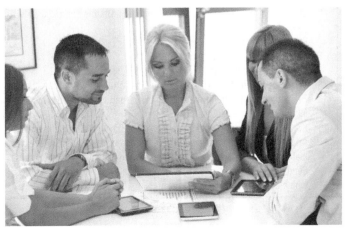

Fig. 14.1 The Instructional Methods Need to Meet the Learning Needs of the Learners. (© 2012 Photos.com, a division of Getty Images. All rights reserved. Image 150854734.)

BOX 14.2   How to Effectively Teach Clients

Use the TEACH mnemonic:

Tune in. Listen before you start teaching. The client's needs should direct the content.

Edit information. Teach necessary information first. Be specific.

Act on each teaching moment. Teach whenever possible. Develop a good relationship.

Clarify often. Make sure your assumptions are correct. Seek feedback.

Honor the client as a partner. Build on the client's experience. Share responsibility with the client.

Modified from Hansen M, Fisher J: Patient-centered teaching from theory to practice, *Am J Nurs* 98:56–60, 1998.

---

description than those with no sight impairment. Persons who have hearing impairments or language limitations need more visual material and speakers or translators who can use sign language or speak their native language. In addition, when the learners have limitations in attention and concentration, educators can use creative methods and tools to keep them focused. For example, you might include frequent breaks; provide simple surroundings with few or no distractions; use small-group interactions to keep learners involved and interested; and use hands-on equipment, such as mannequins, models, interactive games, and other materials and devices the learner can physically manipulate. Involve the learner appropriately, actively, and creatively in learning. Interactive educational programs often are more effective than noninteractive ones. Interactive strategies include discussion, small group work, games, and role playing, whereas noninteractive strategies are lectures, videos, or demonstrations. The Internet and social media have created a new way for providing health information. Platforms such as Facebook, YouTube, Snapchat, and Instagram provide access to and sharing of information, including health information. Box 14.3 details descriptions of learning formats.

The Centers for Disease Control and Prevention (CDC) has created some helpful information about health communication. For example, in the site entitled "Health Communication Basics," health communication is defined as the "study and use of communication strategies to inform and influence decisions and actions to improve health" (January 2020a). They blend health communication and social marketing practices to answer the question of "How do I do it?" with a six-step process that includes: (1) describe the problem; (2) perform market research; (3) define market strategy; (4) develop interventions; (5) evaluate your plan; and (6) implement your plan. These six steps correlate with the nursing process. Although the steps are organized somewhat differently, these six steps are consistent with the six steps in the Clinical Judgment plan described in the preface. The CDC defines health marketing as a multidisciplinary area of public health practice that draws from marketing theories and adds strategies for prevention, health promotion, and health protection (CDC, 2020a). When we consider that marketing is a process designed to meet human or social needs, we can see the relationship to public health. There are four fundamental elements in the marketing mix that can be used in public health. They are often called the "four Ps" and are:

Product: the item, good or service

BOX 14.3 Examples of Learning Formats

Presentation: This method can be used when the group is large and you want to be consistent in the message that is delivered to all participants. Remember, people tend to have a short attention span. So what can you do to keep them engaged? You might ask them to spend some time talking with one another in small groups and then have the group respond to questions or ask attendees to write answers to questions and invite several to share their answers. The presentation can take many forms, ranging from a health seminar to a town hall meeting.

Demonstration: This technique is often used to show attendees how to perform a task. For example, insulin injection demonstration, heart-healthy food preparation, and breastfeeding may be demonstrated.

Small informal group: Because learners often learn as much from one another as from the instructor, small groups can be valuable. This is especially true when the content lends itself to members sharing their own experiences. For example, in working with women in a shelter for abused women, participants may be able to share with one another actions they took to remove themselves safely from the violent environment. They might also be able to jointly plan how each might move to the stage of independent living outside the shelter.

Health fair: See the How To box on ways to plan, implement, and evaluate a health fair. For example, you might offer a health fair in a senior center and have displays, such as posters; videos; live demonstrations; handouts on such topics as reducing fat in selected recipes (including samples) and age-appropriate exercises for flexibility; as well as screenings for elevated blood pressure, glucose, or cholesterol or for osteoporosis and vision.

Nonnative language sessions: You could adapt the health fair approach for a Hispanic group by holding the session in Spanish and providing all of the materials in Spanish. Then ask Spanish-speaking nurses to staff each of the stations for health learning.

Price: both monetary and nonmonetary costs to the market

Place: channels and locations where the product can be obtained

Promotion: direct communication, publicity, and advertising

Develop a brief case related to testing that was initiated in early 2020 to determine who was positive and who was negative for COVID-19 (Fig. 14.2). What was the product, price, and place, and how was the product promoted?

It is important to consider the ethical issues involved in the teaching tools that you use, and this is particularly important with social media. Not all websites are developed by health care professionals, and not all sites are peer reviewed. Consider also the guidelines of the Health Insurance Portability and Accountability Act (HIPAA), *ANA's Principles for Social Networking and the Nurse* (American Nurses Association [ANA], 2011), the

National Council of State Boards of Nursing's White Paper: A *Nurse's Guide to the Use of Social Media (2011)*.

LEVELS OF PREVENTION

Primary Prevention

Education at health fairs regarding immunizations for children, older adults, and people with chronic illnesses.

Secondary Prevention

Education at health fairs regarding early diagnosis and treatment of diabetes and hypercholesterolemia, along with providing health screenings, with the goal of shortening disease duration and severity.

Tertiary Prevention

Education in rehabilitation centers or adult daycare centers to help individuals who have had a stroke maximize their functioning.

Health fairs have been a popular way to provide primary and secondary health education. These types of health education were put on hold during the COVID-19 pandemic. The objectives of holding health fairs are to increase awareness by providing health screenings, activities, information and educational materials, and demonstrations. A health fair can target a specific population or focus on a specific health issue, as well as target a range of groups and cover a variety of health education and health promotion topics. The fair can be held in many locations and can be either inside or outside. The How To box lists guidelines to assist nurses who chair, co-chair, or serve on a planning committee for a health fair.

HOW TO PLAN, IMPLEMENT, AND EVALUATE A HEALTH FAIR

1. Form a planning committee with 2–12 people who represent the groups who will be part of the health fair (i.e., health professionals, representatives from health agencies, schools, churches, employers, the media, and the target audience).
2. Develop a budget.
3. Identify the target group. Develop a theme.
4. Establish goals, expected outcomes, and screening activities consistent with the needs and wishes of the target group.
5. Develop a timeline and schedule.
6. Choose a site and consider the site logistics. Do this approximately 1 year ahead.
7. Plan for the needed supplies.
8. Recruit and manage exhibitors.
9. Publicize the health fair.
9. On the day of the fair, arrive early and greet attendees.
10. Evaluate the health fair by having exhibitors, participants, and volunteers fill out a specific evaluation form.
11. Stay after the event concludes to thank the committee and volunteers.
12. After the event, analyze the evaluations and develop a list of lessons learned. Include any recommendations for the next health fair. Pay bills. Send thank-you notes to the committee, volunteers, sponsors, and others who made the health fair a success.

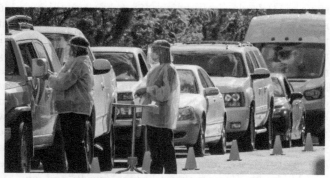

Fig. 14.2 COVID-19 Drive Through Testing Station. (© 2021 iStock by Getty Images. All rights reserved. Image # 1254924307.)

There are many guides on the web for planning health fairs. These helpful guides often are developed by health insurers or hospital systems. Start your search by typing in "Plan a health fair."

Skills of the Effective Educator

The educator needs to understand the basic sequence of instruction. The following steps are useful in planning an educational program. Begin by (1) *gaining the attention* of the learners and helping them understand that the information being presented is important and beneficial to them; then (2) *tell the learners the objectives of the instruction;* (3) *ask* learners to recall previous knowledge related to the topic of interest so they link new knowledge with previous knowledge; (4) *present the essential material* in a clear, organized, and simple manner and in a way consistent with the learners' strengths, needs, and limitations; (5) *help learners apply* the information to their lives and situations; (6) *encourage learners to demonstrate* what they have learned, which will help you correct any errors and improve skills; and (7) *provide feedback* to help learners improve their knowledge and skills. By using these steps, nurses may help clients maximize learning experiences. If steps of this process are omitted, superficial and fragmented learning may occur.

❓ CHECK YOUR PRACTICE

Consider the client, Anna, and examine her motivation to change her eating and activity patterns. Anna says that her family will eat only fried foods, so to get her husband and children to eat dinner, she fries their meats and vegetables. The family does eat fresh fruit and drink milk. Anna says that she gets exercise by walking to the bus stop en route to work and cleaning her home. She has not considered other forms of regular exercise. What are some of the ways in which you could design your nursing plan for Anna?

1. Expressing empathy by trying to see the world through Anna's eyes
2. Building on Anna's strengths and helping her believe that she has the ability to make a change (self-efficacy)
3. Rolling with resistance when Anna is ambivalent about her ability to change
4. Help Anna to recognize that her current actions conflict with her expressed goals of eating healthy foods and exercising regularly

In your intervention with Anna, consider how you could use open-ended questions which invite elaboration; affirmations designed to recognize her strengths; reflections that convey to her that you were listening and understood what she said; and summaries where you summarize what you heard her say and what you believe she plans to do. How would you apply the six steps in the Clinical Judgment process defined in the preface?

HOW TO USE PLAIN LANGUAGE IN HEALTH EDUCATION

1. Organize the audience.
   - Know your audience and purpose before you begin.
   - Put the most important message first.
   - Present other information in order of importance to the audience.
   - Break text into logical chunks and use headings.
2. Choose words carefully.
   - Write in the active voice.
   - Choose words and numbers the audience knows
   - Keep words, sentences, and paragraphs short.
   - Include "you" and other pronouns.
3. Make information easy to find.
   - Use headings and text boxes.
   - Delete unnecessary words sentences and paragraphs.
   - Create lists and tables (CDC, 2019b.).

The Quad Council Practice Competences for Public Health Nursing in Domain 3 list competencies related to communication skills. They begin with assessing the health literacy of the individuals, families, groups, and communities being served. They emphasize the importance of effective written, oral, and electronic communication, as well as communication delivered in a culturally responsive and relevant fashion (Quad Council Coalition, 2018, p. 19).

The type of learning format you select will depend on the learners. If they are young, you will want an interactive format, and many of your options will include the use of technology. You could use a game, such as developing a bingo game with food groups to teach about healthy eating. The old adage "A picture is worth a thousand words" still holds true. People tend to remember what they see or hear; a lively format rather than a passive one encourages learning. Most people have a short attention span, so you need to make your point quickly and directly. It may help to provide take-home written or electronic materials for further reminders and follow-up of what is taught. People often learn better when they are actively engaged in the learning; thus small-group discussion, role-playing, use of a computer-based program, and question-and-answer sessions may reinforce learning.

A patient education tool that is being increasingly used is "teach-back." Teach-back is a health literacy tool that allows nurses to immediately assess what the individual, family, or group has learned by having the person or group immediately say or demonstrate what they learned during the session. It is considered to be a "show me" approach whereby the nurse can clarify immediately any misunderstandings (Caplin and Saunders, 2015). Nurses can also use **ACTS** (assess, collaborate, train, and survey) with clients and client groups. Assess the client's main concern (can be a person, family, or community group); then assess learning needs and baseline level of knowledge, how they prefer to learn, their core values, and potential influential language, cultural, social or physical influences. Next compare the assessed needs with the resources available. The next step is to use Teach 3 or teach-back strategies. Teach 3 means that you teach the audience three or fewer key actions, pieces of information, or skills. Attendees then restate or demonstrate what was taught. Just as with teach-back, any misunderstandings can be immediately corrected. The key point in the two teaching strategies is to teach a small amount at any one time, and then immediately have the attendees provide feedback on what they heard or saw (French, 2015).

Fig. 14.3 shows a community group being educated, and Box 14.4 lists ways to design clear educational programs.

Educational Issues and Barriers to Learning

There are three important educational issues to consider when you are planning educational programs. First, different populations of learners require different teaching strategies. Second, be prepared to overcome barriers to learning. And third, consider the appropriateness of using technology in the programs.

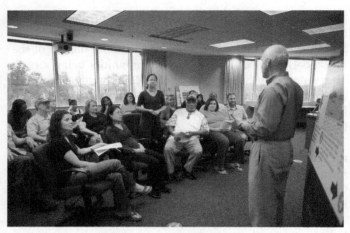

Fig. 14.3 A Nurse Educates a Community Group About Environmental Health Issues and Gathers Their Concerns. (From Centers for Disease Control and Prevention, 2009, courtesy Dawn Arlotta.)

BOX 14.4   Designing Clear Educational Programs

1. Develop the content for your message.
2. Identify the most appropriate format and location for your program, taking into account your budget, location, and other available resources and constraints. See Box 14.3 for examples of formats.
3. Organize the learning experience to suit the audience; consider how to engage the learners in the process.
4. Plan how you will deliver the material using the following points:
   - Limit the number of points you wish to cover to the most important ones.
   - Begin with a strong opening and close with a strong ending; people remember most what is said first and last.
   - Fit your use of language to the learners; use an active voice and emphasize the positive. For example, "Many people are able to lose weight by reducing their intake by 500 calories a day and exercising 45 minutes at least four times a week."
   - Use examples, stories, and other vivid messages. Limit statistics and complex terminology.
   - Refer to trustworthy sources. In general, government, educational, or professional association sources are peer reviewed by professionals and are dependable. The Centers for Disease Control and Prevention, National Cancer Institute, American Association of Public Health, and the American Academy of Pediatrics are four examples of organizations whose sites offer useful information.
   - Use aids to highlight your message. For example, you might have posters, handouts, or CDs to give to attendees. You might also incorporate a clip from a website, such as http://www.YouTube.com, to emphasize your point.
5. Do not forget to plan the evaluation when you are initially planning the program.

Population Considerations Based on Age and Cultural and Ethnic Backgrounds

Nurses are a trusted source of health education in the community; nurses continue to be rated via the Gallup Poll as the highest professional group in terms of honesty and ethics. According to Reinhart (2020) reporting on the Gallup Poll "For the 18th year

in a row, Americans rate the honesty and ethics of nurses highest among a list of profession…" For this reason, nurses are in ideal positions to teach people how to promote their health via health education.

The increase in populations of varying cultural and ethnic backgrounds and the aging of Baby Boomers require that community health education cross age and cultural boundaries. In terms of age, children, adults, and older adults have different learning needs and respond to different educational strategies. In each age group, learners also vary in their cognitive ability, personality, and prior knowledge. Some people learn better with more direct instruction, supervision, and encouragement than do other people. As discussed in Chapter 7, culture can be "defined by group membership, such as racial, ethnic, linguistic or geographical groups, or as a collection of beliefs, values, customs, ways of thinking, communicating, and behaving" (CDC, 2019a). Nurses need to tailor their education to the cultural group(s) they are teaching. The Quad Council Practice Competences for Public Health Nursing in Domain 4 discuss Cultural Competency Skills. They say that the public health nurse uses the social and ecological determinants of health to work effectively with diverse individuals, families, and groups and to develop culturally responsive interventions with communities and populations (Quad Council Coalition, 2018, p. 21).

Learning strategies for children and individuals with little knowledge about a health-related topic are characterized as **pedagogy**. In the pedagogic model of learning, the teacher makes decisions about what will be learned and how and when it will be learned. This form of learning is teacher directed. Learning strategies for adults, older adults, and individuals with some health-related knowledge about a topic are called **andragogy**. In the andragogic model, learners influence what they need and want to learn. Andragogy is a more transactional way of learning than the pedagogic model. Each model has useful elements (Knowles et al., 2015). For example, when learners are dependent and entering a totally new content area, they may require more pedagogic experiences. Consider both the age of the learner population and their learning needs as you choose the pedagogic or andragogic principles for the program. In educational programs for children, provide information that matches the developmental abilities of the group. Nurses can use the following age-specific strategies to tailor educational programs for children.

- **With younger children, use more concrete examples and word choices.** You might tell 3-year-olds to brush their teeth two times per day; for 10-year-olds, you can explain to them the benefits of brushing their teeth and the risks in not brushing and talk about issues such as the care of the teeth with braces.
- **Use objects or devices, rather than just discuss ideas to increase attention.** When teaching a group of children with asthma how to use inhalers, hand out inhalers to each one so he or she can practice proper technique with the inhalers rather than just giving them a handout with instructions or demonstrating how to use an inhaler while they watch you.
- **Incorporate repetitive health behaviors into games to help children retain knowledge and acquire skills.** Singing songs

while acting out healthy activities such as washing hands before eating helps children to get into the habit of hand washing and makes this health promotion activity fun. Most people, including adults and children, wash their hands too hastily to remove germs. The actual physical activity of washing hands is more beneficial in germ control than the soap used or sanitizers.

CHECK YOUR PRACTICE

Assume that you are trying to teach a group of 5-year-olds how to effectively wash their hands before meals or after they have done an activity or touched items. You know that an activity often helps young children to learn. So you:

- Ask each child to wash his or her hands while completely singing a favorite song.
- The song "Twinkle, Twinkle Little Star" takes about the exact amount of time to sing as is recommended for effective hand washing.
- Other songs can be used when they are appropriate to the season, such as "Jingle Bells." Or as was taught during the COVID-19 pandemic, you could count to 20 while you wash your hands with soap and water.
- By singing a song as a group or one child at a time, learning the appropriate length to wash hands can be fun and easy to accomplish.
- Schools have direct contact with approximately 95% of children between 5 and 17 years, and this makes them an excellent place to teach health promotion. Healthy students are better learners. (See Figure 31.1 for an illustration on the whole child approach to education).

It is also important to consider characteristics of learners that depend on the generation to which they belong. People born after 1980 are considered the *net generation* because they have always had digital media and access to the Internet, use mobile devices to access and process information and to stay in contact with their friends, and are "always on and connected to their devices." During the social isolation and physical distancing phase of the COVID-19 virus, meetings, classes, and other forms of gathering were often carried out using an Internet platform. This format helped members of all generations stay connected with work, school, friends, and the groups to which they belonged. People of different ages have different learning styles, and it is important to know which style fits the person(s) being taught.

In thinking about culture, it is important to know that by 2050 approximately 50% of the US population will consist of ethnic minorities, such as Asians, African Americans, Hispanic Americans, Native Americans, and Pacific Islanders. Culture influences family structure and interactions, as well as views about health and illness. These demographic changes present new challenges to nurse educators. Nurses need to understand the health belief systems of the ethnic populations being served and be familiar with populations who are prone to develop certain health problems. When presenting seminars or using written, audio, or visual information, provide the information in a culturally competent manner.

For example, in a rural farming area, there might be a large population of Mexican migrant crop workers. Knowing that this Spanish-speaking group is more likely to have tuberculosis than other segments of the community, nurses may visit the migrant worker camp to present information on tuberculosis, such as prevention, symptom identification, early diagnosis, and treatment. An interpreter may accompany the nurses and provide oral content in Spanish. Written handouts can be in Spanish and designed to be read and understood on the level at which the group comprehends.

Barriers to learning fall into two broad categories: one concerning the educator and the other concerning the learner.

Educator-Related Barriers

Some common educator-related barriers to learning, together with strategies to minimize them, are as follows:

- **Fear of public speaking.** Be well prepared, use icebreakers, recognize and acknowledge the fear, and practice in front of a mirror or video camera or with a friend.
- **Lack of credibility with respect to a certain topic.** Increase your confidence by carefully preparing for the talk so that the information is useful and you understand the information. Avoid apologizing for lack of expertise and instead convey the attitude of an expert by briefly sharing your personal and professional background.
- **Limited professional experiences related to a health topic.** You may want to describe personal experiences (brief ones), share experiences of others, or use analogies, illustrations, or examples from movies, current news, or famous people. Be certain the examples fit the audience.
- **Inability to deal with difficult learners.** One strategy is to confront the problem learner directly. Other strategies include using humor, using small groups to foster the participation of timid people, and asking disruptive people to give others a chance to speak, or, if this does not work, asking them to leave.
- **Lack of knowledge about how to gain participation.** Foster participation by asking open-ended questions, inviting participation, and planning small-group activities in which a person responds based on the group rather than presenting individual information.
- **Lack of experience in timing a presentation so that it is neither too long nor too short.** Plan ahead and practice the presentation at the same pace that you will speak to the group.
- **Uncertainty about how to adjust instruction.** You can more easily adjust instruction when you know the participants' needs, request feedback, and redesign the presentation during breaks based on what you have learned about the participants.
- **Discomfort when learners ask questions.** Try to anticipate questions, concisely paraphrase questions to be sure that you correctly understood the question, and recognize that it is appropriate to admit that you do not know the answer to a question.
- **Desire to obtain feedback from learners.** Solicit informal feedback during the program and at the end with program evaluation.

- **Concern about whether media, materials, and facilities will function properly.** Test the equipment before the program to make sure it runs and also that you know how to use it. Have back-up plans for how to get help if you have a problem.
- **Difficulty with openings and closings.** Strategies to foster successful openings and closings include developing several examples of openings and closings, memorizing the opening and closing, concisely summarizing information, and thanking participants for attending.
- **Overdependence on notes.** You may wish to use note cards or visual aids as prompts, and practicing in advance is a proven way to increase skill at presenting.

Learner-Related Barriers

Two of the most important learner-related barriers are low literacy and lack of motivation to learn information and make needed behavioral changes. Nurses often deal with individuals and populations who are illiterate or who have *low literacy levels.* These individuals may be embarrassed to admit this deficit to health care providers and educators and may try to appear to understand when they really do not. Specifically, they may not ask questions to clarify information even when they do not understand it. As society becomes more multicultural, the problem of low literacy can increase because of limited use of the primary language and limited education. It is essential to assess the literacy, especially health literacy of the learners. The *Plain Writing Act of 2010* requires the federal government to write all new publications, forms, and publicly distributed documents in a "clear, concise, well-organized" manner and according to plain writing guides (see Public Law 111-274 at http://www.gpo/gov). The next paragraphs discuss the significance of this problem and the need for nurses to address health literacy.

The National Assessment of Adult Literacy (NAAL) is the largest literacy assessment study done in the United States. This assessment was first conducted in 1992. At that time, of the five levels in the assessment, 50% of American adults were in the top two levels and 50% were in the bottom three levels of literacy. The minimal standard needed to function in the workplace is level 3 proficiency. In 2003 the tool measured literacy in four levels: *below basic, basic, intermediate,* and *proficient.* The literacy scales used in 2003 were prose literacy, document literacy, and quantitative literacy. Prose examples include searching, comprehending, and using information from editorials, news stories, brochures, and instructional materials. Document literacy refers to searching, comprehending, and using information from documents such as job applications, payroll forms, transportation schedules, maps, tables, and drug and food labels. Quantitative literacy is the ability to identify and perform computations such as balancing a checkbook, completing an order form, or determining the interest on a loan from an advertisement. The 2003 test is more than just a survey and actually asks the test takers to perform tasks to demonstrate their literacy level (Kutner et al., 2006).

The 2003 NAAL included information about health literacy, which is an important topic for nurses. The 2003 NAAL used the Institute of Medicine's definition of health literacy: "The degree to which individuals have the capacity to obtain, process, and understand basic health information and services needed to make appropriate health decisions" (Ratzan and Parker, 2000). Kutner et al. (2006) found that the majority of participants had an intermediate (53%) literacy level, 12% were proficient, 22% were basic, and 14% had below basic levels of literacy. The assessment was given to more than 19,000 adults in households or prisons. Interestingly, women had a higher literacy level than men; White and Asian/Pacific Islander adults had higher scores than African American, Hispanic, American Indian/Alaska Native, and multiracial adults; and adults 65 years of age or older and persons living below the poverty line had a lower average literacy level than others surveyed. The Health Resources and Services Administration (HRSA) added medically underserved people to the list of individuals who were more likely to have low health literacy (HRSA, n.d.). In addition, the National Action Plan to Improve Health Literacy (US Department of Health and Human Services [USDHHS], Office of Disease Prevention and Health Promotion, 2010) adds recent refugees and immigrants to the list of people who may have low health literacy, including nonnative English speakers.

Since the NAAL was developed and used, another major assessment has been implemented. The Program for the International Assessment of Adult Competencies (PIAAC) is a large-scale assessment of adult skills. This program began in 2011 to 2012 and is the most current indicator of the nation's progress in literacy, numeracy, and problem solving in technology-rich environments (NCES, n.d.). During collection cycle 1, adults were surveyed in 24 countries in 2012, 9 countries in 2014, and 5 additional countries in 2017.

Individuals with limited literacy may be unable to understand instructions on prescription bottles, seek preventive care, understand the relationship between risky behavior and health, manage chronic health conditions, interpret health appointment cards, fill out health insurance forms, and read and understand self-care or hospital discharge instructions. In addition, individuals may have weak literacy and numeracy skills in their native language, and even translated materials may be difficult for them to understand because not all languages have words that directly translate into English. Nine out of 10 adults have difficulty using and understanding health information, when it is unfamiliar, complex, or jargon filled (CDC, 2019a) (Fig. 14.4). The following may happen when someone has health illiteracy. The person may:

- Have a limited vocabulary and general knowledge and not ask for clarification
- Focus on details and deal in literal or concrete concepts versus abstract concepts
- Select responses on a survey or questionnaire without necessarily understanding them
- Be unable to understand math (which is important in calculating medications)
  - Not be familiar with medical terms or how their bodies work
  - Have been diagnosed with a serious illness and is scared and confused

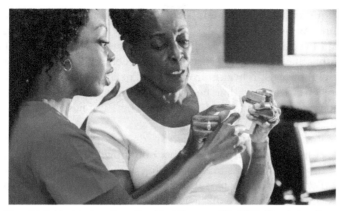

Fig. 14.4 Understanding Health Literacy. (© 2021 iStock by Getty Images. All rights reserved. Image #1297322811.)

- Have to interpret statistics and evaluate risks and benefits that affect their health and safety (CDC, 2019d).
- Have sight problems

Health illiteracy is expensive when people cannot understand their health care treatment or follow directions correctly. This inability can lead to increased numbers of emergency room visits, hospitalizations, and health care complications resulting from those hospitalizations, poorer health care outcomes, and decreased life expectancy (National Network of Libraries of Medicine [NNLM], n.d.). Some reasons for low health literacy are:

1. Lack of educational opportunity—people with a high school education or lower
2. Learning disabilities
3. Cognitive decline in older adults
4. Use it or lose it. Reading levels are typically three to five grade levels below the last year of school completed (NNLM, n.d.).

Some people are not motivated to learn. Although adults respond to some external motivators, the most powerful motivators are internal. People are motivated to learn if they value and feel they will benefit from the outcome of the learning, if they think they can follow through on what is being taught, and if it will improve their situation in life or increase their self-esteem (Wlodkowski and Ginsberg, 2017).

Another area in which some people have low literacy is in relation to foods. They may choose unhealthy foods due to lack of knowledge as well as lack of time, access, and funds to buy healthier food. See the following case study.

CASE STUDY

Food Literacy

Alice Doback is a single mother who works two jobs; one is full-time during the day in a call center, and the second is part-time in the evenings cleaning office buildings. When not at school, her two children, Erik (age 13) and Jason (age 7), spend most of their time next door with their neighbor, who looks after them while Alice works. In addition to having some concerns about making ends meet, Alice was newly diagnosed with hypercholesteremia.

Before Alice and her husband divorced, the family ate most meals together and there was always a variety of healthy foods to eat. Since Alice has been on her own, it has become difficult to ensure a variety of foods, especially fresh fruits and vegetables, due to the limited grocers in her geographic area. The nearest "chain" grocery store is 20 miles away and the family mainly has access to a few local quick mart gas/convenient shops. In addition to the lack of access of stores that carry a wide variety of healthy options, Alice rarely has time to cook and eat dinner with her children. She microwaves some food for herself and her kids before she leaves for her second job in the evening.

Erik and Jason will often eat unhealthy snacks and candy throughout the day. Their neighbor drinks nothing but soda, and that is what they are drinking when under their neighbor's care. Erik's body mass index (BMI) is 17.6 (35th percentile) and Jason's BMI is 21.3 (98th percentile). Their activity levels are low, and most of their free time is spent in sedentary activities playing video games and watching television. There is not much green space outside for them to be able to engage in activities.

Alice has become concerned that her choices are negatively impacting her health and the health of her children. She has become very stressed and depressed about this, but she has few social supports to turn to and continues to work both jobs because she needs the income. The neighbor's daughter-in-law, Barb (a registered nurse), came for a visit and spent some time talking with Alice. She suggested Alice go and speak to someone about all of this. Alice has health insurance but has no time free to meet with a counselor or a nutritionist.

What Would You Do?

1. If you were Barb, what would be your next course of action to try to help Alice and her children?
2. Describe the determinants of health surrounding Alice and her current nutritional/food habits.
3. Identify the role that social determinants of health can have on nutrition and dietary status.
4. Would you consider Erik and Jason to be underweight, normal weight, or overweight? Explain your reasoning.
5. Alice is newly diagnosed with hypercholesteremia. Describe what this condition is and what it can lead to, in terms of overall health and cardiac disease.
6. What recommendations would you give to this family to help Alice, Erik, and Jason become armed with the knowledge and skills to adopt a healthier lifestyle?
7. Describe the components of food literacy and how they relate to this family's situation.

Developed by: Susan Lowey, PhD, RN, CHPN, CNE, associate professor & advisement coordinator, State University of New York at Brockport.

There are a variety of government websites that regularly update their information about health literacy, including the CDC, Agency for Healthcare Research and Quality, (AHRQ), and National Institutes of Health (NIH).

Now apply the six clinical judgment steps of (1) recognize the cues; (2) analyze the cues; (3) identify and prioritize your hypotheses; (4) develop solutions for each hypothesis; (5) act on your first and primary hypothesis; and (6) evaluate the outcomes that you expect from your actions.

Health Promotion Models

Health promotion is a broader area than health education. Health promotion helps people to increase control over their health. It includes health education and health literacy. A variety of health promotion models can be used to structure health education and health promotion plans. One model, the Health Belief Model (HBM) is an individual-level model that can be used to plan programs if you think the motivation of learners might be a concern. Specifically, the HBM was one of the first theories of health behavior. It began in an interesting way that is still applicable to the behavior of people today. In the 1950s the US Public Health Service sent mobile radiography units to communities to provide free chest radiographs as a way to screen for tuberculosis. The radiography examinations were free, convenient, and painless, yet people did not take advantage of the service. A group of social psychologists were asked to try to explain the failure to use this screening—specifically, to determine what would motivate people to seek health care.

The HBM includes six components that attempt to answer the question of what motivates an individual to do something. These components are (1) perceived susceptibility ("Will something happen to me?"), (2) perceived severity ("If something does happen to me, will it be a big problem?"), (3) perceived benefits ("If I do what is suggested, will it really help me?"), (4) perceived barriers ("Assuming I do what is suggested, will there be barriers that will be unpleasant, costly, and so forth?"), (5) cues to action ("What might motivate me to actually do something?"), and (6) self-efficacy ("Can I really do this?"). This model has been applauded and criticized. It does offer guidance in planning health education programs in that it reminds nurses to think carefully about what motivates people to change. To understand motivation, it is important to learn: (1) how people involved feel about the health problem, (2) whether they think the problem is serious, (3) whether they think that action on their part will make a difference, and (4) whether they think they can both manage the barriers and actually perform the action (Edberg, 2015).

Consider the following example of how the HBM might be applied to a person in the community who has recently been diagnosed with diabetes. The person, June, is 25 years old and was diagnosed 2 months ago with diabetes mellitus. She has found it hard to follow the recommendations of the public health nurse she saw in the community clinic. When the nurse asked June what seemed to be getting in her way of complying, June said that she wondered what might happen to her if she did not follow the advice the nurse had given her about diet, exercise, and taking her insulin. June questioned whether something would really happen to her and, if that was the case, would it really be a problem? Her ambivalence about making this change led her to wonder: If she took her medication, ate a diabetic diet, exercised, and took her insulin correctly, would it really reduce the seriousness of her disease? She also questioned whether she could afford the food and insulin and had the time to cook appropriately and exercise regularly. June was afraid that insulin self-injection might be painful. If the nurse used the information provided about health communication and health literacy to help June develop and commit to a health change plan, what steps would the nurse take? June said that when she saw her friend Sue, who is also a diabetic patient, she noticed that Sue chose her foods carefully, exercised regularly, and looked and felt better than she had in the past. How would the nurse use the information about Sue to help June?

A second set of models is presented. The selection of these three models—the HBM, the Transtheoretical Model (TTM), and Precaution Adoption Process Model (PAPM)—does not imply that they are the best or only models. However, they are useful models in health promotion. The TTM and the PAPM are discussed together because they both deal with change that occurs in stages and over time. The TTM has the following six stages:

1. Precontemplation: The person does not plan to change either because the person does not know there is a problem or does not want to do anything about it (Edberg, 2015). For example, the person may not know that it is better to cook food in olive oil than in lard.
2. Contemplation: The person begins thinking about making a change in the future and examines the pros and cons of doing so. The person might have gone to a class in which he learned that it is better to cook food in olive oil rather than in lard and is beginning to wonder if his food would taste as good if he made that change.
3. Preparation: The person intends to do something. In the cooking example, the person might put olive oil on the shopping list.
4. Action: The person actually buys the oil and cooks a chicken with it instead of the lard.
5. Maintenance: The person decides that he can get used to eating chicken cooked in oil and begins preparing his food in that way on a regular basis.
6. The person terminates the change process because he is able to continue the new, more health-conscious way of cooking.

Although the terms used are slightly different, the intent of the PAPM is much like that of the TTM. The stages are (1) unaware of the issue, (2) unengaged by the issue, (3) deciding about acting, (4) deciding not to act, (5) deciding to act, (6) acting, and (7) maintenance. You can apply the earlier cooking example to these stages as well.

Use of Technology in Health Education

As has been mentioned earlier in the chapter, many kinds of technologies, such as computer games and programs, videos, CDs, and Internet resources, can increase learning. These technologies may enable the learner to control the pace of instruction, offer flexibility in the time and location of learning, present an appealing form of education, and provide immediate feedback. During the COVID-19 pandemic of 2020, many schools ceased meeting in classrooms, and classes were conducted for all grades and college level via online platforms. People used the Internet for school, work, other types of meetings, and socialization and as a source of health information. In a 2019 update of a 2015 post, analysts at the Pew Research Center found that 10% of US adults said they did not use the Internet, and the group most likely to not use the Internet were individuals 65 years old and older. All of the 18- to 29-year-olds who participated in the study said they used the Internet. The percentage of non-Internet users ages 65 and older declined from 2018 to 2019 by 7%. However, in 2019, 27% of individuals in this age group did not use the Internet. They also found that adults with less than a high school education and who earned less than $30,000 per year were less likely to use the Internet (Anderson M, Perrin A, Jiang J, and Kuman M, 2019).

When the Pew Research Center began tracking social media use in 2005, only 5% of American adults used at least one of these platforms. That number grew to 50% in 2011 and 72% in 2019. The most widely used platforms are YouTube and Facebook, and approximately three-fourths of Facebook users visit the site at least once a day. Young adults were the early adopters of social media and continue to use these sites at high levels; however, older adult usage has increased in recent years (Pew Research Center, June 2019).

Why do people use the Internet? A major benefit is its convenience: It is available 24 hours per day, 7 days per week, and there is no need to drive there, take public transportation, or find a parking place. Is the Internet a good source of health information? The answer depends on the site you use to find your information.

Clients may ask nurses to provide them with information about ways to evaluate the quality and reliability of this information. According to the NNLM, there are several things to consider when evaluating health information on the Internet (NNLM, 2018):

- *Accuracy*: Is the information accurate and from a reputable site (i.e., CDC; National Institutes of Health). Is there an editorial review? Do you see spelling or grammatical errors?
- *Authority*: Are there references or citations? Are the authors, their credentials, and affiliations listed, and are they credible?
- *Bias/Objectivity*: Does the information come from a source that is biased? Does the site market products?
- *Currency/Timeliness:* Are there dates when the information was updated? Do the links work?
- *Coverage:* Is the information complete?

The following Evidence-Based Practice box describes the effective use of a smartphone app for health promotion.

EVIDENCE-BASED PRACTICE

The use of technology as a way to provide health education and intervene in the progress of a chronic illness, hypertension, was presented in a case study. The authors used TXT2DASH, which is an mHealth program designed to improve self-management and increase nutritional self-efficacy in patients who sought care at free health care clinics and who had hypertension. In this program the patients were sent weekly educational text messages on the Dietary Approaches to Stop Hypertension (DASH) diet. This diet has been shown to reduce and control blood pressure. Messages were sent 3 days a week for 4 weeks; each week, a different food category was discussed. Three health care clinics providing free care participated in the project, and 13 patients completed the final data collection and demonstrated dietary behavior improvements, especially in the areas of drinking soda and using fats and oils.

Nurse Use

It is important in any health education program to consider the readability and user friendliness of the program. The cost of the program to the participants or to the clinic must be considered. If a text messaging program is used, it is important to determine whether there is any support to the patients to enable them to have cellular devices.

Welsh, P: Strategies in development of an mHealth technology for low socioeconomic groups in free healthcare clinics, *Comput Inform Nurs* 34(1):3–5, January 2016.

Evaluation of the Educational Process

Evaluation is important in both the educational process and the nursing process. Evaluation is a systematic and logical way to make decisions to improve the educational program. You will need to evaluate the educator, the process, and the product. Feedback to the *educator* provides the educator an opportunity to modify the teaching process and better meet the learner's needs. The educator may receive written feedback from learners, such as with an evaluation sheet. The educator also may ask for verbal feedback, as well as get nonverbal feedback by using return demonstrations to see what learners have mastered and by observing facial expressions when feedback is being given. Increasingly evaluations are done on a computer platform.

Process evaluation examines the dynamic components of the educational program. It follows and assesses the movements and management of information transfer and attempts to make sure that the objectives are being met. Process evaluation is necessary *throughout* the educational program to determine whether goals and objectives are being met and the time required for their accomplishment. Ongoing evaluation also allows the teacher to correct misinformation, misinterpretation, or confusion and to periodically reconsider the goals and objectives of the program. Periodically review program goals and objectives to determine if the health behavior change is really necessary.

The *educational product,* an outcome of the educational process, is measured both qualitatively and quantitatively (Bastable, 2014). For example, a qualitative assessment should answer the question, "How well does the learner appear to understand the content?" A quantitative assessment should answer the question, "How much of the content does the learner retain?" Thus the quality of the product is measured by improvement and increase, or the lack thereof, in the learner's knowledge, skills, and abilities related to the content of the educational program. Selected outcomes for the population of interest need to be identified when the educational program is designed so you can measure the program's effectiveness.

Evaluation of Health and Behavioral Changes

Various approaches, methods, and tools can be used to evaluate health and behavioral changes. These include questionnaires, rating scales, surveys, checklists, skills demonstrations, testing, subjective client feedback, and direct observation of improvements in client mastery of materials. Qualitative or quantitative strategies may be used to measure changes in knowledge, skills, abilities, attitudes, behavior, health status, and quality of life. Choose the method of evaluation based on the situation. For example, when evaluating a person's ability to perform a psychomotor skill such as changing a dressing, it is best to watch the person perform the skill.

Also evaluate both short-term and long-term effects of the health teaching. A short-term evaluation of whether a client can perform a return demonstration of breast self-examination requires minimal energy, expense, or time and shows skill mastery within a matter of minutes. If the short-term objective is not met, the nurse determines why and identifies possible solutions so that successful learning can occur. If the short-term objective is met, the nurse then focuses on long-term evaluation designed to assess the lasting effects of the education program.

Long-term follow-up with clients is challenging, and it focuses on following and assessing the status of an individual, family, community, or population over time to determine whether specific goals and objectives were met. Often, for nurse educators, the goal of long-term evaluation is to analyze the effectiveness of the education program for the entire community, not the health status of a specific client. Nurses track the achievement of community objectives over time but not that of the individual community members. Thus in a changing population, long-term evaluation of the results of an education program is still possible. The percentage of objectives and goals met by sampling the target population gives valid statistics for program assessment, even though the population of individuals may have experienced a complete turnover.

For example, a nurse notes that according to annual health department data, 60% of the pregnant women in the nurse's catchment area received some prenatal care. Wanting to increase this percentage to 100%, the nurse tries an educational intervention in which radio and television stations make public service announcements about the importance and availability of prenatal services.

After 1 year, the nurse discovers that 80% of all pregnant women now receive prenatal care. The nurse continues to use public service announcements the following year because good results are evident. However, the long-term goal of the education program to influence the behavior of 100% of the pregnant women in the community has not yet been met. Therefore the nurse enlists volunteers to put informational posters in shopping malls, grocery stores, public transportation stops, laundries, and public transportation vehicles. In the second year after implementing the revised educational program, again using the statistics from the health department, the nurse finds that 95% of all pregnant women in the target area now receive prenatal care. The nurse can thus evaluate and modify a community educational program over time to increase the rate, range, and consistency of progress made toward meeting the long-term goals of the project.

It may be hard to keep track of the clients to complete the evaluation; some will move, and others will lose interest and fail to keep appointments or return calls, text messages, or e-mails. During the COVID-19 pandemic, contact tracing was a challenging way to locate people exposed to the virus. The virus was spread rapidly and via minute particles; it was challenging to know who came into contact with the person who had the virus.

A considerable amount of health education is carried out in the community in groups rather than provided to one person at a time. For this reason, the following section discusses how groups can be used as a tool for health education and the promotion of health.

HEALTH EDUCATION FOR COMMUNITY GROUPS

Nurses often provide health education to groups. Members of the group may support either beneficial or poor health practices. For example, a young person may be part of a group that abuses substances. Another youth might be part of a group that runs marathons. The health-oriented goals of each of these two groups are different. A group is an effective and powerful medium to initiate and implement changes for individuals, families, organizations, and the community. Groups form for various reasons. They may form for a clearly stated purpose or goal, or they may form naturally as shared values, interests, activities, or personal characteristics attract individuals to each other.

Community groups represent the collective interests, needs, and values of individuals; they provide a link between the individual and the larger social system. Throughout life, group membership influences thoughts, choices, behaviors, and values as people socialize and interact. Through groups, people may express personal views and relate them to the views of others. Groups serve as communication networks and can help to organize various aspects of communities.

Community groups may be informal or formal. Formal groups have a defined membership and a specific purpose. They may or may not have an official place in the community's organization. In informal groups, the ties among members are multiple, and the purposes are unwritten yet understood by members. These groups often form spontaneously when participants have a common interest or need. You can find out about what formal and informal groups exist in a community by reading the local newspaper or local Internet sites, listening to public service information on the radio or television, and asking residents about the groups to which they belong. Nurses can help to form new groups or create linkages among existing groups.

Group support often helps people to make needed changes for health that they are unable to accomplish on their own or with the help of just one individual. For example, groups may support physical activity and fitness, sound nutrition, conquering smoking or drug abuse, getting out of abusive relationships, and safe sexual practices. One of the core competencies for public health professionals is to "use group processes to advance community involvement" (Council on Linkages, 2014, p 9).

Group: Definitions and Concepts

A group is a collection of interacting individuals who have common purposes. To some extent, each member influences and is in turn influenced by every other member. Groups form for a variety of reasons. Families, an example of a community group, share kinship bonds, living space, and economic resources. There are many group purposes, such as teaching the members and providing psychological support and socialization.

Groups also form in response to community needs, problems, or opportunities. For example, community residents may form a neighborhood association to protect their health and welfare. Community groups occur spontaneously because of mutual attraction between individuals and to meet personal needs such as those for socialization and recreation. Health-promoting groups may form when people meet in community and health care settings and discover common challenges to their physical and emotional well-being.

Groups need to identify a clear purpose so they can establish criteria for member selection and determine an action plan. A clear statement of purpose proved valuable in forming a new group in one city's housing development. The local department of social services had received numerous reports of child abuse and neglect. Routine home visits for well-child care documented high stress between parents and their offspring, and some parents asked the nurse to teach them about child discipline. The nurse proposed that a parent group address this community need, and she chose this purpose for the group: *dealing with kids for child and parent satisfaction.* The purpose indicated both the process (to help parents deal with children) and the desired outcome (satisfaction for parents and children). Having a group purpose stated enabled parents to decide if they wanted to join.

Cohesion is the attraction among individual members and between each member and the group. Individuals in a highly cohesive group identify themselves as a unit, work toward common goals, endure frustration for the sake of the group, and defend the group against outside criticism. Attraction increases when members feel accepted and liked by others, see similar qualities in one another, share similar attitudes and values, and work together to meet group goals. Member traits that increase group cohesion and productivity include: (1) compatible personal and group goals, (2) attraction to group goals, (3) attraction to members of the group, and (4) a mix among members with problem solving, leading, and following skills.

Groups have both task and maintenance functions. A task function is anything a member does that deliberately contributes to the group's purpose. Members with task-directed abilities tend to attractive to the group. These traits include strong problem-solving skills, access to material resources, and skills in directing. Maintenance functions help members to affirm, accept, and support one another, resolve conflicts, and create social and environmental comfort. Groups need members with both task and maintenance functions. In contrast, some member traits can decrease cohesion and productivity, such as (1) conflicts between personal and group goals, aversion to some members of the group, and not understanding the behaviors and attributes of one another; (2) lack of interest in group goals and activities; (3) poor problem-solving and communication abilities; and (4) lack of both leadership and supporter skills and (5) disagreement about types of leadership. Usually, the more alike group members are, the stronger is a group's attraction. Differences tend to decrease attractiveness and may lead to competition and jealousy among members. At the same time, personal differences can increase group cohesion if they support complementary functioning or provide contrasting viewpoints necessary for decision making. Cohesive factors are complex, and many factors influence member attraction to each other and to the group's goal. High group cohesion positively affects productivity and member satisfaction. The following example illustrates factors that influence group cohesion.

A nurse initiated a group for clients who had been treated for burns. Ten residents from the same town had been discharged after a month in the local burn unit. The stated purpose of the group was to teach coping skills to assist members in the transition from hospital to home. Each person had been treated for extensive burns in an intensive care treatment center; each had relied heavily on health care workers for physical, social, and emotional rehabilitation; and each had faced the challenge of resuming work and family roles. Individuals shared some similar experiences and hopes for the future but varied in the amount of trauma and stress experienced. They also differed widely in psychological readiness for return to ordinary daily routines. One woman in the group was able to return quickly to her job as a cashier in a large supermarket. The strength of her determination to overcome public reaction to her scars, coupled with an ability to "use the right words" and an empathy for others, distinguished her from others in the group. These differences proved attractive to other members, inspiring them to work toward a return to their own roles in life. These members saw her differences as attainable.

This group's cohesion was provided by the members' attraction to the common purpose of returning to successful life patterns and managing relationships with others. Members also thought that interaction with others with similar burn experiences could help them reach that goal. This example shows that certain member experiences, such as crises or traumas, may help individuals identify with each other and increase member attraction.

Being different from the general population and similar to the other group members is, for some, a compelling force for membership in the group. Other members may not want to be identified by an aversive characteristic such as disfigurement. Empathy for another's pain, learned only through mutual experience, may provide each individual with a required perspective for problem solving or affirming another's view. This group was effective, and the nurse helped members use common experiences and learn from their differences.

Member' attraction to the group is influenced by factors such as. the group programs, size, type of organization, and position in the community. Attraction to the group is increased when individuals understand the goals and see group activities as effective. Cohesive groups tend to be more productive and able to accomplish their goals; cohesion can be increased as members better understand the experiences of others and identify common ideas and reactions to various issues. Nurses facilitate this process by pointing out similarities, contrasting supportive differences, or helping members redefine differences in ways that make those dissimilarities compatible.

Norms are standards that guide, control, and regulate individuals and communities. Group norms set the standards for group members' behaviors, attitudes, and perceptions. Group norms suggest what a group believes is important, what it finds acceptable or objectionable, or what it perceives is of no consequence. The task norm is the commitment to return to the central goals of the group. The strength of the task norm determines the group's ability to adhere to its work.

Maintenance norms create group pressures to affirm members and maintain their comfort. Maintenance behaviors include identifying the social and psychological tensions of members and taking steps to support those members at high-stress times. For example, maintenance norms often refer to things such as scheduling meetings at convenient times and in an accessible and comfortable space with parking as well as seating, refreshments, and toilets.

Groups also have reality norms, whereby members reinforce or challenge and correct their ideas of what is real. Groups can examine the life situations facing members and help to make sense of them. As individuals gather information, attempt to understand that information, make decisions, and consider the facts and their implications, they can take responsible action, not only in relation to themselves and their group but also for the community. Group (task, maintenance, and reality) norms combine to form a group culture. Reality norms influence each member to see relevant situations in the same way the other members see them. For example, suppose a group of individuals with diabetes defines an uncontrolled diet as harmful; members may try to influence one another to maintain diet control. The nurse can provide accurate information about diet and the disease process while continually conveying an assurance that health through diet control is attainable and desirable.

Group members with similar backgrounds may have a limited scope of knowledge. For example, women members of a spouse abuse group may think that men are exploitative and harmful based on their childhood and marriage experiences. Such a stereotypical view of men could be reinforced by similar perceptions in other members; this might lead to continuing anger, fear of interactions with men, and a hostile or helpless approach to family affairs. Nurses or group members who have known men in loving, helpful, and collaborative ways can describe these perceptions of men and offer positive examples. Nurses bring an important perspective to groups in which similar backgrounds limit the understanding and interpretation of personal concerns.

Groups have role structures that define the expected ways in which members behave toward one another. The role that each person assumes serves a purpose in the group. Roles might be as leader, follower, task specialist, maintenance specialist, evaluator, peacemaker, and gatekeeper. Box 14.5 includes descriptions of each of these group roles. Because leadership is an especially complex role, it will be discussed in greater detail.

Leadership is a complex concept. It consists of behaviors that guide or direct members and determine and influence group action. Positive leadership defines or negotiates the group's purpose, selects and helps implement tasks that accomplish the purpose, maintains an environment that affirms and supports members, and balances efforts between task and maintenance. An effective leader pays attention to communications and interactions among the members, including spoken words and body language, and this information provides continuous feedback about the members and the group process. By paying close attention to communications and interactions, members detect changing group needs and can take responsibility and pride in their own involvement. One or more members may lead the group, or many may share leadership. Shared leadership may increase productivity, cohesion, and satisfying interactions among members.

After initiating or establishing a group, nurses may facilitate leadership within and among members, frequently relinquishing central control and encouraging members to determine the ultimate leadership pattern for their group. In some settings and circumstances, a single authority is necessary (e.g., when members have limited skills or time or are uncomfortable with shared responsibility for leading). A leadership style that shares leading functions with other group members is effective when there are many alternatives and when issues of values and ethics are involved in the group's action. Leadership can be described as patriarchal (paternal) or democratic. Each of these styles has a particular effect on members' interaction, satisfaction, and productivity. Groups may reflect one or a combination of styles.

A patriarchal or paternal style is seen when one person has the final authority for group direction and movement. A person using patriarchal leadership may control members through rewards and threats, often not informing them about the goals and rationale behind prescribed actions. Patriarchal and paternal styles of leadership are authoritarian; they can be used in a disaster team, in which immediate task accomplishment is the goal. Group morale and cohesiveness are typically low under sustained authoritarian styles of leadership, and members may not learn how to function independently. In addition, issues of authority and control may disrupt productivity if the group members challenge the power of the leader. Democratic leadership is cooperative and promotes and supports member involvement in all aspects of decision making and planning. Members influence each other as they explore goals, plan steps toward the goals, implement those steps, and evaluate progress.

Choosing Groups for Health Change

Nurses choose the type of group to use after considering the overall needs of the community and its people, including client contacts, expressed concerns of community spokespersons, health statistics for the area, available health resources, and the

---

BOX 14.5   Examples of Group Role Behavior

There are many examples; this is a representative list of the types of roles members may use.

Follower: Seeks and accepts the authority or direction of others
Gatekeeper: Controls outsiders' access to the group
Leader: Guides and directs group activity
Maintenance specialist: Provides physical and psychological support for group members, thereby holding the group together
Peacemaker: Attempts to reconcile conflict between members or takes action in response to influences that disrupt the group process and threaten its existence
Task specialist: Focuses or directs movement toward the main work of the group

community's general well-being. These data point to the community's strengths and critical needs.

The nurse can identify goals for the community and for various groups through media reports and from community informants and colleagues. Community members should be involved in setting the goals and in planning the interventions. Alliances or coalitions unite diverse interest groups whose members share a common interest in perceived threats to community health to both analyze the community and develop the plan for change. Nurses and other professionals are active in groups formed to address community issues.

Nurses may work with existing groups or form new groups. Deciding whether to work in established groups or to begin new ones is based on client needs, the purpose of existing groups, and the membership ties in existing groups. The advantages to using established groups for individual health change are that membership ties already exist, the existing structure can be used, and it is not necessary to find new members because compatible individuals already form a working group. Established groups usually have operating methods that have proved successful; an approach for a new goal is built on this history. Members are aware of each other's strengths, limitations, and preferred styles of interaction and may be comfortable working together, and they may be able to influence one another. If you choose to work with an established group, be sure to determine whether the new focus is compatible with the existing group purposes. Fig. 14.5 shows a breakout session during a community forum.

Nurses can use existing community groups as a source of information to conduct a community assessment. Many community groups, such as health-planning groups, better business clubs, women's action groups, school boards, and neighborhood councils, are excellent resources for information because part of

their purpose is to determine and respond to community needs. In addition, they are already established as part of the community structure. When a group representing one community sector is selected for community health intervention, the total community structure is studied. Groups reflect existing community values, strengths, and norms.

How might nurses help established groups work toward community goals? The same interventions recommended for groups formed for individual health change can be used for groups focused on community health. Such interventions include the following:

- Build cohesion through clarifying goals and individual attraction to groups
- Build member commitment and participation
- Keep the group focused on the goal
- Maintain members through recognition and encouragement
- Maintain member self-esteem during conflict and confrontation
- Analyze forces affecting movement toward the goal
- Evaluate progress

When nurses enter established groups, they need to assess the leadership, communications, and normative structures. This facilitates group planning, problem solving, intervention, and evaluation. The steps for community health changes parallel those of decision making and problem solving in other methodologies.

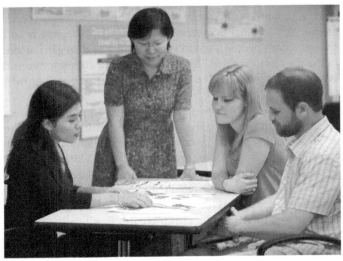

Fig. 14.5 Breakout Session in a Community Forum on Environmental Health Concerns. (From Centers for Disease Control and Prevention, 2009, courtesy Dawn Arlotta.)

CASE EXAMPLE

A nurse was asked to meet with a neighborhood council to help them study and "do something about" the number of homeless living on the streets. Residents knew the nurse from a local clinic and from his consulting work at a shelter for the homeless in an adjacent community. When the council invited him, they said, "Our intent is to be part of the solution rather than part of the problem." The nurse agreed to meet, and he learned that the neighborhood council had addressed concerns of the neighborhood for 20 years—protecting zoning guidelines, setting up a recreational program for teens, organizing an after-school program for latchkey children, and generally representing the homeowners of the area. The neighborhood was composed of low-income families who took great pride in their homes. After meeting with the council and listening to their description of the situation, the nurse agreed to help, and he joined the council.

As the first step in addressing the problem, the council conducted a comprehensive problem analysis on the homeless situation. All known causes and outcomes of homeless persons on the street were identified, and the relationships between each factor and the problem were documented from literature and from the local history. The nurse brought expertise in health planning and knowledge of the homeless and their health risks. He suggested negotiation between the council and the local coalition for the homeless, recognizing that planning would be most relevant if homeless individuals participated. The council was cohesive and committed to the purpose, had developed working operations, and did not need help with group process. They made adjustments in their usual group operation to use the knowledge and health-planning skills of the nurse. Interventions for the homeless included establishing temporary shelters at homes on a rotating basis, providing daily meals through the city council or churches, and joining the area coalition for the homeless.

This example shows how an established, competent group addressed a new goal successfully by building on existing strengths in partnership with the nurse. Community groups, because of their interactive roles, are logical and natural vehicles for people who work together for community health change. As the decision-making and problem-solving capabilities of community groups are strengthened, the groups become more able representatives for the whole community. Nurses improve the community's health by working with groups toward that goal.

When it is neither desirable nor possible to use existing groups, the nurse can initiate a selected membership group. Choose members who have common health needs or concerns. For instance, individuals with diabetes can meet to discuss diet management and physical care and to share problem-solving remedies; community residents can meet for social support and rehabilitation after treatment for mental illness; or isolated older adults can meet to socialize, eat nutritious meals, and exercise. Consider members' attributes when composing a new group. Members are attracted to others from similar backgrounds, with similar experiences, and with common interests and abilities.

The size of the group influences effectiveness; between 8 and 12 is useful for group work focused on individual health changes. Groups of up to 25 members may be effective when their focus is on community needs. Large groups often divide and assign tasks to the smaller subgroups, with the original large groups meeting less frequently for reporting and evaluation. Setting member criteria can facilitate recruitment and selection of the most appropriate members for any group. The criteria usually suggest a mixture of member traits, allowing for balance for the processes of decision making and growth.

Beginning Interactions and Dealing with Conflict

Begin to work on the stated purpose as soon as the group forms. Help members interact by paying attention to maintenance tasks of attending, eliciting information, clarifying, and recognizing contributions of members. Discuss what brought each member to the group. Encourage each person to participate; recognize and support them as they take on leadership functions. The new group begins to take shape in the early sessions as members try out familiar roles and test their individual abilities. The core competency skills for communication recommended by the Public Health Foundation (Council on Linkages, 2014) are useful to nurses who work with groups in the community. Box 14.6 lists these competencies. Subsequent steps are then planned not only according to the nurse's skill and preference but also according to the group composition and the skills brought by members.

Conflict is normal in human relations. People may see conflict as the opposite of harmony and try to guard against it. This is an unfortunate view because the tensions of difference and potential conflict actually help groups work toward their purposes. It is important to understand common causes

BOX 14.6 **Core Competencies for Communication Skills of Educators**

Communication Skills
- Communicates effectively both in writing and orally, including via e-mail.
- Solicits input from individuals and organizations.
- Advocates for public health programs and resources.
- Leads and participates in groups to address specific issues.
- Uses the media, various technologies, and community networks to convey information.
- Effectively presents accurate demographic, statistical, programmatic, and scientific information for professional and lay audiences.

Attitudes
- Listens to others in an unbiased manner.
- Respects points of view of others.
- Promotes the expression of diverse opinions and perspectives.

of conflict and conflict management and resolution approaches. Conflict signals that antagonistic points of view must be considered and that one must reexamine beliefs and assumptions underlying relationships. Some people are concerned about security, control of self and others, respect between parties, and access to limited resources. In groups, members may express frustrations about trust, closeness and separation, and dependence and independence. These themes of interpersonal conflict operate to some extent in all interactions and are not unique to groups. Conflict can be overwhelming, especially when members think that expressing controversy is unacceptable or unremitting or when it is suppressed over time and builds up to an explosive stage. A group that repeatedly avoids expressing conflict becomes fragile, unable to adapt, and helpless to face challenges. Conflict may be destructive if contentious parties fail to respect the rights and beliefs of others.

Approaches for acknowledging conflict and solving problems that respect others and represent self-concerns are first learned in families and other small groups. These lessons teach people that conflict is natural and can support growth and change. Other people learn to avoid conflict or disregard others in the promotion of self. Teams that try to be harmonious and avoid conflict may hinder collaboration and personal growth (Fogler et al., 2018.).

It is important to evaluate individual and group progress toward meeting health goals. Early in the planning, specify the action steps that should be taken to meet the goals. These small steps may be responses to learning objectives (listed as action steps designed to support facilitative forces and deal with resistive forces), or they may reflect the group's problem-solving plan. The action steps and the indicators of achievement are discussed and written in a group record. Build recognition of accomplishments into the evaluation system. Recognition may include concrete rewards, such as special foods and drinks, or it may be the personal expression of joy and member-to-member approval. Celebration of group accomplishments marks progress, rewards members, and motivates each person to continue.

⟩⟩ APPLYING CONTENT TO PRACTICE

Just as objectives in *Healthy People 2030* (USDHHS, 2020) recommend that health education and promotion be used to provide public health care, so do other key documents, such as the ANA's *Scope & Standards of Practice: Public Health Nursing* second edition, Standard 5b, labeled Health Education and Health Promotion, which says that the "public health nurse employs multiple strategies to promote health, prevent disease, and ensure a safe environment for populations" (ANA, 2013, p 23). Similarly, the *Core Competences for Public Health Professionals* of the Council on Linkages between Academia and Public Health Practice (2014) lists eight competencies related to communication skills; seven of them relate directly to this chapter. These competencies, which are discussed and illustrated throughout the chapter, are as follows:

1. Assesses the health literacy of populations served
2. Communicates in writing and orally, in person, and through electronic means, with linguistic and cultural proficiency
3. Solicits input from individuals and organizations
4. Uses a variety of approaches to disseminate public health information
5. Conveys data to professionals and to the public using a variety of approaches
6. Communicates information to influence behavior and improve health
7. Facilitates communication among individuals, groups, and organizations
8. Describes the roles of governmental public health, health care, and other partners in improving the health of the community

▮ PRACTICE APPLICATION

During Kristi's BSN student public health practicum at a local health department, the health department got many calls from people wanting information about the COVID-19 virus. For Kristi's community health intervention project, she decides to do a community educational piece on this topic. *What is her best course of action?*

A. Develop a poster presentation to have on display at the health department.

B. Assemble an educative pamphlet to mail to anyone calling with questions.

C. Work with the health department staff to develop a community forum–style presentation and information brochures on this virus.

D. Develop an in-service program for health department staff on the potential spread of the virus and ways to prevent its spread.

Answers can be found on the Evolve website.

▮ REMEMBER THIS!

- Health education is essential in nursing because the promotion, maintenance, and restoration of health rely on clients' understanding of health care topics.
- Nurse educators identify learning needs, consider how people learn, examine educational issues, design and implement educational programs, and evaluate the effects of the educational program on learning and behavior.
- Nurses often use the *Healthy People 2030* educational objectives as a guide to identifying community-based learning needs.
- Education and learning are different. Education is the establishment and arrangement of events to facilitate learning. Learning is the process of gaining knowledge and expertise and results in behavioral changes.

- There are cognitive, affective, and psychomotor domains of learning. Depending on the needs of the learner, one or more of these domains may be important for the nurse educator to consider as learning programs are developed.
- Nine principles associated with community health education are gaining attention, informing the learner of the objectives of instruction, stimulating recall of prior learning, presenting the stimulus, providing learning guidance, eliciting performance, providing feedback, assessing performance, and enhancing retention and transfer of knowledge.
- Often, theory can guide the development of health education programs. Two useful ones are the Health Belief Model and the Transtheoretical Model, which are discussed in connection with the Precaution Adoption Process Model.
- Principles that guide the effective educator include message, format, environment, experience, participation, and evaluation.
- Educational issues include population considerations, barriers to learning, and technologic issues.
- Two important learner-related barriers are low literacy level, especially health literacy, and lack of motivation to learn information and make the needed changes.
- The five phases of the educational process are identifying educational needs, establishing educational goals and objectives, selecting appropriate educational methods, implementing the educational plan, and evaluating the educational process and product.
- Evaluation of the product includes the measurement of short-term and long-term goals and objectives related to improving health and promoting behavioral changes.
- Working with groups is an important skill for nurses. Groups are an effective and powerful vehicle for initiating and implementing healthful changes.
- A group is a collection of interacting individuals with a common purpose. Each member influences and is influenced by other group members to varying degrees.
- Group cohesion is enhanced by commonly shared characteristics among members and diminished by differences among members.
- Cohesion is the measure of attraction between members and the group. Cohesion or the lack of it affects the group's function.
- Norms are standards that guide and regulate individuals and communities. These norms are unwritten and often unspoken and serve to ensure group movement to a goal, to maintain the group, and to influence group members' perceptions and interpretations of reality.
- Some diversity of member backgrounds is usually a positive influence on a group.
- Leadership is an important and complex group concept. Leadership is described as patriarchal or democratic.
- Group structure emerges from various member influences, including members' understanding and support of the group purpose.
- Conflicts in groups may develop from competition for roles or member disagreement about the roles ascribed to them.
- Health behavior is greatly influenced by the groups to which people belong and for which they value membership.

- Understanding group concepts provides a basis for identifying community groups and their goals, characteristics, and norms. Nurses use their understanding of group principles to work with community groups toward needed health changes.

EVOLVE WEBSITE

http://evolve.elsevier.com/Stanhope/foundations
- Case Study, with Questions and Answers
- NCLEX® Review Questions
- Practice Application Answers

REFERENCES

American Nurses Association: *ANA's principles for social networking and the nurse,* Silver Spring, MD, 2011. ANA.

American Nurses Association: *Scope & standards of practice: public health nursing,* ed 2, Silver Spring, MD, 2013, ANA.

Anderson M, Perrin A, Jiang J and Kuman M: *10% of Americans don't use the internet. Who are they?"* Pew Research Center, April 22, 2019, www.pewresearch.org/fact-tank, retrieved May 2020.

Bastable SB: *Nurse as educator,* ed 4, Boston, 2014, Jones and Bartlett.

Bloom BS, Englehart MO, Furst EJ, et al: *Taxonomy of educational objectives: the classification of educational goals—handbook. I. cognitive domain,* White Plains, NY, 1956, Longman.

Caplin M, Saunders T: Utilizing teach-back to reinforce patient education: A step-by-step approach, *Orthopaedic Nursing* 34(6): 365–368, 2015.

Centers for Disease Control and Prevention: *Tools for cross-cultural communication and language access can help organizations address health literacy and improve communication effectiveness,* Atlanta, October 2019a, Centers for Disease Control and Prevention. Retrieved May 2020 from http://www.cdc.gov/healthliteracy/culture.html.

Centers for Disease Control and Prevention: *Health literacy: plain language communication,* October 2019 b, Atlanta, Retrieved May 2020 from http://www.cdc.gov.healthliteracy.

Centers for Disease Control and Prevention: *Understanding health literacy,* October 22, 2019d, Atlanta, Retrieved November 2020 from http://www.cdc.gov.understanding health literacy.

Centers for Disease Control and Prevention: *Health communication basics,* 2020a, www.cdc/gov/healthcommunicationbasics, retrieved May 2020.

Council on Linkages between Academia and Public Health Practice: *Core competencies for public health professionals,* Washington, DC, 2014, Public Health Foundation. Retrieved May 2020 from http://www.phf.org.

Cronenwett L, Sherwood G, Barnsteiner J, et al: Quality and safety education for nurses, *Nurs Outlook* 55:122–131, 2007.

Edberg M: *Essentials of health behavior: Social and behavioral theory in public health,* ed 2, Burlington, MA, 2015, Jones and Bartlett.

Fogler J, Poole MS, Stutman RK: Communication & conflict. In *Working through conflict: strategies for relationships, groups and organizations,* New York, NY, 2018, Routledge/Taylor & Francis.

French KS: Transforming nursing care through health literacy *Nurs Clin N Am* 50:87-98, 2015. ACTS,

Graff M, Scott RA. Justice AE, et al: Genome-wide physical activity interactions in adiposity—A meta-analysis of 200,452 adults, *PLOS, Genetics,* 13(8): e1006972. Accessed May 2020.

Health Resources and Services Administration: *Health literacy,* n.d. Retrieved February 2016 from http://www.hrsa.gov/publichealth/healthliteracy/.

Knowles MS, Holton EF III, Swanson RA: *The adult learner: the definitive classic in adult education and human resource development,* ed 8, New York, 2015, Routledge.

Kutner M, Greenberg E, Jin Y, Paulsen C: *The health literacy of America's adults: results from the 2003 National Assessment of Adult Literacy.* NCES 2006-483, Washington, DC, 2006, US Department of Education, Center for Education. Retrieved May 2020 from www. NCES.gov.

Ratzan SC, Parker RM: Introduction. In Selden CR, Zorn M, Ratzan SC, et al, editors: *National*

National Center for Education Statistics (NCES): *What is PIAAC?* www.nces.ed.gov, n.d.

National Council of State Boards of Nursing: (NCSBN): *A nurse's guide to the use of social media,* 2011, NCSBN. Retrieved from https://www.ncsbn.org, Mary 2020.

National Network of Libraries of Medicine (NNLM): *Evaluating health websites,* 2018, https://nnlm.gov/initiates/topics/health-websites. Retrieved May 2020.

National Network of Libraries of Medicine (NNLM): *Health literacy,* n.d. https://www.nnlm.gov, Retrieved May 2020.

Pew Research Center: *Social media fact sheet,* 2019, www.pewresearch-center.org>topics/social media, Retrieved May 2020.

Quad Council Coalition Competency Review Task Force, 2018, Community/Public Health Nursing Competencies.

Reinhart RJ: *Nurses continue to rate highest in honesty, ethics,* 2020, Gallup Poll, https://news.gallup.com/poll, Retrieved May 2020.

US Department of Health and Human Services: *Healthy People 2030,* Washington, DC, 2020, DHHS. http://www.healthypeople.

US Department of Health and Human Services, Office of Disease Prevention and Health Promotion: *National action plan to improve health literacy,* Washington, DC, 2010, Author.

Wlodkowski RJ, Ginsberg MB: What motivates adults to learn? *Enhancing adult motivation to learn: A comprehensive guide to teaching all adults,* San Francisco, 2017, Jossey Bass, pp. 81-106.

Welsh P: Strategies in development of an mHealth technology for low socioeconomic groups in free healthcare clinics, *CIN: Computers, Informatics, Nursing* 34(1):3–5, January 2016.

15

Case Management

Ann H. Cary

OBJECTIVES

After reading this chapter, the student should be able to:

1. Define continuity of care, care management, case management, care coordination, population health management, transitional care, integrated care, social determinants of health, and advocacy.
2. Describe the scope of practice, roles, and functions of a case manager.
3. Compare and contrast the nursing process with the process of case management and advocacy
4. Identify methods to manage conflict, as well as the process of achieving collaboration.
5. Define and explain the legal and ethical issues confronting case managers.

CHAPTER OUTLINE

KEY TERMS

Since the Patient Protection and Affordable Care Act (ACA) was initiated in 2010 and has evolved throughout implementation, the health care industry continues to reevaluate systems and processes that attempt to integrate financing, management, quality, and service delivery models that will ultimately improve population health. Challenges abound for clients and providers as they attempt to coordinate care, transition clients among providers and systems, access and share information and documentation about clients and communities, and navigate the complexity of integrated care to optimize quality and access while managing costs and achieving value-based health care. The new models of health care financing provide incentives to value care outcomes over the volume of care provided. Delivery of care is now organized through a network of providers, such as negotiated contracts with hospitals and other levels of care, physicians, nurse practitioners, pharmacies, ancillary health services, outpatient centers, and home health care.

Managing the health of populations served by any integrated system is essential, whether the definition includes a geographic area or shared characteristics of the population such as age, race, gender, occupation, education, or health status, as examples (National Advisory Council on Nurse Education and Practice [NACNEP], 2016). These include accountable care organizations (ACOs). Nurse case managers and nurse care managers play a pivotal role in population health delivery. Population management includes the following:

- Wellness and health promotion
- Illness prevention
- Acute and subacute care
- Chronic disease
- Rehabilitation
- End-of-life care
- Care coordination
- Community engagement

Case managers and care coordination are at the core of population health strategies to improve the community outcomes (Kimmel, 2016). Population health management can maintain and improve the physical and psychosocial status of clients through cost-effective and customized solutions, such as coordinating and transitioning care to reduce gaps and costs; supporting evidence-based practices; selecting quality care that is culturally competent; and providing disease management and self-management educational programming (Case Management Society of America [CMSA], 2016). Examples include planning and delivery strategies for adolescents in a school-based clinic system or the chronic disease management of elderly in a rural community to avoid nursing home placement (Huber, 2018; McKesson Corporation, 2014; Sebelius, 2011).

The ACA endorses the use of integrated systems to attain the following objectives:

- Emphasis is on population health management across the continuum, rather than on episodes of illness for an individual.
- Management has shifted from inpatient care as the point of management to primary care providers as points of entry.
- Care management services and programs provide access and accountability for the continuum of health.

- Successful outcomes are measured by systems performance and pay for performance for providers to meet the needs of populations.

The contemporary focus of integrated health systems defines the nature of the client as a population in addition to that as an individual. In these systems, population management involves the following activities:

- Assessing the needs of the client population through health histories (and, in the future, genograms), claims, use-of-service patterns, and risk factors, and communicating through interoperable information systems to ascertain patterns, trends, and responses to health programming in a population
- Creating benefits and network designs to address these needs
- Selecting dashboard indicators to measure performance
- Prioritizing actions to produce a desired outcome with available resources
- Selecting evidence-based programs related to wellness, prevention, health promotion, and demand management; patient/client engagement; and educating the population about them
- Instituting evidence-based care management processes that ensure transitional and coordinated care across the health continuum for a population aggregate
- Deploying case managers within a variety of delivery and insurance systems to clients and providers
- Evaluating provider patterns of performance and client dashboard indicators for impact

Establishing a relationship between financing, managing, delivering, and coordinating services is critical to reach the goal of population health management (i.e., achieving health outcomes at the population level). The *Healthy People 2030* goals are a social mandate for health care. In the coming decade, care coordination and planned transitional care will be an essential intervention provided by nurses. Many of the interventions nurses use with clients and health care systems will further the *Healthy People 2030* objectives. These include case management and care coordination interventions to minimize fragmented care and promote quality transitions of care; incorporate standardized practice tools and adherence guidelines; improve safety of care; and use interprofessional teams to deliver services.

Establishing evidence-based strategies for all functions is critical to the success of case management and care coordination for individuals and populations. Using the current best evidence blended with clinical expertise is a critical skill of the case manager (American Nurses Association [ANA], 2013; CMSA, 2016; Lamb and Newhouse, 2018). In their practice, nurse case managers and community/public health nurses have the following core values:

- Increasing the span of healthy life
- Reducing disparities in health among Americans
- Promoting access to care and to preventive services

In the Intervention Wheel model for public health nursing practice, the nursing actions of case management, collaboration, and advocacy are 3 of 17 evidence-based interventions for individuals, families, and populations served by public health nurses (Keller et al., 2004; Minnesota Department of Health, 2019). Case management incorporates many of the Council of Public Health Nursing Organizations (CPHNO) of *Community/Public*

Health Nursing Competencies (Quad Council, 2018) because it involves individual and family care as well as community resources, population health, interprofessional teams, and policy implementation.

 HEALTHY PEOPLE 2030

Access to Care

> Case management strategies offer opportunities for nurses to help meet the following *Healthy People 2030* objectives for target populations:
> - **AHS-04:** Reduce the proportion of people who can't get medical care when they need it.
> - **AHS-06:** Reduce the proportion of people who can't get prescription medications when they need them.
> - **AHS-07:** Increase the proportion of people with a usual primary care provider.
> - **AHS-08:** Increase the proportion of adults who get recommended evidence-based preventive health care.
> - **HC/HIT-03:** Increase the proportion of adults whose health care providers involved them in decisions as much as they wanted

From U.S. Department of Health and Human Services: *Healthy People 2030.* HHS, 2020. Available at https://health.gov/healthypeople.

DEFINITIONS

Care management is a health care delivery process that helps achieve better health outcomes by anticipating and linking populations with the services they need more quickly (CMSA, 2016). It is an enduring process in which a population manager establishes systems and processes to monitor the health status, resources, and outcomes for a targeted aggregate of the population. Care management strategies were initially developed by health maintenance organizations (HMOs) in the late 1970s to manage the care of different populations. The purpose then and now is to promote quality and ensure appropriate use and costs of services. Care management strategies include utilization management, critical pathways, case management, disease management, and demand management (Box 15.1).

Case management, in contrast to care management, involves activities implemented with individual clients in the system. The case manager builds on the basic functions of the traditional nurse's role and adapts new competencies for managing the transition from one part of the system to another or to home. Case management is provided by the disciplines of nursing, social work, and rehabilitation counseling, to name a few.

This chapter describes the nature and process of case management for individual and family clients. Case management has a rich tradition in public health nursing as practiced by Lillian Wald and now is frequently found in hospitals, transitional and long-term care, home and hospice care, and health insurance companies.

CONCEPTS OF CASE MANAGEMENT

A historical focus on collaboration is seen in the Commission for Case Manager Certification definition:

> *A collaborative process that assesses, plans, implements, coordinates, monitors, and evaluates the options and services required to meet the client's health and human services*

> **BOX 15.1 Additional Definitions of Case Management Strategies**
>
> - **Utilization management** attempts to redirect care and monitors the appropriate use of provider care and treatment services for both acute and community and ambulatory service
> - **Critical pathways** are tools that name activities that can be used in a timely sequence to achieve the desired outcomes for care. The outcomes are measurable, and the critical path tools strive to reduce differences in client care.
> - **Case management** is "a collaborative process of assessment, planning, facilitation, care coordination, evaluation, and advocacy for options and services to meet client needs. It uses communication and available resources to promote safety, quality of care, and cost-effective outcomes" (Minnesota Department of Health, 2019, p 104). The focus is on improving care coordination and reducing the fragmentation of the services.
> - **Disease management** are systematic activities to coordinate health care interventions and communications for populations with disease conditions, such as diabetes and asthma, in which client self-care efforts are significant (Case Management Society of America [CMSA], 2016). These programs work with providers and consumers to educate on self-care, shared decision making, and knowledgeable use of medicines.
> - **Demand management** seeks to control use by providing clients with correct information to empower them to make healthy choices, use healthy and health-seeking behaviors to improve their health status, and make fewer demands on the health care system (Pawson et al., 2016).

needs. It is characterized by advocacy, communication, and resource management and promotes quality and cost-effective interventions and outcomes (Mullahy, 2017).

Case management is defined in public health nursing as "a collaborative process of assessment, planning, facilitation, care coordination, evaluation, and advocacy for options and services to meet client needs. It uses communication and available resources to promote safety, quality of care, and cost-effective outcomes" (Minnesota Department of Health, 2019, p 104). In 2018 the *Community/Public Health Nursing Competencies* were updated, and case management for populations can be assumed in Domain 5 (Community Dimensions of Practice Skills) and Domain 8 (Leadership and Systems Thinking Skills) (Quad Council, 2018). The following knowledge and skills are required to achieve this competency (Mullahy, 2017):

- Knowledge of community resources and financing mechanisms
- Written and oral communication and technology-enhanced documentation
- Proficient negotiating and conflict-resolving practices
- Critical-thinking processes to identify and prioritize problems from the provider and client viewpoints
- Application of evidence-based practices and outcomes measures
- Advocacy for patients, populations, and policy (Tahan, 2016a)

Case management practice is complex because of the need to coordinate activities of multiple providers, payers, and settings throughout a client's continuum of care. Care provided must be assessed, planned, implemented, adjusted, and evaluated on the basis of mutually agreed-upon goals. The nurse employed and located in one setting will be influencing the selection, monitoring, and evaluation of care provided in other settings by formal and informal care providers. With the increased use of electronic care delivery through telehealth activities and robotics, case management activities are now handled via tablets like iPads, phones, e-mail, fax, and video visits in the client's residence from a case manager who is located elsewhere. They may also deliver care to a global network of clients located in different countries. Health information technology (HIT) interoperability and electronic health records (EHRs) are benefiting collaborative care team communication, real-time data, and timely adjustments in care (American Association of Ambulatory Care Nurses and Academy of Medical Surgical Nurses [AAACN/AMSN], 2017).

Although the activities in case management may differ among providers and clients, the goals are as follows (Mullahy, 2017):

- To promote quality services provided to clients
- To reduce institutional care while maintaining quality processes and satisfactory outcomes
- To manage resource use through protocols, evidence-based decision making, guideline use, and disease management programs
- To control expenses by managing care processes and outcomes

A particularly challenging problem is the fragmenting of services, which can result in overuse, underuse, gaps in care, and miscommunication. This may ultimately result in costly client outcomes. The Transitional Care Model was developed and led by APRN providers for care coordination for chronic diseases or patients with complex needs at risk for poor outcomes at discharge to the home (Naylor and Sochalsik, 2010). This work resulted in Medicare payment for transitional care within the first 30 days of discharge (CMS, 2016). Another model of care coordination that has produced positive outcomes, cost effectiveness, and lower costs is the Aging in Place model by Rantz et al. (2014) (http://www.agingmo.com). Transitional care services bridge the gaps among diverse services, providers, and settings through the systematic application of evidence-based interventions that improve communication and transfer of information within and across services, enhance post–acute care follow-up, and decrease gaps in care by using a single consistent provider (cited in ANA, 2013). The Transitional Care Bundle includes seven essential interventions (Lattimer, 2013):

- Medication management
- Transition planning
- Client/family engagement and education
- Information transfer
- Follow-up care
- Provider engagement
- Shared accountability across providers

Case management in rural settings is more complex because of the following:

- Fewer organized community-based systems
- Geographic distance to delivery
- Population density
- Finances
- Pace and lifestyle
- Values
- Social organization differences from the urban setting

👤 CHECK YOUR PRACTICE

As an employee of the school system, you have been asked to become the case manager for the population of asthmatic children in the school system. What will this involve? What will you be responsible for doing? See if you can apply these steps to this scenario. (1) Recognize the cues, looking at available data about rates of child asthma in the school system and your community; (2) analyze the cues looking at the numbers of children in this population and what it means to be the case manager for this population; (3) state several and prioritize the hypotheses you have stated; (4) generate solutions for each hypothesis; (5) take action on the number one hypothesis you think best reflects the asthmatic issues and the schools involved; and (6) evaluate the outcomes you would expect as a result of the work you will do as case manager for these children.

Case Management and the Nursing Process

Case management activities with individual clients and families reveal the broader picture of health services and health status of the community. *Community assessment, policy development,* and *assurance activities* that frame core functions of public health actions are often the logical next step for a nurse's practice. The nurse views the process of case management through the broader health status of the community. Clients and families receiving service represent the microcosm of health needs within the larger community. Through a nurse's case management activities, general community deficiencies in quality and quantity of health services are often discovered. When observing lack of care or services at the individual and family intervention levels, the nurse can, through case management, intervene at the community level to make changes. For example, the management of a severely disabled child by a nurse case manager may uncover the absence of respite services or parenting support and education resources in a community. While managing the disability and injury claims within a corporation, the nurse may discover that alternative care referrals for home health visits and physical therapy are generally underused by the acute care providers in the community. Through a nurse's case management of brain-injured young adults, the absence of community standards and legislative policy for helmet use by bicyclists and motorcyclists may be revealed, stimulating advocacy efforts for changing community policy. Clearly, the core components of case management and the nursing process are complementary (Table 15.1).

Although Secord's classic illustration of case management (1987) remains an appropriate picture of the process, the CMSA model (2016) is a contemporary illustration of the case manager's process in the continuum of care (Fig. 15.1); Table 15.1 also compares the case management process and nursing process.

Characteristics and Roles

Case management can be labor intensive, time consuming, and costly. Because of the rapid growth in complexity in clients' problems managed by the case manager, the intensity and duration of activities required to support the case management function may soon exceed the demands of direct caregiving. Managers and clinicians in community health are exploring methods to make case management more efficient, including the use of providers who can perform to the limit of

TABLE 15.1	The Nursing Process and Case Management	
Nursing Process	**Case Management Process**	**Activities**
Assessment	• Case finding • Identification of incentives and barriers for target population • Screening, selection, and intake • Determination of eligibility • Assessment of challenges, opportunities, and problems	• Develop networks with target population • Disseminate written materials • Seek referrals • Apply screening tools according to program goals and objectives • Use written and on-site screens • Apply comprehensive assessment methods (physical, social, emotional, cognitive, economic, and self-care capacity) • Obtain consent for services if appropriate
Diagnosis	• Identification of problem/opportunity and challenges	• Hold interprofessional, team, family, and client conferences • Determine conclusion on basis of assessment • Use interprofessional team
Planning for outcomes	• Problem prioritizing • Planning to address care needs • Identification of resource match	• Validate and prioritize problems with all participants • Select evidence-based interventions • Develop goals, activities, time frames, and options • Create case management plan • Gain client's consent to implement • Have client choose options
Implementation	• Advocating for client interests • Frequent monitoring to assess alignment with goals and changing nature of client needs • Facilitation for executing right services, right time, right patient, right place	• Contact providers • Coordinate care activities • Negotiate services and price • Adjust as needed during implementation • Document processes and monitor progress
Evaluation	• Measuring attainment of activities and goals of service delivery plan • Continued monitoring and follow-up of client status during service • Reassessment • Bringing closure to care when client needs are achieved or change • Appropriate discharge to ensure effective transitional care and termination of case management processes	• Ensure quality of transitional communication and coordination of service delivery • Monitor for changes in client or service status • Follow up as needed • Examine outcomes and metrics against goals • Examine needs against service • Examine costs • Examine satisfaction of client, providers, and case manager • Examine best practices and outcomes for this client • Examine readmissions, Emergency Department visits

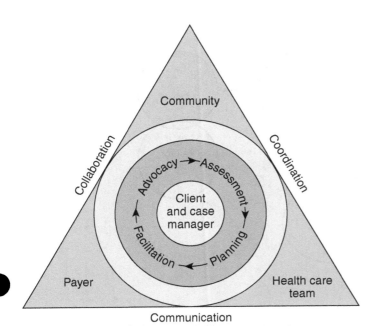

Fig. 15.1 The Continuum of Care–Case Management Model.

their licenses, auxiliary case management providers/services, and evidence-based practices.

In 1998, Cary described the roles of case managers in the practice setting. These roles are clearly affirmed now by the CMSA (2016) (Box 15.2) (assessor, planner, facilitator, coordinator, monitor, evaluator, and advocate). The roles demanded of the nurse as case manager are greatly influenced by the forces that support or detract from the role. Fig. 15.2 presents factors that demand the attention of both the nurse and the system during the case management process.

Knowledge and Skill Requisites

Adopting the case management role for a nurse does not happen automatically with an agency position. Knowledge and skills that are developed and refined are essential to success. Knowledge domains useful for nurses in systems desiring to implement quality case management roles are found in Box 15.3 (Cary, 1998; Stanton and Dunkin, 2009; Treiger, 2013, Tahan and Treiger, 2017). If a nurse seeks a case manager position, some of the skills and knowledge will need to be acquired through academic and continuing education

---

BOX 15.2   Case Manager Roles

- **Broker:** Acts as an agent for provider services that are needed by clients to stay within coverage according to budget and cost limits of health care plan
- **Client advocate:** Acts as advocate, provides information, and supports benefit changes that assist member, family, primary care provider, and capitated systems
- **Consultant:** Works with providers, suppliers, the community, and other case managers to provide case management expertise in programmatic and individual applications
- **Coordinator:** Arranges, regulates, and coordinates needed health care services for clients at all necessary points of services. Effectively participates and leads interprofessional teams
- **Educator:** Educates client, family, and providers about case management process, delivery system, community health resources, and benefit coverage so that informed decisions can be made by all parties
- **Facilitator:** Supports all parties in work toward mutual goals
- **Liaison:** Provides a formal communication link among all parties concerning the plan of care management
- **Mentor:** Counsels and guides the development of the practice of new case managers

- **Monitor/reporter:** Provides information to parties on status of member and situations affecting client safety, care quality, and client outcome, and on factors that alter costs and liability
- **Negotiator:** Negotiates the plan of care, services, and payment arrangements with providers; uses effective collaboration and team strategies
- **Researcher:** Accesses and applies evidence-based practices for programmatic and individual interventions with clients and communities; participates in protection of clients in research studies; initiates/collaborates in research programs and studies; accesses real-time evidence for practice
- **Standardization monitor:** Formulates and monitors specific, time-sequenced critical path and care map plans as well as disease management protocols that guide the type and timing of care to comply with predicted treatment outcomes for the specific client and conditions; attempts to reduce variation in resource use; targets deviations from standards so adjustments can occur in a timely manner; uses dashboards and predictive modeling to anticipate outcomes
- **Systems allocator:** Distributes limited health care resources according to a plan or rationale

---

programs, literature reviews, onboarding, orientation, and mentoring experiences.

Tools of Case Managers

The six "rights" of case management are right care, right time, right provider, right setting, right price/value, and right outcomes. How does the nurse judge the effectiveness of case management? Three tools are useful for case management practice: case management plans, disease management, and life care planning tools. An underlying principle for the use of each of these tools is to use robust evidence as the basis for the selection of activities; technology, health information systems (HISs) and EHRs, and analytics are currently the drivers of these tools.

Technology and technology-enabled information and decision support such as artificial intelligence—still in early development—can optimize the delivery of processes used by the case manager. The technology sector is refining software in the areas of documentation, decision support, dashboard tools, predictive modeling, workflow automation, reporting capabilities, EHRs, patient engagement strategies and social media, and remote monitoring (Carneal and Pock, 2014; Lamb and Newhouse, 2018; Stricker, 2014; Treiger, 2013). For

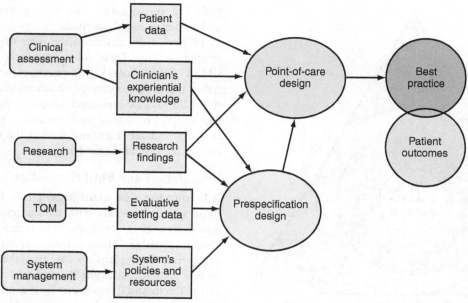

Fig. 15.2 Factors That Require the Attention of the Nurse and the System in the Case Management Process.

BOX 15.3 Knowledge Domains for Case Management

- Standards of practice for case management
- Evidence-based practice guidelines for specific health and disease conditions and communities
- Knowledge of health care financial environment and the financial dimension of client populations managed by nurses
- Clinical knowledge, skill, and maturity to direct quality timing and sequencing of care activities
- Care resources for clients within institutions and communities: facilitating the development of new resources and systems to meet clients' needs
- Transition planning for ideal timing, sequencing, and levels of care
- Management skills: communication, delegation, persuasion, use of power, consultation, problem solving, conflict management, confrontation, negotiation, management of change, marketing, group development, accountability, authority, advocacy, ethical decision making, and profit management
- Teaching, counseling, and education skills
- Program evaluation and research
- Performance improvement techniques
- Peer and team consultation, collaboration, and evaluation
- Requirements of eligibility and benefit parameters by third-party payers
- Legal and ethical issues
- Information management systems: clinical and administrative
- Health care legislation/policy
- Technical information skills, interoperable information systems, dashboard monitoring, data management and analysis, predictive modeling software, facile use of EHRs
- Outcomes management and applied research

EHR, Electronic health record.

example, HIT allows the case manager to access real-time data to improve timeliness of decisions or program changes for any number of adjustments in care protocols to ensure optimal outcomes. Data analytic software and dashboards allow for rapid decisions for clinical, administrative, and financial outcomes.

Case management plans have evolved through various titles and methods (e.g., critical paths, critical pathways, care maps, multidisciplinary action plans, nursing care plans). Regardless of the title given, standards of client care, standards of nursing practice, and clinical guidelines using evidence-based practices for case management serve as core foundations of case management plans. Likewise, in interprofessional action plans, core professional standards of each discipline guide the development of the standard process.

Adaptation of any standardized case management plan to each client's characteristics is a crucial skill for the process and outcome of care. These plans link multiple provider interventions to client responses and social determinants of health factors and offer reasonable predictions to clients about health outcomes. Institutions report that engaging patients in the case management plans empowers clients to assume responsibility for monitoring and adhering to the plan of care and ensures the plan is culturally sensitive. Self-responsibility by clients incorporates the values of autonomy and self-determination as the core of case management. For the nurse employed as a

case manager, ample opportunity exists to apply and revise critical path/map care guidance prototypes for a target population experiencing acute and chronic health problems within their unique cultural, social determinants, and population needs.

Disease management is an organized program of coordinated health care interventions that use consensus-driven performance measures and scientifically based evaluations in clinical outcomes for populations with conditions in which client self-care efforts are critical (utilization review accreditation commission [URAC], 2018). This approach focuses on the natural progression of diseases in high-risk populations. Due to comorbidities, a whole person model is the basis for a disease management program (Population Health Alliance, 2016).

Disease management programs may contain many of the following components (Hisashige, 2012):

- Selection of high-risk patients, with a focus on a singular disease state (diabetes, asthma, congestive heart failure [CHF])
- Financial and risk-sharing arrangements between payers and providers
- Programs for monitoring the use of clinical paths and evidence-based guidelines to assess outcomes and costs
- Protocols for clinical and administrative processes as well as cost allocations
- Services to educate clients and promote self-management skills
- Enhanced quality through evidence-based decision support and other registry technologies
- Support for provider-client relationships and plans of care
- Evaluation of clinical, humanistic, and economic outcomes to address the goal of improving overall health

Disease management can give clients the tools needed to better manage their lives (CMSA, 2016; Newman et al., 2014). Clients with chronic diseases may benefit from a disease management approach. The goals are to interrupt the continued development of a disease and prevent future disease and complications through secondary and tertiary prevention interventions. Promotion of wellness is necessary for success. For specific client populations that consume a disproportionate share of resources, disease management programs allocate the correct resources in an efficacious manner. Disease management programs may reduce emergency department visits and result in fewer inpatient days and rehospitalizations, greater client satisfaction, and reduced school absences (NTOCC, 2011; Sidorov, 2010; URAC, 2018). As the science of disease management evolves to predict direct relationships between outcomes and protocols of care, case managers will need to demonstrate cost-effective, optimal clinical care across the continuum—a goal of care management for populations. In fact, disease management is viewed as a top strategy by employers. The Joint Commission (TJC) certifies and URAC accredits disease management organizations and programs on the basis of their respective standards (see websites www.jointcommission.org and www.urac.org). This may influence the choice of programs a case manager selects to use with clients.

Life care planning is another tool used in case management. It assesses the current and future needs of a client for catastrophic or chronic disease over a life span. The life care plan is a customized, medically based, organized plan to estimate reasonable and necessary current and future medical and nonmedical needs of clients with associated costs and frequencies of goods and services. Typically, these needs incorporate medical, financial (income), psychological, vocational, built environment, and social costs during the remaining life of the client (Sambucini, 2013). Life care plans are typically used for clients experiencing catastrophic illness or adverse events resulting from professional malpractice or accidents/injuries, or those who have sustained an injury when younger and subsequently have changes in resource requirements as they age. For example, conditions may include spinal cord injury, traumatic brain injury, chronic pain, amputation, cerebral palsy, and burns. Life care plans are also used to set financial awards, which can be used to secure resources for care in the future and create a lifetime care plan. A systematic process like the nursing process is used and interprofessional input is required.

The first phase of the plan includes a thorough assessment of the client, financial/billing agreements, an information release signed by the client, and a targeted date for report completion. Development of the plan is the second phase. Plans are based on a number of factors: social and cultural situation, leisure activities, educational and employment status, medical history, physical and psychological abilities, current status, assistance required for completing activities of daily living, and regulatory requirements.

The execution of a life care plan is typically managed by a case manager who will work with the life care planner, especially when reevaluation of the plan is necessary (American Association of Nurse Life Care Planners [AANLCP], 2013).

All of these tools/programs, in coordination, constitute individual and population health management strategies to educate clients, promote self-management and wellness, provide nurse coaching support, promote safe care transitions, improve care management and coordination, and enhance quality.

HOW TO ENSURE HIGH-QUALITY CARE

The following actions can ensure high-quality care for clients and have implications for case managers in their practice:

- Provide access to easily understood information for each client based on his or her needs and health literacy level.
- Remember that the client is the source of control and that patient/family engagement is critical.
- Provide access to appropriate specialists with coordination and communication transparency.
- Ensure continuity of care for those with chronic and disabling conditions (transition care).
- Provide access to emergency services when and where needed.
- Disclose financial incentives that could influence medical decisions and outcomes.
- Prohibit "gag clauses" (which mean that providers cannot inform clients of all possible treatment options).
- Provide antidiscrimination protections.
- Provide internal and external appeal processes to solve grievances of clients.
- Make decisions on the basis of evidence.

EVIDENCE-BASED PRACTICE

The Effectiveness of a Registered Nurse Case Manager

This retrospective case-control study sought to assess the effectiveness of a registered nurse case managers (RNCMs) certified diabetes educator (CDE) quality improvement case management program. The RNCMs provided chronic care interventions, particularly for high-risk diabetes populations with glycosylated hemoglobin (HbA_{1c}) of 9% or higher. The RNCMs used protocols to titrate medications and assess patients for medication adherence, diabetes knowledge, and barriers to care. Researchers Watts and Sood (2016) reviewed computerized patient records over a period of 10 years for patients seen at 11 different community outpatient clinics. Results indicated that a large portion of high-risk patients with a baseline HbA1C of 9% or higher were seen by the RNCM. Patients who were seen by an RNCM had a statistically significant reduction in HbAIC after 14–26 months of intervention (t-test, $P < .001$). The RNCMs clinical intervention demonstrated a significant A1C reduction of approximately 2%.

Nurse Use

Nursing case management can improve health outcomes for high-risk diabetes populations. These finding may have additional implications for health care policy makers for planning interventions with respect to long-term management of diabetes mellitus.

From Watts SA, Sood A: Diabetes nurse case management: improving glucose control: 10 years of quality improvement follow-up data, *Appl Nurs Res* 29(1):202–205, 2016.

ESSENTIAL SKILLS FOR CASE MANAGERS

Three skills are essential to the role performance of the case manager: advocacy, conflict management, and collaboration.

Advocacy

Case managers report that they are first and foremost client advocates (CMSA, 2016; Tahan, 2016a). The definition of nursing includes advocacy: "Nursing is the protection, promotion and optimization of health and abilities, prevention of illness and injury, alleviation of suffering through the diagnosis and treatment of human response, and advocacy in the care of individuals, families, communities and populations" (ANA, 2015a, p 1). For nurses, advocacy involves various activities, ranging from exploring self-awareness to lobbying for health policy. Advocacy is essential for practice with clients and their families, communities, organizations, and colleagues on an interprofessional team. The functions of advocacy require scientific knowledge, expert communication, facilitating skills, and problem-solving and affirming techniques.

As the *Guide to the Code of Ethics for Nurses* (ANA, 2015b) states, "The nurse practices with compassion and respect for the inherent dignity, worth, and unique attributes of every person" (p. v). This means the nurse has the obligation to move beyond his or her own personal feelings of agreement or disagreement to respond compassionately. However, this goal is a contemporary one; the perspective regarding the advocacy function has shifted through history. The nurse advocate has been described in earlier writings as one who acted on behalf of or interceded for the client. An example of the nurse interacting on behalf of the client is the nurse who calls for a well-child appointment for a mother visiting the family planning clinic when the mother is capable of making an appointment on her own. The contemporary goal of advocacy would direct the nurse to move clients toward making the call themselves.

The advocate role evolved to that of mediator and is described as a response to the complex configuration of social change, reimbursement, and providers in the health care system (Tahan, 2016b). Mediating is an activity in which a third party attempts to provide assistance to those who may be experiencing a conflict in obtaining what they desire. The goal of the nurse advocate as mediator is to assist parties to understand each other on many levels so that agreement on an action is possible. In the example of a nurse as case manager for an HMO, mediating activities between an older adult client and the payer (the HMO) could accomplish the following results: The client may understand the options for community-based skilled nursing care, and the payer may understand the client's desires for a less restrictive environment for care, such as the home. The case manager as mediator does not decide the plan of action but facilitates the decision-making processes between the client and the payer so that the desired care can be reimbursed within the options available or new options created.

In today's practice, nurse advocates place the client's rights as the highest priority. The goal of promoter for the client's autonomy and self-determination may result in an optimal degree of patient engagement and empowerment and independence in decision-making. For example, when a group of young pregnant women is the collective "client" (the aggregate), the nurse advocate's role may be to inform the group of the benefits and consequences of breastfeeding their infants. However, if the new mothers decide on formula feeding, the nurse advocate should support the group and continue to provide parenting, infant, and well-child services. This example shows a different perspective of the nurse as advocate. It notes that the nurse's role as advocate may demand a variety of functions that are influenced by the client's physical, psychological, social, and environmental abilities. Advocacy can result in clients becoming their own "client expert" in problem solving, decision making, maximization of resources, partnership development with providers, and ultimately using appropriate interventions (Burton et al., 2010; Tahan, 2016a).

The advocacy role aims to achieve engagement—a process in which clients are invested in their health and care through programs that provide information and tools to empower them to take control and evaluate their care (ANA, 2013; Tahan, 2016a). The nurse adapts the advocacy function to the client's dynamic capabilities as the client moves from one health state to another.

Process of Advocacy

The goal of advocacy is to promote self-determination and patient empowerment in a client (Tahan, 2016a). The client may be an individual, family, peer, group, or community. The classic process of advocacy has been historically defined by Kohnke (1982), Mallik and Rafferty (2000), and Smith (2004) to include informing, supporting, and affirming. All three activities are more complex than they may initially seem, and they require self-reflection by the nurse as well as skill development. It is often easier for the nurse to inform, support, and affirm another person's decision when it is consistent with the nurse's values. When clients make decisions within their value systems that are different from the nurse's values, the advocate may feel conflict about contributing to the process of informing, supporting, and affirming those decisions. Promoting self-determination in others demands that the nurse have a philosophy of free choice once the information necessary for decision making has been discussed.

Informing

Knowledge is essential, but it is not sufficient to make decisions that affect outcomes. Interpreting knowledge is affected by the client's values and the meanings assigned to the knowledge. Interpreting facts is the result of both objective and subjective processing of information. Subjective processes greatly influence client decisions, as prior experiences, myths, and fears can influence patients' decisions. Informing clients about the nature of their choices, the content of those choices, and the consequences to the client is not a one-way activity. More active participation of clients in conversations with providers has been linked to better treatment compliance and health outcomes (Hibbard and Greene, 2013). Although the exchange may be initiated at the factual level, it will likely proceed to include the opinions of both parties—the client and the nurse (see the How To box in information exchange).

HOW TO PROVIDE FOR INFORMATION EXCHANGE BETWEEN NURSE AND CLIENT

1. Assess the client's present understanding of the situation. Have you considered your client's literacy level? Health literacy level? Cultural and ethnic values? Age and any disabilities that would interfere with learning? Do they endorse myths, legends, and/or previous experiences that would influence their understanding?
2. Provide correct information.
3. Communicate on the client's literacy level, making the information as understandable as possible. Use interpreters and translators where needed.
4. Use a variety of media sources and teach-back methods to increase the client's comprehension.
5. Discuss other factors that affect the decision, such as financial, legal, and ethical issues.
6. Discuss the possible consequences of a decision.

Supporting

Upholding a client's right to make a choice and to act on it involves supporting. People who become aware of clients' decisions fall into three general groups: supporters, dissenters, and obstructers. Supporters approve and support clients' actions. Dissenters do not approve and do not support clients. Obstructers cause difficulties when clients try to implement their decisions. There is a need for the nurse advocate to assure clients that they have the right and responsibility to make decisions, and reassuring them that they do not have to change their decisions because of others' objections.

Affirming

Affirming is based on an advocate's belief that a client's decision is consistent with the client's values and goals. The advocate validates that the client's behavior is purposeful and consistent with the choice that was made. The advocate expresses a dedication to the client's mission, and a purposeful exchange of new information may occur so that the client's choice remains possible. Recognizing that a client's needs may fluctuate with changing resources, the affirming activity must encourage a process of reevaluation and rededication to promote client self-determination.

The importance of affirming activities cannot be emphasized strongly enough. Many advocacy activities stop with assuring and reassuring, but affirming is often critical in promoting a client's self-determination. Table 15.2 compares the nursing process with the advocacy process.

It is not the advocate's role in the decision-making process to tell the client which option is "correct" or "right"; instead, the advocate's role involves the following:

- Providing the opportunity for information exchange and arming clients with tools that can empower them in making the best decision from their point of view.
- Enabling the clients to make an informed decision. This is a powerful tool for building self-confidence. It gives clients the responsibility for selecting the options and experiencing the success and consequences of their decisions.
- Empowering clients in their decision making when they recognize that although some events are beyond their control, other events are predictable and can be affected by decisions they can make. Ultimately, patient engagement brings improvements in patients' lives (Tahan, 2016a).

Nurses can promote client decision making in the following ways:

- Using the information exchange process
- Promoting the use of the nursing process
- Incorporating written techniques (e.g., contracts, lists)

TABLE 15.2 Comparison of Nursing Process and Advocacy Process

Nursing Process	Advocacy Process

Assessment/diagnosis	• Exchange information
	  • Gather data
	  • Illuminate values

Planning/outcome	• Generate alternatives and consequences
	  • Prioritize actions
	  • Engage the client

Implementation	• Empower the client to make decisions as possible
	  • Support the client
	  • Assure
	  • Reassure

Evaluation	• Affirm
	  • Evaluate
	  • Reformulate
	  • Close client case

- Using reflecting and prioritizing techniques
- Using role playing and sculpturing to "try on" and determine the "fit" of different options and consequences for the client
- Helping clients recognize the progression of activities they experience as they build their informed decision-making base
- Empowering clients with skills that can strengthen their autonomy and confidence in the future

Advocacy is a complex process that maintains a delicate balance between doing for the client and promoting autonomy. The process is influenced by the client's physical, emotional, and social capabilities. The goal of advocacy is to promote the maximal degree of client self-determination, given the client's current and potential status; for most clients, this goal can be realized.

Skill Development

Skills needed by the nurse advocate are not unique to their profession. Nursing demands scientific, technical, relationship, and problem-solving knowledge and skills. Advocacy applies nursing skills of communication and competency to promote client self-determination.

Knowledge of nursing and other disciplines as well as of human behavior is essential for the advocacy role in establishing authority, promoting authenticity, and developing skills. The capacity to be assertive for personal rights and the rights of others is essential.

Systematic Problem Solving

The nursing process—assessment, diagnosis, planning, implementing, and evaluating—is an example of a method of problem solving that can be used in the advocacy role. Advocates can be particularly helpful with clients in identifying values and generating alternatives as described in the following sections.

Illuminating Values

People's values affect their behavior, feelings, and goals. The advocate seeks to understand a client's values. The role of the advocate is to assist clients in discovering their values, which can be particularly demanding in the information exchange and affirming process. One way to help clients state their values is through a process called *clarification*. A simple way to do this is to ask questions such as the following:

- What are 10 things you enjoy doing?
- What are the most important things to you in life (e.g., family, money, happiness, health, comfort, pleasure, recognition)?
- How do you spend a typical day?

Generating Alternataives

Clients and advocates may feel limited in their options if they generate solutions before completely analyzing the problems, needs, desires, and consequences. Several techniques can be used to generate alternatives, including brainstorming and a technique known as the problem-purpose-expansion method (Box 15.4).

BOX 15.4 Techniques of Generating Alternatives for Problem Solving

Brainstorming

1. The nurse, client, professionals, or significant others generate as many alternatives as possible, without critical evaluation.
2. They examine the list for the critical elements the client seeks to preserve (e.g., environmental preferences, degree of control).
3. They analyze the list for consequences, the probability of chance events occurring, and the effect of the alternatives on self and others.

Problem-Purpose-Expansion Method

1. Restate the problem.
2. Expand the problem statement so different solutions can be generated. For example, if the purpose of the problem statement is to convince the insurance company to approve a longer hospital stay, the nurse and client have narrowed their options. If the purpose of the problem statement is to make the client's convalescence as beneficial and safe as possible, several solutions and options are available, as follows:
   * Obtaining skilled nursing facility placement
   * Obtaining home health skilled services
   * Arranging physician home visits
   * Paying for custodial care
   * Paying for private skilled care
   * Obtaining informal caregiving

Impact of Advocacy

Advocacy empowers clients to participate in problem-solving processes and decisions about health care. Clients try to understand changing opportunities in the health care system for access, use, and achieving continuity of care. Nurse advocates promote client engagement and self-determination and management of behavior as it relates to health and the adherence to therapeutic regimens. Clients are part of larger systems: the family, the work environment, and the community. Each system interacts with the client to shape the available options through resources, needs, and desires. Each system also exhibits both confirming and conflicting goals and processes that need to be understood for client self-determination to be successful. For example, the practice of advocacy among minority groups may involve the ability to focus attention on the magnitude of problems caused by diseases affecting minority clients. Whether the client is an individual, family, group, or community, the advocacy function can promote the interest of self-determination, which influences the progress of societies.

Advocacy is not without opposition. Clients and advocates may find barriers to services, vendors, providers, and resources. A community may experience a shortage in nursing home beds or providers, a childcare facility may experience staffing shortages, a family may not have the money to keep a child at home, and a client may find that the school system cannot fund a full-time nurse for its clinic. The reality of scarce resources creates a difficult barrier for advocates. However, events such as these often stimulate a community's self-determination and lead to innovative actions to correct gaps in service (see the Levels of Prevention box).

LEVELS OF PREVENTION

Primary Prevention

Use information exchange process to increase health literacy as a requisite to impact wellness and to use the health care system, adopt health promotion strategies that will maintain health, and engage in health education to create and maintain healthy lifestyles.

Secondary Prevention

Use case finding and dashboard data to identify existing health problems in your caseload and the population served by your agency. Timely, holistic assessments and interventions can slow disease trajectories and promote healing and health.

Tertiary Prevention

Monitor and adjust the use of prescription medications and adherence to treatment to reduce the risk of complications. Institutionalize this approach in your agency.

Conflict Management

Case managers help clients manage conflicting needs and scarce resources. Mutual benefit with limited loss is a goal of conflict management. Techniques for managing conflict include the following:

* Using a range of active communication skills directed toward learning all parties' needs and desires
* Detecting areas of agreement and disagreement
* Determining abilities to collaborate
* Assisting in discovering alternatives and activities for reaching a goal

Negotiating is a strategic process used to move conflicting parties toward an outcome. Parties must see the possibility of agreeing and the costs of not agreeing (Lee and Lawrence, 2013). Preparations must be made as to time, place, and ground rules concerning participants, procedures, and confidentiality. In a conflict situation, parties engage in behaviors that reflect the dimensions of assertiveness and cooperation. Assertiveness is the ability to present one's own needs. Cooperation is the ability to understand and meet the needs of others. Each person uses a primary and secondary orientation to engage in conflict (Box 15.5).

BOX 15.5 Categories of Behaviors Used in Conflict Management

* **Competing:** An individual pursues personal concerns at another's expense.
* **Accommodating:** An individual neglects personal concerns to satisfy the concerns of another.
* **Avoiding:** An individual pursues neither personal concerns nor another's concerns.
* **Collaborating:** An individual attempts to work with others toward solutions that satisfy the work of both parties.
* **Compromising:** An individual attempts to find a mutually acceptable solution that partially satisfies both parties.

Modified from Thomas KW, Kilmann RH: *Thomas-Kilmann conflict mode instrument*, New York, 1974, Xicom. *History and validity of the Thomas-Kilmann Conflict Mode Instrument (TKI)*. Mountain View, CA, CPP, Inc. From: https:// www.cpp.com/products/tki/tki_info.aspx. Retrieved January 2015.

Clearly, flexibility in conflict management behavior can facilitate an outcome that meets the client's goals. Helping parties navigate the process of attaining a goal requires effective personal relations, knowledge of the situation and alternatives, and a commitment to the process.

Collaboration

In case management, the activities of many disciplines (social workers, nurses, physicians, insurers, physical therapists, etc.) are needed for success. Clients, the family, significant others, payers, and community organizations contribute to achieving the goal. Collaboration can include working with communities; local, state, and federal resources; providers; team members; payers; and family, to name a few. It can include the techniques of motivational interviewing, mediation, and negotiation to facilitate communication and relationships (CMSA, 2016). Collaboration is achieved through a developmental process. Collaboration is a dynamic, highly interactive, and interdependent process in which people work together, sharing resources and even a vision for a goal (Morales Arroyo, 2003). Androwich and Cary (1989) found that collaboration occurs in a sequence and is reciprocal.

The goal of communication in the collaborative development process is to amplify, clarify, and verify all team members' points of view. Although communication is essential in collaboration, it is not sufficient to result in or maintain collaboration. Although the collaboration model recognizes the contributions of joint decision making, one member of the team should be accountable to the system and to the client. This team member should be responsible for monitoring the entire process (see the following QSEN box).

QSEN FOCUS ON QUALITY AND SAFETY EDUCATION FOR NURSES

Targeted Competency: Teamwork and Collaboration

Function effectively within nursing and interprofessional teams, fostering open communication, mutual respect, and shared decision making to achieve quality client interventions and outcomes.

Important aspects of teamwork and collaboration include:

- **Knowledge:** Describe scopes of practice and roles of health care team members
- **Skills:** Clarify roles and accountabilities under conditions of potential overlap in team member functioning. Use negotiation when disputes exist.
- **Attitudes:** Value the perspectives and expertise of all health team members

Teamwork and Collaboration Question

Observe a typical workday of a nurse case manager in an acute care, community health or public health setting, noting the types of activities that are done in coordination and handoffs, the team members involved, and the amount of time spent in these areas. Interview several staff members to determine whether they perceive that the amount of their time spent in case management is changing. To what degree are the staff members involved in care management activities? Ask about colleagues with whom case managers collaborate. Besides primary care physicians, which health care team members are often involved in managing clients' care across time and across settings? Reflect and state the skills that are needed by the case management nurse to best facilitate these interdisciplinary teams.

Prepared by Gail Armstrong, ND, DNP, MS, PhD, Professor and Assistant Dean/DNP program, Oregon Health and Sciences University, and adapted by Ann Cary, 2018.

Teamwork and collaboration clearly demand knowledge and skills about the following:

- Clients
- Health status
- Resources
- Treatments
- Community providers
- Clients' and families' complex needs
- Intrapersonal, interpersonal, medical, nursing, and social dimensions
- Team member and leadership skills

It is unlikely that any single professional possesses the expertise required in all dimensions. However, it is likely that the synergy produced by all can result in successful outcomes.

ISSUES IN CASE MANAGEMENT

Legal Issues

Liability concerns of case managers exist when the following three conditions are met:

1. The provider had a duty to provide reasonable care,
2. A breach of contract occurred through an act or an omission to act, and
3. The act or omission caused injury or damage to the client.

Case managers must strive to reduce risks, practice wisely within acceptable practice standards, and limit legal defense costs through professional insurance coverage (Box 15.6).

Legal citations relevant to case management and managed care include the following:

- Negligent referrals
- Provider liability
- Payer liability
- Breach of contract
- Denial of care
- Bad faith

As in any scope of nursing practice, proactive risk-management strategies can lower the provider's exposure to legal liability (Box 15.7). When courts find that cost considerations affect decisions related to medical care, all parties to the decision, such as the nurse, the agency, and all other health care providers, will be liable for any resulting damages.

Ethical Issues

Case managers as nursing professionals are guided in ethical practice by the *Code of Ethics for Nursing* (ANA, 2015b) and *Code of Professional Conduct for Case Managers* (Commission for Case Management Certification [CCMC], 2015), by performance indicators for ethics in the *Standards of Practice for Case Management* (CMSA, 2016), and by the contract expressed in *Nursing's Social Policy Statement* (ANA, 2015c).

By integrating these guidelines and philosophies, nursing practice is ideally suited to preserve the ethical principles of autonomy, beneficence, fidelity, justice, nonmaleficence, and veracity in case management processes. Numerous authors, notably Hendricks and Cesar (2003), McCollom (2004), Llewellyn and Leonard (2012 and 2016), Fink-Samnick and Muller (2010) and Fink-Samnick, (2018), Apuna-Grummer and Howland (2013),

---

BOX 15.6   Five General Areas of Risk for Case Managers

1. Liability for managing care (Leonard and Miller, 2012; Sminkey and LeDoux, 2016)
   - Inappropriate design or implementation of the case management system
   - Failure to obtain all pertinent records on which case management actions are based
   - Failure to have cases evaluated by appropriately experienced and credentialed clinicians
   - Failure to confer directly with the treating provider at the onset of and throughout the client's care
   - Substituting a case manager's clinical judgment for that of the medical provider
   - Requiring the client or provider to accept case management recommendations instead of any other treatment
   - Harassment of clinicians, clients, and family in seeking information and setting unreasonable deadlines for decisions or information
   - Claiming orally or in writing that the case management treatment plan is better than the provider's plan
   - Restricting access to otherwise necessary or appropriate care because of cost
   - Referring clients to treatment furnished by providers who are associated with the case management agency without proper disclosure
   - Connecting case managers' compensation to reduced use and access
2. Negligent referrals (Leonard and Miller, 2012; Sminkey and LeDoux, 2016)
   - Referral to a practitioner known to be incompetent
   - Substituting inadequate treatment for an adequate but more costly option
   - Curtailing treatment inappropriately when curtailment caused the injury
   - Referral to a facility or practitioner inappropriate for the client's needs
   - Referral to another facility that lacks care requirements

3. Experimental treatment and technology (Sminkey and LeDoux, 2016)
   - Failure to apply the contractual definition of "experimental" treatment found in the client's insurance policy
   - Failure to review sources of information referenced in the client's insurance policy (e.g., US Food and Drug Administration determination, published medical literature)
   - Failure to review the client's complete medical record
   - Failure to make a timely determination of benefits in light of **timelines** of treatment
   - Failure to communicate to the insured client or participant how coverage was determined
   - Improper financial considerations determining the coverage
4. Confidentiality (Leonard and Miller, 2012)
   - Failure to deny access to sensitive information awarded special protection by state law
   - Failure to protect access allowances to computerized medical records
   - Failure to adhere to regulations, such as the Health Insurance Portability and Accountability Act of 1996 (HIPAA) and the Americans with Disabilities Act
5. Fraud and abuse (Leonard and Miller, 2012)
   - Making false statements on claims or causing incorrect claims to be filed
   - Falsifying the adherence to conditions of participation of Medicare and Medicaid
   - Submitting claims for excessive, unnecessary, or poor-quality services
   - Engaging in payment, bribes, kickbacks, or rebates in exchange for referral
   - Coding intervention requirements improperly

BOX 15.7   Elements That Reduce Risk Exposure

1. Clear documentation of the extent of participation in decision making and the reasons for decisions
2. Records demonstrating accurate and complete information on interactions and outcomes
3. Use of reasonable care in selecting referral sources, which may include verification of the provider licensure
4. Written agreements when arrangements are made to modify benefits other than those in the contract
5. Good communication with clients
6. Informing clients of their rights of appeal

---

and Tahan (2016a), describe how case managers may confront dilemmas in these areas:

- Case management may hamper a client's **autonomy**, or the individual's right to choose a provider, if a particular provider is not approved by the case management system. If a new provider must be found who can be approved for coverage, continuity of care may be disrupted.
- Beneficence, or doing good, can be impaired when excessive attention to containing costs supersedes the nurse's duty to improve health or relieve suffering.
- Fidelity is defined as faithfulness to the obligation of duty (www.merriam-webster.com), in this case to the client by keeping promises and remaining loyal within the nurse-client

relationship. Duty to clients to secure benefits on their behalf and to limit unnecessary expenditures can create dilemmas when the goals are not uniform.

- Justice as an ethical principle for case managers considers equal distribution of health care with reasonable quality. Tiers of quality and expertise among provider groups can be created when quality providers refuse to accept reimbursement allowances from the managed system, leaving less experienced or lower quality providers as the caregiver of choice for clients being managed.
- Nonmaleficence is defined as doing no harm. When case managers incorporate outcomes measures, evidence-based practice, and monitoring processes in their plans of care, this principle is addressed.
- Veracity, or truth telling, is absolutely necessary to the practice of advocacy and building a trusting relationship with clients. Clients particularly complain that in the changing health care system, payers do not seem to be able to provide comprehensive yet inexpensive options Maintaining familiarity with ethical issues published in the case management literature can offer specific assistance for practicing case managers.

Important guidance in developing a community-based case management program can be found in the United States. Case management is a key component of federally financed and many state-financed health delivery options. The experiences of states over the past two decades provide testimony to the importance of case management for populations at risk. For older clients, state-derived case management provides objective advice and assistance with care needs. It also provides access to interprofessional providers and services. For payers (federal, state, clients), case management serves as a way to ensure that funds are allocated appropriately to those in greatest need. Case management serves a policy assurance and accountability function for communities. The PACE (Program of All-Inclusive Care for the Elderly) program addresses the needs of chronically ill seniors who wish to remain in their homes rather than be admitted to nursing homes. PACE participants are enrolled in a managed care model of medical, nursing and support services, case management, medications, respite, hospital, and nursing home care when necessary. These services are financed by Medicare and Medicaid, and some seniors will pay a monthly premium. The PACE model uses interdisciplinary care teams to provide services. PACE prevents institutionalization in nursing homes, uses a strong social model of health care delivery, and case manages transitions of clients between delivery systems and providers. Studies (Fretwell and Old, 2011; On Lok, 2017; Sebelius, 2011; Wieland et al., 2013) have demonstrated cost savings with PACE programs in both urban and rural areas compared with nursing home costs. The PACE model has been permanently recognized as a provider type under both Medicare and Medicaid and operates in the majority of the states (On Lok, 2017).

The clinical practice skill of advocacy is an inherent concept in the practice of case management. Of the 16 interventions by public health nurses described in the Wheel of Intervention model, both advocacy and case management are described in accordance with best practices and operational definitions of 3 of the 16 interventions. Advocacy can be applied at the community, systems, individual, or family level. In fact, when a public health nurse advocates for clients at any of these levels, the source of conflict and collaboration will likely come from competing values (i.e., those of the client and any of the other levels of population values). For example:

- A client may want access to unlimited treatment, but financial values may pose a source of conflict as the system attempts to justify the comparative effectiveness or costs.
- Family members may pose conflicting values for the nature of care they wish a family member to receive, even as the client refuses care.
- Communities can divert budget allotments to needs that are in competition for other population services such as community policing, health care access, and environmental services.

PRACTICE APPLICATION

During her regularly scheduled visit to a blood pressure clinic in a local apartment cluster, a Hispanic resident, Mrs. B., 45 years old, complained of feeling dizzy and forgetful. She could not remember which of her six medications she had taken during the last few days. Her blood pressure readings on

> ## ▶▶ APPLYING CONTENT TO PRACTICE
>
> The clinical practice skill of advocacy is an inherent concept in the practice of case management. Of the 16 interventions by public health nurses described in the Wheel of Intervention model, both advocacy and case management are described in accordance with best practices and operational definitions of 3 of the 16 interventions. Advocacy can be applied at the community, systems, individual, or family level. In fact, when a public health nurse advocates for clients at any of these levels, the source of conflict and collaboration will likely come from competing values (i.e., those of the client and any of the other levels of population values). For example:
>
> - A client may want access to unlimited treatment; financial values may pose a source of conflict as the system attempts to justify the comparative effectiveness or costs.
> - Family members may pose conflicting values for the nature of care they wish a family member to receive, even as the client refuses care.
> - Communities can divert budget allotments to needs that are in competition for other population services such as community policing, health care access, and environmental services.
>
> The nurse as advocate must listen carefully to his or her client to truly represent the interest of the client and encourage "win-win" processes and outcomes for the client. Advocacy occurs in all three of the core functions of public health: assessment, policy development, and assurance.

reclining, sitting, and standing revealed gross elevation. The nurse and Mrs. B. discussed the danger of her present status and the need to seek medical attention. Mrs. B. called her physician from her apartment and agreed to be transported to the emergency department.

In the emergency department, Mrs. B. manifested the progressive signs and symptoms of a cerebrovascular accident (a CVA, or stroke). During hospitalization, she lost her capacity for expressive language and demonstrated hemiparesis and loss of bladder control. Her cognitive function became intermittently confused, and she was slow to recognize her physician and neighbors who came to visit. The utilization review/discharge planning nurse at the hospital contacted the case manager from the home health agency to screen and assess for the continuum of care needs as early as possible because Mrs. B. lived alone and family members resided out of town.

It became apparent that family caregiving in the community could only be intermittent because family members lived too far away. Mrs. B. had residual functional and cognitive deficits that would demand longer-term care.

As the case manager contracted by the plan, place the following actions in the correct sequence to construct a case management plan:

A. Discuss with the family their schedule of availability to offer care in the client's home.
B. Discuss their cultural values in caring for family members.
C. Call the client and introduce yourself, as a prelude to working with her.
D. Obtain information on the scope of services covered by the benefit plan for your client.
E. Arrange a skilled nursing facility site visit for the client and family.

Answers can be found on the Evolve website.

■ REMEMBER THIS!

- An important role of the nurse is that of client advocate.
- The goal of advocacy is to promote the client's engagement in the plan and self-determination.
- When performing in the advocacy role, conflicts may emerge about the full disclosure of information, territoriality, accountability to multiple parties, legal challenges to clients' decisions, and competition for scarce resources.
- Information systems and interoperability are critical to communication and successful handoffs from provider to provider and patients during the case management process
- Skills important to fulfilling the role of client advocate include the helping relationship, assertiveness, and problem solving.
- Problem solving is a systematic approach that includes understanding the values of each party and generating alternative solutions.
- Brainstorming and the problem-purpose-expansion method are two techniques to enhance the effectiveness of problem-solving skills.
- During conflict, negotiations can move conflicting parties toward an outcome.
- Care management is a strategic program to maintain the health of a population enrolled in a delivery system.
- Continuity of care is a goal of nursing practice. It requires making linkages with services and information systems to improve the client's health status.
- As the structure of the health care system moves toward delivering more services in the community, the achievement of continuity of care will present a greater challenge.
- Case management is typically an interprofessional process in which the client is the focus of the plan.
- Documentation and use of dashboards for case management activities and outcomes are essential to nursing practice.
- Case management is a systematic process of assessment, planning, service coordination, referral, monitoring, and evaluation that meets the multiple service needs of clients.
- Nurses functioning as advocates and case managers need to be aware of the ethical and legal issues confronting these components of their practice.
- Standardization of care for predictable outcomes can be achieved through critical paths, disease management protocols, dashboards, data analytics, clinical guidelines, interprofessional action plans, and a caring-based practice in which processes of diagnosis and treatment are applied to the human experiences of health and illness.
- Telehealth application provides expansive alternatives within resource delivery options but must be customized for clients.

EVOLVE WEBSITE

http://evolve.elsevier.com/Stanhope/community/
- Answers to Practice Application
- Case Study
- Review Questions

REFERENCES

American Association of Ambulatory Care Nurses and Academy of Medical Surgical Nurses (AAACN/AMSN): Care Transition Hand-off Tool Task Force Evidence Table, 2017, AAACN.org. Retrieved from https://www.aaacn.org.

American Association of Nurse Life Care Planners (AANLCP): *A core curriculum for nurse life care planners,* Bloomington Indiana, October 2013, Universe LLC.

American Nurses Association (ANA): *Framework for measuring nurses' contributions to care coordination,* Silver Spring, MD, 2013, ANA.

American Nurses Association (ANA). *Nursing scope and standards of practice,* ed 3, Silver Spring, MD: 2015a, ANA.

American Nurses Association (ANA): *Guide to the Code of Ethics for Nurses with interpretative statements,* Silver Spring, MD, 2015b. Retrieved from Nursesbooks.org.

American Nurses Association (ANA): *A guide to Nursing's Social Policy Statement: from social contract to social covenant,* ed 1, Silver Spring, MD, 2015c. Retrieved from Nursesbooks.org.

Androwich I, Cary AH: A Collaboration Model: A Synthesis of Literature and a Research Survey. Paper presented at the Association of Community Health Nurse Educators Spring Institute. Seattle, June 1989.

Apuna-Grummer D, Howland WA, editors: *A Core Curriculum for Nurse Life Care Planning,* Bloomington, IN, 2013, iUniverse.

Burton J, Murphy E, Riley P: Primary immunodeficiency disease: a model for case management of chronic disease, *Prof Case Manag* 15:5–14, 2010.

Carneal G, Pock R: Six year of study reveals the impact of IT on the practice of case management, *CMSA Today* 2:16–17, 2014.

Cary AH: Advocacy or allocation, *Nurs Connect* 11:1–7, 1998.

Case Management Society of America (CMSA): *Standards of practice for case management,* Little Rock, AR, 2016, CMSA. Retrieved from http://www.cmsa.org.

Centers for Medicare and Medicaid Services (CMS). Transitional care management services, 2016. Retrieved from https://www.cms.gov.

Commission for Case Management Certification (CCMC): *Code of Professional Conduct for Case Managers with standards, rules, procedures, and penalties,* Mt. Laurel, 2015, Author.

CPP: *History and validity of the Thomas-Kilmann Conflict Mode Instrument (TKI),* Mountain View, CA, CPP, Inc. Retrieved from https://www.cpp.com.

Fidelity [Def. 2]: Merriam-Webster Online. In *Merriam-Webster,* n.d. Retrieved from http://www.merriam-webster.com.

Fink-Samnick E, Muller LS: Case management across the life continuum: ethical obligations versus best practice, *Prof Case Manag* 15:153–156, 2010.

Fink-Samnick E: Managing social determinants of health: Part I: Fundamental knowledge for case managers, *Prof Case Manag* 23(3):107–129, 2018.

Fretwell MD, Old JS: The PACE program: home-based care for nursing home-eligible individuals, *N C Med J* 72:209–211, 2011.

Hendricks AG, Cesar WJ: How prepared are you? Ethical and legal challenges facing case managers today (CEU), *Case Manager* 14:56–62, 2003.

Hibbard JH, Greene J: What the evidence shows about patient activation: better health outcomes and care experiences; fewer data on costs, *Health Aff,* 32:207–214, 2013.

Huber DL: *Leadership & nursing care management,* ed 6, St Louis, MO, 2018, Elsevier Saunders.

Institute of Medicine (IOM): *Crossing the quality chasm: a new health system for the 21st century, Washington,* DC, 2011, National Academies Press.

Keller LO, Strohschein S, Schaffer MA, Lia-Hoagberg B, et al.: Population-based public health interventions: innovations in practice, teaching and management, Part II, *Public Health Nurs* 21:469–487, 2004.

Kimmel KC: Current Health IT Challenges and opportunities in population health. Presentation at the 133rd meeting of the National Advisory Council for Nurse Education and Practice, Rockville, MD, January 2016.

Kohnke MF: Advocacy: *risk and reality,* St. Louis, 1982, Mosby.

Lamb G, Newhouse R: Care Coordination—a blueprint for action for RNs, Silver Spring, MD, 2018, ANA.

Lattimer C: Working to improve transitions of care, *CMSA Today* 5:12–14, 2013.

Lee R, Lawrence P: *Organizational behavior: politics at work,* New York, NY, 2013, Routledge.

Llewellyn A, Leonard M: Patient: Transfer (intrahospital) [Monograph] Evidence Summaries. Retrieved from the Joanna Briggs Institute Library Database, 2016, AAACN/AMSN Care Transition Hand-Off Tool Table.

Llewellyn A, Leonard M: *Case management review and resource manual,* ed 4, Silver Spring, MD, 2012, Nursesbooks.org.

Leonard M, Miller E: *Nursing case management: review and resource manual,* ed 4, Silver Spring, MD, 2012, American Nurses Credentialing Center.

Mallik M, Rafferty AM: Diffusion of the concept of patient advocacy, *J Nurs Scholarsh* 32:399–404, 2000.

McCollom P: Advocate versus abdicate, *Case Manager* 15:43–45, 2004.

McKesson Corporation: How Care Management Evolves with Population Management—A White Paper, 2014. Retrieved from http://www.healthleadersmedia.com.

Minnesota Department of Health: *Public health interventions: applications for public health nursing practice,* ed 2, St. Paul, Minn, 2019, Minnesota Department of Health.

Morales Arroyo MA: *The physiology of collaboration: an investigation of library-museum-university partnerships.* Dissertation, August 2003. Retrieved from http://digital.library.unt.edu.

Mullahy C: *The case manager's handbook,* ed 6, Sudbury, MA, 2017, Jones & Bartlett.

National Advisory Council on Nurse Education and Practice (NACNEP): Preparing Nurses for New Roles in Population Health Management, Rockville, 2016, HRSA.

National Transitions of Care Coalition (NTOCC): Improved Transitions of Patient Care Yield Tangible Savings, 2011. Retrieved from http://www.ntocc.org.

Naylor MD, Sochalski JA: Scaling up: Bringing the transitional care model into the mainstream, Issue Brief (Commonw Fund) 103:1–12, 2010.

Newman MB, Kowlsen T, Beckworth V: An integrated approach: the impact of health care reform from a managed care perspective, *CMSA Today* 1:20–23, 2014.

On Lok: Annual Report, San Francisco, On Lok Inc. 2017.

Pawson R, Greenhalgh J, Brennan C: Demand management for planned care: a realist synthesis, *Health Services and Delivery Research* 4:1–21, 2016.

Population Health Alliance PHM Glossary: Disease Management, Washington DC, 2016, Population Health Alliance. Retrieved from http://www.populationhealthalliance.org.

Quad Council Coalition Competency Review Task Force: Community/Public Health Nursing Competencies, 2018. Retrieved from http://www.quadcouncilphn.org.

Rantz M, Popejoy LL, Galambos C, et al.: The continued success of registered nurse care coordination in a state evaluation of aging in place in senior housing, *Nurs Outlook* 62:237–246, 2014.

Sambucini A: History and evolution of the nurse life care planning specialty. In Apuna-Grummer D, Howland WA, eds: *A core curriculum for nurse life care planners,* Bloomington, IN, 2013, iUniverse.

Sebelius K: Report to Congress-Evaluation of the rural PACE provider grant program, 2011. Retrieved from https://www.cms.gov.

Secord LJ: *Private case management for older persons and their families,* Excelsior, MN, 1987, Interstudy.

Sidorov J: TRICARE saves taxpayers millions on chronic illness disease management [Disease Management Care Blog], 2010. Retrieved from http://diseasemanagementcareblog.blogspot.com.

Sminkey PV, LeDoux J: Case management ethics: high professional standards for health care's interconnected worlds, *Prof Case Manag* 21:193–198, 2016.

Smith AP: Patient advocacy: roles for nurses and leaders, *Nurs Econ* 22:88–90, 2004.

Stanton MP, Dunkin J: A review of case management functions related to transitions of care at a rural nurse managed clinic, *Prof Case Manag* 14:321–327, 2009.

Stricker P: Data analytics: a critical tool, *CMSA Today* 4:20–23, 2014.

Tahan HA: Essentials of advocacy in case management: Part 1: Ethical underpinnings of advocacy-theories, principles, and concepts, *Prof Case Manag* 21:163–179, 2016a.

Tahan HA: Essentials of advocacy in case management: Part 2: Client advocacy model and case manager's advocacy strategies and competencies, *Prof Case Manag* 21:217–232, 2016b.

Tahan HM, Treiger TM: *Case Management Society of America (CMSA) Core curriculum for case management,* ed 3, Philadelphia, PA, 2017, Wolters Kluwer.

Treiger TM: Case management today and its evolution into the future, *CSMA Today* 7:16–20, 2013.

URAC: Disease Management. Retrieved from https://www.urac.org.

URAC: Transitions of Care—Proven strategies to close care gaps, 2018. Retrieved from http://URAC.org.

U.S. Department of Health and Human Services: *Healthy People 2030.* HHS, 2020. Available at https://health.gov/healthypeople.

Wieland D, Kinosian B, Stallard E, Boland R: Does Medicaid pay more to a program of all-inclusive care for the elderly (PACE) than for fee-for-service long term care? *J Gerontol A Biol Sci Med Sci* 68:47–55, 2013.

16

Disaster Management

Sherry L. Farra, Sherrill J. Smith, and Roberta Proffitt Lavin

OBJECTIVES

After reading this chapter, the student should be able to:

1. Discuss how disasters, both natural and human-made, affect people and their communities.
2. Describe the disaster management phases of prevention (mitigation and protection), preparedness, response, and recovery.
3. Examine the nurse's role in each phase of the disaster management cycle.
4. Identify how community groups and other organizations such as the American Red Cross can work together to prepare for, respond to, and recover from disasters.

CHAPTER OUTLINE

KEY TERMS

Around the world, people are experiencing unprecedented disasters from natural causes such as hurricanes, volcano eruptions, earthquakes, and tsunamis (which can lead to nuclear power plant meltdowns) and human-made disasters such as oil spills, mass shootings, and acts of terrorism. Many would consider the COVID-19 pandemic a disaster due to its effects on people and economies. Disasters occur suddenly and unexpectedly, and they often cannot be prevented. However, communities can be helped to prepare for, respond to, and recover from disaster. This chapter describes management techniques to be used in the prevention, preparedness, response, and recovery phases of disaster. The nursing role is discussed for each phase.

DISASTERS

A disaster is any natural or human-made incident that causes disruption, destruction, or devastation requiring external assistance. Disasters can affect a single family or a small group, as

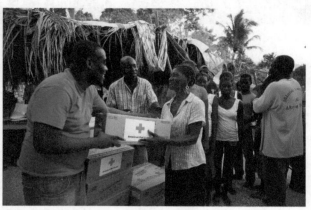

Fig. 16.1 The American Red Cross is a Major form of Support and Assistance to People Affected by Disasters. (Courtesy of the American Red Cross Disaster Online Newsroom, Washington, DC. Retrieved January 2015 from http://newroom.redcross.org).

in a house fire, or they can kill thousands and have economic losses in the millions, as with floods, earthquakes, tornadoes, hurricanes, viruses, and bioterrorism. Disasters are expensive in terms of lives affected and property lost or damaged. Although natural events such as earthquakes or hurricanes often trigger disasters, predictable and preventable human-made factors can increase the effects of the disaster. Each year, hurricanes in the United States batter the coasts and inland areas. A 9.0 magnitude earthquake struck northeastern Japan on March 11, 2011, and it was quickly followed by a tsunami (Fig. 16.1). These dual natural disasters caused an estimated death toll of 20,000, but there was a third, human-made component to complete the incident triad: a nuclear reactor crisis. An independent parliamentary investigation later found the Fukushima nuclear disaster to be the result of a mix of several human-made factors (Inajima et al., 2012). Box 16.1 lists examples of natural and human-made disasters.

Unfortunately, developing countries experience a disproportionate burden from natural disasters. These countries are usually poor and have limited resources for dealing with the effects of the disaster. To add to the misery, the governments of some countries thwart the efforts of international aid workers to bring relief to their people, as seen in recent years in Syria. Disasters have political aspects in addition to the enormous losses to the people; for example, some countries will not accept aid from nations they do not consider to be allies or supporters.

In recent years, we have learned more about what is called a "complex humanitarian emergency" (CHE). These emergencies result from a "humanitarian crisis in a country, region or society where there is total or considerable breakdown of authority resulting from internal or external conflict and which requires an international response that goes beyond the mandate or capacity of any single and/or ongoing UN country programme" (Downes, 2015, p 12).

The urbanization and overcrowding of cities have increased the danger of natural disasters because communities have been built in areas that are vulnerable to such disasters, as in known tornado zones or near rivers or flood plains. Increases in population and development for habitation of areas vulnerable to natural disasters have led to major increases in insurance payouts in the United States every decade. Projections suggest that by 2050, at least 46% of the world's population will live in areas vulnerable to natural floods, earthquakes, and severe storms.

Overcrowding and urban development have also increased human-made disasters. The stress of overcrowding has caused civil unrest and riots. In some parts of the world, modern wars waged over land rights and space have markedly increased the risk for injury and death from disaster. In the United States and other countries, school violence, a human-made disaster, has increased in intensity and magnitude. Disaster recovery efforts are expensive, and the costs are growing because of the number of people involved as well as the amount of technology that must be restored. People in industrialized countries are becoming less

---

BOX 16.1   Types of Disasters

Natural	Human-Made
• Hurricanes	• Conventional warfare
• Tornadoes	• Nonconventional warfare (e.g., nuclear, chemical)
• Hailstorms	• Transportation accidents
• Cyclones	• Structural collapse
• Blizzards	• Explosions and bombings
• Droughts	• Fires
• Floods	• Hazardous materials incident
• Mudslides	• Pollution
• Avalanches	• Civil unrest (e.g., riots)
• Earthquakes	• Terrorism (e.g., chemical, biological, radiological, nuclear, explosives)
• Volcanic eruptions	• Cyberattacks
• Communicable disease epidemics	• Airplane crashes
• Lightning-induced forest fires	• Radiological incidents
• Tsunamis	• Nuclear power plant incidents
• Thunderstorms and lightning	• Critical infrastructure failures
• Extreme heat and cold	• Water supply contamination

From US Department of Health and Human Services: *Healthy People 2020: a roadmap to improve all Americans' health*, Washington, DC, 2010, USDHHS.

self-sufficient because they rely heavily on technology as well as social and economic systems within their community. People who live on the brink of disaster every day physically, emotionally, or economically are among the first to be affected when disaster strikes.

Disasters that have little or no advance notice, such as earthquakes or bioterrorism, often have more casualties due to the lack of time to prepare or obtain treatment. Individuals can also be injured while attempting to prepare for the disease or while evacuating. Public health disasters can create needs across a large region or around the globe. In a pandemic, urgent and competing health needs can occur within a close time frame, producing a public health surge. This was clearly evident in the COVID-19 pandemic; in the disaster recovery phase, the immediate threat shifts to adjusting to a new normal in the affecting areas.

Although the number of disasters worldwide continues to grow, the number of lives lost has decreased. The increase in the number of lives saved may be due to better disaster forecasting and early warning systems that help people better prepare for the impending disaster. Disaster disproportionately strikes at-risk individuals, whether their day-to-day risk is physical, emotional, or economic. Disasters in less developed communities can also destroy decades of progress in a matter of hours, in a manner that rarely happens in more developed countries. The poor, elderly, ethnic minorities, people with disabilities, and women and children in developing communities are excessively affected and least able to rebound (World Health Organization, 2017). Economic losses from disasters such as tsunamis, cyclones, earthquakes and flooding now reach an annual average of US $250 to $300 billion and are expected to rise to $415 billion in 2030; this does not include the global costs of COVID-19. As the United Nations Development Programme said in mid-2020, "The coronavirus COVID-19 pandemic is the defining global health crisis of our time and the greatest challenge we have faced since World War Two." Further, this source said, "The pandemic is moving like a wave—one that may yet crash on those least able to cope. But COVID-19 is much more than a health crisis. By stressing every one of the countries it touches, it has the potential to create devastating social, economic and political crises that will leave deep scars" (United Nations Development Programme, 2020). The mortality and economic loss associated with risk in low- and middle-income countries is increasing. Unfortunately, by 2050, the percentages of population areas more vulnerable to disasters will increase. Eighty percent of the world's population will live in developing countries, with 46% living in tornado and earthquake zones, near rivers, and on coastlines (UNDDR, 2015; United Nations Development Programme, 2016). The costs of disasters in more developed countries are higher than in developing countries because of the costs of labor, materials, and complex infrastructures including technology.

Although natural disasters cannot be prevented, much can be done to prevent further increases in accidents, death, and destruction after impact. A concise, realistic, and well-rehearsed disaster plan is essential. Open, clear, and ongoing communication among involved workers and organizations is critical. Many of the human-made disasters listed in Box 16.1 can be prevented (e.g., major transportation accidents and fires resulting from substance abuse).

NATIONAL DISASTER PLANNING AND RESPONSE: A HEALTH-FOCUSED OVERVIEW

As the single largest health care professional group, nurses need to understand the national disaster management cycle. The US Department of Homeland Security (DHS) was created through the Homeland Security Act of 2002 (DHS, 2002), consolidating more than 20 separate agencies.

Presidential Policy Directive 8: National Preparedness (PPD-8) was signed and released by President Barack Obama on March 30, 2011. PPD-8 replaced Homeland Security Presidential Directive 8 (HSPD 8) from the Bush era, and guides how the nation, from the federal level to private citizens, can "prevent, protect against, mitigate the effects of, respond to, and recover from those threats that pose the greatest risk to the security of the Nation" (DHS, 2008 and updated 2011). The National Preparedness Guidelines (NPG) (DHS, 2014) and the National Response Plan (NRP), which provide a national doctrine for preparedness that includes the National Response Framework (NRF), was promulgated in January 2008. The fourth edition of the NRF, updated in 2019, reorganizes and streamlines the previous version, expanding principles and concepts to more fully integrate government and private sector response efforts and introducing the community lifelines concept and terminology. Community lifelines are those services that support the continuous operation of critical government and business functions essential to health, safety, or economic security (DHS, 2019). Community lifelines include: (1) safety and security, (2) food, water, and shelter, (3) health and medical, (4) energy (power and fuel), (5) communications, (6) transportation, and (7) hazardous materials.

The National Preparedness Goal was first released in September 2011, and the second edition in 2015 maintains the goal of "a secure and resilient nation with the capabilities required across the whole community to prevent, protect against, mitigate, respond to, and recover from the threats and hazards that pose the greatest risk" (FEMA, 2015, p.1).

Homeland Security Presidential Directive 5 (HSPD 5) directed the Secretary of Homeland Security to develop and administer the National Incident Management System (NIMS)—a unified, all-discipline, and all-hazards approach to domestic incident management (FEMA, 2018a). The NIMS was established to provide a common language and structure to help those involved in disaster response to communicate more effectively and efficiently.

Two national preparedness documents specifically guide disaster health preparedness, response, and recovery: HSPD 21: Public Health and Medical Preparedness, and the National Health Security Strategy (NHSS). HSPD 21 established a national strategy that enables a level of public health and medical preparedness sufficient to address a range of possible disasters. It does so through four critical components of public health and medical preparedness: (1) biosurveillance, (2) countermeasure stockpiling and distribution, (3) mass casualty care, and (4) community resilience (NPS, 2020). The NHSS emphasizes "protecting the nation's physical and psychological health, limit economic losses, and preserve confidence in government, and the national will to pursue its interests when threatened by incidents that result in serious health consequences whether natural, accidental, or deliberate" (NHSS 2019-2022, 2019). The latest plan has three overarching objectives:

1. Prepare, mobilize, and coordinate the Whole-of-Government to bring the full spectrum of federal medical and public health capabilities to support state, local, tribal, and territorial authorities in the event of a public health emergency, disaster, or attack.
2. Protect the nation from health effects of emerging and pandemic infectious diseases as well as chemical, biological, radiological, and nuclear (CBRN) threats.
3. Leverage the capabilities of the private sector.

The NHSS was directed by the 2006 Pandemic and All-Hazards Preparedness Act (PAHPA). The goal of this act is to improve the nation's ability to detect, prepare for, and respond to a variety of public health emergencies. The PAHPA was reenacted in both 2013 and 2019 and is now called the Pandemic and All-Hazards Preparedness and Advancing Innovation Act (PAHPIA). The PAHPIA funds public health and hospital preparedness programs as well as medical countermeasures under the BioShield Project (USDHHS, 2019).

Healthy People 2030 Objectives

Because disasters affect the health of people in many ways, they have an effect on almost every *Healthy People 2030* objective. Disasters clearly affect the objectives that relate to unintentional injuries, occupational safety and health, environmental health, food and drug safety, immunization and infectious disease, and mental health. Disasters affect many of the objectives in the areas of access to health services and public health infrastructure (USDHHS, 2020). In the past few years, with the many incidents and scares related to possible bioterrorism, people have become even more aware of the importance of disaster preparedness and how the things they take for granted such as safe food, water, and housing can be threatened. Public health professionals study the effect that disasters have on population health and develop new prevention strategies. Other organizations, such as the American Red Cross (ARC), work with communities in the preparedness, response, and recovery phases of a disaster. The *Healthy People 2030* box provides examples of objectives related to disaster mitigation.

THE DISASTER MANAGEMENT CYCLE AND THE NURSING ROLE

Disaster management includes four stages: prevention (including mitigation and protection), preparedness, response, and recovery. Fig. 16.2 shows the disaster management cycle. Nurses have skills that enable them to work in all aspects of disasters, such as assessment, priority setting, collaboration, health education, disease screening, and mass clinic expertise. Nurses also have the ability to provide essential public health services, make referrals, serve as liaisons among organizations, health care, and social service providers, and provide psychological first aid, triage, and rapid needs assessment.

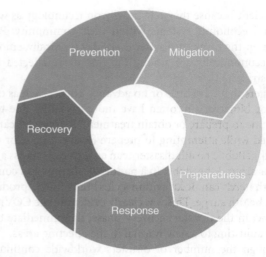

Fig. 16.2 Disaster Management Cycle. The original work for the disaster management cycle comes from National Governors' Association Center for Policy Research: Comprehensive emergency management: a governor's guide, Washington, DC, 1979, National Governors' Association. (Image from Ontario Agency for Health Protection and Promotion [Public Health Ontario]: Public health emergency preparedness: an IMS-based workshop. Base scenario. Toronto, ON, July 2015, Queen's Printer for Ontario, p. 7.)

♥ HEALTHY PEOPLE 2030

Examples of Objectives Related to Disaster Mitigation

- **PREP-003:** Increase the proportion of adults who know how to evacuate in case of a hurricane, flood, or wildfire.
- **PREP-D01:** Increase the proportion of parents and guardians who know the emergency or evacuation plan at their children's school.
- **PREP-D02:** Increase the proportion of adults who prepare for a disease outbreak after getting preparedness information.

From Department of Health and Human Services (DHHS): *Healthy People 2030*. Retrieved September 2020 from http://www.healthypeople.gov.

Prevention (Mitigation and Protection)

All-hazards mitigation (prevention) is an emergency management term for reducing risks to people and property from natural hazards before they occur. Prevention can include structural measures, such as protecting buildings and infrastructure from the forces of wind and water, and nonstructural measures, such as land development restrictions. Prevention also includes human-made hazards and the ability to deter potential terrorists, detect terrorists before they strike, and take action to eliminate the threat (DHS, 2016). Prevention activities may include heightened inspections, improved surveillance and security operations, public health and agricultural surveillance and testing, immunizations, isolation, or quarantine, and halting chemical, biological, radiological, nuclear, and explosive (CBRNE) threats.

Nurses are involved in many aspects of prevention, including the following:
- Awareness and education: Holding or attending community meetings on disaster preparedness, including informing the

community about the many educational resources available to them. One resource is an in-depth citizen guide for preparing for a disaster, called "Are You Ready?" The guide is available at http://www.fema.gov.

- Organization and participation: Organizing and participating in mass prophylaxis and vaccination campaigns to prevent, treat, or contain disease.
- Advocacy: Identifying environmental hazards, serving on the public health team for mitigation work, and supporting actions and efforts for effective building codes and proper land use.

Because disasters are both natural and human-made, nurses need to assess for and report environmental health hazards, such as unsafe equipment and faulty structures. They must be aware of high-risk targets and current vulnerabilities, as well as what can be done to eliminate or mitigate these vulnerabilities. Targets may include military and civilian government facilities, health care facilities, international airports and other transportation systems, large cities, and high-profile landmarks. Terrorists might also target large public gatherings, water and food supplies, banking and finance, information technology, postal and shipping services, utilities, or corporate centers.

Preparedness

Personal Preparedness

Nurses who are disaster victims themselves and must provide care to others will experience considerable stress. Conflicts between family and work-related duties are inevitable. For example, a nurse who is also the mother of a young child will not be able to participate fully, if at all, in disaster relief efforts until she has made arrangements for her child. Personal and family preparation in advance can help ease some of the conflicts that arise and allow nurses to attend to client needs sooner. In addition, nurses assisting in disaster relief efforts must be as healthy as possible, both physically and mentally, to serve clients, families, and other disaster victims. During the COVID-19 pandemic, some schools, including day care and preschools, were closed—yet nurses had to work. Schools reopened in fall 2020; some allowed in-person classes, others did all virtual learning, and others allowed students to combine in-person and virtual learning. Managing these competing obligations was challenging. In some instances, nurses could work from home, but that was not appropriate when direct patient care was required. There was a large increase in telehealth and electronic group meetings.

Disasters require nurses to respond quickly. Public health nurses need to have their own personal plans in place before a disaster. Preparedness is multifaceted; the family of each nurse must be included and informed about the disaster plan. One way a nurse can ensure that his or her family is protected is by providing them with the skills and knowledge to help them cope with a disaster. Long-term benefits will come by involving children and adolescents in activities such as writing preparedness or response plans, rehearsing the plan, preparing disaster kits, becoming familiar with their school emergency plan and where families should reunite in the event of an emergency, finding out where the evacuation shelters are located, identifying the evacuation routes, and learning about the range of potential hazards in their vicinity. Natural and human-made hazards, including terrorism, should be discussed. Vulnerable types of infrastructure such as dams, chemical plants, bridges, and transportation should be pointed out. Discussion offers children and adolescents an opportunity to express their feelings. The ability to control as much as they can during each phase of a disaster provides them with the ability to bounce back (Fig. 16.3). The How

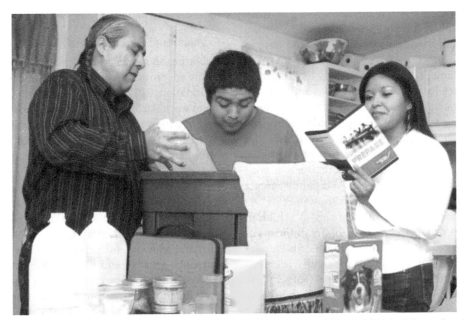

Fig. 16.3 Personal Preparedness. Participants in National Preparedness Month, 2015, building a disaster kit. (Available at https://www.fema.gov.)

HOW TO BE RED CROSS READY

1. Get a Kit

   Consider the following when assembling or restocking your kit to ensure that you and your family are prepared for any disaster:

   - Store at least 3 days of nonperishable food and water (1 gallon per person per day) for drinking and hygiene purposes
   - Battery-powered or hand-crank radio (NOAA weather radio if possible)
   - Flashlight and extra batteries
   - First aid kit, medications, and medical items
   - Copies of all important documents (proof of address, deed/lease to home, passports, birth certificates, insurance policies, etc.)

2. Make a Plan: Talk with household members about what you would do during emergencies. Plan what to do in case you are separated and choose two places to meet—one right outside your home in case of a sudden emergency such as a fire, and another outside your neighborhood in case you cannot return home or are asked to evacuate.

   - Choose a contact person out of the area and make sure all household members have this person's phone number and email address. It may be easier to call long distance or text if local phone lines are overloaded or out of service.
   - Tell everyone in the household where emergency information and supplies are kept.
   - Practice evacuating your home twice a year. Drive your planned evacuation route and plot alternative routes on a map in case main roads are impassable.
   - Don't forget your pets. If you must evacuate, make arrangements for your pets. Keep a phone list of "pet-friendly" motels/hotels and animal shelters that are along your evacuation route.

3. Be informed. Know the risks where you live, work, learn, and play.

   - If you live or travel often to areas near a fault line, learn how to prepare and what to do during an earthquake. If summer brings to mind not just beaches and picnics but also tropical storms and hurricanes, arm yourself with information about what to do in case one occurs. Remember that emergencies like fires and blackouts can happen anywhere, so everyone should be prepared for them.
   - Find out how you would receive information from local officials in the event of an emergency.
   - Learn first aid and CPR/AED so that you have the skills to respond in an emergency before help arrives, especially during a disaster in which emergency responders may not be as available. (American Red Cross: *Be "Red Cross Ready"—It's as Easy as 1-2-3,* May 2018, www.redcross.org)

What nurses need to add to their "be ready" emergency kit:

- Identification badge and driver's license
- Proof of licensure and certification
- Pocket-size reference book (or electronic versions on a smartphone)
- Blood pressure cuff (adult and child) and stethoscope
- Gloves, mask, and other personal protective equipment (PPE) for general care
- First aid kit with mouth-to-mouth cardiopulmonary resuscitation (CPR) barrier and tourniquet
- Crank radio and cell phone charger
- Cash, credit card
- Important papers and contact information in hard copy
- Sun protection and insect repellant
- Sturdy shoes with socks
- Medical identification of allergies, blood type
- Medications for self
- Weather-appropriate clothing, including rain gear
- Toiletries
- Watch, cell phone with charger and preentered emergency numbers
- Flashlight, extra batteries
- Record keeping materials, including pencil/pen
- Map of area

Note: Some of the items in the kit for nurses might also be useful in anyone's kit.

Courtesy of the American Red Cross. Retrieved May 2020 from http://www.redcross.org

---

To box is an excellent guide for developing and putting together the supplies needed for a disaster plan. This plan can work for you and the clients for whom you provide care. The second box lists the additional information that nurses should have in their kits.

In addition to the items in the How To box, include these items: manual can opener, list of your medications and dosages; list of allergies and physician names; candles and matches; sanitation supplies including toilet paper, soap, feminine hygiene items, and plastic garbage bags; special items for infants, older adults, or disabled family members; an extra pair of eyeglasses, pet supplies if you have animals; and documents such as your passport, birth certificate, insurance policies, and family contact information. Store documents in a waterproof container.

Nurses should consider several contingencies for children and seniors, and plan to seek help from neighbors in the event of being called to aid in a disaster. Many special-needs shelters encourage preregistration for physically or mentally challenged people. Because most shelters do not allow pets other than "pocket" pets, other arrangements will need to be made for animals, such as going to a special pet shelter or placing the pet in a bathroom with sufficient food and water. A note should be placed on the front door for emergency personnel as to where the pet might be found. Currently, many local emergency management offices are considering incorporating pets into the local disaster plans.

Professional Preparedness

Public health nurses are leaders in coordinating interprofessional teams to promote community health (Robert Wood Johnson Foundation, 2017). These nurses take time to read and understand workplace and community disaster plans and participate in disaster drills and community mock disasters. Adequately prepared nurses can serve as leaders and enable others to have a smoother recovery phase.

Disaster management in the community is about population health, and the three core public health functions are used just as in day-to-day operations: assessment, policy development, and assurance. Although disaster work is not highly technological, there is increasing information provided in a wireless format. Fieldwork, including shelter management, requires that nurses be creative and willing to improvise in delivering care. All workers should be certified in first aid and CPR. In addition, the ARC provides a comprehensive program of disaster training for health professionals to enable them to provide assistance within their own communities and to other affected communities and countries. The courses teach nurses how to adapt their existing nursing skills to a disaster setting and to the scope of

ARC disaster nursing. Note that the knowledge a nurse will need for chemical, biological, radiological, nuclear, and explosive (CBRNE) disasters and those involving weapons of mass destruction (WMD) requires a base of specialized information. Box 16.2 describes competencies for all public health workers in the event of a disaster.

Nurses who want to know more about disaster management and be more active can become involved in several community organizations. The National Disaster Medical System (NDMS) enables nurses to work on specialized teams such as the Disaster Medical Assistance Team (DMAT). In a presidentially declared disaster, including overseas war, the US Public Health Service can activate disaster medical assistance teams (DMATs) to an area to supplement local and state medical care needs. These teams can also be activated by the Assistant Secretary for Health if requested by a state health officer. Teams of specially trained civilian physicians, nurses, and other health care personnel can be sent to a disaster site within hours of activation. DMATs can provide triage and continuous medical care to victims until they can be evacuated to a national network of hospitals prearranged by the NDMS (DHS, 2014). Because of the nature of this country's disasters since the initiation of DMATs, these teams have been used primarily to staff community health outpatient clinics in the affected areas. The Medical Reserve Corps (MRC) and the Community Emergency Response Team (CERT) provide opportunities for nurses to support emergency preparedness and response in their local jurisdictions. The ARC offers training in disaster health services and disaster mental health for both local response and national deployment opportunities. After participation in disaster training, nurses can take the following steps: join a local disaster action team, act as a liaison with local hospitals, determine health-services support for shelter sites, plan on a multidisciplinary team for optimal client service delivery, address the logistics of health and medical supplies, and teach disaster nursing in the community. A list of education and training opportunities is shown in Box 16.3.

The importance of being adequately trained and properly associated with an official response organization to serve in a disaster cannot be overstated. In a disaster, many untrained and ill-equipped individuals rush in to help. Spontaneous volunteer overload creates added burden on an already tense situation that now includes role conflict, anger, frustration, and helplessness.

Community Preparedness

The level of community preparedness for a disaster is only as good as the people and organizations in the community make it. Some communities stay prepared for a possible disaster by having a written disaster plan and participating in yearly disaster drills, while other communities are less prepared and depend on luck and the fact that they are unlikely to experience a disaster. Some organizations within the community may be more prepared than others. For example, most health care facilities have

---

BOX 16.2 Core Competencies for Disaster Medicine and Public Health

1.0: Demonstrate personal and family preparedness for disasters and public health emergencies.

2.0: Demonstrate knowledge of one's expected role(s) in organization and community response plans activated during a disaster or public health emergency.

3.0: Demonstrate situational awareness of actual/potential health hazards before, during, and after a disaster or public health emergency.

4.0: Communicate effectively with others while in a disaster or public health emergency.

5.0: Demonstrate knowledge of personal safety measures that can be implemented in a disaster or public health emergency.

6.0: Demonstrate knowledge of surge capacity assets, consistent with one's role in organization, agency, and/or community response plans.

7.0: Demonstrate knowledge of principles and practices for the clinical management of all ages and populations affected by disasters and public health emergencies, in accordance with professional scope of practice.

8.0: Demonstrate knowledge of public health principles and practices for the management of all ages and populations affected by disasters and public health emergencies.

9.0: Demonstrate knowledge of ethical principles to protect the health and safety of all ages, populations, and communities affected by a disaster or public health emergency.

10.0: Demonstrate knowledge of legal principles to protect the health and safety of all ages, populations, and communities affected by a disaster or public health emergency.

11.0: Demonstrate knowledge of short- and long-term considerations for recovery of all ages, populations, and communities affected by a disaster or public health emergency.

From National Center for Disaster Medicine and Public Health (NCDMPH): *Core Competencies Project*, 2014. Available at: https://www.usuhs.edu/ncdmph/research-education/competencies/core-competencies-project.

BOX 16.3 Websites Providing Education and Training Opportunities

Public Health Workforce Development Centers
- Centers for Disease Control and Prevention: https://www.slu.edu/public-health-social-justice/training/center_heartlandphp
- Heartland Centers for Public Health and Community Capacity Development: http://www.heartlandcenters.slu.edu/
- National Public Health Training Centers Network, HRSA: http://bhpr.hrsa.gov/grants/publichealth/trainingcenters/index.html
- Northwest Center for Public Health Practice: http://www.nwcphp.org/training

Government and Other Nurse-Specific Courses
- American Red Cross Disaster Health and Sheltering Course for Nursing Students: http://www.drc-group.com/library/exercise/osc/OSC-DHS-Fact-Sheet.pdf
- Emergency Management Institute: http://training.fema.gov/
- Federal Emergency Management Agency (FEMA) Training: http://www.fema.gov/prepared/train.shtm
- National Nurse Emergency Preparedness Initiative: http://www.nnepi.org/

Public Health Organizations
- American Public Health Association (APHA): http://www.apha.org
- Association of Public Health Nurses (APHN): http://www.phnurse.org/
- Association of Schools and Programs of Public Health (ASPPH): http://www.aspph.org/
- National Association of County and City Health Offices (NACCHO): http://www.naccho.org
- Public Health Foundation (PHF): http://www.phf.org

written disaster plans and require employees to perform annual mock drills, but many businesses lack these requirements. In recent years, hospitals and health departments in cities with nursing, medical, and other health professional schools include their faculty in the disaster planning work so that if a disaster occurs, faculty and students can easily be mobilized to assist.

Presidential Policy Directive (PPD)-8 emphasizes that true preparedness is a whole community event. PPD-8 urges the strengthening of our nation's security and resilience through an integrated set of guidance, programs, and processes to implement the national preparedness goal, described earlier in this chapter (DHS, 2008, 2011).

This planning and implementation require a coordinated response that involves many stakeholders, including first and foremost the general public. Community preparedness also involves all levels of government, public health agencies, hospitals, first responders, emergency management, health care providers within the community, schools and universities, the private sector, and business and nongovernmental organizations (NGOs) such as the ARC. Mutual aid agreements and prior planning help to bridge perceived and actual barriers, establish relationships before the incident at the local, regional, state, and national levels, and ensure seamless service. Sometimes barriers involve regulatory authority and jurisdictional boundaries; sometimes the barriers involve organizational control versus the common good.

Emergency management is responsible for developing and coordinating emergency response plans within their defined area, whether local, state, federal, or tribal. The Federal Emergency Management Agency (FEMA) coordinates comprehensive, all-hazard planning at the national level, assuring a menu of exercises and plan templates to address plausible incidents in any given community. Emergency management personnel at the state and local level works closely with their communities and response partners, providing opportunities to train, exercise, evaluate, and update disaster plans. Stronger predisaster partnerships which include all stakeholders produce a more coordinated response.

Disaster planning involves simplicity and realism with backup contingencies because (1) the disaster will never be an "exact fit" for the plan, and (2) all plans must be implementation ready, no matter who is present to start them (DHS, 2014). The following Quality and Safety Education for Nurses box describes safety guidelines for the nurse's family.

Finally, the community must have an adequate warning system and a backup evacuation plan to remove individuals who are hesitant to leave from areas of danger. Some people refuse to leave their homes because they are afraid their possessions will be lost or destroyed either by the disaster or from looting after the disaster. Law enforcement personnel or others in authority may have to speak directly to these reluctant residents to

---

QSEN FOCUS ON QUALITY AND SAFETY EDUCATION FOR NURSES

Targeted Competency: Safety—Minimize risk for harm to clients and providers through both system effectiveness and individual performance. Selected knowledge, skills, and attitudes are cited here to develop a disaster safety plan.

- **Knowledge:** Examine human factors and other basic safety design principles as well as commonly used unsafe practices (such as workarounds and dangerous abbreviations). Specific steps might be:
  1. Learn how you can get information during the disaster or emergency.
     - Determine what types of disasters are most likely to happen.
     - Learn about warning signals in your community.
     - Ask about post disaster pet care (shelters usually will not accept pets).
     - Review the disaster plans at your workplace, school, and other places where your family spends time.
     - Determine how to help older or disabled family members or neighbors.
     - What should you do?
- **Skills**: Demonstrate effective use of strategies to reduce risk of harm to yourself or others.
  1. Create a disaster plan:
     - Talk with your family and create two places to meet: one outside your home and one outside your neighborhood. Give each member of the family a copy of the plan.
     - Discuss the types of disasters that are most likely to happen and review what to do in each case and make a plan.
     - Choose an out-of-state friend to be your family contact; this person will verify the location of each family member. After a disaster, it may be easier to call long distance than to make local calls.
     - Review evacuation plans, including care of pets. Have alternative routes for evacuation.
  2. Complete this checklist:
     - Post emergency phone numbers next to telephones.
     - Teach everyone how and when to call 9-1-1.

- Determine when and how to turn off water, gas, and electricity using the main switches.
- Check adequacy of insurance coverage for yourself and your home.
- Locate and review the use of fire extinguishers.
- Install and maintain smoke detectors.
- Conduct a home hazard hunt and fix potential hazards.
- Stock emergency supplies and assemble a disaster supplies kit.
- Acquire first aid and cardiopulmonary resuscitation (CPR) certification.
- Locate all escape routes from your home. Find two ways out of each room.
- Find safe spots in your home for each type of disaster.
  3. Practice and maintain your plan:
     - Review the plan every 6 months.
     - Conduct fire and emergency evacuation drills.
     - Replace stored water every 3 months and stored food every 6 months.
     - Test and recharge fire extinguishers according to manufacturer's instructions.
     - Test your smoke detectors monthly and change the batteries at least once a year.
  4. What more should you do?
- **Attitudes**: Appreciate the cognitive and physical limits of human performance.
- Monitor your personal reactions to the disaster. Seek assistance if the stress of the losses and the potential work to reestablish a new normal seem overwhelming. Monitor the reactions of your colleagues and the clients you serve, and provide or refer to others anyone who needs stress management intervention.

Safety Question
To prepare more effectively for the event of a future disaster, list the steps that you would take to ensure the safety of your family, including any pets you may have.

convince them to leave their homes and go to safer quarters. Also, some people mistakenly believe that experience with a particular type of disaster is enough preparation for the next one. They must be convinced that predisaster warnings are official, serious, and personally important before they are motivated to take action.

The National Health Security Strategy

As previously discussed, the purpose of the National Health Security Strategy was to build community resilience and to strengthen and sustain health and emergency response systems. Outcomes of the NHSS include community strengthening, integration of response and recovery systems, and seamless coordination among all levels of the public health and medical system (USDHHS, 2017a). Community resilience has become a central theme in disaster planning and is defined as the sustained ability of a community to withstand and recover from adversity (Links et al., 2018). Healthy individuals, families, and communities with access to health care and protective, preventive knowledge that can be used to launch timely action become some of our nation's strongest assets in disaster incidents. Preincident capacity has a direct impact on resilience (Links et al. (2018). The prefunctioning domains are communication, economy, education, food and water, government, housing, health care, public health, nurturing care, transportation, and well-being. Strengths or deficits in these domains either increase or decrease resilience. Population factors that contribute to resilience include vulnerability, inequity, and deprivation. Prevention/mitigation factors include natural systems, engineered systems, and countermeasures. The nurse works to build on the strengths and mitigate areas of weakness to build resiliency in their communities. Healthier communities are better able to bounce back.

Disaster and mass casualty exercises. Although practice will not ensure a perfect response to disaster, disaster and mass casualty drills and exercises are extremely valuable components of preparedness. After the exercise, the lessons learned through after-action reports are used to update disaster plans and subsequent operations. Exercise categories include discussion-based simulations, or "tabletops," and operations-based events, such as drills and functional, full-scale exercises (FEMA, 2018b). Operations-based events involve escalating the scope and scale testing of the disaster preparedness and response network using a specific plan.

The National Exercise Program (NEP) serves to test and validate core capabilities. Participation in exercises, simulations, or other activities (such as real-world incidents) helps organizations validate their capabilities and identify shortfalls, pulling in their partners and stakeholders including citizen participation (FEMA, 2018b). An annual Capstone Exercise, formerly titled the National Level Exercise (NLE), is conducted every 2 years as the final component of each NEP progressive exercise cycle. The 2020 exercise was scheduled to focus on cybersecurity; however, in light of COVID-19, the focus was changed to that of the pandemic (FEMA, 2020).

The Homeland Security Exercise and Evaluation Program (HSEEP) was developed to help states and local jurisdictions improve overall preparedness with all natural and human-made disasters. It provides a standardized methodology and terminology for exercise design, development, conduct, evaluation, and improvement planning, and assists communities in creating exercises that will make a positive difference before a real incident (FEMA, 2018b). HSEEP is the national standard for all exercises.

Whether conducted as drills, tabletops, functional scenarios, or full-scale scenarios, and whether the scope is local or national, nurses and other health care providers must be included as a part of the exercise's planning, response, and after-action activities. Nurses, as client and community advocates, are essential players in the exercise and preparedness arena.

CASE STUDY

Use of the Mock Attack Strategy to Prepare for Potential Disasters

The Saber city disaster preparedness (DP) team wanted to coordinate a mock terrorist attack to study the effectiveness of its disaster management plan. The goal of the mock attack was to promote confidence, develop skills, coordinate activities, and coordinate participants of the disaster management team. The DP team planned a commonly seen terrorist attack: A bus carrying important politicians would explode outside the federal courthouse in downtown Saber. All participating organizations (including the health department, hospital, police department, and fire department) were notified of the date the mock attack would be held. Volunteers were found to play victims on the scene.

After months of planning, the day of the mock attack came. The members of the DP team watched how well the organizations worked together during the events of the mock attack. At noon, reports of an exploded bus in front of the courthouse came across police scanners: "Several people are dead and many more injured." Emergency medical response teams and hazardous material response crews were called to the scene to care for the injured and attend to the potential hazardous exposure. Police officers quickly cleared the area of people and established a barrier around the scene. Firefighters put out the fire on the burning bus.

From the mock attack, the DP team learned that the city of Saber was prepared for a terrorist attack. Communication among organizations flowed smoothly, and the disaster management team was skillful in controlling the situation. Participants in the mock attack stated they were happy to have the practice and felt more confident in their ability to provide care in the case of a major disaster.

Response

The first level of disaster response occurs at the local level with the mobilization of responders such as the fire department, law enforcement, public health, and emergency services. If the disaster needs exceed local resources, the county or city emergency management agency will coordinate activities through an emergency operations center. Generally, local responders within a county sign a regional or statewide mutual aid agreement which allows the sharing of needed personnel, equipment, services, and supplies.

The initial scope of disaster assessment is usually measured in dollars, health risk and injury, and/or lives lost. The more destruction and lives at risk, the greater is the degree of attention and resources provided at the local, regional, and state levels. When state resources and capabilities are overwhelmed, governors may request federal assistance under a presidential disaster or emergency declaration. If the event is considered an incident of national significance (a potential or high-impact disaster), appropriate response personnel and resources are provided.

National Response Framework

Once a federal emergency has been declared, the NRF may take effect, depending on the specific needs arising from the disaster. As discussed, the NRF was written to provide an approach to domestic incidents in a well-coordinated manner, enabling all responding entities the ability to work together more effectively and efficiently. The online component of the NRF Resource Center (http://training.fema.gov/nrfres.aspx) contains supplemental materials, including annexes, partner guides, and other supporting documents and learning resources. This information is dynamic and is designed to change with lessons learned from real-world events. The framework involves the entire community (individual families, community leaders, nongovernmental agencies, and the private sector) and is scalable, flexible, and adaptable to the given situation. It is a living document that is revised every 18 months in response to evolving conditions and real-world applications (DHS, 2019).

The NRF includes Emergency Support Functions (ESFs). The 15 ESFs provide a mechanism to bundle federal resources and capabilities in order to support the nation. Functions include transportation, communications, public works and engineering, firefighting, information and planning, mass care, emergency assistance, temporary housing and human services, logistics, public health and medical services, search and rescue, oil and hazardous materials, agriculture and natural resources, energy, public safety and security, energy, and long-term community recovery, and external affairs/standard operating procedures (FEMA, 2019). Each ESF includes a coordinator function, and both primary and support agencies work together to coordinate and deliver the full breadth of federal capabilities. The ESFs provide the structure for coordinating federal interagency support for a federal response to an incident.

ESF-8, Public Health and Medical Services, provides guidance for medical and mental health personnel, medical equipment and supplies, assessment of the status of the public health infrastructure, and monitoring for potential disease outbreaks. The ESF-8 primary coordinating agency is the USDHHS; supporting agencies include the USDHS, the ARC, the Department of Defense, and the Department of Veterans Affairs. The NDMS is part of ESF-8 and includes the DMATs. These teams of specially trained civilian physicians, nurses, and other health care personnel can be sent to a disaster site within hours of activation (FEMA, 2019).

National Incident Management System

The NIMS is the national platform for disaster response, and it includes universal protocols and language. NIMS identifies concepts and principles that answer how to manage emergencies from preparedness to recovery regardless of their cause, size, location, or complexity. "NIMS provides a consistent, nationwide approach and vocabulary for multiple agencies or jurisdictions to work together to build, sustain and deliver the core capabilities needed to achieve a secure and resilient nation" (FEMA, 2018a, p 1).

No matter what type of nursing practice or which agency a nurse chooses, they will come into direct contact with NIMS, which includes the Incident Command System (ICS). NIMS includes varying levels of education and training, with many organizations requiring a base level of familiarization to comply with federal funding requirements. A well-developed training program promotes nationwide NIMS implementation. The training program also grows the number of adequately trained and qualified emergency management/response personnel.

? CHECK YOUR PRACTICE

Nurses working as members of a disaster assessment team need to provide accurate information to others in the National Incident Management System (NIMS) environment. A part of that communication involves the rapid and ongoing needs assessment. Accurate information helps in providing the most appropriate and necessary resources. In a time of crisis or great uncertainty, there is a crucial need for accurate and timely information. Health care personnel are the best sources of essential health information, especially technical information. The NIMS approach uses public affairs spokespersons for formal communication. The Public Information Officer (PIO) is a person with the authority and responsibility to communicate information to the public. Because nurses are considered highly trustworthy, they are often asked to do media interviews. If the nurse is asked for an interview, what is the best first approach?

1. Set up a time for the interview later in the day after you prepare your notes.
2. Refer the media to the PIO representing the agency.
3. Politely say that you are extremely busy dealing with victims of the disaster and you do not have time for an interview.

Response to Biological Incidents

Biological agents pose a high risk to public health because only a small amount of the agent is needed to affect thousands of people, and some of the agents are easy to conceal, transport, and disseminate. Chemical terrorist attacks require a very different response. An unannounced dissemination of a biological agent may easily go unnoticed, and the victims may have left the area of exposure long before the act of terrorism is recognized. The first signs that a biological agent has been released may not be apparent for days or weeks, until the victims become ill and seek a health evaluation. In this case, the health care professionals are considered the "first on the scene." The five components of a comprehensive public health response to outbreaks of illness are (1) detecting the outbreak, (2) determining the cause, (3) identifying factors that place people at risk, (4) implementing measures to control the outbreak, and (5) informing the medical and public communities about treatments, health consequences, and preventive measures (Rotz et al., 2000).

Identifying the chemical or biological agent is the first priority. The CDC is an excellent source of information on biological agents; the fact sheet lists specific agents. Information includes the methods of transmission and the communicability period (CDC, 2018a). Rapid identification is vital to protect health care workers and any others affected. Results of a biological release are hard to recognize because many biological agent symptoms mimic influenza or other viral syndromes. Pathogens such as bacteria, viruses, and toxins can be used to create biological weapons. Although an aerosol release may be a likely vehicle for dissemination, certain biological agents could also be released through the water and food supply. Only about a dozen pathogens pose a major threat, even though there are thousands of pathogens, some highly contagious. Quarantine of those exposed to contagious agents may be considered in some instances. A few vaccines have been developed to combat bacterial pathogens. The Centers for Disease Control and Prevention (CDC) provide an excellent source of biological agent information that includes the latest agent fact sheets for health practitioners (CDC, 2018a, 2018b). Important information provided includes the methods of transmission and communicability period. Through the Pandemic and All-Hazards Preparedness Reauthorization Act (PAHPRA), several biodefense programs exist to help public health professionals mount a proactive response to these events (USHHS, 2017b):

- BioWatch is an early warning system for biothreats; it uses an environmental sensor system to test the air for biological agents in several major metropolitan areas.
- BioSense is a data-sharing program to facilitate surveillance of unusual patterns or clusters of diseases in the United States. It shares data with local and state health departments and is a part of the BioWatch system.
- Project BioShield is a program that develops and produces new drugs and vaccines as countermeasures against potential bioweapons and deadly pathogens.
- Cities Readiness Initiative is a program that aids cities to increase their capacity to deliver medicines and medical supplies during a large-scale public health emergency such as a bioterrorism attack or a nuclear accident.
- Strategic National Stockpile (SNS) is a CDC-managed program with the capacity to provide large quantities of medicine and medical supplies to protect the American public in a public health emergency which may include bioterrorism. The SNS is deployed through a combination of state level request and the public health system.

Some of the most common lessons from exercises as well as live incidents involve communication. In an effort to keep the public health community informed, the CDC developed the Public Health Information Network (PHIN). The PHIN provides for the electronic exchange of information among governmental agencies. It focuses on six components that help ensure information access and sharing: early event detection, outbreak management, connecting laboratory systems, countermeasure and response administration, partner communications and alerting, and cross-functional components. It is critical to information exchange (CDC, 2020).

How Disasters Affect Communities

The pain and suffering of people who lose their possessions, are injured, or lose loved ones is immeasurable. When disaster hits, people in a community will be affected physically and emotionally, depending on the type, cause, and location of the disaster, the magnitude and extent of damage, the duration, and the amount of prewarning provided.

The first goal of any disaster response is to reestablish sanitary barriers as quickly as possible (Aronson-Storrier, 2017). Water, food, waste removal, vector control, shelter, and safety are all basic needs. Difficult weather conditions such as extreme heat or cold can hamper efforts, especially if electricity is affected. Continuous monitoring of the environment proactively addresses potential hazards. Disease prevention is an ongoing goal, especially if there is an interruption in the public health infrastructure. Infectious disease outbreaks occur in the recovery phase of disasters, and occasionally disaster workers introduce new organisms into the area.

People in a community will be affected physically and emotionally, depending on the type, cause, and location of the disaster; its magnitude and extent of danger; the duration; and amount of prewarning provided. Reflect on the COVID-19 pandemic; this was a unique type of disaster as everyone was affected differently. Some people were able to continue their jobs by working at home rather than at their usual workplace, others kept their jobs but were forced to take pay cuts, and others still were furloughed, laid off, or terminated. New jobs were created in many areas including transportation, contact tracing, and technology to name a few. Schools met electronically and this was more successful for some children and youth than for others. These are only a few examples of how this pandemic affected people.

Stress reactions in individuals. A traumatic event can cause moderate to severe stress reactions. Individuals react to the same disaster in different ways depending on their age, cultural background, health status, social support structure, and general ability to adapt to crisis. Symptoms that may require assistance are listed in Box 16.4.

People who are affected by a disaster often have an exacerbation of an existing chronic disease. For example, the emotional stress of the disaster may make it difficult for people with diabetes to control their blood glucose levels. Grief results in harmful effects on the immune system, reducing the function of cells that protect against viral infections and tumors. Hormones produced by the body's fight-or-flight mechanism also play a role in mediating the effects of grief.

Older adults' reactions to disaster depend a great deal on their physical health, strength, mobility, independence, and income. They can react deeply to the loss of personal possessions because of the sentimental value attached to the items and their irreplaceable value. Their need for relocation depends on the extent of damage to their home or their compromised health, and they may try to conceal the seriousness of their health conditions or losses if they fear the loss of independence. Box 16.5 lists other populations at higher risk for serious disruption after a disaster. Many of them are the same populations who are also at risk for adverse health effects before a disaster.

The effect of disasters on young children can be especially disruptive (National Institute of Mental Health [NIMH], n.d.) (Fig. 16.4). Regressive behaviors such as thumb sucking, bedwetting, crying, and clinging to parents can occur. Children tend to reexperience images of the traumatic event or have recurring

BOX 16.4   Know When to Seek Help: Tips for Survivors of a Disaster or Other Traumatic Event: Managing Stress[a]

You may feel emotionally:
- Anxious, fearful, or sad
- Extreme sense of urgency or panic
- Angry, especially if the event involved violence
- Guilty, even when you had no control over the traumatic event
- Heroic, like you can do anything
- Like you have too much energy or no energy
- Disconnected, not caring about anything or anyone
- Numb, unable to feel either joy or sadness

You may have physical reactions such as:
- Stomachaches and diarrhea
- Headaches or other physical pains for no obvious reason
- Eating too much or too little
- Sweating or having chills
- Having tremors or muscle twitches/being jumpy or easily startled

Behavior reactions may include:
- Trouble remembering things, thinking, making decisions, or concentrating
- Feeling confused or numb
- Worrying excessively
- Trouble talking about what happened and listening to others
- Trouble sleeping
- Increase or decrease in energy or activity levels
- Feeling sad or crying often
- Using alcohol, tobacco, illegal drugs, or prescription medicines to reduce distress
- Having outbursts of anger, or feeling irritated and blaming others or to forget
- Having difficulty helping others and accepting help or making decisions when around people
- Being reluctant to abandon property

Children
- Regressive behaviors (e.g., bedwetting, thumb sucking, crying, clinging to parents)
- Fantasies that disaster never occurred
- Nightmares
- School-related problems, including inability to concentrate and refusal to go back to school

[a]The tips in Box 16.4 are not an entire list. For further details, see Substance Abuse and Mental Health Services Administration. *Tips for survivors of a disaster or other traumatic event: Managing stress,* 2013. Retrieved from http://www.disasterdistress.samhsa.gov.

BOX 16.5   Populations at Greatest Risk for Disruption After Disaster

- Older adults
- Women
- Pregnant women
- Children
- Persons with disabilities
- Hearing impaired
- Visually impaired
- Individuals with chronic disease
- Individuals with chronic mental illness
- Low income
- Homeless
- Non–English-speaking
- Rural populations
- Tourists; persons new to an area
- Single-parent families
- Substance abusers
- Undocumented residents

Based on US Department of Health and Human Services Outreach Activities and Resources: *Special populations: emergency and disaster preparedness,* 2017. Available at http://sis.nlm.nih.gov.

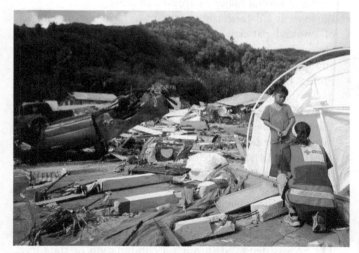

Fig. 16.4 The Effects of Disaster on Children Can Be Especially Disruptive. In 2013, one week after Typhoon Haiyan made landfall, residents of Tanauan, the Philippines, struggled to cope amid the devastation. Every house in the city of 50,000 was badly damaged or destroyed. The effects of a disaster on young children can be especially disruptive. (Courtesy of the American Red Cross Photo Library. Photo by Patrick Fuller/International Federation of Red Cross and Red Crescent Societies, Geneva, Switzerland. Retrieved January 2015 from: http://media.redcross.org/sites/.)

thoughts or sensations, or they may intentionally avoid reminders, thoughts, and feelings related to disaster events. Children may have arousal or heightened sensitivity to sights, sounds, or smells, and may experience exaggerated responses or difficulty with usual activities. Children not immediately affected by a disaster can also experience effects from it; the constant bombardment of disaster stories on television can cause fear in children. They may believe that the event could happen to them or their family, believe someone will be injured or killed, or think they will be left alone. It is best to turn off the news and engage in activities with family, friends, and neighbors, as parents' reaction to a disaster greatly influences their children's (NIMH, n.d.). The National Institute of Mental Health document titled "Helping children and adolescents cope with violence and disasters: What parents can do" is an excellent resource; it provides

guidance according to age groups five and under, 5 to 11, and 12 to 17. It also provides helplines and other sources of support.

One special population that may be overlooked is children in childcare facilities. Children are cared for in many different locations, ranging from freestanding buildings to provider homes. They tend to have little, if any, security against a disaster, and people come and go out of the facility all day. If a disaster occurs, a plan must be in place for how the children can be reunited with their parents. Because of their small size, someone may have to help them leave the facility. They are more vulnerable to chemical and biological agents because of their immature physiological and psychological development, and they have a smaller fluid reserve than adults, so are more susceptible to dehydration. With all populations, review individual strategies, including available specific resources, in the event of an emergency. The following actions are recommended regarding childcare emergency supplies: in addition to the family readiness kit, add copies of the child's medical information; comfort items such as games, toys, blanket, crayons, markers, and paper; and if the facility is putting the kit together, they should include the attendance list of children.

Public health nurses should help those in the affected community talk about their feelings, including anger, sorrow, guilt, and perceived blame for the disaster or the outcomes of the disaster. Community members should be encouraged to engage in healthy eating, exercise, rest, daily routine maintenance, limited demanding responsibilities, and time with family and friends.

Stress reactions in the community. Communities reflect the individuals and families living in them, both during and after a disaster incident. Four community phases are commonly recognized: (1) heroic, (2) honeymoon, (3) disillusionment, and (4) reconstruction. The first two phases—the heroic and honeymoon phases—are most often associated with response efforts. The latter two phases—disillusionment and reconstruction—are most often linked with recovery. For purposes of continuity, all phases will be discussed in this response section.

During the heroic phase, there is overwhelming need for people to do whatever they can to help others survive the disaster. First responders, including health and medical personnel, will work hours on end with no thought of their own personal or health needs. They may fight needed sleep and refuse rest breaks in their drive to save others. Moreover, imported responders may be unfamiliar with the terrain and inherent dangers; those with oversight responsibilities may need to order helpers to take necessary breaks and attend to their health needs. Exhausted, overworked responders present a danger to themselves and the community served.

In the honeymoon phase, survivors may be rejoicing that their lives and the lives of loved ones have been spared. Survivors will gather to share experiences and stories. The repeated telling to others creates bonds among the survivors. A sense of thankfulness over having survived the disaster is inherent in their stories.

The disillusionment phase occurs after time elapses and people begin to notice that additional help and reinforcement may not be immediately forthcoming. This results in a sense of despair, and exhaustion starts to take its toll on volunteers, rescuers, and medical personnel. The community begins to realize that a return to the previous normal is unlikely and that they must make major changes and adjustments. Nurses need to consider the psychosocial impact and the consequent emotional, cognitive, and spiritual implications of this stage. Public health nurses should identify groups and population segments particularly at risk for burnout and exhaustion, including responders and volunteers involved in rescue efforts. They may need breaks and reminders for nourishment. In addition, those in shock and those consumed by grief related to loss of loved ones will need compassionate care, with possible referrals to mental health counseling resources.

The last phase—reconstruction—is the longest. Homes, schools, churches, and other community elements need to be rebuilt and reestablished. The goal is to return to a new state of normalcy. Because the scope of human need may still be extensive, the nurse will continue to function as a member of the interprofessional team to provide and ensure provision of the best possible coordinated care to the population.

Role of the Nurse in Disaster Response

The nurse's role during a disaster depends largely on the nurse's experience, professional role in a community disaster plan, specialty training, and special interest. Flexibility is essential because the only certainty is that there will be continuing changes. Nurses serve in many roles in the community; they advocate for a safe environment and know that disasters are both natural and human-made, so they assess for and report environmental health hazards. The nurse should be aware of and report unsafe equipment, faulty structures, and the beginning of disease epidemics such as measles or influenza. The public health nurse brings leadership, policy, planning, and practice expertise to disaster preparedness and response (Association of Public Health Nurses [APHN], 2014).

Assessment is a major nursing role during a disaster. In completing an assessment, they should use the skills of interview, observation, individual physical examinations, health and illness screening, surveys (i.e., sample and special health), and records (i.e., census, school, vital statistics, disease reporting). The traditional model of community assessment presents the foundation for the rapid community assessment process. The acute needs of a population in disaster turns the community assessment into rapid appraisal of a sector or region's population, social systems, and geophysical features. Elements of a rapid needs assessment include determining the magnitude of the incident, defining the specific health needs of the affected population, establishing priorities and objectives for action, identifying existing and potential public health problems, evaluating the capacity of the local response, including resources and logistics, and determining the external resource needs for priority actions (Stanley et al., 2008). Assessments in sudden-impact disasters, such as tornadoes and earthquakes, are more concerned with ongoing hazards, injuries and deaths, shelter requirements, and clean water. Triage should begin immediately and is the process of separating casualties and allocating treatment on the basis of an individual's potential for survival. Highest priority is given to individuals with life-threatening injuries, but also those who have a high probability of survival once they are stabilized (Veenema, 2019). Second priority is given to victims with injuries that have systemic complications that are not yet life threatening and could wait 45 to 60 minutes for treatment. Last priority is given to those victims with local injuries without immediate complications and who can wait several hours for medical attention.

Assessments in gradual-onset disasters, such as famines, are most concerned with mortality rates, nutritional status, immunization status, and environmental health.

Nurses should understand what the available community resources will be after a disaster strikes, and, most importantly, how the community will work together. A community-wide disaster plan serves as a roadmap for what "should" occur before, during, and after the response, as well as the role of each participant in the plan.

There may be times when the nurse is the first to arrive on the scene of a disaster. If so, the more usual skills of community assessment, case finding and referring, prevention, health education, surveillance, and working with aggregates will be put aside temporarily so that the nurse can deal with life-threatening problems. Once rescue workers arrive on the scene, plans for triage should begin immediately.

Nurses can help initiate or update an agency's disaster plan, provide educational programs and materials regarding disasters specific to the area, and organize disaster drills. They can also provide an updated record of vulnerable populations within the community; when calamity strikes, disaster workers must know what kinds of populations they are attempting to assist. For example, if a tornado strikes a retirement village, the needs are quite different from those seen after a tornado hits a church filled with families or a center for the physically challenged. In addition to knowing where special populations exist, the nurse can educate groups about what effect the disaster might have on them. Nurses should review individual strategies, including available specific resources, in the event of an emergency.

Lack of or inaccurate information regarding the scope of the disaster and its initial effects contributes to the misuse of resources. Often, too many volunteers who lack official sponsorship convene at the site of disaster and are disappointed when their help cannot be used. Similarly, well-meaning people may send clothes and food to disaster sites that lack storage and distribution abilities. Contributions that add to the stress of coping with the disaster can be a burden. Local and regional emergency management and public health resources need to be readjusted as assessment reports continue to come in. Establishing a priority of needs that benefit the largest aggregate of affected individuals with the most correctable problems is consistent with the basic tenets of triage.

Ongoing assessments or surveillance reports are just as important as initial assessments. Surveillance reports indicate the continuing status of the affected population and the effectiveness of ongoing relief efforts. They continue to inform relief managers of needed resources. Nurses are involved in ongoing surveillance and their work continues into the recovery phase of a disaster.

Nursing Role in Sheltering

Shelters are generally the responsibility of the local ARC chapter, although in massive disasters, the military may set up "tent cities" or bring in trailers for the masses who need temporary shelter. Nurses, because of their comfort with delivering aggregate health promotion, disease prevention, and emotional support, make ideal shelter managers and team members. Each person who comes to the shelter is assessed to determine what type of facility is most appropriate for their needs. Although initially physical health needs may be the priority, especially among older adults and the chronically ill, many of the predominant problems in shelters revolve around stress. The shock of the disaster itself, the loss of personal possessions, the fear of the unknown, living in proximity to total strangers, and even boredom can cause stress.

In addition to providing assessments, nurses working in shelters also provide referrals and meet health care needs such as helping clients get prescription glasses, medications, first aid, and appropriate diet adjustments, keeping client records, ensuring emergency communications, and providing a safe environment (ARC, 2012). The ARC provides training for shelter support and use of appropriate protocols. It partners with other agencies such as the MRC and local public health agencies to ensure adequate health care is given to those in shelters. Nurses can use common-sense approaches to help shelter residents; these measures include listening to victims tell and retell their disaster story and current situation, encouraging residents to share their feelings with one another if it seems appropriate to do so, helping residents make decisions, delegating tasks (e.g., reading, crafts, playing games with children) to teenagers and others to help combat boredom, providing basic necessities (i.e., food, clothing, rest), attempting to recover or obtain needed items (e.g., prescription glasses, medication), providing basic compassion and dignity (e.g., privacy when appropriate and if possible), and referring to a mental health counselor or other source of help.

> ## EVIDENCE-BASED PRACTICE
>
> Labrague et al. performed a systematic review of the literature exploring nurses' preparedness for response to disasters (17 articles). A major finding from the literature review was the low level of preparedness reported by nurses. It was found that prior disaster experience and participation in disaster-related training enhanced disaster preparedness. The findings highlight the need for opportunities for both nursing students and practicing nurses to take part in disaster-related training experiences. An example of a training program that promotes training for both nursing students and health care practitioners in an interprofessional environment is the National Disaster Health Consortium (NDHC) training course (https://nursing.wright.edu). These types of training programs promote nurses' readiness to work in interprofessional teams in order to best promote positive outcomes. Training opportunities, like NDHC, can also help prepare nurses for the unique interprofessional disaster certification from the American Nurses Credentialing Center, documenting their expertise in disaster (https://www.nursingworld.org).
>
> Data from Labrague LJ, Hammad K, Gloe DS, et al: Disaster preparedness among nurses: a systematic review of the literature. *Int Nurs Rev* 65:41–53, 2018.

Nurses need to be aware of the surrounding medical facilities and services provided in their area, including special needs shelters. Individuals who are medically dependent and not acutely ill but have varied physical, cognitive, and psychological conditions should be directed to a special needs shelter. The federal government provides assistance to special needs shelters through one of the emergency support functions (ESF 8) of the NRP, which provides assessment of public health and medical needs, health surveillance, supplies, and medical care personnel such as teams from the NDMS (DHS, 2014).

Special needs shelters reduce the surge demands on hospitals and long-term care facilities that often occur during disasters. Although helpful in reducing surge, too many referrals can create tension among the special needs shelters, the regular shelters, and the health care facilities as roles and responsibilities become blurred and overall resources and personnel limited. Careful preplanning for a community's special needs population is essential.

International Relief Efforts

Disasters occur throughout the world, and people suffer from natural disasters and human-made disasters on a global scale. Civil strife leads to war, famine, and communicable disease outbreaks. Sometimes disaster or relief workers are sent to these international disasters at the request of the affected country's government. At other times, workers are not welcomed but may go with the support of the United Nations. When workers are not welcomed, their lives may be in danger, even though they go as peacekeeping agents of the Federation of the Red Cross and Red Crescent societies and the International Committee of the Red Cross or as health representatives from the World Health Organization. International disaster or relief workers generally have intensive training and preparation before embarking on a mission.

Psychological Stress of Disaster Workers

Disaster relief work can be rewarding because it provides an opportunity to have a profound and positive impact on the lives of those who may be experiencing their greatest time of need. However, the work is also challenging and stressful; during an assignment, responders may be exposed to chaotic environments, long hours, rapidly changing information and directives, long wait times before getting to work, noisy environments, and living quarters that are less than ideal. According to the National Institute of Occupational Health and Safety (NIOSH, 2013), responders may not recognize the need for self-care and neglect monitoring their own emotional and physical health. As recovery efforts span time frames of weeks to months, there is increasing risk for adverse effects to responders.

No one who experiences a disaster either personally or in a professional capacity is untouched by it. Nurses who work with survivors of disasters may be at risk for stress reactions. Self-care is as important as the care that is provided to community members. Symptoms that may signal a need for stress management assistance include being reluctant or refusing to leave the scene until the work is finished, denying needed rest and recovery time, feeling overriding stress and fatigue, engaging in unnecessary risk-taking activities, having difficulty communicating thoughts, remembering instructions, making decisions, or concentrating, engaging in unnecessary arguments, having a limited attention span, and refusing to follow orders (ARC, 2012). Physical symptoms such as tremors, headaches, nausea, and cold or flulike symptoms can also occur. Suppressing feelings of guilt, powerlessness, anger, and other signs of stress will eventually lead to symptoms such as irritability, fatigue, headaches, and distortions of bodily functions. It is normal to experience stress, but it must be dealt with. The worst thing anyone can do is to deny that it exists.

The nurse should understand that everyone reacts differently after a disaster assignment. Most reactions are considered normal and are temporary, resolving in days or a few weeks. For some workers, disasters bring forth strong thoughts and emotions, both positive and negative. Others may experience a mild reaction or hardly any reaction at all. There are some common strategies that will help individuals returning from the incident, including rest and recovery time, focusing on accomplishments, using calming strategies such as relaxation techniques or working on hobbies, taking deep breaths, listening to music, concentrating on self-care through healthy food and drink, exercise, and sleep, and talking to others, such as a trusted friend, family member, faith-based leader, or a professional counselor (SAMSHA, 2013). Delayed stress reactions, or those that occur once the disaster is over, can include exhaustion and an inability to adjust to the slower pace of work or home.

Workers may be disappointed if family members and friends do not seem as interested in what they have been through or if coming back home in general does not live up to expectations. They may feel frustration and conflict if their needs seem inconsistent with those of their family and co-workers, or if they have left the disaster site thinking that much more could have been done (Bryce, 2001). Issues or problems that once seemed pressing may now seem trivial. Anger may emerge as others present problems that seem trivial in contrast to those faced by the victims who were left behind. Disaster workers may fantasize about returning to the disaster site if they think their actions are appreciated more there than at home or the office. Mood swings are common and serve to resolve conflicting feelings. Feelings or actions that persist or that the worker perceives are interfering with daily life should be dealt with by a trained mental health professional.

Recovery

Recovery is about returning to a new normal with the goal of reaching a level of organization that is as near the predisaster level as is possible. This is often the hardest part of the disaster; during the recovery period, all involved agencies pull together to restore the institutions and properly rebuild. For example, the government takes the lead in rebuilding efforts, whereas the business community tries to provide economic support. Many religious organizations help with rebuilding efforts as well, while the Internal Revenue Service educates victims as to how to write off losses, and the Housing and Urban Development Department provides grants for temporary housing. The CDC provides continuing surveillance and epidemiological services, and voluntary agencies continue to assess individual and community needs and meet them when possible. When housing is destroyed, groups such as Habitat for Humanity play a valuable role in the rebuilding.

The best time to start thinking about the lessons learned from a recent disaster is during the recovery phase of the disaster cycle. The National Disaster Recovery Framework is a guide that enables effective recovery support to disaster-impacted states, tribes, territorial and local jurisdictions; it provides a flexible structure that enables disaster recovery managers to operate in a unified and collaborative manner.

Role of the Nurse in Disaster Recovery

The role of the nurse in the recovery phase of a disaster is as varied as in the three levels of prevention (see the Levels of Prevention box), preparedness, and response phases. Flexibility is essential in the recovery operation. Community cleanup efforts can cause many physical and psychological problems; for example, the physical stress of moving heavy objects can cause back injury, severe fatigue, and even death from heart attacks. Nurses must also continue to teach proper hygiene and make sure immunization records are current, given the threat of disease.

The reality of the recovery effort is that the rapid needs assessment continues into an ongoing community needs assessment. In order to determine effective interventions to ensure the best possible outcomes, it is essential to have ongoing accurate data about the population, as some conditions manifest only after time elapses. A major advantage of the recovery community assessment efforts is that they can be more in-depth, with greater confidence in the results. Some examples of community data points in the recovery phase include ongoing illness and injuries related to the disaster; diseases related to disruption of environmental or health services; health facility infrastructure in terms of adequate personnel, beds, and medical and pharmaceutical supplies; and environmental health assessment to include water quantity and quality, sanitation, shelter, solid waste disposal, and vector populations.

 LEVELS OF PREVENTION

Related to Disaster Prevention Management

Primary Prevention
Participate in developing a disaster management plan for the community.

Secondary Prevention
Assess disaster victims and triage for care.

Tertiary Prevention
Participate in home visits to uncover dangers that may cause additional injury to victims or cause other disasters (e.g., house fires from faulty wiring).

Disruption of the public health infrastructure, including water and food supply, the sanitation system, the vector control program, and access to primary and mental health care can lead to increased disease and community dysfunction. Nurses will engage in ongoing community assessments during the recovery phase. It is important to be alert for environmental health hazards during the recovery phase of a disaster. During home visits, nurses may uncover situations such as a faulty housing structure or lack of water or electricity. Objects that have been blown into the yard by a tornado or that floated in from a flood may be dangerous and must be removed. The nurse should also assess the dangers of living or dead animals and rodents that may be harmful to a person's health. For example, poisonous snakes may be found in and around homes once the waters from a flood start to recede. Case finding and referral are critical during the recovery phase and may continue for a long time.

Other examples of community data points to watch for during the recovery phase include ongoing illnesses and injuries related to the disaster, disease and acute respiratory infections related to disruption of environmental health services, and health facility infrastructure in terms of adequate personnel, beds, and medical and pharmaceutical supplies (Landesman, 2012).

The hurricanes, tornadoes, fires, and other natural disasters in the United States over the past several years changed how the health care system prepares for, responds to, and recovers from a disaster. People have learned how critical it is for communities to have a well-organized plan and for key players to know their roles and be flexible and collaborative. The value of an electronic medical record became more apparent in recent years when hospitals, clinics, and health departments lost records during a disaster and when people were relocated for substantial periods of time without access to their medications or medical records.

It is important to have a realistic perspective related to how long recovery may take. It will take months or years to return to a semblance of normal, and this new normal may be different from the predisaster state. Post disaster cleanup may also lead to unintentional injuries, including those resulting from falls, contact with live wires, accidents while cutting items, heart attacks from overexertion and stress, and auto accidents caused by road conditions or absent traffic signals. Nurses need to educate the community about the hazards described earlier, as well as hazards related to carbon monoxide poisoning from using lanterns, gas ranges, generators, or from burning charcoal to heat an enclosed area.

Nurses play a key role in helping survivors by providing psychological support. Acute and chronic illness may become worse after a disaster. The psychological stress of loss, cleanup, or moving can lead to feelings of hopelessness, depression, and grief in the disillusionment phase. Referrals to mental health professionals should continue throughout the recovery phase and as long as the need exists. The role of the nurse in case finding and referral remains critical during this phase. In the end, it is the concept of community resilience that will lead the community to its new normal. The public health nurse is the community and client advocate who ensures that resilience is supported in partnership with the population.

FUTURE OF DISASTER MANAGEMENT

In the last several years, the 2010 H1N1 pandemic, the earthquake in Haiti, the earthquake and tsunami in Japan, the civil war in Syria, and the 2020 global COVID-19 pandemic underscore the need for nursing involvement at every step of the disaster management cycle. To fully participate in this mission, nurses must continue to plan and train in an all-hazards environment, regardless of their specialty practice. Public health nurses are critical members of the multidisciplinary disaster health team due to their population-based focus and specialty knowledge in epidemiology and community assessment. Although sophisticated technology and surveillance will continue to advance in response to both human-made and natural disasters, disasters will continue to be unpredictable. Unpredictability and the medical and public health surge requirements in disaster makes prevention and preparedness activities on the part of individuals and communities even more important. Disaster information changes rapidly because of the learning that occurs during and after each incident, producing new best practices. Staying current in disaster training requires the public health nurse's commitment in community planning activities, exercise participation, and actual disaster work.

►► APPLYING CONTENT TO PRACTICE

Throughout this chapter, how nurses work in disaster management is applied to standards of public health nursing and the core competencies of health professionals in disaster work. Other applicable areas include discussion about the continuous processes of assessment, planning, implementation, evaluation, collaboration, and cooperation. The role of the nurse in disaster management relates to both standards of nursing and public health practice. Specifically, the nurse must first assess, then plan, implement, and evaluate, while simultaneously working with a variety of other concerned and involved agencies and individuals.

▌ PRACTICE APPLICATION

Paula Miller, a nurse in a medium-sized public health department in Lincoln, Nebraska, was called to serve on her first national disaster assignment. Her disaster skills were tested when a fire destroyed most of the town of Paradise, California. Ms. Miller left Lincoln to help manage a shelter in an elementary school cafeteria in a nearby town.

The devastation that she saw en route to the school upset her. Assigned to help with client intake, she patiently listened to the disaster victims, referred many of her most distraught clients to the mental health counselor, and set priorities for other needs as they arose. For example, she found that many of her clients left their medications behind and needed therapy. Other needs included diapers and formula for infants, prescription eyeglasses, and clothing. By identifying their needs, Ms. Miller helped ensure that the master "needs list" was complete.

As the days went on, the stress level in the shelter grew. The crowded living conditions and lack of privacy took its toll on the residents. Around the tenth day of her assignment, Ms. Miller began to experience pounding headaches and had difficulty concentrating. She thought she would be fine, but the mental health counselor said that she was experiencing a stress reaction.

Which of the following actions would probably be the most useful for this nurse to take?

A. Share her feelings with the onsite mental health counselor on a regular basis.
B. Call home to share her feelings with family members.
C. Meet the needs of her clients to the best of her ability, and accept the fact that stress is a part of the job.

Answers can be found on the Evolve website.

▌ REMEMBER THIS!

- The number and types of disasters, both human-made and natural, continues to increase, as does the number of people affected by them.

- The cost to recover from a disaster has risen sharply because of the amount of technology that must be restored, the businesses that closed, and the jobs lost.
- Professional preparedness involves an awareness and understanding of the disaster plan at work and in the community.
- Nurses are increasingly getting involved in disaster planning, response, and recovery through their local health department or local government.
- Disaster health and disaster mental health training from an official agency such as the ARC can prepare nurses for the many opportunities and challenges that await them in disaster prevention, preparedness, response, and recovery.
- It is important to be knowledgeable about community resources available to vulnerable populations before a disaster incident to ensure a more coordinated response and recovery.
- During all phases of disaster management, it is important for nurses to help clients maintain a safe environment and to advocate for environmental safety measures in the community.
- Community residents react differently to disasters depending on the type, cause, and location of the disaster, its magnitude and extent of damage, its duration, and the amount of warning that was provided.
- People also react differently to disasters depending on factors such as their age, cultural background, health status, social support structure, and general adaptability to crisis.
- The stress of nurses is compounded if they are both victims and caregivers in a disaster, or in the example of the COVID-19 pandemic, are asked to care for patients who have a virus that they may contract or transmit to another person, such as a family member.
- Disaster shelter nurses are exposed to a variety of physical and emotional problems, including stress. Stress may be instigated by the shock of the disaster, the loss of personal possessions, the fear of the unknown, living in proximity to strangers, and boredom.
- The degree of worker stress during disasters depends on the nature of the disaster, the worker's role in the disaster, individual stamina, noise level, adequacy of workspace, potential for physical danger, availability of needed equipment, stimulus overload, and, especially, being exposed to death and trauma.
- Symptoms of worker stress during disasters include minor tremors, nausea, decreased concentration, difficulty thinking and remembering, irritability, fatigue, and other somatic disorders.
- Flexibility is important when aiding disaster victims.
- The recovery stage of a disaster occurs as all involved agencies work together to restore the economic and civic life of the community.

EVOLVE WEBSITE

http://evolve.elsevier.com/Stanhope/foundations
- Case Study, with Questions and Answers
- NCLEX Review Questions
- Practice Application Answers

REFERENCES

American Red Cross: Be "Red Cross Ready"—It's as Easy as 1-2-3, May 2018, www.redcross.org. Accessed May 2020.

American Red Cross: Disaster sheltering services handbook, Washington, DC, 2012, ARC.

Association of Public Health Nurses: The Role of the Public Health Nurse in Disaster Preparedness Response and Recovery: A position paper, 2014. Retrieved May 6, 2020 from http://www.quadcouncilphn.org

Aronsson-Storrier M: Sanitation, human rights and disaster management, Disaster Prev Manag, 25:514-525, 2017.

Bryce CP: Stress management in disasters, Washington, DC, 2001, Pan American Health Organization.

Centers for Disease Control and Prevention: Emergency preparedness and response: bioterrorism agents and diseases, 2018a, Retrieved May 7, 2020 from http://www.bt.cdc.gov.

Centers for Disease Control and Prevention (CDC): Emergency preparedness and response: Coping with a disaster or traumatic event, 2018b. Available at https://emergency.cdc.gov. Accessed May 7, 2020.

Centers for Disease Control and Prevention: Public Health Information Network (PHIN), 2020, Retrieved May 6, 2020 from http://www.cdc.gov/phin/.

Department of Homeland Security: National disaster medical system: DMAT, Washington, DC, 2014, USDHS. Retrieved May 6, 2020 from http://www.phe.gov.

Department of Homeland Security: Homeland Security Act of 2002: Title 1—Department of Homeland Security, Washington, DC, 2002, USDHS.

Department of Homeland Security: Homeland security presidential directives, Washington, DC, 2008, updated March 2011. USDHS.

Department of Homeland Security: National Preparedness Guidelines, 2014. Retrieved May 7, 2020 from http://www.fema.gov.

Department of Homeland Security (DHS): National disaster prevention framework (2nd ed.), 2016. Available at: https://www.fema.gov/media-library/assets/documents/117762. Accessed June 2018.

Department of Homeland Security: National Response Framework (NRF), ed 4, 2019. Retrieved May 7, 2020 from http://www.fema.gov/national-response-framework.

Downes E: Nursing and complex humanitarian emergencies: Ebola is more than a disease, Nurs Outlook 63:12–15, 2015.

Federal Emergency Management Agency: National Preparedness Goal, Second Edition—What's New, 2015. Retrieved May 5, 2020 from http://www.fema.gov>media-library-data>national-prepar.

Federal Emergency Management Agency: National Incident Management System (NIMS), 2018a. Retrieved May 7, 2020 from http://www.fema.gov/national-incident-management-system.

Federal Emergency Management Agency: Homeland Security Exercise and Evaluation Program (HSEEP), Washington, DC, 2018b,. Retrieved May 7, 2020 from http://www.fema/gov/hseep.

Federal Emergency Management Agency: Emergency Support Function#8-Public Health and Medical Services Annex, 2019. Retrieved May 7, 2020 from http://www.fema.emergencysupportfunction8.

Federal Emergency Management Agency (FEMA): Emergency Management Institute (EMI), 2020. Available at: https://training.fema.gov. Accessed May 7, 2020.

Federal Emergency Management Agency: National Level Exercise Program (NLE)—2020, Retrieved May 7, 2020 from http://www.fema.gov.national-exercise.

Inajima T, Adelman J, Okada Y: Fukushima disaster was manmade, investigation finds, Bloomberg Businessweek, July 5, 2012. Retrieved January 2015 from http://www.bloomberg.com/news/2012-07-05/fukushima-nuclear-disaster-was-man-made-investigation-rules.html.

Labrague LJ, Hammad K, Gloe DS, et al: Disaster preparedness among nurses: a systematic review of the literature. Int Nurs Rev, 65: 41-53, 2018

Landsman L: Public health management of disasters: the practice guide, 3rd ed., Washington DC, 2012, American Public Health Association.

Links JM, Schwart BS, Lin S, et al: COPEWELL: a conceptual framework and system dynamics model for predicting community functioning and resilience after disasters, Disaster Med Public Health Prep 12(1):127–137, 2018.

National Institute of Occupational Health and Safety: Traumatic incident stress, 2013. Retrieved May 6, 2020 from http://www.cdc.gov/niosh/topics/traumaticincident/.

National Institute of Mental Health: Helping children and adolescents cope with violence and disasters: What parents can do, n.d. Retrieved May 7, 2020 from http://www.nimh.nih.gov.

Naval Postgraduate School (NPS): Directives, instructions, specifications, and standards, Monterey, 2020, Dudley Knox Library. Available at: http://libguides.nps.edu Accessed May 6, 2020.

Robert Wood Johnson Foundation: Ten ways public health nurses (PHNs) improve health, 2017. Available at: http://www.phnurse.org. Accessed May 7, 2020.

Rotz LD, Koo D, O'Carroll PW, et al: Bioterrorism preparedness: planning for the future, J Public Health Manag Pract 6:45, 2000.

Substance Abuse and Mental Health Services Administration: Tips for survivors of a disaster or other traumatic event: Managing stress, 2013. Retrieved from http://www.store.samhsa.gov. Accessed May 5, 2020.

Stanley S, Polivka B, Gordon D, et al: The ExploreSurge trail guide and hiking workshop: discipline specific education for public health nurses, Public Health Nurs 25:166–175, 2008.

United Nations Development Programme: Disaster recovery: challenges and lessons, 2016. New York, Author.

United Nations Office for Disaster Risk Reduction: Making development sustainable: The future of disaster risk management. Global Assessment Report on Disaster Risk Reduction, Geneva, Switzerland, 2015, UNDRR.

United Nations Development Programme, 2020: COVID-19 pandemic, Retrieved 2020 from www.undp.org.

US Department of Health and Human Services: National Health Security Strategy of the United States of America, 2017a. Retrieved May 5, 2020 from http://www.phe.gov/nhss.

US Department of Health and Human Services: Public Health Emergency Pandemic and All-Hazards Preparedness Reauthorization Act of 2013, 2017b. Retrieved May 6, 2020 from https://www/phe.gov.

US Department of Health and Human Services: National health security strategy 2019-2022, 2019, Retrieved November 2020 from http://www.phe.gov.

US Department of Health and Human Services: Pandemic and All-Hazards Preparedness and Advancing Innovation Act. 2019, Retrieved May 7, 2020 from https://www.phe.gov.

US Department of Health and Human Services: Healthy People 2030, Washington, DC, 2020, US Government Printing Office. Retrieved from http://www.healthypeople.gov.

Veenema TG: Disaster nursing and emergency preparedness for chemical, biological, and radiological terrorism and other hazards, New York, 2019, Springer Publishing.

World Health Organization (WHO): Emergency response framework, 2017. Retrieved from http://www.who.int.

17

Public Health Surveillance and Outbreak Investigation

Laura H. Clayton

OBJECTIVES

After reading this chapter, the student should be able to:

1. Define public health surveillance.
2. List types of surveillance systems.
3. Identify steps in planning, analyzing, interviewing, and evaluating surveillance.
4. Recognize sources of data used when investigating a disease or condition outbreak.
5. Describe the role of the nurse in surveillance and outbreak investigation.
6. Relate the nurse's role in investigation to the national core competencies for public health nurses.

CHAPTER OUTLINE

KEY TERMS

Disease surveillance has been a part of public health protection since the 1200s, during the investigations of the bubonic plague in Europe. The Constitution of the United States provides for "police powers" necessary to preserve health safety as well as in other events (see Chapter 4. These powers include public health surveillance. State and local "police powers" also provide for surveillance activities. Health departments usually have legal authority to investigate unusual clusters of illness as well (Gostin and Wiley, 2018).

Florence Nightingale first demonstrated the nurse's role in responding to disasters. Public health nurses bring specific skills to events that require emergency responses. They are prepared for conducting and evaluating disaster response drills, exercises, and trainings. Public health nurses are first responders in emergency situations in the community, they can lead and manage in the field and in the incident command center, and they are able to collaborate with others to sustain the emergency infrastructure (Association of Public Health Nurses [APHN], 2014). It is important for nurses to be prepared to lead and be a team member if an unusual occurrence or event strikes a community, like the COVID outbreak in 2020 (USA Facts, 2020).

DISEASE SURVEILLANCE

Definitions and Importance

Disease surveillance is the ongoing systematic collection, analysis, interpretation and dissemination of specific health data for use in public health (Blazes and Lewis, 2016; World Health Organization, 2018a). Surveillance provides a means for nurses to monitor disease trends in order to reduce morbidity and mortality and to improve health (McNabb et al., 2016; Veenema, 2018). The CDC indicates that public health surveillance is the foundation of public health practice (CDC, 2015).

Surveillance is a critical role function for nurses practicing in the community. A comprehensive understanding and knowledge of the surveillance systems and how they work will help nurses improve the quality and the usefulness of the data collected about a disease or for an event outbreak (including timing, geographic distribution, and those populations who are susceptible). Box 17.1 provides the features of the surveillance process.

Surveillance is built on understanding of epidemiologic principles of agent, host, and environmental relationships and on the natural history of disease or conditions (see Chapter 10. Surveillance systems make it possible to engage in effective continuous quality improvement activities within organizations and to improve quality of care (Kimble et al., 2017; Veenema, 2018).

Surveillance focuses on the collection of process and outcome data. Process data focus on what is done (i.e., services provided or protocols for health care delivery). Outcome data focus on changes in health status. The activities generated by analyses of these data aim to improve public health response systems. An example of process data is collection of data about the proportion of the eligible population vaccinated against influenza in any one year. Outcome data in this case are the incidence rates (new cases) of influenza among the same population in the same year.

Although surveillance was initially devoted to monitoring and reducing the spread of infectious diseases, it is now used to monitor and reduce chronic diseases and injuries, as well as environmental and occupational exposures (Latshaw et al., 2017; Perlman et al., 2017; Veenema, 2018) as well as personal health behaviors. Surveillance systems help nurses and other professionals monitor emerging infections and bioterrorist outbreaks (Veenema, 2018). Bioterrorism is one example of an event creating a critical public health concern that involves environmental exposures that must be monitored. This event also requires serious planning in order to be able to respond quickly and effectively. Bioterrorism is defined as "the intentional use of microorganisms or toxins derived from living organisms to cause death or disease in humans or the animals and plants on which we depend" (Ryan, 2016, p. 26). The CDC's bioterrorism website provides emergency preparedness and response information for the general public and health care professionals, as well as information on specific bioterrorism agents (http://emergency.cdc.gov) (CDC, 2017a).

Chemical terrorism is the intentional release of hazardous chemicals into the environment for the purpose of harming or killing (CDC, 2016a; Ryan, 2016). The CDC (2016b) provides chemical emergency preparedness and response information to health care professionals and the public, along with information about specific chemical agents (https://emergency.cdc.gov). In the event of a bioterrorist attack, imagine how difficult it would be to control the spread of biological agents such as botulism or anthrax or chemical agents such as sarin or ricin if no data were available about these agents, their resulting diseases or symptoms, and their usual incidence (new cases) patterns in the community.

Uses of Public Health Surveillance

Public health surveillance can be used to facilitate the following (Brownson et al., 2018; McNabb et al., 2016):

- Estimate the magnitude of a problem (disease or event)
- Determine geographic distribution of an illness or symptoms
- Portray the natural history of a disease
- Detect epidemics; define a problem
- Generate hypotheses; stimulate research
- Evaluate control measures

BOX 17.1   Surveillance Features

The surveillance features indicate it:
- Is organized and planned
- Is the principal means by which a population's health status is assessed
- Involves ongoing collection of specific data
- Involves analyzing data on a regular basis
- Requires sharing the results with others
- Requires broad and repeated contact with the public about personal health issues
- Motivates public health action as a result of data analyses to:
  - Reduce morbidity
  - Reduce mortality
  - Improve health

- Monitor changes in infectious agents
- Detect changes in health practices and health behaviors
- Facilitate planning
- Guide public health policy and programs

Purposes of Surveillance

Surveillance helps public health departments identify trends and unusual disease patterns, set priorities for using scarce resources, and develop and evaluate programs for commonly occurring and universally occurring diseases or events (Box 17.2).

Surveillance activities can be related to the core functions of public health: assessment, policy development, and assurance. Disease surveillance helps establish baseline (endemic) rates of disease occurrence and patterns of spread. Surveillance makes it possible to initiate a rapid response to an outbreak of a disease or event that can cause a health problem. In the past over a 24-month period, the CDC responded to 750 health threats (CDC, 2018c). For example, surveillance made it possible to respond quickly to outbreaks of Ebola (2014–2018), Zika (2016–2017), water contamination (2016), hepatitis A (2017), the opioid epidemic in the United States, and numerous foodborne outbreaks predominately related to salmonella and *Escherichia coli (E. coli)* in recent years (CDC, 2018c, 2018f). The CDC (2018b) maintains an active list of disease outbreak investigations and provides guidance for health care professionals regarding symptoms and treatment options. In 2020 the CDC responded to the COVID-19 health threat to the citizens of the United States. Visit the CDC website to see the exact process used for this response (www.CDC.Gov).

Surveillance data are analyzed, and interpretations of these data analyses are used to develop policies that better protect the public from problems such as emerging infections; bioterrorist, biological, and chemical threats; and injuries from problems such as motor vehicle accidents. In 2006 a great deal of emphasis was placed on developing disaster management policies in health care organizations, industries, and homes so that the US population could be prepared in the event of an emergency. Surveillance within individual organizations, such as infection control systems in hospitals, can be used to establish policies related to clinical practice that are designed to improve quality of care processes and outcomes. An example is documented by Sorour et al. (2016), where the standard of care of patients with Foley catheters was expanded to include the use of cranberry-containing products and antimicrobial metal care, resulting in a reduced incidence of catheter-associated urinary tract infections.

Surveillance makes it possible to have ongoing monitoring in place to ensure that disease and event patterns improve rather than deteriorate. They can also make it possible to study whether the clinical protocols and public health policies that are in place can be enhanced, based on current science, so that disease rates actually decline (World Health Organization, 2018). For example, the ongoing monitoring of obesity in children in a community may show that new clinical and effective protocols need to be developed to be used in school-based clinics to reduce the prevalence of obesity among the school populations.

Surveillance data are very helpful in determining whether a program is effective. Such data make it possible to determine whether public health interventions are effective in reducing the spread of disease or the incidence of injuries. By determining the change in the number of cases at the beginning of a program (baseline) with the number of cases after program implementation, it is possible to estimate the effectiveness of a program. One could then compare the effectiveness of different approaches to reducing the problem or to improving health.

Collaboration Among Partners

A quality surveillance system requires collaboration among a number of agencies and individuals: federal agencies, state and local public health agencies, hospitals, health care providers, medical examiners, veterinarians, agriculture, pharmaceutical agencies, emergency management, and law enforcement agencies, as well as 911 systems, ambulance services, urgent care and emergency departments, poison control centers, nurse hotlines, schools, and industry. Such collaboration promotes the development of a comprehensive plan and a directory of emergency responses and contacts for effective communication and information sharing. It is sometimes essential to include collaboration with international agencies as well. The type of information to be shared using algorithms is shown in the How To box.

HOW TO USE ALGORITHMS TO IDENTIFY WHICH EVENTS SHOULD BE INVESTIGATED
- That is, this means using a precise step-by-step plan outlining a procedure that in a finite number of steps helps to identify the appropriate event
- How to investigate?
- Whom to contact?
- How and to whom information is to be disseminated?
- Who is responsible for appropriate action?

Nurses are often in the forefront of responses to be made in the surveillance process, whether working in a small rural agency or a large urban agency; within the health department, school, or urgent care center; or on the telephone performing triage services during a disaster. It is the nurse who sees the event first (Association of Public Health Nurses, 2014).

Nurse Competencies

The national core competencies for public health nurses were developed from the Core Competencies for Public Health

---

BOX 17.2 Purposes of Surveillance

- Assess public health status
- Respond to unusual disease spread and terrorism
- Define public health priorities
- Plan public health programs
- Evaluate programs
- Stimulate research
- Improve health

TABLE 17.1   Phases of Nursing Process Linked to Preparedness

DEFINITION OF:				
Preparedness	**Assessment**	**Planning**	**Implementation**	**Evaluation**
Assure capacity to respond effectively to disasters and emergencies	Assess the populations at risk for special needs during a disaster	Develop plans to care for special needs populations during a disaster	Conduct training, drills, and exercises related to care of special needs persons	Evaluate plans for serving populations with special needs

Excerpted from Association of Public Health Nurses: *The role of public health nurses in emergency preparedness and response: position paper* [Table 1: The Phases of Disaster Linked to the Nursing Process], 2013. Retrieved from https://www.resourcenter.net.

Professionals (Council on Linkages between Academia and Public Health Practice, 2014) and by the Quad Council of Public Health Nursing Organizations in 2011and revised in 2018). These competencies are divided into eight practice domains: assessment and analytical skills; policy development/program planning; communication; cultural competence; community dimensions of practice; public health sciences; financial planning, evaluation, and management; and leadership and system thinking (Quad Council Coalition Competency Review Taskforce, 2018).

To be a participant in surveillance and investigation activities, the staff nurse must have the following knowledge related to the core competencies (Quad Council Coalition Competency Review Taskforce, 2018):

1. Assessment and analytical skills
   - Defining a problem
   - Determining a cause
   - Identifying and understanding relevant data
   - Using data to address community health problems
   - Developing community health assessments
   - Incorporating evidence in decision making
   - Identifying risks
2. Policy development/program planning skills
   - Planning, implementing, and evaluating policies and programs aimed at improving community health and strategic plans
3. Communication
   - Assessing and addressing population literacy levels
   - Providing effective oral and written reports
   - Soliciting input from others and effectively presenting accurate demographic, statistical, and scientific information to other professionals and the community at large
4. Community dimensions of practice
   - Establishing and maintaining links during the investigation
   - Collaborating with partners
   - Developing, implementing, and evaluating an assessment to define the problem
5. Basic public health science skills
   - Identifying individual and organizational responsibilities
   - Identifying and retrieving current relevant evidence-based practice
6. Leadership and systems thinking
   - Identifying internal and external issues that have an effect on the investigation

- Promoting team and organizational efforts
- Contributing to developing, implementing, and monitoring of the investigation

While the staff nurse participates in these activities, the advanced practice public health nurse should be proficient in applying these competencies. In addition, the nurse applies the nursing process in preparedness as illustrated in Table 17.1.

The Minnesota model of *Public Health Interventions: Applications for Public Health Nursing Practice* (Minnesota Department of Health, 2018), suggests that surveillance is one of the interventions related to public health nursing practice. The model gives seven basic steps of surveillance for nurses to follow:

1. Consider whether surveillance as an intervention is appropriate for the situation.
2. Organize the knowledge of the problem, its natural course of history, and its aftermath.
3. Establish clear criteria for what constitutes a case.
4. Collect sufficient data from multiple valid sources.
5. Analyze data.
6. Interpret data and disseminate to decision makers.
7. Evaluate the impact of the surveillance system.

EVIDENCE-BASED PRACTICE

A systematic qualitative review was conducted by Klinger et al. (2017) to identify ethical issues in public health surveillance. The researchers noted that ethical issues sometimes arise in public health surveillance, particularly around informed consent and study design, yet there is a lack of clear ethics guidance and training for public health surveillance programs. In this systematic review, ethical issues were defined based on principlism, searching PubMed and Google Books for relevant publications. The search identified 525 references, of which 83 met the inclusion criteria and were reviewed. Most of the publications reviewed were journal articles (78%); the rest were books or book chapters (22%). The researchers identified 86 distinct ethical issues that come up over the surveillance life cycle. The researchers also identified 20 conditions in which forgoing informed consent procedures was more or less justifiable. From the systematic review, a comprehensive ethics matrix was developed which may be used to inform guidelines, reports, strategy papers, and educational material, and raise awareness among practitioners.

Nurse Use

In this example of using evidence to promote quality practice, the nurse can use this systematic review to change practice if necessary to adhere to the ethics matrix. Quality and ethical practices are essential components of surveillance.

Data Sources for Surveillance

Clinicians, health care agencies, and laboratories report cases to state health departments. Data also come from death certificates and administrative data such as discharge reports and billing records (McNabb et al., 2016; Veenema, 2018). The following are select sources of mortality and morbidity data:

1. Mortality data are often the only source of health-related data available for small geographic areas. Examples include the following:
   - Vital statistics reports (e.g., death certificates, medical examiner reports, birth certificates)
   - Mortality data can be obtained from the National Vital Statistics System. These data are one of the few sources of health-related data that are available for a long time period for small geographic areas (CDC, 2018g).
2. Morbidity data include the following:
   - Notifiable disease reports
   - Laboratory reports
   - Hospital discharge reports
   - Billing data
   - Outpatient health care data
   - Specialized disease registries
   - Injury surveillance systems
   - Environmental surveys
   - Sentinel surveillance systems

An example of a process in place to collect morbidity data is the National Program of Cancer Registries (NPCR) (CDC, 2018b). This program provides for monitoring of the types of cancers found in a state and the locations of the cancer risks and health problems in the state. Information about the health of a state or community can also be found at County Health Rankings and Roadmaps, a Robert Wood Johnson Foundation program (http://www.countyhealthrankings.org/).

Each of the data sources has the potential for underreporting or incomplete reporting. However, if there is consistency in the use of surveillance methods, the data collected will show trends in events or disease patterns that may indicate a change needed in a program or a needed prevention intervention to reduce morbidity or mortality. Underreporting or incomplete reporting may occur for the following reasons: social stigma attached to a disease (such as human immunodeficiency virus [HIV]/acquired immunodeficiency syndrome [AIDS]); ignorance of required reporting system; lack of knowledge about the case definition, procedural changes in reporting, or changes in a database; limited diagnostic abilities; or low priority given to reporting (CDC, 2010; McNabb et al., 2016; Ryan, 2016).

Mortality data assist in identifying differences in health status among groups, populations, occupations, and communities; monitoring preventable deaths; and examining cause-and-effect factors in diseases (CDC, 2018c). Vital statistics can be used to plan programs and to monitor programs to meet *Healthy People 2030* goals. The National Notifiable Diseases Surveillance System (NNDSS), as well as local public health laboratories, hospital discharge data, and billing data provide mechanisms for classifying diseases and events and calculating rates of diseases within and across groups, populations, and communities (CDC, 2018i).

The *Healthy People 2030* objectives related to global health surveillance and disease outbreaks are as follows:

HEALTHY PEOPLE 2030

- **GH-D01:** Increase the number of individuals trained globally to prevent, detect, or respond to public health threats
- **GH-D02:** Increase the number of globally important public health events that are tracked and reported
- **GH-D03:** Increase laboratory diagnostic testing capacity, surveillance, and reporting globally

US Department of Health and Human Services: *Healthy People 2030*, Washington, DC, 2020, US Government Printing Office.

The sentinel surveillance system provides for the monitoring of key health events when information is not otherwise available or for calculating or estimating disease morbidity in vulnerable populations (McNabb et al., 2016). Registries monitor chronic disease in a systematic manner, linking information from a variety of sources (health department, clinics, hospitals) to identify disease control and prevention strategies. Surveys then provide data from individuals about prevalence of health conditions and health risks. Such surveys allow for monitoring changes over time and assessing the individual's knowledge, attitudes, and beliefs (see QSEN box). This information can be used to assist health care professionals in providing education and planned interventions (Gostin and Riley, 2018).

QSEN FOCUS ON QUALITY AND SAFETY EDUCATION FOR NURSES

Targeted Competency: Safety—Minimizes risk of harm to clients and providers through both system effectiveness and individual performance.

- **Knowledge:** Discuss potential and actual impact of national client safety resources, initiatives, and regulations.
- **Skill:** Use national client safety resources for development and to focus attention on safety in the community and health care settings.
- **Attitude:** Value relationship between national safety campaigns and implementation in practices and practice settings.

Safety Question:

The Quad Council Coalition competency for communication skills indicates that the public health nurse uses a variety of methods to disseminate public health information to individuals, families, and groups within a *population* within a community, and provides a presentation of targeted health information to multiple audiences at a local level: groups, professionals, peers and agency peers (2018).

How would the nurse use the national sentinel surveillance system to identify health conditions and risks in a population or in the community? What types of data sources in this system would the nurse collect? After careful analysis of the data sources, what would the nurse include in a presentation to multiple audiences, at the local health department, the local government, or a community gathering?

NOTIFIABLE DISEASES

Before 1990, state and local health departments used many different criteria for identifying cases of reportable diseases.

Using different criteria made the data less useful than it could have been because it could not be compared across health departments or states. For this reason, some diseases may have been underreported and others may have been overreported. In 1990 the CDC and the Council of State and Territorial Epidemiologists assembled the first list of standard case definitions. This list was revised in 1997, and more information may be found at the CDC Division of Public Health Informatics and Surveillance website (CDC, 2018d). This site contains information about the National Notifiable Disease Surveillance System (NNDSS), and the standard case definitions which are updated on a case-by-case basis or otherwise remain the same. New case definitions are added as new diseases are identified.

National Notifiable Diseases

Box 17.3 shows the national notifiable infectious diseases. Reporting of disease data by health care providers, laboratories, and public health workers to state and local health departments is essential if trends are to be accurately monitored.

"The data provide the basis for detecting disease outbreaks, for identifying person characteristics, and for calculating incidence, geographic distribution, and temporal trends. They are used to initiate prevention programs, evaluate established prevention and control practices, suggest new intervention strategies, identify areas for research, document the need for disease control funds, and help answer questions from the community" (CDC, 2018d).

The CDC and the Council of State and Territorial Epidemiologists have a policy that requires state health departments to report selected diseases to the CDC National Notifiable Disease Surveillance System (NNDSS). The data for nationally notifiable diseases from 50 states, the US territories, New York City, and the District of Columbia are published weekly in the *Morbidity and Mortality Weekly Report* (MMWR). Data collection about these diseases and revision of statistics is ongoing. Annual updated final reports are published in CDC WONDER (CDC, 2018b).

State Notifiable Diseases

Requirements for reporting diseases are mandated by law or regulation. Although each state and Washington, DC, differ in the list of reportable diseases, the usefulness of the data depends on "uniformity, simplicity, and timeliness." Because state requirements differ, not all nationally notifiable diseases are legally mandated for reporting in a state. For legally reportable diseases, states compile disease incidence data (new cases) and transmit the data electronically (weekly) through the National Electronic Disease Surveillance System (CDC, 2018h).

Ongoing analysis of this extensive database has led to better diagnosis and treatment methods, national vaccine schedule recommendations, changes in vaccine formulation, and the recognition of new or resurgent diseases. Selected data are reported in the CDC MMWR report (https://www.cdc.gov). Adverse health data for the calendar year are documented on the reportable disease form, entitled EPID, to the local health department or the state department for public health. Local health department surveillance personnel investigate case reports and proceed with recommended public health measures, requesting assistance from the state's department assigned to monitor the reports when needed. Reports are forwarded by mail or fax or, in urgent circumstances, by telephone 24 hours a day, 7 days a week. When reports are received, they are scrutinized carefully and, when appropriate, additional steps are initiated to assist local health departments in planning interventions.

To determine which of the national notifiable diseases are reportable in your state, go to your state health department website.

Case Definitions
Criteria

Criteria for defining cases of different diseases are essential for having a uniform, standardized method of reporting and monitoring diseases. A case definition provides understanding of the data that are being collected and reduces the likelihood that different criteria will be used for reporting similar cases of a disease. Case definitions may include clinical symptoms, laboratory values, and epidemiologic criteria (e.g., exposure to a known or suspected case). Each disease has its own unique set of criteria based on what is known scientifically about that particular disease. Cases may be classified as *suspected*, *probable*, or *confirmed*, depending on the strength of the evidence supporting the case criteria.

Although some diseases require laboratory confirmation, even though clinical symptoms may be present, other diseases do not have laboratory tests to confirm the diagnosis. Other cases are diagnosed on the basis of epidemiologic data alone, such as exposure to contaminated food. If a case definition has been established by the CDC or another official source, it should be used for reporting purposes. The case definition should not be used as the only criterion for clinical diagnosis, quality assurance, standards for reimbursement, or taking public health action. Action to control a disease should be taken as soon as a problem is identified, although there may not be enough information to meet the case definition.

Case Definition Examples

The CDC (2018k) identified a clinical case definition for hepatitis A as a "discrete onset of symptoms consistent with hepatitis (e.g., fever, headache, malaise, anorexia, nausea, vomiting, diarrhea, and abdominal pain) AND either jaundice or elevated serum aminotransferase levels." The clinical symptoms of patients with all types of acute viral hepatitis are the same; therefore a person with acute hepatitis A must (1) have a positive immunoglobulin M (IgM) antibody for hepatitis A or (2) meet the clinical symptoms and "occur in a person who has an epidemiologic link with a person who has laboratory-confirmed hepatitis A (i.e., household or sexual contact with an infected person during the 15 to 50 days before the onset of symptoms)" (https://www.cdc.gov).

BOX 17.3   Infectious Diseases Designated as Notifiable at the National Level During 2018

- Anthrax
- Arboviral diseases, neuroinvasive and non-neuroinvasive
- California serogroup virus diseases
- Chikungunya virus disease
- Eastern equine encephalitis virus disease
- Powassan virus disease
- St. Louis encephalitis virus disease
- West Nile virus disease
- Western equine encephalitis virus disease
- Babesiosis
- Botulism
- Botulism, foodborne
- Botulism, infant
- Botulism, wound
- Botulism, other
- Brucellosis
- Campylobacteriosis
- Carbapenemase producing carbapenem-resistant Enterobacteriaceae (CP-CRE)
- CP-CRE, *Enterobacter* spp.
- CP-CRE, *Escherichia coli* (*E. coli*)
- CP-CRE, *Klebsiella* spp.
- Chancroid
- Chlamydia trachomatis infection
- Cholera
- Coccidioidomycosis
- Congenital syphilis
- Syphilitic stillbirth
- Cryptosporidiosis
- Cyclosporiasis
- Dengue virus infections
- Dengue
- Dengue-like illness
- Severe dengue
- Diphtheria
- Ehrlichiosis and anaplasmosis
- Anaplasma phagocytophilum infection
- *Ehrlichia chaffeensis* infection
- *Ehrlichia ewingii* infection
- Undetermined human ehrlichiosis/anaplasmosis
- Giardiasis
- Gonorrhea
- Haemophilus influenzae, invasive disease
- Hansen's disease
- Hantavirus infection, non-Hantavirus pulmonary syndrome
- Hantavirus pulmonary syndrome
- Hemolytic uremic syndrome, postdiarrheal
- Hepatitis A, acute
- Hepatitis B, acute
- Hepatitis B, chronic
- Hepatitis B, perinatal virus infection
- Hepatitis C, acute
- Hepatitis C, chronic
- Hepatitis C, perinatal infection
- HIV infection (AIDS has been reclassified as HIV stage III)
- Influenza-associated pediatric mortality
- Invasive pneumococcal disease
- Latent TB infection (TB infection)
- Legionellosis
- Leptospirosis
- Listeriosis
- Lyme disease
- Malaria
- Measles
- Meningococcal disease
- Mumps
- Novel influenza A virus infections
- Pertussis
- Plague
- Poliomyelitis, paralytic
- Poliovirus infection, nonparalytic
- Psittacosis
- Q fever
- Q fever, acute
- Q fever, chronic
- Rabies, animal
- Rabies, human
- Rubella
- Rubella, congenital syndrome
- Salmonellosis
- Severe acute respiratory syndrome-associated coronavirus disease
- Shiga toxin-producing *Escherichia coli*
- Shigellosis
- Smallpox
- Spotted fever rickettsiosis
- Streptococcal toxic shock syndrome
- Syphilis
- Syphilis, primary
- Syphilis, secondary
- Syphilis, early nonprimary/nonsecondary
- Syphilis, unknown duration or late
- Tetanus
- Toxic shock syndrome (other than streptococcal)
- Trichinellosis
- Tuberculosis
- Tularemia
- Typhoid fever
- Vancomycin-intermediate *Staphylococcus aureus* and vancomycin-resistant *Staphylococcus aureus*
- Varicella
- Varicella deaths
- Vibriosis
- Viral hemorrhagic fever
- Crimean-Congo hemorrhagic fever virus
- Ebola virus
- Lassa virus
- Lujo virus
- Marburg virus
- New World arenavirus—Guanarito virus
- New World arenavirus—Junin virus
- New World arenavirus—Machupo virus
- New World arenavirus—Sabia virus
- Yellow fever
- Zika virus disease and Zika virus infection
- Zika virus disease, congenital
- Zika virus disease, noncongenital
- Zika virus infection, congenital
- Zika virus infection, noncongenital

The World Health Organization (2020) issued a clinical case definition of COVID-19 as a person who meets the clinical criteria: Acute onset of fever AND cough; OR Acute onset of ANY THREE OR MORE of the following signs or symptoms: fever, cough, general weakness/fatigue, headache, myalgia, sore throat, coryza, dyspnea, anorexia/nausea/vomiting, diarrhea, altered mental status.

TYPES OF SURVEILLANCE SYSTEMS

Informatics is essential to the mission of protecting the public's health. Surveillance systems are designed to assist public health professionals in the early detection of disease and event outbreaks in order to intervene and reduce the potential for morbidity or mortality, or to improve the public's health status (Blazes and Lewis, 2016; CDC, 2018e,CDC, 2018j). Surveillance systems in use today are defined as *passive, active, sentinel,* and *special.*

Passive System

In the passive system, case reports are sent to local health departments by health care providers (e.g., physicians, public health nurses), or laboratory reports of disease occurrence are sent to the local health department. The case reports are summarized and forwarded to the state health department, national government, or organizations responsible for monitoring the problem, such as the CDC or an international organization such as the WHO.

The National Electronic Disease Surveillance System (NEDSS) is a voluntary system monitored by the CDC and includes a total of 682 infectious diseases or conditions with case definitions that are considered important to the public's health (CDC, 2018d). Each state determines for itself which of the diseases and conditions are of importance to the state's health and legally requires the reporting of those diseases to the state health department by health care providers, health care agencies, and laboratories. This system has the ability to provide disease-specific demographic, geographic, and seasonal trends over time for reported events. An example is a cancer registry system in which cases of cancer are required to be reported to the state on the basis of the type of cancer, the demographics of the client, and the geographic location. Because the system has limits, a disease outbreak may be occurring before all reports are received by the state health department (CDC, 2018d).

Active System

In the active system, the nurse, as an employee of the health department, may begin a search for cases through contacts with local health care providers and health care agencies. In this system, the nurse names the disease or an event and gathers data about existing cases to try to determine the magnitude of the problem (how widespread it is).

For example, the CDC defines a foodborne disease outbreak as occurring when two or more people get the same illness after ingesting the same contaminated food or drink. Numerous examples of multistate foodborne illness occur annually in the United States. In 2018, foodborne outbreaks were linked to ingestion of contaminated coconut, raw sprouts, lettuce, fast-food chain salads, and precut melon (CDC, 2018d). Bacteria most commonly associated with the outbreaks included various strains of *E. coli* and salmonella.

Sentinel System

In the sentinel system, trends in commonly occurring diseases or key health indicators are monitored. A disease or event may be the sentinel, or a population may be the sentinel. In this system a sample of health care providers or agencies, like state governors, are asked to report the problem. The system is useful because it helps to monitor trends in community occurring diseases and events.

Questions that may be asked include the following:

- What really happened?
- What are the consequences?
- What was different in this event?
- What was the outcome?
- Could the occurrence have been prevented?
- Did providers follow procedures?
- Did providers know what to do?
- Has this happened before?
- If so, how was it fixed or can it be fixed?
- Who reported the event?
- What might prevent it from happening again?

For example, certain providers and/or agencies in a community may be asked to report the number of cases of influenza seen during a given time period in order to make projections about the severity of the flu season.

Special Systems

Special systems are developed for collecting particular types of data and may be a combination of active, passive, and/or sentinel systems. As a result of bioterrorism, newer systems called syndromic surveillance systems are being developed to monitor illness syndromes or events. This approach requires the use of automated data systems to report continued (real-time) or daily (near-real time) disease outbreaks (CDC, 2020a) (Box 17.4).

BOX 17.4   Bioterrorism and Response Networks

Integrating of training and response preparedness can be supported by the following networks:

- Health Alert Network (http://emergency.cdc.gov)
- The Emerging Infections Program (http://www.cdc.gov)
- Epidemiology and Laboratory Capacity program (ELC) (http://cdc.gov)
- Hazardous Substances Data Bank (TOXNET.gov)
- Influenza surveillance in the United States
- Community emergency response systems (check local health department)

The National Syndromic Surveillance Program (NSSP) promotes timely exchange and monitoring of syndromic data, including client encounter data from emergency departments, urgent care, ambulatory care, and inpatient health care settings, as well as pharmacy and laboratory data. The real-time data are used as potential indicators of an event, disease, or outbreak concern (CDC, 2018j). For example, syndromic surveillance data were useful in tracking influenza trends in New York City through monitoring emergency department visits, detecting clusters of carbon monoxide poisoning due to power outages after a windstorm. This occurred in Louisiana from the use of generators after a hurricane (2020). Most recently this system has tracked the COVID-19 outbreak in the United States and worldwide. An example of a use of the NSSP system occurred in 2020, when persons on cruise ships or when visiting other countries were found to be infected with the COVID-19 virus (CDC, 2020a).

Although all of the systems are important, the public health nurse is most likely to use the active or passive systems. An example of when one might use a passive system is the use of the state reportable disease system to complete a community assessment or Mobilizing for Action through Planning and Partnerships (MAPP). The active system is used when several schoolchildren become ill after eating lunch in the cafeteria or following up on contacts of a newly diagnosed tuberculosis or sexually transmitted disease (STD) client at the local homeless shelter.

THE INVESTIGATION

Investigation Objectives

Any unusual increase in disease incidence (new cases) or an unusual event in the community should be investigated. The system used for investigation depends on the intensity of the event, the severity of the disease, the number of people or communities affected, the potential for harm to the community or the spread of disease, and the effectiveness of available interventions (CDC, 2020a). The objectives of an investigation are as follows:

- To control and prevent disease or death
- To identify factors that contribute to the outbreak of the disease and the occurrence of the event
- To implement measures to prevent occurrences

Defining the Magnitude of a Problem/Event

The following definitions provide a way to describe the level of occurrence of a disease or event for purposes of communicating the magnitude of the problem. A disease or an event that is found to be present (occurring) in a population is defined as endemic if there is a persistent (usual) presence with low to moderate number of cases of the disease or event. The endemic levels of a disease or an event in a population provide the baseline for establishing a public health problem. For example, foodborne botulism is endemic to Alaska. The baseline must be known to determine the existence of a change or increase in the number of cases from baseline. If a problem is considered hyperendemic, there is a persistently (usually) high number of

cases. An example is the high cholera incidence rate among Asian and Pacific Islanders. Sporadic problems are those with an irregular pattern, with occasional cases found at irregular intervals.

Epidemic means that the occurrence of a disease within an area is clearly in excess of expected levels (endemic) for a given time period. This is often called the outbreak. Pandemic (CDC2017b) refers to the epidemic spread of the problem over several countries or continents (e.g., COVID-19] outbreak). Holoendemic in a population implies a highly prevalent problem that is commonly acquired early in life. The prevalence of this problem decreases as age increases (Nmadu et al., 2015). Outbreak detection, or identifying an increase in the frequency of disease above the usual occurrence of the disease, is the function of the investigator (CDC, 2020a).

Patterns of Occurrence

Patterns of occurrence can be identified when investigating a disease or event. These patterns are used to define the boundaries of a problem to help investigate possible causes or sources of the problem. A common source outbreak refers to a group exposed to a common noxious influence such as the release of noxious gases (e.g., ricin in the Japanese subway system several years ago and in a water system in the United States [Merrill, 2017]). In a point source outbreak, all persons exposed become ill at the same time, during one incubation period. A mixed outbreak is "when a victim of a common source epidemic has person-to-person contact with others and spreads the disease, further propagating the health problem" (Merrill, 2017, p. 316), as in the spreading of influenza. Intermittent or continuous source cases may be exposed over a period of days or weeks, as in the recent food poisonings at a restaurant chain throughout the United States as a result of the restaurant's purchase of contaminated green onions. A propagated outbreak does not have a common source and spreads gradually from person to person over more than one incubation period, such as the spread of tuberculosis from one person to another.

Causal Factors from the Epidemiologic Triangle

Factors that must be considered as causes of an outbreak are categorized as agents, hosts, and environmental factors (see Chapter 10. The belief is that these factors may interact to cause the outbreak and therefore the potential interactions must be examined. Box 17.5 presents definitions used to classify agents in an attack. Box 17.6 lists the types of agent factors that may be present.

BOX 17.5 Classification of Agents

- **Infectivity**: Refers to the capacity of an agent to enter a susceptible host and produce infection or disease
- **Pathogenicity**: Measures the proportion of infected people who develop the disease
- **Virulence**: Refers to the proportion of people with clinical disease who become severely ill or die

---

BOX 17.6　Types of Agent Factors

- **Host factors:** age, sex, race, socioeconomic status, genetics, and lifestyle choices (e.g., cigarette smoking, sexual practices, contraception, eating habits)
- **Environmental factors:** weather, temperature, humidity, physical surroundings, and biological (e.g., insects that transmit the agent)
- **Socioeconomic factors:** behavior (e.g., terrorist behaviors), personality, cultural characteristics of group, crowding, sanitation, and availability of health services

---

CHECK YOUR PRACTICE

You have joined the community response team to investigate the COVID-19 disease outbreak in the university now that students have returned from summer break. How would you determine the existence of an unusual outbreak of COVID-19 at the university? See if you can apply these steps to this scenario. (1) Recognize the cues, looking at available data about rates of COVID-19 in the university and your community; (2) analyze the cues, looking at the numbers of students in this population and what it means to investigate the disease in this population.; (3) state several and prioritize the hypotheses you have stated; (4) generate solutions for each hypothesis; (5) take action on the number one hypothesis you think best reflects the impact of the outbreak of COVID-19 cases involved; and (6) evaluate the outcomes you would expect as a result of the work you will do to determine how unusual this outbreak is in the school and community.

When to Investigate

An unusual increase in disease incidence should be investigated. The amount of effort that goes into an investigation depends on the severity or magnitude of the problem, the numbers in the population who are affected, the potential for spreading the disease, and the availability and effectiveness of intervention measures to resolve the problems. Most of the outbreaks of diseases (or increased incidence rates) occur naturally and/or are predictable when compared with the consistent patterns of previous outbreaks of a disease, such as influenza, tuberculosis, or common infectious diseases. When a disease or an event outbreak occurs as a result of purposeful introduction of an agent into the population (like COVID-19), then predictable patterns may not exist. See How To box below.

HOW TO CONDUCT AN INVESTIGATION

- Confirm the existence of an outbreak.
- Verify the diagnosis and/or define a case.
- Estimate the number of cases.
- Orient the data collected to person, place, and time.
- Develop and evaluate a hypothesis.
- Institute control measures and communicate findings.

Centers for Disease Control and Prevention: *Steps to investigation,* 2020b. Retrieved September 2020 from http://www.cdc.gov.

While the community response team does not anticipate a bioterriorism attack, the team prepares the team members in the event that such an attack may occur. Such attacks may be caused by poisons like ricin recently sent via mail to the U.S. president: food or water contaminates, or viruses and bacteria like COVID-19 virus, or the anthrax bacteria (CDC, 2020a). Sobel and Watson (2009) provide clues to be used when trying to determine the existence of bioterrorism. These clues are simplified and appear in the How To box.

HOW TO RECOGNIZE THE EPIDEMIOLOGIC CLUES THAT MAY SIGNAL A COVERT BIOTERRORISM ATTACK

- Large number of ill persons with similar disease or syndrome
- Large number of unexplained disease, syndrome, or deaths
- Unusual illness in a population
- Higher morbidity and mortality than expected with a common disease or syndrome
- Failure of a common disease to respond to usual therapy
- Single case of disease caused by an uncommon agent
- Multiple unusual or unexplained disease entities coexisting in the same person without other explanation
- Disease with an unusual geographic or seasonal distribution
- Multiple atypical presentations of disease agents
- Similar genetic type among agents isolated from temporally or spatially distinct sources
- Unusual, atypical, genetically engineered, or antiquated strain of agent
- Endemic disease with unexplained increase in incidence
- Simultaneous clusters of similar illness in noncontiguous areas, domestic or foreign
- Atypical aerosol, food, or water transmission
- Ill people presenting at about the same time
- Death or illness among animals that precedes or accompanies illness or death in humans
- No illness in people not exposed to common ventilation systems but illness among those people in proximity to the systems

LEVELS OF PREVENTION

Surveillance Activities

Primary Prevention
Develop an approach for mass screening and vaccinations for citizens to reduce the occurrence of COVID-19 in the community.

Secondary Prevention
Investigate an outbreak of flulike illness in a local school to determine the cause of the symptoms.

Tertiary Prevention
Provide health care and treatment for those infected by COVID-19

PRACTICE APPLICATION

As a clinical project, the health department has asked the public health nursing class at the university to develop a community service message to air on local radio about how to protect individuals, families, and populations during a pandemic crisis. What does the message need to contain to help the community prepare and to understand the urgency for protecting self and others from continuing the spread of the biologic agent causing the crisis? What would the message say that other public service messages have not emphasized?

Answers can be found on the Evolve website.

▶▶ APPLYING CONTENT TO PRACTICE

Remember that disease and event surveillance systems exist to help improve the health of the public through the systematic and ongoing collection, distribution, and use of health-related data. A nurse can contribute to such systems and best use the data collected through such systems to help manage endemic health problems and those that are emerging, such as evolving infectious diseases and bioterrorist (human-made) health problems. Functions of surveillance and investigation include detecting cases, estimating the impact of disease or injury, showing the natural history of a health condition, determining the distribution and spread of illness, generating hypotheses, evaluating prevention and control measures, and facilitating planning (CDC, 2018g; McNabb et al., 2016). Response to bioterrorism or large-scale infectious disease outbreak may require the use of emergency public health measures such as quarantine, isolation, closing public places, seizing property, mandatory vaccination, travel restrictions, and disposal of the deceased. In 2020 in preparation for the COVID-19 outbreak, information was distributed about the use of several of these interventions, including isolation and closure of public places. Suggestions for protecting health care providers from exposure included use of standard precautions when coming into contact with broken skin or body fluids, the use of disposable nonsterile gowns and gloves followed by adequate hand washing after removal, and the use of a mask or face shield (CDC, 2020c).

The chapter applies this by looking at trends of occurrences and events before investigating the situation and deciding on an intervention. It is also important to be able to use the databases and the tools of investigation to ensure safe processes of care. The attitude of engaging in continuous learning and the development of new technology skills is essential. In the case of a pandemic and to assist community residents in being safe during such an outbreak, Appendix A provides steps for assisting individuals and families in preparation for such an occurrence.

▌ REMEMBER THIS!

- Disease surveillance has been a part of public health protection since the 1200s during the investigations of the bubonic plague in Europe.
- Surveillance provides a means for nurses to monitor disease trends to reduce morbidity and mortality and to improve health.
- Surveillance is a critical role function for nurses practicing in the community.
- Surveillance is important because it generates knowledge of a disease or event outbreak patterns.
- Surveillance focuses on the collection of process and outcome data.
- Although surveillance was initially devoted to monitoring and reducing the spread of infectious diseases, it is now used to monitor and reduce chronic diseases and injuries, as well as environmental and occupational exposures.
- Surveillance activities can be related to the core functions of public health assessment, policy development, and assurance.
- A quality surveillance system requires collaboration among agencies and individuals.
- The Minnesota model of *Public Health Interventions: Applications for Public Health Nursing Practice* (Minnesota Department of Health, 2018) suggests that surveillance is one of the interventions related to public health nursing practice.
- Clinicians, health care agencies, and laboratories report cases to state health departments.

- Data also come from death certificates and administrative data such as discharge reports and billing records.
- Each of the data sources has the potential for underreporting or incomplete reporting. However, if there is consistency in the use of surveillance methods, the data collected will show trends in events or disease patterns that may indicate a change needed in a program or a needed prevention intervention to reduce morbidity or mortality.
- The sentinel surveillance system provides for the monitoring of key health events when information is not otherwise available or for calculating or estimating disease morbidity in vulnerable populations.
- Reporting of disease data by health care providers, laboratories, and public health workers to state and local health departments is essential if trends are to be accurately monitored.
- Requirements for reporting diseases are mandated by law or regulation.
- Surveillance systems in use today are defined as passive, active, sentinel, and special.
- Any unusual increase in disease incidence (i.e., new cases) or an unusual event in the community should be investigated.
- Patterns of occurrence can be identified when investigating a disease or event. These patterns are used to define the boundaries of a problem to help investigate possible causes or sources of the problem.
- Factors that must be considered as causes of outbreak are categorized as agents, hosts, and environmental factors.
- An unusual increase in disease incidence should be investigated.
- Functions of surveillance and investigation include detecting cases, estimating the impact of disease or injury, showing the natural history of a health condition, determining the distribution and spread of illness, generating hypotheses, evaluating prevention and control measures, and facilitating planning.

EVOLVE WEBSITE

http://evolve.elsevier.com/Stanhope/foundations
- NCLEX Review Questions
- Practice Application Answers

REFERENCES

Association of Public Health Nurses (APHN): *The role of the public health nurse in disaster preparedness, response, and recovery: a position paper*, APHN Public Health Preparedness Committee, 2014. Retrieved from http://www.achne.org.

Blazes DL, Lewis SH: Disease surveillance—technology contributions to global health security, Boca Raton, 2016, CRC Press.

Brownson RC, Baker EA, Deshpande AD, Gillespie KN: *Evidence-based public health*, ed 3, New York, 2018, Oxford University Press.

Centers for Disease Control and Prevention (CDC): *Public health preparedness and response core competency model, 2010*. Retrieved from https://www.cdc.gov.

Centers for Disease Control and Prevention (CDC): *National Notifiable Disease Surveillance System (NNDSS)*, 2015. Retrieved from https://www.cdc.gov.

Centers for Disease Control and Prevention (CDC): *Chemical emergencies,* 2016a. Retrieved from https://emergency.cdc.gov.

Centers for Disease Control and Prevention (CDC): *Nationally notifiable infectious diseases: United States,* 2016b, CDC. Retrieved from https://www.cdc.gov.

Centers for Disease Control and Prevention: *Get your household ready for pandemic,* 2017b. Available at https://cdc.gov. Accessed July 2018.

Centers for Disease Control and Prevention (CDC): *Preparation & planning. Emergency Preparedness and Response,* 2020c. Retrieved from https://emergency.cdc.gov.

Centers for Disease Control and Prevention (CDC): *National Biomonitoring Program: Chemical threat agents,* 2017a. Retrieved from https://www.cdc.gov.

Centers for Disease Control and Prevention (CDC): *CDC WONDER,* 2018b. Retrieved from https://wonder.cdc.gov/.

Centers for Disease Control and Prevention (CDC): Division of Health Informatics and Surveillance, 2018c. Retrieved from https://www.cdc.gov.

Centers for Disease Control and Prevention (CDC): *Foodborne outbreaks: List of selected multistate foodborne outbreak investigation,* 2018d. Retrieved from https://www.cdc.gov.

Centers for Disease Control and Prevention (CDC): *Improving public health surveillance data,* 2018e. Retrieved from https://www.cdc.gov.

Centers for Disease Control and Prevention (CDC): National Center for Health Statistics. *National Vital Statistics Reports,* 2018f. Retrieved from https://www.cdc.gov.

Centers for Disease Control and Prevention (CDC): *National Notifiable Diseases Surveillance System (NNDSS),* 2018g. Retrieved from https://wwwn.cdc.gov.

Centers for Disease Control and Prevention (CDC): *National Notifiable Diseases Surveillance System (NNDSS): Data collection and reporting,* 2018h. Retrieved from https://wwwn.cdc.gov.

Centers for Disease Control and Prevention (CDC): *National Notifiable Disease Surveillance System (NNDSS): Why we do notifiable disease surveillance,* 2018i. Retrieved from https://wwwn.cdc.gov.

Centers for Disease Control and Prevention (CDC): *National Syndromic Surveillance Program (NSSP): NSSP Overview,* 2018j. Retrieved from https://www.cdc.gov.

Centers for Disease Control and Prevention (CDC): *The National Institute for Occupational Safety and Health (NIOSH),* 2018k. Retrieved from https://www.cdc.gov.

Center for Disease Control and Prevention(CDC): CDC's *Role in Outbreak Investigation,* 2020a. Retrieved from from https://www.cdc.gov.

Centers for Disease Control and Prevention: *Steps to investigation,* 2020b. Retrieved Sept 2020 from http://www.cdc.gov.

Council on Linkages between Academia and Public Health Practice: *Core competencies for public health professionals,* Washington, DC, 2014, The Council. Retrieved from http://www.phf.org.

Gostin LO, Wiley LF: *Public health law and ethics: a reader,* ed 3, Oakland, 2018, University of California Press.

Latshaw MW, Degeberg R, Patel SS, et al: Advancing environmental health surveillance in the US through a national human biomonitoring network, *Int J Hyg Environ Health,* 220(2, PT A):98–102, 2017.

McNabb S, Conde JM, Ferland L, et al: *Transforming public health surveillance—proactive measures for prevention, detection, and response,* Jordan, 2016, Elsevier.

Merrill RM: *Introduction to epidemiology,* ed 7, Burlington, Mass, 2017, Jones & Bartlett.

Minnesota Department of Health: Division of Community Health Services, Public Health Nursing Section: *Public Health Interventions—Applications for Public Health Nursing Practice,* 2018. Retrieved from http://www.health.state.mn.us.

Nmadu PM, Peter E, Alexander P, et al: The prevalence of malaria in children between the ages 2–15 visiting Gwarinpa General Hospital Life-Camp, Abuja, Nigeria, *J Health Sci* 5:47–51, 2015.

Perlman SE, McVeigh KH, Thorpe LE, Jacobson L, Greene CM, Gwynn RC: Innovations in population health surveillance: using electronic health records for chronic disease surveillance, *Am J Public Health* 107(6):853–857, 2017.

Quad Council Coalition Competency Review Task Force: *Community/Public Health Competencies,* 2018. Retrieved from http://www.quadcouncilphn.org.

Ryan J: *Biosecurity and bioterrorism,* ed 2, Cambridge, 2016, Elsevier.

SanDiego County: Health and Human Services: *San Diego Hepatitis A Outbreak,* 2018. Retrieved from https://www.sandiegocounty.gov.

Sobel J, Watson JC: Intentional Terrorist contamination of food and water. In: Lutwick SM, Lutwick LI, eds.: *Beyond anthrax: The weaponization of infectious diseases,* ed 2, New York, 2009, Springer.

Sorour K, Nuzzo E, Tuttle M, et al: Addition of bacitracin and cranberry to standard Foley care reduces catheter-associated urinary tract infections, *Can J Infect Control* 3:166–168, 2016.

USA Facts. *COVID-19 Impact and Recovery,* 2020. USAFACTS.gov

US Department of Health and Human Services: *Healthy People 2030,* Washington, DC, 2020, US Government Printing Office.

Veenema TG: *Disaster nursing and emergency preparedness for chemical, biological, and radiological terrorism and other hazards,* ed 3, New York, 2018, Springer.

World Health Organization (WHO): *Integrated disease surveillance and response,* 2018. Retrieved from http://www.who.int.

18

Program Management

Catherine Carroca, Lisa M. Turner, and Marcia Stanhope

OBJECTIVES

After reading this chapter, the student should be able to do the following:

1. Compare and contrast the program management process and the nursing process.
2. Describe the application of the program planning process to nursing in the community.
3. Identify the benefits of program planning and evaluation.
4. Describe the types of program evaluation measures.
5. Apply the components of a program evaluation method in practice.

CHAPTER OUTLINE

KEY TERMS

Program management consists of assessing, planning, implementing, and evaluating a program. This chapter focuses primarily on planning and evaluation. Although presented in separate discussions, these factors are related and interdependent processes that work together to bring about a successful program. This chapter does not address implementing programs because other chapters in this text focus on implementation.

The program management process is like the nursing process. One process is applied to a program that addresses the needs of a specific population, whereas the other process is applied to the clients in public health. The process of program management, like the nursing process, consists of a rational decision-making system designed to help nurses:

- in making a decision to develop a program (assessment),
- where they want to be at the end of the program (goal setting),
- how to decide what to do to have a successful program (planning),
- how to develop a plan to go forward from where they start to where they want to be (implementing),
- how to know that they are getting there (formative evaluation),
- and what to measure to know that the program has successful outcomes (summative evaluation).

Today there is a greater need for the nurse to be accountable for nursing actions and client outcomes. Prospective and retrospective payment systems, pay for performance, health care reform, and integrated care delivery models have changed the focus of nursing. Planning for nursing services is necessary today if the nurse is to survive in the health care delivery field. Nurses are expected to demonstrate leadership in addressing community-based health problems.

This chapter examines how nurses can *act* instead of *react* by planning programs that can be evaluated for their effectiveness. These programs may be single health-promotion programs for a client group, an ongoing program to provide health care services to a client group, or a program designed to address a population problem at the community level.

DEFINITIONS AND GOALS

Community health planning is population focused, and it positions the well-being of the public to promote health equity, community empowerment, and social justice above private interests (American Planning Association, 2018; American Public Health Association, 2020). A program is an organized approach to meet the assessed needs of individuals, families, groups, populations, or communities by reducing the effect of or eliminating one or more health problems. Community health programs are planned to meet the needs of designated populations or subpopulations in a community. Many programs exist as specific efforts within the umbrella of large, complex organizations such as state health departments, universities, health systems, and private organizations such as insurance companies. Unlike these complex organizations, smaller programs are endeavors that focus on more specific services and communities or groups. Specific examples in population-focused nursing are

- home health,
- immunization and infectious disease programs,
- health-risk screening for industrial workers, and
- family planning programs.

These are usually conducted under the direction of the total plan of a local health department, a managed care agency, or, in some instances, an insurance company.

Examples of more complex broadly based group and community programs are

- school health,
- occupational health and safety,
- environmental health,
- community programs directed at preventing specific illnesses through special-interest groups (e.g., American Heart Association, American Cancer Society, March of Dimes), and
- disaster preparedness programs through collaborative efforts of several community organizations or agencies.

Programs are ongoing organized activities that become part of the continuing health services of a community or organization, whereas projects are smaller, organized activities with a limited time frame. A health fair and a blood pressure screening day at the mall are examples of projects that nurses may implement.

Planning is defined as the selecting and carrying out of a series of activities designed to achieve desired improvements (Issel and Wells, 2018). The *goal* of planning is to ensure that health care services are acceptable, equal, efficient, and effective. Planning provides a blueprint for coordination of resources to achieve these goals.

Evaluation is determining whether a service is needed and can be used, whether it is conducted as planned, and whether the service actually helps communities and populations in need. (Royse, 2016). Evaluation is a process of accountability

---

BOX 18.1   Two Levels of Program Evaluation

- **Formative evaluation:** Evaluation for the purpose of assessing whether objectives are met or planned activities are completed. This type of evaluation begins with an assessment of the need for a program and is ongoing as the program is implemented.
- **Summative evaluation:** Evaluation to assess program outcomes or as a follow-up of the results of the program activities and usually occurs when a program is completed or at a specific point in time (e.g., at the end of 1 year or 5 years).

---

and done for the purpose of assessing whether objectives are met or planned activities are completed *and* to assess program outcomes or as a follow-up of the results of the program activities (Box 18.1).

QSEN   FOCUS ON QUALITY AND SAFETY EDUCATION FOR NURSES

Targeted Competency-Program Planning and Policy Development— Uses data to monitor outcomes of the program planning model and use the outcomes to design and test changes to policies to improve quality and safety of health care systems.

- **Knowledge:** Describe approaches for implementing program planning
- **Skill:** Identify gaps between local programming and best practice
- **Attitude:** Value measurement and its role in delivering programs and developing policy to improve client care

QI Question

The Quad Council Coalition of Public Health Nursing Organizations (2018) has identified a beginning public health nurse (PHN) competency as policy development and program planning skills. The beginning PHN participates in developing organizational plans to implement programs and policies and participates as a team member. How could the new PHN best contribute to program management? What type of activity might the PHN participate in to determine gaps in policies to improve existing programs?

？ CHECK YOUR PRACTICE

As a student assigned to the local mayor's office, you have been asked to participate in completing a plan to develop programs to address the needs of the community identified through an assessment of the characteristics of the population of the community. What would you do? How would you approach this assignment? (1) Recognize the cues, looking at available data which identifies the needs in your community; (2) analyze the cues offered about the characteristics of the population; (3) state several and prioritize the hypotheses you have stated; (4) generate solutions for each hypothesis; (5) take action on the number one hypothesis you think best reflects the type of programs needed to address the population needs; and (6) evaluate the outcomes you would expect as a result of the contributions you have made to the plan.

BENEFITS OF PROGRAM PLANNING

Systematic planning for meeting client needs does the following:
- Benefits clients, nurses, employing agencies, and the community
- Focuses attention on what the organization and health provider are attempting to do for clients

- Assists in identifying the resources and activities that are needed to meet the objectives of client services
- Reduces role ambiguity (uncertainty) by giving responsibility to specific providers to meet program objectives
- Reduces uncertainty within the program environment
- Increases the abilities of the provider and the agency to cope with the external environment
- Helps the provider and the agency anticipate events
- Allows for quality decision making and better control over the actual program results

Today this type of planning is referred to as strategic planning, and it involves the successful matching of client needs with specific provider strengths and competencies and agency resources. Everyone involved with the program can anticipate the following:

- What will be needed to implement the program
- What will occur during implementation
- What the program outcomes will be

PLANNING PROCESS

Program planning is affected by governments, and by the culture and belief system of the population in which the program must function. Program planning is required by federal, state, and local governments; by philanthropic organizations; and by the employing agency. Planning programs and planning for the evaluation of programs are two very important activities, whether the program being planned is a national health insurance program such as Medicare, a state health care program such as an early childhood development screening program, a local program such as vision screening for elementary school children, or a health education program. Regardless of the type of program, the planning process is the same.

Nutt (1984) described a basic planning process that is reflected in the steps of most planning methods and remains a great influence on strategic planning for population health and health programs today (Issel and Wells, 2018). The process includes five planning stages: formulating, conceptualizing, detailing, evaluating, and implementing. (See the How To box below.)

HOW TO DEVELOP A PROGRAM PLAN

A. Describe the problem.
B. Formulate the plan.
   1. Assess population need.
      - Who is the program population?
      - What is the need to be met?
      - How large is the client population to be served?
      - Where are they located?
      - Are there other programs addressing the same need? (Describe)
      - Why is the need not being met?
   2. Establish program boundaries.
      - Who will be included in the program?
      - Who will not be included? Why?
      - What is the program goal?
   3. Assess program feasibility.
      - Who agrees that the program is needed (i.e., stakeholders: administrators, providers, clients, funders)?
      - Who does not agree?
   4. Assess resources (general).
      - What personnel are needed? What personnel are available?
      - What facilities are needed? What facilities are available?
      - What equipment is needed? What equipment is available?
      - Is funding available to support the project? Is additional funding needed?
      - Are resources being donated (e.g., space, printing, paper, medical supplies)?
         (1) Type
         (2) Amount
   5. Determine tools used to assess need.
      - Census data
      - Key informants
      - Community forums
      - Existing program surveys
      - Surveys of the client population
      - Statistical indicators (e.g., demographic and morbidity/mortality data)
C. Conceptualize the problem.
   1. List the potential solutions to the problem.
   2. What are the risks of each solution?
   3. What are the consequences?
   4. What are the outcomes to be gained from the solutions?
   5. Draw a decision tree to show the problem-solving process used.
D. Detail the plan.
   1. What are the objectives for each solution to meet the program goal?
   2. What activities will be done to conduct each of the alternative solutions listed under C1 and based on objectives?
   3. What are the differences in the resources needed for each of the alternative solutions?
   4. Which of the alternative solutions would be chosen if the resources described under B4 were the only resources available?
   5. Who would be responsible or accountable for implementing the plan?
E. Evaluate the plan.
   1. Which of the alternative solutions is most acceptable to:
      - The client population
      - The agency administrator
      - You
      - The community
   2. Which of the alternative solutions appears to have the most benefits to the following:
      - The client population
      - The agency administrator
      - You
      - The community
   3. Based on costs, which alternative solution would be chosen by:
      - The client population
      - The agency administrator
      - You
      - The community
F. Implement the program plan.
   1. On the basis of data collected, which of the solutions has been chosen?
   2. Why should the agency administrator approve your request? Give your rationale.
   3. Will additional funding be sought?
   4. When can the program begin? Give date.

Basic Program Planning

Definition of Problem and Need

The initial and most critical step in health program planning is defining the problem and assessing client need. The target population, or client, to be served by any program must be identified and involved in designing the program to be developed. Program planners must verify that a current health problem exists and is being ignored or is being unsuccessfully treated in a client group within a population. *Needs assessment* is defined as a systematic appraisal of type, depth, and scope of problems as perceived by clients, health providers, or both (Box 18.2).

Needs assessment includes the steps in section B. 1. of the How To box on the previous page. The client may be identified as a community or group, as families, or as individuals. The client should be defined by biological and psychosocial characteristics, by geographic location, and by the problems to be addressed. For example, in a community with a large number of preschool children who require immunizations to enter school, the client population may be described as all children between 4 and 6 years of age residing in Central County who have not had up-to-date immunizations. This example identifies the client, specifies the need, and states the population size and where they are located.

A health education program may be necessary to alert the population to the existing need. In an example of the need for immunizing preschool children, public service announcements on television and radio and in newspapers may be used to alert parents to laws requiring immunizations, to the continuing problems with communicable diseases, and to the outcomes of successful immunizing programs, such as vaccination programs that have been successful in eliminating smallpox worldwide. A good example of the use of media occurred during an outbreak of rubella in Los Angeles. Local and national television was used to bring attention to the problem, to encourage parents to have children immunized, and to encourage other communities to launch campaigns to prevent additional outbreaks. More recent campaigns related to the pandemic of COVID-19 in the United States (USA Facts, 2020).

During the process of formulating a plan to address the problem identified, the nurse attempts to determine type, size and distribution of the population. These data assist in developing the program goal. More is involved than counting the number of persons in the community who may be eligible for the program. It involves determining the number of persons with the problem who are not being served by existing programs and the numbers of eligible persons who have and have not taken advantage of existing services. For example, consider again the community need for a preschool immunization program. In planning the program, the size of the population of preschool children in the county may be obtained from census data or state vital statistics. The nurse then must determine the number of children unserved and the number of children who have not used services for which they are eligible. Today there are many opportunities to locate the unserved children through early start programs for preschool children.

The populations' perspective of the need for a program might be interpreted differently by health care providers, agency administrators, policy makers, and potential clients. These groups are considered the stakeholders in the program. Collecting data on the opinions and attitudes of all persons, whether directly or indirectly involved with the program, is necessary to determine if the program is feasible, if there is a need to redefine the problems, or if a new program should be developed or an existing program should be expanded or modified. If a new or changed program is to be successful, it must not only be *available*, but also be *accessible* and *acceptable* to the people who will use it. For example, policy makers in the 1970s decided that neighborhood health clinics were the answer to providing services for low-income residents. They discovered that their perspective was not the same as those of most health providers and clients, who did not support development of neighborhood clinics.

The neighborhood health clinics have evolved over time to better reflect clients' perspectives. It is important for policy makers to explore the perspectives of the clients when planning the program. Clients might choose another type of service to offer rather than the one the policy maker or provider thinks best for them. Today community health centers have replaced the concept of the neighborhood health centers, and these centers are being supported and increased in number by health care reform (Rosenbaum et al., 2018).

Before implementing a health program, the nurse must also identify available resources. *Program resources* include financing, personnel, facilities, and equipment and supplies. The source and amount of funds must be adequate to support the program. The number and kinds of personnel required and available must be determined. There must be a place for the program to operate, and up-to-date equipment and supplies are essential. If any one of the four categories of resources is unavailable, the program is likely to be inadequate to meet the needs of the client population. If planners consider the problem to be a critical one, funding may be sought by seeking donations or by writing a proposal for grant funds to support the program. A well-done assessment provides direction and suggests strategies for appropriate interventions. The How To box on the previous page (B5) identifies needs assessment tools the nurse can use. The evidence-based practice box below provides an example of the application of a needs assessment tool.

BOX 18.2　Stages Used in Assessing a Client Need

- **Preactive:** Projecting a future need
- **Reactive:** Defining the problem based on past needs identified by the client or the agency
- **Inactive:** Defining the problem based on the existing health status of the population to be served
- **Interactive:** Describing the problem using past and present data to project future population needs

EVIDENCE-BASED PRACTICE

Thorland et al. (2017) evaluated the impact of the Nurse-Family Partnership (NFP) program on status of breastfeeding and child immunization outcomes of the program participants. The needs assessment tool used to identify the program was a survey of existing data. This home-visiting program was developed to serve first-time, low-income mothers, identified as the population to be served, who are regularly visited by a specially trained registered nurse from the program. The nurse helps the mother receive the care and support needed for a healthy pregnancy, teaches responsible, competent child care (up to 2 years old), and supports the mother in becoming economically self-sufficient. The program participant data were compared to National Survey of Children's Health data and National Immunization data. The researchers found that NFP clients were significantly more likely to have ever breastfed and maintain breastfeeding at 6 and 12 months, but less likely exclusively breastfeed at 6 months, compared to the national data. NFP clients were also significantly more likely to be up to date on immunizations at 6, 18, and 24 months (no significant difference at 12 months). The researchers concluded that NFP clients had more beneficial breastfeeding and immunization outcomes than children of mothers with similar demographic profiles; however, further improvement with exclusive breastfeeding at 6 months could be sought after.

Nurse Use

Nurse home-visiting programs for new, low-income mothers can positively impact breastfeeding and immunization outcomes of client populations. Evaluating a program's impact on health outcomes provides evidence for continuing or discontinuing/changing the program in question. Nurses can teach leaders in the community how to identify and evaluate evidence-based prevention programs. By educating key stakeholders, community mobilization on priority health needs is strengthened.

From Thorland W, Currie D, Wiegand ER, et al.: Status of breastfeeding and child immunization outcomes in clients of the Nurse-Family Partnership, *Matern Child Health J* 21:439–445, 2017.

The need and demand for a program are determined. The conceptualizing stage of planning creates options for solving the problem and considers several solutions. Each option for program solution is examined for its uncertainties (risks) and consequences, leading to a set of outcomes. The outcomes sought are improvements in the health status of the population served by the program.

A first step in the conceptualizing process is a review of the literature to determine what approaches have been used in other places with similar problems, and with what success. Such review can assist nurses to improve the quality, effective, and appropriate outcomes of health programs by combining the evidence and translating it into practice (evidence-based practice). Review of the literature should be guided by the following question: What can be learned from the experience of others in similar circumstances?

Some alternative solutions to the problem will have more risks or uncertainties than others. The nurse must decide between a solution that involves more risk and a solution that is free of risk. A "do nothing" decision is always the decision with the least risk to the provider. When choosing a solution, the nurse looks at whether the desired outcome can be achieved. After careful thought about each possible solution to the problem, the nurse rethinks the solutions. The assessment data compiled during the formulation stage should be used to develop alternative solutions.

Decision trees are useful graphic aids that give a picture of the solutions and the risks of each solution. Such a picture graph of the process of identifying a solution helps clients and administrators rank the consequences of a decision (Issel and Wells, 2018). Fig. 18.1 shows an example of a decision tree.

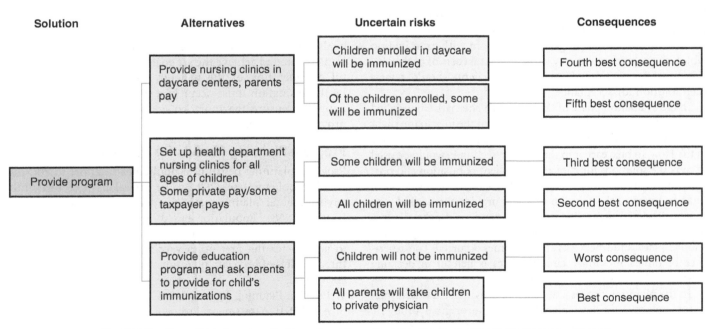

Fig. 18.1 Ranking of Solutions to a Problem: Providing a Preschool Immunization Program to Low-Income Children Using a Decision Tree to Rank Solutions to the Problem.

As shown in Fig. 18.1, the best consequence would be for each low-income child to be given flu immunization by their private physician. One must consider the value of this action to the person, the odds that immunizations will be obtained, the cost to families as opposed to the taxpayer, and the cost to the community. Costs to the community include the possibility of increased incidence of communicable disease or mortality and increased need for more expensive services to treat the diseases if vulnerable people are not immunized. Conversely, if families self-pay for the immunizations, costs to the taxpayer and to the community are low.

In the next phase, the provider, with client input, considers the possibilities of solving a problem using one of the solutions identified. The provider details (or is specific about) the costs, resources, and program activities needed to choose one of the solutions from the conceptualizing phase. For each of the three proposed alternatives shown in the immunization scenario in Fig. 18.1, the program planner lists the activities that would need to be implemented. Using the proposed solution of encouraging families to see their private physicians for the vaccine (the best consequence), examples of activities include developing a script for a health education program and implementing a television program to encourage parents to see a physician. If an alternative that produced the second, third, fourth, or fifth best consequence was chosen, offering a clinic at the health department or providing a mobile clinic to each daycare center to provide the immunizations would be possible activities.

For each alternative, the nurse lists the resources needed to implement each activity. The resources to be considered include all costs of personnel, supplies, equipment, and facilities, and the potential acceptance by the clients and the administrators of the program. In the example, personnel could include nurses, volunteers, and clerks; supplies might include handouts, Band-Aids, vaccines, records, and consent forms; equipment might include syringes, needles, stethoscopes, and blood pressure cuffs; and facilities might include a television studio for a media blitz on the education program and a room with examination tables, chairs, and emergency carts. The total costs of each solution must be considered. As indicated, clients should review each solution for acceptance.

In the evaluation phase of the plan, each alternative is weighed to judge the costs, benefits, and acceptance of the idea to the client population, community, and providers. The information outlined in the How To box, earlier in the chapter, section E, would be used to rank the solutions for choice by the client population and provider on the basis of cost, benefit, and acceptance. Consideration must be given to the solution that will provide the desired outcomes. Review of the literature or interviews might disclose whether someone else had previously tried each of the options in another place, and what costs and outcomes occurred. The experience of others in similar circumstances is helpful in deciding whether a chosen solution would be useful.

In the planning process, the clients, providers, and administrators selected the best plan to solve the original problem. Providing reasons why a particular solution was chosen will help the provider get the approval of the agency administration for the plan. Once approved, the plan is implemented.

Implementation requires obtaining and managing the resources required to operationalize the program in a way that is consistent with the plan. Program implementation requires accountability and responsibility (Issel and Wells, 2018). Change theory can be useful to help create an environment in which the program is supported.

Community members may participate in implementing the program either as volunteers or as paid staff. Program success will be increased if community residents are included in the work of the program and if they are on advisory boards and participate in program evaluation. The greater the participation of community members in developing a program, the greater the sense of ownership of that program by members of the target population, and therefore the greater the probability that the program will achieve its objectives and result in positive changes in health (Issel and Wells, 2018).

The Program Planning Process and the Nursing Process

Program planning may be compared with the nursing process (Table 18.1). The nursing process is a standardized and systematic process utilized by nurses to ensure quality client care. The first and second steps of the nursing process involve accurate assessment and nursing diagnosis of the client. The client is then involved in the next step of planning and outcome identification with the nurse to ensure that realistic and appropriate goals are formulated. Nurses must then choose suitable interventions and implement them to achieve the goals that were set. The last step involves evaluation of the plan and goal achievement.

Program management utilizes similar steps as the nursing process. Creating a successful program relies on careful assessment of the population or community to identify needs. All stakeholders should then be involved in the formulation of goals and outcomes. Appropriate interventions should be implemented to achieve the set goals and outcomes after careful consideration of the benefits, risks, and consequences. Lastly, evaluation must occur in a formative and summative nature to ensure the intended goals and objectives for the program were met.

Program Planning Models for Public Health

Program planning began as a public health effort to address health problems (Issel, 2021). The first plans were related to environmental planning for city water and sewer services (Rosen, 1958). Population-based program planning began with the need for mass immunizations, such as the program to administer the first polio vaccine. The following are the three models of program planning used in public health today (Box 18.3):

1. **PATCH:** Planning Approach to Community Health
2. **APEXPH:** Assessment Protocol for Excellence in Public Health
3. **MAPP:** Mobilizing for Action through Planning and Partnership

TABLE 18.1 Comparison of the Nursing Process and Program Planning

Nursing Process	Basic Planning Process
Assessment Subjective and objective data are systematically collected.	**Formulation** Assess the client's need and define the problem.
Nursing Diagnosis Client's problem is defined by using the assessment data to guide the nurse in looking for similar patterns in the systematically collected subjective and objective data.	**Conceptualization** Provider group identifies solutions; each solution is examined for its risks, consequences, and expected outcomes.
Nursing Intervention Any direct care treatment or nursing action based on the nursing diagnosis is performed by a nurse and includes rationale that justifies the treatment or nursing action. Treatment or action is evaluated by the nurse for its appropriateness and acceptability to the client before implementation.	
Implementation Direct care treatment or nursing action established in the intervention is implemented.	**Detailing** Client and provider analyze solutions proposed in the conceptualizing phase for costs, resources, and program activities.
Evaluation Implementation of the nursing intervention is evaluated.	**Evaluation of the Plan** Client, providers, and administrators select best plan based on costs, benefits, and acceptability of the plan to the client and provider.
	Implementation Best plan (solution) based on input from the client and provider is presented to administration and implemented.
	Program Evaluation Implemented best plan (solution) is evaluated.

BOX 18.3 Elements of Three Public Health Program Planning Models

PATCH (Planning Approach to Community Health)	APEXPH (Assessment Protocol for Excellence in Public Health)	MAPP (Mobilizing for Action Through Planning and Partnership)

1. Mobilize the community to act
2. Collect data
3. Choose health priorities
4. Develop a comprehensive intervention plan
5. Implement plan
	1. Assess internal organizational capacity
	2. Assess priorities for health problems
	3. Set priorities for health problems
	4. Implement the plan
		1. Mobilize community members and organizations
		2. Generate shared visions and common values
		3. Develop a framework for long-range planning
		4. Conduct needs assessments in four areas:
		  Community strengths
		  Local public health system
		  Community health status
		  Forces of change
		5. Evaluate the process

PATCH, Planning Approach to Community Health; *APEXPH*, Assessment Protocol for Excellence in Public Health; *MAPP*, Mobilizing for Action through Planning and Partnership.
From Issel LM: *Health program planning and evaluation: a practical, systematic approach for community health*, Burlington, 2021, Jones & Bartlett Learning.
Websites: PATCH: http://www.cdc.org; APEXPH/MAPP: http://www.NACHO.org.

The PATCH model of program planning was developed using Green's PRECEDE model of health education (Sharma, 2017). The PATCH model does the following (Issel, 2021):
- Considers health education a process that helps people be more in control of their health
- Provides ways for people to be in control of their health
- Incorporates clients viewed as essential to planning success through the following:
  - Community participation
  - Use of data to develop a comprehensive health promotion strategy

- Evaluation for improvement
- Setting long-term goals on increasing community capacity

APEXPH addresses the three core competencies of public health: assessment, assurance, and policy development. This model provides a framework to assess the organization and management of health departments and to work with communities in assessing the health status of the community (Issel, 2021).

MAPP is the newer approach of the three models and is a strategic planning model that helps community health workers be facilitators as communities establish priorities in their public health issues and identify resources to address the issues (Issel,

2021). The process using MAPP is often referred to as the community health assessment and improvement process (CHIP). Box 18.3 provides the elements of the three program planning models.

PROGRAM EVALUATION

Benefits of Program Evaluation

The major benefit of program evaluation is that it shows whether the program is meeting its purpose. It should answer the following questions:

- Are the needs for which the program was designed being met?
- Are the problems it was designed to solve being solved?

Quality assurance audits are prime examples of formative program evaluation in health care delivery. Evaluation data are used to justify continuing programs in community health. Program records—including client evaluations, community indexes, and case registers—serve as the major source of information for program evaluation. Surveys, interviews, observations, and diagnostic tests are ways to assess consumer and client responses to health programs. Planning for the evaluation process is an important part of program planning. When the planning process begins, program evaluation begins with the needs assessment (formative evaluation).

Evaluation Process

A framework for evaluation in public health has been developed by the Centers for Disease Control and Prevention (CDC) to guide understanding about program evaluation and facilitate integration of evaluation in the public health system. This framework defines program evaluation as a systematic way to improve and to account for public health actions by using methods that are useful, feasible, ethical, and accurate. Six interdependent steps are identified that must be part of an evaluation process (CDC, 2018):

1. **Engage stakeholders**—including those involved in program operations; those served or affected by the program; and primary users of the evaluation.
2. **Describe the program**—including the need, expected effects, activities, resources, stage, context, and logic model.
3. **Focus the evaluation design**—to assess the issues of greatest concern to stakeholders while using time and resources as efficiently as possible. Consider the purpose, users, uses, questions, methods, and agreements.
4. **Gather credible evidence**—to strengthen evaluation judgments and the recommendations that follow. These aspects of evidence gathering typically affect perceptions of credibility: indicators, sources, quality, quantity, and logistics.
5. **Justify conclusions**—by linking them to the evidence gathered and judging them against agreed-upon values or standards set by the stakeholders. Justify conclusions on the basis of evidence using these five elements: standards, analysis/synthesis, interpretation, judgment, and recommendations.
6. **Ensure use and share lessons learned**—with these steps: design, preparation, feedback, follow-up, and dissemination.

It should be noted that the steps are very similar to the steps in the planning process.

Formulation of Objectives

The most important step in the planning and evaluation process is the writing of program objectives. The objectives provide direction for conducting the program, and they provide the mechanism for evaluating specific activities and the total program. The following discussion addresses the development of well-written objectives. Development of program objectives begins with the initial phases of program planning.

Specifying Goals and Objectives

A program may begin with a mission statement. This is a broad general statement of the overall conceptual framework or philosophy of the program. The mission statement clarifies the values and overall purpose of the program and provides a framework for the goals and objectives that follow.

A goal is a statement that describes the general direction of logical response to a demonstrated need. One or two goals are often sufficient for a program to state how it will resolve or lessen the problem defined in the need statement. The goals should be consistent with the values and overall intent set forth in the mission statement. Their purpose is to focus on the major reason for the program—to support the mission. The goals are also the basis for writing the objectives for the program and the action steps that reflect the overall goal accomplishment.

- Mission—statement of values
- Goal—overall aim
- Objectives—specific measurable outcomes
- Action steps—explicit actions to accomplish objectives
- Evaluation measures—the operational indicator that shows the objectives have been met.

Objectives are concise statements describing in measurable and time-bound terms precisely what specific outcome is to be accomplished. *Measurable* means that the objective contains the specific outcome anticipated that could be documented with collectable data. *Time-bound* means that the objective contains the target date when the specific outcome will be accomplished. Objectives should be realistic and attainable means to meet the program goal (The Community Toolkit, 2018; UNCHSL, 2017).

The *objectives* identified in the planning process set the stage for conducting the program and provide the method for evaluating the activities of the program. The following discussion helps in the development of clear, concise objectives.

Specifying Objectives to Meet Program Goals

If the objectives are too general, program evaluation becomes impossible. The objectives must be specific and stated so that anyone reading them could conduct the program without further instruction. To be truly effective, the program plan should begin with a general program goal and move on to specific objectives that will help meet the program goal. Useful program objectives include the following:

- A statement of the specific behaviors
- Accomplishments
- Success criteria or expected result, for the program

Each program objective requires the following:
- A strong, action-oriented verb to specify the behavior
- A statement of a single purpose
- A statement of a single result (an *outcome*)
- A time frame for achieving the expected result

In the example about childhood immunizations, a program objective that meets these criteria may be as follows: to decrease (action verb) the incidence of early childhood disease in Center County (outcome) by providing immunization clinics in all schools (purpose) between August and December of 2022 (time frame).

As objectives are developed, an operational indicator for each objective should be considered so the evaluator knows when and if the objective has been met. For instance, an operational indicator for the previous objective would be a 10% to 25% decrease in the incidence rates of the most frequently occurring childhood vaccine–preventable illnesses in Center County. Such indicators provide a target for persons involved with program implementation. A review of *Healthy People 2030* objectives will give the reader examples of objectives that include all the elements just listed. (See the *Healthy People 2030* Box below.)

Sources of Program Evaluation

Major sources of information for program evaluation are program clients, program records, and *community indexes*. The program participants, or clients of the service, have a unique and valuable role in program evaluation. Whether the clients for whom the program was designed accept the services will determine to a large extent whether the program achieves its goal. Thus their reactions, feelings, and judgments about the program are important to the evaluation.

To assess the response of participants in a program, the evaluator may use the following:
- Written survey in the form of a questionnaire
- Attitude scale
- Interviews
- Observations

Attitude scales are probably used most often and are usually phrased in terms of whether the program met its objectives. The client satisfaction survey is an example of an attitude scale often used in the health care delivery system to evaluate the program objectives.

The second major source of information for program evaluation is *program records,* especially clinical records. Clinical records provide information about the health interventions of clients and the results of interventions on the total population. Whether a program goal has been met can be determined by summarizing the data from the records for the total population who received the intervention. For example, if one overall goal is to reduce the incidence of low-birth-weight babies through prenatal care, records would be reviewed to obtain the number of mothers who received prenatal care and the number of low-birth-weight babies born to them.

A third major source of evaluation is *epidemiological data*. Mortality and morbidity data measuring health and illness indicators are likely to be cited more frequently than any other single index for program evaluation. Incidence and prevalence are valuable indexes used to measure program effectiveness and impact, and these data are readily available on the Internet. (See Chapter 10 for a further discussion of rates and ratios.)

An example of a national program based on a needs assessment of the United States population is the national health objectives program *Healthy People 2030* (US Department of Health and Human Services [USDHHS], 2020). *Healthy People* documents have been published every 10 years since 1980. The data gathered from each 10-year period have been used to evaluate the community, the health care system, and population needs met. The data are used to focus the direction for the next *Healthy People* document.

A person's community can have a major impact on their health and well-being. *Healthy People 2030* focuses on ways organizations, businesses, schools, and residents can help build healthier communities. The example shown in the *Healthy People 2030* box below highlights the need to build more infrastructure to make community's healthier. This box shows that objectives include an action verb, a purpose, an outcome, an operational indicator, and a time frame for implementing the objective over a number of years, with the implementation begun in 2020.

♥ HEALTHY PEOPLE 2030

Goals for Program Planning and Evaluation

Focus Area	Overall Goal	Objective	Measuring the Objective
Community, Public Health Infrastructure	**Increase the proportion of local public health jurisdictions that have developed a community health improvement plan**	By 2030 increase the percent of public health agencies who have a CHIP	An overall percent increase from 67.2% to 72.8% who have a CHIP

US Department of Health and Human Services: *Healthy People 2030,* Washington, DC, 2020, US Government Printing Office.

The Levels of Prevention box provides examples of applying levels of prevention to program planning and evaluation.

Aspects of Evaluation

The aspects of program evaluation include the following (CDC, 2018; Issel and Wells, 2018):
1. *Relevance*——Need for the program
2. *Adequacy*—Program addresses the extent of the need
3. *Progress*—Tracking of program activities to meet program objectives
4. *Efficiency*—Relationship between program outcomes and the resources spent
5. *Effectiveness*—Ability to meet program objectives and the results of program efforts

LEVELS OF PREVENTION

Program Planning and Evaluation

Primary Prevention

Plan a community-wide program with the local school system and health department to serve healthy meals and snacks in all schools to promote good childhood nutrition.

Secondary Prevention

Develop screening programs for all school children to determine the incidence/prevalence of childhood obesity before implementing the program.

Tertiary Prevention

Evaluate the incidence/prevalence of obesity among school children after the implementation of the program and provide programs to reduce complications from the condition.

6. *Impact*—Long-term changes in the client population
7. *Sustainability*—Enough resources to continue the program

The How To box suggests questions that may be asked about program evaluation using this process.

The following paragraphs provide an explanation of each step in program evaluation.

Relevance. Evaluation of relevance is an important component of the initial planning phase. As money, providers, facilities, and supplies for delivering health care services are more closely monitored, the needs assessment done by the nurse will determine whether the program is needed.

Adequacy. Evaluation of adequacy looks at the extent to which the program addresses the entire problem defined in the needs assessment. The magnitude of the problem is determined by vital statistics, incidence, prevalence, and expert opinion.

HOW TO DO A PROGRAM EVALUATION

To do a program evaluation, first choose the type of evaluation you wish to conduct. Second, identify the goal and objectives for the evaluation. Third, decide who will be involved in the evaluation. Fourth, answer the questions related to the type of evaluation as follows:

A. Program relevance: needs assessment (formative)
1. Use answers to all questions listed in section B of How To Develop a Program Plan.
2. On the basis of the needs assessment, was the program necessary?

B. Adequacy
1. Is the program large enough to make a positive difference in the problem/need?
2. Are the boundaries of the services defined so that the problem/need can be addressed for the target population?

C. Program progress (formative)
1. Monitor activities (circle which this reflects: daily, weekly, monthly, annually).
   a. Name the activities provided.
   b. How many hours of service were provided?
   c. How many clients have been served?
   d. How many providers are there?
   e. What types of clients have been served?
   f. What types of providers were needed?
   g. Where have services been offered (e.g., home, clinic, organization)?
   h. How many referrals have been made to community sources?
   i. Which sources have been used to provide support services?
2. Budget
   a. How much money has been spent to carry out activities?
   b. Will more/less money be needed to conduct activities as outlined?
   c. Will changes to objectives and activities be needed to sustain the program?
   d. What changes do you recommend and why?

D. Program efficiency (formative and summative)
1. Costs
   a. How do costs of the program compare with those of a similar program to meet the same goal?
   b. Do the activities outlined in C1 compare with the activities in a similar program?
   c. Although this program costs more/less than expected, is it needed? Why?

2. Productivity (may use national or state averages for comparison)
   a. How many clients, populations, or community groups does each type of staff see per day (e.g., registered nurses, clinical nurse specialists, nurse practitioners)?
   b. How does this compare with similar programs?
   c. Although the productivity level of this program is low/high, is the program needed? Why?
3. Benefits
   a. What are the benefits of the program to the clients served?
   b. What are the benefits to the community?
   c. Are the benefits important enough to continue the program? Why? (Look at cost, productivity, and outcomes of care.)

E. Program effectiveness (summative)
1. Satisfaction
   a. Is the client satisfied with the program as designed?
   b. Are the providers satisfied with the program outcomes?
   c. Is the community satisfied with the program outcomes?
2. Goals
   a. Did the program meet its stated goal?
   b. Are the client needs being met?
   c. Was the problem solved for which the program was designed?

F. Impact (summative)
1. Long-term changes in health status (1 year or more)
   a. Have there been changes in the community's health?
   b. What are the changes seen (e.g., in morbidity or mortality rates, teen pregnancy rates, pregnancy outcomes)?
   c. Have there been changes in individuals' health status?
   d. What are the changes seen?
   e. Has the initial problem been solved or has it returned?
   f. Is new or revised programming needed? Why?
   g. Should the program be discontinued? Why?

G. Sustainability
1. Was the program funded as a demonstration or by an external agency?
2. Can money and resources be found to continue the program after the initial funding is gone?

Depending on the answers to the questions, the program can be found to be successful or unsuccessful.

Developed by Marcia Stanhope.

Progress. The monitoring of program activities, such as hours of services, number of providers used, number of referrals made, and amount of money spent to meet program objectives, provides an evaluation of the progress of the program. This type of evaluation is an example of formative or process evaluation, which occurs on an ongoing basis while the program exists. This provides an opportunity to make effective day-to-day management decisions about the operations of the program. Progress evaluation occurs primarily while implementing the program. The nurse who completes a daily or weekly log of clinical activities (e.g., number of clients seen in clinic or visited at home, number of phone contacts, number of referrals made, number of community health promotion activities) is contributing to progress evaluation of the nursing service.

Efficiency. If the reason for evaluation is to examine the efficiency of a program, it may occur on an ongoing basis as formative evaluation or at the end of the program as a summative evaluation. The evaluator may be able to determine whether the program provides better benefits at a lower cost than a similar program, or whether the benefits to the clients, or number of clients served, justify the costs of the program.

Effectiveness and impact. An evaluation of program effectiveness may help the nurse evaluator determine both client and provider satisfaction with the program activities, as well as whether the program met its stated objectives. However, if evaluation of impact is the goal, long-term effects such as changes in morbidity and mortality must be investigated. Both effectiveness and impact evaluations are usually summative evaluation functions primarily performed as end-of-program activities.

Sustainability. A program can be continued only if there are resources for the program. Ongoing evaluation of sustainability is important! As an example, in past research the combination of prenatal care programs delivered by nurses and the Special Supplemental Nutrition Program for Women, Infants, and Children (WIC) produces better pregnancy and postnatal outcomes for mothers and babies than does traditional medical care. Looking at the program evaluation process in the How To box on the previous page and given this example, how would you determine whether this program could be sustained.

▶ APPLYING CONTENT TO PRACTICE

Program planning skills and knowledge are essential for public health nurses. In *Public Health Nursing: Scope and Standards of Practice* (ANA, 2013), the first standard is that of assessment. This addresses the issue of conducting needs assessments and having the ability to collect multiple sources of data, analyze population characteristics, problem solve, and set priorities based on the data collected. Standard 2 speaks to using the assessment data to diagnosis health problems with input from the client population. Standards 3 through 5 address the nurses' roles in identifying health status outcomes, planning and implementing processes to address the health problem, and directing strategies to meet the outcomes. Standard 6 discusses the nurses' role in evaluation including participating in process and outcome evaluation by monitoring activities in programs.

The four professional organizations dedicated to public health nursing—The Association of Public Health Nurses, The Association of Community Health Nursing Educators, the Public Health Nursing section of the APHA, and the Alliance of Nurses

for Healthy Environments—have banded together in an organization called the Quad Council Coalition. This council, which at one time included the ANA, developed a document identifying the domains of practice for public health nurses. One of the domains is Policy Development and Program Planning Skills. The competencies the nurse needs for this domain of practice related to program management are:

* Determining needed policies and programs
* Advocating for policies and programs
* Planning, implementing and evaluating policy and programs
* Developing and implementing strategies for continuous quality improvement
* Developing and implementing community health improvement plans (CHIP)
* and strategic plans (Quad Council, 2018)

New baccalaureate nurses will want to be knowledgeable and be able to participate in program management; graduate nurses will want to be able to direct programs.

▮ PRACTICE APPLICATION

The following is a real-life example of the application of the program management process by an undergraduate nursing student. This activity resulted in the development and implementation of a nurse-managed clinic for the homeless. This example shows how students as well as providers can make a difference in health care delivery. It also illustrates that no mystery surrounds the program management process.

Eva was listening to the radio one Sunday afternoon and heard an announcement about the opening of a soup kitchen within the community for the growing homeless population. She was beginning her public health nursing course and wanted to find a creative clinical experience that would benefit herself as well as others. The announcement gave her an idea. Although it mentioned food, clothing, shelter, and social services, nothing was said about health care.

Eva was interested in finding a way to provide nursing and health care services at the soup kitchen. Which of the following should she do? Select all that apply.

A. Talk with key leaders to determine their interest in her idea.
B. Review the literature to find out the magnitude of the problem.
C. Survey the community to determine if others are providing services.
D. Discuss the idea with members of the homeless population.
E. Consider potential solutions to the health care problems.
F. Consider where she would get the resources to open a clinic.
G. Talk with church leaders and nursing faculty members to seek acceptance for her idea.

Answers can be found on the Evolve website.

REMEMBER THIS!

- Planning and evaluation are essential elements of program management and vital to the survival of the nursing discipline in health care delivery.
- The program management process is population focused and is parallel to the nursing process. Both are rational decision-making processes.
- The health care delivery system has grown in the past century, making health planning and evaluation very important.
- Comprehensive health planning grew out of a need to control costs.
- A program is an organized approach to meet the assessed needs of individuals, families, groups, populations, or communities by reducing or eliminating one or more health problems and addressing health disparities.
- Planning is defined as selecting and carrying out a series of actions to achieve a stated goal.
- Evaluation is defined as the methods used to determine if a service is needed and will be used, whether a program to meet that need is carried out as planned, and whether the service actually helps the people it intended to help.
- To develop quality programs, planning should include four essential elements: assessment of need and problem diagnosis, identification of problem solutions, analysis and comparison of alternative methods, and selection of the best plan and planning methods.
- The initial and most critical step in planning a health program is assessment of need. Assessment focuses on the needs of the population or the community to determine who will use the services planned.
- Some of the major tools used in needs assessment are census data, community forums, surveys of existing community agencies, surveys of community residents, and statistical indicators about demographics, morbidity, and mortality of the population.
- The major benefit of program evaluation is to determine whether a program is fulfilling its stated goals.
- Quality assurance programs are prime examples of program evaluation.
- Plans for implementing and evaluating programs should be developed at the same time.
- Program records and community indexes and health data serve as major sources of information for program evaluation.
- Planning programs and planning for their evaluation are two of the most important ways in which nurses can ensure successful program implementation.
- Program planning helps nurses and agencies focus attention on services that clients need.
- Planning helps everyone involved understand their role in providing services to clients.
- The assessment of need process provides an evaluation of the relevance that a new service may have to clients.
- A decision tree is a useful tool to choose the best alternative for solving a problem.
- Setting goals and writing objectives to meet the goals are necessary to evaluate program outcomes.
- *Healthy People 2030* is an example of a national program based on needs assessment that has stated goals and objectives on which the program can be evaluated.
- Program evaluation includes assessing structure, process, and outcomes of care.
- Grant writing is a tool used by nurse managers to provide resources for needed services.
- Grant proposals are documents that incorporate principles of program planning and evaluation.

EVOLVE WEBSITE

http://evolve.elsevier.com/Stanhope/foundations
- Case Study, with Questions and Answers
- NCLEX Review Questions
- Practice Application Answers

REFERENCES

American Nurses Association (ANA): *Public Health Nursing: Scope and Standards of Practice*, 2nd ed., Silver Spring, 2013, American Nurses Association.

American Planning Association (APA): *What is planning?* 2018. Available at: https://www.planning.org/. Accessed August 14, 2018.

American Public Health Association (APHA): Community Health Planning and Policy Development, Washington, DC, 2020, APHA.

Centers for Disease Control and Prevention (CDC): Framework for program evaluation in public health, *MMWR Recomm Rep* 48(RR-11):1–40, 2018.

Issel LM, Wells R: *Health program planning and evaluation: a practical, systematic approach for community health*, 4th ed., Burlington, 2018, Jones and Bartlett Learning, LLC.

Issel LM, Wells R: *Health program planning and evaluation: a practical, systematic approach for community health*, 5th ed., Burlington, 2021, Jones and Bartlett Learning, LLC.

Nutt P: Planning *methods for health and related organizations*, New York, 1984, Wiley.

Quad Council Coalition of Public Health Nursing Organizations: *Community/Public Health Nursing Competencies*, 2018, Quad Council Coalition Competency Review Task Force. Available at: http://www.quadcouncilphn.org/documents-3/2018-qcc-competencies/. Accessed August 14, 2018.

Rosenbaum S, Tolbert J, et al. Community Health Centers: Growing Importance in a Changing Health Care System, Mar 09, 2018, Kaiser Family Foundation, Retrieved at www.KFF.org

Rosen G. *A history of public health*, Baltimore, 1958, Johns Hopkins University Press.

Royse D, Thyer BA, Padgett DK: *Program evaluation: an introduction to an evidence-based approach*, 6th ed., Boston, 2016, Cengage Learning.

Sharma S: *Theoretical foundations of health education and health promotion*, 3rd ed., Burlington, 2017, Jones & Bartlett Learning.

The Community Tool Box. Toolkits, 2018. The Center for Community Health and Development, University of Kansas, Lawrence, Kansas.

Thorland W, Currie D, Wiegand ER, Walsh J, Mader N: Status of breastfeeding and child immunization outcomes in clients of the Nurse-Family Partnership, *Matern Child Health J* 21:439–445, 2017.

University of North Carolina Health Services Library: *Finding information for a community health assessment*, 2017. Available at: https://guides.lib.unc.edu. Accessed July 2, 2018.

USA Facts: COVID-19 Impact and Recovery. Retrieved September 2020 at USAFACTS.org.

USDHHS: *Healthy People 2030*. Washington, DC, 2020, US Government Printing Office.

19

Health Care Improvement in the Community

Marcia Stanhope

OBJECTIVES

After reading this chapter, the student should be able to:

1. Describe the role of health care improvement programs in the community.
2. Understand the historical development of the quality process in nursing.
3. Evaluate approaches and techniques used in Community Health Improvement Processes.
4. Identify the purpose for required quality measures and voluntary quality measures.
5. Assess nursing contributions to community health care improvement.

CHAPTER OUTLINE

KEY TERMS

Although the concept of **quality** has been a part of the health care arena for many years, it is only in the past few years that a major movement to improve health care quality has begun in the United States (Knickman and Ebel, 2018). Knowledge about quality of care in this country has been limited for the following two reasons:

1. A variety of definitions of *quality* being used.
2. It is difficult to obtain comparable data from all providers and health care agencies.

The Institute of Medicine has defined health care quality as "the degree to which health care services for individuals and populations increase the likelihood of desired health outcomes and are consistent with current professional knowledge" (AHRQ, 2018). To be of quality, the level of health care to the population must contribute to improving access to care, a stable economy, educational outcomes, improving social and community participation and relationships, as well as improving neighborhoods and physical environments (*Healthy People 2030*).

In a changing health care market, the demand for quality has become a rallying point for health care consumers, and, in public health, that is the population. Other consumers, including private citizens, insurance companies, industries, the federal government, state, and local, are concerned about achieving the highest quality outcomes at the lowest possible cost. Moreover, consumers want information about quality. Information is empowering to the consumer. With the expanded use of Internet, access to information on the quality of health care is readily available on topics ranging from talking to consumers about quality health care (https://talkingquality.ahrq.gov) to clinical practice guidelines that promise to improve care for all (http://www.guideline.gov).

Both consumers and providers have a vested interest in the quality of the health care system, as follows (National Quality Forum 2017):

1. Improving safety of care saves lives
2. Costs reduction by using effective interventions
3. Increases in client (population) confidence in health care delivery regardless of setting

In health care, a direct link has been known to exist between doing a good job and individual and professional survival. Health care providers pride themselves on individual achievement and responsibility for good client outcomes (Knickman and Ebel, 2018). Health care organizations are natural extensions of health care providers and thus can demonstrate their responsibility for optimal outcomes through a rigorous quality improvement (QI) process. The application of QI strategies in the following six areas of performance could result in better outcomes (USDHHS, 2016):

1. Consistently providing appropriate and effective care
2. Reducing unjustified geographic variation in care
3. Eliminating avoidable mistakes
4. Lowering access barriers
5. Improving responsiveness to clients
6. Eliminating racial/ethnic, gender, socioeconomic, and other disparities and inequalities in access and treatment (USDHHS, 2016)

US MILESTONES IN QUALITY

Total quality management (TQM) was a management philosophy, introduced in the 1950s that included a focus on client, continuous quality improvement (CQI), and teamwork. Although relatively new in health care and even a newer concept in public health, TQM/CQI was tried and proven in the health care industry and public health as leading the way in governmental efforts to improve health care services (Claxton et al., 2015). By the 1990s, TQM was being replaced by a new concept, health care performance improvement.

Beginning in the 1970s, the United States entered a new era of population-centered, community-controlled delivery of care in which managed care organizations (MCOs) played an integral role. MCOs are integrated entities in the health care system, which endeavor to reduce costs associated with health care expenditures. Since the 1970s, MCOs have shaped health care delivery in the United States through preventive medicine strategies, financial provisioning, and treatment guidelines (Heaton and Prasanna, 2020). MCOs are agencies such as health maintenance organizations (HMOs), preferred provider organizations (PPOs), exclusive provider organizations (EPOs), and point of service organizations (POS) which are designed to monitor and deliver health care services within a specific budget. Currently, providers, clients, payers, and policymakers all have input into the quality measurement process. The Health Plan Employer Data and Information Set (HEDIS), a data-collection arm of the National Committee for Quality Assurance (NCQA, 2017), provides performance information, or report cards, for 90% of America's Health Plans.

In the Affordable Care Act of 2010 (KHN, 2015) accountable care organizations (ACOs) were being promoted. However, important differences exist between ACOs and MCOs. ACOs are not insurance companies and their providers are financially rewarded for coordinating all aspects of client care. Primary care providers needed to increase their reliance on nurse practitioners, pharmacists, and other members of the health care team to track appointment compliance, manage medication schedules, and oversee lifestyle changes.

ACO clients can be seen by any physician of their choice. Participation in ACOs is strictly voluntary, there are no enrollment or lock-in provisions. Clients who are unhappy with their care are free to seek treatment elsewhere. Consistent with traditional Medicare rules, there are no gate-keeping or pre authorization provisions in the ACO model and clients are not required to obtain a referral before consulting with another provider.

The growth of the managed care industry changed the face of health care in the United States, both in how health care was delivered and how it was received by consumers. Consumers form partnerships in their communities to counteract the power of MCOs by holding them accountable for the quality of health outcomes in relation to costs. Partnerships are using data-based community assessments to improve health and ensure that communities receive quality services and the establishing of quality indicators for ACOs. Consumers are no longer willing to have care just given to them. Instead, they want to be partners in making decisions on their care. The ACO concept under the Affordable

Care Act did not work out as planned and has lost money for the government and was being overhauled in 2018 (KHN, 2018).

Although introduced in the 1990s, report cards for public health agencies have been used to measure quality health care in communities. The term *community health report card* refers to different types of reports, community health profiles, needs assessments, scorecards, quality of life indicators, health status reports referred to as community health status indicators, and progress reports (http//:www.cdc.gov). All of these reports have been critical components of community-based approaches to improving the health and quality of life of communities (Community Tool Box, 2018). Community health report cards can be a useful tool in efforts to help identify areas in which change is needed, to set priorities for action, and to track changes in population health over time. The CDC had an interactive website referred to as the CHSI so that states and communities could download data collected through the report card process for comparison of progress within the state and across the United States. The report card was used to track leading causes of morbidity and mortality in a community, looking at trends over time to see if public health interventions had improved health care outcomes Beginning in 2017, the CHSI was replaced by the County Health Rankings and Roadmaps program. This program is a collaboration between Robert Wood Johnson Foundation and the University of Wisconsin Population Health Institute. Data about any county in the United States can be found at http://www.countyhealthrankings.org.

As a part of a movement to provide quality health care in communities, health departments began examining their place in promoting quality (CDC, 2017). It was in 2011 that the public health accreditation board was established "to improve and protect the health of the public by advancing and transforming the quality and performance of governmental public health agencies and the US and abroad" (PHAB, 2020). In 2020, 36 states and 269 health departments had been accredited. It is recognized that public health and quality health care improvement are connected because of the use of the systems approaches that public health takes in identifying problems and developing interventions. Public health cannot ensure services that improve health if those services lack quality. Public health works to maintain the quality in its workforce and continually evaluates the effectiveness of its services whether the service is delivered to the individual, the community, or the population.

Nurses in community practice are in a perfect position to implement strategies to improve community level health care including strategies to improve population-centered health care. Community assessments, identification of high-risk individuals, use of targeted interventions, case management, and management of illnesses across a continuum of care are strategies suggested as part of the focus in improving the health of communities. These strategies have long been used by nurses (Quad Council Coalition of Public Health Nursing Organizations, 2018).

The strategies are gaining attention because they are cost-effective and healthy consumers obviously use fewer health care resources than do sick people. Thus, everyone—consumers, providers, and those who pay the health care bills—benefit if people stay healthy. The competencies for public health leadership developed by the Council on Linkages (2001, updated 2010 and 2014) are crucial to ensure the quality and performance of the public health workforce (Rowitz, 2014; See Appendix C for a list of the competencies). Records are maintained on all health care system clients to provide complete information about the client and indicate the quality of care being given to the client within the system. Records are a necessary part of a health care performance improvement process, as are the tools and methods for evaluating services quality.

In 1972 the Social Security Act (PL 92-603) was amended to establish the Professional Standards Review Organization (PSRO) and to mandate the process for the review of the delivery of health care to clients of Medicare, Medicaid, and maternal and child health programs. The PSRO program later became the Professional Review Organization (PRO) under the 1983 Social Security Amendments. The purpose of the PRO was to monitor the implementation of the prospective reimbursement system for Medicare clients (the diagnosis-related groups [DRGs]). Although PSROs were intended for physicians, PROs have made quality performance a primary issue for all health care professionals. The PRO has been renamed the Quality Improvement Organization (QIO) and is mandated to improve the quality and efficiency of Medicare funded services (CMS, 2014). Some public health agencies provide home health services and other individual client services funded by Medicare, Medicaid, and governmental funding of maternal and child health programs. Thus, these agencies must adhere to the standards of care related to these services.

In response to increasing charges of malpractice claims, the government passed the National Health Quality Improvement Act of 1986. Although it was not funded until 1989, its two major goals were to (1) encourage consumers to become informed about their practitioner's practice record and (2) create a national clearinghouse of information on provider malpractice records. The emphasis of this act continued to be on the structure of care rather than the process or outcomes of care (National Association for Healthcare Quality, 1993; Oster and Braaten, 2016).

HEALTH CARE QUALITY AND NURSING PRACTICE

Improving the quality of care has been a part of nursing since the days of Florence Nightingale. In 1860, Nightingale called for the development of a uniform method to collect and present hospital statistics to improve hospital treatment. Nightingale was a pioneer in setting standards for nursing care (Karimi and Alavi, 2015). The movement to establish nursing schools in the United States came in the late 1800s from a desire to set standards that would upgrade nursing care. In the early 1900s, efforts were begun to set similar standards for all nursing schools. From 1912 to 1930, interest in quality nursing education led to the development of nursing organizations involved in accrediting nursing programs. Licensure has been a major issue in nursing since 1892. By 1923, all states had permissive or mandatory laws directing nursing practice (Benefiel, 2011).

After World War II, the attention of the emerging nursing profession focused on establishing a scientific method of practice. The nursing process was the chosen method and included evaluation of how nursing activities helped clients (Maibusch, 1984). Quality assurance (QA) and QI were the evaluative steps in the nursing process.

QA measurement tools were developed in the 1950s. One of the first tools was Phaneuf's nursing audit method (1965), which has been used extensively in population-centered nursing practice.

In 1966, the American Nurses Association (ANA) created the Divisions on Practice. As a result, in 1972 the Congress for Nursing Practice was charged with developing standards to institute QA programs. The Standards for Community Health Nursing Practice (now public health nursing practice) were distributed to ANA Community Health Nursing Division members in 1973, in 1986, 1999, and 2005, with updates in 2007. In 2013 the scope and standards were again revised to strengthen the focus on the population as client and on evidence based practice.

Efforts to strengthen nursing practice in the community have been carried out by several nursing organizations, including the ANA, the Public Health Nursing Section of the American Public Health Association (APHA), the Association of State and Territorial Directors of Nursing (now APHN), the Association of Community Health Nursing Educators (ACHNE) and the Alliance of Nurses for Healthy Environments. Other than ANA, the other organizations are called the *Quad Council Coalition for Public Health Nursing*. The quality of nursing education is a major concern of the ACHNE, which was established in 1978. In 1993, 2000, 2003, 2007, and 2009, five reports published by this organization identified the curriculum content required to prepare nurses for practice in the community (Association of Community Health Nursing Educators, 1993, 2000a, 2000b, 2003, 2007, 2009). In 2005 and again in 2007, the Quad Council organizations reviewed scopes and standards of population-focused (public health) and community-based nursing practice and developed new standards to guide the profession in obtaining the best health outcomes for the populations they served. These Scopes and Standards of Public Health Nursing Practice were updated and published in 2013 (ANA, 2013).

The Council on Linkages between Academia and Public Health Practice (the Council) is a coalition of representatives from 23 national public health organizations in 2020. Since 1992, the Council has worked to further academic and practice collaboration to ensure a well-trained, competent workforce and a strong, evidence-based public health infrastructure. The Council is funded by the Centers for Disease Control and Prevention and staffed by the Public Health Foundation. The most recent core competencies were updated in 2014. These competencies are used as performance measurements of providers to ensure quality of services (Council on Linkages, 2020). In 2003 and using the work of the Council on Linkages, the Quad Council of Public Health Nursing developed a set of core competencies for public health nurses. This was updated in 2009, 2011 and again in 2018 and can be used as a performance measure for public health nursing practice (Quad Council Coalition, 2018).

DEFINITIONS AND GOALS

What is Quality?

Quality is a hard term to define. To some extent, quality has to be defined in relation to the product and service under consideration. Also, quality is often determined differently by the provider than by the person receiving the product or service. Quality is defined by the client as the improvement in health status. The Institute of Medicine, now known as the Health and Medicine Division of the National Academies of Science, defined quality as "the degree to which health services for individuals and populations increase the likelihood of desired health outcomes and are consistent with current professional knowledge" (IOM, 2011, p 1000). The Agency for Healthcare Research and Quality (AHRQ, 2016) defined quality health care as doing the right thing, for the right client, and having the best possible results. Quality in public health has been defined as "the degree to which policies, programs, services, and research for the population increase desired health outcomes and conditions in which the population can be healthy" (IOM, 2013, p 3).

However, a definition of quality rests largely on the perception of the client, the provider, the care manager, the purchaser, the payer, or the public health official. Whereas the physician views quality in a more technical sense, the client may look at the personal outcome; the manager, purchaser, or payer may consider the cost effectiveness; and the public health official looks at performance improvement in population health care, and the appropriate use of health care resources (USDHHS, 2016).

AHRQ (2018) described quality in terms of six priorities: client safety, person-centered care, care coordination, effective treatment, healthy living, and care affordability. Between 2000 and 2017 AHRQ noted improvement in health care quality. The variation in service quality was getting smaller between population groups except for the poor and uninsured clients. The variation was also seen among regional, state, and local health care services and stemmed from lack of evolutionary health care practice and not keeping abreast of the constant changes taking place in health care (evidence-based practice) (AHRQ, 2018). Disparities in quality refer to racial, ethnic, and socioeconomic in accessibility and affordability of health care (AHRQ, 2018).

The term *health services* applies to a wide range of health delivery institutions. Of particular interest to public health are the following:

- The question of access to appropriate and needed services
- A well-prepared workforce
- Improvement in the status of the population's health
- Client satisfaction and well-being
- The processes of client-provider interaction

The goals of QI are on a continuum of quality, and in public health they are (1) to continuously improve the timeliness, effectiveness, safety, and responsiveness of programs, and (2) to optimize internal resources to improve the health of the community, which in this case is the client (PHF, 2020).

QI in public health can help teams use resources more effectively. It has been demonstrated to improve service delivery and customer service, and help meet national public health standards, such as those for voluntary public health department accreditation

(PHF, 2020). Many agencies use concepts, such as client satisfaction questionnaires, or the plan-do-check-act approach to see if improvement has occurred in health care delivery.

APPROACHES TO QUALITY IMPROVEMENT

Two basic approaches exist to assure QI in health care: required and voluntary. The voluntary approach involves a large governing or official body's evaluation of a person's or an agency's ability to meet criteria or standards through processes like accreditation or certification. Required approaches to QI are methods used to manage a specific health care delivery system in an attempt to deliver care with outcomes that are acceptable to the consumer, such as state licensure of a health department, licensing of health care providers, like boards of nursing. See Table 19.1 for examples of each approach.

Quality Improvement in Public Health

In public health care, the customers are clients, individual, populations, or communities. Public health care agencies have recently begun using an approach entitled Community Assessment-Community Health Improvement Plans.

The CHA/CHIP is a long-term systematic approach to address public health problems based on the results of a community assessment and the development of an improvement plan to address the problems defined (CDC, 2018). This approach is focused on the customer (client) and everyone in the organization must be committed to quality. There are both internal and external customers. Internal customers are employees in departments or work units, such as nurses, business staff, outreach workers, environmental health workers, sanitation workers, statisticians, or physicians. External customers are regulators, accrediting bodies, clients, families, populations, and communities. The internal

---

TABLE 19.1 Approaches to Quality Improvement

Voluntary Approaches	Required Approaches
1. Credentialing is generally defined as the formal recognition of a person as a professional with technical competence or of an agency that has met minimum standards of performance.	1. Licensure is one of the oldest required approaches in the United States and Canada. Individual licensure is a contract between the profession and the state whereby the profession is granted control over who can enter into and who exits from the profession. Licensure controls entry into a profession. Exit is generally punitive for some infraction.
2. Accreditation is a voluntary approach used for institutions. a. The American Association of Colleges of Nursing (AACN) through the Commission on Collegiate Nursing Education accredits baccalaureate and higher degree nursing programs (Commission on Collegiate Nursing Education, 2020). b. The National League for Nursing also accredits associate degree programs and all other programs. c. State boards of nursing accredit basic nursing education programs so that their graduates are eligible for the licensing examination. d. The Public Health Accreditation Board, located in Washington, DC, voluntarily accredits public health departments.	2. Accreditation is also considered required because it is often linked to governmental regulations that encourage programs to participate in the accrediting process to be reimbursed for services. For example, only accredited public health and home health agencies are eligible for reimbursement for Medicare clients.
3. Certification may be voluntary if a nurse wishes to be recognized as having a certain set of skills beyond basic nursing education.	3. Certification combines features of licensure and accreditation. Educational achievements, experience, and performance on an examination determine a person's qualifications for functioning in an identified specialty area, such as nursing in the community. Nurse practitioners are required to take examinations to be recognized or licensed to practice per state laws.
4. Charter is the mechanism by which a state governmental agency grants corporate status to institutions with or without rights to award degrees (e.g., university-based nursing programs).	
5. Recognition is defined as a process by which one agency accepts the credentialing status of and the credentials conferred by another agency. A recent approach to recognition is the Magnet Health Care Organization Recognition program, which emphasizes status given by the ANCC to organizational nursing services that, after an extensive review, are considered excellent.	
6. Academic degrees are titles awarded by degree-granting institutions to individuals who have completed a predetermined program of studies. Students voluntarily enter such programs of study.	4. Academic degrees can be required to enter specific professions. For example, to obtain a position in nursing, one must have one or more of the following degrees: Associate of Arts or Sciences; Bachelor of Science in Nursing; master's degrees, such as Master of Science in Nursing and Master of Nursing; and doctoral degrees, such as Doctor of Philosophy and Doctor of Nursing Practice.

customer has often been overlooked. Employees forget that their professional colleagues are often customers for their services. For example, nurses working in community settings are often customers of the agency's laboratories or data offices. It is easy to take co-workers for granted and forget that they deserve efficient, effective service, as do clients, families, and other service recipients. Several key determinants that can lead to customer satisfaction are listed in the "How To" box.

HOW TO ENSURE CUSTOMER SATISFACTION WITH SERVICES PROVIDED

Tangibles
- Facility attractiveness when visiting the public health department
- Employee appearance
- Characteristics of other customers

Reliability
- Dependability
- Consistency of service delivery

Responsiveness
- Employee willingness
- Promptness in service delivery

Competence
- Employee knowledge

Understanding the Customer
- Effort to learn customer needs
- Individualized attention

Access
- Distance to health care facility or community meeting facility
- Waiting time or appointment times in the community
- Hours of operation

Courtesy
- Staff politeness and mannerisms

Communication
- Ability of employees to explain the material in an understandable way
- Openness to questions

Credibility
- Trustworthiness of staff

Security
- Physical safety
- Confidentiality

Customer satisfaction for both internal and external users of services can be assessed through the use of focus groups (of clients or employees), surveys (written or telephone), and response cards. Personnel policies that are motivating and provide continuous training and learning opportunities are important parts of a performance improvement process. In QI, people are not blamed for failures in the system and therefore are supported in their efforts to look for problems and seek ways to improve system performance. Guidelines from the *NCQA* provide approaches for population health management and quality of care (NCQA, 2018). **Population Health Management** (PHM) has

been defined by NCQA as a model of care that addresses individuals' health needs at all points along the continuum of care, including in the community setting, through participation, engagement and targeted interventions for a defined population. The goal of PHM is to maintain or improve the physical and psychosocial well-being of individuals and address health disparities through cost-effective and tailored health solutions. *Healthy People 2030* also provides objectives with their stated targets, measurement tools, and reflected intended performance expectations.

PERFORMANCE MONITORING

As health care reform continues, especially with the implementation of the Patient Protection and Affordable Care Act, public health agencies face competition and are trying to reform themselves. A promising outcome of reform is private health care and public health coming together in a community-level effort to monitor performance and improve health.

Recognizing the many factors that cause health problems and the fragmenting that continues to exist in the health care system, this public–private collaborative framework supported by the *Healthy People* documents involves many stakeholders, including those in public health, in monitoring the health of entire communities. Performance monitoring is defined as "a continuing community-based process of selecting indicators that can be used to measure the process and outcomes of an intervention strategy for health improvement (making the results available to the community as a whole) to inform assessments of an effective intervention and the contributions of accountable agencies to this" (Community Tool Kit, University of Kansas, 2018).

Home health care agencies have increasingly adopted QI programs because of the competition that exists (see Chapter 30 for more information).

Finally, in the area of standards and guidelines, consistency in providing appropriate and effective care is applicable to all health care practitioners, including nurses. Evidence-based practice guidelines are one way to deliver consistent, up-to-date care and improve outcomes for individuals, communities, and populations. The use of guidelines helps gather data on the effectiveness and outcomes of nurse interventions.

Guidelines are protocols or statements of recommended practice developed by governmental and health care agencies and professional organizations; they are based on the distilling of scientific evidence and expert opinion that guide a clinician in decision making. Guidelines provide research-based evidence for interventions and promote improved health outcomes. Using research findings as guidelines or frames of reference can improve nurses' awareness of new or better ways to practice, allow for documentation of nurse interventions, and improve outcomes at all levels of public health nursing practice (Puri and Tadi, 2020). Keystones of evidence-based practice guidelines arise from client concerns, clinical experience, best practices, and clinical data and research (Boswell and Cannon, 2017). Clinical practice guidelines are systematically developed statements to assist practitioner and client decisions about appropriate health care for specific clinical circumstances. See the Evidenced-Based Practice box for an example.

EVIDENCE-BASED PRACTICE

This mixed-methods study sought to identify factors that support or hinder the development of a quality improvement culture in public health agencies. The researchers conducted case studies of 10 agencies that participated in early quality improvement efforts. Agency staff who participated in National Association of County and City Health Officials (NACCHO)-sponsored quality improvement trainings were invited to complete a survey. Health directors and quality improvement teams from these agencies were also interviewed. The investigators found that agencies that were successful in creating a positive quality improvement culture had the following characteristics: had leadership support, had participated in national quality improvement initiatives, had a greater number of staff trained in quality improvement, had quality improvement teams that met regularly with decision-making authority, reported that accreditation was a major driver to quality improvement work, and had a history of evidence-based decision making and use of quality improvement to address emerging issues. The investigators reported that the role of accreditation preparation was a driving force in quality improvement and appeared to diminish as an agency developed a quality improvement culture. The researchers noted that common barriers to creating a quality improvement culture included lack of time and resources and relevance of quality improvement to daily work. However, they also reported that staff used quality improvement to overcome these barriers.

Nurse Use

Leadership and teamwork within an organization plays a key role in creating a positive quality improvement environment. Public health nurses are in a prime position to be leaders in their organizations in developing a quality improvement environment.

Modified from Davis MV, Mahanna E, Joly B, et al: Creating quality improvement culture in public health agencies, *Am J Public Health* 104(1):e98–e104, 2014.

CHECK YOUR PRACTICE

One approach useful for measuring the performance improvement of care to populations of an agency is the plan-do-check-act process. You have been asked to suggest the best approach to conducting a plan-do-check-act process for the school health program at the health department. How would you do it? See if you can apply these steps to this scenario: (1) Recognize the cues, look at the literature to see how an RN could be helpful in applying the plan-do-check-act (PDCA) method; (2) analyze the cues; (3) state several and prioritize the hypotheses you have stated; (4) generate solutions for each hypothesis; (5) take action on the number one hypothesis you think best reflects an approach to take to implement the PDCA in the school health program; and (6) evaluate the PDCA outcomes and changes to be made in the program.

METHODS FOR EVALUATING HEALTH CARE PERFORMANCE IMPROVEMENT

Three key models have been used over time to evaluate performance improvement: Donabedian's structure-process-outcome model, the tracer method, and the sentinel method. One model is gaining more attention for evaluating performance improvement, the plan do check (study) act model.

Donabedian's model (1981, 1985, 2003, Gardner, 2014) introduced three major methods for evaluating quality performance improvement:

1. Structure: Evaluating the setting and instruments used to provide care. Examples of structures include facilities, equipment,

characteristics of the administrative organization, client mix, and the qualifications of health providers
2. Process: Evaluating activities as they relate to standards and expectations of health providers in the management of client care
3. Outcome: The net change or result that occurs as a result of health care

The three methods may be used separately to evaluate a part of care. However, to get an overall picture of the quality of care, they should be used together.

The tracer method described by Kessner and Kalk (1973; Wetsman, 2020) is currently used and is a measure of both process and outcome of care and is used today. This method is more effective in evaluating the health care of groups or population than of individual clients. It is also more effective in evaluating care delivered by an institution than care delivered by an individual provider. The following are essential characteristics for implementing the tracer method (The Joint Commission, 2016):

- A tracer, or a problem, that has a definite impact on the clients' (group or populations level of functioning
- Well-defined and easily diagnosed characteristics
- Population prevalence high enough to permit adequate data collection
- A known variation resulting from use of effective health care
- Well-defined management techniques in prevention, diagnosis, treatment, or rehabilitation
- Understood (documented) effects of nonmedical factors on the tracer

Groups or populations selected for tracer outcome studies in nursing would have the following:

1. A shared health care issue
2. A similar intervention used to solve the issue
3. Similar needs
4. Be located in the same community
5. A similar lifestyle
6. Be at the same disease stage, like diabetes, arthritis, asthma.

The tracer method provides nurses with data to show the differences in outcomes as a result of nursing care standards. See Box 19-1 for types of problems studied.

BOX 19.1 Types of Problems Studied in a Quality Improvement Program

- Client death (population mortality)
- Client injury (population morbidity)
- Personnel and client safety
- Agency liability
- Increased costs
- Denied reimbursement by third-party payers (decreased program funding by government)
- Client complaints
- Inefficient service
- Staff noncompliance with standards of structure
- Lack of resources
- Unnecessary staff work and overtime
- Documenting of care
- Client health status (population health status)

The sentinel method of quality evaluation is based on epidemiological principles. This method is an outcome measure for examining specific diseases and the impact on the health and economics of a population, such as COVID-19 (WHO, 2020, Ross, 2014). Changes in the sentinel indicate potential problems for others. For example, increases in encephalitis in certain communities may result from increases in mosquito populations. Data may be collected at the health department through a state or local required disease reporting system. The health department would be notified, and an immediate mosquito control strategy would be put into place. Such an intervention could include nurses notifying the population to remove standing water around the outside of homes, such as animal water bowls, rain barrels, and gutter downspout water collection pools. Flyers may be sent home with school children or given to clients visiting the public health clinics, and media announcements may be used. In addition, the environmental office at the health department may inspect local swimming pools and also may implement a nighttime mosquito spraying program throughout the community.

The characteristics of the sentinel method are described in the "How To" box.

HOW TO CONDUCT A SENTINEL EVALUATION

- Identify cases of unnecessary disease, disability, and complications. Example: tuberculosis (TB).
- Count the deaths from these causes.
- Examine the circumstances surrounding the unnecessary event (or sentinel) in detail.
- Review morbidity and mortality rates as an index for comparison; determine the critical increase in the untimely event, which may reflect changes in quality of care. Example: compare the incidence and prevalence of TB cases before the increased population occurred.
- Explore health status indicators, such as changes in social, economic, political, and environmental factors that may have an effect on health outcomes. Example: overcrowding in the shelter in which migrant workers stay (environmental) and the inability to follow up on testing because of the transient nature of the population (social).

The **Plan-Do-Check-Act (PDCA)/Plan-Do-Study-Act (PDSA) model** originated in 1920 with a statistician named Walter Shewhart. This later became known as the Deming cycle, with four repetitive steps to be applied to a continuous improvement process. The four steps were described in sequence as PLAN: Plan ahead for change and analyze and predict the results; DO: Execute the plan, taking small steps in controlled situations; CHECK: Study the results of the plan; and ACT: Take action to standardize or improve the performance process. A similar version became known as the PDSA. Both approaches were useful in small - scale testing of performance improvements and can prevent recurring mistakes from occurring in the workplace. The method for applying PDC(S)A follows:

1. The first step in use of the model is PLAN.
   - A team will be assembled, and roles, responsibilities, timelines, and meeting schedules will be established.
   - Next is drafting an 'aim statement' to answer the following questions:
     - What will be accomplished?
     - How will it be known that any changes made are improvements?
     - What changes can be made that will result in an improvement?
   - Then brainstorming: A SWOT analysis may be implemented during this step. The team may examine the agency's strengths, weaknesses, opportunities, and threats. In this step, the team will want to gather input from the community about needs and expectations from the agency, the scope of services provided by the agency, the technologies used, the available staff to provide the services, and outcome data from past performance improvement projects.
   - Describe the problem to be addressed using data from the three aim statement questions above and write the problem statement to summarize team consensus.
   - Identify causes of the problem. There are many tools that can be used to describe the causes. The simplest would be a flow chart or diagram.
   - Develop an action plan for solving the problem or providing improvement.
2. The second step in the model is DO.
   - Begin implementing the action plan and document problems implementing, unexpected effects, and note any observations from the team members
3. The third step is CHECK or STUDY.
   - Discuss as a team: Did improvements occur? Were the improvements substantial? Was the investment of time and money worth the changes noted? Were there unintended consequences?
   - In this stage, you may gather information to check the outcomes of changes or you may study the changes more thoroughly: Will the team use the CHECK approach and simply analyze what happened when changes were introduced and make the changes, or will the team choose to do more in-depth study of the changes over a longer time period to determine whether the changes are worth pursuing?
4. The fourth stage is ACT.
   - If change from the performance improvement plan seems successful, then the changes will be permanent until the PDCA cycle is implemented again.
   - If it does not seem a different approach to improving performance would be better, then return to step 1 (Minnesota Department of Health, 2020).

The CHA/CHIP Model of Quality Improvement— A Long-Term Approach to Quality Improvement at the Health Agency Level

The Community Health Assessment/Community Health Improvement Model (CHA/CHIP) is a more recent model that is being used to monitor the outcomes of health agency services over a 3- to 5-year period. This plan is used by health, governmental, and human services in collaboration with the community partners to set priorities and coordinate efforts to improve the health of the communities. First, a community health assessment is conducted to gather information about the target community's health status, needs, and issues. This data then is used to develop a community health improvement plan to address the community's needs. The outcomes of this approach include an improved health agency; community coordination and collaboration; increased knowledge about public health activities in the community; improved partnerships between agency and community; improved knowledge about current performance of the health agency, which helps with accreditation and identifies the benchmarks within the community and the health agency, which are used to improve public health practice (CDC, 2018).

The Mobilizing for Action through Planning and Partnerships (MAPP) model is often used for the strategic planning process to prioritize community public health issues and needed resources to address those issues. Nurses and other health care workers may be a part of the public health agency's team and are trained in the process and participate in the community health assessment.

EVALUATION, INTERPRETATION, AND ACTION

Interpreting the findings of a quality evaluation is an important part of the process. It allows differences between the quality standards of the agency and the actual practice of the nurse or other health care providers. These patterns reflect the total agency's functioning over time and generate information for decisions to be made about the strengths and limitations of the agency. Regular intervals for evaluation should be established within the agency, and periodic reports should be written so that the combined results of performance improvement efforts can be analyzed and health care delivery patterns and problems identified. These reports should be used to establish an ongoing picture of changes that occur within an agency to justify nursing services.

Identification and choices of possible courses of action to correct the weaknesses within the agency should involve both the administration and the staff. The courses of action chosen should be based on their importance, cost, and timeliness. For example, if there is a nursing problem in the records of a population health issue the agency administration and staff may analyze the problem to see why it is occurring. Reasons for lack of recordkeeping given by the nurses include a lack of time to properly do paperwork, workloads that reduce the amount of time spent with clients, and lack of available resources for health care interventions. If such reasons are given, it would not be appropriate to deal with the problem by providing a staff development program on the importance of doing and recording their services. It would be more important to assess how to provide the time and resources necessary for the nurses to offer needed services to the clients. Economically, it may be more beneficial to provide smartphones, tablets, or laptop computers and clerical assistance so that nurses can make notes at the point of implementation, thereby providing more client contact time, or it may be more beneficial economically to employ an additional nurse and reduce workloads.

QSEN FOCUS ON QUALITY AND SAFETY EDUCATION FOR NURSES

Targeted Competency: Quality Improvement—Use data to monitor the outcomes of intervention processes, and use improvement methods to design and test changes to continuously improve the quality and safety of health care systems.

Important aspects of quality improvement include:

- **Knowledge:** Recognize that nursing and other health professions students are parts of systems and intervention processes that affect outcomes for populations.
- **Skills:** Identify gaps between local practices and best practice.
- **Attitudes:** Value own and others' contributions to outcomes in local community settings.

Quality Improvement Question:

You are working as a public health nurse and are discovering a trend of an increase in the numbers of children arriving the first day of school without required vaccinations. Using the quality improvement approach, consider the following questions:

- What is being done now?
- Why is it being done?
- Is it being done well?
- Can it be done better?
- Should it be done at all?
- Are there improved ways to deliver service?
- How much is it costing?
- Should certain activities be abandoned or replaced?

To which aspects of your clients' quality of life and care transitions will you apply these questions?

Answer: It would be helpful to look at an elementary school population that is reflective of your community. Are parents receiving adequate information about school entry requirements and how are they receiving it? You could also gather data about the number of children being managed by the public health agency and how many are missing the beginning of school due to lack of compliance by parents. How often the children are being followed by the school health nurse.

Prepared by Gail Armstrong, ND, DNP, MS, PhD, Professor and Assistant Dean/DNP program, Oregon Health and Sciences University.

Taking action is the final step in a QI model. Once the alternative courses of action are chosen to correct problems, actions must be implemented for change to occur in the overall operation of the agency. Follow-up and evaluation of the actions taken must occur for performance improvement. Although health provider evaluation will continue to be included in a QI effort, the focus on the effort is the population of health providers and not the person. It is assumed that health care professionals and other employees want to do the best job possible for the client, and problems or differences in a process should not be automatically attributed to their behavior. Although frequent feedback should be given to all employees, the hallmark of QI is continuous learning. Staff development must be ongoing for all employees (see the Levels of Prevention box).

LEVELS OF PREVENTION

Related to Quality Management

Primary Prevention

The nurse participates in a parent education program to improve the immunization level of children in the local elementary school and develops a strategy for follow-up.

Secondary Prevention

Agency evaluation, using a retrospective audit of records of the immunization program, determines that the vaccine-preventable infectious disease rates have declined in the elementary school after the implementation of the parent education program.

Tertiary Prevention

A review of the public health report card indicated that community incidence of complications from vaccine-preventable diseases have declined over a 2-year period after the implementation of the parent education program.

DOCUMENTATION

Documentation is essential to evaluate the quality improvement in any organization. The following text focuses on the kinds of documentation that normally occur in a community agency.

Records

Records are an important part of the communication structure of the health care organization. Accurate and complete records are required by law and must be kept by all agencies, both governmental and nongovernmental. In most states, the state departments of health stipulate the kinds of records to be kept and their content requirements for community agencies. Records provide complete information about the client (whether a family, group, population, or community), indicate the extent and quality of services being given, resolve legal issues in malpractice suits, and provide information for education and research.

Public Health Agency Records

Within the community or public health agency, many types of records are kept and used to predict population trends in a community, to identify health needs and problems, to prepare and justify budgets, and to make administrative decisions. The kinds of records the agency keep can include reports of accidents, births, census, chronic disease, communicable disease, mortality, life expectancy, morbidity, child and spouse abuse, occupational illness and injury, and environmental health.

Agencies also keep records to maintain administrative contact and control the organization. These records are clinical, provider service, and financial. The *clinical record* is the client's health record. The *provider service records* include information about the numbers of clients seen daily, the immunizations given, home visits made daily, transportation and mileage, the provider's time spent with the client, and the amount and kinds of supplies used. The service record is completed on a daily basis by each provider and is summarized monthly and annually to indicate trends in health care activities and costs relative to personnel time, transportation, maintenance, and supplies. The *financial records* include salaries, overhead, and transportation costs, and they serve as the basis for the cost accounting system. These records are basic to performance improvement processes.

 APPLYING CONTENT TO PRACTICE

Healthy People 2030 provides examples of how health care quality can be improved. One of the goals of *Healthy People 2030* is to engage leadership, key constituents, and the public across multiple sectors to take action and design policies that improve the health and well-being of all. This will be accomplished by helping individuals of all ages increase their life expectancy and improve their quality of life. According to *Healthy People 2030,* there are substantial differences in life expectancy among population groups within the nation. This is influenced by gender, race, and income. Quality of life reflects a sense of happiness and personal satisfaction. Health-related quality of life reflects a personal sense of physical and mental health and the ability to react to the physical and social environments. Basically, all the objectives are directed toward meeting this goal(USDHHS, 2020).

PRACTICE APPLICATION

Oscar, a male nursing student, has been working in the migrant farmworker clinic and has noted that each practitioner uses a different educational method for teaching good nutrition practices to clients with newly diagnosed diabetes. The clinic has seen a substantial increase in the number of new clients with diabetes in the Hispanic farmworker population. Oscar knows that practice guidelines for teaching nutrition practices exist in his clinical facility and that charts have an area in which to note nutrition education information. He is also aware that for nurses to be most effective and ensure quality client outcomes, research-based practice guidelines should be used by all nurses in the health department.

As part of his course, Oscar must prepare a teaching plan and conduct a class on a health care problem. He obtains permission from his instructor and the director of the clinic to conduct an in-service program. The purpose of Oscar's in-service program is to instruct the nursing staff in how to teach good nutrition practices to clients with newly diagnosed diabetes. He obtains and studies the guidelines about teaching good nutrition practices and researches the methodological background for the development of the guidelines. Oscar's native language is Spanish, so this will help him determine whether brochures regarding good nutrition for clients with newly diagnosed diabetes convey the appropriate message.

As part of his in-service program, Oscar maintains demographic records on attendees and conducts before-and-after tests of knowledge, adding questions about the present use of the guidelines. He plans to follow up with the nurses in 6 months with a further test and questions about use of the guidelines. The director will help him determine an outcome measure that can be used with the client population to show effective use of the guidelines.

A. What outcome measure would be useful in this project?

B. How will this help in determining a quality improvement approach to be used in the nursing service?

Answers can be found on the Evolve website.

REMEMBER THIS!

- The health care delivery system is the largest employing industry in the United States; society is demanding increased efficiency and effectiveness from the system.
- Quality improvement is the approach used to ensure effectiveness and efficiency.
- The managed care industry changed the face of the American health care delivery system.
- The objective and systematic evaluation of nursing care is a priority within the profession for several reasons, including the effects of cost on health care accessibility, consumer demands for quality, and the increasing involvement of nurses in public and health agency policy formulation.
- The concept of quality includes community involvement and customer satisfaction.
- Efforts are being made by the public and private sectors to form partnerships to monitor the performance of all players in health care delivery for the purpose of improving the health of communities.
- Quality improvement is the monitoring of the activities of health care delivery to determine the degree of excellence attained in implementation.
- Quality has been a concern of the profession since the 1860s, when Florence Nightingale called for a uniform format to gather and disseminate hospital statistics.
- Licensure has been a major issue in nursing since 1892.
- Two major categories of approaches exist in quality assurance and improvement today: required approaches and voluntary approaches.
- Accreditation is an approach to quality used for institutions, whereas licensure is used primarily for individuals.
- Certification combines features of both licensing and accreditation.
- Four major models have been used to evaluate quality: Donabedian's structure-process-outcome model, the sentinel model, the tracer model, and the PDC(S)A model.
- Records are an integral part of the communication structure of a health care organization.
- Accurate and complete records are required by law of all agencies, whether governmental or nongovernmental.
- Quality improvement mechanisms in health care delivery are the mechanisms for controlling the system and requesting accountability from individual providers and health care agencies within the system.
- Records help establish a total picture of the contribution of the agency to the client community.

EVOLVE WEBSITE

http://evolve.elsevier.com/Stanhope/foundations
- NCLEX Review Questions
- Case Study, with Questions and Answers
- Practice Application Answers

REFERENCES

Agency for Healthcare Research and Quality [AHRQ]: *Provide a framework for understanding health care quality,* Rockville, MD, 2018.

Agency for Healthcare Research and Quality [AHRQ]: *2015 national healthcare quality and disparities report and 5th anniversary update on the national quality strategy,* AHRQ Pub. No. 16-0015, Rockville, MD, 2016, AHRQ, National Quality Strategy.

American Nurses Association: *Public health nursing: scope and standards of practice,* Silver Spring, Md, 2013, ANA.

Association of Community Health Nursing Educators: *Perspectives on doctoral education in community health nursing,* Lexington, Ky, 1993, ACHNE.

Association of Community Health Nursing Educators: *Graduate education for advanced practice education in community/public health nursing,* Chapel Hill, NC, 2000a, ACHNE.

Association of Community Health Nursing Educators: *Essentials of baccalaureate nursing education for entry level community health nursing practice,* Chapel Hill, NC, 2000b, ACHNE.

Association of Community Health Nursing Educators: *Graduate education for advanced practice in community public health nursing,* New York, 2003, ACHNE.

Association of Community Health Nursing Educators: *Graduate education for advanced practice public health nursing: at the crossroads,* Chapel Hill, NC, 2007, ACHNE.

Association of Community Health Nursing Educators: *Essentials of baccalaureate nursing education for entry level community health nursing practice,* Chapel Hill, 2009, ACHNE.

Benefiel D. The history of nurse licensure. *Nurse educator,* 36(10, pg 16-20, 2011, Wolters Kluwer Health, Lippincott Williams & Wilkins.

Boswell C, Cannon S: *Introduction to nursing research: incorporating evidence-based practice,* ed. 4, Burlington, MA, 2017, Jones & Bartlett Learning.

Centers for Disease Control and Prevention [CDC]: *Community Health Assessment/Community Health Improvement Process.* Centers for Disease Control and Prevention [CDC]: Atlanta, GA, 2018, CDC. Retrieved August 2020 from http://wwwn.cdc.gov.

Claxton G, Cox C, Gonzales S, Kamal R, Levitt L: *Measuring the quality of healthcare in the US,* Kaiser Family Foundation Insight Brief, 2015. Retrieved August 2016 from http://www.healthsystemtracker.org.

Centers for Disease Control and Prevention: *Performance and Quality Improvement, 2017,* Washington, DC. Retrieved 2020 at www.cdc.gov.

Centers for Medicare and Medicaid Services: *Quality Improvement Organizations 2014.* Retrieved 9/10/2020 at www.cms.gov.

Community Tool Box: Creating and using community report cards, 2018, University of Kansas: The community tool kit. retrieved from edu.ku.edu, Sept, 2020.

Council on Linkages between Academia and Public Health Practice: *Core competencies for public health professionals,* Washington, DC, 2020, The Public Health Foundation.

Davis MV, Mahanna E, Joly B, et al: Creating quality improvement culture in public health agencies, *Am J Public Health,* 104(1): e98-e104, 2014.

Donabedian A: *Explorations in quality assessment and monitoring*, vol 2, Ann Arbor, Mich, 1981, Health Administration Press.

Donabedian A: *Explorations in quality assessment and monitoring*, vol 3, Ann Arbor, Mich, 1985, Health Administration Press.

Donabedian A: *An introduction to quality assurance in health care*, New York, 2003, Oxford University Press.

Gardner G., Gardner A. O'Connell, J. The Donabedian Framework to examine the quality and safety of nursing service innovation. Journal of Clinical Nursing, Jan. 2014,: 23(1-2), 145-55.

Heaton J & Prasana T.: *Managed care organizations.* StatPearls Publishing, Treasure Island Fla, 2020.

Institute of Medicine: Health matters, Washington, DC, 2011, National Academy Press.

Institute of Medicine [IOM]: *Toward quality measures for population health and the leading health indicators*, Washington DC, 2013, The National Academies Press.

Kaiser Health News,(KHN): *Accountable Care Organizations Explained, 2015.* Gold J., Kaiser Family Foundation. Retrieved from https:// khn.org.

Kaiser Health News,(KHN): Medicare To Overhaul ACOs But Critics Fear Less Participation, Galewitz, P, August 9, 2018, Gold, J. & Kaiser Family Foundation. Retrieved from https:// khn.org.

Karimi H, Masoudi Alavi N. Florence Nightingale: The Mother of Nursing. *Nurs Midwifery Stud.* 2015 Jun;4(2)nmsjournal. Epub 2015 Jun 27.

Kessner DM, Kalk CE: Assessing health quality: the case for tracers, *New Engl J Med* 288:189-194, 1973.

Knickman JR & Elbel, B., eds. *Jonas and Kovner's health care delivery in the United States*, ed 12, New York, 2018, Springer Publishing Company.

Maibusch RM: Evolution of quality assurance for nursing in hospitals. In: Schrolder PS, Maibusch RM, eds.: *Nursing quality assurance*, Rockville, 1984, Aspen.

Minnesota Department of Health: PDSA, St. Paul, 2020, Rapid Cycle Improvement.

National Association for Healthcare Quality: *Risk management: NAHQ guide to quality management*, Skokie, 1993, NAHQ.

National Committee for Quality Assurance: *HEDIS 2017 measures: summary table of measures, product lines and changes*, Washington, DC, 2017, NCQA. Retrieved August 2020 from http://www.ncqa.org.

National Committee for Quality Assurance: Population Health Management. Rockville, 2018, AHRQ, USDHHS.

National Quality Forum: *Patient safety 2017*, Washington, DC, 2018, USDHHS.

organizations: a healthcare handbook for patient safety and quality, Indianapolis, IN, 2016, Sigma Theta Tau International.

Phaneuf M: A nursing audit method, *Nurs Outlook* 5:42-45, 1965.

Public Health Accreditation Board: *About PHAB*, 2020. Retrieved in 2020 from http://www.phaboard.org.

Public Health Foundation: *National Public Health Performance Standards*, Washington, DC, 2020, NACCHA, ASTHO.

Puri I, Tadi P. Quality Improvement. In: StatPearls [Internet]. Treasure Island (FL): StatPearls Publishing; 2020 Jan-. Available from: https://www.ncbi.nlm.nih.gov.

Quad Council Coalition of Public Health Nursing Organizations: *Quad Council competencies for public health nurses*, Washington, DC, 2018, Public Health Foundation. Retrieved August 2020 from http://www.phf.org.

Ross TK: *Health care quality management: tools and applications*, San Francisco, 2014, Jossey-Bass.

Rowitz L: *Public health leadership: putting principles into practice*, ed 3, Burlington, 2014, Jones & Bartlett Learning.

The Joint Commission: *Facts about the tracer methodology*, 2016. Retrieved August 2016 from https://www.jointcommission.org.

US Department of Health and Human Services: *Healthy People 2030*, Washington, DC, 2020, US Government Printing Office.

US Department of Health and Human Services, *Quality Improvement* Washington, DC, 2016, Health Resources and Services Administration.

Wetsman, N.: Contact Tracing Programs have to work with local communities to be successful, 2020, Retrieved Nov. 2020 from The Verge.com.

World Health Organization: Surveillance for Vaccine Preventable Diseases. Geneva, Switzerland, 2020 Retrieved Nov. 2020 from http:// www.who.int.

20

Family Development and Family Nursing Assessment and Genomics

Jacqueline F. Webb

OBJECTIVES

After reading this chapter, the student should be able to:

1. Explain the multiple ways public health nurses work with families and communities.
2. Identify challenges to working with families in the community.
3. Describe family function and structure.
4. Describe family demographic trends and demographic changes that affect the health of families.
5. Work with families using a strength-based approach to assess, develop, and evaluate family action plans.

CHAPTER OUTLINE

KEY TERMS

Family nursing is practiced in all settings. The trend in the delivery of health care has been to move health care to community settings; thus, family nursing is pertinent to nurses in community health. Public health nurses need skills that enable them to move between working with individual families, bridge relationships between family and the community, advocate for family and community legislation, and influence policies that promote and protect the health of populations. Family nursing is a specialty area that has a strong theory base and blends both public health and family-based nursing. Family nursing consists of nurses and families working collaboratively and with other members of health, educational, and social service teams to ensure the success of the family and its members in adapting to responses to health and illness. The purpose of this chapter is to present a current overview of families and family nursing, theoretical frameworks, and strategies for assessing and intervening with families in the community.

Nurses practicing in the community use the core competencies for public health professionals (Quad Council Coalition, 2014), and the core public health functions of assessment, assurance, and policy development to promote the interconnectedness of individual health with the health of families and communities (Eddy et al., 2018).

CHALLENGES FOR NURSES WORKING WITH FAMILIES IN THE COMMUNITY

Many challenges exist that influence the practice of family nursing in the community. The definition of what constitutes a family has changed over time; there are single-parent families, same-gender families, two parents of different gender families, multigenerational families living together, grandparents raising grandchildren. To make this more complex, there is no single agreed-upon definition of family.

Many policies related to families assume legal marriage and that children will be raised by married-couple families. For example, Social Security benefits are based on earnings of a spouse to determine retirement security for the living survivor. According to the US Census Bureau, 4 million out of about 12 million single-parent families have children under the age of 18, and more than 80 percent are headed by single mothers (Cohen, 2018). In the current health care system, families are significant members of health care teams because they are the consistent person or people involved in the care.

Nurses are responsible for the following:
- Helping families promote their health
- Meeting family health needs
- Coping with health problems within the context of the existing family structure and community resources
- Collaborating with families to develop useful interventions

Nurses must be knowledgeable about family structures, functions, processes, and roles. In addition, nurses must be aware of and understand their own values and attitudes pertaining to their own families, as well as being open to different family structures and cultures. Nurses are often the link between the family and the services that a member or members need. Nurses need excellent communication and negotiation skills because they often must advocate for the family as well as explain to the family what another agency representative is telling them.

FAMILY FUNCTIONS AND STRUCTURES

Knowledge of family functions and structures is essential for understanding how families influence health, illness, and well-being. Family functions are the ways in which families meet the needs of (1) each family member, (2) the family as a whole, and (3) their relationship to society. Historically families have performed these functions: (Kaakinen, 2018a):

1. *Economic function:* Family income is a substantial part of family economics, but it is also related to family consumerism,

money management, housing decisions, insurance choices, retirement, and savings. Family economics affect and reflect the nation's economy.
2. *Reproductive function:* The survival of a society is linked to patterns and rates of reproduction. The family has been the traditional structure in which reproduction was organized. Today, the reproductive function of family has become more separated from traditional family structure as more children are born outside of marriage and into nontraditional family structures.
3. *Socialization function:* A major expectation of families is that they are responsible for raising their children to fit into society and take their place in the adult world. In addition, families disseminate their culture, including religious faith and spirituality. However, some families choose to teach their children to try to change or rebel against society, which typically causes community problems.
4. *Affective function:* Families establish boundaries and structure that provide a sense of belonging and identity of who the family members are individually and to their family. The purpose of the affective function is to learn about intimate reciprocal caring relationships, to learn about dependency and how to nurture future generations.
5. *Health care function:* Families teach members the concepts of health, health promotion, health maintenance, disease prevention, and illness management. Family members provide informal caregiving to ill family members and are primary sources of support.

Family structure refers to the characteristics and demographics (e.g., sex, age, number) of individual members who make up family units. More specifically, the structure of a family defines the roles and the positions of family members (Box 20.1).

Family structures have changed over time to meet the needs of the family and society. The great speed at which changes in family structure, values, and relationships are occurring makes working with families in the twenty-first century exciting and challenging. According to Kaakinen (2018a), the following aspects need to be addressed when determining the family structure:
1. The individuals that compose the family
2. The relationships between them
3. The interactions between the family members
4. The interactions with other social systems

The family structure changes and modifies over time. An individual may participate in a number of family life experiences over a lifetime (Fig. 20.1). For example, a child may spend the early, formative years in the family of origin (mother, father, siblings); experience some years in a single-parent family because of divorce or death; and participate in a stepfamily relationship when the single parent who has custody remarries.

This same child as an adult may experience several additional family types: cohabitation while completing a desired education, and then a commuter marriage while developing a career. As an adult, the individual may divorce and become a custodial parent. The custodial parent may live with another partner and later marry a partner who also has children. As couples age, they have to address issues of the aging family, and subsequently the woman may become an older single widow. Thus nurses work with families representing different structures and living arrangements.

BOX 20.1 Family and Household Structures

Married Family
- Traditional nuclear family
- Dual-career family
- Spouses reside in the same household
- Commuter marriage
- Husband or father is away from the family
- Stepfamily
- Stepmother family
- Stepfather family
- Adoptive family
- Foster family
- Voluntary childlessness

Single-Parent Family
- Never married
- Voluntary singlehood (with children, biological or adopted)

- Involuntary singlehood (with children)
- Formerly married
- Widowed (with children)
- Divorced (with children)
- Custodial parent
- Joint custody of children
- Binuclear family

Multiadult Household (With or Without Children)
- Cohabitating couple
- Commune
- Affiliated family
- Extended family
- New extended family
- Home-sharing individuals
- Same-sex partners

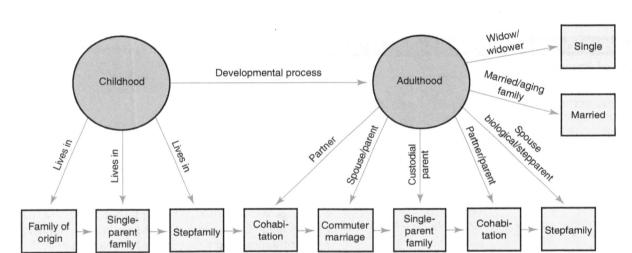

Fig. 20.1 An Individual's Family Life Structure Over Time.

Prospects for families in the 21st century are numerous. New family structures that are currently experimental will emerge as everyday "natural" families (e.g., families in which the members are not related by blood or marriage, but who provide the services, caring, love, intimacy, and interaction needed by all persons to experience a quality life). Also, some individuals choose not to have children.

At times it is helpful to understand families through a narrow framework of family function and structure. However, a family is a system within itself as well as the basic unit of a society. Some would argue that the traditional concept of family is disintegrating based on how the structure and functions of the family have changed over time. On the other side of that debate, families change in response to the societal changes and are ever evolving and thriving as they seek different ways of interconnectedness (Kaakinen, 2018a).

Families depend on a variety of agencies to provide safety, such as law enforcement, and other agencies, such as churches, synagogues, and other religious organizations, are involved in the passing on of religious faith. Education (socialization function) is relegated to the schools. Family names are no longer needed to confer status as in the past, when names were important in a community.

FAMILY HEALTH

Despite the focus on family health in nursing, the meaning of family health lacks consensus and is not precise. The term family health is often used interchangeably with the concepts of family functioning, healthy families, or familial health. Hanson (2005, p 7) defines family health as "a dynamic changing relative state of well-being, which includes the biological, psychological, spiritual, sociological, and cultural factors of individual members and the whole family system."

This holistic approach refers to individual members as well as the family unit as a whole. An individual's health affects the entire family's functioning, and in turn the family's functioning affects the health of individuals. Thus assessment of family health involves simultaneous assessment of individual family members and the family system as a whole, and the community in which the family is embedded.

Health professionals have tended to classify clients and their families into two groups: healthy families and nonhealthy families, or those in need of psychosocial evaluation and intervention. A popular term for nonhealthy families is dysfunctional families, also called noncompliant, resistant, or unmotivated—terms that label families who are not functioning well with each other or in their communities. Box 20.2 provides a description of healthy families. Families are neither all good nor all bad; rather, all families have both strengths and difficulties. Families with strengths, functional families, or balanced families are often referred to as healthy families. All families have seeds of resilience.

Families with strengths, functional families, and resilient families are terms often used to refer to healthy families. Research has been conducted about healthy families, but it is clear that the issues examined all concern relational needs. These families tend to be affectionate in their relationships with one another. This means that in healthy families, the basic survival needs are met. Balanced families also are able to adapt to situations; they are flexible in terms of leadership, relationships, rules, control, discipline, negotiation, and role sharing (Kaakinen, 2018a). The Levels of Prevention box and Evidence-Based Practice box provide information related to one physical health problem of obesity in one or more members of the family.

 LEVELS OF PREVENTION

Levels of Prevention

Primary Prevention
- Educate parents about healthy nutritional choices for young children and the risks associated with obesity.
- Provide counseling and weight management for overweight children and teens.
- Help mothers who qualify for the Special Supplemental Nutrition Program for Women, Infants and Children (WIC) complete the extensive paperwork.

Secondary Prevention
- Screen teens for obesity with body mass index (BMI) greater than or equal to 30 for obesity.
- Analyze children's height and weight growth as part of annual health assessments.

Tertiary Prevention
- Work with schools to improve the quality of food offered in school lunches.
- Help communities establish local farm-to-school networks, create school gardens, and ensure that more local foods are used in the school setting.

BOX 20.2   **Characteristics of Healthy Families**

1. The family tends to communicate well and listen to all members.
2. The family affirms and supports all of its members.
3. The family values teaching respect for others.
4. The family members have a sense of trust.
5. The family plays together, and humor is present.
6. All members interact with each other, and a balance in the interactions is noted among the members.
7. The family shares leisure time together.
8. The family has a shared sense of responsibility.
9. The family has traditions and rituals.
10. The family shares a religious core.
11. The family honors the privacy of members.
12. The family opens its boundaries to admit and seek help with problems.

From Kaakinen JR, Hanson SMH: Family health care nursing: an introduction. In Kaakinen JR, Coehlo DP, Steele R, et al., eds: *Family health nursing: theory, practice & research,* ed 5, Philadelphia, 2015, FA Davis, pp. 3–32.

EVIDENCE-BASED PRACTICE

Reducing obesity in the United States is a *Healthy People 2030* objective. Data collected by the Centers for Disease Control and Prevention (2020) found that the prevalence of obesity among adults in the United States in 2017–18 was 42.4%. Obesity is more prevalent in some groups. Specifically, non-Hispanic blacks (49.6%) had the highest age-adjusted prevalence of obesity, followed by Hispanics (44.7%), non-Hispanic whites (42.2%), and non-Hispanic Asians (17.4%). The study also found that men and women with college degrees had lower obesity prevalence compared to a similar age and gender group with less education. It is not surprising that among youth, the prevalence of childhood obesity decreased with increasing level of education of the head of the household. The study did not find a correlation in youth obesity and income.

Nurse Use

Nurses can advocate for social policies that improve the health of families and educate parents of young children to make healthy food choices for them and their children. Public health nurses should be actively involved in helping to decrease childhood and adult obesity. The Levels of Prevention box provides information on reducing childhood obesity.

From Centers for Disease Control and Prevention: Overweight & obesity: adult obesity facts. https://cdc/gov/obesity/. Accessed February 27, 2020; Ogden CL, Carroll MD, Fakhouri TH, et al: *MMWR, MorbMortalWkly* 67:186–189, 2018.

Four Approaches to Family Nursing

Central to the practice of family nursing is conceptualizing and approaching the family from four perspectives. Each approach has an implication for nursing assessment and intervention (Figs. 20.2 and 20.3). Which approach nurses use is determined by many factors, including the health care setting, family circumstances, and resources available to the nurse:

- **Family as a context or structure.** The family has a traditional focus that places the individual first and the family second. The family as context serves as either a resource or a stressor to individual health and illness issues. A nurse using this focus might ask an individual client, "How has your diagnosis of type 1 diabetes affected your family?" or, "Can your son help you get up and down the stairs?"
- **Family as client.** The family is the primary focus, and individual members are second. The family is seen as the *sum* of individual family members. The focus is concentrated on each individual as he or she affects the family as a whole. From this perspective, a nurse might say to a family member who has just become ill, "Tell me about what has been going on with your own health and how you perceive each family member responding to your diagnosis of liver cancer." Or, "How has your diagnosis of diabetes affected your family?"
- **Family as a system.** The focus is on the family as a client, and the family is viewed as an interacting system in which the whole is more than the sum of its parts. This approach simultaneously focuses on individual members and the family as a whole at the same time. The interactions among family members become the target for nursing interventions (e.g., the direct interactions between the parents, or the indirect interaction between the parents and the child).

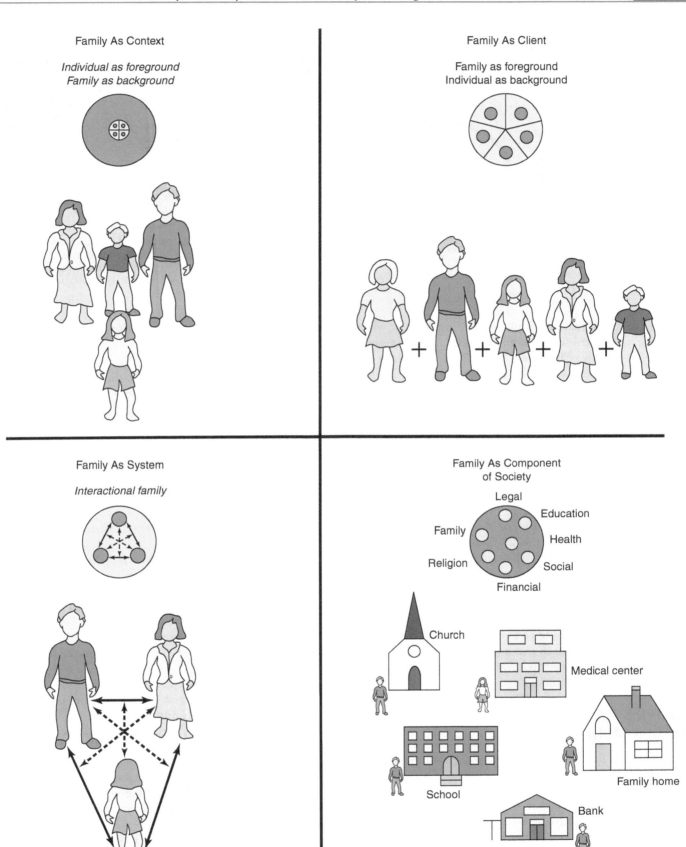

Fig. 20.2 **Approaches to Family Nursing.** (From Kaakinen JR, Hanson SMH: Family health care nursing: an introduction. In Kaakinen JR, Coehlo DP, Steele R, et al., eds.: *Family health nursing: theory, practice & research,* ed 5, Philadelphia, 2015, FA Davis, p 11.)

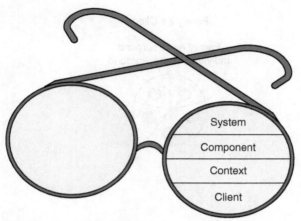

Fig. 20.3 Four Views of the Family. (From Kaakinen JR, Hanson SMH: Family health care nursing: an introduction. In Kaakinen JR, Coehlo DP, Steele R, et al., eds.: *Family health nursing: theory, practice & research*, ed 5, Philadelphia, 2015, FA Davis, p. 12.)

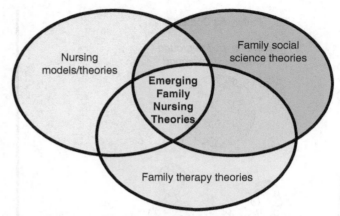

Fig. 20.4 Theory-based Family Nursing. (Modified from Kaakinen JR, Hanson SMH: Family health care nursing: an introduction. In Kaakinen JR, Coehlo DP, Steele R, et al., eds.: *Family health nursing: theory, practice & research*, ed 5, Philadelphia, 2015, FA Davis, pp. 3–32.)

The systems approach to family always implies that when something happens to one family member, the other members of the family system are affected. Questions nurses ask when approaching a family as system are, "What has changed between you and your spouse since your child's head injury?" or, "How do you feel about the fact that your son's long-term rehabilitation will affect the ways in which the members of your family are functioning and getting along with one another?"

- **Family as a component of society.** The family is seen as one of many institutions in society, along with health, education, religious, or financial institutions. The family is a basic or primary unit of society, as are all the other units, and they are all a part of the larger system of society. The family as a whole interacts with other institutions to receive, exchange, or give services and to communicate. Nurses have drawn many of their tenets from this perspective as they focus on the interface between families and community agencies. Using this framework, the nurse might use these questions: "How do you protect your family from the COVID-19 virus when your husband has to go to work for the transit authority?" This is the approach that a public health nurse would use to implement population-centered strategies to improve the health of the community.

THEORIES FOR WORKING WITH FAMILIES IN THE COMMUNITY

Family nursing theory is an evolving synthesis of the scholarship from three different traditions: family social science, family therapy, and nursing (Fig. 20.4). Of the three categories of theory, the family social science theories are the most well developed and informative with respect to how families function, the environment-family interchange, interactions within the family, how the family changes over time, and the family's reaction to health and illness. Therefore, in this chapter, three family social science theories that blend well with public health nursing are reviewed. These social science theories are

the family systems theory, family developmental and life cycle theory, and the bioecological systems theory.

Family Systems Theory

Families are social systems, and much can be learned from the systems approach. A system is composed of a set of organized, complex, interacting elements. Nurses use family systems theory to understand how a family is an organized whole as well as a collection of individuals (Kaakinen, 2018b). The purpose of the family system is to maintain stability through adaptation to internal and external stressors that are created by change (Kaakinen, 2018b; White et al., 2015). Assumptions of family systems theory include the following:

- Family systems are greater than and different from the sum of their parts.
- There are many hierarchies within family systems and logical relationships between subsystems (e.g., mother-child, family-community).
- Boundaries in the family system can be open, closed, or random.
- Family systems increase in complexity over time, evolving to allow greater adaptability, tolerance to change, and growth by differentiation.
- Family systems change constantly in response to stresses and strains from within and from outside environments.
- Change in one part of a family system affects the total system.
- Family systems are an organized whole; therefore, individuals within the family are interdependent.
- Family systems have homeostatic features to maintain stable patterns that can be adaptive or maladaptive.

An excellent way to understand family systems theory is to visualize a mobile that consists of different members of a family suspended from each arm of the mobile; this represents the family as a whole. The parts of the mobile move about in response to changes in the balance. The amount of movement and length of time it takes to achieve a calm, balanced state depends on the severity of the imbalance. The family is a system similar to that of the mobile. When one member is affected by a health event, the whole family and each member of the family is affected differently by this change in balance. Imagine what would happen to the mobile if one of the parts was removed as in the death of a family member, an additional part was added as in the birth or adoption of an infant, an arm of the mobile was extended such as a child moving out of the family home, or one part is yanked really hard and held down for an extended period of time and then suddenly released such as when a family member experiences a life-limiting illness and recovers or proceeds to a chronic illness.

The family systems theory encourages nurses to view the individual clients as participating members of a whole family. The goal is for nurses to help families maintain balance and stability in the family system so that the family can maximize their ability to function and adapt (Kaakinen, 2018b). Nurses using this theory determine the effects of illness or injury on the entire family system. Emphasis is on the whole rather than on individuals. Nursing assessment of family systems includes assessment of individual members, subsystems, boundaries, openness, inputs and outputs, family interactions, family processing, and adapting or changing abilities. Examples of assessment questions nurses could ask a family based on a family systems theory would include the following:

- Who are the members of your family?
- How has one member's illness affected the family?
- Who in the family is or will be affected the most?
- What has helped your family in the past when you have had a similar experience?
- Who outside of your family do you see as being able to help?
- How would your family react to having someone from outside the family come to help?

- How do you think the children, spouse, or parents are meeting their needs?
- What will help the family cope with the changes?

Interventions need to build on the strengths of the family to improve or support the functioning of the individual members and the whole family. Some nursing strategies based on a family systems theory include establishing a mechanism for providing families with information about their family members on a regular basis, helping the family maintain routines and rituals, and discussing ways to provide for everyday functioning when a family member becomes ill.

The major strength of the systems framework is that it views families from both a subsystem and a suprasystem approach. That is, it views the interactions within and between family subsystems as well as the interaction between families and the larger supersystems, such as the community and the world. The major weakness of the systems framework is that the focus is on the interaction of the family with other systems rather than on the individual, which is sometimes more important.

Family Developmental and Life Cycle Theory

Family developmental and life cycle theory provides a framework for understanding normal predicted stresses that families experience as they change and transition over time. In the original theory of family development by Duvall and Miller (1985), they applied the principles of individual development to the family as a unit. The stages of family development are based on the age of the eldest child. Overall family tasks that need to be accomplished for each stage of family development are identified. Table 20.1 shows the stages of the family life cycle

TABLE 20.1	Traditional Family Life Cycle Stages and Family Developmental Tasks
Stages of Family Life Cycle	**Family Developmental Tasks**
Married couple	Establish relationship as a family unit, role development Determine family routines and rituals
Childbearing families with infants	Adjust to pregnancy and then birth of infant Learn new roles as mother and father Maintain couple time, intimacy, and relationship as a unit
Families with preschool children	Understand growth and development, including discipline Cope with energy depletion Arrange for individual time, family time, and couple time
Families with school-age children	Learn to open family boundaries as child increases amount of time spent with others outside of the family Manage time demands in supporting child's interests and needs outside of the home Establish rules, new disciplinary actions Maintain couple time
Families with adolescents	Adapt to changes in family communication, power structure, and decision making as teen increases autonomy Help teen develop as individual and family member
Families launching young adults	As young adult moves in and out of the home, allocate space, power, communication, roles Maintain couple time, intimacy, and relationship
Middle-aged parents	Refocus on couple time, intimacy, and relationship Maintain kinship ties Focus on retirement and the future
Aging parents	Adjust to retirement, death of spouse, and living alone Adjust to new roles (i.e., widow, single, grandparent) Adjust to new living situations, changes in health

and some of the family developmental tasks. One developmental concept of this theory is that families as a system move to a different level of functioning, thus implying progress in a single direction. Family disequilibrium and conflicts occur during these expected transition periods from one stage of family development to another. The family begins as a married couple. Then the family becomes more complex with the addition of each new child until it becomes simpler and less complex as the younger generation begins to leave the home. Finally, the family comes full circle to the original husband-wife pair. Recognizing that families of today are different in structure, function, and processes, McGoldrick and colleagues (2015) expanded the work of Duvall and Miller (1985) to have the family developmental and life cycle theory include different family structures such as divorced families and blended families.

Family developmental and life cycle theory explains and predicts the changes that occur to families and its members over time. Achievement of family developmental tasks helps individual family members to accomplish their tasks. Two of the major assumptions of this theory are as follows:

- Families change and develop over time based on the age of the family members and the social norms of the society. Families have predictable stressors and changes based on changes in the family development and family structure. For example, when a family has their first child, there are predictable stresses and goals to accomplish. Also, families who experience a divorce have some predictable stresses based on when in the life cycle of the family the divorce occurs.
- Families experience disequilibrium when they transition from one stage to another stage. These transitions are considered "on time" or "off time." For example, a couple in their late 20s having their first child would be considered "on time," whereas a teenager having a child or a 30-year-old wife and mother dying from breast cancer would be considered "off-time" transitions.

This theory assists nurses in anticipating stresses families may experience based on the stage of the family life cycle and if the family is experiencing these changes "on time" or "off time." Nurses can also use these predictable stresses to identify family strengths in adaptation to the changes. In conducting an assessment of families, Box 20.3 gives examples of the types of questions nurses can ask based on the family developmental and life cycle theory.

Nursing intervention strategies that derive from the family developmental and life cycle theory help individuals and families understand the growth and development stages and manage the normal transition periods between developmental periods (e.g., tasks of the school-age family member versus tasks of the adolescent family member) with the least amount of stress possible. Family nurses must recognize that in every family there are both individual and family developmental tasks that need to be accomplished for every stage of the individual or family life cycle that are unique to that particular family.

The major strength of this approach is that it provides a basis for forecasting normative stresses and issues that families will experience at any stage in the family life cycle. The major weakness of the model is that it was developed at a time when the traditional nuclear family was emphasized and that some theory development has been conducted on how family life cycles or stages are affected in divorced families, stepparent families, and domestic-partner relationships (McGoldrick et al., 2015).

Bioecological Systems Theory

The bioecological systems theory was developed by Urie Bronfenbrenner (1972, 1979, 1997) to describe how environments and systems outside of the family influence the development of a child over time. Even though this theory was designed around how both nature and nurture shape the development of a child, the same underlying principles can be applied when the client is the family. This theory is useful for public health nurses since it helps identify the stresses and potential resources that can affect family adaptation. Fig. 20.5 depicts the five systems in this theory at different levels of engagement that can affect family development and adaptation. The family as the client is at the center of the concentric circles. Each of the levels contains roles, norms, and rules that influence the current situation of the family.

Microsystems are composed of the systems and individuals that the family directly interacts with on a daily basis. These systems vary for each family, but could include their home,

---

BOX 20.3   Examples of Assessment Questions Nurses Can Ask Based on the Family Developmental and Life Cycle Theory

- How has time that the family spends together been affected?
- How has communication among and between the family members been altered?
- Has physical space in the home been changed to meet the needs of the evolving family?
- In what ways have the informal roles of the family been changed?
- What changes are being experienced in family meals, recreation, spirituality, or sleep habits?
- How are the family finances affected as the family members age?
- Who should be included in the family decision making?

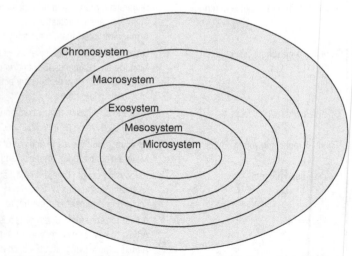

Fig. 20.5 Bioecological Family Systems Model: Level of Systems.

neighborhood, workplace, schools, extended family, health care system, community/public health system, or close friends.

Mesosystems are the systems that the family interacts with frequently but not on a daily basis. These systems vary based on the situation in which the public health nurse is working with a family. Some ideas for systems at this level could be a home health aide who comes to the home twice a week, a hospice nurse who comes to the home once a week, a social worker, church members who come to deliver food to the family, the transportation system, the school system, specialty physicians, pharmacy, or extended family.

Exosystems are external environments that have an indirect influence on the family. Examples of these systems could be the economic system, local and state political systems, religious system, the school board, community/health and welfare services, the Social Security office, or protective services.

Macrosystems are broad overarching social ideological and cultural values, attitudes, and beliefs that indirectly influence the family. Examples include a Jewish religious ethic, a cultural value of autonomy in decision-making, or ethnicity.

Chronosystems refer to time-related contexts in which changes that have occurred over time may influence any or all of the other levels/systems. Examples include the death of a young parent, a divorce and remarriage, war, natural disasters, or a pandemic.

One assumption of this model is that what happens outside of the family is equally as important as what happens inside the family. The interaction between the family and the systems in which it interacts is bidirectional in that the family is affected by the outside systems and the family affects these systems. The strength of this model is that it provides a holistic view of interactions between the family and society. In working with the family, a critical intervention strategy is drawing a family *ecomap* that shows the systems with which the family interacts, including the flow of energy from that system into the family or out of the family. The family ecomap is a visual diagram of the family unit in relation to other units or subsystems in the community. It can serve to organize and present factual information and show the nature of relationships among family members, and between family members, and the community. The weakness of this model is that it does not address how families cope or adapt to the interaction with these systems.

In addition to these three types of theories that describe ways to work with families, the Friedman Family Assessment Model (Friedman et al., 2003) draws on the structure-function framework and on developmental and systems theory. The model with its broad approach to family assessment views families as a subsystem of society. The family is viewed as an open social system. The family's structure (organization) and functions (activities and purposes) and the family's relationship to other social systems are the focus of this approach.

This assessment approach is important for family nurses because it enables them to assess the family system as a whole, as part of the whole of society, and as an interaction system. The general assumptions for this model are (1) the family is a social system with functional requirements; (2) the family is a small group possessing certain generic features common to all small groups; (3) the family as a social system accomplishes functions that serve the individual and society; and (4) individuals act in accordance with a set of internalized norms and values that are learned primarily in the family through socializations.

The guidelines for the Friedman Family Assessment Model consist of the following six broad categories of interview questions:
1. Identifying data
2. Developmental family stage and history
3. Environmental data
4. Family structure, including communication, power structures, role structures, and family values
5. Family functions, including affective, socialization, and health care
6. Family coping

Each category has several subcategories. There are both long and short forms of this assessment tool. In summary, this approach was developed to provide guidelines for family nurses who are interviewing a family to gain an overall view of what is going on in the family. The questions are extensive, and it may not be possible to collect all the data at one visit. All the categories may not be pertinent for every family.

QSEN FOCUS ON QUALITY AND SAFETY EDUCATION FOR NURSES

Targeted Competency: Client-Centered Care—Recognize the client or designee as the source of control and full partner in providing compassionate and coordinated care based on respect for the client's preferences, values, and needs.

Important aspects of client-centered care include:
- **Knowledge:** Describe strategies to empower clients or families in all aspects of the health care process
- **Skills:** Assess the level of the client's decisional conflict, and provide access to resources
- **Attitudes:** Value active partnership with clients or designated surrogates in planning, implementing, and evaluating care

Client-Centered Care Question

Describe how a family assessment is different from an individual client assessment. Beyond immediate family members, who might be included in a client's "family"? Think about the difference between being an advocate for an individual (the client) and an advocate for a family. What different skills are needed?

Prepared by Gail Armstrong, PhD, DNP, ACNS-BC, CNE, Professor and Assistant Dean of the DNP Program, Oregon Health and Sciences University

GENOMICS AND FAMILY HEALTH

The mapping of the human genome created a major shift in how professionals provide care and approach public health. April 2020 marked the 17th anniversary of the completion of the Human Genome Project (HGP). The terms genetics and genomics are often used interchangeably. However, they are different. Genetics refers to the study of the function and effect of single genes that are inherited by children from their parents. Genomics is the study of all of a person's genes, including their interaction with one another as well as the interaction of a person's genes with the environment (National Human Genome Research Institute [NHGRI], 2015a) and NHGRI, 2015b). The stated goals of the HGP were determining the sequences of the 3 billion chemical base pairs that make up human DNA; storing this information in databases; improving tools for data analysis; transferring related technologies to the private sector; and addressing the ethical, legal, and social issues that may arise. Many genetic tests have implications for families, and it is important for nurses to help individuals, families, and communities understand the purpose, limitations, potential benefits, and potential risks of a test before submitting samples for analysis. Over the years a variety of home tests have been developed, and they are controversial.

At the core of the issues related to genetics and genomics is DNA. DNA is the chemical inside the nucleus of a cell that has the genetic instructions for making living organisms. DNA can be compared to long-term storage or a blueprint or code to construct other components of cells such as proteins and ribonucleic acid (RNA) molecules. The DNA segments that carry the genetic information are called genes. Within cells, DNA is organized into long structures called chromosomes. These chromosomes are duplicated before cells divide, in a process called DNA replication. DNA is composed of four bases: adenine (A), guanine (G), cytosine (C), and thymine (T). Genes are composed of specific sequences of these bases.

Alterations in the usual sequence of bases that form a gene or changes in DNA or chromosomal structures are called mutations. A large number of agents are known to cause mutations. These mutations, which are attributed to known environmental causes, can be contrasted with spontaneous mutations, which arise naturally during the process of DNA replication. Approximately 3 billion DNA base pairs must be replicated in each cell division, and considering the large number of mutagens to which we are exposed, DNA replication is fascinatingly accurate. A key reason for this accuracy is a mechanism called DNA repair, which occurs in all normal cells of higher organisms. It is estimated that repair mechanisms correct at least 99.9% of initial errors (NHGRI, 2018a).

Chemicals produced in industry are now known to be mutagenic in laboratory animals. A mutagen is a chemical or physical phenomenon that promotes errors in DNA replication. Among these are nitrogen mustard, vinyl chloride, alkylating agents, formaldehyde, sodium nitrite, and saccharin. In addition, ionizing radiation, such as those produced by x-rays and from nuclear fallout, can promote chemical reactions that change DNA bases or break the bonds of double-stranded DNA (NHGRI, 2018b).

How does an understanding of DNA and the science of genetics relate to public health nursing and family nursing? The field of genetics shows that human disease comes from the collision between genetic variations and environmental factors. While we cannot change the genes of our fellow human beings, nurses in public health are uniquely poised to advocate for environmental changes (for example, advocating for colorectal cancer screening for those with a family history of colorectal cancer) that can impact the wider health of humankind. As knowledge has evolved with the mapping of the human genome, our understanding of this interaction continues to advance. For example, more than 50 hereditary cancer syndromes have been described. If a person is concerned that he or she may have an inherited cancer susceptibility syndrome in the family, it is generally recommended that when possible, a family member with cancer have genetic counseling and testing first, to identify with more certainty if the cancer in the family is due to an inherited genetic variant. The features of a person's personal or family medical history that particularly in combination may suggest a hereditary cancer syndrome include:

- Cancer was diagnosed at an unusually young age
- Several different types of cancer occurred in the same person
- Cancer in both organs in a set of paired organs, such as both kidneys or both breasts
- Several first-degree relatives (the parents, siblings, or children of an individual) have the same type of cancer (for example, a mother, daughter, and sisters with breast cancer); family members with breast or ovarian cancer; family members with colon cancer and endometrial cancer
- Unusual cases of a specific cancer type (for example, breast cancer in a man)
- The presence of birth defects that are known to be associated with inherited cancer syndromes, such as certain noncancerous (benign) skin growths and skeletal abnormalities associated with neurofibromatosis type 1
- Being a member of a racial or ethnic group that is known to have an increased risk of having a certain inherited cancer susceptibility syndrome and having one or more of the above features as well
- Several family members with cancer (National Cancer Institute, 2019)

Nurses can play a key role both by assisting patients with obtaining their personal family history and also helping patients and families navigate through the disclosure process and uncovering their personal and family health history and understanding specific genetic tests and the costs of these tests. In addition, if patients are willing to make lifestyle changes or health decisions, the appropriate psychosocial support and education can be provided to clients and their families. Nurses can answer questions and assist in challenges these clients and families face with making decisions when there is any suspicion of increased risk for genetically based diseases.

In order to provide appropriate nursing care that includes gathering genetic information in the family health history, it is essential that nurses be knowledgeable. The Centers for Disease Control and Prevention (CDC) recommends that all public health workers need to be aware of the advances in the field of genomics. While various health care professional groups have developed competency lists for their members, the guidelines by the American Nurses Association (ANA, 2008) are useful for nurses who work with families in the community. These competencies have four major sections. Each section has a set of skills the nurse should have. The overall domains are:

- Professional practice: nursing assessment: applying/integrating genetic and genomic knowledge
- Identification

- Referral
- Provision of education, care and support

Help families complete a health history by using these steps:

1. Inform the family that a family health history is a written or graphic record of diseases or health conditions present in their biological family.
2. Encourage the family to develop a three-generation history of biological relatives, their age of diagnosis of a chronic disease, and the age and cause of death of any deceased family members.
3. Explain to the family that this type of history is a useful tool to help them know about their health risks and to prevent disease in themselves and their close relatives.
4. Tell the family that the health history is not a one-time document, but rather one that should be updated periodically.
5. Suggest that the family consider using the CDC online tool "My Family Health Portrait" to collect and organize their family health history. The tool is available free at https://phgkb.cdc.gov/FHH, 2020.

Mapping Out a Pedigree

A *pedigree* is a drawing of a family tree used by health care professionals and genetic counselors to assess families and try to spot patterns or indications that may be helpful in diagnosing or managing an individual's health. The pedigree symbols are used globally. A useful example of how to develop a pedigree can be found at the Iowa Institute of Human Genetics (www.medicine.uiowa.edu, 2021). This site gives step-by-step instructions for drawing a pedigree. Steps to take when helping a family or member of a family draw a pedigree are:

- Talk to the client and/or family, and ask questions and collect all information, including biological parents, brothers and sisters, including half-siblings, children, grandparents, aunts and uncles, cousins, nieces and nephews, and include the family member giving the history.
- Draw a basic outline of the family tree using pedigree symbols.
- Next to each family member's name, write down everything you know about his or her health and medical history. You can also ask family members if you are uncertain. If a family member is adopted, you can possibly collect information on either or both the adopted and birth families.
- Include the following information: (1) age or date of birth, (2) age or date of death and cause of death for family members who have passed away, (3) medical conditions and how old the person was when diagnosed with the condition, and (4) where each side of the family comes from originally and pertinent cultural heritage (e.g., England, Iceland, Mexico, Ashkenazi or Eastern European Jewish).

WORKING WITH FAMILIES FOR HEALTHY OUTCOMES

Family nurses should transcend the traditional nursing approach as a service model and change their practice to a capacity-building model (Bomar, 2004; Kim-Godwin and Bomar, 2015). In a capacity-building model, nurses assume the family has the most knowledge about how their health issues affect the family, supports family decision making, empowers the family to act, and facilitates actions for and with the family. The goal of family nursing is to focus care, interventions, and services to optimize the self-care capabilities of families and to achieve the best possible outcomes.

Nurses work with all types of family structures in a variety of settings. Each family is unique in how it responds to the stresses that evolve when a family member experiences a health event. Public health nurses are in a unique position to help families by providing direct care, removing barriers to needed services, and improving the capacity of the family to take care of its members (Kaakinen, 2018c).

Preencounter Data Collection

Nurses need to use excellent communication skills to help families prioritize the issues they are confronting, identify their needs, and develop a plan of action. Family members are experts in their own health. They know the family health history, their health status, and their health-related concerns (Pelletier and Stichler, 2013). Nurses gather information about the family from many sources as well as directly from the family. Data collection begins when an actual or potential problem is identified by a source, which may be the family, the health care provider, a school nurse, or a caseworker.

The assessment process and data collection begin as soon as the referral occurs or the appointment is made. Sources of preencounter data the nurse gathers include the following:

- *Referral source.* This would be information that led to the identification of a family problem and could include demographic information and subjective and objective information.
- *Family.* A family may identify a health care concern and seek help. During the initial intake or screening procedure, valuable information can be collected from the family. Information is collected during phone interaction with the family member, even when calling to set up the initial appointment. This information might include family members' views of the problem, surprise that the referral was made, reluctance to set up the meeting, avoidance in setting up the interview, or recognition that a referral was made or that a probable health care concern exists.
- *Previous records.* Previous records may be available for review before the first meeting between the nurse and the family. Often, a record release for information is necessary to obtain family or individual records. However, one challenge may be that many of the electronic health records are premade templates that ignore family information.

Determining Where to Meet the Family

Before contacting the family to arrange for the initial appointment, the nurse decides the best place to meet with the family, which might be in the home, clinic, or office. The following list identifies questions nurses need to consider before meeting the family. The type of agency in which the nurse works may determine where the family meeting is held (e.g., home health is conducted in the home, and mental health agencies meet the family in the clinic).

Assessment of families requires an organized plan before you see the family. This plan is developed through the following questions:

1. Why are you seeing the family?
2. Are there any specific family concerns that have been identified by other sources?
3. Is there a need for an interpreter?
4. Who will be present during the interview?
5. Where will you see the family and how will the space be arranged?
6. What are you going to be assessing?
7. How are you going to collect the data?
8. What services do you anticipate the family will need?
9. What are the insurance sources for the family?
10. What cultural factors need to be considered in working with this family?

One major advantage to meeting in the family home is seeing the everyday family environment. Family members are likely to feel more relaxed in their home, thereby demonstrating typical family interactions. Meeting with a family in their home emphasizes that the whole family and not one family member is the client. This approach allows the whole family to participate in the identification and resolution of the health problem. Conducting the interview in the home may increase the probability of having more family members present. There are two important disadvantages of meeting in the family home: (1) the family home may be the only sanctuary or safe place for the family or its members to be away from the scrutiny of others, and (2) meeting with a family on their ground requires the nurse to be highly skilled in communication by setting limits and guiding the interaction.

Conducting the family appointment in the office or clinic allows easier access to other health care providers for consultation. An advantage of using the clinic may be that the family situation is so intense that a more formal, less personal setting may be necessary for the family to begin discussion of emotionally charged issues. A disadvantage of not seeing the everyday family environment is that it may reinforce a possible culture gap between the family and the nurse.

Making an Appointment with the Family

After the decision is made regarding where to meet the family, the nurse contacts the family. It is important to remember that the family gathers information about the nurse from this initial phone call to arrange a meeting, so the nurse should be confident and organized. After the introduction, the nurse concisely states the reason for requesting the family visit and encourages all family members to attend the meeting. The How To Make an Appointment With the Family box reviews steps for making an appointment with the family. Determine if you need an interpreter with you or if you need to arrange to have one available by phone during the visit. Several possible times for the appointment can be offered, including late afternoon or evening, which allows the family to select the most convenient time for all members to be present. It is important to remember that families ultimately retain control of the situation and they do not have to let the nurse enter their home.

HOW TO MAKE AN APPOINTMENT WITH THE FAMILY

Data collection starts immediately upon referral to the nurse. The following are suggestions that will make the process of arranging a meeting with the family easier:

1. Remember that the assessment is reciprocal and the family will be making judgments about you when you call to make the appointment.
2. Introduce yourself and state the purpose for the contact.
3. Do not apologize for contacting the family. Be clear, direct, and specific about the need for an appointment.
4. Arrange a time that is convenient for the greatest possible number of family members.
5. If appropriate, ask if an interpreter will be needed during the meeting.
6. Confirm the place, time, date, and directions.

Planning for Personal Safety

It is critical to plan for your own safety when you make a home visit. Learn about the neighborhood you will be visiting, anticipate the needs you may have, and determine whether it is safe for you to make the home visit alone or if you need to arrange to have a security person with you during the visit. Always have your cell phone fully charged and readily available. The following strategies will help to ensure your safety when you visit families in their homes (Smith, 2009, p. 316; Loftus, 2020):

1. Leave a schedule at your office and stay in touch with the office.
2. Plan the visit during safe times of the day and know exactly where you are going.
3. Dress appropriately; wear little or no jewelry and take little money.
4. Put any valuables in your trunk before you leave for an appointment.
5. Avoid secluded places if you are alone; keep a buffer zone of a car length between you and the car in front of you so you can maneuver if you are in danger.
6. Obtain an escort, a coworker or volunteer if you think there is a need to do so. If you feel unsafe, do not visit.
7. Sit between the client and the exit.
8. Check in with your office at the end of the day.
9. Establish parameters; that is, make it clear that you have a schedule to keep in case you have to leave for any reason.
10. Be aware of who else is in the apartment or house for both confidentiality and safety.
11. Ask about pets if you have allergies; find out if they are friendly or not.
12. Guard your own privacy and pay attention to what you put on social media.

Interviewing the Family: Defining the Problem

It is important to build a trusting family-nurse relationship. Working with families requires nurses to use therapeutic communication efficiently and skillfully by moving between informal conversation and skilled interviewing strategies. Prepare your family questions before your interview based on the best family theory given what is known about the family situation.

Remember that it is important to introduce yourself to the family and initiate conversation with each member present. Spending some initial time on informal conversation helps put the family at ease, allows them time to assess the person or nurse, and disperses some of the tension surrounding the visit (Wright and Leahey, 2019). Involving each family member in the conversation, including children, the elderly, or a disabled family member, demonstrates respect and caring and sends the message that the purpose of the visit is to help the whole family and not just the individual family member.

Shifting the conversation into a more formal interview can be accomplished by asking the family to share their story about the current situation. If the nurse focuses only on the medical aspect or illness story, much valuable information and the priority issue confronting the family may be missed in the data collection. The purpose of the interview is to gather information and help the family focus on their problem and determine solutions. The specific therapeutic questions listed below have been found to provide important family information (Leahey and Svavarsdottir, 2009, p 449):

1. What is the greatest challenge facing your family right now?
2. Who in the family do you think the illness has the most impact on?
3. Who is suffering the most?
4. What has been the most and least helpful to you in similar situations?
5. If there is one question you could have answered, what would it be?
6. How can we best help you and your family?
7. What are your needs/wishes for assistance now?

Box 20.4 lists a variety of additional questions that you might ask. Encourage several members of the family to provide input into the discussion. One strategy is to ask the same question of several different family members. It is critical for the nurse to not take sides in the family discussion and to focus on guiding them in their decision making. In addition to the family story, the nurse will likely need to ask specific assessment questions about the family member who is in need of services.

Designing Family Interventions

Nurses will be challenged to help families identify the primary problem confronting them and to step aside and accept the family priority as they work in partnership with the family to keep their interventions simple, specific, timely, and realistic. It is essential that the family participate in determining the primary need and in designing interventions. As the nurse designs interventions for the family, it is important to consider the health literacy of the client. See Chapter 14 for a discussion of health literacy for individuals and families.

It is important to view the family with an open approach because the central issue identified by the referral source may not be the actual problem the family is experiencing. See the following case study.

❓ CHECK YOUR PRACTICE

The nurse works with the family to help them design realistic steps or a plan of action based on their ability to successfully adapt to the health issue given the strengths of the family. Working with the family, the following action plan approach helps focus the family on things they can do immediately to help address the problem:

1. We need the following type of help.
2. We need the following information.
3. We need the following supplies.
4. We need to involve or tell the following people.
5. We need to list five things in the order in which they need to happen to make our family action plan. Provide examples of these five things.

Using knowledge and evidence-based practice, you would guide the family in outlining ways to prevent a potential problem, minimize the problem, stabilize the problem, or help the family recognize it as a growing problem. How would you use the clinical judgment steps with the Raggs family described below? (1) Recognize the cues; (2) analyze the cues; (3) state several and prioritize hypotheses; (4) generate solutions for each hypothesis; (5) take action on your highest-priority hypothesis; and (6) evaluate the outcomes that you would expect, as well as the outcomes that were achieved.

BOX 20.4 Family Interview Questions

- What do you believe is the most important or pressing issue right now?
- What have you done to improve the situation?
- Share with me your primary goal in the immediate situation.
- What are the main problems you are having related to ____?
- What is causing you the most stress?
- How has this stress affected you and the members of your family?
- How are the everyday needs of the family getting done (e.g., cooking, shopping, cleaning, laundry, transportation, sleeping)?
- How well is your family managing this stress?
- What results or outcomes do you hope for?
- What do you feel you need to help solve this situation?
- What can your family do for you?
- Who do we need to involve in this situation?
- What information do you need to know?
- Walk me through a typical 24-h day in your home.

- During times of need, where can you go for support and resources?
- What do you think would help me better understand what you are experiencing?
- How does your family anticipate caring for ____?
- How does this situation affect you financially?
- Where, how, and from whom do you receive your support, inspiration, and energy to maintain the responsibilities required of you?
- What has been the biggest surprise to you about all of this?
- How do you think your family roles and routines are going to change in this situation?
- How have you and your family prepared to provide care for ____?
- What are your family plans for when you have to return to work?
- What does your family do to feel relief or take a break?
- What are some specific changes that you and your family members have had to make?
- What do you fear the most about ____?

CASE STUDY

A physician refers the Raggs family to the home health clinic for medication management. Sam, the 73-year-old husband, has had diabetes for 13 years and has developed type 1 diabetes mellitus. He is being discharged from the hospital. The potential area of concern that prompted the referral was the administration of insulin. After the initial meeting with the family, the primary problem the family uncovers is really not the administration of the medication, but managing his nutrition. The inference of the referral source was that the family knew how to manage the dietary aspects of diabetes because Sam has had a form of diabetes for 13 years.

If the primary family issue is not accurately identified, the family and the nurse will collect data, design interventions, and implement plans of care that do not meet the most pressing family needs. The importance of identifying the family issue of concern and accurately making the **family nursing diagnosis** is demonstrated by comparing the following two scenarios:

Scenario 1: The hypothesized central issue for the Raggs family was identified by the referral source: Is insulin being administered correctly? Based on this question from the referral source, the nurse asked only for information pertaining to this specific problem. The nurse asked questions that elicited information about the following:

Concerns of giving injections including drawing up the exact amount of insulin and how to store the insulin.

The nurse focused the interventions on:

1. The psychomotor skills of family members necessary to give the insulin injection
2. The correct amount of insulin to give according to blood glucose level
3. The correct storage and handling of the medication and the equipment. By not looking at the whole family, the care was based on the nurse's perception of the problem confronting the family.

Scenario 2: The central question asked by a nurse who knows how to integrate family theory into practice was, "What is the best way to ensure that the Raggs family understands how to manage the new diagnosis of type 1 diabetes mellitus?" By asking the family to share their story of the situation together, they determined that the primary issue was not medication administration but rather a lack of family knowledge related to health care management of a family member who has been newly diagnosed with type 1 diabetes mellitus.

Asking broader-based questions uncovers the whole picture of the family dealing with this specific health concern and directs a more comprehensive holistic data-collection process. More evidence was collected in this case scenario because more options for possible interventions were considered concurrently. Areas of data collection based on the whole family story were as follows:

1. Administration of medication
2. Nutritional management
3. Blood glucose monitoring
4. Activity/exercise
5. Coping with a changed diagnosis
6. Knowledge of pathophysiology of diabetes

The following scenario shows how nurses work with families to determine their strengths, identify the problem, and design interventions.

Scenario 3: The home hospice nurse has been working with the Brush family for 3 weeks. The Brush family consists of Dylan (father), Myra (mother), William (10 years of age), Jessica (7 years of age), and Beatrice (maternal grandmother, 73 years of age).

Beatrice was diagnosed with terminal liver cancer 4 weeks ago. The Brush family—Beatrice, Dylan, Myra, William, and Jessica—agreed that Beatrice should live with them and be cared for until her death in their home. Beatrice has other children who live in the same city. The hospice nurse, in collaboration with the Brush family, identified that the primary problem is that Myra is experiencing role stress, strain, and overload in her new role as the family caregiver. Myra showed her role conflict by stating, "Sometimes I do not know who I am— daughter, nurse, mother, or wife." Myra took a family leave from her job to stay home to care for her mother. Some family members were surprised by her statement because they did not realize she was so overwhelmed. The family worked with the nurse to find ways to minimize Myra's role strain by spreading the caregiver role among the extended family members.

By understanding family systems theory, you know that what affects one family member affects all family members. One of the strengths this family has is the shared belief that caring for the dying grandmother in their home is the "right" ethical choice for them. The nurse brings knowledge and evidence into this situation because the nurse knows that the disruption to the family and their expected roles will be short term because the grandmother will probably not live for more than 4 months. However, experience with families also supports the nurse's knowledge that Myra's role conflict may likely increase when her caregiver role becomes more intense as her mother's health declines. A strength of this family is uncovered: It has a strong internal and external support system. The family determines that the extended family is willing to be involved in the care of Beatrice. The intervention is aimed at mobilizing resources to minimize Myra's role conflict. Using the simple action plan outlined previously, the family determined the following:

1. We need the following type of help:
   - Other family members will come every day to relieve Myra.
   - Every other weekend, one of Beatrice's other daughters (Sally or Peggy) will provide care through the night to relieve Myra.
   - Jobs in the family will be shared to relieve Myra. Dylan will do the shopping, William will clear the table and put dishes in the dishwasher, and Jessica will help fold the clothes and put them away. William and Jessica agreed to help by spending some time each evening with Beatrice, such as reading to her or watching TV with her.
2. We need the following information:
   - How to call the hospice nurse when Beatrice gets worse or when we need immediate help
   - A list of who to call when an emergency occurs
   - A list with names and numbers of Beatrice's health care team
3. We need the following supplies: None at this time
4. We need to involve or tell the following people: Sally and Peggy
5. To make our family action plan happen, we need to . . . (list five things in the order in which they need to happen):
   - Invite Sally and Peggy over for a family meeting and include the home hospice nurse.
   - Make a list of what weekends Sally and Peggy will help with Beatrice.
   - Make a calendar with whose turn it is to spend time with Beatrice every evening, which will relieve Myra of the care.

Based on the family story just described, as viewed through the frame of family systems theory, the following interventions were implemented:

1. Assisting the family in the role negotiation of tasks and who performs them.
2. Educating family members so they can safely care for Beatrice now and when she enters the stage of active dying.
3. Determining what additional resources the family needs. After a plan is put into place, it needs to be evaluated periodically.

Of all of these problems, the nurse worked with the family to help them identify that their major concern centered on nutritional management, which ultimately affects the administration of medication.

The major difference between the two scenarios presented here was the way in which the nurse framed questions while listening to the family story. In the first scenario, the nurse asked questions that allowed for consideration of only one aspect of family health. This type of step-by-step, nurse-led, linear problem-solving process is tedious and time consuming, and will likely cause errors in the identification of the most pressing family concern. In the second scenario, the nurse asked questions that allowed for critical thinking about the family view of their challenges. The nurse gathered information from the referral source, conducted an assessment of the impact of the new diagnosis on the whole family, and collaboratively the nurse and family identified the critical family issue that had a more far-reaching effect on the health of the whole family.

Evaluation of the Plan

In evaluating the outcome, nurses use critical thinking to determine whether the plan is working. When the plan is not working, the nurse and the family work together to determine the barriers interfering with the plan or determine if something changed in the family story. Family apathy and indecision are known to be barriers in family nursing (Friedman et al., 2003). Friedman and colleagues also identified the following nurse-related barriers that can affect achievement of the outcome:

1. Nurse-imposed ideas
2. Negative labeling
3. Overlooking family strengths
4. Neglecting cultural or gender implications

Family apathy may occur when there are value differences between the nurse and family; the family is overcome with a sense of hopelessness; the family views the problems as too overwhelming; or family members fear failure. Additional factors must be considered because family members may be indecisive for the following reasons:

- They cannot determine which course of action is better.
- They have an unexpressed fear or concern.
- They have a pattern of making decisions only when faced with a crisis.

An important part of the judgment step in working with families is the decision to terminate the relationship between the nurse and family. Termination is phasing out the nurse from family involvement. When termination is built into the interventions, the family benefits from a smooth transition process. The family is given credit for the outcomes of the interventions that they helped design. Strategies often used in the termination component are as follows: (1) decreasing contact with the nurse; (2) extending invitations to the family for follow-up; and (3) making referrals when appropriate. The termination should include a summative evaluation meeting in which the nurse and family put a formal closure to their relationship.

When termination with a family occurs suddenly, the nurse needs to determine the forces bringing about the closure. The family may be initiating the termination prematurely, which requires a renegotiating process. The insurance or agency requirements may be placing a financial constraint on the amount of time the nurse can work with a family. Regardless of how termination comes about, it is important to recognize the transition from depending on the nurse on some level to having no dependence. Strategies that help with the termination are as follows: (1) increase the time between the nurse's visits; (2) develop a transition plan; (3) assess the family support systems; (4) make referrals to other resource; and (5) provide a written summary to the family.

SOCIAL AND FAMILY POLICY CHALLENGES

National, state, and local social and family policies provide challenges to nurses' practice. As professionals, public health nurses are accountable for participating in the three core public health functions: assessment, policy development, and assurance.

National family policy refers to government actions that have a direct or indirect effect on families. The range of social policy decisions that affect families is vast, such as health care access and coverage, low-income housing, Social Security, welfare, food stamps, pension plans, affirmative action, and education. Although all government polices affect families in both negative and positive ways, the United States has little overall explicit family policy (Coehlo et al., 2018). Most government policy indirectly affects families. The Family Medical Leave legislation passed in 1993 by the US Congress is an example of a type of family policy that has been positive for families. A family member may take a defined amount of leave for family events (e.g., births, deaths) without fear of losing his or her job. Despite its controversial introduction, many programs exist for families, such as Social Security, Head Start, and the Healthy Marriage Initiative. Another beneficial program is Temporary Assistance to Needy Families. Not all programs are available to all families. State assistance for families varies by state. Also, learn how the Affordable Care Act affects families.

The challenges of social policy for families are numerous. Given the ongoing debate as to what constitutes a family, social policies may specify a definition that is not consistent with the family's own definition. Examples include same-sex partnerships and marriage, legal definition of parents, reproductive and fertility issues (e.g., a surrogate mother decides she wants to keep the baby), or issues involving care of older adults (e.g., a niece wants to institutionalize an older aunt with dementia because her children are not available). Besides how families define themselves, governments define health care services that affect families.

Teen pregnancy prevention is a monitored health status throughout the United States and a good example of the challenges of family health policy. In some states, any child who is sexually active may have access to reproductive health services. This is a family policy to which some families object, yet the sexually active teenager is protected by laws, both state and federal. The teenager who requests confidential services is protected by Title X and the Health Insurance Portability and Accountability Act (HIPAA) federal regulations, given the state law allowing access to services. Providers can encourage teens to talk with their parents, but ultimately it is the teen's decision. Nurses need to know about these policies because they participate in carrying out family policy and have a responsibility to inform state policy regarding the services they provide.

Nurses participate in enforcing laws and regulations that affect the family, such as state immunization laws. Most states have some school immunization laws that exclude from school children who are not vaccinated. If the child does not have that particular set of immunizations and the parents do not want the child vaccinated, two sets of laws are in conflict—the immunization laws and the school attendance laws. The state could provide a mechanism for a waiver or the child could be excluded from school, thus making home schooling the only option.

Health care insurance is a social and family policy issue. Medicare and Medicaid, enacted in 1965, provide some health care for the elderly and low-income families. Today Medicare covers nearly 44 million beneficiaries with enrollments expected to rise to 79 million by 2030 (CMS, 2018). Both living wills and durable powers of attorney for health care, legal contracts that designate a person to make health care decisions when the individual is incapacitated, are more commonplace today than in the past. However, without these legal instruments, families are faced with making end-of-life decisions for their loved ones. Although Medicare and Medicaid provide health care to many, a significant population is still uninsured. Emergency departments continue to be the only access to health care for the uninsured and a convenient and accessible source of health care for many without access to a health care provider (Marco et al., 2012).

The H1N1 pandemic was an excellent example of mobilizing community partnerships to solve health problems. In one county health department, space for storing vaccines was insufficient in the county health clinics, so arrangements were made with the law enforcement departments to store vaccines in their secure evidence refrigerators. Other examples of partnering included collaboration with Health and Human Services departments and homeless programs to get at-risk populations and the homeless vaccinated. County health departments and pediatricians worked together to vaccinate members of families who had infants under six months of age, since these infants were too young to receive the H1N1 vaccine.

Similarly, during the COVID-19 pandemic, many for-profit companies partnered with state or national governments to provide testing for the virus. For example, CVS, the drug store chain, partnered early in the pandemic to provide highly organized drive-through testing centers. Also, many hospitals partnered with local health departments to give the vaccines. Often firefighters and members of the military worked beside nurses to provide injections.

These are only a few examples of social and family policy in which nurses are involved. Population-focused nurses need to be involved at the state, local, and national level in making policy that affects families. Using the core public health functions as a framework allows the population-focused nurse to view the broad spectrum of activities that improve the lives of communities, families, and the individuals within those families.

HEALTHY PEOPLE 2030 AND FAMILY IMPLICATIONS

Although *Healthy People 2030* emphasizes individual and community issues, some objectives relate specifically to families or homes, as shown in the *Healthy People 2030* box.

 HEALTHY PEOPLE 2030

Objectives Specific to Families and Family Nursing

- AH-03: Increase the proportion of adolescents who have an adult they can talk to about serious problems.
- MICG-17: Increase the proportion of children who receive a developmental screening.
- FP-09: Increase the proportion of women who get needed publicly funded birth control services and support.

From US Department of Health and Human Services: *Healthy People 2030*, Washington, DC, 2020, US Government Printing Office.

▶▶ **APPLYING CONTENT TO PRACTICE**

This chapter describes how nurses and families work together to ensure the success of the family and its members in adapting to responses to health and illness. Family nursing is linked to several foundational public health nursing documents. The Quad Council's Coalition of Public Health Nursing Organizations (2018) *Community/Public Health Nursing Competencies* clarifies that one of the assumptions of the document is that although PHNs engage in population-focused practice, they can and often do apply public health concepts at the individual and family level. The Public Health Nurse Intervention Wheel identifies "Individuals/Families" as one of the three levels of public health practice (Public Health Nursing Section, 2001). Within that level, the focus of nursing practice is to change knowledge, attitudes, beliefs, practices, and behaviors of individuals, either alone or as part of a family, class, or group. The American Nurses Association's (2013) *Public Health Nursing: Scope and Standards of Practice* lists the following competencies related to family nursing:

- The public health nurse incorporates individual and/or family care management to include broad community coordination of public health services (Standard 5A: Coordination of Care).
- The public health nurse describes how individual, family, group, and community-focused programs contribute to meeting the core public health foundations and the 10 essential public health services (Standard 8: Education).
- The public health nurse abides by the vision, the associated goals, and the plan to implement and measure progress of an individual, family, community, or population (Standard 12: Leadership).

■ PRACTICE APPLICATION

The idealized family portrayed in the media during the 20th century consists of a working father, a mother who stays home, and their children. Many families today compare their turbulent, hectic lives with those of the fictionalized past and find their situations wanting.

A. Did the idealized version of the traditional family ever really exist?
B. Some people believe that American families are in decline, whereas others believe that families are healthy. What do you think?

C. What seems to be happening with the definition of American families?

D. How does a definition of family influence our care and society's support of families?
Answers can be found on the Evolve website.

REMEMBER THIS!

- Families are the context within which health care decisions are made. Nurses are responsible for assisting families in meeting health care needs.
- Family nursing is practiced in all settings.
- Family nursing is a specialty area that has a strong theoretical base.
- Family demographics is the study of structures of families and households, as well as events that alter the family, such as marriage, divorce, births, cohabitation, and dual careers.
- Demographic trends affecting the family include the age of individuals when they marry, an increase in interracial marriages with subsequent children, an increase in the number of divorced individuals remarrying, an increase in dual-career marriages, an increase in the number of children from families in which marriage is disrupted, a large increase in the divorce rate, a dramatic increase in cohabitation, an increase in the number of children who spend time in a single-parent family, a delay of childbirth, an increase in the number of children born to women who are single or who have never married, and an increase in the number of children who live with grandparents.
- Traditionally, families have been defined as a nuclear family: mother, father, and children. A variety of family definitions exist, such as a group of two or more, a unique social group, and two or more individuals joined together by emotional bonds.
- The six historical functions performed by families are economic survival, reproduction, protection, cultural heritage, socialization of young, and conferring status. Contemporary functions involve relationships and health.
- Family structure refers to the characteristics, gender, age, and number of the individual members who make up the family unit.
- Family health is difficult to define, but it includes the biological, psychological, sociological, cultural, and spiritual factors of the family system.
- The four approaches to viewing families are family as context, family as a client, family as a system, and family as a component of society.
- Nurses should ask clients whom they consider to be family and then include those members in the health care plan.
- The purpose of the initial family interview is based on the identified issue.
- It is important for the nurse to recognize that the family has the right to make its own health care decisions.
- Nurses who work with families must evaluate the family outcomes and response to the plan, not the success of the interventions.
- The future of the family, health care, and nursing is not an exact science. However, all areas are changing and many challenges are to be understood and overcome in this new century.

EVOLVE WEBSITE

http://evolve.elsevier.com/Stanhope/foundations
- Case Study, with Questions and Answers
- NCLEX Review Questions
- Practice Application Answers

REFERENCES

American Nurses Association: *Public health nursing: scope and standards of practice*, ed 2, Silver Spring, MD, 2013, ANA.

American Nurses Association: *Essential of genetic and genomic nursing: Competences, curricula guidelines, and outcome indicators*, 2 ed, 2008, Silver Spring, MD, author.

Bomar PJ: *Nurses and family health promotion: concepts, assessment, and interventions*, ed 3, Philadelphia, PA, 2004, Saunders.

Bronfenbrenner U: *Influences on human development*, Hinsdale, Ill, 1972, Dryden Press.

Bronfenbrenner U: *The ecology of human development*, Cambridge, Mass, 1979, Harvard University Press.

Bronfrenbrenner U: Ecology of the family as a context for human development: research perspectives. In Paul JL, Churton M, Rosselli-Kostoryz H, et al: *Foundations of special education*, Pacific Grove, Calif, 1997, Brooks/Cole.

Centers for Disease Control and Prevention: Overweight & Obesity: Adult obesity facts, Retrieved May 2020 at https://www.cdc.gov/obesity/

Centers for Medicare & Medicaid Services (CMS): *CMS fast facts*, July 2018. Available at: https://www.cms.gov/Research-Statistics-Data-and-Systems/Statistics-Trends-and-Reports/CMS-Fast-Facts/index.html. Accessed September 11, 2018.

Coehlo DP, Henderson TL, Lester C: Family policy: the intersection of family policies, health disparities, and health care policies. In Kaakinen JR, Coehlo DP, Steele R, Robinson M, eds: *Family health care nursing: theory, practice, and research*, ed 6, Philadephia, PA, 2018, F.A. Davis, pp. 83–112.

Cohen PN: *The family: diversity, inequality, and social change*, New York, 2018, Norton.

Duvall EM, Miller BL: *Marriage and family development*, ed 6, New York, 1985, Harper & Row.

Eddy L, Bailey A, Doutrich D: Families and community and public health nursing. In Kaakinen JR, Coehlo DP, Steele R, Robinson M, editors: *Family health care nursing: theory, practice, and research*, ed 6, Philadelphia, PA, 2018, F.A. Davis.

Friedman MM, Bowden VR, Jones EG: *Family nursing: research, theory and practice*, ed 5, Upper Saddle River, NJ, 2003, Prentice Hall.

Hanson SMH: Family health care nursing: an overview. In Hanson SMH, Gedaly-Duff V, Kaakinen JR, eds: *Family health care nursing: theory, practice and research*, ed 3, Philadelphia, PA, 2005, F.A. Davis.

Kaakinen JR: Family health care nursing: an introduction. In Kaakinen JR, Coehlo DP, Steele R, Robinson M, eds: *Family health care nursing: theory, practice, and research*, ed 6, Philadephia, PA, 2018a, F.A. Davis.

Kaakinen JR: Theoretical foundations for the nursing of families. In Kaakinen JR, Coehlo DP, Steele R, Robinson M, eds: *Family health care nursing: theory, practice, and research*, ed 6, Philadelphia, PA, 2018b, F.A. Davis.

Kaakinen JR: Family nursing assessment and intervention. In Kaakinen JR, Coehlo DP, Steele R, Robinson M, eds: *Family health care* nursing: theory, practice, and research, ed 6. Philadelphia, PA, 2018c, F.A. Davis.

Kim-Godwin YS, Bomar PJ: Family health promotion. In Kaakinen JR, Coehlo DP, Steele R, Robinson M, eds: *Family health care nursing: theory, practice, and research*, ed 5, Philadelphia, PA, 2015, F.A. Davis.

Leahey M, Svavarsdottir EK: Implementing family nursing: how do we translate knowledge into clinical practice? *J Fam Nurs* 15: 445–460, 2009.

Loftus TD: *How to stay safe during home visits*, Retrieved May 11, 2020 at https://www.crisisprevention.com/blog.how-to-stay-safe

Marco CA, Moskop JC, Schears RM, et al: The ethics of health care reform: impact on emergency medicine, *Acad Emerg Med* 19(4):461–468, 2012.

McGoldrick M, Preto NAG, Carter BA, eds: *The expanded family life cycle: individual, family and social perspectives*, ed 5, New York, 2015, Pearson.

National Human Genome Research Institute: *A brief guide to genomics: DNA, Genes and Genomes*, 2015a. Retrieved from https://www.genome.gov/18016863/a-brief-guide-to-genomics/

National Human Genome Research Institute: *All about the human genome project(HGP)*, 2015b. Retrieved from https://www.genome.gov/10001772/all-about-the—human-genome-project-hgp/

National Human Genome Research Institute: *Specific genetic disorders*, 2018a. Retrieved from https://www.genome.gov, May 2020.

National Human Genome Research Institute: *Genetic terms: Mutagen*, 2018b. Retrieved from https://www.genome.gov, May 2020.

National Cancer Institute: *Genetic testing for hereditary cancer susceptibility syndromes*, 2019. Retrieved from https://www.cancer.gov, May 2020.

Ogden CL, Carroll MD, Fakhouri TH, et al., *MMWR Morb Mortal Wkly Rep*, 2018:67:186-188.

Pelletier LR, Stichler JF: Action brief: patient engagement and activation: a health reform imperative and improvement opportunity for nurses, *Nurs Outlook* 61:51–54, 2013.

Public Health Nursing Section: *Public Health Interventions: applications for public health nursing practice*, St. Paul, Minnesota, 2001, Minnesota Department of Health.

Quad Council Coalition of Public Health Nursing Organizations: *Community/public health nursing competencies*, Washington, DC, 2014, Public Health Foundation.

Smith CM: Home visit: opening the doors for family health. In Maurer FA, Smith CM, eds: *Community public health nursing practice: health for families and populations*, ed 4, St. Louis, MO, 2009, Saunders, pp 302–326.

White JM, Klein DN, Martin TF: *Family theories: an introduction*, ed 4, Thousand Oaks, Calif, 2015, Sage Publications.

Wright LM, Leahey M: *Nurses and families: a guide to family assessment and intervention*, ed 7, Philadelphia, 2019, F.A. Davis.

21

Family Health Risks

Mollie E. Aleshire, Kacy Allen-Bryant, and Debra Gay Anderson

OBJECTIVES

After reading this chapter, the student should be able to:

1. Analyze the various approaches to defining and conceptualizing family health.
2. Determine the major risks to family health.
3. Identify the interrelationships among individual health, family health, population health, and a community's health.
4. Explain the relevance of knowledge about structures, roles, and functions for family- and population-focused nursing.
5. Discuss the implications of policy and policy decisions, at all government levels, on families and populations.
6. Explain the application of the nursing process and the use of clinical judgment to reducing family health risks and promoting family health.

CHAPTER OUTLINE

KEY TERMS

What is a "family?" Is there one definition that fits all families? Is there a new normal? Was there ever a true "normal" family? Rather than settling for a universal definition, it seems more appropriate to define families according to the particular issue involved (Purdue University, 2015).

Since the 1960s there has been an evolution of family structure, which includes "more unmarried couples raising children; more gay and lesbian couples raising children; more single women having children without a male partner to help raise them; more people living together without getting married; more mothers of young children working outside the home; more people of different races marrying each other; and more women not ever having children" (Livingston, Pew Research Center, 2018).

A nation's family health care policy is a primary determinant of family health. Family policy means anything done by the government that directly or indirectly affects families. Family health policy and its relative effectiveness demonstrates a government's understanding of families and its role in promoting their health, with an important desired outcome being that families derive a sense of empowerment and are able to take responsibility for their own health (KFF, 2018). The responsibility for family health programs is shared by the federal government with state and local governments. Each state, as well as each region within states, has programs and laws related to family services. Although the United States is an affluent and technologically advanced country, many disparities remain in health status between different populations of families (Families USA, 2015). These disparities have resulted, at least in part, from previous attempts to develop and implement "family policies" that either directly or indirectly affect specific issues related to family health but which have failed to take a comprehensive system-wide approach.

Although many disparities and inequities continue in the United States, the health care disparities related to health insurance coverage have decreased as a result of the Patient Protection and Affordable Care Act (ACA) as more low-income families and families of color have gained health insurance coverage (Artiga et al., 2017). At the 2014 Health Action Conference, Families USA, then-Vice President Joe Biden spoke of the importance of the ACA (discussed throughout this text) and the importance of the ACA for families in the United States. The specific benefits he highlighted were the coverage of pre-existing conditions, mental health coverage, the disparity in the cost of insurance for women and men, the more than three million young adults on their parents' insurance policies, and not receiving medical care simply because one does not have insurance (Biden, 2014). In 2017, federal legislation eliminated the ACA's individual health insurance mandate, which is predicted to negatively affect the health insurance coverage and cost of insurance for families (Congressional Budget Office, 2017). Nursing has a rich history in social activism and social justice which should be continued, emphasizing advocacy and policy work to help families and communities become healthier for all populations.

The United States could benefit from a cohesive family policy designed to improve the health and well-being of all families. Such a policy could help prevent future crises in vulnerable family populations, such as those in or on the verge of poverty or families overwhelmed with abuse and neglect, by providing a safety net to help families maintain their health in times of disaster, economic downturns, unemployment, health crises, and other situations. An effective family health policy might begin with developing an infrastructure of programs designed to provide access to primary and preventive health care. Nurses would be key builders of this process. Nurses who are educated in community assessment, planning, development, and evaluation activities that can help promote and maintain primary family health should be key builders in this process.

In establishing health objectives for the nation, an emphasis has been placed on both health promotion and risk reduction. Reducing the risks to segments of the population is a direct way to improve the health of the general population. Objectives have been identified related to specific health risks for families. The family is an important aggregate that affects the health of individuals, as well as a social unit whose health is basic to that of the community and the larger population. It is within the family that health values, health habits, and health risk perceptions are developed, organized, and carried out. Individuals' health behaviors are affected by and acted out within the family environment, the larger community, and society. Family health habits are developed in the same manner in the context of community norms and values and on the basis of availability and accessibility. For example, in a television commercial for an over-the-counter stimulant, a man is featured who is able to coach his child's basketball team, work at a rehabilitation center, and work as a borough inspector for the city, all while pursuing a college degree at night. The commercial credits the drug for providing the man with the energy needed to be successful in all of these areas. The message is clear: You can, and must, do it all, and taking drugs to succeed is a viable option. The health risks to individual and family health are affected by societal norms—in this example, the norm is increasing productivity through drugs, and this is not a message that is conducive to good family health care.

To intervene effectively and appropriately with families to reduce their health risk and thereby promote their health, it is necessary to understand family structure and functioning, family theory, nursing theory, and models of health risk. Additionally, it is necessary to go beyond the individual and the family and understand the complex environment in which the family exists. Increasing evidence of the effects of social, biological, economic, and life events on health requires a broader approach to addressing health risks for families. Chapters in this book address these risk factors.

In this chapter, family health risks and approaches to reducing these risks are discussed. Options for structuring nursing interventions with families to decrease health risks and promote health and well-being are discussed.

EARLY APPROACHES TO FAMILY HEALTH RISKS

Health of Families

Historically, studies of the family in health and illness focused on the following three major areas: (1) the effect of illness on families, (2) the role of the family in the cause of disease, and (3) the role of the family in its use of services. In his classic review of the family as an important unit, Litman (1974) pointed out the important role that the family (as a primary unit of health care) plays in health and illness and emphasized that the relationships among health, health behavior, and family "is a highly dynamic one in which each may have a dramatic effect on the other" (p. 495). Mauksch (1974) proposed the idea of distinguishing between family health and individual health.

Pratt's (1976) examination of the role of the family in health and illness included the role of the family in promoting healthy behavior. Pratt proposed the *energized family* as being an ideal family type that was most effective in meeting health needs. The energized family is characterized as one that promotes freedom and change, is actively engaged with a variety of other groups and organizations, has flexible role relationships and an equal power structure, and exhibits a high degree of autonomy in family members. Doherty and McCubbin (1985) proposed a family health and illness cycle comprising six phases beginning with family health promotion and risk reduction and continuing through the family's vulnerability to illness, their illness response, their interaction with the health care system, and finally their ways of adapting to illness. This framework continues to be relevant today in caring for families.

Health of the Nation

Increased attention has been given to improving the health of everyone in the United States. As a result of major public health and scientific advances, the leading causes of morbidity and mortality have shifted from infectious diseases to chronic diseases, accidents, and violence, all of which have strong lifestyle and environmental components. A population-focused study in Alameda County, California (Belloc et al., 1972) demonstrated relationships between the following seven lifestyle habits and decreased morbidity and mortality. These habits that were identified in 1972 remain beneficial today for health promotion. They include (1) sleeping 7 to 8 hours a day, (2) eating breakfast almost every day, (3) never or rarely eating between meals, (4) being at or near the recommended height-adjusted weight, (5) never smoking cigarettes, (6) never or rarely drinking alcohol, and (7) regularly participating in physical activity.

The Alameda study has been supported by Dan Buettner's (2009) work with the National Geographic Society and their examination of communities around the world who have not only longevity, but quality of life. Public health nurses (PHNs) will want to read *The Blue Zones: 9 Lessons for Living Longer* for in-depth case studies. The nine lessons include the following:

1. Move naturally: Be active without thinking about it;
2. Hara Hachi Bu: Painlessly cut calories by 20%;
3. Plant slant: Avoid meat and processed foods;
4. Grapes of life: Drink red wine in moderation;
5. Purpose now: Take time to see the big picture;
6. Downshift: Take time to relieve stress;
7. Belong: Participate in a spiritual community;
8. Loved ones first: Make family a priority; and
9. Right tribe: Be surrounded by those who share Blue Zone values (Buettner, 2008–2018).

Considerable evidence supports the belief that lifestyle and the environment interact with heredity to cause disease. In response to these findings and the limited effect of medical interventions on the growing numbers of injuries and chronic disease, the government launched a major effort to study the health status of the population. Part of this effort was a report by the Division of Health Promotion and Disease Prevention of the Institute of Medicine that examined how the physical, socioeconomic, and

family environments related to decreasing risk and promoting health (Nightingale et al., 1978). The Surgeon General's Report on Health Promotion and Disease Prevention (Califano, 1979) described the risks to good health. Health objectives for the nation were established and then evaluated and restated for the years 2000, 2010, 2020, and 2030.

The concept of risk, which refers to a factor predisposing or increasing the likelihood of ill health, is important in family health. It is important to pay attention to the environmental and behavioral factors that lead to ill health with or without the influence of heredity. Reducing health risks is a major step toward improving the health of the nation. Although the family is considered an important environment related to achieving important health objectives, limited attention has been given to (or research done on) family health risk and the role of society in promoting healthy families.

 HEALTHY PEOPLE 2030

These objectives are related to housing and homes and promoting healthy and safe home environments:

TU 18: Increase the proportion of smoke-free homes

DH 04: Increase the proportion of homes that have an entrance without steps

MICH 19: Increase the proportion of children and adolescents who receive care in a medical home

MHMD R01: Increase the proportion of homeless adults with mental health problems who get mental health services

EH 04: Reduce blood lead levels in children aged 1–5 years

SDOH 04: Reduce the proportion of families that spend more than 30% of income on housing

From US Department of Health and Human Services: *Healthy People 2030,* Washington, DC, 2020, US Government Printing Office.

CONCEPTS IN FAMILY HEALTH RISK

The Health Promotion Model developed in 2019 states that two factors motivate individuals to engage in positive health behaviors. One is a desire to promote one's own health using behaviors that can increase the well-being of the individual, family, community, and populations, and in the process, be able to move toward not only individual self-actualization but also population actualization. The second factor is a desire to protect health, using those same behaviors in an effort to decrease the probability of ill health and provide active protection against illness and dysfunction in families (Murdaugh, 2019). A person can reduce health risk by participating in health-protecting and health-promoting behavior. It is important to understand the following seven concepts: family health, family health risk, risk appraisal, risk reduction, life events, lifestyle, and family crisis. These concepts will be defined and discussed. It is important to remember that *health* can be defined in various ways and that it is defined by individuals based on their own culture and value system.

Family Health

Family theorists refer to healthy families but generally do not define family health (White et al., 2015). Based on the variety of perspectives of family, definitions of healthy families can be seen within the guidelines of any one framework. For example, within the developmental framework, family health can be defined as having the abilities and resources to accomplish family developmental tasks. Thus the accomplishment of stage-specific tasks is one indicator of family health.

❓ CHECK YOUR PRACTICE

As a student in public health nursing, you have been assigned to work with a group of families in a low-income community in your city. Your assessment indicates that these families are not accomplishing their stage-specific tasks, which may affect their family health. What would you do to assist these families as a community to work toward improved family health? The following are the steps to use in making a clinical judgment. See if you can apply these steps to this scenario. (1) Recognize the cues from the family on how to improve their health; (2) analyze the cues; (3) state several and prioritize the hypotheses you have stated; (4) generate solutions for each hypothesis; (5) take action on the number one hypothesis you think will work; and (6) evaluate the outcomes you will be looking for improvements in the family's health.

Because the family unit is a part of many societal systems, the systems perspective can explain many family health concepts and actions. Using the Neuman Systems Model (Beckman and Fawcett, 2017), family health is defined in terms of system stability as characterized by five interacting sets of factors: physiological, psychological, sociocultural, developmental, and spiritual. The client family is seen as a whole system with the five interacting factors. The Neuman Systems Model is a wellness-oriented model in which the nurse uses the strengths and resources of the family to maintain system stability while adjusting to stress reactions that may lead to health change and affect wellness. In other words, this model focuses on family wellness in the face of change. Because change is inevitable in every family, the Neuman Systems Model proposes that families have a flexible external line of defense, a normal line of defense, and an internal line of resistance. When a life event is big enough to contract the flexible line of defense (a protective mechanism) and breaks through the normal line of defense, the family feels stress. The degree of wellness is determined by the amount of energy it takes for the system to become and remain stable. When more energy is available than is being used, the system remains stable. Examples of energy-building characteristics in this system are social support, resources, and prevention (or avoidance) of stressors. Nurses can use preventive health care to both reduce the possibility that a family encounters a stressor and help strengthen the family's flexible line of defense. The following clinical example illustrates the application of the Neuman Systems Model to one family's situation.

The Harris family consists of Ms. Harris (Gloria), 12-year-old Kevin, 8-year-old Leisha, and Ms. Harris's mother, 75-year-old Betty. Kevin was recently diagnosed with type 2 diabetes mellitus, and the family was referred by the endocrinology clinic to the local health department to work with the family in adjusting to the diagnosis.

The focus of the Neuman Systems Model would be to assess the family's ability to adapt to this stressful change (the diagnosis of type 2 diabetes mellitus) and then focus on their strengths to stabilize the family reaction. The answers to questions about the following *five interacting variables* would be an important component of the assessment:

1. **Physiological:** Is the Harris family physically able to deal with Kevin's illness?
   Is everyone else in the family currently healthy? Are there current health stressors?
2. **Psychological:** How well will the family be able to deal with the illness psychologically?
   Are their relationships stable and healthy? Are there any memories of other family members with diabetes?
3. **Sociocultural:** How will the sociocultural variable come into play in Kevin's illness?
   Does the family have social support? Are the treatment and diagnosis culturally sensitive? Can family members support each other?
4. **Developmental:** How will Kevin's development as a preadolescent be affected by diabetes? How will the family's development change? How will Kevin's diagnosis affect Leisha?
5. **Spiritual:** How will the family's spiritual beliefs be affected by the diagnosis? What effect will they have on Kevin's treatment and willingness to adhere to therapy?

Health Risk

Several factors contribute to the development of healthy or unhealthy outcomes. Clearly, not everyone exposed to the same event will have the same outcome. The factors that determine or influence whether disease or other unhealthy results occur are called health risks. Control of health risks is done through disease prevention and health promotion efforts. Health risks can be classified into three general categories: (1) inherited biological risks (including age-related risks), (2) environmental risks (composed of social factors, economic, and physical environments), and (3) behavioral risks (USDHHS, 2010). These three categories of risk are discussed later in terms of family health risk, under Major Family Health Risks and Nursing Interventions (USDHHS, 2010).

Although single risk factors can influence outcomes, the combined effect of accumulated risks is often greater than the sum of the individual effects. For example, a family history of cardiovascular disease is a single biological risk factor that is exacerbated by smoking (a behavioral risk that is more likely to occur if other family members also smoke). This risk factor can also be affected either positively or negatively by diet and exercise. Diet and exercise are influenced both by family and society's norms. Although the demographics may be changing, residents of the Northwest and West have historically been more likely to eat heart-healthy diets and to exercise compared with people who live in the Midwest and South; thus, communities in the Northwest and West are often more supportive of exercise programs, bicycle paths, and diets lower in fat than communities in other parts of the United States. This example illustrates how the combined effect of a family history, family behavioral risks, and society's influences is more than just the sum of the three individual behavioral risk factors (smoking, diet, and exercise) and demonstrates how a nurse working with populations of families and intervening within a community is more likely to reduce the effects of the health risks overall and produce a healthier community as well as a healthier family unit.

Health Risk Appraisal

Health risk appraisal refers to the process of assessing for the presence of specific factors in each of the categories that have been identified as being associated with an increased likelihood of an illness, such as cancer, or an unhealthy event, such as an automobile accident. Several techniques have been developed to accomplish health risk appraisal, including computer software programs and paper-and-pencil instruments. One technique is the Youth Risk Behavior Surveillance System instrument (YRBSS) of the Centers for Disease Control and Prevention (2017). This system monitors priority health-risk behaviors and the prevalence of obesity and asthma among youth and young adults. The general approach is to determine whether a risk factor is present and to what degree. On the basis of scientific evidence, each factor is weighted and a total score is derived. This appraisal method provides an individual score that can be examined as a whole within the family, thus appraising the health risks likely to be experienced by other members of the family.

Health Risk Reduction

Health risk reduction is based on the assumption that decreasing the number or the magnitude of risks will decrease the probability of an undesired event occurring. For example, to decrease the likelihood of adolescent substance abuse, family behaviors such as parents not drinking, alcohol not available in the home, and family contracts related to alcohol and drug use may be useful. Also, family discussions about the pros and cons of drinking and the potential adverse effects of excessive drinking or consuming other substances can influence risks. Health risks can be reduced through a variety of approaches, such as those just described. It is important to note the specific risk and the family's tolerance of it. Murdaugh et al. (2019) cites the following examples of different kinds of risks:

- Voluntarily assumed risks, such as overeating, are tolerated better than those imposed by others.
- Risks about which scientists debate and are uncertain are more feared than risks about which scientists agree, such as the causes of colon cancer.
- Risks of natural origin, such as hurricanes, are often considered less threatening than those created by humans.

Risk reduction is a complex process that requires knowledge of the specific risk and the family's perceptions of the nature of the risk. A public health approach to risk reduction would say that it is always more effective to prevent disease or health disruption than to treat, cure, or rehabilitate.

Family Crisis

A family crisis occurs when the family is not able to cope with an event and becomes disorganized or dysfunctional. Some life events can lead to stress and increase risk for health disruptions.

Examples include when a child leaves home to go to college or to work and live independently, divorce or death in the family, job loss or job change, or relocation. Price et al. (2017) differentiate between family resources and family coping strategies. A family crisis exists when the demands of the situation exceed the resources of the family. When families experience a crisis or a crisis-producing event, they try to gather their resources to deal with the demands created by the situation. Examples of family resources are money and extended family members. Families cope by using known processes and behaviors to help them manage or adapt to the problem. Thus, if the primary wage earner has an unexpected illness, family resources might include financial assistance from relatives or emotional support. Family coping strategies, in contrast, would include being able to ask a relative to loan them emergency funds or being able to talk with relatives about the worries they were experiencing.

It is important to note that the amount of support available to families in times of crisis from government and nongovernment agencies varies in different locales. In addition, the rules and conditions of support often differ and may inhibit families from seeking support, particularly if the conditions are demeaning.

MAJOR FAMILY HEALTH RISKS AND NURSING INTERVENTIONS

As mentioned previously, risks to a family's health typically come from these three major areas: biological and age-related risks, environmental risks, and behavioral risks. In most instances, a risk in one of these areas may not be enough to threaten family health, but a combination of risks from two or more categories could threaten health. For example, there may be a family history of cardiovascular disease, but often the health risk is increased by an unhealthy lifestyle. An understanding of each of these categories provides the basis for a comprehensive approach to family health risk assessment and intervention.

Healthy People 2030 targets areas related to health conditions, health behaviors, populations, settings and systems, and social determinants of health. Each of these topics addresses age-related objectives (USDHHS, 2020). A variety of preventive services designed to reduce risks for illness have been identified for various health-related situations. These include maternal and infant health, heart disease and stroke, cancer, diabetes, and other chronic disabling conditions such as human immunodeficiency virus (HIV) infection and other sexually transmitted diseases. These preventive services consist of immunization for infectious diseases, and other clinical preventive services. The interrelationships among the various groups of risk are clear when the objectives for the nation are considered. Most of the national health objectives are based on risk factors of groups or populations in a variety of categories as described above. However, it is important to recognize that some of these factors have been recognized as relating to and having potential effects on the individuals' families, work, school, and communities, such as those described in the topic area of systems and settings.

Family Health Risk Appraisal

Assessment of family health **risk** requires many approaches. As in any assessment, the first and most important task is to get to know the family, their strengths, and their needs (see Chapter 20). This section focuses on appraisal of family health risks in the areas of biological and age-related risk, social and physical environmental risk, and behavioral risk. Box 21.1 includes several definitions related to family health.

Biological and Age-Related Risk

The family plays an important role in both the development and management of a disease or condition. Several illnesses are associated with either genetics or lifestyle patterns. These factors contribute to the biological risk for certain conditions. Patterns of cardiovascular disease, for example, often can be traced through several generations of a family. Such families are said to be at risk for cardiovascular disease. How or whether cardiovascular disease is found in a family is often influenced by the lifestyle of the family. Research findings support the positive effects of diet, exercise, and stress management on preventing or delaying cardiovascular disease. The development of hypertension can be managed by consuming a low-sodium diet, maintaining a normal weight, exercising regularly at the age-appropriate type and amount, and practicing effective stress management techniques, such as meditation (Vooradi and Mateti, 2016).

Diabetes mellitus is another disease with a strong correlation with a family's genetic pattern; the family also plays a major role in the management of the condition. Family patterns of obesity increase individuals' risks for heart disease, hypertension, diabetes, some types of cancer, and gallbladder disease. It is often difficult to separate biological risks from individual lifestyle factors (USDHHS, Healthy People 2030, 2020).

Transitions that occur when individuals or families move from one stage or condition to another are times of potential risk for families. Examples of these are age-related or life-event risks. See Table 21.1 for a list of family stages and the developmental tasks associated with each stage. Transitions present new situations and demands for families. These experiences often require families to change behaviors, schedules, and patterns of communication; make new decisions; reallocate family roles; learn new skills; and identify and learn to use new resources. The demands that transitions place on families have

TABLE 21.1   Family Life Cycle Stages

Stages	Tasks
Launching: single young adult leaves home	Coming to terms with the family of origin Development of intimate relationships with peers Establishment of self: career and finances
Marriage: joining of families	Formation of identity as a couple Inclusion of spouse in realignment of relationships with extended families Parenthood: making decisions
Families with young children	Integration of children into family unit Adjustment of tasks: child rearing, financial, and household Accommodation of new parenting and grandparenting roles
Families with adolescents	Development of increasing autonomy for adolescents Midlife reexamination of marital and career issues Initial shift toward concern for the older generation
Families as launching centers	Establishment of independent identities for parents and grown children Renegotiation of marital relationship Readjustment of relationships to include in-laws and grandchildren Dealing with disabilities and death of older generation
Aging families	Maintenance of couple and individual functioning while adapting to the aging process Support role of middle generation Support and autonomy of older generation Preparation for own death and dealing with the loss of spouse and/or siblings and other peers

Wright LM, Leahey M: Nurses and families: a guide to family assessment and intervention, 6th ed. Philadelphia, 2013, F.A. Davis & Company.

implications for the health of the family unit and individual family members and can be life-event risks. The nature of a transition event influences how prepared families are to deal with that particular transition. If the event is normative, or anticipated, families may be able to identify needed resources, make plans to cope with the change, learn new skills, and prepare for the event and its consequences. This kind of anticipatory preparation can increase the family's coping ability and decrease stress and negative outcomes. However, when the event is non-normative, or unexpected, families have little or no time to prepare and the outcome can be increased stress, crisis, or even dysfunction.

Several normative events have been identified for families. The developmental model organizes these events into stages and identifies important transition points. It provides a useful framework for identifying normative events and preparing families to cope successfully with related demands. The developmental tasks associated with each stage identify the types of skills families need. The kinds of normative events families experience are usually related to the addition or loss of a family member, such as the birth or adoption of a child, death of a grandparent, a child moving out of the home to go to school or take a job, or the marriage

BOX 21.1   Definitions Related to Family Health

- **Determinants of health:** An individual's biological makeup influences health through interactions with social and physical environments, as well as behavior.
- **Behaviors:** These may be learned from other family members.
- **Social environment:** This includes the family; it is where culture, language, and personal and spiritual beliefs are learned.
- **Physical environment:** Hazards in the home may affect health negatively, and a clean and safe home has a positive influence on health.

of a child. Health-related responsibilities are associated with each of these tasks. For example, the birth or adoption of a child requires that families learn about human growth and development, parenting, immunizations, management of childhood illnesses, normal childhood nutrition, and safety issues. Adding a new person to the family also requires that members learn new ways to manage all of their roles and partner with one another to meet the changing needs of the family.

Non-normative events present different kinds of issues for families. Unexpected events can be either positive or negative. A job promotion or inheriting a substantial sum of money may be unexpected but is usually a positive event. However, for some families, a new job for one member may include more responsibility, stress, or travel, which could affect all members of the family. Likewise, inheriting money can change family dynamics in a variety of ways, including who decides how the money will be used. More often, non-normative events are unpleasant, such as when a family member has a major illness, or when there is a divorce, a new marriage or partner living arrangement, the death of a child, or the family income substantially decreases because of loss of a job or other changes in the ways the family gets income.

Conger et al. (2014) supported a systems-oriented concept of family stress. They pointed out that families develop a series of processes to manage or transform inputs to the system (e.g., energy, time) to outputs (e.g., cohesion, growth, love), known as *rules of transformation*. Over time, families develop these patterns in enough quantity and variety to handle most changes and challenges. However, when families do not have an adequate variety of rules to allow them to respond to an event, the event becomes stressful. Rather than being able to deal with the situation, they fall into a pattern of trying to figure out what they need to do, and the usual tasks of the family are not adequately addressed. Rules that were implicit in the family are now reconsidered and redefined.

The family stress theory of Conger et al. (2014) proposes three levels of stress:

- Level I is change in the more specific patterns of behavior and transforming processes, such as change in who does which household chores.
- Level II is change in processes at a higher level of abstraction, such as changes in what are considered as family chores.
- Level III is change in highly abstract processes, such as family values.

Coping strategies can be identified to address each level of stress that families go through in sequence, if necessary.

Biological Health Risk Assessment

One of the most effective techniques for assessing the patterns of health and illness in families is the genogram. Briefly, a genogram is a drawing that shows the family unit of immediate interest and includes several generations using a series of circles, squares, and connecting lines. Basic information about the family, relationships in the family, and patterns of health and illness can be obtained by completing the genogram with the family (Fig. 21.1). Note that the symbols are depicted in this way: squares indicate

---

CASE STUDY

The six members of the Mitchell family are Mr. Mitchell, Mrs. Mitchell, 18-year-old Annie, 15-year-old Michelle, 13-year-old Sean, and 7-year-old Bobby. Mr. Mitchell has been the pastor of Faith Baptist Church for the last 15 years. Mrs. Mitchell is a homemaker and primary caretaker for the children.

For the past year, Mrs. Mitchell has felt tired and "run down." At her annual physical, she describes her symptoms to her physician. After several tests, Mrs. Mitchell is diagnosed with stomach cancer. She starts to cry and says, "How will I tell my family?"

Mrs. Mitchell's primary physician refers the family to Trisha Farewell, a nurse in community health. Ms. Farewell calls the household and speaks with Mrs. Mitchell. Ms. Farewell tells Mrs. Mitchell that she was referred by the physician and she can help Mrs. Mitchell cope with the diagnosis. Mrs. Mitchell confides in Ms. Farewell that it has been 2 weeks since she received the diagnosis but she has yet to tell her husband and children. Mrs. Mitchell asks Ms. Farewell if she can help her tell her family and explain what it all means. Ms. Farewell makes an appointment to go to the Mitchell household and facilitate the family meeting. As seen in this case, the nurse often can help a family talk about a difficult subject and help the family examine ways in which they will cope with the difficulty.

---

males, circles indicate females, an X through either a square or a circle indicates a death, marriage is indicated by a solid horizontal line, and offspring and children are noted by a solid vertical line. A broken horizontal line indicates a divorce or separation. The dates of birth, marriage, death, and other important events can be indicated where appropriate. Major illnesses or conditions can be listed for each individual family member. Patterns can be quickly assessed and provide a guide for the health interviewer about health areas that need further exploration.

The genogram in Fig. 21.1 was completed for the fictional Graham family. Some of the interesting health patterns that can be seen from the genogram are the repetition of the following chronic health conditions: hypertension, type 2 diabetes mellitus, cancer, and hypercholesterolemia. Completing a genogram requires interviews with as many family members as possible. It is important to develop a family chronology, a timeline of family events over three generations, to extend the genogram for a better description of family patterns.

A more intensive and quantitative assessment of a family's biological risk can be achieved using a standard family risk assessment. Because such assessments involve other areas in addition to biological risk, one will be described later, after the description of the assessment of other types of risk.

As discussed earlier, both normative and non-normative life events pose potential risks to the health of families. Even events that are generally viewed as being positive require changes and can place stress on a family. The normative event of the birth of a child, for example, requires considerable changes in family structures and roles. Furthermore, family functions are expanded from previous levels, requiring families to add new skills and establish additional resources. These changes in turn can result in strain and, if adequate resources are not available, stress. Therefore, to adequately assess life risks, both normative and non-normative events occurring in the family need to be considered. Community-level support groups can help families deal

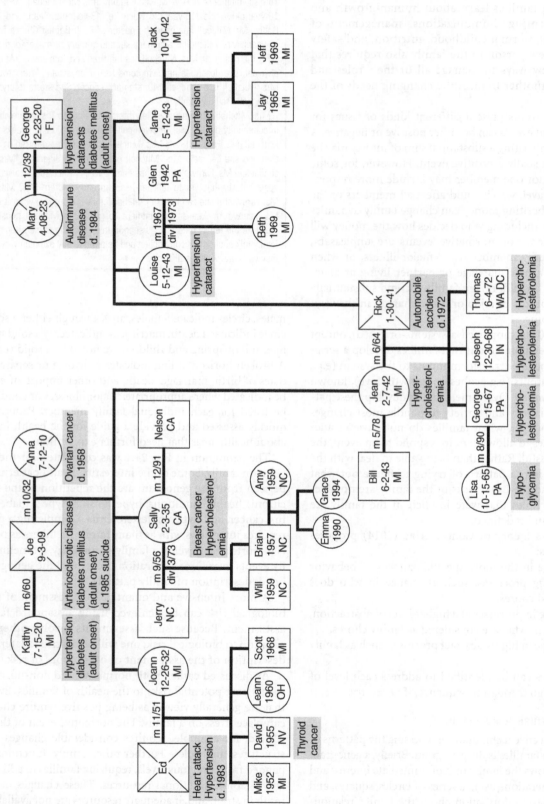

Fig. 21.1 Family Genogram of the Graham Family. (Developed by Carol Loveland-Cherry. In: Stanhope M, Lancaster J: *Public health nursing*, 8th ed. St Louis, 2012, Mosby.)

with a variety of stressful situations and crises (e.g., Families Anonymous, Bereaved Parents, Parents and Friends of Lesbian and Gay Persons, Single Parents) that arise from both life events and age-related events. Nurses can develop and moderate such groups.

Environmental Risk

The importance of environmental risks include several indentified risks. Social risks to family health are gaining increased recognition. A family's health risk increases if they are living in high-crime neighborhoods, communities without adequate recreation or health resources, communities with major noise pollution or chemical pollution, or other high-stress environments. One social risk is discrimination, whether racial, cultural, or other (Artigia, 2018). For example, consider the stress of a mother with children 6, 8, and 12 years of age who are unable to play outside their one-bedroom apartment because the area lacks parks or other green areas, the apartment is on a busy street, and the area has two aggressive youth gangs who are known to bully younger children. The psychological burden resulting from discrimination is itself a stressor, and it adds to the effects of other stressors. The implication of these examples of risky social situations is that they contribute to the stressors experienced by the families. If adequate resources and coping processes are not available, breakdowns in health can occur.

The poor are at greater risk for health problems. Economic risk, which is related to social risk, is determined by the relationship between the financial resources of a family and the demands on those resources. Having adequate financial resources means that a family is able to purchase the necessary services and goods related to health. These include environmental issues such as adequate housing, clothing, food, education, and health or illness care. The amount of money that a family has available is related to situational, cultural, and social factors. A family may have an income well above the poverty level, but because of a devastating illness of a family member, they may not be able to meet current financial demands. Likewise, families from ethnic populations or families with same-sex parents may experience discrimination in finding housing. Even if they find housing, they may not be welcome and may be harassed, resulting in increased stress.

Unfortunately, not all families have access to health care insurance. For families at the poverty level, programs such as Medicaid are available to pay for health and illness care. Families in the upper income brackets usually have health insurance through an employer, or they can afford to either purchase health insurance or pay for health care out of pocket. An increasing number of middle-income families have major wage earners in jobs that do not have health benefits. These people often do not have enough income to purchase health care but earn too much money to qualify for public assistance programs. The economic downturn in recent years has affected many families. Some of these families have lost their homes, jobs, automobiles, and health insurance. Other families have financial resources that allow them to maintain themselves but that limit the quality of their purchasing power for preventive health

care or fresh, healthy, nutritious food. Families with limited resources may qualify for programs such as Medicaid; Special Supplemental Nutrition Program for Women, Infants, and Children (WIC); or Temporary Assistance to Needy Families (TANF). The WIC program and the family participation in WIC affects Medicaid costs and use of health care services. A family's children who participated in WIC were more linked to the health care system than children who were not. Children in WIC were more likely to receive both preventive and curative care more often than children not participating in WIC (Thomas et al., 2014). Nurses play an important role in teaching families about the resources available to them and giving them clear directions about how and where to apply for needed services (Carlson and Neuberger, 2017; USDA, 2018).

Environmental Risk Assessment

Assessment of environmental health risk is less defined and developed. Information on relationships the family has with others, such as relatives and neighbors; their connections with other social units (e.g., church, school, work, clubs, organizations); and the flow of energy—positive or negative—can be assessed through the use of an ecomap (Holtslander et al., 2014).

An ecomap represents the family's interactions with other groups and organizations, accomplished by using a series of circles and lines. The family illustrated in Fig. 21.2 is represented by a *circle* in the middle of the page; other groups and organizations are indicated by other *circles*. *Lines*, representing the flow of energy, are drawn between the family circle and the circles representing other groups and organizations. An *arrowhead* at the end of each line indicates the direction of the flow of energy (into or out of the family), and the *darkness* of the line indicates the intensity of the energy.

The Graham family ecomap demonstrates that much of the family energy goes into work (also a source of stress for the parents). Major sources of energy for the Grahams are their immediate and extended families and friends.

In addition to the support network shown by the ecomap, other aspects of social risk include characteristics of the neighborhood and community in which the family lives. A nurse who has worked in the general geographic area may already have done a community assessment and have a working knowledge of the neighborhood and community. It is helpful for the nurse to obtain certain information from the family to understand how the family views the community. For example, information about the origins of the family is useful to understand other social resources and stressors. Information about how long the family has lived in their current location and the immigration patterns of the family and their ancestors helps the nurse understand some of the pressures they may experience.

Economic risk is a key predictor of health. Families often consider financial information private, and both the nurse and the family may be uncomfortable when discussing finances. The nurse would only need to know the actual family income to help the family determine whether they are eligible for programs or benefits. It is helpful to know if the family's resources are adequate to meet their needs. It is important to remember that the family may have a standard of living different from

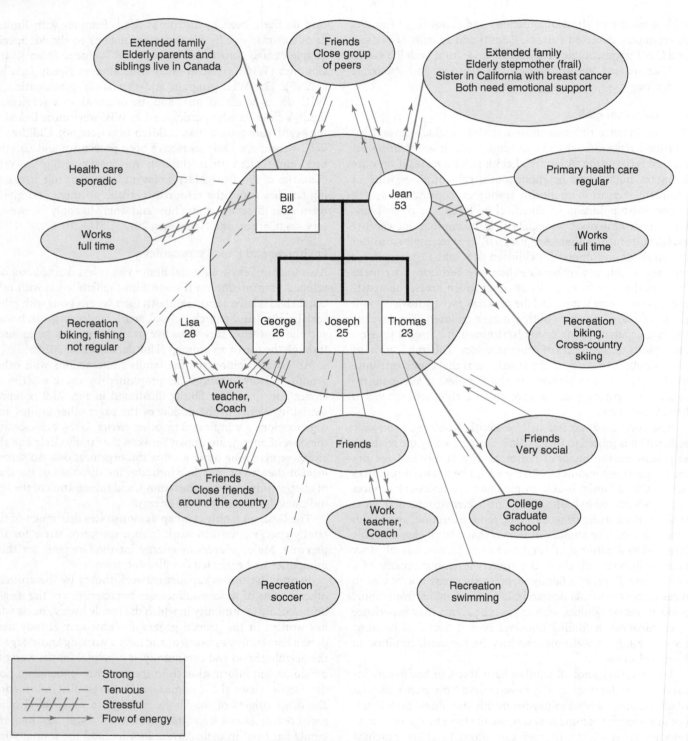

Fig. 21.2 Ecomap of the Graham Family. (Developed by Carol Loveland-Cherry. In Stanhope M, Lancaster J: *Public health nursing*, 8th ed. St. Louis, 2012, Mosby.)

that of the nurse, and they may be comfortable or at least accepting of their standard of living. Be careful to avoid imposing your financial values onto the family. In terms of health risk, be aware that the resources available to the family need to be used to obtain health and illness care; adequate shelter, clothing, and food; and access to recreation. As mentioned earlier, in an increasing number of families, the main wage earner is employed but receives no medical benefits and the salary is insufficient for health promotion or illness-related care. This is a **policy** issue for which nurses can help draft legislation and provide testimony using stories of families in their caseloads.

Behavioral (Lifestyle) Risk

Personal health habits continue to contribute to the major causes of morbidity and mortality in the United States. The pattern of personal health habits and behavioral risk defines individual and family lifestyle risk. The family is the basic unit within which health behavior—including health values, health habits, and health risk perceptions—is developed, organized, and performed. Families maintain major responsibility for determining what food is purchased and prepared, setting sleep patterns, planning family activities, setting and monitoring norms and expected behaviors about health and health risks, determining when a family member is ill, deciding when health care should be obtained, and carrying out treatment regimens.

In 2016 more than half of all deaths in the United States were attributed to heart disease or cancer, both of which identify diet as a causative factor (NCHS, 2017). General guidelines from the US Department of Health and Human Services and the US Department of Agriculture include eating a variety of foods; maintaining healthy weight; choosing a diet low in fat and cholesterol, including plenty of vegetables, fruits, and grain products; limiting use of sugars, salt, and sodium; and consuming alcohol only in moderation (USDA, 2015).

Multiple health benefits of regular physical activity have been identified. Regular physical exercise is effective in promoting and maintaining health and preventing disease (CDC, 2018).

Benefits of regular physical activity include increased muscle strength, endurance, and flexibility; management of weight; prevention of colon cancer, stroke, and back injury; and prevention and management of heart disease, hypertension, diabetes, osteoporosis, and depression. Families can structure time and activities for family members. It is helpful when the community in which they live promotes exercise by having accessible parks and walking or biking paths that help families select activities that provide moderate, regular physical exercise, rather than sedentary activities in the home setting.

Substance use and abuse are major contributors to morbidity and mortality in the United States. When caring for a family in which one or more members smokes, consider not only talking with them about smoking cessation, but also provide education about the effects of secondhand smoke. Passive or secondhand smoke has been associated with several types of cancer, heart disease, chronic obstructive pulmonary disease, low birth weight, premature births, and sudden infant death syndrome (USDHHS, 2010).

Similarly, drug use, including alcohol, is a major social and health problem that affects individuals, families, and communities. Drug use is associated with transmission of HIV, fetal alcohol syndrome, liver disease, unwanted pregnancy, delinquency, school failure, violence, and crime (NIDA, 2014).

The literature consistently identifies the following family factors that decrease the risk for substance use in children:

- Family closeness
- Families doing activities together
- Behavior modeled in the family

Although violence and abusive behavior are not limited to families, the amount of intrafamilial violence is thought to be underestimated. It is difficult to collect data and obtain accurate statistics on family violence because the issue is so sensitive for families. Evidence supports the intergenerational nature of violence and abuse—that is, abusers were often abused as children (USDHHS, 2018). It is important for nurses to be watchful and observant for signs of neglect and abuse. This is not a topic that clients and families readily bring up in a visit. Often it is what is not said as much as what is said that will provide a clue to violent behavior in the family. Observe closely for nonverbal behavior and listen carefully to what families say when they describe their interactions with one another.

EVIDENCE-BASED PRACTICE

In the Environmental Risk Reduction through Nursing Intervention and Education (ERRNIE) study, public health nurses sought to educate rural low-income families about potential or actual environmental risks in homes, along with a home inspection for risk reduction. Following this study, researchers (Oneal et al., 2015) explored how these families processed health information following the intervention. The researchers used grounded theory methodology, conducting 10 semistructured interviews of primary child caregivers in rural low-income families who had participated. Three phases emerged, explaining the core process of understanding health information: (a) visiting my perception, (b) weighing the evidence, and (c) making a new meaning. Together, the three make up the core category of "Re-Forming the Risk Message." Although this process did not always lead to engaging the behavior to reduce or eliminate risk, it did lead to making a decision to engage on some level. To understand whether people are ready to engage in positive behaviors through interventions or if needed changes to the information must be made, nurses need to discover and explore reasons for the re-formed risk messages.

Nurse Use

Nursing interventions designed to improve health behaviors and reduce risks are often based on stage theories that explain how change occurs through steps leading to positive actions through delivery of risk messages. Family health promotion and risk reduction interventions may be more effective if the nurse can assess and tailor the health message to the family for optimal motivation for positive behavior change.

From Oneal GA, Eide P, Hamilton R, et al.: Rural families' process of re-forming environmental health risk messages, *J Nurs Scholarsh* 47(4):354–362, 2015.

Behavioral (Lifestyle) Health Risk Assessment

Families are the major source of factors that can promote or inhibit positive lifestyles. They regulate time and energy and the boundaries of the system. Various tools exist for assessing individuals' lifestyle risks, but few are available for assessing family lifestyle patterns. Although assessment of individual lifestyles contributes to determining the lifestyle risk of a family, it is important to look at risks of the family as a unit. Lifestyle can be assessed in several dimensions. From the literature on health behavior research, the critical dimensions include the following:

- Value placed on the behavior
- Knowledge of the behavior and its consequences
- Effect of the behavior on the family
- Effect of the behavior on the individual
- Barriers to performing the behavior
- Benefits of the behavior

It is important to assess the frequency, intensity, and regularity of specific behaviors. It is also important to evaluate the resources available to the family for implementing the behaviors. Physical activity as a family has many positive outcomes, including health benefits from the activity, the potential for quality time spent with one another, and the chance to be outside and active. You could assess physical activity in a family by looking at the value a family places on physical activity; the hours a family spends in exercise; the kinds of exercise the family does; the resources available for exercise; and the family's description and self-report of the activity.

NURSING APPROACHES TO FAMILY HEALTH RISK REDUCTION

Home Visits

Nurses work with families in a variety of settings, including clinics, schools, support groups, and offices. However, an important aspect of the nurse's role in reducing health risks and promoting the health of populations has been providing services to families in their homes.

Purpose

Home visits, in contrast to clinic visits, give a more accurate assessment of the family structure, the natural or home environment, and behavior in the home environment. Home visits also provide opportunities to identify both barriers and supports for reaching family health promotion goals. The nurse can work with the client directly to modify interventions to match resources. Visiting the family in the home may also contribute to the family's sense of control and active participation in meeting its health needs.

Home visiting provides a broad range of services to achieve a variety of health-related goals. Long-term effects of home visits are positive and can be cost effective for society in contrast to caring for individuals in hospitals or other in patient sites. As a result, several states have reinstituted home visits for high-risk families. If the home visit is to be a valuable and effective intervention, careful and systematic planning must occur (Avellar et al., 2016; Robling et al., 2016). It is important to remember that a home visit is more than just taking care of people in a different setting. Instead, it is a useful intervention format.

Advantages and Disadvantages

The effectiveness of health promotion services in the home has been critically reexamined by agencies such as health departments and visiting nurses associations. Advantages include the convenience for clients, especially those with mobility issues or those who are unable or unwilling to travel; client control and comfort of the setting; the ability to individualize services; and a natural, relaxed environment for the discussion of concerns and needs. Costs, on the other hand, are a major disadvantage. The cost is high because of preparation for the previsit, travel time and expense to and from the home, the amount of time

spent with one client, and postvisit follow-up. Many agencies have considered alternative modes of providing services to families, such as group education, counseling, or other interventions. The important issue is determining which families would benefit the most and how home visits can most effectively be structured and scheduled. With increasing demands for home health care, the home visit is again becoming a prominent mode for delivery of nursing services. When looking at cost versus effectiveness, it is not always the least costly service that is the most effective (Sewell and Marczak, 2014); rather the social value produced may be more compelling. An example is that of home visits. Although more costly in the short term, some services are more effective in family health outcomes using home visitation rather than visits to the health department or clinic.

Process

The components of a home visit are summarized in Table 21.2. The phases include the initiation phase, the previsit phase, the in-home phase, the termination phase, and the postvisit phase. Building a trusting relationship with the family client is the cornerstone of successful home visits. The following five skills are fundamental to effective home visits: observing, listening, questioning, probing, and prompting. The need for these skills is evident in all phases of the home visit process.

Initiation phase. Usually, a home visit is initiated as the result of a referral from a health care or social agency. However, a family may request services, or the nurse may initiate the home visit as a result of case-finding activities. The initiation phase is the first contact between the nurse and the family. It provides

TABLE 21.2 Phases and Activities of a Home Visit

Phase	Activity
I. Initiation	Clarify the source of referral for the visit Clarify the purpose for the home visit Share information on the reason and purpose of the home visit with the family
II. Previsit	Initiate contact with the family Establish a shared perception of purpose with the family Determine the family's willingness for a home visit Schedule the home visit Review the referral and/or family record
III. In-home	Introduce self and professional identity Interact socially to establish rapport Establish the nurse–client relationship Implement the nursing process
IV. Termination	Review the visit with the family Plan for future visits
V. Postvisit	Record the visit Plan for the next visit

Wright LM, Leaghy M: Nurses and families: a guide to family assessment and nursing intervention, 6th ed. Philadelphia, 2013, F.A. Davis & Company.

the foundation for an effective therapeutic relationship. Subsequent home visits should be based on need and mutual agreement between the nurse and the family. Frequently, nurses are not sure of the reason for the visit. As a result, the visit may be compromised and come aimlessly or abruptly to a premature halt. The nurse must be clear about the purpose of the home visit, and this purpose or understanding must be shared with the family.

HOW TO PREPARE FOR THE HOME VISIT: INITIATION PHASE

- First, if at all possible, nurses should contact the family by telephone before the home visit to introduce themselves, to identify the reason for the contact, and to schedule the home visit. A first telephone contact should be a maximum of 15 min. Nurses should give their name and professional identity—for example, "This is Karen Smith. I'm a nurse from the Fayette County Health Department."
- The family should be informed of how they came to the attention of the nurse—for example, as the result of a referral or a contact from observations or records in the school. If a referral was received, it is important and useful to learn if the family is aware of the referral.
- A brief summary of the nurse's knowledge about the family's situation will allow the family to clarify their needs. For example, the nurse might say, "I understand that your baby was discharged from the hospital yesterday and that you requested some assistance with learning more about how to care for your baby at home."
- A visit should be scheduled as soon as possible. Letting the family know agency hours available for visits, the approximate length of the visit, and the purpose of the visit is helpful to the family in determining when to set the visit. Although the length of the visit may vary, depending on circumstances, approximately 30–60 min is usual.
- If possible, the visit should be arranged when as many family members as possible will be available for the entire visit. It is important to tell clients about any fee for the visit and subsequent visits and possible methods for payment.
- The telephone call can terminate with a review by the nurse of the time, place, and purpose for the visit and a means for the family to contact the nurse in case they need to verify or change the time for the visit or to ask questions. If the family does not have a telephone, another method for setting up the visit can be used. A note can be dropped off at the family home or sent by mail informing the family of when and why the home visit will occur and providing a way for the family to contact the nurse if necessary.

Previsit phase. The previsit phase has several components. For the most part, these are best accomplished in order, as presented in the How To box. Be aware that the family may refuse a home visit. Do not immediately interpret this as a personal rejection. Families may have a variety of reasons when they make decisions about when and which outsiders are allowed entry into their homes. The nurse needs to explore the reasons for the refusal. For example, there may be a misunderstanding about the reason for a visit or there may be a lack of information about services, including payment for them. The contact for a visit may be terminated as requested (1) if the nurse determines that either the situation has been resolved or services have been obtained from another source, and (2) if the family understands that services are available and how to contact the agency if desired. However, the nurse should leave open the possibility of future contact. In some instances, the nurse will be mandated to persist in requesting a home visit because of legal obligations, such as follow-up of certain communicable and infectious diseases. The agency will make the decision whether home visits will occur if a family member has diagnosed COVID-19.

Before visiting a family, the nurse should review the referral or, if this is not the first visit, the family record. If time has lapsed between the contact and the visit, a brief telephone call to confirm the time often ensures that someone will be at home.

Personal safety is an issue that may arise either in approaching the family home or once the family has opened the door to the nurse. Nurses need to examine personal fears and objective threats to determine if safety is indeed an issue. Certain precautions can be taken in known high-risk situations. Agencies may provide escorts for nurses or have them visit in pairs; readily identifiable uniforms may be required; or a sign-out process indicating the timing and location of home visits may be used routinely. Home visits are generally safe; however, as with all worksites, the possibility of violence exists. Therefore, the nurse needs to use caution and exercise good judgment. If a reasonable question exists about the safety of making a visit, the nurse should not make the visit. While most safety issues relate to the home environment, please note that COVID-19 has also become a safety issue for the nurse. If the nurse or agency is aware of family members(s) affected by COVID-19, the nurse can take precautions before entering the home.

The nurse should be aware that families may think the nurse is checking up on them, that the nurse views them as being inadequate or dysfunctional, or that the nurse is impinging on their privacy. Nursing services, especially those from health departments, have been identified by the public as being "public services" for needy families or those with inadequate funds to pay for care. These potential areas of concern underlie the need for sensitivity on the part of the nurse, the need for clarity in information regarding the reason for the visits, and the need to establish collaborative, trusting relationships with the family.

Another factor that may affect the nature of the home visit is whether the visit is viewed as voluntary or required. A *voluntary* home visit (a visit requested by the client) is characterized by easier entry for the nurse, client-controlled interaction, a more informal tone, and a mutual discussion of the frequency of future visits. For example, a voluntary visit would be when a new mother requests that the nurse come to the home and assist her with effective breastfeeding for the infant. In contrast, the client may feel little need for *required* home visits (often legally mandated). When a visit is required, entry into the home may be more difficult than during a voluntary visit. The interaction is often more nurse controlled, and there may be a more formal, investigatory tone to the visit, with distorted nurse–client communication. There may not be any mutual discussion of the frequency of future visits. An example of a required visit might be when a family member has been diagnosed with tuberculosis and the nurse needs to verify that the client is taking medication regularly, or the family is using quarantine measures when COVID-19 is an issue.

The changing nature of the American family can make it difficult to schedule visits during what have been traditional agency hours. The number of working single-parent or dual-income, two-parent families is increasing, which means that families have more demands on their time. Even if one parent is at home during the usual workday, the ideal is to visit when the entire family is present. This often is not possible because of conflict between agency hours and school or work schedules. It may be possible to schedule a visit at the beginning or end of a day to meet with working or school-age members. In some parts of the country, agencies are reconsidering traditional hours and Monday through Friday visits. These issues are important to assess and address during the previsit phase so the nurse and the family will be better prepared for the visit.

Culture influences a person's interpretation of and response to health care (Shi and Singh, 2019). It is impossible, given the diversity of the United States and the diversity within cultural groups, to cover every group extensively. Instead, practitioners need to take the responsibility to learn about their client's culture as they prepare for visits with families or communities.

In-home phase. The actual visit to the home is the in-home phase and gives the nurse the opportunity to assess the family's home, lawn, neighborhood, and community resources, as well as the family interactions. When making the home visit, once at the home, the nurse provides personal and professional identification and tells the client where the agency is located. Next, a brief social period allows the client to assess the nurse and establish rapport. The next step is for the nurse to describe his or her role, responsibilities, and limitations. Another important component of this phase is to determine the client's expectations.

The major portion of the home visit involves establishing the relationship and implementing the nursing process. Assessment, intervention, and evaluation are ongoing. The reason for the visit then determines what will occur in the home visit. Keller et al. (2004a, 2004b) recommend using the Intervention Wheel to guide nursing practice during home visits. The Intervention Wheel provides guidelines for the purpose of home visits. Some reasons for visits are listed in Box 21.2.

It is important that the nurse be realistic about what can be accomplished in a home visit. In some situations, one visit may be all that is possible or appropriate. In this instance, the nurse needs to discuss with the family their needs and the resources available to meet them and determine whether further services are desired or indicated. If further services are indicated and the nurse's agency is not appropriate, the nurse can help the family identify other services available in the community and help initiate referrals. Although it is not unusual to have only one home visit with a family, often multiple visits are made. The frequency and intensity of home visits vary not only with the needs of the family but also with the eligibility of the family for services as defined by agency policies and priorities.

Families may or may not be able to control interruptions during the visit. Telephones ring, pets join in the visit, people

---

BOX 21.2   Reasons for the Home Visit

Nursing interventions may include some or all of the following 17 resources identified by the Minnesota Department of Health, Section of Public Health Nursing:
- Advocacy
- Case management
- Coalition building
- Collaboration
- Community organizing
- Consultation
- Counseling
- Delegated medical treatment and observations
- Disease and other health investigation
- Health teaching
- Outreach
- Policy development and enforcement
- Case finding
- Referral and follow-up
- Screening
- Social marketing
- Surveillance

From Keller LO, Strohschein S, Lia-Hoagberg B et al.: Population-based public health interventions: practice-based and evidence-supported. I, *Public Health Nurs* 21:453–468, 2004a.

---

come and go, and televisions are left on. The nurse can ask that for a limited time, televisions be turned off or that other disruptive activities be limited. Families may be so used to the background noises and routine activities that they do not recognize them as being potentially disruptive.

Home visits are important for families to help them effectively manage their health.

Termination phase. When the purpose of the visit has been accomplished, the nurse reviews with the family what has occurred and what has been accomplished. This is the major focus of the termination phase, and it provides a basis for planning further home visits.
- Ideally, termination of the visit and, ultimately, termination of service begin at the first contact with the establishment of a goal or purpose.
- If communication has been clear to this point, the family and nurse can now plan for future visits, specifically the next visit.
- Planning for future visits is part of setting goals and planning service.
- Contracting is a constructive approach to working with clients and is receiving increasing attention by health professionals (Duiveman and Bonner, 2012).
- The purpose and components of contracting with clients are discussed in more detail later in the chapter.

Postvisit phase. Even though the nurse has concluded the home visit and left the client's home, responsibility for the visit is not complete until the interaction has been recorded. A major task of the post-visit phase is documenting the visit and services provided. It is important to consider

QSEN FOCUS ON QUALITY AND SAFETY EDUCATION FOR NURSES

Targeted Competency: Safety—Minimizes risk for harm to clients and providers through both system effectiveness and individual performance.

Important aspects of safety include:
- **Knowledge:** Examine human factors and other basic safety design principles as well as commonly used unsafe practices (e.g., workarounds and dangerous abbreviations)
- **Skills:** Use national client safety resources for own professional development and to focus attention on safety in care settings
- **Attitudes:** Value the contributions of standardization/reliability to safety

Safety Question: Assume that you are a home care nurse, planning a predischarge visit to the home of your client, Bill Jones. Mr. Jones is 78 years old and has recently suffered a left-sided cerebrovascular accident (CVA). This CVA affected his cognitive, motor, and sensory functioning. You know that individuals who suffer a left-sided stroke may experience memory deficits. Mr. Jones is experiencing moderate expressive aphasia and right-sided weakness, which make it difficult for him to carry out simple tasks of daily living.

Mr. Jones lives with his wife, Helen Jones, who is in good health. Their 45-year-old daughter lives an hour away and visits monthly. The family is concerned about Mr. Jones's safety and asks for assistance in setting up safety systems in the home. Specifically, the family has asked for aid in setting up a safe system for the complex medication regimen, adjusting the physical environment to minimize the risk for Mr. Jones falling, and a communication system to accommodate his aphasia. You are aware that Mr. Jones is concerned about maintaining his autonomy.

Use the phases and activities outlined in contracting (Table 21.3) in outlining how to address the concerns of the client and his family.

1. Which data will you collect to address the three requests of the family? What data will you collect from Mr. Jones?
2. What might be some mutually agreeable goals related to medications, the home environment, and a communication system?
3. How might you involve Mr. Jones in the development of a plan for these goals?
4. How might you guide his wife and daughter in exploring the division of responsibilities?
5. What processes might be effective in evaluation of goals and renegotiation?
6. How will you, Mr. Jones, and his family know when the time is right to terminate your contract with this family?

Answer

1. As you begin contracting with this family, determine Mr. Jones's baseline functioning after the CVA. Review evaluation and plans of care by physical and occupational therapy. How much can Mr. Jones contribute to his own care? What have been Mr. Jones's habits around his medications before the CVA? Did he use pill boxes? How many of these medication administration habits can be maintained with his new medication regimen? Having a physical therapist evaluate the home environment for fall risks would be helpful. Is the client able to write? If so, having dry erase boards handy throughout the home would be an effective means of communication. Otherwise, Mr. and Mrs. Jones will need to develop effective sign language so Mr. Jones can contribute to conversations.
2. Goals around medication administration management might be for Mr. Jones to initiate taking his own medications at the correct time each day, with assistance from his wife only when needed. This approach will allow him to maintain some autonomy, which he has stated is important to him.

   A goal around adjustment of the physical environment might be to have the home environment evaluated and the suggested alterations implemented within a week of Mr. Jones returning home. It would also be a helpful goal to monitor near-falls so that Mr. and Mrs. Jones can continue to monitor the effectiveness of the environmental adjustments. Subtle alterations may continue to be needed as they adjust to Mr. Jones's lack of balance.

   A goal around communications systems might be for you and the family to check in with Mr. Jones weekly to ensure that he thinks he has adequate opportunity to contribute to family communication and processes.
3. Use alternative communication strategies so Mr. Jones can actively participate in care decisions.
4. Depending on the degree of Mr. Jones's care, it would be easy for his wife to become overwhelmed. As the health care professional most in touch with the family dynamics on a regular basis, it is important to discuss how the daughter's visits can provide respite for Mrs. Jones. Are the monthly visits adequate? Does Mrs. Jones need more support when Mr. Jones first comes home? Are there responsibilities (e.g., refilling medication prescriptions) that the daughter can assume?
5. Facilitate regular communication among the family members about new routines and care rhythms.
6. At what point does the family feel independent and autonomous in their care of Mr. Jones? This point would be a good time to begin discussing termination of your contract with this family.

Prepared by Gail Armstrong, ND, DNP, MS, PhD, Professor and Assistant Dean/DNP program, Oregon Health and Sciences University.

that agencies may organize their records by families. That is, the basic record may be a "family" folder with all members included. However, this often does not occur, although it is useful for the family history and background. More often, in agencies, each family member has a separate record, and other family members' records are cross-referenced. This is because the focus often shifts from the family to the individual. Consequently, nursing diagnoses, goals, and interventions are directed toward individual family members rather than the family unit. This approach has its shortcomings and it is important for the nurse to recognize these limitations. It is important for the nurse to focus on the continuing assessment of the individual behaviors, responses, and work health status, and the impact on the

family. Interventions at the family level may become necessary, such as educating all family members on hygiene and cleanliness or on the appropriate disposal of supplies of the client with tuberculosis in the home.

Record systems and formats vary from agency to agency, including computerized record systems. The nurse needs to become familiar with the particular system used in the agency. All systems should have a database; list a nursing diagnosis and problem list; specify a plan, including specific goals, actual actions, and interventions; and have an evaluation. These are the basic elements needed for legal and clinical purposes. The format may consist of narratives; flow sheets; a problem-oriented medical record (POMR); a subjective, objective, assessment plan (SOAP); or a combination of formats. It is important that recording be current, dated, and signed.

The nurse should use theoretical frameworks appropriate to the family-centered nursing process. For example, a nursing diagnosis of *ineffective mothering skill* related to lack of knowledge of normal growth and development is an individual-focused nursing diagnosis. *Inability of a family to accomplish the stage-appropriate task of providing a safe environment for a preschooler related to lack of knowledge and resources* is a family-focused nursing diagnosis based on knowledge of the developmental approach to families. At times, it may be necessary to present information for a specific family member. However, the emphasis should be on the individual as a member of, and within the structure of, the family.

Contracting with Families

Increasingly, health professionals look at working with clients in an interactive, collaborative style. This approach is consistent with a more knowledgeable public and the recent self-care movement in the United States. However, it may not be consistent with other cultures that look to health care providers for more direct guidance; therefore, it is important to determine the family's value system before assuming that contracting will work.

Contracting, which is making an agreement between two or more parties, involves a shift in responsibility and control toward a shared effort by the client and professional as opposed to an effort by the professional alone. The premise of contracting is family control. It is assumed that when the family has legitimate control, its ability to make healthful choices is increased.

Purposes

The nursing contract is a working agreement that is continuously renegotiable and may or may not be written. It may be either a contingency or a noncontingency contract. A *contingency contract* states a specific reward for the client after completion of the client's portion of the contract. In contrast, a *noncontingency contract* does not specify rewards. Instead, the implied rewards are the positive consequences of reaching the goals specified in the contract.

For family health risk reduction, it is essential that the contract be made with all responsible and appropriate members of the family. Involving only one individual is not sufficient if the goal is family health risk reduction, which requires a total family system effort and change. Scheduling a visit with all family members present may require extra effort. If meeting with the entire family is not possible, each family member can review a contract, give input, and sign it. This allows active participation by all family members without the necessity of finding a time when everyone involved can be present.

Process of Contracting

Contracting is a learned skill on the part of both the nurse and the family. All persons involved need to know the purpose and process of contracting. The three general phases are *beginning, working,* and *termination.* The three phases can be further divided into eight sets of activities, as summarized in Table 21.3.

TABLE 21.3	Phases and Activities in Contracting
Phase	**Activity**
I. Beginning phase	Mutual data collection and exploration of needs and problems
	Mutual establishment of goals
	Mutual development of a plan
II. Working phase	Mutual division of responsibilities
	Mutual setting of time limits
	Mutual implementation of a plan
	Mutual evaluation and renegotiation
III. Termination	Mutual termination of a contract

First, collect and analyze the data. This activity involves both the family and the nurse. An important aspect of this step is obtaining the family's view of the situation and its needs and problems. The nurse can present his or her observations and validate them with the family and then obtain the family's view.

It is important that goals be mutually set and realistic. At times, nurses and clients who are new to contracting may set overly ambitious goals. The nurse should recognize that there may be discrepancies between professional priorities and those of the client and decide if negotiating is required. The goals of contracting are not static because the process includes renegotiating when appropriate.

Throughout the process, the nurse and family continually learn and recognize what each can contribute to meeting the health needs of the family. By exploring resources, both the nurse and the family learn about their own and one another's strengths, which requires a review of the nurse's skills and knowledge, the family support systems, and community resources.

Developing a plan to meet the goals involves specifying activities, prioritizing goals, and selecting a starting point. Next, the nurse and the family decide who will be responsible for which activities. Setting time limits involves deciding on a deadline for accomplishing (or evaluating progress toward accomplishing) a goal and the frequency of contacts. At the agreed-on time, the nurse and family together evaluate the progress in both process and outcome. The contract can be modified, renegotiated, or terminated on the basis of the evaluation.

Advantages and Disadvantages of Contracting

Contracting takes time and effort and may require the family and nurse to reorient their roles (Duiveman and Bonner, 2012). Increased control on the part of the family also means increased responsibility. Some nurses may have difficulty relinquishing the role of the controlling expert professional. Contracts are not always successful, and contracting is neither appropriate nor possible in every case. Some clients do not want to have this kind of involvement; they prefer to defer to the "authority" of the professional. Clients who may not choose to contract include persons with minimal cognitive skills, those who are involved in an emergency situation, persons who are unwilling to be more active in their own care, and those who do not see control or authority for health concerns as being within their domain. Some of these clients may learn to contract; others never will be able to do so.

The nursing process does not necessarily provide an active role for the family as a client; the assumption that a need exists is based on professional judgment only, and it is also assumed that changes can and should be made within the family unit. Contracting is one alternative approach that depends on the value of input from both the nurse and family, the competency of the family, the family's ability to be responsible, and the dynamic nature of the process. Contracting not only allows for but also requires continual renegotiating. Although it may not be appropriate in all situations or with all families, contracting can provide direction and structure to health risk reduction and health promotion in families.

Empowering Families

Approaches for helping individuals and families assume an active role in their health care should focus on empowerment rather than enabling or help-giving (Chen et al., 2018). Help-giving interventions do not always have positive outcomes for clients. If families do not perceive a situation as a problem or need, offers of help may cause resentment. Help-giving also may have negative consequences if there is not a match between what is expected and what is offered. A nurse's failure to recognize a family's competencies and to define an active role for them can lead to the family's dependency and lack of growth. This can be frustrating for both the nurse and the family. For families to become active participants, they need to feel a sense of personal competence and a desire for and willingness to take action. Definitions of empowerment reflect the following three characteristics of the empowered family seeking help:

- Access and control over needed resources
- Decision-making and problem-solving abilities
- The ability to communicate and to obtain needed resources

The last characteristic refers to the fact that families may need to learn how to identify sources of help, how to contact agencies, how to ask critical questions, and how to negotiate with agencies to meet family needs. These characteristics often reflect a process by which people (i.e., individuals, families, organizations, and communities) take control of their own lives. The outcomes of empowerment can be positive self-esteem, the ability to set and reach goals, a sense of control over life and change processes, and a sense of hope for the future (Chen et al., 2018).

The Levels of Prevention box shows prevention strategies applied to families.

Empowerment requires a viewpoint that often conflicts with the views of many helping professions, including nursing. Empowerment's underlying assumption is one of a partnership between the professional and the client as opposed to one in which the professional is dominant. Families are assumed to be either competent or capable of becoming competent. This implies that the professional is not an unchallenged authority who is in control. Empowerment promotes an environment that creates opportunities for competencies to be used. Finally, families need to determine that their actions result in behavior change. A nursing intervention that incorporates the principles of empowerment is

directed toward the building of nurse–family partnerships and emphasizes health risk reduction and health promotion. The nurse's approach to the family should be positive and focused on competencies rather than on problems or deficits. The interventions need to be consistent with family cultural norms and the family's perception of the problem. Rather than making decisions for the family, the nurse supports the family in their decision making and bolsters their self-esteem by recognizing and using family strengths and support networks. Interventions that promote desired family behaviors increase family competency, decrease the need for outside help, and result in families seeing themselves as being actively responsible for bringing about desired changes. The goal of an empowering approach is to create a partnership between the nurse and the family characterized by cooperation and shared responsibility.

LEVELS OF PREVENTION

Strategies for Prevention Related to Families

Primary Prevention
Complete a family genogram and assess health risks with the family to contract for family health activities to prevent diseases from developing.

Secondary Prevention
Use a behavioral health risk survey to identify the factors leading to health problems, such as obesity in the family.

Tertiary Prevention
Develop a contract with the family to change nutritional patterns to reduce further complications from the specified health problem.

Vulnerable Populations at Risk: Lesbian, Gay, Bisexual, Transgendered Families and Teenage Parent Families

The following listing is just a beginning of terms for persons who do not identify as heterosexual, such as lesbian, gay, bisexual, transgender, queer/questioning, intersexual, ally/asexual, and a plus sign to designate those who are not included (LGBTQIA+) (Gold, 2018). It is ever evolving, along with the scope of familial and other relationships and groupings to which these persons belong. Over the past decade, there has been an explosion of visibility for this population. Debates and legal battles centering on LGBTQIA+ rights have taken place nationally and in states across the country. Notable examples include same-sex marriage, which was established in a civil rights case in 2015 by the US Supreme Court; adoptions by same-sex couples; opening of the military to gays, lesbians, and transgendered individuals (although the debate continues in the administrative branch of government); and a plethora of antidiscrimination laws. However, antidiscrimination laws often are not clearly written or adhered to, as shown in the 2018 Supreme Court decision that ruled in favor of a Christian baker who refused to bake a wedding cake for a gay couple while at the same time voicing support for gay rights (Savage, 2018).

As noted in the introduction to this section, nurses have an ethical obligation to provide culturally competent care to

LGBTQIA+ families. To fulfill this obligation, nurses should first seek to provide a safe environment for clients to discuss their sexual orientation. Although some nurses may feel a degree of discomfort discussing sexual orientation with their clients, it is important to develop learning strategies to help overcome this barrier to care for LGBTQIA+ families.

Just as there is great variation among heterosexual families, all LGBTQIA+ families are not the same. Nurses are well prepared to learn to better assess and contribute to a growing understanding of the dynamics of LGBTQIA+ families and their associated health care needs as well as the obstacles to care which they may face. Same-sex couples have historically had special barriers within the health care system. Although the Supreme Court settled the issue of same-sex marriage, there continues to be a great variation in LGBTQIA+ adoption rights. The lack of legal recognition for LGBTQIA+ relationships in most areas of the country has resulted in barriers that often present challenges for LGBTQIA+ families seeking to access the health care system as well. Despite the Supreme Court's recognition of same-sex marriage nationwide, there continues to be discrimination (Wordon, 2014).

On April 15, 2010, President Obama signed a directive instructing hospitals that accept Medicaid and Medicare to allow adult clients the right to designate specific individuals who can visit them in the hospital or make medical decisions on their behalf. This helped to alleviate some issues that LGBTQIA+ partners face when interacting with the health care system. (See https://obamawhitehouse.archives.gov for more information.)

Nurses are in an optimal position to fulfill a vital role in helping LGBTQIA+ families achieve equitable access to health care. Nurses can assist with assessing the implementation of health care policy such as Obama's directive. In addition, nurses can help to advocate for more policies designed to reduce barriers within the health care system for LGBTQIA+ families, such as the inclusion of culturally competent care and the education of all health care providers in providing culturally appropriate health care.

Another type of family at risk is the more "traditional" family with a nonheterosexual member. After a family member declares his or her sexual preferences, families may need initial support to process the information. Nurses may be in a position to provide support during this time. Nurses may also refer families to community resources, such as Parents and Friends of Lesbians and Gays (www.pflag.org). Check within your local community for other appropriate resources.

In addition to providing support for the family unit as a whole, nurses may also be in a position to assess LGBTQIA+ individuals. As in all family units, the health of individual members of a family affects the entire family unit. Sexual and gender minorities face a higher risk for depression, anxiety, substance abuse, thoughts of suicide, and suicide. Addressing mental health issues in these populations may help reduce the mental health disparities the LGBTQIA+ population faces.

A vulnerable family group may be one that includes a pregnant teen. This family structure faces multiple health-related and social challenges, especially affordable and accessible health care and the recruitment and development of mentors to help teen parents acquire health care. Teenage parents may feel humiliation and uncertainty and have little confidence in handling adult responsibilities other than actual parenting. Teenage-instructional literature on family health policy information and health care service accessibility written from the perspective of teenagers is needed. Single teenage parents need to understand welfare and how to apply for it, as well as how to find support communities. Teenage parents who decide not to be involved in a child's life need to understand child support, adoption, and legal visitation and involvement issues. Education, vocational opportunity, and social acceptance are "luxuries" often missed by adolescent parents. Although the last of these issues can be solved only by eventual cultural assimilation, schooling and careers should be made possible.

Although it is not advisable to simply hand out opportunities to teenagers with children, it is important to offer assistance, not only so that they may have a second chance at a successful life but for their children as well. Children of teenage parents often make the same mistakes as their parents because of factors of poor living conditions, low socioeconomic status, and a difficult childhood. Adequate family health care can help break the cycle of teen parents. Today many people are advocating for sex education and prevention, but it is also time *now* for postpregnancy programs that accept that there is a child born to two teenagers. Although they may have made a poor choice, these teenagers now have *no* choice but to accept parental responsibility and be shown the tools to do so.

In addition to providing support for the family unit as a whole, nurses may also be in a position to assess LGBTQIA+ individuals. As in all family units, the health of individual members of a family affects the entire family unit. Sexual minorities face a higher risk for depression, anxiety, substance abuse, thoughts of suicide, and suicide. Addressing mental health issues in this population may help reduce the mental health disparities the LGBT and teen parent populations face.

COMMUNITY RESOURCES

Families have varied and complex needs and problems. The nurse is often involved in mobilizing several resources to effectively and appropriately meet family health promotion needs. Although the specific resources vary from community to community, general types include state and national government resources, such as Medicare, Medicaid, TANF, WIC, Supplementary Security Income, food stamps, and State Children's Health Insurance Program (SCHIP). These programs primarily provide support for basic needs (e.g., illness or health care, nutrition, funds for housing, clothing) and funds are based on meeting eligibility criteria (Families USA, 2012, 2013, 2018).

In addition to government agencies providing health-related services to families, most communities have voluntary (nongovernment) programs. Local chapters of such organizations provide education, support services, and some direct services to individuals and families. Examples are the American Cancer Society, American Heart Association, American Lung Association, and Muscular Dystrophy Association. These agencies provide primary prevention and health promotion services, as well as screening programs and assistance after the disease or condition is diagnosed. Local social service agencies (e.g., Catholic Social Services) provide direct services such as counseling to families. Other voluntary organizations provide direct services (e.g., shelters for homeless or battered individuals, substance abuse counseling and treatment, Meals on Wheels, transportation, clothing, food, furniture).

Health resources in the community may be *proprietary, voluntary,* or *public*. In addition to private health care providers, nurses should be aware of voluntary and public clinics, screening programs, and health promotion programs. Identifying resources in a community requires time and effort. The telephone book and the Internet are good places to begin the search for local community resources. Also, community service organizations, such as the local chamber of commerce and health department, publish community resource listings. Brochures listing services are often available in clinics and health care providers' offices. Regardless of how the resource is identified, the nurse needs to be familiar with the types of services offered and any requirements or costs involved. If this information is not available, the nurse can contact the resource.

Locating and using these systems often requires skills and patience that many families lack. Nurses work with families to identify community resources and, as client advocates, they help families learn to use resources. This may involve sharing information with families, rehearsing with families what questions to ask, preparing required materials, making the initial contact, and arranging transportation. The appropriateness and effectiveness of resources should be evaluated with families afterward. It is important to remember that navigating the maze of resources is often difficult for the nurse. If a family is in crisis or does not have a phone or a home base from which to call or receive return calls, this process is even more difficult and their sense of helplessness may be increased. Therefore the nurse's assistance, while promoting the family's sense of empowerment, is a necessary and often complex undertaking.

Telehomecare

Another resource and type of service that is growing in acceptance and availability is telehomecare, which may be called *telehealth* or *telemedicine*. The goal is for clients to communicate with and transfer information to providers from their home. Telehomecare monitoring requires less time per client interaction, so it allows nurses to feasibly care for more clients per day. In addition, clients (including elderly individuals), as well as their caregivers, report few technological problems. Telehomecare can be a particularly useful option in situations in which ongoing and frequent monitoring of a family member's condition is necessary; however, it should be recognized that it is not a substitute for the in-home trust and relationship building and assessment of both family and community resources that can be accomplished only by an attentive and engaged nurse spending time with the family in their home environment. This kind of health care delivery is well suited to areas of the country where the distance between the client and the source of health care is either a large distance or might take a long time because of traffic patterns or when the client does not have transportation.

Policies

I With an influence on family health care, one national policy passed to strengthen and support the family is the *Family Medical Leave Act* (FMLA). On February 5, 1993, President Clinton signed the FMLA (PL 103-3). This act allows covered employees to take up to 12 weeks of leave each year for certain family and medical reasons (National Partnership for Women and Families, 2016). Many states have added more leave time and benefits for employees in their state. Under the FMLA, employees may take an unpaid leave of absence for many reasons: for their own serious illness; for the illness of their child, parent, or spouse; and for the birth or adoption of a child (PL 103-3). While on leave, employees still receive their medical benefits and are guaranteed that their position or one similar to it will be available to them on returning to work. The FMLA was needed to help Americans meet the needs of their families while maintaining employment. Women in particular were experiencing hardship in keeping a job while having a family. A relatively recent emerging family policy issue is paid leave for fathers. Internationally, paternity leave policies vary greatly from country to country. Family policies such as these reflect a growing recognition and valuing of the healthy family unit as a key factor and contributor to the health of not only individuals, but our communities and society at large.

> ### ▶▶ APPLYING CONTENT TO PRACTICE
>
> This chapter focuses on means to define family health. There are risk factors to family health including biological, environmental, behavioral, and health care risks. Health care risks are a result of the family involvement with the health care system which the family is usually unable to control. The overall health of the nation is dependent upon the health of families and reflects the causes of morbidity and mortality rates within the nation's population. Understanding family genetics and family dynamics provide the health care system with data upon which to develop a family health care plan. An approach used in nursing is the home visit, which offers an opportunity to develop a family health plan and better understand the roles and responses to health and illness within the family structure.

■ PRACTICE APPLICATION

The initial contact between a nursing service and a family provides limited information, and the situation that develops may be much more complex than anticipated. The following example, based on an actual case, illustrates the issues and approaches outlined in this chapter.

The Fayette County Health Department was notified that Amy Cress, age 16 years, had been referred by the school counselor at the local high school for prenatal supervision. Amy was 4 months pregnant, in apparently good health, in the 10th grade, and living at home with her mother, stepfather, and younger sister. The family lived in a rural area outside of a small farming community. The father of the baby also lived in the community and continued to see Amy on a regular basis. The referral information provided the nurse with a beginning, but limited, assessment of the family situation.

A. What would you do first as the nurse assigned to this family?

B. How would you help this family learn to take responsibility for this situation?

C. After the initial contact, how would you extend the assessment to the entire family system?

D. Would you contract with this family? How? What would be the terms of the contract?

Answers can be found on the Evolve website.

■ REMEMBER THIS!

- The importance of the family as a major client system for nurses in reducing health risks and promoting the health of individuals and populations is well documented.

- The family is a basic unit within which health behavior, including health values, health habits, and health risk perceptions, is developed, organized, and performed.

- Knowledge of family structure and functioning is fundamental to implementing the nursing process with families in the community.

- Nurses need to go beyond the individual and family and to understand the complex environment in which the family functions to be effective in reducing family health risks. Categories of risk factors that are important to family health are biological, environmental (including economic factors), and behavioral risk.

- Several factors contribute to the experience of healthy or unhealthy outcomes. Not everyone exposed to the same event will have the same outcome. The factors that influence whether disease or other unhealthy results occur are called *health risks*. The accumulated risks are synergistic; their combined effect is more important than individual effects.

- An important aspect of nursing's role in reducing health risk and promoting the health of populations has been providing services to individual families in their homes.

- Home visits offer the opportunity to gain a more accurate assessment of the family structure and behavior in the natural environment. They also provide opportunities to observe the home environment and identify both barriers and supports to reducing health risks and increasingly look toward working with clients in an interactive, collaborative style.

- Contracting, which is making an agreement between two or more parties, involves a shift in responsibility and control from the professional alone to a shared effort by client and professional.

- Families have varied and complex needs and problems. The nurse often mobilizes several resources to effectively and appropriately meet family health needs.

EVOLVE WEBSITE

http://evolve.elsevier.com/Stanhope/foundations
- NCLEX® Review Questions
- Case Study, with Questions and Answers
- Practice Application Answers

REFERENCES

Artiga S, Hinton E: *Beyond Health Care: The Role of Social Determinants in Promoting Health and Health Equity.* May 10, 2017. Retrieved from: www.kff.org.

Artiga S, Ubri P, Foutz J: *What is at stake for health and health care disparities under ACA repeal?* Henry J. Kaiser Family Foundation, 2018. Available at: https://www.kff.org. Accessed June 24, 2018.

Avellar S, Paulsell D, Sam-Miller E, et al.: *Home visiting evidence of effectiveness review: executive summary,* OPRE Report #2015-85a, Mathematica Policy Research, 2016

Beckman S, Fawcett J, editors: *Neuman Systems Model: celebrating academic-practice partnerships,* Fort Wayne, 2017, Neuman Systems Model Trustee Group, Inc.

Belloc NB, Breslow L, Hochstim JR: Measurement of physical health in a general population survey, *Am J Epidemiol* 93:328–336, 1972.

Biden J: Speaker at 2014 Health Action Conference, Washington, DC, 2014, Families USA.

Buettner D: *The blue zones: 9 lessons for living longer,* 2nd ed. Washington, DC, 2009, National Geographic.

Buettner D: *Blue zones, 2008-2018: Power 9, reverse engineering longevity,* 2008-2018, Washington, DC, National Geographic.

Califano JA Jr: *Healthy People: The Surgeon General's Report on Health Promotion and Disease Prevention,* Washington, DC, 1979, US Government Printing Office.

Carlson, S and Neuberger, Z. *WIC Works: Addressing the Nutrition and Health Needs of Low-Income Families for 40 Years.* Center on Budget and Policy Priorities, 2017, Washington, DC.

Centers for Disease Control and Prevention (CDC): *Physical Activity and Health,* 2018. Available at: https://www.cdc.gov. Accessed June 20, 2018.

Chen L, Chen Y, Chen X, et al.: Longitudinal study of effectiveness of a patient-centered self-management empowerment intervention during predischarge planning on stroke survivors, *Worldviews Evid Based Nurs* 15(3):197–205, 2018.

Conger RD, Lorenz FO, Wickrama KAS, editors: *Continuity and change in family relations: theory, methods, and empirical findings,* reprint, New York, 2014, Taylor and Francis.

Congressional Budget Office: *Repealing the Individual Health Insurance Mandate: An Updated Estimate,* Washington, DC, 2017, Congressional Budget Office. Available at: www.cbo.gov. Accessed June 24, 2018.

Doherty WJ, McCubbin HI: Family and health care, *Family Relat* 34:5, 1985

Duiveman T, Bonner A: Negotiating: experiences of community nurses when contracting with clients, *Advances Contemp Nurse* 41:120–125, 2012.

Families USA: *A 50-state look at Medicaid expansion,* 2018. Available at: http://familiesusa.org. Accessed June 25, 2018.

Families USA: *Help is at hand: new health insurance tax credits,* 2013. Available at: http://familiesusa.org. Accessed June 25, 2018.

Families USA: *Medicaid leads to better education,* 2012. Available at: http://familiesusa.org/blog/medicaid. Accessed June 25, 2018.

Families USA: *To tackle health disparities, make care more affordable,* 2015. Available at: http://familiesusa.org. Accessed June 25, 2018.

Gold M: The ABCs of L.G.B.T.Q.I.A. The *New York Times,* June 21, 2018. Available at: https://www.nytimes.com. Accessed June 25, 2018.

Holtslander L, Solar J, Smith NR: The 15-minute family interview as a learning strategy for senior undergraduate nursing students, *J Fam Nurs* 19:230–248, 2014.

Keller LO, Strohschein S, Lia-Hoagberg B et al.: Population-based Public Health interventions: practice-based and evidence-supported. I. *Public Health Nurs* 21:453-468, 2004a.

Keller LO, Strohschein S, Schaffer MA et al.: Population-based public health interventions: innovations in practice, teaching, and management. II. *Public Health Nurs* 21:469-487, 2004b.

Kaiser Family Foundation: Beyond Health Care, 2018, Available at: www.Kff.org.

Litman TJ: The family as a basic unit in health and medical care: a social-behavioral overview, *Soc Sci Med* 8:495–519, 1974.

Mauksch HO: A social science basis for conceptualizing family health, *Soc Sci Med* 8:521–528, 1974.

Livingston G: Family life is changing in different ways in the US, Washington, DC, 2018, Pew Foundation.

Murdaugh CL, Parsons MA, Pender NJ: *Health promotion in nursing practice,* 8th ed. Upper Saddle River, 2019, Pearson.

National Center for Health Statistics (NCHS): *Health, United States, 2016: with chartbook on long-term trends in health,* Hyattsville, 2017, NCHS.

National Institute on Drug Abuse (NIDA): *Addiction and health.* Washington, DC, 2014, USDHHS. Available at: http://www.drugabuse.gov. Accessed June 25, 2018.

Nightingale EO, Cureton M, Kalmar V, et al.: *Perspectives on health promotion and disease prevention in the United States.* Washington, DC, 1978, Institute of Medicine, National Academy of Sciences.

Oneal GA, Eide P, Hamilton R, et al.: Rural families' process of re-forming environmental health risk messages, *J Nurs Scholarsh* 47(4):354–362, 2015.

Pratt L: Family Structure and effective health behavior, Boston, 1976, Houhton Mifflin.

Price CA, Bush, KR, Price SJ: Families and change: coping with stressful events and transitions, 5th ed. Thousand Oaks, 2017, Sage.

Purdue University: What is a family? July 2015. Retrieved from: https://www.purdue.edu/.

Robling M, Butler CC et al.: Effectiveness of a nurse-led intensive home visitation program for first-time teenage mothers (Building Blocks): a pragmatic randomized controlled trial, *Lancet*, 387:146-155, 2016.

Savage DG: Supreme Court rules for Christian cake baker but voices support for gay rights too. *Los Angeles Times,* June 4, 2018. Available at: http://www.latimes.com/. Accessed June 26, 2018.

Sewell M, Marczak M: *Using cost analysis in evaluation,* 2014. Available at: http://ag.arizona.edu. Accessed June 25, 2018.

Shi L, Singh D: *Delivering health care in America: a systems approach,* 7th ed. Burlington, 2019, Jones & Bartlett Learning.

National Partnership for Women and Families: *Guide to Family Medical Leave Act,* ed 8, Washington, DC, 2016, National Partnership for Women and Families.

PL 103-3, The Family Medical Leave Act, 1993.

Thomas TN, Kolasa MS, Zhang F, et al.: Assessing immunization interventions in the Women, Infants, and Children (WIC) program, *Am J Prev Med* 47(5):624–628, 2014.

US Department of Agriculture, Food and Nutrition Service: Women, Infants and Children. *About WIC—how WIC helps,* 2018. Available at: http://www.fns.usda.gov. Accessed June 20, 2018.

US Department of Health and Human Services, Administration for Children and Families: Administration on Children, Youth and Families, Children's Bureau: *Child maltreatment 2016,* 2018. Available at: https://www.acf.hhs.gov. Accessed June 15, 2018.

US Department of Health and Human Services (USDHHS): *Healthy People 2030.* Washington, DC, 2020, USDHHS, Public Health Service.

US Department of Health and Human Services (USDHHS): *Healthy People 2020.* Washington, DC, 2010, US Government Printing Office.

US Department of Agriculture (USDHHS): *Dietary guidelines for Americans 2015-2020,* 8th ed. 2015. Available at: https://health.gov. 2015.

Vooradi S, Mateti UV: A systemic review on lifestyle interventions to reduce blood pressure, *J Health Res* Rev 3:1–5, 2016.

Worden A, Couloumbis A: Pennsylvania governor won't appeal gay marriage ruling, 2014. Available at: http://www.governing.com.

White JM, Klein DM, Martin TF: *Family theories: an introduction,* 4th ed. Thousand Oaks, 2015, Sage Publications.

22

Health Risks Across the Life Span

Cynthia Rubenstein, Monty Gross, Andrea Knopp, Hazel Brown, and Lynn Wasserbauer

OBJECTIVES

After reading this chapter, the student should be able to:

1. Discuss major health problems of children and adolescents.
2. Describe nursing measures to promote child and adolescent health within the community.
3. Discuss risk factors for adults, including those factors that are different in men and women.
4. Describe risk factors for older adults.
5. Discuss risk factors for persons in the community who have special health needs.
6. Explain nursing measures designed to reduce risks for adults in the community.

CHAPTER OUTLINE

KEY TERMS

This chapter examines the health status of individuals across the life span and describes nursing community interventions for these groups. Emphasis is on the health status, leading causes of death and disease, and health risks of children and adolescents, adults, older adults, and selected at-risk populations. Consideration is also given to special needs populations in the community on how to assess health risks. This chapter also discusses major public health problems of populations across the life span as identified in *Healthy People 2030* (US Department of Health and Human Services [USDHHS], 2020a). Nurses who work in the community using a population-centered approach can significantly influence individuals of all ages by teaching how to increase their health promotion activities and reduce risk for disease and disability.

STATUS OF CHILDREN

To provide population-centered nursing care, it is important to understand the changing demographics of American children. The number of children determines the need for schools, health care, and other services. In 2018 there were 73.4 million children in the United States between the ages of 1 to 17. Of this number, 65% lived in a home with two married parents; 17% lived in poverty, and 17% experienced food insecurity (Federal Interagency Forum on Child and Family Statistics, 2019). In 2016, of the children in the US under 18 years of age, 41% were considered low income and 19% were poor. According to the National Center for Children in Poverty (Jiang and Koball, 2018) "Being a child in a low-income or poor family does not happen by chance" (p. 1). Examples of factors associated with children's economic insecurity include education of parents, employment, and race/ethnicity. In 2020, the federal poverty level (FPL) for a family of four was $26,200, and for a family of eight was $44,120. The FPL is higher for residents of Hawaii due to their higher cost of living (US Department of Health and Human Services, 2020b). The percentages of low-income and poor children under 18 vary by race and ethnicity with Hispanics comprising the largest share. Black, American Indian, and children of immigrants are more likely to be in low-income families. Interestingly, in 2016, the largest percentage of low-income children lived in the South. Children of immigrants face more health barriers than native-born children, including a lack of health insurance, poverty, language barriers, and substandard housing (Jiang and Koball, 2018). Because so many of these percentages changed due to the COVID-19 pandemic and its enormous effects on the economy, it is important to look at the current year data on the key sites used.

CHILDREN'S HEALTH AND MAJOR PUBLIC HEALTH ISSUES

The health and well-being of children have a significant impact on the future of any country. Effective health care includes getting immunizations and having regular dental and primary care visits that include health education. Children with health insurance, whether public or private, are more likely to have regular access to health care than are children without insurance. Access to quality health is one of the focus areas of *Healthy People 2030*. Both Medicaid and the State Children's Health Insurance Plan (SCHIP) are federal and state plans that provide publicly funded health care to children. Because physical, cognitive, and emotional changes occur more rapidly during childhood and adolescence than at any other time in the life span, access to regular health visits at key ages is important in monitoring these changes. Nursing assessments include evaluation of growth, development, health status, quality of the parent–child relationship, and family support systems.

Obesity

Obesity rates in American children have risen to epidemic levels over the past few decades. These increases are noted for all children aged 2 to 18 years regardless of gender or ethnicity. The Centers for Disease Control and Prevention (CDC) defines overweight as a body mass index (BMI) at or above the 85th percentile and lower than the 95th percentile, and obesity is defined as a BMI at or above the 95th percentile for children of the same age and sex when plotted on the CDC growth charts (Table 22.1) (CDC, 2016a). In 2015 to 2016, the prevalence of obesity was 13.9% in children aged 2 to 5 years, 18.4% in children aged 6 to 11 years, and 20.6% in adolescents aged 12 to 19 years. The prevalence of obesity is higher in non-Hispanic African American and Hispanic children and teens as compared to non-Hispanic White, and non-Hispanic Asian children and teens (Hales et al., 2020).

Many factors contribute to the likelihood that a child will become overweight or obese, including genetics, family eating and physical activity patterns, and time spent watching television, using digital media, including computer/tablet, phone, or using other electronic devices. The environment in which children live influences obesity. For example, if the area is heavily built up and does not allow space for parks, walking paths, or recreation sites, children have reduced areas to expend energy in games, sports, and play. At least 70% of overweight children will become overweight adults. Many children live in households that are unable to provide adequate amounts of nutritious food. Food insecurity increased during the COVID-19 pandemic when many people lost their jobs.

TABLE 22.1 Classification of the Body Mass Index in Children Aged 2 Years and Above

Plotted Percentile for Age and Gender	BMI Interpretation
<5th percentile	Underweight
5th–85th percentile	Normal
85th–95th percentile	Overweight
≥95th percentile	Obese

BMI, Body mass index.
From Centers for Disease Control and Prevention: Classification of body mass index, 2015. Available at www.CDC.gov

The physiological consequences of childhood obesity are significant and have long-term effects. Specifically, an obese child has an increased disease risk for these health problems: cardiovascular, due to high blood pressure (HBP) and high cholesterol; metabolic, due to increased or impaired glucose tolerance, insulin resistance, and type 2 diabetes; musculoskeletal; respiratory, due to asthma and sleep apnea; and renal problems, due to fatty liver disease, gallstones and gastroesophageal reflux (Chandrasekhar et al., 2017; CDC, 2016a). Childhood obesity is also related to anxiety, depression, low self-esteem, and social problems such as bullying and stigma (CDC, 2016a).

Of particular concern is the rising association between childhood obesity and type 2 diabetes mellitus. Approximately 210,000 US children and adolescents under the age of 20 years had diabetes in 2018 (CDC, 2020a). Whites and males between the ages of 10 to 14 are more likely than other groups to be diagnosed with type 1 diabetes although the rate since 2011 has significantly increased among Asians and Pacific Islanders. There are no known ways to prevent type 1 diabetes (Divers et al., 2020).

Screening for type 2 diabetes mellitus is recommended for children with a BMI from the 85th to the 95th percentile with two or more of the following risk factors:

- Family history of type 2 diabetes in a first- or second-degree relative
- Native American, African American, Latino, Asian American, or Pacific Islander descent
- Signs of insulin resistance or conditions associated with insulin resistance
- Maternal history of diabetes or gestational diabetes mellitus (GDM) during the child's gestation (American Diabetes Association [ADA], 2016).
- The CDC says these factors contribute to childhood obesity: genetics; metabolism, eating and physical activity behavior; community and neighborhood design and safety; short sleep duration; and negative childhood events (CDC, 2018). Excessive body fat at a young age is likely to persist into adulthood and is associated with physical and psychosocial comorbidities, as well as lower cognitive ability, retardation in school, and later life achievement (CDC, 2016a).

High-fat diets and inactivity are the major contributors to obesity. The American diet in general tends to be high in fat, calories, and sugar, with generous serving sizes. School lunches and "fast-food" meals tend to be oversized and nutritionally poor. Vending machines with non-nutritious food choices can be found in schools. Colas and sugary fruit drinks add calories without nutritional value. Also, the increasing popularity among children of using gadgets and watching television contribute to a sedentary lifestyle, and schools do not consistently have physical education on a regular basis.

Interventions need to be based on goals of family lifestyle changes. The goal is to modify the way the family eats, exercises, and plans daily activities. Strategies for working with families for obesity prevention are discussed in Box 22.1. The goal of managing weight in children and adolescents is to normalize weight. This may involve slowing the rate of weight gain and allowing

BOX 22.1   Family Recommendations for Obesity Prevention

- Breastfeeding is associated with a lower risk for developing childhood obesity.
- Parents' responsibilities include providing healthy meals and snacks for their children.
- Limit 100% fruit juices and avoid all other sugary beverages. These are empty calories and fill children up so they are not hungry at meals. Appropriate beverages are milk and water.
- For toddlers and preschoolers, it sometimes takes 10–15 tastes of a new food before learning to like that food. Be persistent!
- Parents should role model good eating behaviors—lots of fruits and vegetables, no sugary beverages, and little to no "junk food" or "fast food."
- Family meals are important for teaching manners, listening to hunger cues, and having quality family time together.
- Encourage children to help with food selection and preparation as appropriate to developmental skills. Allow them to select new foods to try in the produce section of the grocery store.
- Avoid using food as a punishment or reward. Do not expect your child to "clean the plate." These feeding techniques have been associated with increased risk for obesity.
- Turn off the television during meals and do not let your child eat in front of the television. Children do not listen to their cues of satiety when distracted.
- Cook meals at home. Broil, bake, stir-fry, or poach foods rather than frying.
- Modify family eating habits to include low-fat food choices. Serve calorically dense foods that incorporate the food guide pyramid: whole grains, fruits, vegetables, lean protein foods, and low-fat dairy products.
- Encourage family members to stop eating when they are satisfied. Encourage recognizing hunger and satiation cues.
- Schedule regular times for meals and snacks. Include breakfast and do not skip meals.
- Have low-calorie, nutritious snacks ready and available. Avoid having empty-calorie junk foods in the home. Plan for healthy snacks when eating "on the run"—granola, fruits, and nuts.
- Decrease salt, sugar, and fat. Increase complex carbohydrates—whole grains.
- Maintain regular activity (e.g., exercise, sports) and limit television viewing.
- Select family activities and vacations that include or focus on physical activity (hiking, bicycling, swimming).

children to "grow" into their weight, improving dietary habits, increasing physical activity, improving self-esteem, and improving parent relationships. The "Let's Move!" campaign promoted by former First Lady Michelle Obama is a comprehensive initiative to prevent childhood obesity. It has four primary components: healthy schools, access to affordable and healthy food, raising children's physical activity levels, and helping parents make healthy choices. It offers easy-to-understand information on how to eat healthfully, get active, and take action to prevent obesity on the website at http://www.letsmove.gov. See Table 22.2 for daily guidelines for food for children and adolescents.

Healthy People 2030 objectives include improving the nutritional status and physical activity patterns of the nation's youth. The American Academy of Pediatrics (AAP) recommends 60 minutes of moderate aerobic physical activity per day for every child and adolescent (AAP, 2015). It is important for families to be active together because this promotes both physical exercise and family engagement. Schools can be a

TABLE 22.2	Daily Dietary Recommendations: Childhood and Adolescence			
Food Group[a]	2–3 Years	4–8 Years	9–13 Years	14–18 Years
Milk: Try to select low-fat sources of milk, cheese, yogurt	2 cups	2–2½ cups	3 cups	3 cups
Meat and Beans: Lean meats, beans, eggs, seafood	2 oz	4 oz	5 oz	5–6½ oz
Vegetables: Fresh vegetables best choice	1 cup	1–1½ cups	2–2½ cups	2½–3 cups
Fruits: Limit fruit juices	1 cup	1–1½ cups	1½ cups	2 cups
Grains: Half of grains should be whole grains; cooked pasta or rice, bread, cereals	3 oz	5 oz	5–6 oz	6–8 oz

[a]Recommendations are per day for each group.
Modified from US Department of Agriculture: Choose my plate, 2015. www.USDA.gov.

source of physical activity when they have regularly scheduled recess that promotes activity, as well as when they have structured activity for the students.

Injuries and Accidents

Injuries and accidents are the most common causes of preventable disease, disability, and death among children. Unintentional injuries are any injuries sustained by accident, such as falls, fires, drowning, suffocation, poisoning, sports, or recreation or motor vehicle accidents. Reducing injuries from unintentional causes, as well as from violence and abuse, is a goal of *Healthy People 2030*. More than 22,200 children are seen in emergency departments daily for treatment from a nonfatal unintentional injury (Ballesteros et al., 2018). Most injuries are predictable and preventable. Because of their size, growth and development, inexperience, and natural curiosity, children and teens are especially at risk for injury. The key to changing behaviors is teaching age-appropriate safety. The National Action Plan for Child Injury Prevention provides an overarching framework to guide those working to prevent injuries and promote the safety of children and adolescents (CDC, NCIPC, 2012) (Fig. 22.1).

The leading causes of unintentional injuries in children are motor vehicle accidents, suffocation, drowning, poisoning, fire, and falls (CDC, 2016b). Motor vehicle injuries are a leading cause of death among children in the United States (CDC, 2016b). During 2018 in the United States, 1196 children ages 15 years and younger died as occupants in motor vehicle crashes, and more than 198,000 were injured (National Highway Traffic Safety Administration [NHTSA], 2020). Many of these deaths can be prevented by having children of all ages buckle up in age- and size-appropriate car seats, booster seats, and seat belts. This reduces serious and fatal injuries by more than half (CDC, 2016b). The National Highway Traffic Safety Administration provides guidance on the how to provide adequate support to children under the age of 12 years. Drowning, poisoning, and burns account for most of the other deaths for children. For infants, the leading cause of death is suffocation.

Age-related development is an important issue in identifying risks to children. Table 22.3 lists the five leading causes and number of nonfatal unintentional injuries among children treated in emergency departments, by age group.

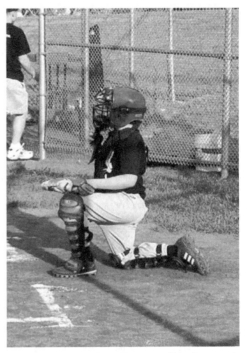

Fig. 22.1 Involvement in Developmentally Appropriate Sports Promotes Physical Activity and Skills Acquisition.

Developmental Considerations

Infants. Infants have the second highest injury rate of all children groups; their small size contributes to some types of injury. The small airway may be easily occluded. The small body fits through places where the head may be entrapped. In motor vehicle crashes, having a small size is a great disadvantage and increases the risk for crushing or being propelled into surfaces.

The second half of infancy brings major accomplishments in gross motor activities. Rolling, sitting, pulling up, and walking bring safety concerns. Their developing motor skills remain immature, which limits their ability to escape from injury and places them at risk for drowning, suffocating, and burns (CDC, NCIPC, 2012).

Toddlers and preschoolers. This population experiences a large number of nonfatal falls and being struck by or against an

TABLE 22.3   Leading Causes of Unintentional Injury Death Among US Children Aged 0 to 19 Years, 2016

Rank	0–1 Years	1–4 Years	5–9 Years	10–14 Years	15–19 Years
1	Suffocation	Drowning	MVT-related[a]	MVT-related[a]	MVT-related[a]
2	Homicide	MVT-related[a]	Drowning	Suicide	Poisoning
3	MVT-related[a]	Suffocation	Burns/fire	Drowning	Homicide
4	Drowning	Homicide	Homicide	Homicide	Suicide
5	Adverse effects from injury	Fire/burns	Suffocation	Burns/fire	Drowning

[a]MVT-related: Motor vehicle traffic-related accidents includes motor vehicle injuries, pedestrian injuries.
Data from National Center for Health Statistics (NCHS), National Vital Statistics System, 2018. Retrieved from www.CDC.gov.

QSEN   FOCUS ON QUALITY AND SAFETY EDUCATION FOR NURSES

Targeted Competency: Client-Centered Care—Recognize the client or designee as the source of control and full partner in providing compassionate and coordinated care based on respect for the client's preferences, values, and needs.

Important aspects of client-centered care include the following:

- **Knowledge:** Describe strategies to assist clients and their families in all aspects of the health care process.
- **Skills:** Communicate client values, preferences, and expressed needs to other members of the health care team.
- **Attitudes:** Willingly support client-centered care for individuals and groups whose values differ from your values.

Client-Centered Care Question: You are making a home visit to the Jones family—Mr. and Mrs. Jones and their children, John (10 years), Sally (6 years), and Tommy (3 years). Mr. and Mrs. Jones are considered obese using the body weight index measures of the American Heart Association. John is considered overweight by this same measure, and you note that both Sally and Tommy are at the upper range for weight for their age. You observe during the visit that the family appears to eat a lot of processed food, including lunch meats, chips, and carbonated drinks with sugar. What steps would you take to help this family (1) understand the importance of maintaining an average weight, (2) learn about the different ways in which foods can be prepared, and (3) learn about the relationship among calorie consumption, physical activity, and weight?

Answer: First, you would need to assess their knowledge about weight management. Next, you would need to determine whether they have the skill and funds to purchase and prepare lower-calorie, nutritious food, and if they are capable of engaging in physical activities. You would also need to evaluate their attitude toward body size and image. Their willingness to change their behavior will be influenced by whether they view themselves as needing to change. If there is a willingness to make weight management behavior change, you can refer them to a nutrition expert for a consultation or to attend a class(es). The class might be a virtual or in-person class. You can find out how they spend their leisure time and what options they can identify that would include the entire family in a physical activity such as a walk, a game, or a trip to the park.

---

object. They are active and lack an understanding of cause and effect, and their increasing motor skills make supervision difficult (CDC, NCIPC, 2012). They are inquisitive and have relatively immature logic abilities.

School-age children. The school-age group has the lowest injury death rate. At this age, it is difficult to judge speed and distance, placing them at risk for pedestrian and bicycle accidents. Boys are twice as likely as girls to sustain a nonfatal bicycle injury, and the highest injury rate is at 10 to 14 years of age. Universal use of bicycle helmets would prevent most deaths. Peer pressure and lack of parental role modeling often inhibit the use of protective devices such as helmets and limb pads (CDC, NCIPC, 2012).

Adolescents. Motor vehicle–related injuries and violence are the leading causes of morbidity and mortality for adolescents. Risk-taking becomes more conscious at this time, especially among boys. The injury death rates for boys are twice as high as those for girls. Adolescents are at the highest risk of any age group for motor vehicle deaths and fatal poisonings. Use of weapons and drug and alcohol abuse play an important role in injuries in this age group. Homicides are the third leading cause of death of US adolescents between the ages of 10 and 19 (Kann et al., 2018). Suicides are the second leading cause of death for US adolescents. Poor social adjustment, psychiatric problems, and family disorganization increase the risk of suicide (Ballesteros et al., 2018). In a survey of adolescents, 23.6% reported being in a physical fight at least one time in the previous 12 months, and 6,7% reported missing school at least 1 day in the previous month because they felt unsafe at school or on their way to school (Kann et al., 2018).

Sports injuries are of particular concern. Children who engage in sports should have annual sports physicals, and guidelines for sports safety should be discussed as follows: Children should be grouped according to weight, size, maturation, and skill level; qualified and competent persons should be available for supervision during games and practices; adequate and appropriate-size equipment should be used; and goals should be developmentally and physically appropriate for the child. For all ages, families should be given anticipatory guidance on the high-risk areas for each age group to promote safety and injury prevention. Nurses can use community centers, schools, workplaces, and health centers to provide teaching to families on how to prevent injuries in their children.

Most states have enacted laws allowing health care providers to treat adolescents in certain situations without parental consent. These include emergency care, substance abuse, pregnancy, and birth control. All 50 states recognize the "mature minors doctrine." This allows youths 15 years of age and older to give informed medical consent if it is apparent that they are capable of understanding the risks and benefits and if the procedure is medically indicated.

Injury Prevention

Nurses play a role in the prevention of accidents and injuries. Nurses can identify risk factors by assessing the characteristics of the child, family, and environment. Interventions include anticipatory guidance, environmental modification, and safety education. Education focuses on age-appropriate interventions based on knowledge of the leading causes of death and the leading risk factors. Topics to consider are listed in Box 22.2. Health care provider offices, schools, and daycare facilities provide opportunities to teach children, adolescents, and their families how to prevent injuries. Safety can be incorporated into required health education courses. *Healthy People 2030* has a range of objectives related to safety (USDHHS, 2020a). Community-sponsored car seat and seat belt safety checks, and safety fairs are another way to educate families, as are early home visitation programs to high-risk families. Injury prevention should be addressed at all health visits. Schools, day care centers, and community groups often need guidance toward developing safe places for children to play.

The US Consumer Product Safety Commission (2015) has published comprehensive guidelines for playground safety that cover structure, materials, surfaces, and maintenance of equipment. The developmental skills of specific ages are incorporated, as well as recommendations for physically challenged children. Nurses can use these guidelines to help the community establish standards for play areas.

Gun violence is another risk factor for children who may be curious and pick up guns without understanding the danger involved. Characteristics associated with gun violence include history of aggressive behaviors, poverty, school problems, substance abuse, and cultural acceptance of violent behavior. A significant number of accidental firearm injuries and deaths in children occur in the homes of friends and family members (AAP, 2017). Interventions must begin early and address each of these factors.

The *Healthy People 2030* objectives seek to reduce the number of high school students who carry guns. Nurses can actively

participate in efforts to reduce gun violence among young people in the following ways (AAP, 2017; McBride, 2018):

- Urge legislators to support gun control legislation, assault weapons bans, and eliminate gun show loopholes.
- Collaborate with schools to develop programs to discourage violence among children.
- Encourage families to remove guns from their homes. If unable to do this, educate families to (1) store all firearms unloaded and uncocked in a securely locked container, with only the parents knowing where the container is located; (2) store the guns and ammunition in separate locked locations; (3) never leave a gun unattended when handling or cleaning it, even for a moment; it should be in the parent's view at all times.
- Initiate community programs focusing on gun storage and safety at school.
- Educate parents on communicating with the homeowners of the homes their children visit about gun access and safety.
- Children and adolescents learning to hunt in rural areas should take gun safety courses.
- Identify populations at risk for violence and target aggression or anger management.
- Discourage mixing alcohol or drugs with guns.
- Encourage families to avoid gun violence in media sources at home

Child Maltreatment

According to the Administration for Children and Families (USDHHS, ACF, 2020c), in 2018, there were an estimated 678,000 victims of abuse and neglect nationally, resulting in a rate of 9.2 victims per 1000 children in the population. Children in their first year of life have the highest rate of victimization at 26.7 per 1000 children; the rate for girls (9.6) is higher than that for boys (8.7), and American Indian or Alaska Native children have the highest rate of victimization at 15.2 per 1000 children of the same rate of race or ethnicity, followed by African Americans at 14.0 per 1000 children (USDHHS, ACF, 2020c). Children with special needs are also at higher risk.

Child maltreatment as defined by the Child Abuse Prevention and Treatment Act (CAPTA) is "any recent act or failure to act on the part of a parent or caretaker which results in death, serious physical or emotional harm, sexual abuse or exploitation; or an act or failure to act, which present an imminent risk of serious harm: to a child or teen under the age of 18" (USDHHS, ACF 2020, p. 16). Acts of commission (abuse) include physical abuse, sexual abuse, and psychological abuse; acts of omission (neglect) include failure to provide (physical neglect, emotional neglect, medical or dental neglect, educational neglect) and failure to supervise (inadequate supervision, exposure to violent environments) (USDHHS, ACF, 2020c).

Children are most likely to be maltreated by their parents, and common parental characteristics include a poor understanding of child development and children's needs, history of abuse in the family of origin, substance abuse in the household, and nonbiological transient caregivers in the home (e.g., mother's boyfriend). Families at highest risk for maltreatment are those experiencing social isolation, family violence, parenting stress, and poor parent–child relationships (USDHHS, ACF, 2020c).

BOX 22.2 Injury Prevention Topics

- Car restraints, seat belts, air-bag safety
- Preventing fires, burns
- Preventing poisoning
- Preventing falls
- Preventing drowning, water safety
- Bicycle safety
- Safe driving practices
- Sports safety
- Pedestrian safety
- Gun safety
- Decreasing gang activities
- Preventing substance abuse

Alterations of Behavior and Mental Health Problems

Behavioral problems in children and adolescents are highly variable and may include eating disorders; attention problems, including attention deficit disorder with or without hyperactivity (ADD/ADHD); substance abuse; elimination problems; conduct disorders and delinquency; sleep disorders; anxiety disorders; autism spectrum disorder; depression; bipolar disorder; or school maladaptation (American Academy of Child and Adolescent Psychiatry [AACAP], 2018). The *Diagnostic and Statistical Manual of Mental Disorders,* 5th edition (American Psychiatric Association, 2013), is the most comprehensive and up-to-date source of information for practitioners who care for children with or suspected of having mental health issues. Early recognition and coordinated management of pediatric mental health issues are critical to the child's functioning in school, at home, and in the community.

Psychosocial stressors for children have increased over the years. There are many underlying causes for mental health problems in children, ranging from lead poisoning to exposure to violence in the home. Some of these causes or precipitating factors are discussed in other chapters in the text.

Many families do not understand the behaviors or symptoms they observe in their child. Embarrassment may prevent parents from seeking help. Nurses can promote community awareness about common mental health problems in children and identify resources for families. The use of the medical home to coordinate management of mental health problems is important to provide oversight of subspecialties, medications, and therapies.

A healthy self-concept is supported by positive interactions with others. Problem behaviors may provide negative feedback, which may generate a low self-esteem. A child's coping mechanisms are influenced by the individual developmental level, temperament, previous stress experiences, role models, and support of parents and peers. Maladaptive coping mechanisms may be seen as problem behaviors. Inappropriate behaviors may lead to further physical or developmental problems.

Acute Illnesses

Many of the acute health problems of children also affect adults and are discussed in detail in other chapters of this book. Many of the communicable diseases discussed in Chapter 12 affect children, and their transmission can be reduced by prevention strategies. For example, colds, influenza, viruses (including COVID-19) and many other communicable diseases seem to be transmitted by droplets or direct contact, so effective handwashing and covering one's nose and mouth when coughing or sneezing can reduce risk. It is important for children to learn how to effectively cough or sneeze into their elbow rather than directly into the air, and for children 2 years and old to learn how to wear a face mask when needed. Nurses can focus on preventive measures and promote high vaccination rates, good handwashing hygiene, use of hand sanitizer and early identification to prevent the spread of disease. See the How To Box for ways in which germs can spread from other people or surfaces.

HOW TO PREVENT GERMS SPREADING

Germs can spread from another person or a surface when you:
- Touch your eyes, nose, and mouth with unwashed hands
- Prepare or eat food and drinks with unwashed hands
- Blow your nose, cough, or sneeze into hands and then touch other people's hands or common objects (CDC, 2020b).

See Box 22.3 for guidelines about teaching families good handwashing techniques. If a child or adolescent is diagnosed with influenza, parents can be instructed to keep the child at home until symptoms have improved and fever absent for 24 hours. Nurses can help develop community-based policies in the event of a pandemic, and this may include plans for mass immunizations, specific flu clinics, and protocols for school closures.

One acute illness, sudden infant death syndrome (SIDS) is discussed here. SIDS is defined as the sudden death of an infant younger than 1 year of age which remains unexplained after a thorough case investigation, including performance of a complete autopsy, examination of the death scene, and review of the clinical history (AAP, 2016). The peak age for SIDS deaths occurs between one and four months of age, although SIDS may occur up to 1 year of age. The rate of SIDS in non-Hispanic African American and American Indian infants is more than twice that of White infants, and that in Alaska Native infants is two to three times the national average. Its incidence has decreased dramatically since the "Back to Sleep" campaign promoted in 1994 (Moon et al., 2016). There is no test to identify infants who may die, making this a frustrating clinical problem. When an infant dies from SIDS, the family requires tremendous support. The nurse provides empathetic support, assists the

---

BOX 22.3 Teaching Families About Handwashing

Key times to wash hands:
- Before, during, and after preparing foods
- Before eating food
- Before and after caring for someone at home who is sick with vomiting or diarrhea
- Before or after treating a cut or wound
- After using the toilet
- After changing diapers or cleaning up a child who has used the toilet
  - *After* blowing your nose, coughing, or sneezing
  - *After* touching an animal, animal feed, or animal waste
  - *After* handling pet food or pet treats
  - *After* touching garbage

How to wash your hands:
- Wet your hands with clean warm or cold running water, turn off the tap, and apply soap.
- Lather your hands by rubbing them together with soap. Lather the back of your hands, between your fingers, and under your nails.
- Rub your hands for at least 20 s (sing the "Happy Birthday" song from beginning to end twice).
- Rinse your hands well under clean running water.
- Dry your hands with a clean towel, or air dryer.

CDC. When and how to wash hands, 2020b.

family as they progress through the grief process, and provides guidance for siblings and other family members. Referral to support groups may be helpful.

Chronic Health Conditions

Improved medical technology has increased the number of children surviving with chronic health problems. In addition, environmental factors are leading to an increase in certain chronic health conditions (Perrin et al., 2014). Examples of common chronic conditions in children are Down syndrome, spina bifida, cerebral palsy, asthma, ADHD, diabetes, congenital heart disease, cancer, hemophilia, bronchopulmonary dysplasia, and acquired immunodeficiency syndrome (AIDS).

Despite the differences in the specific diagnoses, all of these families have complex needs and face similar problems. Several variables exist to assess for each child and family:

- What is the actual health status? Is the condition stable or life threatening?
- What is the degree of impairment to the child's ability to develop?
- What types of treatments and therapy are required and with what frequency?
- How often are health care visits and hospitalizations required?
- To what degree are the family routines disrupted?

The common issues nurses will want to evaluate for these families include the following:

- All children and adolescents with chronic health problems need routine health care. The same issues of pediatric health promotion and acute health care need to be addressed with this group. The use of the medical home, in which one provider or clinic has all of the child's records, is important for this population.
- Ongoing medical care specific to the health problem needs to be provided. Examples include monitoring for complications of the health problem, medications management, dietary adjustments, and coordination of therapies. Evaluation of the effectiveness of the treatment plan is critical.
- Because care is often provided by multiple specialists, it is important to coordinate the scheduling of visits, tests or procedures, and the treatment regimen.
- Skilled care procedures are often necessary, such as suctioning, positioning, medications, feeding techniques, breathing treatments, physical therapy, and use of appliances.
- Equipment needs are often complex and may include monitors, oxygen, ventilators, positioning or ambulation devices, infusion pumps, and suction machines.
- Educational needs are often complex. Communication among the family, the team of health care providers, school administrators, and teachers is essential to meet the child's health and educational needs.
- Safe transportation to health care services and school must be available. Several barriers may exist, including family resources, location, and the burden of supportive equipment.
- Financial resources may not be adequate to meet the needs.
- Behavioral issues include the effect of the condition on the child's behavior, as well as on other family members.

The ultimate goal is for children with chronic health conditions to achieve optimal health and functioning. Nurses can work to identify barriers for individual families and overall community barriers. Developing support groups, advocating for improved community access to resources, and educating those working with these children on their conditions and needs will promote the family's functioning.

Many children with chronic health conditions have physical limitations requiring adaptive devices and the use of wheelchairs. All children love to play, but most playgrounds are designed with equipment that is not safe for children with physical disabilities. Should communities be required to adapt or build playgrounds with wheelchair access and swings for disabled children so that all children can enjoy outdoor play?

Asthma is a chronic disease that is on the rise. In 2017, an estimated 5.5 million children under the age of 18 were affected (NCHS, 2017). Asthma is characterized by excessive lung sensitivity to various stimuli, including viral infection to allergies, irritating gases, and particles in the air. Secondhand smoke can worsen asthma, and asthma is the third leading cause of hospitalization in children under the age of 15 years. Asthma is a major cause of school absenteeism. In 2017, there were 3564 deaths and 1.6 million emergency department visits due to asthma (NCHS, 2017). Preschool children are increasingly among the newly diagnosed cases. Low-income and minority groups are more likely to be hospitalized for or to die of asthma. Population-focused strategies for asthma management include the following:

- Education programs for families of children and adolescents who have asthma
- Development of home and environmental assessment guides to identify triggers
- Education and outreach efforts in high-risk populations to aid in case finding (e.g., in areas with low income, high unemployment, and substandard housing, where there is exposure to secondhand smoke)
- Development of community clean air policies (e.g., no burning of leaves, use of smoke-free zones)
- Improved access to care for asthmatic patients (e.g., developing clinic services with consistent health care providers to decrease emergency department use)
- Assessment of schools and daycare centers for lack of asthma triggers

TARGET AREAS FOR PREVENTION WITH CHILDREN

In addition to the prevention of acute illnesses, selected areas, including smoking, nutrition, immunizations, and environmental health, will be discussed briefly. Many of these topics are discussed in depth in other chapters in the book.

Smoking

Smoking and the effects of tobacco affect both children and adults. Many times, parents do not understand the effects of smoking on children. There are adverse effects from smoking both to the person who smokes as well as those who inhale the smoke.

EVIDENCE-BASED PRACTICE

The purpose of this descriptive research study was to investigate parental perception and childhood obesity. The report focused on the perception of weight status in relationship to actual obesity. Parents participated in a telephone survey to describe their child's weight, as well as their own weight status. Participants answered questions such as, "What would you say best describes your own weight?" and "What would you say best describes (your child's) weight?" The body mass index (BMI) category options were as follows: underweight, healthy weight, overweight, or obese. Parents reported the weights as falling in one of the aforementioned categories, then height and weight were calculated for BMI score. The primary investigator would check parental perception of category with the BMI results for accuracy. The study participants consisted of a random sample of public school parents between 2009 and 2012. Study results revealed that more than two out of five parents misperceived the weight status of their children. Parents who misperceived their child's weight were nearly 12 times more likely to have an obese child.

Nurse Use

Nurses can play an important role in educating parents and children, as only 54.5% of children in this study had a healthy weight. It is imperative that nurses partner with nutritionists, social workers, teachers, and school health councils in assisting families to recognize an unhealthy weight. Practice implications that were learned from the study included that parental misperception of their child's weight was the strongest predictor of childhood obesity.

Data from McKee C, Long L, Southward L, et al.: The role of parental misperception of child's body weight in childhood obesity, *J Pediatr Nurs* 31:196–203, 2016.

Environmental tobacco smoke (ETS) is exhaled smoke, smoke from burning tobacco, or from the mouthpiece or filter end of a cigarette, cigar, or pipe. These effects are particularly harmful to children under 5 years and those living in poverty. An added risk has been the introduction of electronic nicotine delivery systems (ENDS). These products produce an aerosolized mixture containing flavored liquids that appeal to youth and nicotine. Children exposed to ETS often have increased episodes of middle ear infections, asthma, upper respiratory tract infection, and more missed school days. An initial study by Goniewicz et al. (2013) found cancer-causing substances in all of the e-cigarette samples that were tested. More than 23 million children in the United States, or about 35%, have been exposed to secondhand smoke (American Lung Association [ALA], 2020). Parents may not understand or believe the effects of smoking on children. Children of smokers are more likely to smoke, and it is especially hard for adults to quit smoking if they began as teens.

Interventions to discourage smoking focus on the parent, the child or adolescent, and public policy. Parents should be offered (1) educational programs dealing with the negative effects of smoking on children, (2) interventions to stop smoking, (3) ways to create a smoke-free environment, and (4) behavior modification techniques. Antismoking programs directed toward children and teenagers are more successful if the focus is on short-term effects rather than on long-term effects. Developmentally, children and teenagers cannot visualize the future consequences of smoking. The immediate health risks and the cosmetic effects should be emphasized. Teaching should include how advertising puts pressure on people to smoke. Music, sports, and other activities, including stress-reducing techniques, should be encouraged.

Nutrition

Maintaining child health relies on good nutrition and dietary habits. The first 6 years are the most important for developing sound lifetime eating habits. The quality of nutrition influences growth and development and prevention of disease. Atherosclerosis begins during childhood. Other diseases, such as obesity, diabetes, osteoporosis, and cancer, may also have early beginnings. Low-income and minority families are at increased risk for poor nutrition, but all groups show poor dietary habits. Many variables, including ethnicity, race, culture, and socioeconomic status, influence what a family eats. Also, children have some characteristics that affect their nutrition, such as being slow eaters, having picky food choices, allergies, acute or chronic health problems, and changes in growth patterns. It is important for nurses to help parents learn about the daily requirements of their children. You can find useful information about nutrition in a variety of websites including: the American Academy of Pediatrics (http://www.aap.org): Healthy Children which is sponsored by the American Academy of Pediatrics (http://www.healthychildren.org); and MyPlate (www.choosemyplate.gov). The last site has some excellent sections that provide dietary guidelines as well as a section for children including activity sheets, crossword puzzles, videos, and songs to teach children about nutrition. Because nutritional needs for children vary at each developmental stage, it is important for nurses to understand the difference in what an infant needs versus what a toddler needs, as well as what an active 9-year-old needs versus what a 16-year-old male athlete needs. Nurses can guide families to improve their nutrition by providing information on good nutrition in individual or group sessions, conducting diet assessment, delivering educational activities that focus on the effects of fad foods and diets, giving attendees at educational sessions information about the daily food needs and suggesting healthy snacks, and assessing for risks for eating disorders.

Immunizations

Routine immunization of children has been successful in preventing some diseases. The challenge is making sure that children receive immunizations at the appropriate times and in their entirety. In recent years, more families are choosing not to vaccinate their children, and this has an effect on the community. Not all parents appreciate the seriousness of vaccine-preventable diseases because the prevalence is low in the world. They are confused by media misinformation about the consequences of vaccines, including autism. They have concerns about the data showing the safety of vaccines. They doubt the agencies making recommendations and the companies that manufacture vaccines. It is important to understand their concerns and to educate them about vaccine safety. During the COVID-19 pandemic, many children were not immunized due to closed medical practices and parental fear of taking their children to a medical practice. There may be long-term effects of these missed immunizations if parents do not get their children immunized.

The goal of immunization is to protect the individual by using immunizing agents to stimulate antibody formation. For some people, cost and convenience are critical issues in determining whether children are immunized. In many communities, successful programs combine low-cost or free immunizations provided at convenient times and locations. It is important to repeatedly urge parents to obtain immunizations for their children. Immunization recommendations rapidly change as new information and products are available. The most comprehensive place to look for information about immunizations is at the CDC. They have extensive information including "Recommended child and adolescent schedule for ages 18 year or younger, United States, 2020." Both the American Academy of Pediatrics and the American Academy of Family Physicians refer readers to this site, which was approved by the Advisory Council on Immunization Practices of the CDC (CDC, 2020c). Additional information about immunizations can be found in Chapter 11.

Environmental Health Hazards

The quality of the environment directly affects the health of children and adults. Growth, size, and behaviors place the pediatric population at greater risk for damage from toxins. As discussed in Chapter 8, lead poisoning is the most common environmental health hazard for children. Pesticides and poor air quality also pose serious risks. Indoor air pollutants increased as houses were built "tightly" to conserve energy and as more chemicals were used in production. Growing tissues absorb toxins readily. Developing organ systems are more susceptible to damage. A smaller size means an increased concentration of toxins per pound of body weight. The fact that children are small exposes them to lower air spaces, where heavy chemicals tend to concentrate. Outdoor play, especially during summer months, increases the opportunity for exposure to air pollutants. When they are playing, children often run and breathe hard, which increases the volume of pollutants inhaled. Chewing and mouthing behaviors offer contact to toxins such as lead. Playing on the floor increases exposure to chemicals in rugs and flooring, and rolling in grass can expose children to pesticides. Playground materials may be treated with chemicals. Exposure risks for adolescents are similar to those for adults and are primarily through work, school, and hobbies including participating in sports.

Children at greatest risk are those with respiratory diseases and those from low-income families. Children with asthma and other respiratory problems are at risk from poor air quality and chemical irritants. The problems increase in urban and industrialized areas, where pollutant levels are high. Low-income populations are more likely to have substandard housing. Poor nutritional status increases the risk for complications. Screening and treatment may be delayed if access to health care is limited. Low-income neighborhoods are likely to be located closer to waste areas, and they often have higher levels of contaminants in the water source than the general population. It is critical to assess environmental health hazards during health care visits. Referral for treatment may be necessary, and counseling families on risk reduction is important. Bringing screening programs into neighborhoods at risk may facilitate early

case finding and interventions. It is important to also consider how the built environment affects children. In highly concentrated living areas, they are often few green spaces where children and adolescents can play active games. Children often spend considerable time with electronic devices. Many of the advertisements on television and the Internet are targeted to children and may promote unhealthy food choices.

HEALTH POLICY, LEGISLATION, AND ETHICS RELATED TO ADULT HEALTH

Historically, men have dominated the medical and research professions because of cultural and societal norms. Early research was typically conducted on men, with mental health, reproduction, and the role of women as mothers being the exceptions (McKenzie et al., 2016). In the 1980s, recommendations were made by the US Public Health Services Task Force on Women's Health Issues to increase gender equity in biomedical research and the establishment of guidelines for including women in federally sponsored studies (Alexander et al., 2007). As discussed in other chapters in the book, especially Chapter 4, health policy is action taken by public and private agencies to promote health. It is a reflection of the values held in society and can greatly influence the health of the citizens overall. Legislation consists of laws that regulate health care and promote health. Legislation in the form of acts, laws, and regulations, must be congruent with the constitution being the overarching umbrella for national guidance. Fig. 22.2 depicts a cascading policy framework. Because the care provided by nurses is affected by policy and legislation, this figure provides direction in where nurses may be involved.

Five examples of federal legislation that have influenced the health of adults and their lives in communities include the Older Americans Act of 1965, the Americans with Disabilities Act of 1990, the Family and Medical Leave Act of 1993, the Personal Responsibility and Work Opportunity Reconciliation Act of 1996, and the Patient Protection and Affordable Care Act of 2010.

The Older Americans Act (OAA) established the Administration On Aging (AOA) and state agencies to provide for the social service needs of older people. The mission of the AOA is to help older adults maintain dignity and live independently in their communities through a comprehensive and coordinated network across the United States (AOA, 2017). The stated aim of the OAA is to fund "critical services to keep older adults healthy and independent such as meals, job training, senior centers, health promotion, benefits enrollment, caregiver support, transportation, and more" (National Council on Aging, n.d.). The OAA was reauthorized in 2020 and extended through 2024. The reauthorization added some new provisions for removing barriers and providing states and localities with increased flexibility (Administration for Community Living, 2021).

The Americans with Disabilities Act was passed in 1990, providing protection against discrimination to millions of Americans with disabilities. This legislation requires government and businesses to provide disabled individuals with equal opportunities for jobs, education, access to transportation and public buildings, and other accommodations for both physical

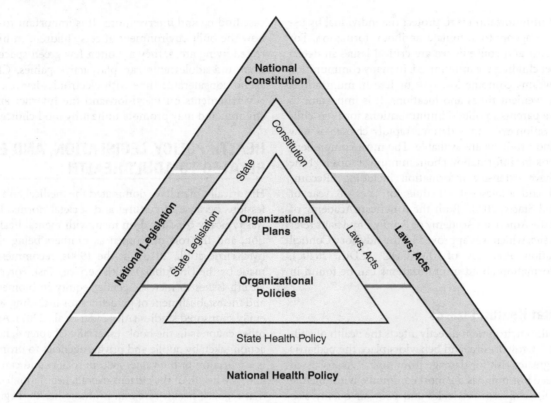

Fig. 22.2 Nest of Cascading Policy Frameworks from National to Organizational Levels Demonstrating the Dependency of the Latter on the Former and the Fractals that Characterize Complex Adaptive Systems. (Developed by Hazel Brown, RN, DNP, June 2018.)

and mental limitations. The disabled as well as the nondisabled and businesses benefit from the changes.

The Patient Self-Determination Act of 1990 (PL 103-43) does not create new rights for patients but reaffirms the common law right of self-determination as guaranteed by the Fourteenth Amendment. This Act requires that providers receiving Medicare and Medicaid funds must ask whether the clients have advance directives and must provide information about their rights under state law (Gerontological Advanced Practice Nurses Association, 2020). A routine discussion of advance medical directives can help ease the difficult discussions faced by health care professionals, family, and clients. The nurse can assist a client in completing a values history instrument. These instruments ask questions about specific wishes regarding different medical situations.

This clarifying process then leads to completion of advance directives to document these preferences in writing. The advance directives have two parts: the living will, which allows the client to express wishes regarding the use of medical treatments in the event of a terminal illness, and a durable power of attorney, which is the legal way for the client to designate someone else to make health care decisions when he or she is unable to do so. A do-not-resuscitate (DNR) order is a specific order from a physician not to use cardiopulmonary resuscitation. State laws vary widely regarding the implementing of these tools, so it is important to consult a knowledgeable source of information. It is also important to involve the family, especially the designated

decision maker or agent, in these discussions so that everyone understands the client's choices (Marco et al., 2012).

Legislated rights of the elderly include individualized care; freedom from discrimination; privacy; freedom from neglect and abuse; control of one's own funds; ability to sue; freedom from physical and chemical restraint; involvement in decision making; the right to vote; access to community services; the right to raise grievances, obtain a will, and enter into contracts; the right to practice the religion of one's choice; and the right to dispose of one's own personal property.

The Family and Medical Leave Act, initially passed in 1993, provides job protection and continuous health benefits where applicable for eligible employees who need extended leave for their own illness or to care for a family member. Frequently, caregivers provide unpaid care for their family members, including aging parents, children, grandchildren, and partners. Adults often find themselves struggling to balance work and caring for a family member. More families find themselves in this struggle as more women enter the workforce and work full time. Caregivers' multiple roles and responsibilities are frequently coupled with financial strain, which can lead them to experience caregiver burden. In 2008, the Family and Medical Leave Act was amended to increase military family entitlements (Rogers et al., 2009).

In 1996, the Congress passed the Personal Responsibility and Work Opportunity Reconciliation Act, commonly known as "welfare reform." This law targeted women who received public assistance and changed the previous Aid to Families with Dependent Children (AFDC) to Temporary Assistance for Needy Families (TANF)—a work program that mandates that women heads of households find employment to retain their benefits. The Administration for Children and Families, within the USDHHS, is responsible for federal programs such as TANF that promote the economic and social well-being of families, children, individuals, and communities (ACF, n.d.).

Nurses can advocate for and support health legislation and policy that support the physical, mental, and social well-being of adults. Advocacy can be accomplished in a variety of ways, such as lobbying, public speaking, participating in grassroots activities, and staying abreast of proposed legislation that influences the health of men and women, their families, and communities.

Ethical and Legal Issues and Legislation for Older Adults

Ethical issues regarding the care and treatment of older adults arise regularly. As the population continues to age and technological advances continue to be developed, complex ethical and legal questions will increase. The most common of these issues involve decision making—assessment of the ability of the client to make decisions, the appropriate surrogate decision maker, disclosure of information to make informed decisions, level of care needed on the basis of function, and termination of treatment at the end of life. A routine discussion of advance medical directives can help ease the difficult discussions faced by health care professionals, family, and clients. The nurse can assist an individual to complete a values history instrument, which asks questions about specific wishes regarding different medical situations.

Elder abuse is an often overlooked concern. Elder abuse encompasses physical, psychological, financial, and social abuse or violation of an individual's rights. The National Center on Elder Abuse, within the AOA, notes that abuse encompasses physical, emotional, and sexual abuse, as well as exploitation, neglect, and abandonment. Abuse consists of the following:

- The willful infliction of physical pain or injury
- Debilitating mental anguish and fear
- Theft or mismanagement of money or resources
- Unreasonable confinement or the deprivation of services

It is estimated that annually one out of six older adults worldwide experience abuse (Yon et al., 2017). Neglect refers to a lack of services or obligations that are necessary for the physical and mental health of an individual by the individual or a caregiver. This can include fiduciary responsibilities. Older persons can make independent choices with which others may disagree. Their right to self-determination can be taken from them if they are declared incompetent. Exploitation is the illegal or improper use of a person or their resources for another's profit or advantage. During the assessment process, nurses need to be aware of conflicts between injuries and explanation of cause, dependency issues between client and caregiver, and substance abuse by the caregiver. Nearly all 50 states have enacted mandatory reporting laws and have instituted protective service programs. The local social services agency or area agency on aging can help with information on reporting requirements.

Many older persons have at least one chronic condition, and many have multiple conditions, putting them at risk for experiencing frailty while living in a community setting. The prevalence of frailty in the older population poses a major public health dilemma because the majority of this group will reside in a community setting, placing new demands on health care systems, family caregivers, and community resources. To improve the health of frail elderly, community-based nursing programs need to address racial/ethnic and socioeconomic disparities.

MAJOR HEALTH ISSUES AND CHRONIC DISEASE MANAGEMENT OF ADULTS ACROSS THE LIFE SPAN

Although there are some similarities in the health threats that adults and children share, some issues are unique to adults. As people live longer, they need to learn ways to promote health to maintain the best possible level of health, and when that is not possible, adults need to learn ways to effectively cope with chronic disease and in some cases disability. In chronic illness, cure is not expected, so nursing activities need to be more holistic, addressing function, wellness, and psychosocial issues. With chronic illness, the focus is on healing (i.e., a unique process resulting in a shift in the body/mind/spirit system) rather than curing (i.e., elimination of the signs and symptoms of disease). Eliopoulos (2018) lists the following goals for chronic care: (1) maintain or improve self-care capacity; (2) manage the disease effectively; (3) boost the body's healing abilities; (4) prevent complications; (5) delay deterioration and decline; (6) achieve the highest possible quality of life; and (7) die with comfort, peace, and dignity.

Chronic illness requires a shift in perspective in contrast to the rapid onset and focus on curing of an acute problem. The focus is on the development of self-management skills. The nurse partners with the client, paying attention to the client's self-concept and self-esteem, as well as to the resources needed to manage the disease outside the medical system. Goals for care are structured to help clients adjust their day-to-day choices to maintain the highest level of functional ability possible within the limits of their conditions. Individuals are often motivated to make lifestyle changes to enable then to cope with chronic illness when they fear death; disability; pain; and negative effects on work, family, or activity.

According to the National Center for Chronic Disease Prevention and Health Promotion (NCCDPHP, 2019), the most common chronic diseases and conditions are heart disease and stroke, cancer, and diabetes. They are not only the most common; they are also the most costly and preventable of all health problems. The major risk factors of these diseases are: excessive alcohol use; poor nutrition; lack of physical exercise; and tobacco use and exposure to secondhand smoke. In 2019, 6 in 10 US adults had one of these chronic diseases and 4 in 10 had two (NCCDPHP, 2019). People with chronic physical and mental health conditions consume approximately 86% of the nation's health care expenditures. They are at risk for the negative effects of drug interactions. In 2017 the leading causes of death for all ages were: heart disease, cancer, unintentional injuries (accidents), chronic lower respiratory diseases, cerebrovascular disease (stroke), Alzheimer's disease and diabetes (NCHS, 2019).

Health Status Indicators

Health status indicators are the quantitative or qualitative measures used to describe the level of well-being or illness present in a defined population or to describe related attributes or risk factors. They can be presented as rates, such as mortality and morbidity, or proportions, such as percentages of a given population who receive immunizations (World Health Organization [WHO], 2016). Life expectancy is a measure that is often used to gauge the overall health of a population. Although the United States spends more money per capita on health than any other country, other developed countries have a longer life expectancy for both genders. In 2017, the life expectancy at birth for all persons in the US was 78.6 years; males had a life expectancy of 76.1 years and females lived until 81.1 years (NCHS, 2019).

When healthy years of life are increased, longer life spans are generally considered desirable. However, chronic diseases and other conditions associated with aging can increase functional limitations and affect the quality of life. Also, being male or female leads to different socialization, expectations, and lifestyles that affect and interact with health in complex ways.

HEALTHY PEOPLE 2030

Selected Objectives Relevant to Major Health Issues in Adults and Youth

- **HDS-D03:** Increase the proportion of adult heart attack survivors who are referred to a rehabilitation program.
- **C-10:** Reduce the proportion of students in grades 9 through 12 who report sunburn.
- **IVP-02:** Reduce emergency department visits for nonfatal injuries.

From US Department of Health and Human Services: *Healthy People 2030*, 2020a. Available at http://health.gov/healthypeople.

Chronic Disease

Cardiovascular Disease

The leading cause of death for both men and women including African Americans, American Indians or Alaska Natives, Hispanics and Whites in the United States is cardiovascular disease (CVD; AHA, 2020). CVD accounted for approximately 17.8 million deaths in 2017, and this number is expected to grow to more than 22.2 million by 2030. Approximately every 40 seconds an American will have a heart attack, and on average in 2016, someone died of stroke every 3 minutes 35 seconds.

The American Heart Association (AHA) works to educate health care providers and consumers about CVD. Their goal, consistent with that of the *Healthy People* 2030 initiative, is to reduce CVD in the United States. They have a variety of consumer- oriented materials on their web site. Two useful ones are: (1) What is heart disease and stroke? (2) What is cardiovascular disease?

Hypertension

In November of 2017, the AHA announced revised guidelines classifying HBP, or hypertension, as a reading of 130 mm Hg for systolic (instead of 140) and 80 mm Hg for diastolic. Blood pressure (BP) should now be categorized as normal, elevated, or stage 1 or 2 hypertension. Normal BP is defined as <120/<80 mm Hg. Elevated BP is 120 to 129/<80 mm Hg. Hypertension stage 1 is defined as a systolic BP of between 130 and 139 mm Hg or a diastolic between 80 and 89 mm Hg. Hypertension stage 2 is defined as a systolic BP of equal to or greater than 140 mm Hg or a diastolic BP equal to or greater than 90 mm Hg (Carey and Whelton, 2018). HBP is estimated to occur in about half of US adults when HBP is defined as a systolic blood pressure at or greater than 130 mm Hg or a diastolic blood pressure at or over 80 mm Hg, or are taking medication for hypertension. About 1 in 4 adults with hypertension have their condition under control. A greater percent of men (47%) have HBP than women (43%); HBP is more common in non-Hispanic Black adults (54%) than in non-Hispanic White adults (46%), non-Hispanic Asian adults 939%) or Hispanic adults (36%) (CDC, 2020d). Because hypertension does not have symptoms, one-third of these people do not know they have the disease. HBP is a major risk factor for CVD, and stroke as uncontrolled hypertension leads to heart attack, stroke, kidney damage, and many other complications. People with elevated blood pressure and other chronic health conditions need routine health care.

Regular physical activity has been found to prevent early death and chronic diseases, including coronary heart disease, stroke, type 2 diabetes mellitus, depression, and some types of cancer. The *2018 Physical Activity Guidelines for Americans* considers physical activity as any form of exercise or movement of the body that uses energy. This can include household chores, yard work, and walking the dog as examples. This second edition of the guidelines provides guidance for people 3 years and older about their need for physical activity. Key guidelines are provided for these age groups: preschool-aged children; children and adolescents; adults; older adults; women during pregnancy and the postpartum period; and adults with chronic health conditions and adults with disabilities. For example, adults should do at least 150 to 300 minutes of moderate intensity or 75 to 150 minutes of vigorous, intensity, aerobic physical activity per week (USDHHS, 2018a).

CHECK YOUR PRACTICE

While at a health fair for your community, you screen a 40-year-old man for hypertension. His vital signs are as follows: BP 200/90, P 77, R 18.

The man tells you, "My dad and grandfather both had high blood pressure. Does that mean I have it too?"

What should you do? How would you apply the six steps of the Clinical Judgment framework described in the Preface? Would this one-time encounter with this man provide you with the information that you need to carry out all six steps? If not, how would you envision doing so if you have continuity with this person?

Stroke

Approximately every 40 seconds, someone in the United States has a stroke, and every 4 minutes someone dies of stroke. The country's highest stroke rates are in the southeastern United States. Stroke is a leading cause of serious long-term disability and reduces mobility in more than half of stroke survivors age 65 and over. While stroke risk varies by age, it can occur at any age. The major risk factors for stroke are HBP, high cholesterol, smoking, obesity and diabetes. About 87% of strokes are ischemic strokes, which occur when the blood flow to the brain is blocked. It is estimated that strokes cost the United States about $4 billion per year. This amount includes the cost of health care, medicines, and missed days of work (CDC, 2020f). Nurses can advocate for smoking cessation because the incidence of ischemic stroke is twice as high in smokers than in adults who do not smoke (Markidan et al., 2018).

Diabetes

Diabetes is a serious public health challenge in the United States. According to the 2020 National Diabetes Statistics Report, 34.2 million people, or 10.5% of the US population, had both diagnosed and undiagnosed diabetes in 2018 (CDC, 2020a). The percentage of people with diabetes increased with age reaching 26% of people aged 65 or older. The prevalence of diabetes varies according to racial groups, with the highest rates in American Indians/Alaska Natives, followed by Hispanics, non-Hispanic Blacks, non-Hispanic Asians and non-Hispanic Whites. People with diabetes are at a higher risk for serious health complications, such as blindness, kidney failure, heart disease, stroke, and loss of toes, feet, or legs. Due to these health complications, medical costs are twice as high for people with diabetes as those without diabetes. Risk factors for diabetes-related complications include smoking, overweight and obesity, physical inactivity, HbA$_1$C levels, HBP, and high cholesterol (CDC, 2020a). The American Diabetes Association (2016) estimates that the cost of diabetes to the nation is $327 billion.

Diabetes is a public health problem. Primary prevention includes educating adults about nutrition and the risks of obesity, smoking, and physical inactivity. Community interventions addressing healthy eating, exercise, and weight reduction also can benefit adults at risk for diabetes. Secondary prevention includes screening for diabetes with finger-stick blood glucose tests or glucose tolerance tests. Screening is also accomplished by thorough history and physical examination. Tertiary prevention targets activities aimed at reducing the complications of the disease. The box in the right column discusses levels of prevention for CVD in women.

Mental Illness

Many adults and children are affected by a mental illness. According to the National Institute of Mental Health (NIMH, 2019) there are two broad categories of mental illness: any mental illness (AMI) and serious mental illness (SMI). AMI is defined as a mental, behavioral, or emotional disorder and can vary in severity. In contrast, SMI is defined as a mental, behavioral, or emotional disorder resulting in serious function impairment. In 2018, 19.1% of US adults experienced mental illness (47.6 million people), and in 2016, 16.5% of US youth

LEVELS OF PREVENTION

Example of Cardiovascular Disease in Women

Primary Prevention
Collaborate with organizations such as the American Heart Association to design and implement interventions to reduce women's risk for cardiovascular disease.

Secondary Prevention
Establish screening clinics in community settings for measuring cholesterol and hypertension.

Tertiary Prevention
Develop a community-based exercise program for a group of women who have cardiovascular disease.

aged 6-17 experienced a mental health disorder (National Alliance on Mental Illness [NAMI], 2019). Mental illness has a ripple effect on the person, the family, and the community.

Mental illness is generally viewed by society in a negative manner and stigmas surrounding mental health are among the barriers that discourage people from seeking treatment (Wu et al., 2017). Because negative stigmas are tied to the decreased utilization of mental health services, public health nurses can take steps to decrease negative stigmas. Community education programs can focus messages that address audiences to educate them and dispel their stereotypes and fears about mental illness. Community education programs can educate attendees and help dispel the stereotypes and fears often applied by society to individuals with mental illness. Local and mass media outlets can broadcast positive aspects of those living with mental disabilities and functioning as a productive part of society. Chapter 25 has more detailed information on mental illness in the community.

Cancer

Cancers of all types are a serious public health concern. Cancers (malignant neoplasms) are the second leading cause of death in the United States, exceeded only by heart disease. A substantial proportion of cancers can be prevented, including those caused by tobacco use and other unhealthy behaviors. Researchers at the American Cancer Society (ACS) estimate that at least 42% of newly diagnosed cancers in the US—about 750,000 in 2020—are possibly avoidable, including those caused by smoking, a combination of excess body weight, alcohol consumption, poor nutrition, and physical inactivity, as well as the many skin cancers caused by excessive sun exposure (ACS, 2020a). Screening can help prevent a variety of cancers including breast, colon, rectum, cervix, lung, skin, and probably prostate. More than 1.8 million new cases of cancer were expected to be diagnosed in 2020, and about 606,520 Americans were expected to die due to cancer in 2020. The cancer death rates have been dropping since they peaked in 1991, and this is driven by reductions in smoking, early detection and treatment, promotion of a healthy lifestyle, access to services, and improved cancer treatments (ACS, 2020a). Men and women need to consistently use sun protection when outside and observe for signs of skin cancer.

Finding cancer lesions in a precancerous state, such as those found in skin, cervical, colorectal, and breast cancer, allows for treatment while in a highly treatable stage. Obesity, physical inactivity, smoking, heavy alcohol consumption, a diet high in red or processed meats, and insufficient intake of fruits and vegetables are risk factors for colorectal cancer. Reducing these risk factors will reduce the incidence of the disease.

Public health agencies, health care providers, and communities must work together to reduce the burden of cancer on society. The *Healthy People 2030* goal is to reduce the number of overall cancer cases, as well as the illness, disability, and death caused by cancer. Education on the hazards of tobacco use and secondhand smoke, eating a healthy diet, and limiting daily consumption of alcohol and exposure to ultraviolet rays are examples of topics for education programs that will reduce the burden of cancer on society.

Sexually transmitted diseases (STDs) or sexually transmitted infections (STIs), human immunodeficiency virus (HIV), and AIDS will not be discussed in detail here because they are covered in depth in Chapter 12. See Chapter 12 for a thorough discussion about these diseases, since they do affect a large number of adults and are amenable to prevention.

Weight Control

Americans spend a great deal of time, energy, and money trying to control their weight. In 1998 the NIH began using the calculation of BMI to define overweight and obesity. BMI is the relationship between body weight and height. A BMI of 25 to 29.9 is defined as overweight, whereas a BMI of 30 and above is considered obese (NHLI, n.d.).

Overweight and obesity are topics addressed numerous times in *Healthy People 2030* and have been discussed earlier in the chapter, especially regarding the association with diabetes. In 2017 to 2018, the age-adjusted prevalence of obesity in the United States was 42.4%, and there were no significant differences between men and women among all adults or by age groups. The prevalence of severe obesity was highest among adults between the ages of 40 and 59. Obesity is associated with serious health risks, and severe obesity increases the risk of heart disease and end-stage renal disease (Hales et al., 2020). Obesity prevalence was lowest among non-Hispanic Asian adults (17.4%) compared with non-Hispanic White (42.2), non-Hispanic Black (41.1), and Hispanic men. Among women, non-Hispanic Asians (17.2%) had the lowest rate of obesity and non-Hispanic Blacks (56.9%) had the highest, with non-Hispanic Whites (39.8%) and Hispanics (43.7%) in between.

Obesity has many effects on health and is linked to major health problems. Nurses can provide education regarding obesity's risks to health. The educational offerings can be fashioned after a community health model using the levels of prevention to establish effective interventions for adults at risk for weight control issues. Although exercise levels have increased in the United States, a community prevention project aimed at increasing activity levels would help in prevention of obesity and the subsequent illnesses of diabetes and heart disease.

Women's Health Concerns

Although there are more commonalities than differences between the health concerns of women and those of men, some notable differences are discussed here. For both sexes, prevention is important, and this includes screening, immunizations, and having a healthy lifestyle.

Eating Disorders

In addition to obesity, other eating disorders have increased among US women. Common eating disorders seen in women include anorexia nervosa and bulimia. Men may exhibit eating disorders, although these are more common in women. Anorexia nervosa is defined as a fear of gaining weight coupled with disturbances in perceptions of the body. Excessive weight loss is the most noticeable clue. Individuals with anorexia rarely complain of weight loss because they view themselves as normal or overweight. Many of these women also struggle with psychological problems, including depression, obsessive symptoms, and social phobias. Bulimia is characterized by a persistent concern with the shape of the body along with body weight, recurrent episodes of binge eating, a loss of control during these binges, and use of extreme methods to prevent weight gain, such as purging, strict dieting, fasting, use of laxatives or diuretics, or vigorous exercise (NIMH, 2019).

Through comprehensive physical and psychosocial assessments, as well as histories of dietary practice, nurses identify women with eating disorders and provide appropriate referrals. Weight control strategies include promoting healthy eating habits and regular physical activity. At a population level, nurses advocate against advertising that promotes exceptionally thin bodies for women. They also promote community-wide exercise and healthy eating programs.

Reproductive Health

Healthy People 2030 objectives address areas related to women's reproductive health. Nurses can advocate for policies that increase women's access to reproductive health services. They can also discuss contraception with women of childbearing age. Contraceptive counseling requires accurate knowledge of current contraceptive choices and a nonjudgmental approach. The goal of contraceptive counseling is to ensure that women have appropriate instruction to make informed choices about reproduction. The choice of contraceptive method depends on many factors, including the woman's health, frequency of sexual activity, number of partners, and plans to have future children. Except for abstinence, no method provides a 100% guarantee against unintended pregnancy or disease (CDC, 2016c). See the CDC discussion about contraception for useful information on methods of birth control. This site was updated in 2020.

Preconceptual counseling addresses risks before conception and includes education, assessment, diagnosis, and intervention. The purpose is to reduce and/or eliminate health risks for women and infants. Neural tube defects, birth defects of the brain and spinal cord, could be significantly affected by preconceptual counseling if the mother is advised to take folic acid vitamins during pregnancy. More than 300,000 babies worldwide annually are born with neural tube defects (anencephaly and spina bifida). Folic acid is a B vitamin that can be found in vitamins and foods. Women of childbearing age are advised to consume 400 mcg of folic acid to prevent neural tube defects. Good food sources are breakfast cereals and some grain products (CDC, 2017).

Another concern critical to preconception awareness is exposure to substances such as alcohol. A major preventable cause of birth defects, mental retardation, and neurodevelopmental disorders is fetal exposure to alcohol during pregnancy. Although fetal alcohol syndrome disorders (FASDs) are declining in the United States, they remain a preventable public health problem. The CDC and the AAP recommend no alcohol during pregnancy. Nurses can be involved in community interventions for women. They can conduct classes and participate in campaigns that print and broadcast advertisements informing women of childbearing age that drinking during pregnancy can cause birth defects. Nurses can serve as advocates not only to encourage their clients to use prenatal care services, but also to work toward establishing services that are accessible, affordable, and available to all pregnant women.

Gestational Diabetes

Gestational Diabetes Mellitus (GDM) GDM is a condition characterized by carbohydrate intolerance that is first identified or develops during pregnancy. Women with GDM are at high risk for pregnancy and delivery complications, including infant macrosomia (extra-large baby), neonatal hypoglycemia, preeclampsia, and cesarean delivery (CDC, 2020e). The incidence of GDM is increasing in the United States, following the trend of the rise in obesity and type 2 diabetes prevalence (DeSisto et al., 2014). The prevalence of GDM increases with maternal age, number of children, and WIC use and decreases with higher education (DeSisto et al., 2014). The CDC offers five tips for women with gestational diabetes: eat healthy foods; exercise regularly; monitor blood sugar often; take insulin, if needed, and get tested for diabetes after pregnancy (CDC, 2020e).

Menopause

During menopause the levels of the hormones estrogen and progesterone change in a woman's body. This change leads to the cessation of menstruation. The decline in these hormone levels can affect the vaginal and urinary tract, cardiovascular system, bone density, libido, sleep patterns, memory, and emotions (Santoro et al., 2015). Women's attitudes toward menopause vary greatly and are influenced by culture, age, support, and the recounted experiences of other women. For decades, however, the prevailing medical view of menopause was a state of deficiency that required hormone replacement to reduce heart disease and osteoporosis. A more positive outlook of menopause encourages women to view it as a transitional and natural stage in the life of a woman.

For decades, many US women used hormone replacement therapy (HRT) or menopausal hormone therapy (MHT), although HRT remained untested by rigorous scientific study. A clinical trial launched in 1991, the Women's Health Initiative, set out to test specific effects of HRT on women's health, especially its effect on heart disease and osteoporosis. Researchers concluded

that HRT did not prevent heart disease and that to prevent heart disease, women should avoid smoking, reduce fat and cholesterol intake, limit salt and alcohol intake, maintain a healthy weight, and be physically active. Long-term studies showed adverse effects of HRT such as increased risk of stroke, coronary heart disease, and thromboembolism (USPSTF, 2018). HRT is still considered useful for management of vasomotor symptoms or "hot flashes" but only for a limited amount of time to avoid the adverse side effects (Martin and Barbieri, 2018). Evidence has been inconclusive about the effectiveness of complementary and alternative therapies in treating menopause symptoms. Information about this can be found on the site for the National Center for Complementary and Integrative Health.

Breast Cancer

The ACS (2020a) reports that breast cancer is the most frequently diagnosed cancer in women. In 2019, the ACS estimated that 268,600 women and 2670 men would be diagnosed with breast cancer. Of this number, 41,760 women and 500 men were expected to die. Although the incidence of breast cancer is higher in White women, the death rate is higher for African American women, which is thought to be due to low screening activity, social determinants such as low income, and poor access (ACS, 2020a). Secondary prevention, which includes screening activities such as mammography every 2 years after age 50, and clinical breast examination, makes a difference in death rates. Early detection can promote a cure, whereas late detection typically ensures a poor prognosis. The ACS "Facts & Figures, 2019–2020," provides detailed information about risk factors, incidence, and treatment.

Osteoporosis

Osteoporosis, or "porous bone," is a disease characterized by low bone mass and structural deterioration of bone tissue, leading to bone fragility and an increased risk for fractures of the hip, spine, and wrist (National Institute of Arthritis and Musculoskeletal and Skin Diseases [NIAMSD], 2018). Women are more likely than men to develop osteoporosis, and age increases the likelihood because of bones becoming thinner and weaker as people age. Small, thin-boned women are at greater risk, and White and Asian women are at highest risk. Hip fractures are a common health problem due to osteoporosis.

Prevention includes diets rich in calcium and vitamin D and avoiding medications that cause bone loss. Always check with the pharmacist and read medication labels to determine which medications to avoid. Exercise also improves bone density, especially weightbearing activities such as walking, running, stair climbing, and weight lifting. Limiting alcohol consumption and avoiding smoking are also important. Finally, several medications are approved for the prevention of osteoporosis in the United States (NIAMSD, 2018). Home assessment and correction of risk factors for falls, bone density testing, and annual height measurements help with fall prevention.

It is important to realize that the health status of one gender affects the health status of the other gender, the family, and society. When the household provider is ill and cannot work, the family and society are affected economically and work productivity is reduced (Giorgianni et al., 2013); the family can suffer from lack of income. If the man dies, the widow generally experiences the loss of companionship and assumes the responsibilities of the lost spouse. Resources to promote and sustain health outcomes of both genders must be balanced for the overall health of the community. However, although a vital aspect of community health, men's health is often overlooked and barriers exist that prevent men from reaching their full health potential (Giorgianni et al., 2013).

Men's Health Concerns

Although health policies, campaigns, and community health organizations offer services for men, women's health is more often emphasized. Several barriers to men reaching their full health potential have been identified. Men do not participate in health care at the same level as women, apparently because of the traditional masculine gender role learned through socialization (Giorgianni et al., 2013). Factors such as "socioeconomic status, access to health care, male acculturation to health issues, harmful perceptions about masculinity, and lack of understanding of male health behaviors contribute to poor health outcomes for men" (Giorgianni et al., 2013, p. 343). Giorgianni et al. (2013) provide examples of why there are different health outcomes for men than for women, including they tend to smoke more, are more likely to be overweight, and less likely to receive routine care or seek out care early in the disease process than are women.

Barriers such as these provide opportunities and challenges for the nurse. The nurse can develop strategies to get men involved in lifestyle changes that prevent illness. Health care providers can reach out to men and offer the guidance and knowledge to improve health. Nurses can actively participate in public policy development and implementation as well as encourage men to identify primary care providers and obtain a physical examination and the recommended screening tests.

Men who establish a working relationship with their health care provider and participate in the recommended screening tests may live healthier, happier, and longer lives. Refer to Box 22.4 for a variety of screening tests with suggested frequencies. Health screenings, as well as other prevention strategies for adults, are regularly updated by the Agency for Healthcare Research and Quality (AHRQ, 2018). Some health screenings are clearly beneficial, and health care providers and researchers debate the benefit of other screening procedures. As a health care professional, it is important to keep up to date on current research and literature to identify the appropriate screenings for the specific population served.

The nurse can assume many roles to fulfill responsibilities to improve the health of men in the community. As an educator, the nurse provides the knowledge and skill for replacing unhealthy behaviors with a healthy lifestyle. As a client advocate, the nurse supports and interacts with those agencies to obtain the needed resources. The nurse acts as a change agent to assess needs and system influences, identify and set priorities, plan and implement programs for men, and evaluate results. Working within groups and communities, nurses can identify needs

---

BOX 22.4   Prevention Strategies for Adults

Dental Health
- Regular dental examinations
- Floss; brush with fluoride toothpaste

Health Screening
- Blood pressure
- Height and weight
- Nutritional screening (obesity)
- Lipid disorders (men 35 and older; women 45 and older)
- Papanicolaou (Pap) test (all sexually active women with a cervix)
- Colorectal cancer (adults 50 and older)
- Mammogram (women 40 and older)
- Osteoporosis (postmenopausal women 60 and older)
- Problem drinking
- Depression screening
- Tobacco use/tobacco-caused diseases
- Rubella serology or vaccination (women of childbearing age)
- Chlamydia (sexually active women age 25 and younger; women older than 25 with new/multiple sexual partners)
- Testicular cancer (symptomatic males)
- Coronary heart disease screening (electrocardiogram, exercise treadmill)
- Syphilis screening (for at-risk population only)
- Diabetes mellitus (adults with hypertension or hyperlipidemia)

Chemoprophylaxis
- Multivitamin, folic acid (women planning or capable of pregnancy)
- Aspirin prevention (adults at risk for coronary artery disease)

Immunizations
- Tetanus-diphtheria boosters
- Rubella (women of childbearing age)
- Pneumococcal vaccine (adults 65 and older)
- Influenza vaccine (adults 65 and older/at risk/annually)

---

and priorities and develop interventions to reduce health risks and improve the health status not only of men, but also of their wives, mothers, daughters, and sisters, and the communities in which they live.

Cancers Unique to Men

Other than skin cancer, prostate cancer is the most common cancer in American men. The ACS estimates that there would be about 191,930 new cases of prostate cancer and about 33,330 deaths from prostate cancer in 2020. About 1 man in 9 will develop prostate cancer during his lifetime (ACS, 2020b). Health disparities are found with African Americans' mortality rate from prostate cancer being nearly twice as high as in any other group (ACS, 2020b). The ACS recommends men be informed about risks and possible benefits of prostate cancer screening. The information should be provided at age 50 for men at average risk for prostate cancer and age 45 for men at high risk, such as African American men and men who have had a father, brother, or son diagnosed with prostate cancer before age 65. Men who have had several of these family members diagnosed with prostate cancer at an early age should be informed about prostate screening at age 40 (ACS, 2020b).

Two screening tests include the prostate-specific antigen (PSA) and the digital rectal examination (DRE). The PSA test is not accurate in terms of sensitivity or specificity. This blood test produces many false-positive results because many factors can elevate the PSA, such as infections, ejaculation, exercise such as bike riding, and benign prostatic hyperplasia (BPH). The DRE is a procedure where the physician inserts a well-lubricated, gloved index finger into the rectum to palpate the prostate gland and examine the rectum for masses. The examiner is unable to palpate the anterior aspects of the prostate, reducing the accuracy of this examination. Men find this examination unpleasant and another reason for avoiding health care (ACS, 2020b).

Testicular cancer is the most common solid tumor diagnosed in males between the ages of 15 and 40 years, with the peak incidence between the ages of 20 and 34 years. The ACS estimated that there would be 9610 new cases of testicular cancer in 2020 and about 440 deaths. About 1 in 250 men will develop testicular cancer. The average age is about 33; 6% of cases occur in children and teens and about 8% occur in men over the age of 55. This form of cancer can often be treated successfully; therefore, the death rate remains low. White men are four to five times more likely than are African American and Asian American men to develop this cancer (ACS, 2020c).

Because painless testicular enlargement is commonly the first sign of testicular cancer, the testicular self-examination has traditionally been recommended for men. However, in 2011 the US Preventive Services Task Force (USPSTF) updated previously published guidelines that significantly altered that tradition for asymptomatic adolescent and adult males (USPSTF, 2014). The new guidelines recommend against screening by self-examination or clinical examination in asymptomatic adult or adolescent males due to insufficient evidence, low incidence rate, and high cure rate even with advanced testicular cancer (USPSTF, 2014). The ACS recommends men be informed about the risks and possible benefits of prostate cancer screening in order make a decision about whether to have the screening (ACS, 2018).

Erectile Dysfunction

Erectile dysfunction (ED), also known as impotence, is the consistent inability to achieve or maintain an erection sufficient for satisfactory sexual performance. Up to 52% of men between the ages of 40 and 70 are affected by ED, and it is associated with decreased quality of life. ED can lead to withdrawal from intimacy, emotional stress, lower self-esteem, and avoidance of physical contact. Although the incidence of ED significantly increases with age, 55% to 70% of men aged 77 to 79 years are sexually active (McMahon, 2014).

Although ED may be discussed more openly with health care providers since the increased publicity generated from the marketing of the medications for ED, many men are embarrassed and reluctant to discuss the subject. Men who respond positively to treatment for ED report significantly better quality of life. With this evidence of positive response, health care providers should be proactive in discussing ED with men.

In summary, regardless of the prevalence differences in the health problems described in this section between men and women, appropriate health care services must be provided, and men and women need to be encouraged equally to take advantage of these services.

HEALTH DISPARITIES AMONG SPECIAL GROUPS OF ADULTS

Health disparities present political implications and influence government action. In the United States health disparities are considered to be differences that exist among specific population groups in the attainment of full health potential that can be measured by differences in incidence, prevalence, mortality burden of disease, and other adverse health condition (National Academies of Sciences, Engineering, and Medicine, 2017). Health inequalities are often due to the unequal distribution of power and resources. Considerable national attention focused on the unequal distribution of power during the riots of 2020. Chapter 23 discusses social determinants of health that can lead to health inequities. See Chapters 23, 24, and 25 for discussions of selected vulnerable groups who are at risk for health disparities.

Certain groups have been recognized as experiencing health disparities and have become a priority for policy efforts. Poverty is a strong and underlying current throughout all of the special groups. Selected groups will be discussed in this chapter to emphasize the importance of understanding and intervening in health disparities.

Adults of Color

In 2000, about 44% of the US population identified themselves as members of racial or ethnic minority groups. By 2050, these groups are projected to comprise almost half of the US population (NHQDR, 2020). In the 2018 National Healthcare Quality and Disparities Report (NHQDR), the priority areas measured were: person-centered care, patient safety, healthy living, effective treatment, care coordination, and care affordability (NHQDR, 2020). Findings indicated that some disparities were decreasing but disparities persist especially for poor and uninsured populations in all priority areas. Blacks, American Indians and Alaska Natives and Native Hawaiians/Pacific Islanders received worse care than Whites for about 40% of the quality measures. Hispanics received worse care than Whites for about 35% of the quality measures. It is currently unclear how disparities will present due to the COVID-19 pandemic and the subsequent levels of unemployment and reduced employment and pay. Although addressing these disparities is complex, the goal is to close the gap with regard to the health disparities in adults of color while at the same time preserving and respecting the richness and unique influences of various cultures. Nurses can advocate for culturally sensitive and gender-sensitive programs necessary in communities where adults of color may reside.

Incarcerated Adults

An estimated 6,613,500 persons were under the supervision of US adult correctional systems on December 31, 2016. The correctional population declined by an average 1.2% annually from 2007 to 2016. However, at year-end 2016, about 1 in 38 persons in the United States were under correctional supervision (Kaeble and Cowhig, 2018). These numbers reflect persons in prisons and jails and those on probation or parole. According to the Bureau of Justice Statistics, "Prisoners in 2018," the combined state and federal imprisonment rate was 431 per 100,000 population, which was the lowest rate since 1996. At the end of 2018, the total prison population in the United States was 1,465,200. This excludes persons on probation or on parole and only includes those in state or federal prisons. The states with the highest rates were in order: Louisiana, Oklahoma, Mississippi, Arkansas and Arizona, and the five with the lowest rates were Minnesota, Maine, Massachusetts, Rhode Island, and Vermont (Bureau of Justice Statistics, 2020).

Lesbian/Gay/Bisexual/Transgender/Queer/Intersexual Adults

Lesbian, gay, bisexual, transgender, queer and intersexual adults (LGBTQI) adults represent a sometimes-hidden special population, in part because of the social stigma associated with homosexuality coupled with the fear of discrimination. Several studies have documented health disparities by sexual orientation in population-based data and have revealed differences in health between LGBTQI adults and their heterosexual counterparts, including higher risks for mental health issues, suicide, and substance abuse (Fredriksen-Goldsen et al., 2013). To improve the health of LGBTQI persons, services need to address their unique needs, and places need to be safe for them to receive health promotion, disease prevention, and treatment.

Adults with Physical and Mental Disabilities

Disability status is based on a person's ability to complete major life activities independently. Major life activities refer to self-care, receptive and expressive language, learning, mobility, self-direction, capacity for independent living, and financial sufficiency.

The Social Security Administration (SSA), which ultimately determines the individual's status for disability benefits, defines disability as the inability "to engage in any substantial gainful activity (SGA) by reason of any medically determinable physical or mental impairments that is expected to result in death, or that has lasted or is expected to last for a continuous period of at least 12 months" (SSA, 2017, p. 5). According to the Americans with Disabilities Act (ADA), the term *disability* means, with respect to an individual, (1) a physical or mental impairment that substantially limits one or more of the major life activities of such an individual, (2) a record of such an impairment, or (3) being regarded as having such an impairment. See http://ada.gov for more information on the ADA. One effect of this legislation is greater emphasis on community care for the disabled, rather than institutionalizations, and there is a growing emphasis on providing care in as "homelike" an environment as possible.

Nurses can develop an awareness of the many health-related issues facing adults with disabilities. In particular, care should be taken to recognize the physical barriers that prevent disabled adults from accessing health care, such as structures that are not accessible despite the ADA recommendations, transportation, or the assistance of family, friends, or caregivers to assist them in getting to a care facility. Developing health promotion programs targeted at this vulnerable, high-risk group is beneficial. There are many technology-based ways in which health promotion and health care can be provided for disabled persons or caregivers who have access to and the skill to use such resources.

Frail Elderly

In the 10 years from 2007 until 2017, the 65 years and over population increased by 34% from 37.8 to 50.9 million. The population is projected to reach 94.7 million in 2060. Also, the 85 years and over population is projected to more than double from 6.5 million in 2017 to 14.4 million in 2024 (123% increase). Older women outnumber older men (28.3 to 22.6 million). In 2018, 32% of older women were widows and about 28% of older men and women lived alone. In 2017, 23% of persons 65 years and older were members of racial or ethnic minority populations: African American (9%), Asian (4%), American Indian and Alaska Native (0.5%), Native Hawaiian/Pacific Islander (0.1%), and Hispanic (8%). The need for caregiving increases with age. From January to June 2018, the percentage of older adults aged 85 and older who needed personal care was 20% compared to 9% in those between 75 and 84 years, and five times that of adults aged between the ages of 65 and 74 (4%) (Administration on Aging, 2018). Also, their major sources of income were Social Security, income from assets, private or government employee pensions, and earnings.

Elders are often the victims of abuse. Chapter 27 discusses violence in the community, including elder abuse. *Elder abuse* encompasses physical, psychological, financial, and social abuse, neglect, or violation of an individual's rights. Abuse consists of the following:

- The willful infliction of physical pain or injury
- Causing debilitating mental anguish and fear
- Theft or mismanagement of money or resources
- Unreasonable confinement or the deprivation of services

Neglect refers to a lack of services that are necessary for the physical and mental health of an individual by the individual or a caregiver. Older persons can make independent choices with which others may disagree. Their right to self-determination can be taken from them if they are declared incompetent. Exploitation is the illegal or improper use of a person or their resources for another's profit or advantage. During the assessment process, nurses need to be aware of conflicts between injuries and explanation of cause, dependency issues between client and caregiver, and substance abuse by the caregiver. Nearly all US states have enacted mandatory reporting laws and have instituted protective service programs. The local social services agency or area agency on aging can help with information on reporting requirements.

A routine discussion of advance medical directives can help ease the difficult discussions faced by health care professionals, family, and clients. The nurse can assist an individual to complete a values history instrument. These instruments ask questions about specific wishes regarding different medical situations.

Legislated rights of the elderly include individualized care, freedom from discrimination, privacy, freedom from neglect and abuse, control of one's own funds, ability to sue, freedom from physical and chemical restraint, involvement in decision making, voting, access to community services, and the right to raise grievances, obtain a will, enter into contracts, practice the religion of one's choice, and dispose of one's personal property.

Many older persons have at least one chronic condition, and many have multiple conditions, putting them at risk for experiencing frailty while living in a community setting. Frailty is a geriatric syndrome that places older adults at risk for adverse health outcomes, including falls, worsening disability, institutionalization, and death. Frailty is a complex state of impairment that signifies loss in areas of physical functioning, physiological resiliency, metabolism, and immune response.

The prevalence of frailty in the older population poses a major public health dilemma because the majority of this group will reside in a community setting, placing new demands on health care systems, family caregivers, and community resources. To improve the health of frail elderly persons, community-based nursing programs need to address racial/ethnic and socioeconomic disparities. For the elderly who do not live in community facilities, the family often provides the care in the home. Female spouses represent the largest group of family caregivers.

Stress, strain, and *burnout* are words that are used to reflect the negative effects of the family caregiver burden. Issues involve the work itself, past and present relationships, effect on others, and the caregivers' lifestyle and well-being. As mentioned above, the need for caregiving increases with the age of the person to whom care is given. For many families the caregiving experience is a positive, rewarding, and fulfilling one. Nursing intervention can facilitate good health for older persons and their caregivers and contribute to meaningful family relationships during this period. Eliopoulos (2018) uses the acronym *TLC* to represent these interventions, as follows:

T = Training in care techniques, safe medication use, recognition of abnormalities, and available resources

L = Leaving the care situation periodically to obtain respite and relaxation and maintain normal living needs

C = Care for the caregiver through adequate sleep, rest, exercise, nutrition, socialization, solitude, support, financial aid, and health management

COMMUNITY-BASED MODELS FOR CARE OF ADULTS

Communities are where people live, work, and socialize. Community health settings include public health departments, ambulatory care clinics, and home health agencies. Nurses are involved in direct care, providing information about self-care, supervising paraprofessionals and collaborating with other disciplines. Knowledge of community resources is essential. The nurse assesses the need for and helps develop or locate the resources.

Most communities have an area agency on aging that is often an excellent resource for information. Older adults need a primary care provider who provides continuity in their care and can make appropriate referrals as needed. The following section describes resources available in many communities.

COMMUNITY CARE SETTINGS

Senior Centers

Senior centers were developed in the early 1940s to provide social and recreational activities (Fig. 22.3). Many centers are multipurpose, offering recreation including exercise classes and other forms of entertainment such as singing or dance classes, education, counseling, therapies, hot meals, and case management, as well as health screening and education. Some even offer primary care services. Nurses have a unique opportunity to provide services to a group of older persons who wish to remain independent in the community. During the COVID-19 pandemic, many senior centers maintained their offerings in an electronic form for members who had access to a computer.

Adult Day Health

Adult day health is for individuals whose mental or physical function requires them to obtain more health care and supervision. It serves as more of a medical model than the senior center, and often individuals return home to their caregivers at night. Some settings offer respite care for short-term overnight relief for caregivers. This provides caregivers the opportunity to work or have personal time during the day. Nurses may provide support groups for caregivers.

Home Health and Hospice

Home health is often provided by multidisciplinary teams. Nurses provide individual and environmental assessments, direct skilled care and treatment, and short-term guidance and instruction. Nurses often function independently in the home and must rely on their own resources and knowledge to improvise or adapt care to meet the client's unique physical and social circumstances.

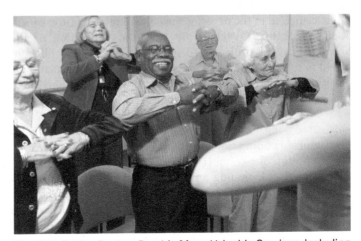

Fig. 22.3 Senior Centers Provide Many Valuable Services, Including Social and Recreational Activities, Exercise, and Often Nutritional Services. (© 2012 Photos.com, a division of Getty Images. All rights reserved. Image 125557433.)

They work closely with the family and other caregivers to provide necessary communication and continuity of care.

Hospice represents a philosophy of caring for and supporting life to its fullest until death occurs. The hospice team encourages the client and family to jointly make decisions to meet physical, emotional, spiritual, and comfort needs. See Chapter 30 for further information on palliative care, home health care and hospice.

Assisted Living

There is a growing trend for continuity of care assisted living arrangements. Persons can choose independent living and many facilities have both assisted living and memory care units in which residents can transition as their health needs change. Assisted living covers a wide variety of choices, from a single shared room to opulent independent living accommodations in a full-service, life-care community. The differences are related to the type and extent of the amenities provided and the contract signed for them. The role of the nurse varies depending on the philosophy and leadership of the management of the facility. The nurse generally provides assessment and interventions, medication review, education, and advocacy. Some facilities have a geriatric physician or nurse practitioner available while others provide transportation for residents to see a physician of their choice.

Long-Term Care and Rehabilitation

Long-term care services and supports (LTSS) include a variety of health and social services to assist individuals who have functional limitations due to physical, cognitive or mental conditions or disability. The goal of LTSS is to improve functioning among those served. Nursing homes, or long-term care facilities, house a growing percent of the older population. Changing family structures and shifting roles for women in the United States affect the need for informal caregivers and the placement of older persons in long-term care facilities. The aging of the population and the growing number of people with disabilities will increase the need for care for older people other than by members of their family. Nursing homes were criticized in the news for the large number of cases of and deaths due to COVID-19. By 2040 the population of the United States is projected to increase from 318.7 million in 2040 to over 380 million people; and the elderly population is expected to increase from 48 million to over 83 million. There are a variety of reasons for this increase, including the aging of the Baby Boom population (those born from 1946 to 1964); increased longevity among Americans; and shifts in health behaviors including smoking, motor vehicle fatality, and excess consumption of alcohol (USDHHS, 2018c). At the same time, risk behaviors including limited physical activity, poor nutrition, and substance use contribute to obesity and chronic health conditions which then lead to greater use of personal health services and LTSS. Adults aged 65 and older are more likely than their younger counterparts to have disability in vision, cognition, mobility, self-care, and independent living (USDHHS, 2018c). Well-managed nursing homes provide a safe environment, special diets and activities, routine personal

care, and the treatment and management of health care needs for those needing rehabilitation, as well as for those needing a permanent supportive residence. Rehabilitation is a combination of physical, occupational, psychological, and speech therapy to help debilitated persons maintain or recover their physical capacities. Rehabilitation is typically needed for older adults after a hip fracture, stroke, or prolonged illness that results in serious deconditioning (Eliopoulos, 2018).

Nursing homes and 24-hour skilled care at home are the most expensive types of long-term care, costing thousands of dollars a month, of which people rely on personal funds, government health insurance programs (such as Medicare and Medicaid), and private financing options (such as long-term care insurance). Medicaid is administrated by the states and this means there is variability in the level of service from one state to another. Medicaid eligibility largely depends on income and assets (USDHHS, 2018c). See Chapters 4 and 5 for more details on government and economics.

⟫ APPLYING CONTENT TO PRACTICE

In this chapter, emphasis is placed on the community health needs of children, adolescents, and adults, including those with disabilities, within the context of the family. The public health care functions of disease prevention, health promotion, and the three levels of health services are important. To meet the core public health competencies, nurses must learn how to assess children and adults using developmental principles to determine safety risks for injury and environmental health exposures. Policy and program development for the specific population is geared toward improving the built environment in which a child grows and in which adults live and educating on health promotion strategies. Nurses develop competencies in communication strategies to help families promote their health at home, in daycare centers, at schools, and at work. This chapter prepares nurses to provide comprehensive, developmentally appropriate education to families; deliver basic health care services in a holistic approach; and develop community programming to improve safety and environmental wellness for children and adults.

▌ PRACTICE APPLICATION

Neighbors and the administrator of the senior high-rise residence where Mrs. Eldridge, a 79-year-old widow, lives reported her to the nurse who visited residents there. Mrs. Eldridge lives alone, and no one had been observed coming or going from her apartment recently. When her neighbors saw her, Mrs. Eldridge appeared self-neglected and did not appear to recognize her neighbors.

When the nurse made a visit to the apartment, Mrs. Eldridge answered the door. She was pleasant, but there was an odor of stale urine. The nurse validated the unkempt appearance of both Mrs. Eldridge and the apartment. Even though Mrs. Eldridge was hesitant and unsure in her answers, the history revealed medical problems. A son and daughter-in-law lived in the next county and phoned at least once a week; their number was taped to the table by the phone.

However, the son is an alcoholic, and the daughter-in-law has beginning symptoms of cardiovascular disease. Mrs. Eldridge's great-grandchild has asthma and is cared for by the son and daughter-in-law. Several pill bottles were observed on the kitchen counter with the names of a local physician and pharmacist.

The nurse noted that both Mrs. Eldridge and her clothes were dirty and that she moved without aids and appeared unsteady on her feet. The kitchen was littered with unwashed dishes and empty frozen-food boxes, which Mrs. Eldridge could not recall being bought or having been delivered. A billfold with several bills was lying open on the kitchen counter, as well as an uncashed Social Security check.

A. What should the nurse do about the situation she found?

1. Call adult protective services and get an emergency order to put Mrs. Eldridge in a nursing home.
2. Call Mrs. Eldridge's son and see if his mother can move in with him because she cannot take care of herself.
3. Complete a physical and mental examination to first determine the cause of Mrs. Eldridge's situation.
4. Call Mrs. Eldridge's pharmacist to see what medications she is taking.
5. Call Mrs. Eldridge's son to discuss the situation with him and to make plans with him and his mother for her future.

B. What factors make this a difficult situation?

Answers can be found on the Evolve website.

REMEMBER THIS!

- Good nutrition is essential for healthy growth and development and influences disease prevention in later life. The adolescent population is at greatest risk for poor nutritional health.
- Immunizations are successful in the prevention of selected diseases. Barriers to immunizing children are cost and convenience. During the COVID-19 pandemic, many children were unimmunized due to the temporary closure of medical practices.
- The family is critical to the growth and development of the child. Social support is one of the most powerful influences on successful parenting.
- Accidents and injuries are the major cause of health problems in the child and adolescent population. Most are preventable. Nurses have a major role in anticipatory guidance and prevention.
- Nurses are involved in strategies to meet the needs of the pediatric population in the community. Home-based service programs have been successful in providing care for at-risk populations. Children of homeless families are at risk for health problems, environmental dangers, and stress. Community programs to provide health care for the homeless may decrease those risks.
- The women's health movement was pivotal in bringing national recognition to women's health issues.
- Women have a longer life expectancy than men. However, women are more likely to have acute and chronic conditions that require them to use health services more than men.
- Women are known as the gatekeepers of health. Women make 75% of the health care decisions in American households.

- Smoking is a risk factor for some major health problems including lung cancer, heart disease, osteoporosis, and poor reproductive outcomes.
- Cardiovascular is the leading cause of death among US adults.
- Diabetes has increased dramatically in the United States in the last decade.
- Overall, White women have a high incidence rate for all cancers, while African American women have high mortality rates.
- In response to the past lack of equality in health-related research and the provision of clinical care, there is now a major national focus on women's health issues.
- Men are more reluctant than women to seek health care.
- Life expectancy of men in the United States is one of the lowest in developed countries.
- Men engage in more risk-taking behaviors, such as physical challenges and illegal behaviors, than do women.
- The population 65 years of age and older in the United States is steadily growing, accompanied by an increase in chronic conditions, a greater demand for services, and strained health care budgets.
- Most older adults live in the community. The last few years of life often represent functional decline. Nurses strive to help elders maximize functional status and minimize costs through direct care and appropriate referral to community resources.
- Nurses address the chronic health concerns of elders with a focus on maintaining or improving self-care and preventing complications to maintain the highest possible quality of life.
- Assessing the elder incorporates physical, psychological, social, and spiritual domains. Individual and community-focused interventions involve all three levels of prevention through collaborative practice.
- Special at-risk populations in the community require nursing interventions at the primary, secondary, and tertiary levels.

EVOLVE WEBSITE

http://evolve.elsevier.com/Stanhope/foundations
- NCLEX Review Questions
- Practice Application Answers

REFERENCES

Administration for Community Living: *Older Americans Act, 2020,* www.acl.gov. modified April 8, 2021. Retrieved June 2021.

Administration on Aging [AOA]: *About AoA*, Washington, DC, 2017, The Administration. Retrieved May 2020 from www.aoa.gov.

Administration on Aging (AOA): 2018 *Profile of Older Americans,* Washington DC, 2018, The Administration for Community Living, Retrieved May 2020 from www.aol.gov.

Agency for Healthcare Research and Quality [AHRQ]: *2018 national healthcare quality and disparities report* www.ahrq.gov. Retrieved April 2020.

Alexander LL, LaRosa JH, Bader H, et al.: *New dimentions in women's health care,* 4th ed. Boston, 2007, Jones and Bartlett.

American Academy of Child and Adolescent Psychiatry [AACAP]: *Facts for Families Guide*, 2018. Retrieved June 2020 from www.aacap.org.

American Academy of Pediatrics [AAP]: *AAP updates recommendations on obesity prevention: it's never too early to begin living a healthy lifestyle*, 2015, Retrieved from https://www.aap.org.

American Academy of Pediatrics [AAP]: Policy statement: SIDS and other sleep-related infant deaths: expansion of recommendations for a safe infant sleeping environment, *Pediatrics* 138(5): 2016.

American Academy of Pediatrics [AAP]: Policy affirmation: firearm-related injuries affecting the pediatric population, *Pediatrics* 139(3), 2017.

American Cancer Society (ACS): *Cancer facts and figures 2018*, Atlanta, 2018, American Cancer Society.

American Cancer Society [ACS]: *Cancer facts and figures 2020*, Atlanta, 2020a, American Cancer Society.

American Cancer Society (ACS): *About prostate cancer, 2020*, Atlanta, 2020b, American Cancer Society.

American Cancer Society (ACS): *Testicular cancer, 2020*, Atlanta, 2020c, American Cancer Society.

American Diabetes Association [ADA]: Standards of medical care in diabetes—2016, *Diabetes Care* 39(Suppl 1):S1–S106, 2016.

American Heart Association [AHA]: *Heart disease and stroke statistical update fact sheet At-A-Glance*, 2020, Retrieved May 2020 from www.heart.org.

American Lung Association [ALA]: *Health effects of secondhand smoke*, 2020. Retrieved May 2020 from www.lung.org.

American Psychiatric Association: *Diagnostic and statistical manual of mental disorders*, 5th ed. Arlington, 2013, American Psychiatric Association Publishing.

Americans with Disabilities Act of 1990, PL 101-336, 1990.

Ballesteros MF, Williams DD, Mack KA, et al.: The epidemiology of unintentional and violence-related injury morbidity and mortality among children and adolescents in the United States, *Int J Environ Res Public Health* 15(4): 616, 2018.

Bureau of Justice: *Prisoners in 2018*, US Department of Justice, 2020, Retrieved June 2020 from www.Bureaujusticestatistics.

Carey RM, Whelton PK, for the 2017 ACC/AHA Hypertension guideline writing committee: Prevention, detection, evaluation, and management of high blood pressure in adults: synopsis of the 2017 American College of Cardiology/American Heart Association Hypertension Guidelines, *Ann Intern Med* 168:351-358, 2018.

Centers for Disease Control and Prevention, National Center for Injury Prevention and Control [CDC, NCIPC]: *National Action Plan for Child Injury Prevention*, Atlanta, 2012, CDC, NCIPC.

Centers for Disease Control and Prevention [CDC]: *Childhood obesity causes & consequences,*:, Atlanta, 2016a, Retrieved May 2020 from www.cdc.gov>obesity>childhood>causes.

Centers for Disease Control and Prevention (CDC): *Child passenger safety: get the facts*, 2016b, Retrieved September 2016 from http://www.cdc.gov.

Centers for Disease Control and Prevention [CDC]: *Contraception: how effective are birth control methods?* 2016c. Retrieved September 2016 from http//:www.cdc.gov.

Centers for Disease Control and Prevention [CDC]: *Folic acid-birth defects count*, Atlanta, 2017, CDC. Retrieved June 2020 from www.cdc.gov/folicacid&neuraltubedefects.

Centers for Disease Control and Prevention (CDC): *Childhood obesity facts*, Atlanta, 2018, CDC. Retrieved June, 2020 from www.cdc.gov.

Centers for Disease Control and Prevention (CDC): *National diabetes statistics report 2020: estimates of diabetes and its burden in the United States*, Atlanta, 2020a.

Centers for Disease Control and Prevention (CDC): *When and how to wash your hands*, Atlanta, CDC, 2020b, Retrieved June 2020 from http://www.cdc.gov>handwashing>when-how-handwashing.

Centers for Disease Control and Prevention [CDC]: *Birth to 18 years immunization schedule*, 2020c, Retrieved June 2020 from www.cdc.gov?schedules/hcp>imz>child-adolescent.

Centers for Disease Control and Prevention (CDC*): Facts about hypertension*,2020d. Retrieved May 2020 from www.cdc.gov>bloodpressure.

Centers for Disease Control and Prevention [CDC]: *Gestational diabetes and pregnancy*, 2020e, Retrieved June 2020 from http://www.cdc.gov/pregnancy/diabetes-gestational.html.

Centers for Disease Control and Prevention [CDC]: *Stroke facts*, 2020f, Retrieved June 2020 from www.cdc.gov/stroke.

Chandrasekhar R, et al.: Social determinants of influenza hospitalization in the United States, *Influenza Other Resp Viruses*, 11(6): 479-488, 2017.

DeSisto CL, Kim SY, Sharma AJ: Prevalence estimates of gestational diabetes mellitus in the United States, pregnancy risk assessment monitoring system (PRAMS), 2007-2010, *Prev Chronic Dis* 11:130415, 2014.

Divers J, Mayer-Davis EJ, Lawrence JM, et al.: Trends in incidence of type 1 and type 2 diabetes among youths-selected counties and Indian reservations, United States, 2002-2015, *MMWR Morb Mortal Wkly Rep* 2020:69:165.

Eliopoulos C: *Gerontological nursing*, 9th ed. Philadelphia, 2018, Lippincott Williams and Wilkins.

Federal Interagency Forum on Child and Family Statistics: *America's children in brief: key national indicators of well-being, 2019*, Washington, DC, 2019, US Government Printing Office.

Fredriksen-Goldsen K, Kim H, Barkan S, et al.: Health disparities among lesbian, gay, and bisexual older adults: results from a population-based study, *Am J Public Health* 103(10):1802–1809, 2013.

Gerontological Advanced Practice Nurses Association: *Patient self-determination act (PSDA)*, 2020, Retrieved June 2020 from www.gapna.org.

Giorgianni S, Porche D, Williams S, et al.: Developing the discipline and practice of comprehensive men's health, *Am J Mens Health* 7(4):342–349, 2013.

Goniewicz ML, Knysak J, Gawron M, et al.: Levels of selected carcinogens and toxicants in vapour from electronic cigarettes, *Tob Control* 2013.

Hales CM, Carroll MD, Fryar CD, et al.: *Prevalence of obesity and severe obesity among adults: United States, 2017-2018*, NCHS Data Brief No. 360, February 2020.

Jiang Y, Koball H: *Basic facts about low-income children: Children under 18 years, 2016*. New York: National Center for Children in Poverty, Columbia University Mailman School of Public Health, 2018.

Kaeble D, Cowhig M: *Correctional populations in the United States, 2016*, US Department of Justice, April 2018, NCJ 251211.

Kann L, McManus T, Harris WA, et al.: Youth risk behavior surveillance, United States, 2017, *MMWR Surveill Summ* 67(8):1-114, 2018.

Marco CA, Moskop JC, Schears RM, et al.: The ethics of health care reform: impact on emergency medicine, *Academic Emergency Med* 19(4):461–468, 2012.

Markidan J, Cole JW, Cronin CA, et al.: Smoking and risk of ischemic stroke in young men, *Stroke*, 49:1276-1278, 2018.

Martin KA, Barbieri RL: *Treatment of menopausal symptoms with hormone therapy,* 2018, Retrieved from, www.uptodate.com.

McBride DL: Pediatric firearm deaths and injuries in the United States, *J Pediatr Nurs* 38:138-139, 2018.

McKenzie SK, Jenkin G, Collings S: Men's perspectives of common mental health problems: a metasynthesis of qualitative research, *Int J Men's Health* 15(91):80–104, 2016.

McMahon C: Erectile dysfunction, *Intern Med J* 44(1):18–26, 2014. doi:10.1111/imj.12325.

Moon RY, Task Force on Sudden Infant Death Syndrome: SIDS and other sleep-related infant deaths: evidence base for 2016 updated recommendations for a safe infant sleeping environment, *Pediatrics,* 138(5):e20162940, 2016.

National Academies of Science, Engineering & Medicine: *Communities in action: pathways to health equity,* Washington, DC, 2017, National Academies Press.

National Alliance on Mental Illness, *Mental health by the numbers, 2019,* www.nami.org.

National Center for Chronic Disease Prevention and Health Promotion [NCCDPHP]: *Chronic diseases: the leading causes of death and disability in the United States,* Atlanta, 2019, CDC. Retrieved June 2020 from http://www.cdc.gov/chronicdisease.

National Center for Health Statistics [NCHS]: *Health, United States, 2018: with special feature on racial and ethnic health disparities,* Hyattsville, 2019, NCHS.

National Center for Health Statistics [NCHS]: *FastStats – statistics by topic,* 2017. Retrieved June 2020 from https://www.cdc.gov/nchs/fastats/default.htm.

National Council on Aging: *Older Americans Act,* n.d. Retrieved June 2020 at www.ncoa.org.

2018 National Healthcare Quality and Disparities Report, Rockville, 2020, Agency for Healthcare Research and Quality.

National Heart, Lung and Blood Institute (NHLI): Calculate your body mass index, n.d., Retrieved June 2020 at www.nhlbi.nih.gov.

National Highway Traffic Safety Administration [NHTSA]: *Traffic safety facts annual report tables,* 2018, Washington, DC, 2020, US Department of Transportation, National Highway Traffic Safety Administration. Available at http://www.cdan.nhtsa.gov. Retrieved November 2020.

National Institute of Arthritis and Musculoskeletal and Skin Diseases [NIAMSD]: *What is osteoporosis?* Bethesda, 2018, National Institutes of Health. Retrieved June 2020 from http://www.niams.nih.gov/Health_Info/Bone/Osteoporosis/osteoporosis_ff.asp.

National Institute of Mental Health [NIMH]: *Mental illness,* 2019. Retrieved June 2020 at www.nimh.gov.

Perrin J, Anderson EL, Van Cleave J: Changing epidemiology of children's health—the rise in chronic conditions among infants, children, and youth can be met with continued health system innovations, *Health Affairs* 33(12):2099–2105, 2014.

Rogers B, Franke J, Jeras J, et al.: The Family and Medical Leave Act: implications for occupational and environmental nursing, *Am Assoc Occup Health Nurses J* 57:239–250, 2009.

Santoro N, Epperson CN, Mathews SB: Menopausal symptoms and their management, *Endocrinol Metab Clin North Am* 44(3):497-515, 2015.

US Consumer Product Safety Commission [USCPSC]: *Public playground safety handbook,* Bethesda, MD, 2015, USCPSC.

US Department of Health and Human Services [USDHHS]: *Physical activity guidelines for Americans,* 2nd edition, Washington, DC, 2018a, USDHHS.

US Department of Health and Human Services (USDHHS): *An overview of long-term services and supports and Medicaid: Final report,* Washington, DC. May 2018b. USDHHS.

US Department of Health and Human Services, Administration for Children and Families, Administration on Children, Youth and Families, Children's Bureau: *Child maltreatment 2018.* Washington, DC, 2020c.

US Department of Health and Human Services [USDHHS]: *Healthy People 2030,* Washington, DC, 2020a, US Government Printing Office.

US Department of Health and Human Services (USDHHS): *Poverty guidelines, 2020,* Retrieved June 2020b from www.aspi.hhs.gov> poverty-guidelines May 2020.

US Preventive Services Task Force [USPSTF]: *Clinical summary: testicular cancer: screening, 2014,* 2014. Retrieved September 2016 from https://www.uspreventiveservicestaskforce.org.

US Preventive Services Task Force (USPSTF): Hormone therapy for the primary prevention of chronic conditions in postmenopausal women: recommendation state, *Am Fam Physician* 97(8), 2018.

US Social Security Administration [USSSA]: *2016 Red Book,* Baltimore, 2017, SSA Office of Research. Retrieved May 2020 from www.ssa.gov/redbook.

World Health Organization [WHO]: *World health statistics 2016: monitoring health for the SDGs,* Geneva, 2016, Publications of the World Health Organization. Available at http://www.who.int/whosis/indicatordefinitions/en/.

Wu IHC, Bathje GJ, Kalibatseva Z, et al.: Stigma, mental health, and counseling service use: a person-centered approach to mental health stigma profiles, *Psychol Serv* 14:490-501, 2017.

Yon Y, Mikton CR, Gassoumis ZD, et al.: Elder abuse prevalence in community settings: a systematic review and meta-analysis, *Lancet Glob Health* 5e:147-e156, 2017.

23

Health Equity and Care of Vulnerable Populations

Carole R. Myers

OBJECTIVES

After reading this chapter, the student should be able to:

1. Describe health equity and its importance to nurses.
2. Describe population health and its application to nursing practice.
3. Define the term vulnerable population and describe selected groups who are more prone to become vulnerable.
4. Describe individual and social factors that can contribute to the development of vulnerability in certain populations.
5. Examine ways in which public policies can lead to health inequities and predispose individuals to become vulnerable.
6. Describe strategies that nurses can use to improve health status and eliminate health inequities in vulnerable populations.

CHAPTER OUTLINE

KEY TERMS

This chapter discusses the concept of health equity and how nurses can advance equity. To understand health equity, it is important to discuss population health, health determinants, and vulnerability. During 2020 with the onset of the COVID-19 pandemic and the demonstrations and riots, the importance of equity and inclusiveness was highlighted in many facets of life, including health care. Selected population groups that are at greater risk than others of poor health outcomes are described briefly in this chapter and in more detail in other chapters of the book. The relationship between health disparities, health equity, and vulnerability is described. A goal in the United States is to eliminate health disparities or health inequities by expanding access to health care for vulnerable or at-risk populations. The document *Healthy People 2030* (US Department of Health and Human Services [USDHHS], 2020a) has as its mission having a society in which all people live long, healthy lives. The overarching goals are:

- Attain healthy, thriving lives and well-being, free of preventable disease, disability, injury, and premature death.
- Eliminate health disparities, achieve health equity, and attain health literacy to improve the health and well-being of all.
- Create social, physical, and economic environments that promote attaining full potential for health and well-being for all.
- Promote healthy development, healthy behaviors, and well-being across all life stages.
- Engage leadership, key constituents, and the public across multiple sectors to take action and design policies that improve the health and well-being of all.

This chapter details the nurse's use of the nursing process with vulnerable population groups and presents case examples to identify how nurses can help individuals, families, groups, communities, and populations meet the goals of *Healthy People 2320* (USDHHS, 2020a).

HEALTH EQUITY

The Robert Wood Johnson Foundation defines health equity as meaning "that everyone has a fair and just opportunity to be healthier. This requires removing obstacles to health such as poverty, discrimination, and their consequences, including powerlessness and lack of access to good jobs with fair pay, quality education and housing, safe environments, and health care" (Braverman et al., 2017). The American Public Health Association (APHA) describes health equity as meaning "everyone has the opportunity to attain their highest level of health" (n.d.). In contrast, health inequities are barriers that prevent individuals and populations from attaining maximum health. Achieving health equity requires a cross-sectoral approach, requiring nurses to partner with a range of stakeholders in public health and across the community.

Population health is the focus of public health nursing. Population health is "an approach to health that aims to improve the health of an entire population and reduce inequities among population groups" (Kindig, 2007; Kindig and Stoddart, 2003). Population health strategies aim to create conditions in which individuals and families can be healthy, and encompasses wellness, prevention, and health promotion. Populations are collections of individuals who have one or more personal or environmental characteristics in common. They can be defined by (1) geography; (2) enrollment in a system (e.g., health plan, accountable care organization; or (3) common characteristic (e.g., older adult, veteran, individual with a disability, pregnant teenager).

DETERMINANTS OF HEALTH

Health determinants include a range of individual characteristics and behaviors, social and economic circumstances, and physical environmental factors that influence health status or outcomes. Health outcomes include mortality, morbidity, life expectancy, health care expenditures, health status, and functional limitations (Artiga and Hinton, 2018). The *County Health Rankings model* (University of Wisconsin Population Health Initiative [UWPHI], 2018) seen in Fig. 23.1 illustrates the many factors that influence population health and that need to be addressed in order to improve the health of the persons being served. The model emphases modifiable determinants because the majority of health outcomes result from actions and behaviors rather than medical care (Hacker and Walker, 2013).

Social determinants of health are the conditions in which people are born, grow, live, work, and age that shape health (Artiga and Hinton, 2018). They include factors such as economic status, education, neighborhood and physical environment, nutrition, stress, employment, social support networks, and prejudice, as well as access to health care (Lathrop, 2013; Artiga and Hinton, 2018). Nursing interventions are designed to help vulnerable populations gain the resources needed for better health and reduction of risk factors.

From an international perspective, the World Health Organization (WHO, 2015) states that many factors in combination affect the health of individuals and communities. Specifically, "whether people are healthy or not is determined by their circumstances and environment." The WHO, consistent with *Healthy People 2030*, describes three overall determinants of health to be (1) the social and economic environment, (2) the physical environment, and (3) the person's individual characteristics and behaviors. The WHO also notes that individuals are unlikely to be able to directly control many of the determinants of health, and this is directly related to vulnerability. That is, when people experience adverse determinants of health that they cannot control, they are predisposed to becoming vulnerable. The WHO (2015) cites seven examples of factors that affect health. There are many more factors that affect health, as noted later in the *Healthy People 2030* information. The seven WHO factors are as follows (WHO, 2015, pp. 1–2):

1. Income and social status: Higher income and social status are associated with better health.
2. Education: Low education is linked with poor health, more stress, and lower self-confidence.
3. Physical environment: Safe water and clean air; healthy workplaces; safer homes, communities, and roads; and good employment and working conditions, especially when the person has more control, all contribute to good health.
4. Social support networks: Family, friends, and community as well as culture, customs, traditions, and beliefs affect health.
5. Genetics, as well as personal behavior and coping skills, affect health.
6. Health services: Access and use of services affect health.
7. Gender: Men and women suffer from different types of diseases at different ages. Fig. 23.2 is a street scene that depicts factors that could influence the determinants of health.

Healthy People 2030 (USDHHS, 2020a) has an increased focus on social determinants of health with an emphasis on how conditions in the environments where people live, learn, work, play, worship, and age influence their health. There are five domains of social determinants of health in *Healthy People 2030*, including economic stability; education access and quality;

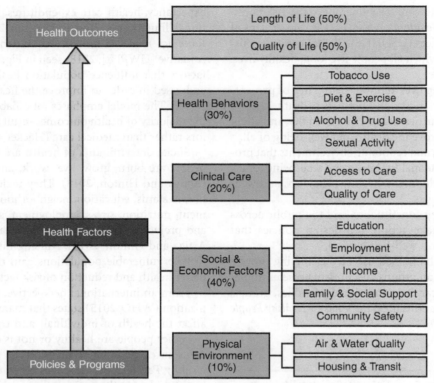

Fig. 23.1 County Health Rankings Model. (University of Wisconsin Population Health Institute. County Health Rankings & Roadmaps 2019. www.countyhealthrankings.org.)

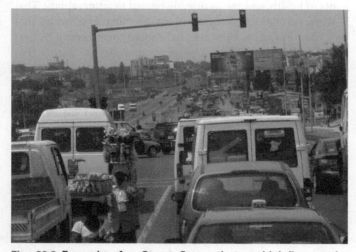

Fig. 23.2 Example of a Street Scene that could Influence the Determinants of Health.

health care access and quality; neighborhood and built environment; and social and community context. Examples of social determinants of health include:

- Safe housing, transportation, and neighborhoods
- Racism, discrimination, and violence
- Education, job opportunities, and income
- Access to nutritious foods and physical activity opportunities
- Polluted air and water
- Language and literacy skills (*Healthy People 2030*)

A useful diagram is also provided that depicts how the five key areas (determinants) of economic stability, education, social and community context, health and health care, and neighborhoods and the built environment serve as a framework for an approach to understanding the social determinants of health (USDHHS, 2020a, p. 4) (Fig. 23.3).

Health disparities are differences that exist among specific population groups that prevent them from attaining their full health potential (Baciu, Negussie, Geller, et al., 2017). Disparities can exist across many dimensions, including race, ethnicity, gender, sexual orientation, age, disability status, socioeconomic status, and geographic location (Baciu, Negussie, Geller, et al., 2017). The most "obstinate" inequities that lead to health disparities continue to be race and ethnicity in the United States. Solutions to reduce these disparities and achieve greater health equity need to take into account social, political, and the historical context of the country and its residents. Examples of groups likely to experience health inequity that leads to health disparities are African Americans, Native Americans, sexual minorities, persons with disabilities, veterans, persons released from being incarcerated, and those who live in rural areas (Baciu, Negussie, Geller, et al., 2017; Albertson, Scannell, Ashtari, and Barnert, 2020).

For more than two decades, *Healthy People* focused on intervening in disparities. Thirty-eight topic areas in *Healthy People 2020* emphasized access, chronic health problems, injury and violence prevention, environmental health, food safety, education and community-based programs, health communication, health

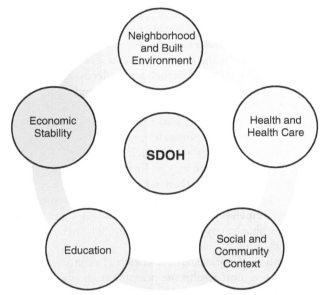

Fig. 23.3 Five Key areas of Social Determinants of Health as Found in *Healthy People 2030*. (From *Healthy People 2030*, US Department of Health and Human Services, Office of Disease Prevention and Health Promotion. Retrieved September 2020, Available at https://health.gov/healthypeople/objectives-and-data/social-determinants-health.)

information technologies, immunization and infectious diseases, and public health infrastructure, among others. *Healthy People 2030* goals have expanded as seen in the following box, but the emphasis on elimination of health disparities and promotion of health equity is unchanged.

> ### ♥ HEALTHY PEOPLE 2030
>
> - AHS-08: Increase the proportion of adults who get recommended evidence-based preventive health care.
> - AHS-06: Reduce the proportion of people who can't get prescription medicines when they need them.
> - HC/HIT-02: Decrease the proportion of adults who report poor communication with their health care provider.

From US Department of Health and Human Services: *Healthy People 2030*, Washington DC, 2020a, USDHHS. Retrieved from http://www.healthypeople.gov/.

As discussed in other chapters, *Healthy People 2020* and *Healthy People 2030* are implementation guides for all federal and most state health initiatives. It is especially relevant to a discussion of vulnerable populations because these underserved and disadvantaged populations have fewer resources for promoting health and treating illness than does the average person in the United States. For example, a family or individual below the federal poverty line is considered disadvantaged in terms of access to economic resources. These groups are thought to be vulnerable because of the combination of risk factors, health status, and lack of resources needed to access health care and reduce risk factors. The health/wealth gradient shows that lower income is related to poorer health.

VULNERABILITY: DEFINITION AND INFLUENCING FACTORS

Vulnerability is defined as susceptibility to actual or potential stressors that may lead to an adverse effect. Vulnerability to poor health does not mean that some people have personal deficiencies. Rather, it results from the interacting effects of many internal and external factors over which people have little or no control. For example, a person may have some biologic limitations, including genetic risks, made more severe by pollution, lead-based paint, excessive noise, or other external factors. Vulnerable populations are those groups which have an increased risk for developing adverse health outcomes.

As discussed in Chapter 10, risk is an epidemiologic term that means some people have a higher probability than others of illness. In the epidemiologic triangle, the agent, host, and environment interact to produce illness or poor health. The natural history of disease model explains how certain aspects of physiology and the environment, including personal habits, social environment, genetic factors, and physical environment, make it more likely that a person will develop particular health problems (Friss, 2018). For example, a smoker or those who are exposed to secondhand smoke are at risk for developing lung cancer because cellular changes occur with smoking. However, not everyone who is at risk develops health problems; not all people who smoke develop lung cancer; and not all people who develop lung cancer have ever smoked. Some individuals are more likely than others to develop the health problems for which they are at risk. These people are more *vulnerable* than others. The web of causation model better explains what happens in these situations. A vulnerable population group is a subgroup of the population that is more likely to develop health problems as a result of exposure to risk or to have worse outcomes from these health problems than the rest of the population. That is, the interaction among many variables creates a more powerful combination of factors that predispose the person to illness. Vulnerable populations often experience multiple cumulative risks, and they are particularly sensitive to the effects of those risks. Risks come from environmental hazards (e.g., lead exposure from lead-based paint from peeling walls or paint used in toy manufacturing), social hazards (e.g., crime, violence, riots), personal behavior (e.g., diet, exercise habits, smoking or use of drugs), or biologic or genetic makeup (e.g., congenital addiction, compromised immune status). Members of vulnerable populations often have multiple illnesses, with each affecting the other. Genetics also plays a role in vulnerability and influences a person's resilience to adverse socioeconomic conditions (Braveman and Gottlieb, 2014). Not all members of vulnerable populations succumb to the health risks that impinge on them. It is important to learn what factors help these people to resist, or have resilience to, the effects of vulnerability.

As described earlier, vulnerable individuals and families often have many risk factors. For example, nurses work with pregnant adolescents who are poor, have been abused, and are substance abusers. Nurses also work with other substance abusers and persons who test positive for human immunodeficiency virus (HIV) and for hepatitis B virus (HBV), those with a communicable

HOW GENETIC FACTORS INFLUENCE A PERSON'S VULNERABILITY TO HEALTH DISRUPTIONS

Some populations become vulnerable due to their genetic risks. An increasing amount of information is being learned about genetic influences on health. For this reason, public health nurses must be able to gather a comprehensive family history, identify family members at risk for genetically influenced factors, and help people to make informed decisions about their health and become more resilient for the possible effects of genetics. Two useful resources for nurses and consumers are: National Human Genome Research Institute at www.genome.gov and Genetics home reference at www.ghr.nlm.nih.gov sponsored by the National Library of Medicine and the National Institutes of Health

disease, and those who are severely mentally ill. Nurses who work in public health provide care to homeless and marginally housed individuals and families. They also provide care for migrant workers and immigrants. Any of these groups may be victimized by abuse and violence. Veterans are often vulnerable to health care risks, as are youth and adults recently discharged from a jail or prison. Chapters 24 to 27 discuss many of the high-risk groups for health disparities.

Vulnerability results from the combined effects of limited resources. Limitations in physical resources, environmental resources, personal resources (or human capital), and biopsychosocial resources (e.g., the presence of illness, genetic predispositions) combine to cause vulnerability (Aday, 2001). Poverty, limited social support, and working in a hazardous environment are examples of limitations in physical and environmental resources. People with preexisting illnesses, such as those with communicable or infectious diseases or chronic illnesses such as cancer, heart disease, or chronic airway disease, have less physical ability to cope with stress than those without such physical problems. Human capital refers to all of the strengths, knowledge, and skills that enable a person to live a productive, happy life. People with little education have less human capital because their choices are more limited than those of people with higher levels of education.

Vulnerability has many aspects. It often comes from a feeling of lack of power, limited control, victimization, disadvantaged status, disenfranchisement, and health risks. Members of vulnerable populations often have multiple illnesses, with each affecting the other. Some of these persons do not succumb to the health risks, and it is important to help them develop resilience. Vulnerability can be reduced or reversed by increasing resilience. Useful nursing interventions to increase resilience include case finding, health education, care coordination, and policy making related to improving health for vulnerable populations.

One aspect of vulnerability, disenfranchisement, refers to a feeling of separation from mainstream society. The person does not seem to have an emotional connection with any group in particular or with the larger society. Some groups such as the poor, the homeless, veterans, persons released from the criminal justice system, and migrant workers often are "invisible" to society as a whole and tend to be forgotten in health and social planning. Vulnerable populations are at risk for disenfranchisement because their social supports are often weak, as are their linkages to formal community organizations such as churches, schools, and other types of social organizations. They also may have few informal sources of support, such as family, friends, and neighbors. In many ways, vulnerable groups have limited control over potential and actual health needs. In many communities, these groups are in the minority and disadvantaged because typical health planning focuses on the majority. Disadvantage also results from lack of resources that others may take for granted. Vulnerable population groups have limited social and economic resources with which to manage their health care. For example, women may endure domestic violence rather than risk losing a place for them selves and their children to live. Women who are among the working poor are more likely to become homeless when they leave an abusive partner. They may not be able to pay for a place to live when they lose their partner's income.

As mentioned, social status influences health in a variety of ways. First, the more wealth the person has, the more likely the person is to have access to better food, more education, a safer community, recreation, and health care. These resources serve as protective barriers again chronic disease, injury, and premature mortality (Lathrop, 2013). Nursing interventions are designed to help vulnerable populations gain the resources needed for better health and reduction of risk factors.

Poverty is a primary cause of vulnerability, and it is a growing problem in the United States. The chronic stress of factors such as poverty, unemployment, and poor education can lead to maladaptive physical responses and disease (Lathrop, 2013). Low income is associated with low life expectancy. A person born in 1960 in the lowest income quintile can expect to live until age 76. In contrast, the life expectancy of those in the highest quintile is 89 years (Stein and Galea, 2018). Poverty is a relative state. The federal definition of poverty is used to develop eligibility criteria for programs such as Medicaid and welfare assistance. In 2020 the federal poverty guideline for a family of four was $26,200 for all states except Hawaii and Alaska. Both Alaska and Hawaii have higher poverty guideline levels due to their higher cost of living (USDHHS, 2020b). Poverty among children is a significant issue. In 2017, 17% of US children from 0 to 17 years lived in poverty (Federal Interagency Forum on Child and Family Statistics, 2020). Children are particularly susceptible to the effects of poverty and more likely to live in poverty if they live in rural America or in the Southeast. In rankings done by Save the Children, data were collected for 180 countries to assess where the most and the fewest children missed out on childhood. They examined variables such as children's health, education, and protection status including such areas as: death, chronic malnutrition, being out of school and being forced into adult roles of work, marriage, and motherhood. Singapore had the highest rating in 2020, with a score of 989 out of 1000. The United States "badly trails nearly all other advanced counties in helping children reach their full potential" (Geoghegan, 2020, p. 1). The United States was ranked 43rd, trailing Canada at 28 and the United Kingdom at 29.

However, many people who earn just a little more than the federal poverty guideline are unable to pay for their living expenses but are ineligible for assistance programs. People who do not have the financial resources to pay for medical care are considered medically indigent. They may be self-employed or work in small businesses and cannot afford health benefits. Other people have inadequate health insurance coverage. This may be either because the deductibles or copayments for their insurance are so high that they have to pay for most expenses or because few conditions or services are covered. In these situations, poverty in its relative sense causes vulnerability; uninsured and underinsured people are less likely to seek preventive health services because of the cost. They are then more likely to suffer the consequences of preventable illnesses. See Chapter 3, which discusses the health care and public health system, and Chapter 5, which discusses the economic influences on health care, for details about people who have health insurance and those who do not, and what impact the Patient Protection and Affordable Care Act of 2010 has and will likely have on helping to insure more of these uninsured persons. The outcomes to persons in the United States due to the COVID-19 pandemic and its effects on employment, loss of income, loss of homes, and so forth are yet to be known. Nurses need to be better prepared for caring for people during a pandemic due to increased urbanization, mass travel and transit, and increased population density (Hassmiller, 2020).

As discussed in Chapter 8, which discusses environmental health, people who are poor are more likely to live in hazardous environments that are overcrowded and have inadequate sanitation, work in high-risk jobs, have less-nutritious diets, and have multiple stressors because they do not have the extra resources to manage unexpected crises and may not even have adequate resources to manage daily life. Poverty often reduces an individual's access to health care. In the developed countries of the world, this is more likely to be a problem for those just above the poverty line who are not eligible for public support, whereas in developing countries, poverty is correlated with decreased access to health care.

Education plays an important role in health status. Although education is related to income, educational level seems to influence health separately. Higher levels of education may provide people with more information for making healthy lifestyle choices. More highly educated people are better able to make informed choices about health insurance and providers. Education also may influence perceptions of stressors and problem situations and give people more alternatives. Finally, education and language skills affect health literacy. Chapter 14 discusses health literacy and its effect on health. In addition, pregnant teens, migrant workers, and homeless persons are often less likely to have adequate education, and this can influence their ability to access health care and to make healthy lifestyle choices.

Access to health care may be more limited for low socioeconomic groups. Barriers to access are policies and financial, geographic, or cultural features of health care that make services difficult to obtain or so unappealing that people do not wish to seek care. Examples include offering services only on weekdays without providing evening or weekend hours for working adults, being uninsured or underinsured, not having reasonably convenient or economical transportation, or providing services only in English and not in the population's primary language. In addition, services for families may be offered in locations that make it difficult for people who do not have reliable forms of transportation. Removing these barriers by providing extended clinic hours, low-cost or free health services for people who are uninsured or underinsured, transportation, mobile vans, and professional interpreters help to improve access to care. The interactions among multiple socioeconomic stressors make people more susceptible to risks than others with more financial resources, who may cope more effectively.

As discussed in Chapter 25, extreme poverty, in the form of homelessness or marginal housing, is related to risk for physical, dental, and mental health problems; food insecurity; and limited access to health care (Baggett et al., 2010). Those who are homeless or marginally housed have even fewer resources than poor people who have adequate housing. Homeless and marginally housed people must struggle with heavy demands as they try to manage daily life. These individuals and families do not have the advantage of consistent housing and must cope with finding a place to sleep at night and a place to stay during the day or moving frequently from one residence to another, as well as finding food, before even thinking about health care. Lack of access to nutritious food on a regular basis poses serious health problems. Mental health problems can increase a person's vulnerability and lead to disability. They may result in high costs to society in the form of loss of productivity and treatment (Hudson et al., 2016). Adverse social and economic conditions contribute to the development of mental health problems; that is, poverty is often associated with depression, and persons who experience considerable stress may develop mental health problems. There is a growing gap between poor and richer children in the world's wealthiest countries, and this gap is at its highest level in three decades.

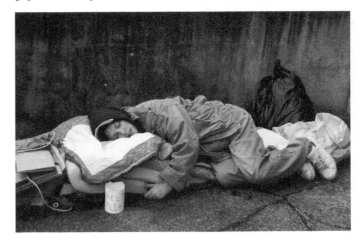

Vulnerability often has a cycle. That is, poor health creates stress as individuals and families who have inadequate resources try to manage health problems. For example, if a person who has acquired immunodeficiency syndrome (AIDS) develops one or more opportunistic infections and is either uninsured or underinsured, that person and the family and caregivers will have more difficulty managing the illness than if the person had adequate insurance. Vulnerable populations often suffer many forms of stress. Sometimes when one problem is solved, another quickly emerges. This can lead to feelings of hopelessness and an overwhelming sense of powerlessness and social isolation. For example, substance abusers who feel powerless over their addiction and who have isolated themselves from the people they care about may see no way to change their situation. Nursing interventions should include strategies that will increase resources or reduce health risks to decrease health disparities between vulnerable populations and populations with more advantages.

HEALTH STATUS AND SPECIAL NEEDS GROUPS

Age is related to vulnerability because people at both ends of the age continuum are often less able physiologically to adapt to stressors. For example, infants of substance-abusing mothers risk being born addicted and having severe physiologic problems and developmental delays. Elderly individuals are more likely to develop active infections from communicable diseases such as the flu or pneumonia and generally have more difficulty recovering from infectious processes than do younger people because of the former group's less effective immune systems. Persons 65 years and older were considered to be high risk for having COVID-19 and also having poorer outcomes from the virus. The older population in the US were the first to be provided with the opportunity to get the COVID-19 vaccine. Older people also may be more vulnerable to safety threats and loss of independence because of their age, multiple chronic illnesses, and impaired mobility.

A person's life experiences, especially those early in life, influence vulnerability or resilience. For example, children who survive disasters may experience difficulties in later life if they do not receive adequate counseling. Higher levels of confidence in one's ability or internal locus of control appear to protect children (particularly adolescents) from the negative effects of disaster and trauma. Persons with an internal locus of control believe that they control their behavior and do not depend entirely on external people, events, or forces to control behavior. It is the person's perception of his or her level of personal control that influences the person's decisions. Persons with a high level of internal locus of control are more likely to participate in health screenings and take responsibility for their health. That is, those who believe they can control their health to some extent were perhaps more likely to follow the Centers for Disease Control and Prevention guidelines. Vulnerable population groups often develop an external locus of control. They may believe that events are outside their control and result from bad luck or fate. People with an external locus of control have more difficulty taking action or seeking care for health problems. They may minimize the value of health promotion or illness prevention because they do not think they have control over their health destinies.

Other population groups that may be considered vulnerable include members of the military and their families, veterans, and persons with disabilities. Family members with a military service member have been found to be more susceptive to domestic violence and child maltreatment, and returning service members may have difficulty reconnecting with their families that have stayed at home. Specifically, children of deployed service members have been found to experience greater psychological difficulties,

anxiety, school and peer problems, depression, and suicidal ideation than children of nondeployed parents (Sullivan, 2015).

The physical and psychological impact of both current and past wartime and military experiences has created a large population of veterans needing health care (Baciu, Negussie, Geller et al., 2018). In the past, there have been large death rates due to combat. More recently due to increased triage, improved trauma treatment, and recovery strategies, more veterans are surviving and returning home with needs.

In 2018 there were 18.0 million veterans; of these, 1.7 million or 9% were female and the number of female veterans is expected to grow to 17% by 2040. The median age of veterans in 2018 was 65 years. Currently, veterans are less likely to be non-Hispanic White and more likely to have attended college than veterans from earlier service periods. The higher levels of education are due to the computer, mathematical, engineering, and mechanical training that is essential to the current armed forces. "Today's veterans have distinctive health issues related to their military service and are more likely to suffer from trauma-related injuries, substance abuse and mental disorders than people who have never served in the armed forces. About one quarter of all veterans had a service-connected disability in 2018 which is an injury, disease or disability that active duty either caused or aggravated" (Vespa, 2020).

It is important for public health nurses to know about the health care issues and needs of veterans. First, learn how many veterans live in your area and where and how they live. That is, do they live with families or significant others? Or do they live alone in adequate housing, or are they homeless?

Persons with a disability often live with limitations in mental or physical functioning that prevent them from having full participation in their communities. Some of the issues related to the vulnerability of persons with a disability include:

1. When youths with disabilities or special health needs move from a pediatric to an adult care system, they may find that there are barriers with health systems not prepared to provide needed care for their complex needs.
2. Health expenditures tend to be high for this group.
3. Despite passage of the Americans with Disabilities Act, many health care facilities do not have accessible examination tables, mammography equipment, and weight scales, nor are their buildings architecturally accessible.
4. Individuals with a disability may also be at increased risk during a disaster.
5. Health care professionals may not be adequately prepared to provide needed care to persons with complex mental and/or physical health needs associated with a disability (Sullivan, 2015).

PUBLIC POLICIES AFFECTING VULNERABLE POPULATIONS

Health in All Policies is a collaborative approach in cities or states that integrates health considerations into policymaking across all sectors to improve health. This strategy is a way to address the complex factors that influence health and equity (i.e., social determinants of health including educational attainment, housing, transportation, and neighborhood safety) (Caplan,

Ben-Moshe, and Dillon, 2013). Examples in the United States from coast to coast can be found on the website of the APHA (apha.org) and include Boston to Oregon and several other localities.

Three pieces of legislation have provided direct and indirect financial subsidies to certain vulnerable groups. The Social Security Act of 1935 created the largest federal support program in history for elderly and poor Americans. This act was intended to ensure a minimal level of support for people at risk for problems resulting from inadequate financial resources. This was accomplished by direct payments to eligible individuals. Later, the Social Security Act Amendments of 1965, Medicare and Medicaid, provided for the health care needs of older adults, the poor, and individuals with a disability who might be vulnerable to impoverishment resulting from high medical bills or poor health status from inadequate access to health care. The Social Security Act and its Amendments created third-party health care payers at the federal and state levels. Title XXI of the Social Security Act, enacted in 1998, created the State Children's Health Insurance Program (SCHIP), which provides funds to insure currently uninsured children. The SCHIP program is jointly funded by the federal and state governments and administered by the states. Using broad federal guidelines, each state designs its own program, determines who is eligible for benefits, sets the payment levels, and decides on the administrative and operating procedures. President Obama signed the Children's Health Insurance Program Reauthorization Act of 2009 (CHIPRA). This legislation provided states with new funding, new program options, and a range of new incentives for covering children through Medicaid and the Children's Health Insurance Program (CHIP) (CHIPRA, 2016). Since the enactment of the Affordable Care Act in 2010, many states have expanded their Medicaid programs.

The Temporary Assistance for Needy Families (TANF) program replaced the previous Aid to Families with Dependent Children (AFDC). TANF is designed to help needy families become self-sufficient. States receive block grants to design and operate programs that accomplish one of the four purposes of this program:

- Provide assistance to needy families so that children can be cared for in their own homes or in the homes of relatives.
- End the dependency of needy parents by promoting job preparation, work, and marriage.
- Prevent and reduce the incidence of out-of-wedlock pregnancies.
- Encourage the formation and maintenance of two-parent families (www.acf.hhs.gov 2019).

See Chapter 5 for detailed information on the economics of health care including the Affordable Care Act (ACA) of 2010.

NURSING APPROACHES TO CARE IN THE COMMUNITY

There is a trend toward providing more comprehensive, family-centered services when treating vulnerable population groups. It is important to provide comprehensive, family-centered, "one-stop" services. Providing multiple services during a single clinic visit is an example of one-stop services. If social assistance and economic assistance are provided and included in interdisciplinary treatment plans, services can be more responsive to the combined effects of social and economic stressors on the health of special population groups. This situation is sometimes referred to as providing wrap around services, in which comprehensive health services are available and social and economic services are "wrapped around" these services. Although this is an excellent approach to care, it is not available in all or even most areas in the United States.

It is helpful to provide comprehensive services in locations where people live and work, including schools, churches, neighborhoods, and workplaces. Comprehensive services are health services that focus on more than one health problem or concern. For example, some nurses use stationary or mobile outreach clinics to provide a wide array of health promotion, illness prevention, and illness management services in migrant camps, schools, and local communities. A single client visit may focus on an acute health problem such as influenza, but it also may include health education about diet and exercise, counseling for smoking cessation, and a follow-up appointment for immunizations once the influenza is over. The shift away from hospital-based care includes a renewed commitment to the public health services that vulnerable populations need to prevent illness and promote health, such as reductions in environmental hazards and violence and assurance of safe food and water. It is important to remember that referring clients to community agencies involves much more than simply making a phone call or completing a form. Nurses should make certain that the agency to which they refer a client is the right one to meet that client's needs. Nurses can do more harm than good by referring a stressed, discouraged client to an agency from which the client is not really eligible to receive services. Nurses should help the client to learn how to get the most from the referral.

Nurses also focus on advocacy and social justice concerns. Advocacy refers to actions taken on behalf of another. Nurses may function as advocates for vulnerable populations by working for the passage and implementation of policies that lead to improved public health services for these populations. For example, a nurse may serve on a local coalition for uninsured people, and another may work to develop a plan for sharing the provision of free or low-cost health care by local health care organizations and providers.

Social justice includes the concepts of egalitarianism and equality. A society that subscribes to the concept of social justice is one that values equality and recognizes the worth of all members of that society Braverman, 2014). Such a society would provide humane care and social supports for all people. Nurses who function in advocacy roles and facilitate change in public policy are intervening to promote social justice. Nurses can be advocates for policy changes to improve social, economic, and environmental factors that predispose vulnerable populations to poor health. The overriding nursing goal for care of all people, including those who come from vulnerable populations, is to provide safe and quality care. See the Quality and Safety Education for Nurses (QSEN) box for information on quality care.

It is important for nurses to provide culturally and linguistically appropriate health care. Linguistically appropriate health care means communicating health-related information in the recipient's primary language when possible and always in a language the recipient can understand. It also means using words that the recipient can understand. The factors that predispose people to vulnerability and the outcomes of vulnerability create a cycle in which the outcomes reinforce the predisposing factors, leading to more negative outcomes. Unless the cycle is broken, it is difficult for vulnerable populations to improve their health. Nurses can identify areas in which they can work with vulnerable populations to break the cycle. The nursing process guides nurses in assessing vulnerable individuals, families, groups, and communities; developing nursing diagnoses of their strengths and needs; planning and implementing appropriate therapeutic nursing interventions in partnership with vulnerable clients; and evaluating the effectiveness of interventions.

The socioecologic model (SEM) is a theory-based framework that takes into account the multiple factors for providing comprehensive health care. This framework was developed by the Centers for Disease Control and Prevention. Similarly, in *Healthy People 2030* (USDHHS, 2020a), social determinants of health are grouped into five domains: (1) economic stability; (2) health care access and quality; (3) social and community context; (4) education access and quality; and (5) neighborhood and built environment. Both the SEM and the *Healthy People 2030* domains help to guide public health nursing practice.

BOX 23.1   Nursing Roles When Working With Vulnerable Population Groups

- Case finder
- Health educator
- Counselor
- Direct care provider
- Community assessor and developer
- Monitor and evaluator of care
- Case manager
- Advocate
- Health program planner
- Participant in developing health policies

---

partnerships between the nurse and client and build on careful assessment. Nurses need to avoid directing and controlling clients' care because this might interfere with their being able to establish a trusting relationship and may inadvertently foster a cycle of dependency and lack of personal health control. The most important initial step is for nurses to demonstrate they are trustworthy and dependable. For example, nurses who work in a community clinic for substance abusers must overcome any suspicion that clients may have of them and eliminate any fears clients may have of being manipulated.

Nurses working with vulnerable populations may fill numerous roles, including those listed in Box 23.1. They identify vulnerable individuals and families through outreach and case finding. They encourage vulnerable groups to obtain health services, and they develop programs that respond to their needs. Nurses teach vulnerable individuals, families, and groups strategies to promote health and prevent illness. They counsel clients about ways to increase their sense of personal power and help them to identify their strengths and resources. Nurses also provide direct care to clients and families in a variety of settings, including storefront clinics, mobile clinics, shelters, homes, neighborhoods, worksites, churches, and schools.

Some examples of care to clients, families, and groups are: (1) a nurse in a mobile migrant clinic might administer a tetanus booster to a client who has been injured by a piece of farm machinery and may also check that client's blood pressure and cholesterol level during the same visit; (2) a home health nurse seeing a family referred by the courts for child abuse may weigh the child, conduct a nutritional assessment, and help the family to learn how to manage anger and disciplinary problems; (3) a nurse working in a school-based clinic may lead a support group for pregnant adolescents and conduct a birthing class; and (4) a nurse may work with people being treated for tuberculosis (TB) to monitor drug treatment compliance and ensure that they complete their full course of therapy.

Public health nurses also serve as population health advocates and work with local, state, or national groups to develop and implement healthy public policy. They also collaborate with community members and serve as community assessors and developers, and they monitor and evaluate care and health programs. Nurses often function as case managers for vulnerable clients, making referrals and linking them to community services. Case management services are especially important

---

QSEN   FOCUS ON QUALITY AND SAFETY EDUCATION FOR NURSES

Targeted Competency: Quality Improvement—Use data to monitor the outcomes of care processes and use improvement methods to design and test changes to continuously improve the quality and safety of health care systems. Important aspects of quality improvement include:

- **Knowledge:** Explain the importance of variation and measurement in assessing quality of care.
- **Skills:** Use quality measures to understand performance.
- **Attitudes:** Value measurement and its role in good client care.

Quality Improvement Question:

Examine health statistics and demographic data in your geographic area to determine which vulnerable groups are predominant. Look on the web for examples of agencies you think provide services to these vulnerable groups. If the agency has a web page, read about the target population they serve, the types of services they provide, and how they are reimbursed for services. Learn about different agencies and share results during class. Based on your findings, identify gaps or overlaps in services provided to vulnerable groups in your community. Which data do these agencies collect to demonstrate the efficacy of their services? How could you deal with these gaps and overlaps to help clients receive needed services?

Prepared by Gail Armstrong, N.D., DNP, MS, PhD, Professor and Assistant Dean of the DNP Program, Oregon Health and Sciences University.

In some situations, the nurse works with individual clients. The nurse also develops programs and policies for populations of vulnerable persons. In both examples, planning and implementing care for members of vulnerable populations involve

for vulnerable persons because they often do not have the ability or resources to make their own arrangements. They may not be able to speak the language, or they may be unable to navigate the complex telephone systems that many agencies establish. They also serve as advocates when they refer clients to other agencies, work with others to develop health programs, and influence legislation and health policies that affect vulnerable populations.

The nature of nurses' roles varies depending on whether the client is a single person, a family, or a group. For example, a nurse might teach an HIV-positive client about the need for prevention of opportunistic infections, may help a family with an HIV-positive member understand myths about transmission of HIV, or may work with a community group concerned about HIV transmission among students. In each case, the nurse teaches individuals how to prevent infectious and communicable diseases. The size of the group and the teaching method for each group differ.

Health education is often used in working with vulnerable populations. The nurse should teach members of populations with low educational levels what they need to do to promote health and prevent illness rather than directing health education to groups that the nurse *thinks* might be at high risk, even though there is no evidence to support the perception. A new concern for nurses in public health is whether the populations with whom they work have adequate health literacy to benefit from health education. It may be necessary to collaborate with an educator, an interpreter, or an expert in health communications to design messages that vulnerable individuals and groups can understand and use. See Chapter 14, which describes health education and health literacy and the nursing roles with each topic.

Levels of Prevention

Healthy People 2030 (USDHHS, 2020a) objectives emphasize improving health by modifying the individual, social, and environmental determinants of health. One way to do this is for vulnerable individuals to have a primary care provider who both coordinates health services for them and provides their preventive services. This primary care provider may be an advanced practice nurse or a primary care physician. Another approach is for a nurse to serve as a case manager for vulnerable clients and, again, coordinate services and provide illness prevention and health promotion services.

One example of primary prevention is to give influenza vaccinations to vulnerable populations who are immunocompromised (unless contraindicated). Secondary prevention is seen in conducting screening clinics for vulnerable populations. For example, nurses who work in homeless shelters, prisons, migrant camps, and substance abuse treatment facilities should know that these groups are at high risk for acquiring communicable diseases. Both clients and staff need routine screening for TB. Screening homeless adults and providing isoniazid to those who test positive for TB are examples of secondary prevention. An example of tertiary prevention is conducting a therapy group with the residents of a group home for severely mentally ill adults. Nurses who work with abused women to help them enhance their levels of self-esteem are also providing tertiary preventive activities.

Levels of prevention changed significantly with the onset of the COVID-19 pandemic, during which people were advised not to gather in groups; to wear masks; and when around other people to maintain a social distance of at least 6 feet and longer in certain settings. These behaviors were changed as the national and state health care advisors learned more about preventing the transmission of the virus.

LEVELS OF PREVENTION

Related to Vulnerable Populations During COVID-19

Primary Prevention
- Provide information about the transmission of COVID-19.

Secondary Prevention
- Conduct screening clinics to assess for persons who are positive for COVID-19.

Tertiary Prevention
- Treat persons who contracted the virus and tell them to self-isolate until they test negative.

Assessment Issues

Nurses who work with vulnerable populations need good assessment skills, current knowledge of available resources, and the ability to plan care based on client needs and receptivity to help. They also need to be able to show respect for the client. The following list provides guidelines for assessing members of vulnerable population groups.

Because members of vulnerable populations often experience multiple stressors, assessment must balance the need to be comprehensive while focusing only on information that the nurse needs and the client is willing to provide. Remember to ask questions about the client's perceptions of his or her *socioeconomic resources*, including identifying people who can provide support and financial resources. Support from other people may include information, caregiving, emotional support, and help with instrumental activities of daily living, such as transportation, shopping, and babysitting. Financial resources may include the extent to which the client can pay for health services and medications, as well as questions about eligibility for third-party payment. The nurse should ask the client about the perceived adequacy of both formal and informal support networks.

When possible, assessment should include an evaluation of clients' *preventive health needs*, including age-appropriate screening tests, such as immunization status, blood pressure, weight, serum cholesterol, Papanicolaou (Pap) smears, breast examinations, mammograms, prostate examinations, glaucoma screening, and dental evaluations. During the COVID-19 pandemic, this might include testing for the virus and providing information in the language the person speaks and about how and where to get a test and if there is any cost involved. People

ASSESSING MEMBERS OF VULNERABLE POPULATION GROUPS

Setting the Stage

- Create a comfortable, nonthreatening environment.
- Learn as much as you can about the culture of the clients you work with so that you will understand cultural practices and values that may influence their health care practices.
- Provide a culturally competent assessment by understanding the meaning of language and nonverbal behavior in the client's culture.
- Be sensitive to the fact that the individual or family you are assessing may have other priorities that are more important to them. These might include financial or legal problems. You may need to give them some tangible help with their most pressing priority before you will be able to address issues that are more traditionally thought of as health concerns.
- Collaborate with others as appropriate; you should not provide financial or legal advice. However, you should make sure to connect your client with someone who can and will help them.

Nursing History of an Individual or Family

- You may have only one opportunity to work with a vulnerable person or family. Try to complete a history that will provide all the essential information you need to help the individual or family on that day. This means that you will have to organize in your mind exactly what you need to ask. You should also understand why you need any information that you gather.
- It will help to use a comprehensive assessment form that has been modified to focus on the special needs of the vulnerable population group with whom you work. However, be flexible. With some clients, it will be both impractical and unethical to cover all questions on a comprehensive form. If you know that you are likely to see the client again, ask the less-pressing questions at the next visit.
- Be sure to include questions about social support, economic status, resources for health care, developmental issues, current health problems, medications, and how the person or family manages their health status. Your goal is to obtain information that will enable you to provide family-centered care.
- Determine whether the individual has any condition that compromises his or her immune status, such as AIDS, or if the individual is undergoing therapy that would result in immunodeficiency, such as cancer chemotherapy.

Physical Examination or Home Assessment

- Again, complete as thorough a physical examination (on an individual) or home assessment as you can. Keep in mind that you should collect only data for which you have a use.
- Be alert for indications of physical abuse, substance use (e.g., needle marks, nasal abnormalities), or neglect (e.g., underweight, inadequate clothing).
- You can assess a family's living environment using good observational skills. Does the family live in an insect- or rat-infested environment? Do they have running water, functioning plumbing, electricity, and a telephone?
- Is perishable food left sitting out on tables and countertops? Are bed linens reasonably clean? Is paint peeling on the walls and ceilings? Is ventilation adequate? Is the temperature of the home adequate? Is the family exposed to raw sewage or animal waste? Is the home adjacent to a busy highway, possibly exposing the family to high noise levels and automobile exhaust?

who needed or wanted to be tested had to know if an appointment was essential and if they needed to fill out any forms in advance to determine their eligibility for testing. It may be necessary to make referrals for some of these tests. Assessment should also include preventive screening for physical health problems for which certain vulnerable groups are at a particularly high risk. For example, people who are HIV positive should be evaluated regularly for T4 cell counts and common opportunistic infections, including TB and pneumonia. Intravenous drug users should be evaluated for HBV, including liver palpation and serum antigen tests as necessary. Alcoholic clients should also be asked about symptoms of liver disease and should be evaluated for jaundice and liver enlargement. Severely mentally ill clients should be assessed for the presence of tardive dyskinesia, indicating possible toxicity from their antipsychotic medications.

Vulnerable populations should be assessed for *congenital* and *genetic predisposition* to illness and either receive education and counseling as appropriate or be referred to other health professionals as necessary. For example, pregnant adolescents who are substance abusers should be referred to programs to help them quit using addictive substances during their pregnancies and, ideally, after delivery of their infants. Pregnant women older than 35 years should receive amniocentesis testing to determine whether genetic abnormalities exist in the fetus.

The nurse should also assess the amount of *stress* the person or family is having. Does the family have healthy coping skills and healthy family interaction? Are some family members able and willing to care for others? What is the level of mental health in each member? In addition, are diet, exercise, and rest and sleep patterns conducive to good health?

The nurse should assess the *living environment* and *neighborhood surroundings* of vulnerable families and groups for environmental hazards such as lead-based paint, asbestos, water and air quality, industrial wastes, and the incidence of crime.

Planning and Implementing Care for Vulnerable Populations

Nurses who work in the community provide services for vulnerable populations. The relationship with the client will depend on the nature of the contact. Some will be seen in clinics and others in homes, schools, testing centers, and at work. Regardless of the setting, the following key nursing actions should be used:

- **Create a trusting environment.** Trust is essential because many of these individuals have previously been disappointed in their interactions with health care and social systems. It is important to follow through and do what you say you are going to do. If you do not know the answer to a question, the best reply is, "I do not know, but I will try to find out."
- **Show respect, compassion, and concern.** Vulnerable people are often defeated by life's circumstances. They may have reached a point at which they question whether they even deserve to get care. Listen carefully, because listening is a form of respect, as well as a way to gather information to plan care.
- **Do not make assumptions.** Assess each person and family. No two people or groups are alike.

CASE STUDY

Felicia is a 22-year-old single mother of three children whose primary source of income is Temporary Assistance for Needy Families (TANF). She is worried about the future because she will no longer be eligible for this funding by the end of the year. She has been unable to find a job that will pay enough for her to afford child care. Her friend Maria said that Felicia and her children can stay in Maria's trailer for a short time, but Felicia is afraid that her only choice after that will be a shelter.

Felicia recently took all three children with her to the health department because 15-month-old Hector needed immunizations. Felicia was also concerned about 5-year-old Martina, who had had a fever of 100°F to 101°F on and off for the past month. Felicia and her friends in the trailer park think that some type of hazardous waste from the chemical plant adjacent to the park is making their children sick. Now that Martina was not feeling well, Felicia was particularly concerned. However, the health department nurse told her that no appointments were available that day and that she would need to bring Martina back to the clinic the next day. Felicia left discouraged because it was so difficult for her to get all three children ready and on the bus to go to the health department, not to mention the expense. She thought maybe Martina just had a cold and she would wait a little longer before bringing her back. However, she wanted to take care of Martina's problem before losing her medical card. Felicia is desperate to find a way to manage her money problems and take care of her children.

- **Coordinate services and providers.** Getting health and social services is not always easy. Often people feel like they are traveling through a maze. In most communities, a large number of useful services exist. People who need them simply may not know about them or how to find them. For example, people may need help finding a food bank or a free clinic, or obtaining low-cost or free clothing through churches or in secondhand stores. Clients often need help in determining whether they meet the eligibility requirements. If gaps in service are found, nurses can work with others to try to get the needed services established.
- **Advocate for accessible health care services.** Vulnerable people have trouble getting access to services. Neighborhood clinics, mobile vans, and home visits can be valuable for them. In addition, coordinating services at a central location is helpful. These multiservice centers can provide health care, social services, day care, drug and alcohol recovery programs, and case management. When working with vulnerable populations, try to have as many services as possible available in a single location and at convenient times. This "one-stop shopping" approach to care delivery is helpful for populations experiencing multiple social, economic, and health-related stresses. Although it may seem difficult and costly to provide comprehensive services in one location, it may save money in the long run by preventing illness.
- **Focus on prevention.** Use every opportunity to teach about preventive health care. Primary prevention may include child and adult immunization and education about nutrition, foot care, safe sex, contraception, and the prevention of injuries or chronic illness. It also includes providing prophylactic anti-TB drug therapy for HIV-positive people who live in homeless shelters, or giving flu vaccine to people who are immunocompromised or older than 65 years of age. Secondary prevention

would include screening for health problems such as TB, diabetes, hypertension, foot problems, anemia, or drug use or abuse. People who spend time in homeless shelters, substance abuse treatment facilities, and prisons often get communicable diseases such as influenza, TB, and methicillin-resistant *Staphylococcus aureus* (MRSA). Nurses who work in these facilities should plan regular influenza vaccination clinics and TB screening clinics. When planning these clinics, nurses should work with local physicians to develop signed protocols and should plan ahead for problems related to the transient nature of the population. For example, nurses should develop a way for homeless individuals to read their TB skin test if necessary and transfer the results back to the facility where the skin test was administered. It is helpful to develop a portable immunization chart, such as a wallet card, that mobile population groups such as the homeless and migrant workers can carry with them.

- **Know when to "walk beside" the client and when to encourage the client to "walk ahead."** At times it is hard to know when to do something for people and when to teach or encourage them to do for themselves. Nursing actions range from providing encouragement and support to providing information and active intervention. It is important to assess for the presence of strength and the ability to problem solve, cope, and access services. For example, a local hospital might provide free mammograms for women who cannot pay. The nurse would need to decide whether to schedule the appointments for clients or to give them the information and encourage them to do the scheduling.
- **Know what resources are available.** Be familiar with community agencies that offer health and social services to vulnerable populations. Also follow up after you make a referral to make sure the client was able to obtain the needed help. Examples of agencies found in most communities are health departments, community mental health centers, voluntary organizations such as the American Red Cross, missions, shelters, soup kitchens, food banks, nurse-managed or free clinics, social service agencies such as the Salvation Army or Travelers' Aid, and church-sponsored health and social services. Nurse-managed clinics provide many services to individuals and families.
- **Develop your own support network.** Working with vulnerable populations can be challenging, rewarding, and, at times, exhausting. Nurses need to find sources of support and strength. This can come from friends, colleagues, hobbies, exercise, poetry, music, and other sources.

? CHECK YOUR PRACTICE

The previous case described above is complex; many actions need to be taken to help Felicia get the care she needs for her children. Apply these steps to this case: (1) Recognize the cues; (2) analyze the cues; (3) develop several hypotheses and decide their priority; (4) develop possible solutions to each hypothesis and identify other personnel and resources you would need to include; (5) act on what you determine to be the most critical hypothesis; and (6) evaluate the outcomes that you believe could have occurred based on your actions. Remember your goal is to help Felicia get the care that she needs for her children.

In addition to the nursing actions described, the How To box summarizes goals and interventions and evaluates outcomes with vulnerable populations.

HOW TO INTERVENE WITH VULNERABLE POPULATIONS

Goals

- Set reasonable goals based on the baseline data you collected. Focus on reducing disparities in health status among vulnerable populations.
- Work toward setting manageable goals with the client. Goals that seem unattainable may be discouraging.
- Set goals collaboratively with the client as a first step toward client empowerment.
- Set family-centered, culturally sensitive goals.

Interventions

- Set up outreach and case-finding programs to help increase access to health services by vulnerable populations.
- Do everything you can to minimize the "hassle factor" connected with the interventions you plan. Vulnerable groups do not have the extra energy, money, or time to cope with unnecessary waits, complicated treatment plans, or confusion. As your client's advocate, you should identify possible hassles and develop ways to avoid them. For example, this may include providing comprehensive services during a single encounter, rather than asking the client to return for multiple visits. Multiple visits for more specialized aspects of the client's needs, whether individual or family group, reinforce a perception that health care is fragmented and organized for the professional's convenience rather than that of the client.
- Work with clients to ensure that interventions are culturally sensitive and competent.
- Focus on teaching skills in health promotion and disease prevention. Role play with clients about how and what questions to ask other health care providers.
- Help clients to learn what to do if they cannot keep an appointment with a health care or social service professional.

Evaluating Outcomes

- It is often difficult for vulnerable clients to return for follow-up care. Help your client to develop self-care strategies for evaluating outcomes. For example, teach homeless individuals how to read their own tuberculosis (TB) skin test, and give them a self-addressed, stamped card they can return by mail with the results.
- Remember to evaluate outcomes in terms of the goals you have mutually agreed on with the client. For example, one outcome for a homeless person receiving isoniazid therapy for TB might be that the person returns to the clinic daily for direct observation of compliance with the drug therapy.

In general, more agencies are needed that provide comprehensive services with nonrestrictive eligibility requirements. Communities often have many agencies that restrict eligibility to make it possible for more people to receive services. For example, shelters may prohibit people who have been drinking alcohol from staying overnight and limit the number of sequential nights a person can stay. Food banks usually limit the number of times a person can receive free food. Agencies are often specialized. For vulnerable individuals and families, this means that they must go to several agencies to obtain services for which they qualify and that meet their health needs. This is tiring and discouraging and can be expensive, and people may forgo help because of these difficulties. Imagine having to take a bus and changing buses two times while navigating this trip with two small children.

Nurses need to know about community agencies that offer various health and social services. It is important to follow up with the client after a referral to ensure that the desired outcomes were achieved. Sometimes excellent community resources may be available but prove impractical because of transportation or reimbursement issues. Nurses can identify these potential problems by following through with referrals, and they can also work with other team members to make referrals as convenient and realistic as possible. Although clients with social problems such as financial needs should be referred to social workers, it is useful for nurses to understand the close connections between health and social problems and know how to work effectively with other professionals.

Nurses who work with vulnerable populations often need to coordinate services across multiple agencies for their clients. It is helpful to have a strong professional network of people who work in other agencies. Effective professional networks make it easier to coordinate care smoothly and in ways that do not add to clients' stress. Nurses can develop strong networks by participating in community coalitions and attending professional meetings. When making referrals to other agencies, a phone call can be a helpful way to obtain information that the client will need for the visit. When possible, having an interdisciplinary, interagency team plan of care for clients at high risk for health problems can be quite effective. It is crucial to obtain the clients' written and informed consent before engaging in this kind of planning because of confidentiality issues. The following list of tips can be helpful:

- Involve clients in making decisions about the services they may find beneficial and can use.
- Work with community coalitions to develop plans for service coordination for targeted vulnerable populations.
- Collaborate with legal counsel from the agencies involved in the coalitions to ensure that legal and ethical issues related to care coordination have been properly addressed. Examples of issues to address include privacy and security of clinical data and ensuring compliance with the Health Insurance Portability and Accountability Act (HIPAA), contractual provisions for coordinating care across agencies, and consent to treatment from multiple agencies.
- Develop policies and protocols for making referrals, following up on referrals, and ensuring that clients receiving care from multiple agencies experience the process as smooth and seamless.

When using case management in working with vulnerable populations: (1) know available services and resources; (2) determine what is missing and look for creative solutions; (3) use your clinical skills ; (4) develop long-term relationships with the clients you serve; (5) strengthen the family's coping and survival skills and resourcefulness; (6) be the road map that guides the family to services, and help them get the services; (7) communicate with the family and the agencies that can help them; and (8) work to change the environment and the policies that affect your clients.

Vulnerable people may have personal coping skills and sources of social support. Learn about these skills and supports.

You can work with clients to help them identify their strengths and draw on those strengths to manage their health needs; they may be able to depend on informal support networks. Even though social isolation is a problem for many vulnerable clients, nurses should not assume they have no one who can or will help them. Case management involves linking clients with services and providing direct nursing services to them, including teaching, counseling, screening, and immunizing. Lillian Wald was the first case manager. She linked vulnerable families with various services to help them stay healthy (Buhler-Wilkerson, 1993). Nurses are often the link between personal health services and population-based health care. Linking, or brokering, health services is accomplished by making appropriate referrals and following up with clients to ensure that the desired outcomes from the referral were achieved. Nurses are effective case managers in community nursing clinics, health departments, hospitals, and various other health care agencies. Nurse case managers emphasize health promotion and illness prevention with vulnerable clients and focus on helping them avoid unnecessary hospitalization. Fig. 23.4 illustrates the coordination and brokering aspect of the nurse's role as case manager for vulnerable populations.

As can be seen, many of these nursing actions are in the realm of case management, in which the nurse makes referrals and links clients with other community services. In the case manager role, the nurse often is an advocate for the client or family. The nurse serves as an advocate when referring clients to other agencies, when working with others to develop health

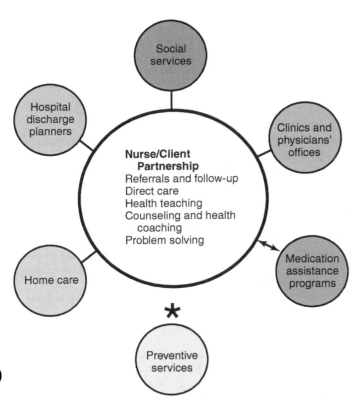

Fig. 23.4 The Nurse as Case Manager for Vulnerable Populations. (© 2012 Photos.com, a division of Getty Images. All rights reserved. Image #135090280.)

programs, and when trying to influence legislation and health policies that affect vulnerable population groups.

APPLYING CONTENT TO PRACTICE

Generalist and staff public health nurses should have competencies in eight domains as defined by the Quad Council Coalition of Public Health Nursing Organizations (2018). Each of the eight competencies is important in working with vulnerable populations. Public health nurses working with vulnerable populations should be able to analyze data and determine when a problem exists with an individual and within a vulnerable population group. They should be able to identify options for programs or policies that could be helpful to these populations and communicate their ideas and recommendations clearly. Public health nurses should be able to provide culturally competent interventions for individuals or for vulnerable populations. As an example, a public health nurse should be able to collect and analyze data related to the prevalence of violence among women in the community, identify key stakeholders, evaluate the cultural preferences of the population, work with others to develop a program to meet a defined need within this population, including preparation of a basic budget for the program, and ensure that the program is culturally appropriate for the population. The Council on Linkages between Academia and Public Health Practice (2014) published a similar list for public health professionals, including but not limited to public health nurses. This list includes an emphasis on evaluation and ongoing improvement of programs. In this example, the nurse would evaluate the program developed for women who are victims of violence and work with others to develop and implement quality improvements on a regular basis.

PRACTICE APPLICATION

Ms. Green, a 46-year-old farm worker pregnant with her fifth child, has come to the clinic requesting treatment for swollen ankles. During your assessment, she said that she saw the nurse practitioner at the local health department 2 months ago. The nurse practitioner gave her some sample vitamins, but Ms. Green lost them. She has not received regular prenatal care and has no plans to do so. Her previous pregnancies were essentially normal, although she said she was "toxic" with her last child. She also said that her middle child was "not quite right." He is in the seventh grade at age 15. Ms. Green is 5 feet 2 inches tall, weighs 180 pounds, and has a blood pressure of 160/90. She has pitting edema of the ankles and a mild headache.

Ms. Green says that she usually takes chlorpromazine hydrochloride (Thorazine) but has run out of it and cannot afford to have her prescription refilled. She says that she has been in several mental hospitals in the past and that she has been more agitated lately and now has problems managing her daily activities. As her agitation grows, she says that she usually hears voices and this really makes her aggressive.

None of her children lives with her, and she has no plans for taking care of the infant. She thinks she will ask the child's father, a racetrack worker, to help her because she usually travels around the country with him.

A. What additional information do you need to help you adequately assess Ms. Green's health status and current needs?

B. What nursing activities are suggested by her history, physical, and psychological descriptions?

Answers can be found on the Evolve website.

REMEMBER THIS

- Every country has population subgroups that are more vulnerable to health threats than the general population is.
- Vulnerable populations are more likely to develop health problems as a result of exposure to risk or to have worse outcomes from those health problems than the population as a whole.
- Vulnerable populations are more sensitive to risk factors than those who are more resilient because they are often exposed to cumulative risk factors.
- Factors leading to the growing number of poor people in the United States include reduced earnings, decreased availability of low-cost housing, more households headed by women, inadequate education, lack of marketable skills, welfare reform, and reduced Social Security payments to children. COVID-19 caused more people to become financially disadvantaged.
- Poverty has a direct effect on health and well-being across the life span. Poor people have higher rates of chronic illness and infant morbidity and mortality, shorter life expectancy, and more complex health problems.
- Child poverty rates are higher than for adults. Children who live in single-parent homes are more likely to be poor than those who live with both parents.
- The complex health problems of homeless people include the inability to obtain adequate rest, sleep, exercise, nutrition, and medication; exposure; infectious diseases; acute and chronic illness; infestations; and trauma and mental health problems.
- Health care is increasingly moving into the community. This began with deinstitutionalization of the severely mentally ill population and is continuing today as hospitals reduce inpatient stays. Vulnerable populations need a wide variety of services, and because these are often provided by multiple community agencies, nurses coordinate and manage the service needs of vulnerable groups.
- Socioeconomic problems predispose people to vulnerability. Vulnerability can become a cycle, with the predisposing factors leading to poor health outcomes, chronic stress, and hopelessness. These outcomes increase vulnerability.
- Nurses assess vulnerable individuals, families, and groups to determine which socioeconomic, physical, biologic, psychological, and environmental factors are problematic for clients. They work as partners with vulnerable clients to identify client strengths and needs and develop intervention strategies designed to break the cycle of vulnerability.

EVOLVE WEBSITE

http://evolve.elsevier.com/Stanhope/foundations
- Case Study, with Questions and Answers
- NCLEX Review Questions
- Practice Application Answers

REFERENCES

Aday LA: *At risk in America: the health and health care needs of vulnerable populations in the United States,* San Francisco, 2001, Jossey-Bass.

Albertson, EM, Scannell C, Ashtari N, Barnett E: Eliminating gaps in Medicaid coverage during reentry after incarceration, *Am J Public Health*, 110(3):317-327, 2020.

American Public Health Association (APHA): Health equity, n.d., Retrieved from https://www.apha.org June 2020.

Artiga S, Hinton E: Beyond health care: the role of social determinants in promoting health & health equity, May 10, 2018, Kaiser Family Foundation Disparities Policy. Retrieved from https://www.kff.org.

Baggett RP, O'Connell JJ, Singer DE, et al.: The unmet health needs of homeless adults: a national study, *Am J Public Health* 100: 1326-1333, 2010.

Baciu A, Negussie Y, Geller A, et al., editors. *Communities in action: pathways to health equity.* Washington D.C.: National Academies Press, 2017.

Braverman P: What are health disparities and health equity? We need to be clear, *Public Health Rep* 129 (Suppl 2):5-8, 2014.

Braveman P, Gottlieb L: The social determinants of health: it's time to consider the causes of the causes, *Public Health Rep* 129(Suppl 2): 19–31, 2014.

Braverman P, Arkin E, Orleans T, Proctor, D, Plough A: What is health equity? May 01, 2017, Robert Wood Johnson Brief. Retrieved from https://www.rwjf.org.

Buhler-Wilkerson K: Bringing care to the people: Lillian Wald's legacy to public health nursing, *Am J Publ Health* 83:1778–1786, 1993.

Caplan RL, Ben-Moshe K, Dillon L. Health in all policies: a guide for state and local governments. Washington D.C. and Oakland CA: American Public Health Association and Public Health Institute, 2013.

CHIPRA: http://www.medicaid.gov/chip/chipra/chipra.htm. March 7, 2016. Retrieved April 9, 2016.

Council on Linkages between Academia and Public Health Practice. *Core competencies for public health professionals, Revised and adopted by the Council on Linkages between Academia and Public Health Practice,* Washington, DC, June 26, 2014, Public Health Foundation.

Federal Interagency Forum on Child and Family Statistics, *America's children: key national indicators of well-being, 2019, 2020,* American Institute of Research; Retrieved at www.air.org, May 2020

Friss RH: *Epidemiology 101,* 2nd ed. Sudbury, 2018, Jones & Bartlett.

Geoghegan T, The hardest places to be a child: Global Childhood Report, Save the Children Foundation, 2020. Retrieved from www. save the children.org, June 2020.

Hacker K, Walker DK: Achieving population health in Accountable Care Organizations, *Am J Public Health* 103:1163-1167, 2013.

Hassmiller S: Health equity and the future of nursing, post-COVID-19, Health Affairs blog, September 30, 2020.

Hudson DL, Kaphingst KA, Croston MA, Blanchard MS, Goodman MS: Estimates of mental health problems in a vulnerable population within a primary care setting, *J Health Care Poor Underserved* 27(2016): 308–326.

Kindig DA: Understanding population health terminology, *Milbank Q* 85(1): 139-161, 2007.

Kindig D, Stoddart G: What is population health? *Am J Public Health* 93(3):380-383, 2003.

Lathrop V: Nursing leadership in addressing the social determinants of health, *Policy Polit Nurse Pract* 14:41–47, 2013.

Quad Council Coalition Competency Review Task Force, 2018, Community/Public Health Nursing Competencies, author.

Stein M, Galea S: Income inequality & our health,, Public Health Post April 11, 2018, Retrieved from https://www.public healthpost.org.

Sullivan K: An application of family stress theory to clinical work with military families and other vulnerable populations, *Clin Soc Work J* 43:89–97, 2015.

US Department of Health and Human Services: *Office of the Assistant Secretary for Planning and Evaluation: Poverty Guidelines,* January 8, 2020b, Washington D.C. Retrieved from www.aspe.hhs.gov/poverty-guidelines, *May 2020.*

US Department of Health and Human Services: *Healthy People 2030,* Washington, DC, 2020a, USDHHS, http://www.healthypeople.gov/.

University of Wisconsin Population Health Initiative (UWPHI): 2018 County Health Rankings key findings report, March 2018. Retrieved from http://www.countyhealthrankings.org.

Vespa JE, Those who served: America's veterans from World War II to the War on Terror, ACH-43, American Community Survey Reports, US Census Bureau, Washington, DC, 2020.

World Health Organization (WHO): *Health impact assessment (HIA): The determinants of health,* 2015. From http://www.who.int/hia/en/. Retrieved June 2020.

24

Rural Health and Migrant Health

Angeline Bushy and Candace Kugel

OBJECTIVES

After reading this chapter, the student should be able to:

1. Compare and contrast definitions for *rural* and *urban*.
2. Describe the health status of rural populations on selected health measures.
3. Discuss access to service issues of rural underserved populations.
4. Define *migrant farmworker* and discuss common health problems of this group and their families and the barriers they experience when seeking health care.
5. Describe the susceptibility to pandemics such as COVID-19 for people in rural areas and for migrant farmworkers.
6. Explain the nursing role for serving persons in rural areas, including migrant farmworkers.

CHAPTER OUTLINE

KEY TERMS

Access to health care is a national priority that remains unsolved. Access is a problem in rural areas, including farms that rely on migrant workers to harvest their crops, and in urban areas, especially in inner cities. This chapter discusses major issues surrounding health care delivery in rural environments as well as issues in providing health care to migrant workers. These issues may differ from those experienced by people living in urban or more populated areas. Recruiting and retraining qualified health care workers can be a problem in both rural and urban areas. These issues have become more challenging during the COVID-19 pandemic when many rural hospitals were financially unable to remain operational. The role of the public health nurse in rural areas is discussed in this chapter.

Formal rural nursing began with the Red Cross Rural Nursing Service (RCRNS), which was organized in November 1912 (Bigbee and Crowder, 1985). Before that time, care of the sick in a small community was provided by informal social support systems. When self-care and family care were not effective in bringing about healing, women who had skills in helping others heal and who lived in the community provided care. Although the health needs of rural people are not all unique, they are different from those of urban populations. Scarcity of health care professionals, poverty, limited access to services, lack of knowledge, and social isolation have plagued many rural communities for generations. A major issue in the rural area is often the distance people must go to find health care services and providers. For migrant workers, a language barrier and cultural differences often exist between them and the farm owners, other area residents, and the health care providers.

RURAL-URBAN CONTINUUM

Each of us has an idea as to what constitutes a rural as opposed to an urban residence. However, the distinctions are becoming blurred as people move further away from cities and towns into less-developed areas. *Rural* is defined generally either in terms of the geographic location and population density or the distance from (e.g., 20 miles) or the time needed (e.g., 30 minutes) to commute to an urban center. Other definitions link rural with farm residency and urban with nonfarm residency.

Some consider rural to be a state of mind. For the more affluent, rural may bring to mind a recreational, retirement, or resort community located in the mountains or in lake country where people can relax and participate in outdoor activities, such as skiing, fishing, hiking, or hunting. For people with limited resources, rural may imply poor and/or crowded housing with lack of adequate facilities for water and sewage.

Just as each city has its own unique characteristics, there is no "typical rural town." For example, rural towns in Florida, Oregon, Alaska, Hawaii, and Idaho are different from one another and quite different from those in Vermont, Texas, Tennessee, Alabama, and California. Descriptions and definitions for rural areas are more subjective and relative than for urban areas.

For example, "small" communities with populations of more than 20,000 have some features that are found in cities. A person who lives in a community with fewer than 2000 people may consider a community with a population of 5000 to 10,000 to be a city. Although some communities may seem geographically remote on a map, the people who live there may not feel isolated. They may think they are within easy reach of services through telecommunication and dependable transportation, although extensive shopping facilities may be 50 to 100 miles from the family home, obstetrical care may be 150 miles away, and nursing services in the district health department in an adjacent county may be 75 or more miles away.

Frequently used definitions to describe rural and urban and to differentiate between them are provided by several federal agencies (RHI-Hub, 2018; USDA, 2018) (Box 24.1). These definitions

---

BOX 24.1 Terms and Definitions

Farm residency: Residency outside area zoned as "city limits"; usually infers involvement in agriculture

Frontier: Regions having fewer than six persons per square mile

Large central: Counties in large (1 million or more population) metro areas that contain all or part of the largest central city

Large fringe: Remaining counties in large (1 million or more population) metro areas

Metropolitan county: Regions with a central city of at least 50,000 residents

Nonfarm residency: Residence within area zoned as "city limits"

Micropolitan county: Counties that do not meet SMSA (see below) criteria

Rural: Communities having fewer than 20,000 residents or fewer than 99 persons per square mile

Small: Counties in metro areas with fewer than 1 million people

Standard metropolitan statistical area (SMSA): Regions with a central city of at least 50,000 residents

Suburban: Area adjacent to a highly populated city

Urban: Geographic areas described as nonrural and having a higher population density; more than 99 persons per square mile; cities with a population of at least 20,000 but less than 50,000

Modified from Rural Health Information Hub (RHI-Hub): *What is rural?* 2018. Available at https://www.ruralhealthinfo.org. Accessed June 25, 2018.

---

fail to take into account the relative nature of "ruralness." Rural and urban residencies are not opposing lifestyles. Rather, the two should be considered as a rural-urban continuum, ranging from living on a remote farm, to a village or small town, to a larger town or city, to a large metropolitan area with a *core inner city*. See Fig. 24.1, which describes the continuum of rural-urban residency. The terms metropolitan area and micropolitan area (metro and micro areas) refer to geographic entities primarily used for collecting, tabulating, and publishing federal statistics. Core-based statistical area (CBSA) is a collective term for both metro and micro areas. A metro area contains a core urban area of 50,000 or more population. A micro area contains an urban core of at least 10,000 people (but fewer than 50,000). Each metro or micro area consists of one or more counties containing the core urban area. Likewise, adjacent counties have a high degree of social and economic integration (as measured by commuting to work) with their urban core.

Demographically, micro areas contain about 60% of the total nonmetro population, with an average of 43,000 people per county. In contrast, non-core areas, with no urban cluster of 10,000 or more residents, have on average about 14,000 residents. In general, lack of an urban core and low overall population density may place these counties at a disadvantage in efforts to expand and diversify their economic base. The designation of micro areas is an important step in recognizing nonmetro diversity. The term also provides a framework to understand population growth and economic restructuring in small towns and cities that have received less attention than metro areas. Nationally and regionally, many measures of health, health care use, and health care resources among rural populations vary by the level of urban influence in a particular region.

Micro areas embody a widely shared residential preference for a small-town lifestyle—an ideal compromise between

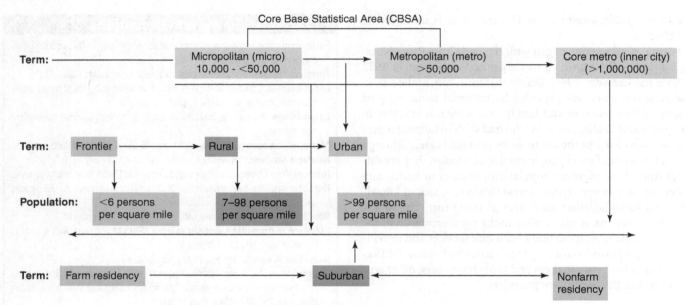

Fig. 24.1 The Continuum of Rural-Urban Residency.

large, highly populated urban cities and sparsely populated rural settings. As information about these places makes its way into government data and publications alongside metro areas in the coming years, hopefully the notion of "micropolitan" will draw increased attention from policy makers and the business community.

In recent years there has been a population shift from urban to less-populated regions of the United States. Demographers refer to this as the "doughnut effect." That is to say, people are moving away from highly populated areas to outlying suburbs of urban centers. Most of the population growth has been in rural counties with a booming economy coupled with the geographic area to expand that is evident in some western and southern states (RHI-Hub, 2018). During 2020 there were news reports saying that many urban residents are relocating to less populated areas during the COVID-19 pandemic in order to separate themselves from other residents.

Clearly, a notable population shift will also affect the health status and lifestyle preferences of communities in which this phenomenon occurs. As beliefs and values change over time, urban-rural differences narrow in some respects while others became more pronounced. Depending on the definition that is used, the actual rural population might vary slightly. In this chapter, rural refers to areas having fewer than 99 persons per square mile and communities having 20,000 or fewer inhabitants.

POPULATION CHARACTERISTICS AND CULTURAL CONSIDERATIONS

Although regional variations exist, in general there are a higher proportion of whites in rural areas than in urban areas. Whites comprise about 80% of the rural population compared to 58% of the urban population. Hispanics comprise 9%, and Blacks comprise 8% (USDA, 2018). Demographically, rural communities have a higher proportion of residents younger than 18 years of age and older than 65 years of age and more residents who are married or widowed than their urban counterparts (CDC, 2018a). Interestingly, the "graying" of rural areas is partly due to the attraction of retirees who choose to live there because of the scenic beauty and slower pace of life (USDA, 2018).

Accompanying the recent population shifts from urban to formerly rural areas, the average income level may change; level of income is a critical factor in whether a family has health insurance or qualifies for public insurance. Consequently, rural families are less likely to have private insurance and more likely to receive public assistance or to be uninsured (RHI-Hub, 2018).

The working poor in rural areas are particularly at risk for being underinsured or uninsured. In working poor families, one or more of the adults are employed but still cannot afford private health insurance. Furthermore, their annual income is such that it disqualifies the family from obtaining public insurance. Several factors help explain why this phenomenon occurs more often in rural settings (Bushy, 2013). For example, a high proportion of rural residents are self-employed in a family business, such as ranching or farming, or they work in small enterprises, such as a service station, restaurant, or grocery store. Also, an individual may be employed in part-time or in seasonal occupations, such as farm or construction work, in which health insurance often is not an employee benefit. A few rural families fall through the cracks and are unable to access any type of public assistance because of other deterrents, such as language barriers, including a low level of health literacy even if they appear comfortable speaking the language, compromised physical status, the geographic location of an agency, lack of transportation, or undocumented worker status. Insurance, or the lack of it, has serious implications for the overall health status of rural residents and the nurses who provide services to them (AHCPR, 2017; NCHS, 2018). The Rural Health Information Hub (2020) identifies nine examples of social determinants

BOX 24.2 Characteristics of Rural Life

- More space; greater distances between residents and services
- Cyclical or seasonal work and leisure activities
- Informal social and professional interactions
- Access to extended kinship systems
- Residents who are related or acquainted
- Lack of anonymity
- Challenges in maintaining confidentiality stemming from familiarity among residents
- Small (often family) enterprises, fewer large industries
- Economic orientation to land and nature (e.g., agriculture, mining, lumbering, fishing, marine related)
- More high-risk occupations
- Town as the center of trade
- Churches and schools as socialization centers
- Preference for interacting with locals (insiders)
- Mistrust of newcomers to the community (outsiders)

From Bushy A: The rural context and nursing practice. In Molinari D, Bushy A, eds.: *The rural nurse: transition to practice*, New York, 2012, Springer, p. 8.

BOX 24.3 Disparities Among US Urban (Metropolitan) and Rural (Micropolitan) Residents' Health Status

Residents of fringe counties near large metro areas have the following:
- Lowest levels of premature mortality, partly reflecting lower death rates for unintentional injuries, homicide, and suicide
- Lowest levels of smoking, alcohol consumption, and childbearing among adolescents
- Lowest prevalence of physical inactivity during leisure time among women
- Lowest levels of obesity among adults
- Greatest number of physician specialists and dentists per capita
- Lowest percent of the population without health insurance
- Lowest percent of the population who had no dental visits
- Residents in the most rural counties have the following:
- Highest death rates for children and young adults
- Highest death rates for unintentional and motor vehicle traffic–related injuries
- Highest death rates among adults for ischemic heart disease and suicide
- Highest levels of smoking among adolescents
- Highest levels of physical activity during leisure time among men
- Highest levels of obesity among adults
- Highest percent of adults with activity limitations caused by chronic health conditions
- Fewest physician specialists and dentists per capita
- Least likely to have seen a dentist
- Highest percentage of the population without health insurance

that are barriers for rural communities in accessing health care. They are:

1. Higher poverty rates
2. Cultural and social norms about health behaviors
3. Low health literacy levels and incomplete perceptions of health
4. Linguistic and educational disparities
5. Limited affordable, reliable, or public transportation
6. Unpredictable work hours or unemployment
7. Lower population densities for program economies of scale coverage
8. Availability of resources to support personnel, use of facilities, and effective program operation
9. Lack of access to healthy foods and physical activity options.

For more discussion on characteristics of rural life, see Box 24.2.

HEALTH STATUS OF RURAL RESIDENTS

Despite the significant number of people who live in rural areas, their health problems and health behaviors are not fully understood. This section summarizes what is known about the overall health status of rural adults and children. The health status measures addressed are perceived health status, diagnosed chronic conditions, physical limitations, frequency of seeking medical treatment, usual source of care, maternal and infant health, children's health, mental health, minorities' health, and environmental and occupational health risks (Bolin and Bellamy, 2015; OSHA, n.d.). As will be noted later in the chapter, rural residents suffer some of the same health problems as migrant farmworkers including exposure to environmental factors and accidents.

In general, people in rural areas have a poorer perception of their overall health and functional status than their urban counterparts. Rural residents older than 18 years of age assess their health status less positively than do urban residents. Studies show that rural adults are less likely to engage in preventive behavior, and this increases their exposure to health risks. Specifically, they are more likely to smoke and report higher rates of alcohol use and obesity. They are less likely to engage in physical activity during leisure time, wear seat belts, have regular blood pressure checks, have Papanicolaou (Pap) smears, perform breast self-examinations, and have colorectal screenings. These omissions affect their overall health (NCHS, 2018). This means that rural residents tend to have more chronic health conditions and limitations in mobility. They are also less likely to seek medical care than urban adults. Rural adults under 65 years of age are more likely than urban adults to view their health status as fair to poor (NCHS, 2018). There are often fewer health care providers in the rural areas which affects their ability to access care in timely ways. See Box 24.3 that discusses rural-urban disparities: lifestyle and health behaviors.

In addition, rural people are less likely to have employer-sponsored health insurance or prescription drug coverage. People living in rural areas have a greater risk than do their urban counterparts for being involved in an accident. More than 50% of vehicle crash-related fatalities occur in rural areas. There is an additional 22% risk of injury-related deaths in rural areas (National Rural Health Association [NRHA], 2020). Also, because of the distances of a farm, ranch, or home from a town and also the likelihood of animals being a possible danger, guns may be more readily found in rural versus urban homes. Nurses can teach people how to prevent accidents, engage in safer and more healthful lifestyle behaviors, and reduce the risk for chronic health problems, and they can help them more effectively manage existing chronic conditions.

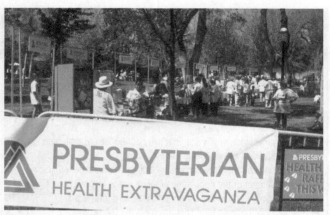

Fig. 24.2 A Hospital-Sponsored Health Fair Is One Example of a Community Event to Provide Health Services to Individuals in a Rural Area.

In general, a person who has a usual source of care is more likely to seek care when ill and to follow prescribed regimens. Rural adults are more likely than urban adults to identify a particular medical provider as their usual source of care. The providers most often seen by rural adults are general practitioners and advanced practice registered nurses (APRNs). In contrast, urban adults are more likely to seek care from a medical specialist. Nurses must be especially thorough in their health assessment of rural and migrant clients who may not receive regular care for chronic health conditions.

Traveling time or distance to ambulatory care services affects access to care for both rural and urban residents. For rural people, it may be the distance they must travel, and for urban people it may be not so much the distance but the amount of traffic they encounter. Both groups tend to wait the same amount of time once they arrive at the clinic or physician's office. There have been differences in seeking health care during the COVID-19 pandemic when patients were reluctant to seek in-person health care or were uncomfortable with telehealth appointments. Nurses provide care in rural areas in a range of locations, including at health fairs that might be conducted at a church, senior center, health care facility, or another readily available location. Fig. 24.2 depicts a health fair at a health care facility.

There is often a maldistribution of health professionals with fewer professionals in rural areas compared to urban areas. The patient-to-primary care physician ratio in rural areas is 39.8 physicians per 100,000 residents, compared to 53.3 physicians per 100,000 residents in urban areas. The gap in providers is even more severe with specialty physicians: 30 per 100,000 in rural areas compared to 263 in urban areas (NRHA, 2020).

Women's Health and Maternal and Infant Health

Overall, rural populations have higher infant and maternal morbidity rates, especially counties designated as HPSAs, which often have a high proportion of racial minorities. Due to the paucity of specialists, there are greater risks for women and infants who have real or potential risk factors. There are extreme variations in pregnancy outcomes from one part of the country to another, and even within states. For example, in several

counties located in the north central and intermountain states, the pregnancy outcome is among the finest in the United States. However, in several other counties within those same states, the pregnancy outcome is among the worst. Particularly at risk are women who live on or near Indian reservations, are migrant workers, and are of African American descent.

Female victims of sexual assault are another at-risk group in rural areas. It is difficult to document the incidence of sexual assault in rural areas because of rural isolation and a higher likelihood that the person who is assaulted knows people in the community. For these reasons, it is thought that the rate is higher than in urban areas (Annan, 2011). Most assaults occur between a woman and someone she knows. Women may be hesitant to report the assault because people who know her may see her car parked at the site where she needs to make the report. Also, the woman may personally know the person(s) to whom the report is made and she would be embarrassed to reveal this incident (Annan, 2011). Because of the closeness of the population in terms of people knowing one another, confidentiality is often an issue in reports of sexual assault. Perpetrators are often family members, so the victim may not be believed or the victim may be threatened to remain silent about the incident.

> ### ? CHECK YOUR PRACTICE
>
> You work in a rural health clinic and although you know many of the clients from seeing them at your children's school, at church, and other locations and events, you do not know Ms. Smith.
> - She comes to the clinic complaining of vague pain in her abdomen and pelvic area.
> - She seems quite anxious and reluctant to describe when her symptoms began.
> - You suspect she may be a victim of a sexual assault.
> - You know that rural women are concerned about confidentiality, and they also worry that they might see the health care provider in a setting outside the clinic and be embarrassed.
> - What would you do? Using the six-step clinical judgment process what cues would you look for? How would you go about analyzing the cues that you note? Once you have made a list of observable cues, list and prioritize the hypotheses you would establish. Next develop possible solutions for each hypothesis and act on what you determine to be the hypothesis of highest priority. Last, evaluate the outcomes of your action(s).
>
> Public health nurses appreciate the effects of socioeconomic factors, such as income level (poverty), education level, age, employment and unemployment patterns, and use of prenatal services, on pregnancy outcomes. There are other, less well-known determinants, such as environmental hazards, occupational risks, and the cultural meaning placed on childbearing and childrearing practices by a community. The effects of these multifaceted factors vary.

Health of Children

Some differences exist between rural and urban children younger than 6 years of age with respect to access to providers and use of services (AHCPR, 2017; Bolin and Bellamy, 2015). For example, urban children are less likely to have a usual provider but are more likely to see a pediatrician when they are ill, and rural adults and children are more likely to have a general practitioner as their regular caregiver. Children who work on farms and ranches are often exposed to noise, organic and inorganic dusts, and the hazards of working with farm equipment. Farm children learn how to work by watching their parents, and some children may not use personal protective equipment. They may also be victims of farm work injuries from using tractors, all-terrain vehicles, working with cattle and horses, using farm hand tools, dealing with barbed wire, and falling from heights, such as in a barn.

School nurses play an important role in the overall health status of children in the United States. The availability of school nurses in rural communities varies across regions. They tend to be scarce in frontier and rural areas of the United States because of (1) a shortage of health care professionals in the area and (2) fewer taxpayers and thus less income to support school nurses.

However, some creative approaches have enabled counties to provide better health care and school nursing services. For example, two or more counties may enter into a partnership in which they share the cost of a "district" health nurse. Other counties have forged partnerships with an agency in an urban setting and contracted for specific health care services. In both of these situations, it is not unusual for the nurse to provide services to all children attending schools in the participating counties. In some frontier states, schools may be more than 100 miles apart and as many miles or more from the district health department office. Because of the number of schools and distances between them, the county nurse may be able to visit each school only once or maybe twice in a school term. Usually the nurse's visit is to update immunizations and perhaps to teach maturation classes to students in the upper grades.

Mental Health

Stress, stress-related conditions, and mental illness are prevalent among populations that have economic difficulties. When the economy in an area is depressed because of slowdowns or federal regulations imposed on agriculture, timber, and marine and mining-related industries as well as trade agreements with other counties, or adverse weather that affects crops, workplaces, and homes, job losses follow. Many job losses occurred during the COVID-19 pandemic of 2020. Farm bankruptcies, mass layoffs of agricultural workers due to low product demand, social distancing, and positive cases affected the farming industry (NCFH, 2020). Economic recession contributes to a family's not having insurance or being underinsured or to their losing their home as a result of mortgage foreclosure. That said, in many communities across the United States, landlords did not evict residents who could not pay their rent due to COVID-19 unemployment. Often, even if mental health services are available and accessible, rural residents delay seeking care when they have an emotional problem until an emergency or a crisis arises. There appears to be a more persistent, endemic level of depression among rural residents. This prevalence may be related to the high rate of poverty, geographic isolation, and an insufficient number of mental health services. Depression may also contribute to the escalating incidence of accidents and suicides, especially among rural male adolescents and young men.

Like many of the indicators in the previous sections, reports on the incidence of domestic violence and alcohol, tobacco, and other drug use and abuse in rural populations are also conflicting. When people are related to one another or know each other well, they are less likely to report these behaviors. After a time, in small, tight-knit communities, destructive coping behaviors often come to be accepted as usual occurrences for a particular family. Family problems also may be ignored if formal social services and public health services are sparse or nonexistent and if the community does not trust the professionals who provide services within a local agency. In underserved rural areas, gaps exist in the continuum of mental health services, which ideally should include preventive education, anticipatory guidance, early intervention programs, crisis and acute care services, and follow-up care. As with other aspects of health care, nurses in rural areas play an important role in community education, case finding, advocacy, and case management of clients experiencing emotional problems and chronic mental health problems (Booth and Graves, 2018; Eisenhauer et al., 2016; Montgomery et al., 2017).

Impact of COVID-19 in Rural America

The National Center for Farmworker Health, Inc. developed a fact sheet related to COVID-19 that they updated weekly. It is believed that rural Americans are more vulnerable to the pandemic than urban Americans due to the proportion of elderly persons, higher smoking rates, and prevalence of certain chronic diseases, and lower numbers of persons covered by health insurance (NCFH, 2020). In addition to a lack of health care professionals, nearly half of rural hospitals operate in a financial deficit and many had to close or lay off or temporarily furlough staff (NCFH, 2020). Many farmworkers fear testing for COVID since a positive test might mean a permanent job loss.

OCCUPATIONAL AND ENVIRONMENTAL HEALTH PROBLEMS IN RURAL AREAS

A community's primary industry or industries are a determinant in the local lifestyle, the health status of its residents, and the number and types of health care services it may need. For example, four high-risk industries identified by the Occupational Safety and Health Administration (OSHA) and found in predominantly rural environments are forestry, mining, marine-related fields, and agriculture. Associated health risks of these industries are machinery and vehicular accidents, trauma, selected types of cancer related to environmental factors, and allergies and respiratory conditions associated with repeated exposure to toxins, pesticides, and herbicides (NCFH, 2018b; OSHA, n.d.; USDA, 2018).

For example, agriculture production industries such as farming and ranching are often owned and operated by a family. Small enterprises with a small number of employees do not fall under OSHA guidelines. For that reason, safety standards are not enforceable on most farms and ranches, since these often are family enterprises. Moreover, small businesses, such as farms, are not covered under workers' compensation insurance.

Additional concerns arise because family members participate in the farm or ranch work. This means that some adults and children may work with animals and operate dangerous machinery with minimal operating instructions on the hazards and on safety precautions. Also, many agriculture workers do not speak or read English. Consequently, agriculture-related accidents result in a sizeable number of deaths and long-term injuries, particularly among children and women. The morbidity and mortality rates associated with agriculture vary from state to state. The rising incidence of these injuries and deaths, however, has become a national concern. Nurses in rural settings can help address this problem by including farm safety content in school and community education programs (Prengaman et al., 2017).

The most common health issues for farmworkers are: (1) pesticide exposure; (2) skin disorders; (3) infectious diseases; (4) musculoskeletal injuries; (6) respiratory illnesses; and (6) hearing and vision disorders (National Center for Farmworker Health, 2018b).

Most of the North American food supply is treated with agricultural chemicals (i.e., pesticides), with the largest group being the organophosphate pesticides. These pesticides are known to be potential hazards. Farmworkers are exposed not only to the immediate effects of working in fields that are foggy or wet with pesticides but also to the unknown long-term effects of chronic exposure to agricultural chemicals. The farmworker's clothing and dwelling also can be major sources of cross-contamination for both the worker and family. The US Environmental Protection Agency (EPA) and OSHA require that farmworkers be given information about pesticide safety. However, migrant farmworkers may not receive this information, may get ineffectual training, or may not be able to read the educational information (Napolitano et al., 2002). Entire families may be at risk for pesticide exposure because of drift from nearby areas, not regularly washing their hands, and bringing contaminated clothes home.

"Mild symptoms of pesticide poisoning include headache, fatigue, dizziness, nervousness, perspiration, loss of appetite, thirst, eye irritation and irritation of the nose and throat. Severe poisoning symptoms include fever, intense thirst, vomiting, muscle twitches, convulsions, inability to breathe and unconsciousness," and exposure to large doses of pesticide can lead to death (NCFH, 2018b, p. 2).

Working for hours in direct sunlight in areas that may have high humidity can generate considerable body heat and can lead to heat stress. The signs and symptoms of heat exhaustion include heavy sweating; cold/pale/clammy skin; fast, weak pulse; nausea and vomiting; and fainting (NCFH, 2018b, p. 2). An added danger is that pesticides are more readily absorbed through hot, sweaty skin than through cool skin. Accidents can occur from being struck by a vehicle or from hand tools, tractors, and other objects and equipment. Infectious diseases among this population are often caused by poor sanitation and crowded conditions. Farmworkers often bend, twist, carry heavy items, and have repetitive motions during long work hours that can lead to musculoskeletal injuries. Farmworkers are often exposed to organic and mineral dusts, animal and plant dusts, toxic gases, molds, and other respiratory irritants. Those who perform the following tasks are at higher risk for respiratory illnesses (NCFH, 2018b, p. 4):

- Working in dusty fields and buildings
- Handling hay
- Feeding or working with feedstuffs
- Working in corn silage
- Cleaning silos or grain bins
- Working around fishmeal
- Working with bird droppings, or dust from animal hair, fur, or feathers
- Applying agricultural chemicals such as fertilizers and pesticides

These same tasks and the environment in which the respiratory illnesses occur can also lead to skin disorders and eye injuries.

📋 LEVELS OF PREVENTION

Related to Rural Health

Primary Prevention
Teach workers how to reduce exposure to pesticides.

Secondary Prevention
Conduct screening such as urine testing for pesticide exposure.

Tertiary Prevention
Initiate treatment for the symptoms of pesticide exposure such as nausea, vomiting, and skin irritation.

RURAL HEALTH CARE DELIVERY ISSUES AND BARRIERS TO CARE

Although each rural community is unique, the experience of living in a rural area has several common characteristics (Bushy and Winters, 2013; Montgomery et al., 2017) (Box 24.4). Barriers to health care in rural areas may be associated with whether services and professionals are available, affordable, accessible, or acceptable to rural consumers. Availability implies that health services exist and have the necessary personnel to provide essential services. Sparseness of population limits the number and array of health care services in a given geographic region. Therefore the cost of providing special services to a few people often is prohibitive, particularly in frontier states, where the number of physicians, nurses, and other types of health care providers is insufficient. Consequently, where services and personnel are scarce, they must be allocated wisely. Accessibility implies that a person has logistical access to needed services, as well as the ability to purchase them. Affordability is associated with both the availability and accessibility of care. It infers that services are of reasonable cost and that a family has sufficient resources to purchase them when they are needed. Acceptability of care means that a particular service is appropriate and offered in a manner that is congruent with the values of a target population. This can be hampered by both the client's cultural preference and the urban orientation of health professions.

BOX 24.4 Barriers to Health Care in Rural Areas

- Lack of health care providers and services and great distances to obtain services
- Lack of personal transportation
- Unavailable public transportation
- Lack of telephone services
- Unavailable outreach services
- Inequitable reimbursement policies for providers
- Unpredictable weather or travel conditions
- Inability to pay for care or lack of health care insurance
- Lack of know-how to procure publicly funded entitlements and services
- Inadequate provider attitudes and understanding about rural populations
- Language barriers (caregivers are not linguistically competent)
- Care and services not culturally and linguistically appropriate

From Bushy A: The rural context and nursing practice. In Molinari D, Bushy A, eds.: *The rural nurse: transition to practice*, New York, 2012, Springer, p. 10.

Providers' attitudes, insights, and knowledge about rural populations are important. A demeaning attitude, lack of accurate knowledge about rural populations, or insensitivity about the rural lifestyle on the part of a nurse can cause difficulties in relating to those clients. Moreover, insensitivity generates mistrust, causing rural clients to view professionals as outsiders to the community. On the other hand, some professionals in rural practice express feelings of professional isolation and lack of community acceptance. To resolve these conflicting views, nursing faculty members can expose students to the rural environment with clinical experiences that include opportunities to provide care to clients in their natural (e.g., rural) setting to gain accurate insight about that particular community.

In developing community health programs that are available, accessible, affordable, and appropriate, nurses must design strategies and implement interventions that mesh with a client's belief system. This implies that a family and a community are actively involved in planning and delivering care for a member who needs it. Essentially, nurses form partnerships with a person, family, agency, or community in order to deliver appropriate care. For example, nursing care can be provided in nutrition, rural health, or migrant health centers, or via a mobile health clinic.

HEALTH OF MINORITIES, PARTICULARLY MIGRANT FARMWORKERS, INCLUDING SUSCEPTIBILITY TO PANDEMICS

Characteristics of Migrant Farmworkers

Migrant and **seasonal farmworker**s (MSFWs) are essential to the agricultural industry in the United States. This is especially true as family farms decrease and the planting of labor-intensive crops such as vegetables, fruit, nuts, and ornamental plants increases. Although the availability and affordability of food in the United States depend on these individuals, their economic status and social acceptance have not reflected the importance of their

work. In 2018, 88.9% of US households were food secure during the year. The remaining 11.1% of households were food insure at least some of the time during that year. Food insecurity rates differ across the United States due to the characteristics of the population and to the state-level policies and economic conditions. The estimated range for food insecurity in 2016–18 was from 7.8% in New Hampshire to 16.8 in New Mexico (USDA, Economic Research Service, 2019). During April 2020 field workers received an average of $15.07 per hour. There were an estimated 688,000 workers hired directly by farm operators to work on farms and ranches during the week of April 12 to 18, 2020 (USDA, 2020a).

Estimates of the number of MSFWs in the United States vary depending on the source of the information. The USDA (2018) estimated that about there were about 1.0 to 2.7 million MSFWs in the United States. A migrant farmworker is a seasonal farmworker who must travel to do farm work and is unable to return to a permanent residence within the same day. A seasonal farmworker returns to his or her permanent residence, works in agriculture seasonally, and does not work year-round exclusively in agriculture. Many hired farmworkers are foreign-born people from Mexico and Central America, and many of them lack authorization to work legally in the United States. Fewer young immigrants are entering agriculture; therefore, the average age of immigrant farmworkers has risen. Also, the share of women farmworkers has risen in recent years, and this may be due to increased mechanical aids in farming, which means that women do not have to carry heavy loads as often or as far as in the past.

Migrant and seasonal farmworkers are one example of an at-risk group. MSFWs are essential to the agricultural industry in the United States. Although the availability and affordability of food in the United States depend on these individuals, their economic status and social acceptance have not reflected the importance of their work. As mentioned, the majority of MSFWs are foreign born (70.7%) with 64.1% born in Mexico (NCFH, 2016). Other workers include Central Americans, African Americans, Jamaicans, Haitians, Laotians, and Thais. Twenty-eight percent said they could not speak English "at all" and 9% said they could speak English "somewhat" (NCFH, 2016). See Table 24.1 for further discussion on some of the groups mentioned above.

An area of growing interest is the difference between documented and undocumented immigrants. Approximately 28% of foreign-born residents in the United States are undocumented immigrants. These are "individuals who either entered or are currently residing in the country without valid immigration of residency documents" (Messias et al., 2015, p. 86). In contrast, documentation "confers legal, social, and physical mobility and facilitates access to information, education, employment, services and legal protections" (Messias et al., 2015, p. 87). See the Evidence-Based Practice box for further discussion of the implications of undocumented immigration on individual and population health in the United States. The issue of undocumented immigrants has been a source of great political debate and considerable fear among those persons who would be affected.

TABLE 24.1	**Select Health Care Needs, Risks, and Conditions of Select Rural Aggregates**	
Rural Aggregates	**Health Care Needs**	**Health Risks/Conditions**
Farmers and ranchers	Advanced life support, emergency services Oral and dental care Obstetrical, perinatal, and pediatric services Mental and behavioral health services Agricultural health nurses Geriatric specialists	Agricultural chemicals and environmental hazards Dermatitis Stress, depression, and anxiety disorders Respiratory conditions (e.g., farmer's lung) Accidents (vehicular, machinery) Trauma-related chronic conditions Dental caries and loss Interpersonal and domestic violence
Native Americans	Advanced life support and emergency services Oral and dental care Obstetrical, perinatal, and pediatric services Mental and behavioral health services Culturally appropriate substance abuse treatment programs Epidemiologists Diabetes screening and educators Community health workers and education	Infectious diseases (e.g., hepatitis, tuberculosis) Sudden infant death syndrome (SIDS) Interpersonal and domestic violence Diabetes Alcohol and substance abuse Cirrhosis of the liver Vehicular accidents Hypothermic and environmental injuries Trauma-related injuries and chronic conditions Dental caries and loss
African Americans	Community nursing health promotion and screening services Diabetes screening and educators Hypertension screening and education Prenatal and perinatal health care services Oncology services (education, screening, follow-up interventions) HIV/AIDS prevention education, screening, and follow-up care Mental and behavioral health services	Diabetes Hypertension Sickle cell anemia Infectious diseases (e.g., hepatitis, HIV/AIDS) Cancer (e.g., prostate, breast) Dental caries and loss Depression Interpersonal and domestic violence
Migrant farmworkers	Environmental protection policies (e.g., safe drinking water, sanitation) Community nursing and migrant health services (primary, secondary, tertiary prevention) Diabetes screening and educators Hypertension screening and education Maternal and child services Oncology services (education, screening, follow-up interventions) Mental and behavioral health services	Infectious diseases (e.g., hepatitis, typhoid, tuberculosis, HIV/AIDS, STDs) Exposure effects of pesticides and herbicides Otitis media (children) Substance abuse (alcohol, recreational drugs, imported medicinal herbs) Dental caries and loss Interpersonal and domestic violence
Native Alaskans	Advanced life support and emergency care services Medical transport services Oral and dental care Obstetrical, perinatal, and pediatric services Mental and behavioral health services Culturally appropriate substance abuse treatment programs Epidemiologists Diabetes screening and educators	Infectious diseases (e.g., hepatitis, tuberculosis) Dental caries and loss Depression Interpersonal and domestic violence Environmental health risks (e.g., exposure to toxic substances, contaminants, hypothermia) Diabetes Alcohol and substance abuse Cirrhosis of the liver Vehicular accidents, trauma, and long-term chronic residual effects
Coal miners	Occupational Safety and Health Administration policy and standards Mental and behavioral health services Emergency and advanced life support services Occupational health nurses Grief counselors	Depression and substance abuse Occupational-related accidents and trauma Respiratory conditions (e.g., black lung, chronic obstructive pulmonary disease) Interpersonal and domestic violence

Data from Meit M, Knudson A, Gilbert T, et al: *The 2014 Update of the Rural-Urban Chartbook.* Accessed from the Rural Health Research Gateway Retrieved July 2020 at http://www.ruralhealthresearch.org/; Migrant Clinicans Network: *FHN key resources for migrant health,* 2017, Available at: https://migrantclinican.org.

Messias and colleagues (2015) described the difficulties that foreign-born individuals who are not documented immigrants have when they work in the United States. They note that being undocumented may not be a permanent state. People can change their status. For example, documented immigrants may let their visas expire and become undocumented, and people who arrive as undocumented immigrants may apply for and be granted permanent status.

Vulnerability and stress are common among undocumented immigrants. They often face a dangerous passage into the United States and once they arrive, they may face rejection, stigmatization, and scapegoating. They constantly worry about potential or actual arrest or deportation. They may fear seeking help due to the worry about deportation if their status is apparent. Their challenges to getting health care are often due to language barriers, social and economic resources, restricted transportation and the distance to services, and fear and mistrust of the health care system. These barriers also lead them to use emergency services more often, which increases the cost of care.

Nurse Use

As the authors eloquently say, "Professional nursing ethics posit the fundamental expectation that nurses provide care of individuals, respecting each person's dignity and worth without regard for the nature of the health issue, social or economic status, or personal attributes or characteristics, including social, economic, or migration status" (p. 92).

Migrant Lifestyle

Migrant farmworkers often have an unpredictable and difficult lifestyle. Many must leave home each year and travel to distant locations to work. They may be uncertain about their work and housing. They may also feel isolated in new communities and lack adequate resources to meet their needs. All of these situations can lead to stress. Many of these workers send some of their earnings to family members in their country of origin. They rarely receive benefits such as workers' compensation, disability compensation, or health or retirement benefits.

Migrant farmworkers traditionally have followed one of three migratory streams: Eastern, originating in Florida; Midwestern, originating in Texas; and Western, originating in California. As workers increasingly travel throughout the country seeking employment, however, these streams are becoming less distinct. Migrant farmworkers are employed in fruit and nut (40%), vegetable (21%), horticultural (23%), field (13%), and miscellaneous (3%) agricultural venues (Carroll, 2016). Eighty-five percent of farmworkers are hired directly and 15% are contract workers. The cyclic nature of agricultural work, along with its dependence on weather and economic conditions, results in considerable uncertainty for migrant farmworkers. These individuals and families leave their homes with the expectation of work at certain sites. Word of mouth from friends or family, newspaper announcements, or previous employment most often influence their choice of a destination. On arrival, however, migrant farmworkers may find that other workers have arrived first or that the crops are late, leaving the farmworkers unemployed.

Migrant farmworkers are vulnerable to forced labor (labor trafficking). According to the Polaris Project (2018), labor traffickers "use violence, threats, lies, debt bondage, or other forms of coercion to force people to work against their will in many different industries." The Polaris Project (2020) defines labor tracking as "the recruitment, harboring, transportation, provision, or obtaining of a person for labor or services, through the use of force, fraud, or coercion for the purposes of subjection to involuntary servitude, peonage, debt bondage, or slavery" (Federal Law 22 USC $ 7102). Trafficked individuals, especially those who are undocumented, need to work but can find themselves in appalling work and housing conditions without means to leave or report due to fear of retaliation. They may owe debt to their employers or recruiters from their home countries.

Federal and state legislation exist against human trafficking, but in isolated agricultural areas enforcement is difficult. Although exact numbers are not available, the agricultural sector is recognized as one of the most common labor markets that involves foreign nationals trafficked in the United States (Urban Institute, 2014). The psychological stress of working in forced labor can lead to physical and mental health problems.

Signs of human labor trafficking include:
- Reports performing work duties in exchange for basic necessities (food, water, housing), rather than money
- Unable to freely choose where they live
- Identification documents are held by employer (Polaris Project, 2020)

Certain questions can identify a victim of forced labor and can be asked as part of a nursing assessment. The National Human Trafficking Hotline (2014) created a set of suggested questions for suspected victims which includes:
- Do you have a debt to your employer or recruiter that you can't pay off?
- Is your job or work different than you were promised?
- Is there verbal or physical abuse at work?

If a minor is identified, then child protective services and law enforcement should be notified. Richards (2014) recommended involving social workers and others in the plan to assist a trafficked minor. The minor should not be left alone until services arrive. For an adult, obtain permission to contact authorities and get a social worker or agency involved. The National Human Trafficking Resource Center hotline (888-373-7888) should be contacted.

The way of life for any migrant farmworker is stressful. Some of the challenges of the migrant lifestyle include leaving one's home every year, traveling, and experiencing uncertainty regarding work and housing, isolation in new communities, and a lack of resources (Fig. 24.3). Farmworkers may be paid an hourly or piece rate, and the specifics for payment differ depending on the location and type of work. Reports of average income for farmworkers have varied. Although many farmworker families meet the income tests for federal and state assistance programs, undocumented workers are not eligible for most of these programs; for others, changing residence from state to state, lack of knowledge, and lack of access to programs impede use of program assistance.

MSFWs often are exempt from the protection of labor laws such as workers' compensation as well as from some OSHA protective provisions due to allowances such as small farm exemptions. Where laws do exist to protect agricultural workers, they may be minimally enforced because of lack of staff and

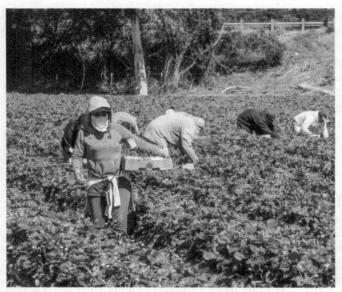

Fig. 24.3 Migrant Farmworkers Pick and Package Strawberries in the Salinas Valley of Central California. (David Litman/Shutterstock.com.)

resources. Laws have been enacted that intend to protect farmworkers (National Farm Worker Ministry, 2018). These include the Fair Labor Standards Act (FLSA) that addresses minimum wage, overtime pay, record keeping, and child labor standards. Farms with fewer than seven workers in a calendar quarter are exempt from minimum wage requirements and farmworkers are not included in overtime pay. The Migrant and Seasonal Agricultural Worker Protection Act mandates that farm contractors, employers, and agricultural associations must disclose employment terms, post information about worker protection at the worksite, pay workers what is due and provide itemized statements, and ensure that housing complies with federal and state safety and health standards. Employers and agricultural associations have made multiple attempts to weaken or void the law.

The Occupational Safety and Health Act's Field Sanitation Standards (US Department of Labor, 2008) ensure drinkable water and accessible sanitation facilities. Another set of regulations apply to H-2A guest workers, which allows agricultural employers to hire temporary workers from other countries. These laws are also difficult to enforce and can place workers in a position where they are unable to protect themselves from abusive working conditions (Farmworker Justice, 2020).

As of January 2017, the EPA implemented revisions to the Agricultural Worker Protection Standard (WPS), regulations that safeguard farmworkers from harmful exposures to pesticides (EPA, 2018). The changes include restrictions related to the age of workers who handle pesticides, training of workers, and other protective practices related to pesticide application (Migrant Clinicians Network, 2017).

Migrant and seasonal agricultural workers are considered a unique vulnerable population because of the factors cited here, including mobility, the physical demands of their work, social and often geographic isolation, language differences, and high rates of financial impoverishment. Although MSFW problems are numerous and creating solutions is difficult, some progress has been made in improving the condition of the farmworker population, such as by improved field sanitation conditions, including providing drinking water, field toilets, and handwashing facilities.

Housing

When migrant workers reach a worksite, housing may not be available, it may be too expensive, or it may be in poor condition. Housing conditions vary among states and localities. Housing for migrant farmworkers may be in camps with cabins, trailers, or houses. Some even live in cars or tents if necessary. National data about the type and quality of housing occupied by farmworkers are limited; however, data indicate that the housing is generally crowded by federal standards (Arcury et al., 2012). Much of the housing is substandard and lacks adequate sanitation and working appliances or may have severe structural defects (NCFH, 2018a). Many workers also support a home and family in their country of origin.

Housing may be located next to fields that have been sprayed by pesticides or where farm machinery is a danger to children. Poor quality and crowded places of residence can contribute to health problems such as tuberculosis (TB), gastroenteritis, and hepatitis and to exposure to high levels of lead. Renting housing in rural areas is nearly impossible because of barriers such as high rent, substantial rental deposits, long-term leases, lack of credit, discrimination, and a lack of rental units. Federal programs provide some funds for farmworker housing, but they are insufficient to meet the demand. Increased funding and better coordination among agencies are needed, as is an increase in the availability of safe public housing.

Issues in Migrant Health

Poor and unsanitary working and housing conditions make farmworkers susceptible to health problems no longer seen as dangers to the general public or seen at a much lower rate. The agriculture industry is one of the most dangerous occupations in the United States. MSFWs have the same health risks and health issues as other farmworkers. See the section above on Occupational and environmental Health Problems in Rural Areas. In general, the most often reported health issues among migrant workers are: overweight/obesity, hypertension, diabetes mellitus, otitis media and eustachian tube disorders, depression and other mood disorders, and substance abuse (NCFH, 2018a). Factors related to their mobility, lifestyle, and racial or ethnic group membership place them at risk for certain health disparities. MSFWs may not know that symptoms such as diarrhea or fever could indicate a serious health problem.

The Migrant Health Act, signed in 1962, provides primary and supplemental health services to migrant workers and their families at migrant health centers. In 2018, 895,789 patients were served at the 174 reporting centers. Of these 324,937 were uninsured (HRSA, 2018). It is estimated that the number served by these clinics represents only a small proportion of migrant workers. The following factors limit adequate provision of health care services:

- **Lack of knowledge about services.** Because of their isolation and lack of fluency in English, migrant farmworkers lack usual sources for information about available services, especially if they are not receiving public benefits.

- **Inability to afford care.** The Medicaid program, which is intended to serve the poor, often is not available to migrant farmworkers, especially undocumented workers. Workers may not remain in a geographic area long enough to be considered for benefits or may lose benefits when they relocate to a state with different eligibility standards. Their salaries may fluctuate monthly, making them ineligible for periods. If they do not work, they are not paid, so many avoid taking time off to get care.

- **Affordable Care Act or health insurance subsidies.** Although it is difficult to determine numbers, many farmworkers do not receive employer-mandated health coverage or subsidies because of the small farm exemption and the exclusion of seasonal workers who are employed less than 120 days in the employer's tax year. Undocumented workers are excluded from any employer and individual insurance mandates (NCFH, 2016).

- **Availability of services.** Immigrants are treated differently depending on whether they were in the United States before the welfare reform legislation of 1966 and depending on the category of their immigration status. Each state determines whether to fill any part of the service's gap to immigrants. As a result, many legal immigrants and unauthorized immigrants are ineligible for services such as Supplemental Security Income (SSI) and the Supplemental Nutrition Assistance Program (SNAP; food stamps).

- **Transportation.** Health care services may be located far from work or home. Transportation may be unavailable, unreliable, or expensive. Many migrant farmworkers do not have access to vehicles. Privacy is compromised when migrant workers depend on employers to provide transportation to clinics (Napolitano, 2008).

- **Hours of services.** Many health services are available only during work hours; therefore, seeking health care leads to lost earnings.

- **Mobility and tracking.** Although migrant families move from job to job, their health care records typically do not go with them. This leads to fragmented services in areas such as treatment for TB, chronic illness management, and immunizations. For example, health departments are known to dispense medications for TB on a monthly basis. Adequate treatment for TB requires 6 to 12 months of medication. When migrant farmworkers move, they must independently seek out new health services to continue their medications. The Migrant Clinicians Network (MCN) TB tracking program makes available to a farmworker's current provider any previous provider information that was entered into the program. This tracking helps maintain continuity of TB care for a mobile population (MCN, 2016).

- **Language barriers.** As discussed in Chapter 7, the inability to speak English presents barriers to getting adequate health care. Often, immigrant adults speak primarily the language of their native country. They may not be able to read or write in English. They also may be embarrassed to admit this inability, so they nod or say yes when their understanding of what is being said is minimal. Although children may be more competent in English, the adults may prefer that children not know about their health needs or conditions. It is important for the nurse to verify whether clients understand what they are being asked or told. Because the majority of seasonal farmworkers are primarily Spanish speakers, the recruitment and retention of bicultural and bilingual health care provider staff are important priorities.

- **Discrimination.** Although migrant farmworkers and their families bring revenue into the community, they are often perceived as poor, uneducated, transient, and ethnically different. These perceptions foster attitudes and acts of discrimination against them.

- **Documentation.** Unauthorized individuals fear that getting services in a federally funded or state-funded clinic may lead to discovery and deportation.

- **Cultural aspects of health care.** See the later discussion of cultural considerations in migrant health care.

Other Specific Health Problems

Dental disease is one of the most common health problems for farmworkers of all ages. Farmworkers may not have dental insurance. They may have long travel times to get dental care, have language problems, and be in an area where there is a shortage of dental providers. Mexican Americans have higher rates of tooth decay and periodontal disease than non-Hispanic whites, and their children are not spared from oral health problems (CDC, 2018a).

Behavioral health issues, including depression, anxiety, posttraumatic stress disorder (PTSD), and stress, are areas of concern for migrants and may be related to isolation, discrimination, trauma, economic hardship, legal status, poor living conditions, and weather conditions that interrupt their work. MSFWs identify themselves as stressed, independently of how they rate their physical health (Carvajal et al., 2014). A survey of California farmworker households (O'Connor et al., 2015) found that 22% of respondents reported *nervios* (a term used by some Western hemisphere Hispanics to refer to increased susceptibility to mental stress and symptoms of nervousness). A study in North Carolina by Pulgar et al. (2016) found that almost a third of the farmworker women in their survey reported significant symptoms of depression, markedly higher than in the overall US population. Related factors cited include job conditions, household responsibilities, taking care of children, and poverty. Farmworkers, especially males, are reluctant to seek mental health care.

Female farmworkers, especially the undocumented, are a vulnerable population suffering harassment and sexual abuse (Fig. 24.4). According to a landmark report by Human Rights Watch (2012), harassment and sexual abuse are so common that female farmworkers see no escape from its occurrence and believe it is part of the job. The report identified sexually charged language, unwanted touching, stalking, and rape as common occurrences. Most victims do not report these abuses, often feeling powerless; however, many who have reported have not seen their perpetrators prosecuted (Yeung and Rubenstein, 2013). Recently, the US Equal Employment Opportunity Commission filed lawsuits against employers in the Northwest as a means to address sexual harassment.

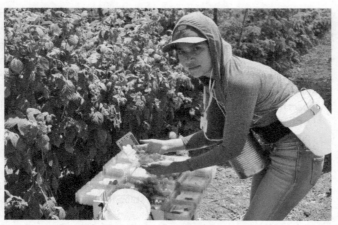

Fig. 24.4 Women Working in Agriculture Face Unique Challenges, Including Sexual Harassment and Reproductive Health Risks. (David Litman/Shutterstock.com.)

Substance use in migrant communities can be a significant source (or result) of stress and injuries. Drinking alcohol poses safety hazards for farmworkers, such as accidents while driving and workplace injuries. Alcohol can also contribute to health problems, greater risk for human immunodeficiency virus (HIV) infection, violence in camps/home sites, domestic violence, and decreased funds for personal and family needs.

The incidence rate for TB is not known for migrant farmworkers; however, Oren et al. (2016, p 630) state that they are "among the highest-risk populations for latent TB infection in the United States." According to CDC statistics (2016), in 2015, Hispanics/Latinos accounted for 28% of the US tuberculosis cases and of the TB cases among foreign-born people, Latinos represented 32% in 2015. Being born outside of the United States is a significant risk factor for TB; in 2016, foreign-born individuals had a rate of 14.7 per 100,000, or 14 times higher than among native-born individuals (CDC, 2017a). The majority of migrant farmworkers are foreign born and Hispanic/Latino. MSFWs are thus at increased risk for TB because of higher rates in their countries of origin (Latin America, Haiti, and Southeast Asia), crowded housing, and malnutrition. Required long-term treatment is difficult to complete because of mobility, fear of deportation, language barriers, and lack of access to services. Incomplete treatment contributes to resistant TB (Tschampl et al., 2016). The MCN Health Network TB tracking program fosters continuity and monitoring of TB treatment as migrant farmworkers move to different work and home sites (MCN, 2016).

Accurate HIV data for migrant farmworkers is also difficult to obtain; however, in the absence of adequate population-based data on farmworkers, useful inferences may be drawn from statistics collected for Latinos in the United States, a group known to be disproportionately affected and infected by HIV. Risk factors for this population include lack of accurate knowledge, barriers to health care services, limited education, poverty, longer time in the United States, sharing needles for common medications such as vitamins and antibiotics, unprotected sexual activity, isolation and separation from families, available prostitution, migration across borders that results in the spread of HIV, and needle sharing through amateur tattooing (NCFH, 2018c).

Among the Latino population in the United States, the prevalence of diabetes is estimated to be three to five times greater than that of the general population, with higher rates of end-stage complications. Data specific to MSFWs are limited, and prevalence statistics for the Hispanic/Latino population are used as a proxy; the CDC (2017a) reported the incidence of diabetes in this population to be 8.4 per 1000 individuals, compared to 5.7 per 1000 for non-Hispanic whites. The lifestyle of migrant farmworkers makes it difficult to obtain proper nutrition, adhere to weight control measures, and procure continuity of health care and medication administration necessary for good diabetes control. The MCN Health Network assists providers with accessing information from farmworkers' previous providers who participated in the tracking program, thereby allowing for better continuity of care for diabetes (MCN, 2017b). Box 24.5 provides a brief description of an assessment with a diabetes focus for migrant farmworkers.

Children of Migrant Workers

Migrant farmworker parents want a better future for their children. In fact, this strong desire is often the catalyst that causes many farmworkers to leave their country of origin. These children often appear to the outsider as happy, outgoing, and inquisitive. On the surface, they may look like children from any other aggregate. However, they often suffer from health care deficits, including malnutrition (e.g., vitamin A, iron), infectious diseases (e.g., upper respiratory tract infection, gastroenteritis), dental caries (caused by prolonged use of the bottle, bottle propping, limited access to fluoride or dental care), inadequate immunization status, pesticide exposure, injuries, overcrowding and exposure to lead in poor housing conditions, and disruption of their social and school life.

Migrant children as young as 8 years of age may stay home to care for younger children. The Migrant and Seasonal Head Start Program is a safe, healthy, and educative option for children 6 months to 5 years of age. However, inadequate funding results in lack of services for all migrant children. The Migrant

Education Program is a state and nationally sponsored summer school program for farmworkers' children older than 5 years of age. However, this program is not available to all eligible migrant youth, and currently is only offered in 38 states. Although the threats to youth from working on farms are similar to those for adults, the most common are as follows (NCFH, 2018d):

- Injuries and fatalities: working with machinery including tractors; use of motor vehicles, including all-terrain vehicles (ATVs) and drownings.
- Heat and sun—there is often a lack of drinking water
- Musculoskeletal injuries characterized by constant bending, twisting, carry heavy items, and repetitive motions during long work hours
- Pesticides
- Educational deprivation

Federal child labor laws have multiple exclusions for agricultural settings. The FLSA in Agriculture includes restrictions based on age and hours worked. Children younger than 12 years can work on a farm with fewer than seven full-time workers. Children as young as 12 years old can work on a farm if they have parental permission or if their parent is also working on the farm. Children ages 14 or 15 may work in nonhazardous positions in agriculture but not during school hours. Minors age 16 and older may work in any farm job at any time, including performing hazardous work with no restrictions on hours (NCFH, 2018d). Federal law does not protect children from overworking or by limiting the hours they work outside of school. Therefore, children may work until late in the evenings or very early in the mornings every day of the week if not protected by state law or if inadequately monitored. Personal communication with Marie Napolitano and adolescent farmworkers in Oregon revealed that they were frequently too tired after working to do homework and to attend classes. They may leave school before the end of the term to travel with their families and arrive late to start school in the fall. Child farmworkers may attend three to five different schools each year as they migrate from one farm to another, and these frequent changes in schools and constant fatigue are obvious obstacles to academic success (Fig. 25.5).

CULTURAL CONSIDERATIONS IN MIGRANT HEALTH CARE

As discussed in Chapter 7, to provide culturally competent care to migrant farmworkers, nurses need to appreciate and understand the cultural backgrounds of these individuals. Because the majority of migrant farmworkers are of Mexican descent, this section focuses on Mexican cultures. Although certain health beliefs and practices have been identified with the Mexican culture, the nurse must remember that beliefs and practices differ among regions and localities of a country and among individuals. Mexico is a multicultural country; therefore, the cultural backgrounds of Mexican immigrants vary, depending on their place of origin. Many indigenous groups in Mexico

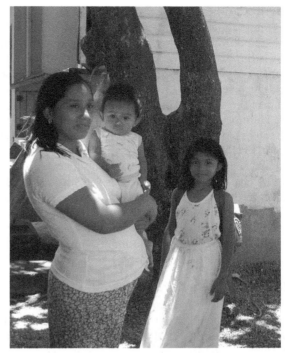

Fig. 24.5 Children of Migrant Farmworkers Experience Many Hardships. They may have to help with the agricultural work or childcare while trying to maintain their schoolwork. (Diana Mary Jorgenson/Shutterstock.com.)

speak their regional dialect. Mexican immigrants may or may not be able to read, understand, or speak Spanish. Mexican immigrants who are less educated, with fewer economic resources, and from the rural areas tend to possess more traditional beliefs and practices.

Folk medicine "is the mixture of traditional healing practices and beliefs that involve herbal medicine, spirituality and manual therapies in order to diagnose, treat, or prevent an ailment or illness" (NCFH, 2018e, p 1). Folk medicine is practiced by the majority of the Mexican population while they are in Mexico. Many will continue to use folk medicine when they work in the United States. The practice of folk medicine is not unique to farmworkers or people from Mexico; people around the world use alternative medicines in addition to or instead of Western, or allopathic, medicine. It is important to know what folk medicine practices clients use so you can determine whether they interfere with the allopathic medical practices that client uses. See the section later in the chapter discussing health values, health beliefs, and health practices for more detail about folk health practices.

Nurse-Client Relationship

The nurse is considered an authority figure who should show respect (respeto) to the individual, be able to relate to the individual on a personal level (personalismo), and maintain the individual's dignity (dignidad). Mexican individuals prefer polite, nonconfrontational relationships with others (simpatia). At times, because of *simpatia*, individuals and families may appear to understand what is being said to them (by nodding their heads) when they do not understand. It is important to validate the understanding in these situations. A Mexican person expects to talk about personal matters (chit-chat) for the first few minutes of an encounter. They expect the nurse not to appear rushed and to be a good listener. Humor is appreciated, and touching as a caring gesture is seen as a positive behavior. However, with the COVID pandemic, touching was no longer appropriate.

Mexican clients may not seek care with health care professionals first. Rather, they may initially consult with knowledgeable individuals in their family or community (the popular arena of care) or with folk healers (the traditional arena of care). Examples of the members of the popular arena are the *señora*, or wise older woman living in the community, one's grandmother (*al abuela*), and the local parish priest.

Health: Values, Beliefs, and Practices

Family, in general, is a significant component of a Mexican individual's health care and social support system. The woman in the household is considered the caretaker, whereas the man is considered the major decision maker. However, Mexican women in certain families have significant influence over most matters, including health decisions. Grandmothers and sisters are highly significant to the wife in the immediate family. They provide advice, care, and support. Even though they communicate regularly with their family in Mexico, they may not have a support system in the United States. The Mexican client may be more willing to follow the advice of another Mexican individual with a similar health problem than the advice of the health care professional.

Love of their children rather than concern for their own health may encourage migrant parents to adopt healthier lifestyles. Many of the children speak better English than their parents. It is often useful to teach the children in school or other community venues healthy behaviors and encourage them to talk with their parents about what they have learned.

In the Mexican culture, health may be considered a gift from God. Another common perception of health is that a healthy person is one who can continue to work and maintain daily activities independent of symptoms or diagnosed diseases. A person may miss a clinic appointment if he or she is able to work that day. Mexican immigrants may believe that illness is a punishment from God and think this is why therapies have not cured them. This more commonly occurs with chronic illnesses. Four common folk illnesses that a nurse may encounter with the Mexican client are (1) *mal de ojo* (evil eye), (2) *susto* (fright), (3) *empacho* (indigestion), and (4) *caida de mollera* (fallen fontanel). Symptoms and treatments may vary depending on the individual's or family's place of origin in Mexico. Other cultural beliefs relate to hot-cold balance, pregnancy, and postpartum behaviors (*cuarentena*). When experiencing a folk illness, the traditional Mexican individual would prefer to seek care with a folk healer. The more common healers are the *curanderos*, *herbalistas*, and *espiritualistas*. The most commonly used herbs are *manzanilla* (chamomile), *yerba buena* (peppermint), aloe vera, *nopales* (cactus), and *epazote* (wormseed).

NURSING CARE IN RURAL ENVIRONMENTS

Rural people, including migrant and seasonal farmworkers, often develop independent and creative ways to cope because of the distance, isolation, and sparse resources they encounter. They may prefer to seek help first through their informal networks, such as neighbors, extended family, church, and civic

---

CASE STUDY

Public health nurse Lynn Smith received a referral to visit 19-year-old primipara, Conchita Garcia, who was near term yet had not received prenatal care. Ms. Smith planned a home visit immediately. Having recently come from Mexico, Ms. Garcia was living in a clean, sparsely furnished apartment with other newly immigrated men and the father of her baby. Rapport was quickly established with the client because Ms. Smith was fluent in Spanish.

Ms. Garcia knew little about the birthing process, so the nurse explained vaginal and cesarean births. Ms. Smith taught her the signs of labor, as well as complications that would merit a visit to the hospital or clinic. Ms. Garcia's physical assessment was normal. Ms. Smith then assessed whether the home environment would be safe for the baby and noted that the young family had bought infant clothes and a crib. The next day, Ms. Garcia gave birth to a healthy baby girl in the hospital.

During the second home visit, the nurse completed a newborn assessment on a well-hydrated, normal newborn that weighed a couple of ounces less than her birth weight. Ms. Garcia reported that the child would not latch on for breastfeeding but denied giving the child formula. The mother's breasts were moderately engorged, and she was feeding the baby breast milk she had pumped. Being far from family, especially female support, Ms. Garcia did not know how to breastfeed well, but she and the baby's father had made good use of the pump and filled bottles with her breast milk. Ms. Smith spent most of the visit teaching breastfeeding techniques.

There was a Band-Aid on the infant's umbilicus. Despite Ms. Smith's warning that the Band-Aid might not allow the umbilicus to dry and fall off, the Band-Aid was always present on each subsequent visit, even after healing was complete; the parents believed the Band-Aid would prevent a protruding umbilicus in later years. (Another tradition in some Hispanic cultures is to put a coin or a piece of thread over the umbilicus.)

Ms. Smith made referrals for postnatal and newborn health care so that the family would have health care at home, avoiding inappropriate use of the emergency department. Because another pregnancy soon would not be optimal, Ms. Smith explained birth control methods that could be used until the mother's postnatal visit. Ms. Garcia's isolation was a concern because she could not drive or speak English, so the nurse suggested attending a church of the family's religious denomination that had a service in Spanish each Sunday and a thriving congregation known to be supportive of young families in need. The health department enrolled the mother and baby in the Special Supplemental Nutrition Program for Women, Infants and Children (WIC), a federal nutrition program for low-income pregnant or breastfeeding mothers and their children younger than 5 years of age. Ms. Smith continued to visit the family, giving anticipatory guidance on the child's needs and advocating for them in the health care system while they learned English and got settled in a new country.

Created by Deborah C. Conway, Assistant Professor (retired), School of Nursing, University of Virginia.

clubs, before seeking a professional's care. Nurses describe some interesting differences when they work in rural areas versus urban ones. The boundaries between one's home and work roles may blur in nurses who go to the same church, shop at the same stores, and have children in the same schools as their clients. Thus many, if not all, clients are personally known as neighbors, as friends of an immediate family member, or perhaps part of one's extended family. There are, then, both social informality and a corresponding lack of anonymity in a small town. Some rural nurses say, "I never really feel like I am off duty because everybody in the county knows me through my work." In part, this may be because nurses are highly regarded by the community and viewed by local people as experts on health and illness. During the COVID pandemic, nurses as well as physicians, first responders, and other health care providers have been seen as essential and compassionate members of society. Residents may ask health-related questions and recommendations about physicians when they see the nurse (who may be a neighbor, friend, or relative) in a grocery store, at a service station, during a basketball game, or at church functions. Nurses in rural areas may also be expected to, in general, know something about everything, and this can be a demanding expectation. Some of the challenges of rural practice are professional isolation, limited opportunities for continuing education, lack of other kinds of health care personnel or professionals with whom one can interact, heavy workloads, the ability to function well in several clinical areas, lack of anonymity, and, for some, a restricted social life (Bushy, 2012). Many nurses value the close relationships with clients and coworkers, along with the diverse clinical experiences that evolve from caring for clients of all ages who have a variety of health problems, caring for clients for long periods (in some cases, across several generations), opportunities for professional development, greater autonomy, and the pleasures of living in a rural area. The nurse can often keep a finger on the pulse of the community by staying active in local political, social, religious, and employment activities that affect their clients. The nurse can be a catalyst for change, act as a community educator, and know how to find resources and services (Box 24.6).

BOX 24.6 Resources for Nurses in Providing Services to Farmworkers, Especially Migrant and Seasonal Farmworkers

1. **National Center for Farmworker Health, Inc. (NCFH):** The NCFH offers vast resources available for both professionals and clients. For professionals, they offer fact sheets on farmworkers, demographics, human immunodeficiency virus and acquired immunodeficiency syndrome, maternal and child health, child labor, occupational health, oral health, tuberculosis, indigenous farmworkers, and folk medicine. These fact sheets are updated periodically and rely on many sources to provide succinct and easy-to-read information.

   The NCFH has developed a series of client health tips. These tips are in both English and Spanish and are distributed in print and electronically to organizations that wish to provide them to clients. They began this service in 2004, and each year the NFCH publishes on four to six topics. Selected topics are nutrition, facts about skin cancer, obesity and children, back pain, and domestic violence. Each Health Tip has photos to supplement the easy-to-read text material. Visit http://www.ncfh.org.

2. **Centers for Disease Control and Prevention (CDC):** The CDC has a national program (Racial and Ethnic Approaches to Community Health [REACH]) designed to eliminate racial and ethnic disparities in health. REACH gives funds to state and local health departments, tribes, universities, and community-based organizations. The funds are to build strong partnerships to guide and support the program's work. Also, the CDC provides expert support to REACH recipients. The program celebrated its 20th anniversary in 2019. In 2018, REACH funded 31 programs. See REACH at http://www.cdc.gov for more details.

3. **The Health Resources and Services Administration within the US Department of Health and Human Services (USDHHS):** The HRSA has a section on rural health that provides a range of resources. Visit http://www.hrsa.gov/ruralhealth.

4. **National Rural Health Association (NRHA):** The NRHA has resources on rural health (visit http://www.ruralhealthweb.org), and the School of Rural Public Health at Texas A&M Health Sciences has "Your Community's Emergency Preparedness Planning: Get Involved" at the e-mail address USACenter@srph.tamhsc.edu.

Nurses working in rural areas, including those working with migrant farmworkers, can use many public health nursing skills. One of the first and most important is that of prevention. Given the barriers to receiving health care in rural areas, the ideal situation is to prevent health disruptions whenever possible. Case management and community-oriented primary health care (COPHC) are two effective models used to address some of those deficits and resolve rural health disparities. The steps of the COPHC process are as follows:

1. Define and characterize the community.
2. Identify the community's health problems.
3. Develop or modify health care services in response to the community's identified needs.
4. Monitor and evaluate program process and client outcomes.

The "Clinical Application" section later in this chapter demonstrates how nursing case management can allow an older adult resident to stay at home in a rural environment if adequate supports can be provided. Outcomes are often remarkably different when case management is used. Additional information on case management is found in Chapter 15. The need for nursing services in the community varies by community. However, there is a need in most rural areas for the following: school nurses; family planning services; prenatal care; emergency care; mental health services; services for children and adults with special needs as well as older adults.

HEALTHY PEOPLE 2030: RELATED TO RURAL AND MIGRANT HEALTH

The goals of 2030 have important implications for nurses who work with rural and migrant populations. Many objectives are relevant to these groups. It is especially important when working in rural areas and with migrant and seasonal farmworker populations to engage the community, including the public, private, and voluntary sectors, to achieve agreed-upon local objectives in planning ways to implement the *Healthy People 2030* objectives.

 HEALTHY PEOPLE 2030

The following selected objectives pertain to rural workers, including migrant workers:

- OSH-01: Reduce deaths from work-related injuries.
- OSH-02: Reduce work-related injuries resulting in missed days of work.
- IVP-03: Reduce unintentional injury deaths.

US Department of Health and Human Services: *Healthy People 2030*, Washington, DC, 2020, USDHHS. Retrieved July 2020 from http://www.healthypeople.gov.

When implementing the objectives of *Healthy People 2030*, consider rural factors, such as sparse population, geographic remoteness, scarce resources, personnel shortages, and physical, emotional, and social isolation. Remember that members of the community must be involved in developing the plan and assume some ownership for it.

HOW TO BUILD PROFESSIONAL, COMMUNITY, AND CLIENT PARTNERSHIPS

1. Gain the local perspective.
2. Assess the degree of public awareness and support for the cause.
3. Identify special interest groups.
4. List existing services to avoid duplication of programs.
5. Note real and potential barriers to existing resources and services.
6. Generate a list of potential community volunteers and professionals who are willing to assist with the project.
7. Create awareness among target groups of a particular program (e.g., individuals, families, seniors, church and recreation groups, health care professionals, law enforcement personnel, and members of other religious, service, and civic clubs).
8. Identify potential funding sources to implement the program.
9. Establish the community's health care priority list, and involve large numbers of community members in considering and selecting their health care options.
10. Incorporate business principles in marketing the program.
11. Measure the health care system's local economic impact.
12. Educate residents about the important role the local health care system plays in the economic infrastructure of the community and the consequences of a system failure.
13. Develop local leadership and support for the community's health care system through training and providing experience in decision making.

Use of Technology

Technology has great potential for connecting rural public health providers and consumers with resources outside their community, as well as with keeping in touch with them. For example, some nurses use text or e-mail messages to stay in close touch with clients and help them remember the details of their health maintenance plan. During the COVID pandemic, the use of electronic meetings for nurses and patients as well as other forms of telehealth were essential. Also, many electronic health care appointments were reimbursed by insurers. Being able to keep in touch in these ways requires that the clients have a cell phone and know how to text and that they have a computer and know how to use e-mail. As found during the COVID pandemic, telehealth uses many forms of communication including email, telephone apps, meetings, and one-on-one appointments.

▶▶ APPLYING CONTENT TO PRACTICE

As discussed, practice in rural areas relies on excellent nursing and public health skills in assessment, communication, cultural competency, problem solving, coalition building, coordination, and policy development, among others. Documents that guide the practice include the American Nurses Association Standards of Nursing Practice, the core competencies as identified by the Council on Linkages between Academic and Public Health Practice (2014), and the Quad Council Coalition: Community/Public Health Nursing Competencies (2018). As one example of the congruence, consider assessment. The Council on Linkages' Core Competency of "Describe factors affecting the health of a community (e.g., equity, income, education, environment" p. 5) under their analytic assessment skills is then elaborated on by the Quad Council as a public health nursing skill of "Utilize an ecological perspective and epidemiological data to identify health risks of a population" (2018, p. 13).

PRACTICE APPLICATION

Ethyl Lewis, a 73-year-old widow, was diagnosed over 10 years ago with progressive Parkinson's disease. Her husband of more than 40 years died suddenly 3 years ago after a serious stroke. Her two married daughters live in California and Illinois. Her small Midwestern town has 1000 residents, and the nearest health care agency is 100 miles away. Her 75-year-old widowed sister, Suzanna Ames, also lives in town. Their brother, Bill Jones, (71 years of age) has recently entered the county nursing home located in a town 20 miles away. Despite her physical rigidity and ataxia, Ms. Lewis manages to live alone in her two-bedroom home with her dog and cat. She insists that she will not relinquish her private, independent lifestyle as her brother has. Yet within this past year she has been hospitalized three times—for a bad chest cold, for a bladder infection, and after a neighbor found her lying unconscious in the garden. Her doctor says that this last episode was related to "a heart problem."

After discharge, a home-health nurse, Liz Moore, was assigned as her case manager. Ms. Moore's office is based at the County Senior Center near the nursing home where her brother is a resident. He is also one of the clients whom the nurse checks on weekly. She provides outreach services to all of the residents in the county who are referred by a large home-health agency in the city. As a case manager, she works closely with the hospital's discharge planners to arrange a continuum of care for clients in the two-county area. Her activities include coordinating formal and informal services for clients, including nutrition, hydration, pharmacological care, personal care, homemaker services, and routine activities, such as writing checks, home maintenance, and emergency backup services.

A. Describe the nursing roles that the nurse assumes in coordinating a continuum of care for Ethyl in terms of nutrition, transportation, and health care.
B. Identify formal health care and support resources that can be accessed for Ms. Lewis.
C. Identify informal support resources that can be used to ensure that Ms. Lewis is safe.
D. Identify three outcomes that have been achieved by using nursing care management.
E. Select a rural community in your geographic area. Create hypothetical situations or select real clients with real health problems (e.g., an older adult with Alzheimer's disease, a middle-aged person with cancer requiring end-of-life care, a child who is dependent on technology as a result of a farm accident). Prepare a list of services and referral agencies in that community that could be used to develop a continuum of care for each of these cases. How are these the same as or different from the case described in this chapter?
Answers can be found on the Evolve website.

REMEMBER THIS!

- Rural environments are diverse and different from those in urban areas.
- The health status of rural populations varies, depending on genetic, social, environmental, economic, and political factors. The availability of health care professionals and the distance to travel for their care also affects the health status of rural residents.
- The incidence of working poor in rural America is higher than in more populated areas.
- Rural adults 18 years of age and older are in poorer health than their urban counterparts; nearly 50% have been diagnosed with at least one major chronic condition. However, they average one less physician visit each year than their healthier urban counterparts.
- More than 26% of rural families live below the poverty level; more than 40% of all rural children younger than 18 years of age live in poverty. These percentages may have changed with the onset of the COVID pandemic.
- A migrant farmworker is a laborer whose principal employment involves traveling from place to place planting or harvesting agricultural products and living in temporary housing situations.
- An estimated one to three million migrant farmworkers are in the United States. These numbers are controversial because of the inconsistency in defining farmworkers and limitations in obtaining data.
- Migrant farmworkers are considered a vulnerable population because of their lifestyle and lack of resources.
- Health problems of migrant farmworkers are linked to their work environment, limited access to health services and education, and lack of economic opportunities.
- Migrant farmworkers are faced with uncertainty regarding work and housing, inadequate wages, unsafe working conditions, and lack of enforcement regarding legislation for field sanitation and safety regulations.
- Farmworkers are exposed not only to the immediate effects in the fields (foggy or wet with pesticides) but also to unknown long-term effects of chronic exposure to pesticides.
- When harvesting is completed, the migrant farmworker becomes simultaneously homeless and unemployed. Forced migration to find employment leaves little time or energy to seek out and improve living standards. Many of them return to their country of origin after the growing season ends.
- Children of migrant farmworkers may need to work for the family's economic survival.
- Nurses must consider the belief systems and lifestyles of a rural population when assessing, planning, implementing, and evaluating community services.
- Barriers to rural health care include the lack of availability, affordability, accessibility, and acceptability of services.
- Partnership models, in particular community health primary health care, are effective models to provide a comprehensive continuum of care in environments with scarce resources.
- Technology offers many options for providing care to people who live in rural areas.

EVOLVE WEBSITE

http://evolve.elsevier.com/Stanhope/foundations
- Case Study, with Questions and Answers
- NCLEX® Review Questions
- Practice Application Answers

REFERENCES

Agency for Health Care Policy and Research (AHCPR): *National healthcare disparities report*, 2017. Available at: https://www.ahrq.gov, Accessed June 25, 2018.

Arcury TA, Weir M, Chen H, et al: Migrant Farmworker Housing Regulation Violations in North Carolina, *American Journal of Industrial Medicine* 55:191-204, 2012.

Annan SL: "It's not just a job. This is where we live. This is our backyard": the experiences of expert legal and advocate providers with sexually assaulted women in rural areas, *J Am Psychiatric Nurs Assoc* 17:139–147, 2011.

Bigbee J, Crowder E: The Red Cross Rural Nursing Service: an innovation of public health nursing delivery, *Public Health Nurs* 2: 109–121, 1985.

Bolin J, Bellamy G: *Rural Healthy People: 2020*, 2015, Southwest Rural Health Research Center, Texas A&M Health Science Center, School of Rural Public Health. Retrieved July 2020 from http://www.sph.tamhsc.edu/srhrc/doc/rhp2020.pdf.

Booth L, Graves BA: Service learning initiatives in rural populations: fostering cultural awareness, *Online J Rural Nurs Health Care* 18(1): 90–111, 2018.

Bushy A: The rural context and nursing practice. In Molinari D, Bushy A, eds.: *The rural nurse: transition to practice*, New York, 2012, Springer.

Bushy A, Winters C: Nursing workforce development, clinical practice, research and nursing theory: Connecting the dots. In Winters C, ed.: *Rural health: best practices and preventive modes*, New York, NY, 2013, Springer.

Bushy A: Health disparities in rural populations across the lifespan. In Winters CA, ed.: *Rural nursing: concepts, theory, and practice*, ed 4, New York, NY, 2013, Springer Publishing.

Carroll D: *Demographic and Employment Characteristics of California's Crop Labor Force: Findings from the National Agricultural Workers Survey 1989-2014* [presentation to the California Agriculture: Water, Labor, and Immigration Conference, U.C. Davis Law School, April 15, 2016]. Available at: https://www.doleta.gov. Accessed March 2018.

Carvajal SC, et al: Stress and sociocultural factors related to health status among US–Mexico border farmworkers, *J Immigrant Minority Health* 16:1176–1182, 2014.

Centers for Disease Control and Prevention (CDC): Disparities in Oral Health. 2018a. Available at: http://www.cdc.gov/OralHealth/oral_health_disparities/. Accessed June 12, 2018.

Centers for Disease Control and Prevention (CDC): *National Diabetes Statistics Report, 2017; Estimates of Diabetes and Its Burden in the United States*, 2017a. Available at: https://www.cdc.gov/diabetes, Accessed June 12, 2018.

Centers for Disease Control and Prevention (CDC): *Trends in Tuberculosis, 2016*, 2017b. Available at: https://www.cdc.gov/tb. Accessed June 13, 2018.

Centers for Disease Control and Prevention (CDC): *Rural health*, 2018a. Available at: https://www.cdc.gov/ruralhealth/. Accessed June 25, 2018.

Council on Linkages Between Academic and Public Health Practice: *Core competencies for public health professionals*, Washington DC, 2014, Public Health Foundation/Health Resources and Service Administration.

Eisenhauer CM, Pullen CH, Nelson T, Kumm SA, Hunter JL: Partnering with rural farm women for participatory action and ethnography, *Online J Rural Nurs Health Care* 16(1): 195–216, 2016.

Environmental Protection Agency (EPA): *Agricultural Worker Protection Standard (WPS)*, 2018. Available at: https://www.epa.gov.

Farmworker Justice, 2020, *The H-2A Temporary agricultural guestworker program: an inherently flawed program*, Retrieved July 2020 at https://www.farmworkerjustice.org.

Health Resources and Services Administration: *2018 National Health Center data, national migrant health centers program grantee data*, Washington, DC, 2018, HRSA. Retrieved Jully 2020 from http://bphc.hrsa.gov/healthcenterdata.

Human Rights Watch: *Cultivating Fear: The Vulnerability of Immigrant Farmworkers in the U.S. to Sexual Violence and Sexual Harassment*, 2012. Available at: https://www.hrw.org.

Messias DKF, McEwen MM, Clark L: The impact and implications of undocumented immigration on individual and collective health in the United States, *Nurs Outlook* 23:86–94, 2015.

Migrant Clinicians Network: *Tuberculosis*, 2016. Retrieved July 2016 from http://www.migrantclinician.org.

Migrant Clinicians Network: A Stronger Worker Protection Standard is Now In Effect What Does It Mean for Workers? Streamline 22:4, 2017a.

Migrant Clinicians Network: *Health network,* 2017b, Retrieved July 2020 at http://www.migrantclinical.org

Molinari D, Bushy A, eds: *The rural nurse: transition to practice*, New York, NY, 2012, Springer Publishing.

Montgomery SR, Sutton AL, Paré J: Rural nursing and synergy, *Online J Rural Nurs Health Care* 17(1):87–99, 2017. Available at: http://rnojournal.binghamton.edu, Accessed June 25, 2018.

Napolitano M: Migrant health issues. In Stanhope M, Lancaster J, eds.: *Public health nursing: population-centered health care in the community*, St. Louis, 2008, Mosby.

Napolitano M, Lasarev M, Beltran M, et al: Un lugar seguro para sus niños: development and evaluation of a pesticide education video, *J Immigr Health* 4:135–145, 2002.

National Center for Farmworkers Health: *Demographics* ,Buda, Tex, 2016, Retrieved May 2016 from http://www.ncfh.org.

National Center for Farmworker Health: Facts about agricultural workers, Buda, Tex, 20018a, NCFH. Retrieved July 2020 from http://www.ncfh.org.

National Center for Farmworker Health: *Occupational safety and health*, Buda, Tex, 2018b, NCFH. Retrieved July 2020 from http://www.ncfh.org.

National Center for Farmworker Health: *HIV/AIDS agricultural worker factsheet*, 2018c, NCFH. Retrieved from http://www.ncfh.org.

National Center for Farmworker Health: *Child labor in agriculture*, Buda, Tex, 2018d, NCFH. Retrieved July 2020 from http://www.ncfh.org.

National Center for Farmworker Health: *Folk medicine and traditional healing*, Buda, Tex, 2018e, NCFH. Retrieved July 2020 from http://www.ncfh.org.

National Center for Farmworker Health: *COVID-19 in rural America: Impact on farms & agricultural workers*, Buda, Tex, 2020. NCFH. Retrieved July 2020 from http://www.ncfh.org.

National Center for Health Statistics (NCHS): *Data visualization gallery*, 2018. Available at: https://www.cdc.gov/nchs/index.htm. Accessed June 25, 2018.

National Farmworker Ministry, 2018, *Farm worker issues: U.S. labor laws for farm workers,* Retrieved July 2020 from http://www.nfwm.org.

National Human Trafficking Hotline: *Labor Trafficking Victim Outreach Card*, 2014. Available at: https://humantraffickinghotline.org.

National Rural Health Association: *About rural health care*, Washington, DC, 2020, NRHA. Retrieved July 2020 from http://www.ruralhealthweb.org.

Occupational Safety and Health Administration: *Safety and health topics: agricultural operations*, Washington, DC, n.d., OSHA. Retrieved July 2020 from https://www.osha.gov.

O'Connor K, Stoecklin-Marois M, Schenker MB: Examining *nervios* among Immigrant male farmworkers in the MICASA study: sociodemographics, housing conditions and psychosocial factors, *J Immigrant Minority Health* 17:198–207, 2015.

Oren E, Fiero MH, Barrett E, Anderson B, Nuñez M, Gonzalez-Salazar F: Detection of latent tuberculosis infection among migrant farmworkers along the US-Mexico border, *BMC Infectious Diseases* 16:630, 2016.

Polaris Project: *Labor Trafficking, 2018.* Available at: https://polarisproject.org/human-trafficking/labor-trafficking Retrieved June 2018.

Polaris Project: *Human trafficking, 2020,* Retrieved July 2020 from http://www.humantraffickinghotline.org.

Prengaman M, Terry DR, Schmitz D, Baker E: The nursing community Apgar questionnaire in rural Australia: an evidence based approach to recruiting and retaining nurses, *Online J Rural Nurs Health Care* 17(2):148–171, 2017.

Pulgar CA, et al: Economic hardship and depression among women in Latino farmworker families, *J Immigrant Minority Health* 18, 497–504, 2016.

Quad Council Coalition (QCC) of Public Health Nursing Organizations: *Community/Public Health Nursing Competencies,* 2018. Available at: http://www.quadcouncilphn.org.

Richards T: Health implications of human trafficking, *Nurs Womens Health* 18:155–162, 2014.

Rural Health Information Hub (RHI-Hub): *What is rural?* 2018. Available at: https://www.ruralhealthinfo.org/topics/what-is-rural Accessed June 25, 2018.

Rural Health Information Hub (RHI-Hub): *Barriers to health promotion and disease prevention in rural areas,* 2020, Retrieved July 2020 at http://www.rural healthinfor.org.

Tschampl CA, Garnick DW, Zuroweste E, Razavi M, Shepard DS: Use of transnational services to prevent treatment interruption in tuberculosis-infected persons who leave the United States, *Emerging Infect Dis* 22(3): 417–425, 2016.

US Department of Agriculture (USDA): *Rural America at a glance: 2018 edition,* 2018. Available at: https://www.ers.usda.gov Accessed July 2020.

US Department of Agriculture (USDA): *Food security and nutrition assistance,* 2019, Economic Research Service, Retrieved July 2020 at http://www.ers.usda.gov.

US Department of Agriculture (USDA): *Farm labor,* 2020, Retrieved July 2020 at http://www.ers.usda.gov.

US Department of Health and Human Services: *Healthy People 2030,* Washington, DC, 2020, USDHHS. Retrieved July 2020 from https://www.healthypeople.gov.

US Department of Labor (DOL): *Fact Sheet #51: Field Sanitation Standards under the Occupational Safety and Health Act,* 2008. Available at: http://www.dol.gov.

Urban Institute: *Understanding the Organization, Operation, and Victimization Process of Labor Trafficking in the United States,* 2014: Owens, C, Dank, M, Breaux, J, et al. Available at: https://www.urban.org/.

Yeung B, Rubenstein G, Center for Investigative Reporting: *Female Workers Face Rape, Harassment in U.S. Agricultural Industry,* 2013. Available at: https://www.revealnews.org.

25

Poverty, Homelessness, Teen Pregnancy, and Mental Illness

Sharon K. Davis, Mary Kay Goldschmidt, and Anita Thompson-Heisterman

OBJECTIVES

After reading this chapter, the student should be able to:

1. Describe the social, economic, political, cultural, and environmental factors that influence poverty.
2. Discuss the effects of poverty on the health and well-being of individuals, families, and communities.
3. Discuss how being homeless affects the health and well-being of individuals, families, and communities.
4. Describe the ways in which teen pregnancies affect the baby, the parents, and their families.
5. Develop nursing interventions for the prevention of pregnancy problems that at-risk adolescents might experience.
6. Explain the extent of the problem of patients who have mental illness or who are at risk for mental illness.
7. Explain nursing interventions for poor and homeless people, pregnant teens and their significant others, and individuals who are mentally ill or at risk for mental illness.

CHAPTER OUTLINE

KEY TERMS

Where you are born, grow, live, work, and age comprise a person's social determinants of health. As discussed in Chapter 23 the social determinants of health are largely responsible for the unfair and avoidable inequities in health in a country or between countries (WHO, 2020). The protests and riots of 2020 and 2021 illustrated the inequities for how people in the United States felt. For the purposes of this chapter, four groups of people who represent members of vulnerable populations and who may experience health inequities are the poor, the homeless, pregnant teens and those with mental illness. Nurses need to understand their own beliefs about these groups as well as the issues surrounding the clients' illness or personal situation. To be able to interact effectively with these groups, it is important for the nurse to identify health care needs, barriers to care, and essential health care services for each of these groups and, in some instances, for their families as well.

This chapter describes the many ways that poverty, homelessness, teen pregnancy, and mental illness affect the health status of individuals, families, and communities and contains effective nursing intervention strategies for these groups. The COVID-19 pandemic has affected especially people who were previously living in poverty, were homeless, or suffered from a mental illness.

UNDERSTANDING VULNERABLE GROUPS

Cultural attitudes are the beliefs and perspectives that a society values. Perspectives on individual responsibility for health and well-being are influenced by prevailing cultural attitudes, and are influenced by the media through print, spoken, and visual means. In recent years, as a result of the economic downturn, and more recently the COVID-19 pandemic, it is difficult to distinguish one's status related to homelessness. Many individuals and families who have been able to take care of themselves have suffered economic setbacks because of job losses and the subsequent loss of homes, health insurance, and other essential resources (Fig. 25.1).

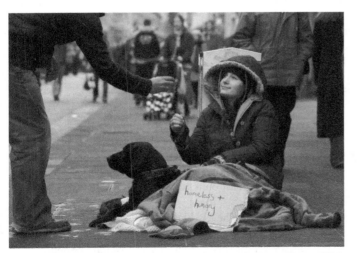

Fig. 25.1 Many Women, Young and Old, as Well as Those With Children Are Homeless. (Copyright © 2013 Thinkstock. All rights reserved. Image #79166814.)

These questions have no easy answers. You might be involved in such clinical encounters in a simulation lab, via virtual reality, or with in-person contact. It is important for nurses to realize that their behavior influences their relationships with their clients. Take one of the clinical scenarios above and apply the six-step clinical judgment process of (1) recognize the cues; (2) analyze the cues; (3) identify possible hypotheses and put them in priority order; (4) develop possible solutions for your highest-priority hypothesis; (5) what action you would take; and (6) given the action that you considered taking, how would you evaluate your effectiveness?

It is important for nurses to value individuals, promote health, respect and restore human dignity, and improve the quality of life of individuals, families, and aggregates. Nursing care needs to be multidimensional and include consideration of biological, psychological, social, cultural, environmental, economic, and spiritual factors. Conflicts in values, beliefs, and perceptions may arise when nurses work with persons from different social, cultural, and economic backgrounds. A lack of awareness between the professional's and the client's perceptions of need can lead to misunderstanding and conflict. When clients do not understand what they are being told or when they disagree, they may not follow the prescribed treatment protocol; the nurse may then inaccurately interpret the client's behavior as resistance, lack of cooperation, or noncompliance. Rather than being resistant, uncooperative, or noncompliant, the person may have low health literacy and may simply not understand what is being said. It is essential to provide the education to clients in a format that allows for them to make appropriate decisions.

POVERTY: DEFINITION AND DESCRIPTION

There are many ways to define and understand poverty. The federal government uses two terms to discuss poverty: *poverty thresholds* and *poverty guidelines*. The Poverty Threshold Guidelines are issued by the US Bureau of the Census and used primarily for statistical purposes. The Federal Poverty Guidelines are issued every year by the USDHHS and are used to determine whether a person or family is financially eligible for assistance or services for certain programs and benefits, including savings on marketplace health insurance, and Medicaid and CHIP (Child Health Insurance Program) coverage.

The federal poverty guidelines are updated annually to be consistent with the Consumer Price Index (CPI). The CPI measures the change in prices paid by consumers for goods and services including food, clothing, shelter, fuels, transportation, doctors' and dentists' services, drugs, and other goods and services that people buy for day-to-day living (US Bureau of Labor Statistics, 2020). See Table 25.1 for the 2020 poverty guidelines for the contiguous states and the District of Columbia (USDHHS, 2020a). In 2018, the official poverty rate was 11.8%. This was the fourth consecutive annual decline in poverty. It is likely that the poverty rate will begin to increase beginning with 2020 due to the effects of the COVID-19 pandemic. In 2018 the median earning of men and women who worked full-time was $55,291 and $45,097 respectively (Semega, Kollar, Creamer, and Mohanty, 2020). The poverty rate for children under 18 years of age was 16.2%, and the poverty rate for people aged 65 and older was 9.7% (Semega, et al 2020). See Chapter 23 for a discussion of poverty in relation to vulnerability.

People who live in poverty are not a homogenous group; therefore, be sure to listen to and learn about each person. In general, poverty refers to having insufficient resources to meet basic living expenses. These expenses include food, shelter, clothing, transportation, and health care. People who are poor are more likely to live in dangerous environments, be underemployed or unemployed or work at high-risk jobs, eat less nutritious foods, and have many stressors. Evidence suggests that poverty levels are higher among African Americans and Hispanics and are associated with disparities in educational level (Stanford Center on Poverty & Inequality, 2017). Single mothers are also at higher risk for poverty. According to the Children's Defense Fund, children are the poorest age group in America. In 2018, nearly 1 in 6 children lived in poverty, and that represented approximately 11.9 million children. The youngest children are the poorest and nearly 73% of poor children in America are children of color. More than 12.5 million children lived in food-insecure households in 2017, with Black and Hispanic households with food-insecure children being nearly two times that of white households (Children's Defense Fund, 2020, p. 6). In fiscal year 2018, the Supplemental Nutrition Assistance Program (SNAP), formerly known as food stamps, helped feed 17 million children. Also both 2017 and 2018 marked the first increases in the number of uninsured US children in a decade (Children's Defense Fund, 2020). A useful resource from the Children's Defense Fund, *The State of America's Children: 2020*, provides state fact sheets on how children are doing in each of the 50 states, in the District of Columbia, and nationwide.

For many years, income level was used as the criterion that determines whether someone is poor. Although income continues to be the measurement of choice, the federal income poverty guidelines have been renamed the federal poverty guidelines.

The terms *persistent poverty* and *neighborhood poverty* are used to describe types of poverty. Persistent poverty refers to individuals and families who remain poor for long periods and who pass poverty on to their descendants. Neighborhood poverty refers to geographically defined areas of high poverty, characterized by dilapidated housing and high levels of unemployment. Multigenerational poverty is common among African Americans in the South, Hispanics along the border of Mexico, and American Indians who live in states with multiple reservations. For nurses, the most significant factor is being able to accept and respect clients and attempt to understand how their life situations influence their health and well-being. Being poor is one variable that must be measured against the presence of other variables that may increase or decrease the negative effects of poverty.

Social Security is keeping fewer seniors out of poverty. However, factors that may cause a senior to enter poverty may be due to a decrease in Social Security or their retirement income or an increase in health care expenses. The US Census Bureau reports poverty according to the official poverty measure and the Supplemental Poverty Measure (SPM). The SPM thresholds vary by geographic area and homeownership status, and these numbers can be higher than the official poverty measure. Under the official poverty measure, in 2017, 4.7 million adults age 65 and older lived in poverty. The rate among seniors increases with age and is higher among women, African Americans, and Hispanics (Cubanski, Koma, Damico, and Neuman, 2018).

The causes of poverty are complex and interrelated. The following factors affect the growing number of poor persons in the United States:

- Decreased earnings
- Increased unemployment rates
- Changes in retirement benefits, particularly when companies move, close, or file for bankruptcy protection and eliminate or reduce retirement benefits
- Changes in the labor force
- Increase in female-headed households
- Inadequate education and job skills
- Inadequate antipoverty programs and welfare benefits
- Weak enforcement of child support statutes
- Dwindling Social Security payments to children
- Increased numbers of children born to single women

TABLE 25.1 Poverty Guidelines for the 48 Contiguous States and the District of Columbia, 2020

Size of Family Unit	Income Guideline ($)
1	12,760
2	17,240
3	21,720
4	26,200
5	30,680
6	35,160
7	39, 640
8	44,120
8 or more	Add $5,600 per person

The poverty guideline is higher for Alaska and Hawaii.
USDHHS: *Poverty guidelines, 2020,* http://www.aspe.hhs.gov,
January 8, 2020.

- Outsourcing of American jobs and during the COVID-19 pandemic, the furloughs, reduced salaries, and loss of jobs
- Trade deficits, debt, and involvement in wars

As the fiscal characteristics of most industrialized nations have changed from industrial economies to service economies, job opportunities have increasingly excluded workers who do not have at least a high school education. Many manufacturing jobs do not pay a sufficient salary to support a family, and many jobs have been moved to foreign countries where lower wages can be paid than in the United States. Also, many jobs at the lower end of the pay scale do not include health care or retirement benefits.

Poverty and Health: Effects Across the Life Span

Poverty directly affects health and well-being, resulting in the following:

- Higher rates of chronic illness
- Higher infant morbidity and mortality
- Shorter life expectancy
- More complex health problems
- More significant complications and physical limitations resulting from the higher incidence of chronic diseases, such as asthma, diabetes, and hypertension
- Hospitalization rates greater than those for persons with higher incomes

The poor health outcomes from poverty are consistent with those that affect rural and migrant populations as discussed in Chapter 24. These poor health outcomes are often secondary to barriers that impede access to health care, such as an inability to pay for health care, lack of insurance, geographic location, language, inability to find a health care provider, transportation difficulties, inconvenient clinic hours, and negative attitudes of health care providers toward poor clients. Access to health care is especially difficult for the working poor. Many employers, especially those paying low or minimum wage, do not provide health care insurance for their employees. Persons working for these employers are ineligible for most public health insurance programs, and they are often unable to obtain affordable health care. The Affordable Health Care Act has positively influenced some, but not all, of these obstacles to getting adequate health insurance.

Poverty, while presenting a significant obstacle to health across the life span, has an especially negative effect on *women of childbearing age*. Women living in poverty have lower levels of physical functioning and higher reported levels of bodily discomfort than women in higher socioeconomic groups. The poverty rate for women was down in 2018 (12.9%) compared to 2017 (13.6%) but still is higher than for men, whose rate was 10.6% in 2018. Full-time, year-round employed women earn $0.82 for each $1.00 a man earns (Semega et al., 2019). Women living in rural areas often face additional barriers. They may have less income, education, transportation, and live in areas with fewer providers.

There are many adverse effects of poverty on the health of children, including increased morbidity and mortality during childhood and a lifelong increased risk of cardiovascular and metabolic disease, much of which can be linked to toxic stress. Box 25.1 describes the impact of poverty on the health and well-being of children.

BOX 25.1 Effects of Poverty on the Health of Children

- Higher rates of prematurity, low birth weight, and birth defects
- Higher infant mortality rates
- Increased incidence of chronic disease
- Increased incidence of traumatic death and injuries
- Increased incidence of nutritional deficits
- Increased incidence of growth restriction and developmental delays
- Increased incidence of iron-deficiency anemia
- Increased incidence of elevated blood lead levels
- Increased incidence of infections
- Increased risk for homelessness
- Decreased opportunities for education, income, and occupation

Younger children are more at risk of poverty-related toxic stress because of their vulnerability and the prevalence of poverty among this age group. The high levels of stress experienced by families living in poverty lead to consistently activated stress hormones and inflammatory mediators in children. High levels and/or prolonged exposure to hormones such as cortisol, norepinephrine, and adrenalin, coupled with mediators such as cytokine, affect the entire body and in particular, a child's developing brain. Poor impulse control and self-regulating behaviors may result from this hypervigilant stress response, which may further impair the relational health between a child and a stressed parent and other family members. As young adults, these children may engage in unhealthy behaviors such as smoking or substance abuse in an effort to provide respite from chronic stress, which can lead to increased morbidity and mortality at a young age. Children who have the benefit of good relational health and a stable family life are better able to minimize the stress response and may not experience the lifelong increased risk of chronic disease. For this reason, interventions that focus on improving parental engagement and good relational health can buffer the harm to a child's developing brain (Pascoe et al., 2016).

EVIDENCE-BASED PRACTICE

Toxic stress among children has been identified as a significant contributor to the development of chronic disease as an adult. Ameliorating the effects of toxic stress among children can be accomplished through stable, supportive relationships with adults during early childhood. Breastfeeding has been suggested as a toxic stress mitigator, beginning with the skin-to-skin contact immediately following birth. This mother-infant contact stimulates a rise in maternal oxytocin and prolactin and decreases cortisol, reducing infant allostatic load and inducing calm. Breastfeeding has been proven to aid in the establishment of maternal-infant attachment and lower the stress response in mothers and infants.

Nurse Use

Interventions that support and promote breastfeeding such as the nurse-family partnership (NFP) address disparities in breastfeeding among communities and work to decrease socioeconomic disparities for mothers and infants. NFP programs have also positively impacted such child/family outcomes as fewer child injuries related to neglect.

Hallowell S, Froh E, Spatz D: Human milk and breastfeeding: an intervention to mitigate toxic stress. *Nurs Outlook* 65(1):58–67, 2017. Available from https://www.nursingoutlook.org.

Under current federal law, noncustodial parents are required to provide financial support to their children. Current child support policies are designed to provide financial security to children, prevent single-parent families from entering the welfare system, help single-parent families get off welfare as quickly as possible, and decrease welfare expenditures. Individual states are responsible for locating nonsupporting custodial parents, establishing paternity, and enforcing financial responsibility. In most states, government involvement in locating noncustodial parents begins when the custodial parent applies for Temporary Assistance to Needy Families (TANF). There are complications in that many parents were never married and have intermittent work histories.

Poverty affects both urban and rural communities. Several characteristics describe poor communities. For example, poorer neighborhoods may have more minority residents and single-parent families, higher rates of unemployment, and lower wage rates. These residents are also more likely to be victims of crime, substance abuse, and racial discrimination. Differences in quality and level of education also exist. Health care is less available to residents of poor neighborhoods. There is evidence about the impact of housing on health. Health is affected by having a stable home; a home that is safe on the inside; and a home in an area that is free from crime and abuse (Health Affairs, *Culture of Health,* 2018). As discussed in Chapter 8: Environmental Health, there can be many health hazards related to environmental conditions both inside and outside the home.

HOMELESSNESS: DEFINING AND UNDERSTANDING THE CONCEPT

Poverty can lead to homelessness. Homelessness, like poverty, is a complex concept. Although people who have never been homeless cannot truly understand what it means to be homeless, nurses can increase their sensitivity toward homeless clients by examining their own personal beliefs, values, and knowledge of homelessness. The Department of Housing and Urban Development defines "homeless" as "a person who lacks a fixed, regular, and adequate nighttime residence" (Henry et al., 2017). This definition can be expanded to cover categories of homelessness such as "chronically homeless individual" or "chronically homeless people in families," the former referring to an individual who has a disability and has either been homeless at least 4 times in 3 years—for a minimum of 12 months—or continuously homeless for a total of 1 year, the latter referring to a family where the head of household meets the definition of chronically homeless individual (Henry et al., 2017).

The concept of homelessness encompasses three categories: chronic homelessness, transitional, and episodic. The episodic homeless are generally marked by hardship and struggle, including chronic unemployment. These individuals move in and out of homelessness, are younger, and often have mental health and substance abuse problems. Transitional homelessness, which can be called crisis poverty, is typically caused by a catastrophic event leading to a short shelter stay, eventually transitioning to permanent housing. This tends to account for the majority of homelessness over time because of the high rates of

turnover among this population, which edges the count higher. Finally, the chronically homeless are usually older individuals who are chronically unemployed, have some type of disability or substance abuse problem, and use the emergency shelter system as a long-term housing solution. This group makes up the smallest percent of the homeless population (National Coalition for the Homeless, 2019).

Those who are homeless sleep at night in shelters that they often must vacate during the day. This means that during the day, they sit or stand on the street; in parks, alleys, shopping centers, and libraries; and in places such as trash bins, cardboard boxes, or under loading docks at industrial sites. Homeless persons may seek shelter in public buildings, such as train and bus stations. Those who do not sleep in shelters may sleep in single-room-occupancy (SRO) hotels, all-night movie theaters, abandoned buildings, and vehicles. Some homeless persons choose to be unsheltered rather than live with family or stay in shelters (Christian and Mukarji-Connollly, 2018). The questions in the How To box can aid in reflection and value clarification.

HOW TO EVALUATE THE CONCEPT OF HOMELESSNESS
- What is it like to live on the streets?
- What issues might confront a young mother and her children inside a homeless shelter?
- How is it that people are so poor that they have no place to go?
- What really causes homelessness?
- How do you respond to the person on the street asking for money to buy a sandwich or catch a bus?
- How is your response different (or not) when a young mother with children asks you for money?
- How do you react to the smell of urine in a stairwell or elevator?

On a single night in 2019, approximately 568,000 people experienced homelessness in the United States. Nearly 63% were staying in sheltered locations such as emergency shelters or transitional housing programs. That left about 37% living on the street, in abandoned buildings, or in other places not suitable for human living (US Department of Housing and Urban Development [HUD], January 2020). Between 2018 and 2019 homelessness increased by 3% in the West Coast states, and this is likely due to the moderate climate. Between 2018 and 2019 the number of homeless veterans declined; there was a small increase in the number of homeless unaccompanied youth (between the ages of 18 and 24). African Americans have remained consistently overrepresented in the US homeless population (HUD, 2020). According to the National Coalition for the Homeless (2018) the numbers provided by HUD may underrepresent the actual number of homeless persons. The HUD definition does not include families who have moved in with friends or family. Others may live in motels, vehicles, or other hidden locations and do not interact with homeless service agencies or volunteers conducting counts. Some homeless people refuse to be interviewed, which may mean that they are not counted.

Poverty and homelessness are affected by the employment rate. When companies close, downsize, or relocate, workers often go long periods without a steady income. All of these factors occurred during the COVID-19 pandemic. Unemployed people often lose their homes and may need to move from the home where they and their family have connections with friends and organizations such as schools, places of worship, or social organizations. Many families move first to rental sites, and some may become unable to afford the rent and move in with family or friends or become homeless. They may also lose their vehicles and become much less able to get to work, school, and appointments.

People who live on the street are the poorest of the poor, and they may be viewed as faceless, nameless, invisible, and inaudible entities. It is important for nurses to respect the individuality of all clients, including those who are homeless. People become homeless for many reasons, and there is no one set of circumstances or patterns that leads to and sustains homelessness. Rural communities are not immune to homelessness. The extent of homelessness in rural areas may be less apparent because these individuals often are hidden from sight, sometimes living in the woods in tents or campers, in barns or ice sheds, or on a friend's couch. Why are so many people living outdoors? "There is not enough affordable housing or shelter available" (National Coalition for the Homeless, 2018).

Consider the situation of Mary Jones and her children, Sam and Julie, ages 6 and 8 years, respectively, and discuss with one or more of your classmates the kinds of nursing interventions that might assist this family.

CASE STUDY

Ms. Jones, a single mother, was able for several years to maintain an apartment, have an older-model car, and purchase an adequate amount of food for her children. She worked for a cleaning service, and although the pay was not especially good, she worked regular hours and had health insurance for her children. She hurt her back at work, and when her workers' compensation payments expired, she found herself unable to afford her rent or keep her car. She was able to stay in a shelter at night with her children, and they were all able to have breakfast and dinner there and take regular showers. By living at the shelter from approximately sunset to sunrise, she was able to get her children to school, and she looked for work that would not aggravate her injured back.

Imagine what the life of the Jones family is now in contrast to the time when they had a home and a car. What are the most pressing issues this family faces? What options do you think are available to the family to improve their living situation? How would you respond if Ms. Jones or one of the children approached you on the street and asked you for money to buy food? Identify services and resources in your community that would help Ms. Jones if she lived there. For example, are there job training programs? Is there other assistance for which she would qualify? How can Ms. Jones keep her children in school? Could the children participate in any extracurricular activities?

As illustrated by the case of Mary Jones, the typical sheltered family is made up of a single mother with two or three children; they are most likely to be people of color, and the mothers may not have a high school diploma and have poor job skills and limited work options that pay a livable wage and offer health care benefits. The mothers have often been victims of domestic violence, and they often have more medical, mental health, and substance abuse problems than women who are housed (Bassuk, 2010).

Homeless children and youth fall into one of two groups: those who are part of a homeless family and those who are "unaccompanied" by homeless family members. As is true for all homeless subpopulations, it is difficult to get an accurate count. According to the 2019 Annual Homeless Assessment Report (AHAR) to Congress, 63% of the people who were homeless were staying in a sheltered location, and 37% were unsheltered, living in places not meant for human habitation, such as streets, parks, vehicles, or abandoned buildings. In five states—Arkansas, California, Hawaii, Nevada, and Oregon—more than half of all homeless people were in unsheltered locations. In contrast, in Maine, Massachusetts, Nebraska, New York, and North Dakota, at least 95% of the homeless population were sheltered. Twenty-seven percent of the homeless population were under age 25; African Americans remain overrepresented in the homeless population, and 8% were veterans (HUD, 2020). Causes of homelessness among youth include unstable family life and domestic violence, fractured social supports, substance abuse, mental illness, and sexual orientation and gender identity and expression (SOGIE).

The US Department of Education's ED Data Express provides an estimate of the rates of homelessness among children under the age of 18 who attend public school, but these data do not capture those who are not in the public-school system or those that attempt to hide their homelessness. Adolescents are particularly reticent about identifying as homeless. They do this in an effort to blend in with their peers, or if they are unaccompanied, they may fear entering into the child welfare or criminal justice system (National Network for Youth, 2018). Another significant factor impacting homelessness among youth is sexual orientation or gender identity expression. An estimated 40% of unaccompanied homeless youth are lesbian, gay, bisexual, transgender, and queer (LGBTQ) young adults (Dashow, 2017).

One in five homeless persons has a severe mental illness, with similar rates of chronic substance abuse. Severe mental illness and substance abuse are often associated with chronic homelessness, which may be caused in part by a lack of adequate engagement with outpatient treatment and long-term follow-up. Historically, the deinstitutionalization of mental health care was thought to be a contributing cause to the high rate of mentally ill persons who are homeless. However, a meta-analysis completed in 2016 showed that other factors may be responsible for the high rate of mentally ill homeless individuals in the United States. These factors include changes in mental health care funding in programs such as Medicaid, restrictions in Social Security and disability payments, a reduction in low-cost housing, and other social and political changes (Winkler et al., 2016; Roche et al., 2018). (Fig. 25.2).

Many homeless persons were mentally ill before becoming homeless, whereas others develop acute mental distress as a result of being homeless. Although treatment options exist, homeless persons are often unable to access mental health treatment facilities. Barriers to treatment include lack of awareness of treatment options, lack of available space in treatment facilities, inability to pay for treatment, lack of transportation, unsupportive or disrespectful attitudes of care providers, and

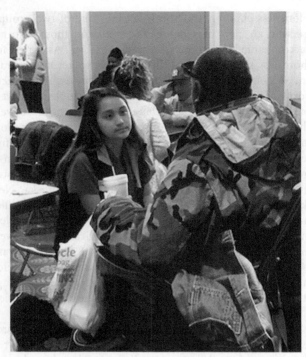

Fig. 25.2 Nurses Must Be Able to Communicate Therapeutically With Homeless Individuals to Assess Their Needs, Create a Plan of Care, and Effectively Advocate for the Patient.

lack of coordination of services (Roche et al., 2017). See the Substance Abuse and Mental Health Services Administration (SAMHSA) website for "Homeless programs and resources," which provides information designed to help prevent and end homelessness among people with mental or substance use disorders (SUD).

Veterans are another at-risk population for becoming homeless. However, the number of homeless veterans decreased between 2018 and 2019 and has dropped nearly 50% since 2009. These decreases are largely due to veterans staying in both sheltered and unsheltered locations (USDHUD, 2020) and to a coordinated effort initiated by the US Department of Veterans Affairs (VA) and HUD to engage public and private housing and service providers and state and federal government agencies to eliminate homelessness among veterans. See information on rapid rehousing through the US Department of Veterans Affairs' "Supportive Services for Veteran Families" (SSVF) program and permanent supportive housing through the HUD-Veterans Affairs Supportive Housing program (HUD-VASH) for more information on housing the nation's homeless (National Alliance to End Homelessness, 2019). On a single night in January 2019, 37,085 veterans were experiencing homelessness. They tend to be veterans without children, and only 2% were part of a family; 90.3% were men and 8.9% were women.

Veterans become homeless for many of the same reasons as nonveterans, but they are overrepresented among the homeless population, and it is thought that the experience of combat and numerous deployments may increase the risk of homelessness. Posttraumatic stress disorder (PTSD), traumatic brain injury with cognitive impairment, and other mental health issues may impair social relational health and/or negatively affect family relationships. In addition, the majority of homeless veterans are unmarried and may be socially isolated, a risk factor for homelessness. About 50% of veterans who are homeless have serious mental illness and 70% have substance use issues.

The VA provides universal screening for all veterans who seek services through the VA health system and can be linked with housing and other appropriate services as needed, although some veterans may not be eligible for VA health services, which is dependent upon their discharge status (Henry et al., 2017; National Alliance to End Homelessness, 2018; United States Interagency Council on Homelessness, 2018).

As mentioned in the previous Case Example, many homeless people sleep at night in shelters but must leave during the day. This means that during the day if they do not attend school or are not looking for work, they may sit or stand on the street, in parks, alleys, shopping centers, or libraries, and in places such as trash bins or cardboard boxes or under loading docks at industrial sites. They may also seek shelter in public buildings, such as train and bus stations. Those who do not sleep in shelters may sleep in SRO hotels, all-night movie theaters, abandoned buildings, and vehicles.

Effects of Homelessness on Health

Homelessness is correlated with poor health outcomes. Homeless persons suffer from multiple health problems at a much higher rate than the general population due to increased exposure to the elements, disease, violence, crowded and unsanitary living conditions, malnutrition, stress, and addictive substances. Additionally, conditions that require regular, uninterrupted treatment, such as tuberculosis (TB) and HIV/AIDS, are extremely difficult to treat or control among those without adequate housing (National Coalition for the Homeless, 2019).

Health care is usually crisis oriented and sought in emergency departments, and this is expensive for the hospital and the government. Homeless people who access health care have a hard time following prescribed regimens. For example, an insulin-dependent diabetic man who lives on the street may sleep in a shelter. His ability to get adequate rest and exercise, take insulin on a schedule, eat regular meals, or follow a prescribed diet is virtually impossible. How does someone purchase an antibiotic without money? How is a child treated for scabies and lice when there are no bathing facilities? How does an older adult with peripheral vascular disease elevate his legs when he must be out of the shelter at 7 am and on the streets all day? These health problems are often directly related to poor access to preventive health care services. Homeless people devote a large portion of their time trying to survive. Health promotion activities are a luxury for them, not a part of their daily lives. *Healthy People 2030* has goals to increase awareness and use of preventive health services (see *Healthy People 2030* box), but this is difficult for the homeless. In addition to mental illness and substance abuse, homeless people can have the following health problems:

- Hypothermia and heat-related illnesses due to their living conditions

- Infestations and poor skin integrity; respiratory conditions or TB due to crowded sleeping conditions
- Peripheral vascular disease and hypertension because they may be on their feet for long hours daily
- Diabetes and nutritional deficits because the food in the shelters and fast-food restaurants often has high sodium content
- HIV/AIDS
- Trauma that could include gunshot or stab wounds, head trauma, suicide attempts, and fractures as well as more minor trauma including bruises, abrasions, concussions, sprains, puncture wounds, eye injuries, and cellulitis
- Barriers to getting adequate health care can include not knowing where to get treated; lack of transportation; lack of identification; embarrassment; nervousness or inability to fill out the forms and answer questions; and self-consciousness about appearance and hygiene if they live on the street (National Coalition for the Homeless, 2019).

Also, homeless people may not have access to dental care, places to bathe, and nutritious food, which makes it important for nursing assessments to consider teeth, skin, and feet.

COVID-19 has presented particular risk to homeless people. The Centers for Disease Control and Prevention has consistently warned that people 65 years and older and those with serious medical conditions are at higher risk for becoming seriously ill from COVID-19. As discussed above, these two risk groups are often part of the homeless population. Crowded shelters and encampments, sleeping outdoors, and housing instability make it difficult for homeless people to engage in the following activities that can help prevent disease: (1) eating sufficient nutritious food; (2) getting adequate sleep and rest; (3) social distancing; and (4) maintaining good hygiene with frequent handwashing (National Alliance to End Homelessness, 2020b.)

 HEALTHY PEOPLE 2030

Objectives Related to Poor and Homeless People, Adolescent Reproductive Health, and Mental Illness

- **MHMD-R01:** Increase the proportion of homeless adults with mental health problems who get mental health services.
- **SDOH-01:** Reduce the proportion of people living in poverty.
- **FP-03:** Reduce pregnancies in adolescents.

From US Department of Health and Human Services: *Healthy People 2030*, Washington, DC, 2020b, US Government Printing Office.

In addition to its effects on physical health, homelessness also affects psychological, social, and spiritual well-being. Becoming homeless means more than losing a home or a regular place to sleep and eat; it also means losing friends, personal possessions, and familiar surroundings. Homeless persons live in chaos, confusion, and fear. Many describe experiencing loss of dignity, low self-esteem, lack of social support, and generalized despair.

Homelessness and At-Risk Populations

Being homeless affects health across the life span. Imagine the effect of homelessness on pregnancy, childhood, adolescence, or older adulthood; each group has different needs. Nurses must be aware of the unique needs of homeless clients at every age.

Homeless pregnant women are at high risk for complex health problems. Richards et al. (2011), in studying homeless pregnant women in 31 states, found them to be younger, unmarried, uninsured, less educated, and less likely to initiate and sustain breastfeeding and to have fewer prenatal and well-child visits than other pregnant women. Outcomes for homeless pregnant women are significantly poorer than for pregnant women in the general population. Pregnant homeless women present several challenges. They have higher rates of sexually transmitted infections (STIs), higher incidences of addiction to drugs and alcohol, poorer nutritional status, more kidney and bladder infections, and poorer birth outcomes (e.g., lower birth weight, preterm labor). Although homeless women who are pregnant are at increased risk for complications of pregnancy, they have less access to prenatal care (Merrill et al., 2011).

The health problems of homeless children, although similar to those of poor children, often have more serious consequences. Homeless children have poorer health than children in the general population, and they experience more symptoms of acute illness, such as fever, ear infections, diarrhea, and asthma, than their housed counterparts. Homeless children living on the streets in urban areas are at greatest risk for poor health as a result of poor nutrition, inconsistent health care, high levels of anxiety, and an inability to practice good health behaviors. Homeless children also experience higher rates of school absenteeism, academic failure, depression, and emotional and behavioral maladjustments. They change schools often, which affects them and the school. They lose their sense of place, friends, pets, possessions, and sometimes their families. There is little stability in their lives. The stress of homelessness can be manifested in behaviors such as withdrawal, depression, anxiety, aggression, regression, and self-mutilation. Homeless children may have delayed communication, more mental health problems, and histories of abuse. They also typically witness more violence than their housed counterparts and are less likely to have attended school regularly (Gerber, 2013).

Homeless adolescents living on the streets exhibit greater risk-taking behaviors, including earlier onset of sexual activity. They also have poorer health status and decreased access to health care than do teens in the general population. They are at high risk for contracting serious communicable diseases, such as AIDS and hepatitis B, and are more likely to use alcohol and illicit substances. Homeless teens often have histories of runaway behavior, physical abuse, and sexual abuse. Once on the streets, many homeless adolescents exchange sex for food, clothing, and shelter. In addition to the increased risk for sexually transmitted diseases (STDs) and other serious communicable diseases, homeless adolescent girls who exchange sex for survival are at high risk for unintended pregnancy.

Homeless older adults are the most vulnerable of the impoverished older-adult population. They have lived in long-standing poverty, have fewer supportive relationships, and are likely to have become homeless as a result of catastrophic events. Life expectancy for homeless older adults is significantly lower than for older housed adults. The average life expectancy for someone who is homeless is 44 years (Gerber, 2013). Permanent physical deformities, often secondary to poor or absent medical care, are common among homeless older adults. They often suffer from untreated chronic conditions, including TB, hypertension, arthritis, cardiovascular disease, injuries, malnutrition, poor oral health, and hypothermia. As with younger homeless persons, older adults who are homeless must focus their energy on survival, leaving little time for health promotion activities.

Homelessness has a negative effect on the health of persons across the life span. Nurses need to identify the precursors to homelessness; anticipate the effects of homelessness on physical, emotional, and spiritual well-being; and learn about resources to assist the homeless.

TRENDS IN ADOLESCENT SEXUAL BEHAVIOR AND PREGNANCY

Teen pregnancy is an area of public concern because of its significant effect on communities. Resources to support the special needs of pregnant teenagers are decreasing. Many teenagers who become pregnant are caught in a cycle of poverty, school failure, and limited life options. Even under the ideal circumstances of adequate finances, loving and supportive families, and good birth outcomes, a teen mother must circumvent her own necessary developmental tasks to raise her child.

There is neither a uniform reason that teens become pregnant nor a universally acceptable solution. The causes of teen pregnancy are diverse and affected by changing moral attitudes, sexual codes, and economic circumstances. Teen pregnancy places an enormous strain on the health care and social service systems. Social concern is also raised about the lost potential for young parents when pregnancy occurs, and the academic and economic disadvantages that their children will experience. Nurses are in a key position to understand how teen pregnancy affects both the individual and the community. This chapter presents a variety of issues associated with teen pregnancy and proposes nursing interventions to promote healthy outcomes for individuals, families, and communities.

Although some specific risk factors are discussed here, there are four social determinants of health that influence teen pregnancy rates: (1) income, (2) education, (3) social support networks, and (4) living environment (Danawi et al., 2016). These four social determinants are discussed for a variety of populations in Chapter 23 in regard to contributing factors to vulnerability.

There have been some improvements in teen risk behaviors and some worsening of others. High school students report significant involvement in sexual intercourse. The Youth Risk Behavior Surveillance System (YRBS) monitors six categories of health-risk behaviors among youth and young adults. One of these categories relates to sexual behaviors related to unintended pregnancy and sexually transmitted diseases, including HIV infection (Centers for Disease Control and Prevention, 2020b). YRBS also reports on health-related behaviors including sexual identify and sex of sexual contacts as well as five other major categories of factors contributing to death and disability among teens. Other health issues associated with the teen years are use of alcohol and marijuana; mental health issues, including feeling sad and hopeless; and behaviors that place teenagers at risk for chronic illnesses and the leading causes of morbidity and mortality, including cardiovascular disease, cancer, and diabetes.

The Adolescent Client

Adolescents have limited experience in independently seeking health care. When they do seek care, it is often to discuss concerns about a possible pregnancy or to find a birth control method. These teens may also need assistance negotiating complex health care systems. Special approaches in both client interview and subsequent client education are often warranted. The behavior of adolescents toward the nurse can range from mature and competent during one visit to hostile, rude, or distant at other times because behavior often reflects intense anxiety over what the teen is experiencing.

Because client interviews usually begin with evaluation of a chief complaint, teens need to know that their concerns are heard. Health care providers may have their own opinions about what teenagers need and may fail to take the chief complaint seriously. For example, when a teen expresses ambivalence about or a desire to become pregnant, this should be discussed in depth even though the nurse may feel uncomfortable when asked to provide information to a teen about how to conceive. During this interview, the nurse can provide preconception counseling and emphasize the need to achieve good health and to establish a health-promoting lifestyle before pregnancy. Health risks to the mother, as well as to fetal development, can be discussed. The nurse can encourage a young person to consider lifetime goals and discuss how parenthood might affect them. Not only does information presented this way demonstrate that the nurse has heard what the teen is saying, but it also allows the nurse to provide useful health information that may encourage the teen to examine her plans carefully, seriously, and maturely.

It is also important to pay attention to what the teen *fails* to verbalize. Knowledge of adolescent health care issues is valuable so that the nurse can anticipate other health concerns and provide an environment in which the adolescent feels safe about discussing other issues. By creating a caring and understanding atmosphere, the nurse can encourage the young person to discuss concerns about family violence, drugs, alcohol, or dating.

Discussing reproductive health care is a sensitive matter for both teens and many adults. Teens may have difficulty expressing themselves because of a limited sexual vocabulary or embarrassment resulting from their lack of knowledge. The nurse must recognize this potential deficit and embarrassment and assist teens by anticipating concerns. It is also important to allow teens to express themselves in their own language, which may include crude or offensive words. Nurses must learn about common slang expressions and common misconceptions so they do not miss important concerns that a teenager might have. The nurse can offer more appropriate terms once trust is established.

Teens may have difficulty discussing topics that provoke a judgmental reaction, such as discussing STDs. See Chapter 12 for a discussion of STDs. The nurse can choose neutral words to evaluate symptoms (e.g., "Has there been a change in your typical vaginal discharge?"). This approach also gives the nurse a chance to educate the young client about normal anatomy and physiology.

Considerable debate exists over whether adolescents should make reproductive health care decisions without their parents' knowledge. The issue of reproductive rights, especially abortion, is controversial in the United States. There are both federal and state laws that affect this issue. The National Abortion and Reproductive Rights Action League Foundation (NARAL) has a comprehensive website that allows readers to examine the status in each state. See prochoiceamerican.org. The 116th Congress "reflects a wave of historical firsts—most significantly the first pro-choice majority in the House of Representatives" (NARAL, 2019). Factors that influence the pro-choice majority are a record number of women serving in Congress; more LGBTQ people serving; a younger freshman class; and record-breaking racial, ethnic, and religious diversity. Obstacles to services do exist, however, and this may result in a teen not receiving contraceptive information and treatment. Obstacles can include lack of transportation to a health care facility, insufficient money to pay for services, or lack of permission to leave school early to attend an appointment (Fig. 25.3).

Although most minor teens can consent to birth control services in the United States, there is great variability in who may access and release their medical records. In recognition of the importance of confidentiality in reproductive health care, federal privacy rules were established in 2002 as follow-up to the Health Insurance Portability and Accountability Act of 1996 (HIPAA). This rule, the HIPAA Privacy Rule (or more correctly, the Standards for Privacy of Individually Identifiable Health Information), established that if a minor consented to care, then only that individual could access and release those medical records. However, the Privacy Rule also deferred to existing state law. No state explicitly requires parental consent or notification for minors to obtain contraceptive services. However, two states (Texas and Utah) require parental consent for contraceptive services paid for with state funds (Guttmacher Institute, 2019),

which limits the confidentiality assurances offered to a teen seeking reproductive health care. Nurses who work with teens should be knowledgeable about state and federal laws so that they can accurately inform teenagers of their rights and limitations in seeking reproductive health care. Since state laws can change regarding reproductive health care, check what the laws and requirements are in your state.

Abortion services for adolescents are not clearly defined. No federal protection is extended to adolescents requesting abortion services, and the adolescent's right to privacy and ability to give consent varies by state. Confidential care to teenagers may mean the difference in preventing an unwanted pregnancy, an abortion, and a birth. This care can influence whether prenatal visits begin in the first trimester or in the second or third trimester. Teens have various reasons for pursuing confidential care, including seeking independence as well as serious and well-founded concerns about a parent's potential reaction (e.g., abuse or abandonment of the teen). Once nurses recognize the reason for confidential care, they can work with teens to discuss reproductive health care needs with the family. To do so, first clarify family values about sexuality and family communication styles with the teen. In a non-healthy family, referral to community agencies (e.g., child protective services, Al-Anon) may be necessary. However, the nurse may need to honor the adolescent's need for confidentiality for an unknown period and proceed with the usual interventions, such as pregnancy testing, options counseling, and referral for clinical care.

Many adults have difficulty understanding why young people would jeopardize their careers and personal potential by becoming pregnant during the teen years. Adolescents, however, do not view the world in the same way as adults. Teens often feel invincible and therefore do not recognize any risk related to their behaviors or anticipate the consequences. That is, they may not think that sexual activity will lead to pregnancy. When teens become pregnant, they do not believe that the negative outcomes they are advised of could come true. Many teens believe that they are unique and different and that everything will work out fine. The developmental circumstances of adolescence, coupled with potential background disadvantages, can magnify the problems facing the pregnant and parenting teen. Pregnant teens often express the unrealistic attitude that they can do it all: school, work, parenting, and socializing. However, compared to their peers, teen girls who have babies are more likely to: rely on public assistance; be poor as adults; and have children who have poorer educational, behavior, and health outcomes over the course of their lives than do children born to older parents (USDHHS, 2019). In regard to the teen mother, a disproportionate number are poor, have limited educational achievements, and have limited opportunities within their communities for positive youth experiences (CDC, 2019).

Most teens report that their pregnancy was unplanned. They typically think that a pregnancy should be delayed until people are older, have completed their education, and are employed and married. Several factors that often contribute to pregnancy are discussed next.

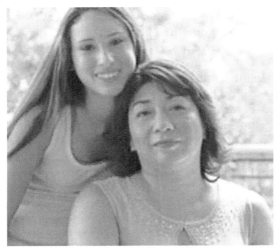

Fig. 25.3 Parents can help teens make healthy choices about sex (From https://www.cdc.gov/teenpregnancy/parent-guardian-resources/index.htm).

Sexual Activity, Use of Birth Control, and Peer and Partner Pressure

The sexual debut, or first experience with intercourse, for a teen has a significant impact on pregnancy risk. In 2019, among high school students who were surveyed, 27.4% were sexually active; approximately half were female and White, and approximately one third were in grade 12. Also 7% had sexual intercourse for the first time before they were 13 years of age. Among those reporting, 20.5% had sexual intercourse with more than two persons during the previous 3 months and 21.2% had drunk alcohol or used drugs before the last sexual intercourse (*MMWR*, Supplement/2020, p. 13). From 2005 to 2015 there was a linear decline in the percent of youth who initiated sexual intercourse: male students dropped from 46.8% to 41.2%, and female students dropped from 45.7% to 39.2%. Ethnicity of the students having sexual intercourse was also reported for the same time period: White students dropped from 43% to 39.9%, Black students dropped from 67.6% to 48.5%, and Hispanic students dropped from 51% to 42.5% (Ethier et al., 2018). The *Healthy People 2030* goal is to increase the proportion of adolescents who have never engaged in sexual intercourse by age 17 (USDHHS, 2020b).

Although more teens have begun using birth control in the past 10 years, there is still progress to be made. *Healthy People 2030* addresses this with goals to increase the proportion of 15- to 19-year-olds who use condoms and a hormonal contraceptive and increase the proportion of teens who receive reproductive health information through formal instruction as well as from their parents or guardians (USDHHS, 2020b). Condoms are the most commonly used method of birth control for adolescents. In 2015-2017, 89% of females and 94% of males aged 15 to 19 reported that they or their partner had used contraceptives the last time they had sexual intercourse, and 77% of females and 91% of males reported contraceptive use the first time they had sexual intercourse (Guttmacher Institute, 2019). The current recommendation for greatest protection against pregnancy and STI is the use of a hormonal contraceptive, preferably long-acting reversible contraception (LARC), and a condom, referred to as dual protection.

In 2012 the American College of Obstetricians and Gynecologists (ACOG) made a strong recommendation to encourage adolescents to use LARC methods—intrauterine devices and contraceptive implants. These methods are reversible and have the highest rates of continuation and prevention of pregnancy, rapid repeat pregnancy, and abortion in young women. Reports from the Contraceptive CHOICE Project, an observational clinical trial, prompted ACOG to strengthen their recommendation in 2015 when it was reported that LARC methods were 20 times more effective at preventing pregnancy in their participants (ACOG, 2015). As noted earlier, the use of alcohol and other substances is common among adolescents and can contribute to unplanned pregnancy. Mood-altering effects may reduce inhibitions about engaging in intercourse and interfere with the proper use of a chosen birth control method.

Peer pressure among teens is not a new phenomenon, but many of the influences have become more serious. Influence has expanded from fashion and language to cigarettes, substance abuse, sexuality, pregnancy, and sexting. Teens are more likely to be sexually active if their friends are sexually active (Gregg et al., 2018). Peers reinforce teen parenting by exaggerating birth control risks, discouraging abortion and adoption, and glamorizing the impending birth of the child.

Both young men and young women may think that allowing a pregnancy to happen verifies one's love and commitment for the other. In addition, young men from socioeconomically disadvantaged backgrounds may be more likely to say that fathering a child would make them feel more manly, and they are less likely to use an effective contraceptive (Farrell et al., 2017).

Other Factors

Other factors influencing teen pregnancy are a history of sexual victimization, family structure, parental influences, and diverse sexual orientations. With a history of poverty only, 16.8% of teens had been pregnant once by age 17. For teens with a history of poverty and reported child abuse or neglect, 28.9% had been pregnant by age 17 (Garwood et al., 2015). Adolescent girls with a history of sexual abuse are at risk for earlier initiation of voluntary sexual intercourse, are less likely to use birth control, are more likely to use drugs and alcohol at first intercourse, and are more likely to have older sexual partners. Adolescents are often the victims of coercive sex or statutory rape. Young women may also become pregnant as a result of forced sexual intercourse. A history of sexual victimization will influence a young woman's ability to exert control over future sexual experiences, which will affect the use of birth control and rejection of unwanted sexual experiences. Teen pregnancy is also more common among sexual minorities compared with heterosexuals, which is thought to be partially due to childhood mistreatment (Charlton et al., 2018). All these factors contribute to an increased risk for becoming pregnant. In addition, young women who have experienced a lifetime of economic, social, and psychological deprivation may think that a baby will bring joy into an otherwise bleak existence. Some mistakenly believe that a baby can provide the love and attention that her family has not provided.

Family structure can influence adolescent sexual behavior and pregnancy. While the number of single-parent families has increased in recent years, it is interesting that recent researchers found that it was not single-parent families with working mothers that had the highest risk for an unplanned teen pregnancy, but that it was adolescents who have girlfriends with early sexual activity who have a 1.63 times greater risk of getting pregnant unintentionally (Vázquez-Nava et al., 2014).

Parents have a major impact on whether teens make healthy decisions. Parenting styles can influence a young woman's risk for early sexual experiences and pregnancy. Parents who are extremely demanding and controlling or neglectful and who have low expectations are least successful in instilling parental values in their children. Parents who have high demands for their children to act maturely and who offer warmth and understanding with parental rules have children more likely to exhibit appropriate social behavior and to delay early sexual experiences and pregnancy. Children of parents who are neglectful are the most sexually experienced, followed by children of parents who are very strict. Teens who talk with their parents about sex, relationships, birth control, and pregnancy: (1) begin to have sex at a later age; (2) use condoms and birth control more often if they do have sex; (3) have better communication with romantic partners; (4) have sex less often (CDC, 2020a). Nurses can teach, coach, and support parents in learning how to talk with their children directly and provide useful, factual information.

Young Men and Paternity

Although there have been declines in the number of pregnant female teens in recent years, the percent of teenage fathers increased. At first, this may seem contradictory, but it may be explained by several factors: teenage males are partnering with older women, females are partnering with older males, paternity is more readily determined by genetic testing and voluntary establishment, child support is enforced, and stigma has decreased (Pirog et al., 2017). About 7% of males become fathers before the age of 20; two-thirds were ages 18 to 19 years when they fathered their first child, and one-third were younger than 18 years. These are conservative numbers because not all of the males are aware that a partner became pregnant, nor do they always know the outcome of the pregnancy. Teen fathers face special challenges because of their own social problems, including delinquency, alcohol or substance use, school problems, and limited future plans or ability to provide support. Paternity, or fatherhood, is legally established at the time of the birth for a married teen. It is more difficult to establish paternity among nonmarried couples. Some of the difficulty lies in the complexity of the specific state system for young men to acknowledge paternity. In some states, a young man may have to work with the judicial system outside of the hospital after the birth, and if he is younger than 18 years, he may need to involve his parents.

Some young couples do not attempt to establish paternity and prefer a verbal promise of assistance for the teen mother and child. Although a verbal commitment may be acceptable when the child is born, the mother may become more inclined to pursue the establishment of paternity later when the relationship ends or for reasons related to financial, social, or emotional needs of the child. Young women who receive state or federal assistance (e.g., TANF, Medicaid) may be asked to name the child's father so the judicial process can be used to establish paternity.

Young men's reactions to learning that their partner is pregnant vary. The reaction often depends on the nature of the relationship before the pregnancy. Many young men will accompany the young woman to a health care center for pregnancy diagnosis and counseling and prenatal visits and will attend the delivery. They may also choose to be involved with their children regardless of changes in their relationships with the teen mother. It is not unusual for a young man to be excluded or even rejected by the young woman's family (usually her mother). He may then begin to act as though he is disinterested when he may really feel

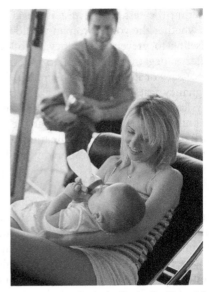

Fig. 25.4 It Is Important to Include Both the Teen Mother and the Father in Teaching About Child Development. (© 2012 Photos.com, a division of Getty Images. All rights reserved. Image #77280263.)

that he cannot provide resources for his child or does not know how to take care of the child. Mothers who report less social support from their child's father are more apt to be unhappy and distressed in the parenting role and consequently more at risk for abuse of the child (Massachusetts General Hospital [MGH], 2016) (Fig. 25.4).

Nurses can acknowledge and support the young man as he develops in the role of father. His involvement can positively affect his child's development and provide greater personal satisfaction for himself and greater role satisfaction for the young mother. The immediate concerns revolve around his financial responsibility, living arrangements, relationship issues, school, and work. The families of both teen parents can help clarify these issues and identify roles and responsibilities.

Early Identification of the Pregnant Teen

Some teens delay seeking pregnancy services because they fail to recognize signs such as breast tenderness and a late period. Most young women, however, suspect pregnancy as soon as a period is late. These young women may still delay seeking care because they falsely hope that the pregnancy will just go away. A teen also may delay seeking care to keep the pregnancy a secret from family members, who may be angry, disappointed, or force her into a decision she does not want to make, or because she does not want to have a gynecological examination.

Pay attention to subtle cues that a teenager may offer about sexuality and pregnancy concerns, such as questions about fertile periods or requests for confirmation that you need not miss a period to be pregnant. Once the nurse identifies the specific concern, he or she should then provide information about how and when to obtain pregnancy testing. The nurse should determine how a teenager would react to the possible pregnancy before completing the test. If the test is negative, the nurse should assess whether the young woman would consider birth control counseling to prevent pregnancy. A follow-up visit is important after a negative test result to determine whether retesting is necessary or if another problem exists.

If the pregnancy test result is positive, the next step is to perform a physical examination and pregnancy counseling. It is useful to do both at the same time so that the counseling is consistent with the findings of the examination. The purpose of the examination is to assess the duration and well-being of the pregnancy, as well as to test for STDs. Pregnancy counseling should include the following:

- Information on adoption, abortion, and childrearing
- Assessment of support systems for the young woman
- Identification of the immediate concerns she might have

The availability of affordable abortion services up to 13 weeks of gestation varies from community to community. Similarly, second-trimester services may be available locally or involve extensive travel and cost. The nurse should know about abortion services and provide information or refer the pregnant teenager to a pregnancy counseling service.

The pregnant teenager needs information about adoption, such as current policies among agencies that allow continued contact with the adopting family. Also, church organizations, private attorneys, and social service agencies provide a variety of adoption services with which the nurse should be familiar.

Pregnancy counseling requires that the nurse and young woman explore strengths and weaknesses for personal care and responsibility during pregnancy and parenting. Young women vary in their interest in including the partner or their parents in this discussion. It is important to discuss education and career plans, family finances and qualifications for outside assistance, and personal values about pregnancy and parenting at this time in their life. It may be difficult to focus on counseling in any depth at the time of the initial pregnancy testing results. A follow-up visit is usually more productive and should be arranged as soon as possible (Fig. 25.5).

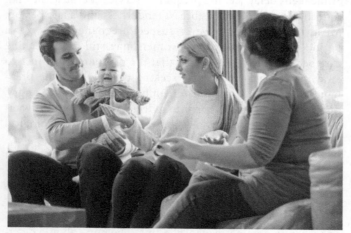

Fig. 25.5 Nurse Teaching a Young Couple Parenting Skills. (Copyright Monkey Business Images, #466375791, iStock, Thinkstock.)

As decisions are made about the course of the pregnancy, the nurse is instrumental in referral to appropriate programs such as Women, Infants, and Children (WIC), Medicaid, and prenatal services. The young woman and her family also need to know about expected costs of care and, if there is a family insurance policy, whether it will cover the pregnancy-related expenses of a dependent child. For those without insurance, the family can apply for Medicaid or determine whether local facilities offer indigent care programs (e.g., Hill-Burton programs for assistance with hospital expenses). The nurse can also begin prenatal education and counseling on nutrition, substance abuse and use, exercise, and special medical concerns.

Special Issues in Caring for the Pregnant Teen

Pregnant teenagers are considered high-risk obstetrical clients. Pregnancy complications can result from poverty, late entry into prenatal care, sporadic prenatal care, and limited self-care knowledge. Teens are more likely to get no prenatal care or to begin the care later in the pregnancy than their older counterparts. Nursing interventions through education and early identification of problems may dramatically alter the course of the pregnancy and the birth outcome. Some of the issues include violence, initiation of prenatal care, low-birth-weight infants and preterm delivery, nutrition, infant care, repeat pregnancy, and schooling and educational needs.

Violence

Teens are more likely to experience violence during their pregnancies than adult women. Age may be a factor in their greater vulnerability to potential perpetrators, who include partners, family members, and other acquaintances. Violence in pregnancy has been associated with an increased risk for substance abuse, poor compliance with prenatal care, and poor birth outcome. In the case of partner violence, young women may be protective of their partners because of fear or helplessness. Eliciting this history from an adolescent is not easy. The nurse must ask about violence at each visit. Frequent routine assessments are more revealing than a single inquiry at the first prenatal visit. Violence that begins in pregnancy may continue for several years after, with increasing severity. See Chapter 27 for a discussion of violence and human abuse.

Initiation of prenatal care. Pregnant adolescents differ remarkably from pregnant adults in initiation and compliance with prenatal care. Inadequate prenatal care has been associated with increased health risks to both the mother and the fetus. Once a teen is enrolled in prenatal care, the nurse becomes an important liaison between personnel at the clinical site and the young woman. Confusion and misunderstandings occur easily when teens do not understand what a health care provider says to them. Often these misunderstandings are based on lack of knowledge about basic anatomy and physiology. For example, a teen may be told as she gets close to term that the head of the baby is down and it can be felt. This is an alarming piece of information for a young woman who imagines the entire baby could just pop out at any time!

Cooperation between the nurse and the clinical staff can also maximize the client's compliance with special health or nutritional needs. For example, a teen who has premature contractions may be restricted to bed rest and instructed to increase fluids. The nurse who makes home visits can provide additional assessment of the teen's condition and can solve problems about self-care, hygiene, meals, and schooling.

Low-Birth-Weight Infants and Preterm Delivery

Teens are more likely than adult women to deliver infants weighing less than 5.5 lb or to deliver before 37 weeks of gestation. These low-birth-weight and premature infants are at greater risk for death in the first year of life and are at increased risk for long-term physical, emotional, and cognitive problems (Marvin-Dowle et al., 2018). For example, low-birth-weight and premature infants can be more difficult to feed and soothe. This challenges the limited skills of the young mother and can further strain relations with other members of the household, who may not know how to offer support or assistance.

The risk for low-birth-weight infants and premature births can be averted by the teen's early initiation into prenatal care. Although such births still occur, it is important to work closely with the teen mother as soon as she is identified as pregnant to try to promote compliance with prenatal care visits and self-care during the pregnancy. After the pregnancy, these infants and their mothers will benefit from frequent nursing supervision to ensure that their care is appropriate and that everyone in the home is coping adequately with the strain of a small infant.

Nutrition

The nutritional needs of a pregnant teenager are especially important. First, the teen lifestyle does not lend itself to overall good nutrition. Fast foods, frequent snacking, and hectic social schedules limit nutritious food choices. Snacks, which account for approximately a third of a teen's daily caloric intake, tend to be high in fat, sugar, and sodium and limited in essential vitamins and minerals. Second, the nutritive needs of both pregnancy and the concurrent adolescent growth spurt require the

adolescent to change her diet substantially. The growing teen must increase caloric nutrients to meet individual growth needs as well as allow for adequate fetal growth. Third, poor eating patterns of the teen and her current growth requirement may leave her with limited reserves of essential vitamins and minerals when the pregnancy begins. The nurse can assess the pregnant teenager's current eating pattern and provide creative guidance. Identifying good choices that a teen can consume "on the run" might include snacks of drinkable yogurt, leftover pizza, string cheese, or energy/granola bars. The teen who eats out can boost her protein at fast-food establishments by ordering milkshakes instead of soft drinks, and cheeseburgers or broiled chicken sandwiches can be ordered instead of hamburgers. Adding lettuce and tomato or other sliced vegetables to burgers will improve nutrition, and fruit smoothies can satisfy a sweet craving (Cornforth, 2018). Table 25.2 describes adolescent nutritional needs during pregnancy.

Weight gain during pregnancy is one of the strongest predictors of infant birth weight. Although precise weight gain goals in adolescence are controversial, pregnant adolescents who gain 25 to 35 lb have the lowest incidence of low-birth-weight babies. Babies born to teenagers may be at risk for being small for gestational age despite adequate weight gain if there is very slow gain in the first 24 weeks. Teenagers who begin the pregnancy at a normal weight should be counseled to begin weight gain in the first trimester and to average gains of 1 lb per week for the second and third trimesters. Younger teen mothers (ages 13 to 16), because of their own growth demands, may need to gain more weight than older teen mothers (ages 17 and older) to have the same birth weight baby.

It is important for the nurse to assess the attitudes of the pregnant teen about weight gain and to monitor her progress, providing feedback on adequate weight gain and counseling if weight gain is excessive. Gaining weight beyond the recommendations raises the risk for infants to be hypoglycemic, to be large for gestational age, and to have low Apgar scores, seizures,

TABLE 25.2 Adolescent Nutritional Needs During Pregnancy

Nutrient	Daily Requirement During Pregnancy[a]	Food Source
Calcium	1300 mg for ages 14–18 and 1000 for ages 19+	Macaroni and cheese; pizza; puddings, milk, yogurt; also fortified juices, water, breakfast bars and fast foods, including Taco Bell's chili cheese burrito, McDonald's Big Mac
Iron	27 (milligrams) mg	Meats; dried beans; peas; dark green, leafy vegetables; whole grains; fortified cereal; absorption of iron from plant foods improved by vitamin C sources taken simultaneously
Iodine	15 mg	Iodized table salt, dairy products, seafood, meats, eggs, some breads
Folic acid	600 micrograms (mcg)	Fortified cereal, enriched bread and pasta, peanuts, dark green vegetables, orange juice, beans
Vitamin A	750 mcg age 18 and younger; 770 mcg for age 19+	Carrots, green leafy vegetables, sweet potatoes
Vitamin B6	1.9 mg	Chicken, fish, liver, pork, whole grain cereals, bananas
Vitamin D	600 IU	Sunlight, fortified milk products, fatty fish
Vitamin C	600 IU	Citrus fruit, broccoli, tomatoes, and strawberries
Vitamin B12	2.6 mcg	Meat, fish, poultry, milk
Choline	450 mg	Meat, beef, liver, eggs, peanuts, soy products

American College of Obstetricians and Gynecologists, *Nutrition during pregnancy*, 2020b. www.acog.org.

polycythemia, and a predisposition to obesity (Restall et al., 2014). Family support of the pregnant teen can be a strong influence in adequate weight gain and good nutrition during the pregnancy. Nutrition education should emphasize what accounts for weight gain and how fetal growth will benefit.

Globally, iron-deficiency anemia is the most common nutritional problem among both pregnant and nonpregnant adolescent females with about 50% of the cases being due to inadequate intake. The metabolic processes involved in tissue oxygenation are dependent upon iron (Abu-Ouf and Jan, 2015). The increased maternal plasma volume and increased fetal demands for iron (especially in the third trimester) can further compromise the adolescent. Iron deficiency in pregnancy may contribute to increased fetal prematurity, low birth weight, and low iron stores for the infant that can last for up to one year. For the mother, iron deficiency may contribute to cardiovascular stress, increased risk of urinary tract infection, sleep difficulties, decreased well-being, postpartum hemorrhage, and slower wound healing (Abu-Ouf and Jan, 2015). The nurse can reinforce the need for the teen to take prenatal vitamins during pregnancy and after the baby's birth. Vitamins should contain 30 to 60 mg of elemental iron daily. The nurse should educate about iron-rich foods and foods that promote iron absorption, such as those containing vitamin C.

Infant Care

Many adolescents have cared for babies and small children and feel confident and competent. Few teens are ever prepared, however, for the reality of 24-hour care of an infant. The nurse can help prepare the teen for the transition to motherhood while she is still pregnant. The trend toward early discharge from the hospital has made prenatal preparation even more important. The nurse can enlist the support of the teen's parents in education about infant care and stimulation. Young fathers-to-be would benefit from this education as well. Adolescents may not know how to communicate with an infant or know about their growth and development, or they may have unrealistic expectations about their children's development (Healthy Children Organization, [HCO], 2017). For example, they may expect their children to feed themselves at an early age or think that their children's behavior is more difficult than an adult mother might think. These skills can be taught and may prevent the child from later developing academic or behavioral problems.

Abusive parenting is more likely to occur when the parents have limited knowledge about normal child development or when they cannot adequately empathize with a child's needs. Younger teens are at risk for being unable to understand what their infant or child needs. This frustration may be exhibited as abusive behavior toward the child. Nurses need to continually assess for child abuse risks when dealing with teens who exhibit greater psychological distress or lack social supports (McHugh et al., 2015).

After the birth of the baby, the nurse should observe how the mother responds to infant cues for basic needs and distress. Specific techniques that the new mother can be instructed to use in early child care are listed in the How To box. Parenting education should begin as early as possible. Adolescents who

feel competent as parents have higher self-esteem, which in turn positively influences their relationship with their child. Recognizing these good parenting skills and providing positive feedback help a young mother gain confidence in her role (Angley et al., 2015).

A useful resource is *How to have a healthy teen pregnancy*, American Pregnancy Association, www.americanpregnancy. org, accessed February 2020. See also "Frequently asked questions," American College of Obstetricians and Gynecologists, August 2020b, www.acog.org, accessed August 2020.

HOW TO PROMOTE INTERACTIONS BETWEEN THE TEEN MOTHER AND HER BABY

The nurse can make the following suggestions to the teen mother:

- Make eye contact with your baby. Position your face 8 to 10 inches from your baby's face and smile.
- Talk to your baby often. Use simple sentences but try to avoid baby talk. Allow time for your baby to "answer." This will help your baby acquire language and communication skills.
- Babies often enjoy when you sing to them, and this may help soothe them during a difficult time or help them fall asleep. Experiment with different songs and melodies to see which your baby seems to like.
- Babies at this age cannot be spoiled. Instead, when babies are held and cuddled, they feel secure and loved.
- Babies cry for many reasons and for no reason at all. If your baby has a clean diaper, has recently been fed, and is safe and secure, he or she may just need to cry for a few minutes. What works to calm your baby may be different from that for other babies you have known. You can try rocking, gentle reassuring words, soft music, or quiet.
- Make feeding times pleasant for both of you. Do not prop the bottle in your baby's mouth. Instead, you should sit comfortably, hold your baby in your arms, and offer the bottle or breast.
- When babies are awake, they love to play. They enjoy taking walks and looking at brightly colored objects or pictures and toys that make noises, such as rattles and musical toys.

Schooling and Educational Needs

Teen parents may have had limited school success before the pregnancy. In addition, the demands of pregnancy and parenting may make completing high school difficult or impossible. Returning to school may reduce the possibility of a closely spaced second birth, which would pose both physical and emotional stresses for the teen. Federal legislation passed in 1975 prohibits schools from excluding students because they are pregnant. Instead it is important to keep the pregnant adolescent in school during the pregnancy and to have her return as soon as possible after the birth. Several factors may positively influence a young woman's return to school. These include her parents' level of education and marital stability, small family size, whether there have been reading materials at home, whether her mother is employed, and whether the young woman is African American.

It may be hard to find affordable quality child care. Young women who have pregnancy complications may choose home instruction. The availability of home education depends on state board of education regulations. If the teen returns to school, be sure to discuss these needs: (1) using the bathroom frequently, (2) carrying and drinking more fluids or eating more snacks to relieve nausea, (3) climbing stairs and carrying heavy book bags, and (4) fitting comfortably behind stationary desks. Schools that are committed to keeping students enrolled are generally helpful and will assist in accommodating special needs.

MENTAL ILLNESS IN THE UNITED STATES

Mental health and illness can be viewed as a continuum. Mental health is being able to engage in productive activities and to have fulfilling relationships with other people, to adapt to change, and to cope with adversity. *Healthy People 2030* (USDHHS, 2020b*)* "focuses on the prevention, screening, assessment, and treatment of mental disorders and behavioral conditions, and says that about half of all people in the United States will be diagnosed with a mental illness at some point in their lifetime." Mental health is an integral part of personal well-being, of both family and interpersonal relationships, and of contributions to community or society. Mental disorders are conditions characterized by alterations in thinking, mood, or behavior associated with distress or impaired functioning. Mental illness refers collectively to all diagnosable mental disorders. Severe mental disorders are determined by diagnoses and criteria that include the degree of functional disability (American Psychiatric Association, 2013). Mental disorders occur across the life span and affect persons of all races, cultures, sexes, and educational and socioeconomic groups. They are common in the United States and internationally.

The SAMHSA of the USDHHS provides considerable information about mental illness. SAMHSA also provides a range of timely publications for practitioners as well as the public related to substance abuse and mental illness. Mental disorders "involve changes in thinking, mood, and/or behavior." To be formally diagnosed as having a mental disorder depends on a reduction in the person's ability to function as a result of the disorder. SAMHSA defines serious mental illness as "someone over 18 having (within the last year) a diagnosable mental, behavior, or emotional disorder that causes serious functional impairment that substantially interferes with or limits one or more major life activities and for people under age 18, the term "Serious emotional disturbance" refers to the above definition with the limitation being able to function in the family, school, or community activities (SAMHSA, 2020). SAMHSA defines any mental illness (AMI) as persons having any mental, behavioral, or emotional disorder in the past year that met DSM-5 criteria. These are criteria in the *Diagnostic and Statistical Manual of Mental Disorders,* fifth edition. The National Institute for Mental Health's Mental Health Information page has information about specific conditions and disorders as well as their symptoms. The National Survey on Drug Use and Health (NSDUH) is the primary source of data on illicit drug use, alcohol use, SUD, and mental health issues for the civilian, noninstitutionalized population in the United States. It is an annual survey of persons 12 years and older (SAMHSA, 2019).

In 2018, an estimated 47.6 million adults aged 18 or older had AMI in the past year. An estimated 11.4 million adults had SMI. Also in 2018, about 1 in 7 adolescents aged 12 to 17 had a major depressive episode (MDE) in the past year. In 2020 an estimated 5.8 million Americans had Alzheimer disease. One in 10 people in the United States age 65 or older had Alzheimer disease in 2020. People younger than age 65 can develop this form of dementia, but it is less prevalent. The risk factors for the disease are older age, genetics, and family history (Alzheimer's Association, 2020). The above provides examples of mental health issues in the community. There are many other forms of mental illness including affective disorders such as major depression, bipolar illness, and anxiety disorders that can impair effective functioning.

The impact of mental illness on overall health and productivity in the United States and throughout the world is not always recognized. In addition to diagnosable mental conditions, there is an increasing awareness and concern about the public health burden of stress. This stress was intensified during the pandemic of 2020 with the enormous uncertainty about the future, the isolation imposed by the need to prevent the spread of the virus, the need to wear face masks in public, and so forth.

Mental health issues are a worldwide public health problem. The WHO reports that there is a sizable global burden of mental health, substance abuse, and neurological diseases at 14%, and in recognition of the lack of resources, the WHO launched a mental health global action program (mhGAP) to begin to address the needs (WHO, 2016). The WHO poster "No Health Without Mental Health" describes the need to integrate physical and mental health services. It is important for nurses to recognize and provide health services for those with mental disorders in a variety of nontraditional community settings.

Although every person is vulnerable to stressful life events and may develop mental health problems, those with chronic and persistent mental illness have numerous problems. Mental illness is misunderstood, and those who suffer from it often experience stigma and lack of social support that is critical to health. Persons with mental illness are often identified by the illness as a "schizophrenic" instead of a person with the illness. The onset of the disruptive symptoms of schizophrenia often occurs just as young persons are attempting to finish schooling and develop a career, shattering lives and driving many into a lifetime of underemployment, poverty, and lack of access to adequate health services, housing, and social supports. Many accessible and coordinated services are needed to enable people with chronic mental illness to live in the community, yet these often are not available. Despite the inadequacy of resources, advances have been made in the treatment of mental illness. Two movements have influenced treatment advances: consumer advocacy and better understanding of the neurobiology of mental illness (Macedo, 2017; Pandya and Jan Myrick, 2013). Naturally, the financing of mental health services affects access to care and influences treatment. The system known as managed care had a significant impact on service delivery for the past 25 years, and passage of mental health parity and national health care reform through the Patient Protection and Affordable Health Care Act will influence mental health care in the future (Mechanic & Olfson, 2016; Pearlman, 2013). It takes many accessible and coordinated services to enable people with chronic mental illness to stay in the community, and these services are not always available. Community mental health nurses (CMHNs) play an important role in identifying stressful events, assessing stress responses, educating communities, and intervening to prevent or alleviate disability and disease resulting from stress. The following descriptions of several key issues and populations at high risk for mental illness illustrate the scope of this public health concern.

Deinstitutionalization

Deinstitutionalization involved moving many people from state psychiatric hospitals to communities. The cost of institutional care was perhaps the main reason for the movement; other influences included the discovery of psychotropic medications and civil rights activism (Boyd, 2018). The goal of deinstitutionalization was to improve the quality of life for people with mental disorders by providing services in the communities in which they lived rather than in large institutions. To change the locus of care, large hospital wards were closed, and persons with severe mental disorders were returned to the community to live. Many were discharged to the care of family members; others went to nursing homes. Still others were placed in apartments or other types of adult housing; some of these were supervised settings and others were not.

Unfortunately, the community-based services were not always in place when persons were released to the community, and continuity of care became a problem. Deinstitutionalization was noble in conception yet bankrupt in implementation. For example, families were not prepared for the treatment responsibilities they had to assume, and few mental health systems offered them education and support programs. Although many older adult clients were admitted to nursing homes and personal care settings, education programs were seldom available for staff. The staff often lacked the skills necessary to treat persons with mental disorders. In addition, some clients found themselves in independent settings such as rooming houses and single-room occupancy hotels with little or no supervision, and others were placed in jails and prisons. These types of issues prompted additional legislation and advocacy efforts.

The development of community mental health centers (CMHCs) was based partially on the principle that persons with mental disorders had a right to treatment in the least restrictive environment (Boyd, 2018). Although CMHCs were less restrictive than institutions, they lacked necessary services. For example, people with severe mental disorders require daily monitoring or hospitalization during acute episodes of illness. Even though hospital services were available, many individuals expressed their rights to refuse treatment and resisted admission. Also, transitional care after discharge for those who were admitted to hospitals was not available in most communities. With the repeal of the Mental Health Systems Act in 1980, federal leadership was reduced, and costs were shifted back to the states from the federal government. This further impeded the implementation and provision of community mental health services. State systems of mental health services developed in varied ways and were often inadequate. In 1990 the Americans

with Disabilities Act (ADA) was passed. The ADA mandated that individuals with mental and physical disabilities not be discriminated against and be brought into the mainstream of American life through access to employment and public services (Boyd, 2018). History reveals that past legislation promoted the rights of persons with mental disorders, but litigation was also responsible for the lack of growth, if not the decline, in community mental health services.

At-Risk Populations for Mental Illness
Children and Adolescents

The goals of the community mental health movement are consistent with the health promotion and disease prevention objectives outlined in *Healthy People 2030*. These objectives aim to increase the number of children screened and treated for mental health problems. Children are at risk for disruption of normal development by biological, environmental, and psychosocial factors that impair their mental health, interfere with education and social interactions, and keep them from realizing their full potential as adults (USDHHS, 2020b). For example, children may become depressed after a loss or may develop behavior problems from abuse or neglect. Examples of environmental factors include crowded living conditions, violence, separation from parents, and lack of consistent caregivers. Exposure to community violence was related to significant stress and depression in children. Depression, anxiety, and attention deficit disorders are often diagnosed in children, and intellectual disabilities, Down syndrome, and autism are examples of chronic disorders. These problems affect growth and development and influence mental health during adolescence.

Suicide was the second leading cause of death for youth ages 10 to 24. Males take their lives about four times more often than do females, yet females are more likely to have suicidal thoughts than males are. Firearms are the most common method of suicide among males, and poisoning among females. *Healthy People 2030* has objectives related to reducing suicide attempts by adolescents; screening for depression in both adolescents and adults; and increasing the number of children and adolescents who have a serious emotional disturbance and who get treatment (USDHHS, 2020b). Some of the risk factors for both adolescents and adults include prior suicide attempts, stressful life events, and access to lethal methods. In addition to depression and substance abuse, adolescent problems include conduct disorders, social anxiety, and eating disorders. See the DSM-5 for a description of conduct disorders and social anxiety (American Psychiatric Association, 2013).

Effective services for children, particularly for those with serious emotional disturbances, depends on promoting collaboration across critical areas of support, including schools, families, social services, health, mental health, and juvenile justice. Better services and collaboration for children with serious emotional disturbance and their families will result in greater school retention, decreased contact with the juvenile justice system, increased stability of living arrangements, and improved educational, emotional, and behavioral development. Children and adolescents require a variety of mental health services, including crisis intervention and both short-term and long-term counseling. Nurses working in community settings, well-child clinics, and home health can help offset this problem through prevention and education and by including parents in program planning. Because many children and adolescents lack services or access to them, community mental health assessment activities are essential. Assessment activities include identifying types of programs available or lacking in places in which children and adolescents spend time. Assessments should be performed in schools and in homes of clients, as well as in day-care centers, churches, and organizations that plan and guide age-specific play and entertainment programs. Assessment data are essential for planning and developing programs that address mental health problems prevalent from the prenatal period through adolescence. Preventing problems during these developmental periods can reduce mental health problems in adulthood. Areas that should be considered include children and adolescents who engage in physical fights and bullying. Families, schools, religious and community organizations, and the media are important influences on the way children and youth view violence. Education and role modeling are important aspects of prevention. During the pandemic of 2020 and 2021, more health care and mental health visits were conducted via telemedicine. Young people with their competency with telecommunications were adept at working with providers online.

Adults

Stress contributes to adults' mental health status. Sources of stress include multiple role responsibilities, job insecurity, lack of or diminishing resources, and unstable relationships. All of these sources of stress were evidenced in many adults beginning in early 2020 when the pandemic began to spread around the world. These and other conditions can undermine mental health and contribute to serious mental illness, depression, anxiety disorders, and substance abuse. Objectives of *Healthy People 2030* (USDHHS, 2020b) are aimed at helping adults access treatment to decrease associated human and economic costs and to reduce rates of suicide.

At some time or another, almost all adults will experience a tragic or unexpected loss, a serious setback, or a time of profound sadness, grief, or distress. Major depressive disorder, however, differs both in intensity and duration from normal sadness or grief. Depression disrupts relationships and the ability to function and can be fatal. In terms of suicide, the diagnosable mental disorder is most likely to be depression. Other risk factors include prior suicide attempts, stressful life events, and access to lethal methods. Also, domestic violence can lead to PTSD and major depression among women. Available medications and psychological treatment can help 80% of those with depression, yet only a few seek help. Those with depression are more likely to visit a physician for some other reason, and the mental health condition may not be noted. Therefore it is important that nurses in all settings recognize and screen for depression.

Anxiety disorders are common both in the United States and elsewhere. An alarming 31.1% of the adult population will experience an anxiety disorder at some time in their lives (NIMH, 2018). Anxiety disorders may have an early onset and are characterized by recurrent episodes of illness and periods of disability.

The lifetime rates of co-occurrence of mental disorders and SUD are high. In 2018 approximately 358,000 adolescents had a SUD and a MDE. That same year an estimated 9.2 million adults aged 18 or older had both an AMI and at least one SUD, and 3.2 million adults had co-occurring SMI and an SUD in the past year (SAMHSA, 2019).

How can nurses intervene? The general medical sector, including primary care clinics, hospitals, and nursing homes, has long been identified as the initial point of contact for many adults with mental disorders; for some, these providers may be the only source of mental health services. Early detection and intervention for mental health problems can be increased if persons seeking primary care are assessed for mental health problems. Nurses are in an ideal position to assess and detect mental health problems. They conduct comprehensive biopsychosocial assessments and are often the professionals whom clients trust most with sensitive information. The use of screening tools for depression, anxiety, substance abuse, and cognitive impairment can assist in early detection and intervention for mental health problems. Suicide can be prevented in many cases by early recognition and treatment of mental disorders and by preventive interventions that focus on risk factors. Thus reduction in access to lethal methods and recognition and treatment of mental and substance abuse disorders are among the most promising approaches to suicide prevention. Nurses, long respected as community health providers, can work with legislators to develop measures to limit access to weapons such as handguns.

Adults with Serious Mental Illness

Healthy People 2030 has a variety of objectives that address tertiary prevention and are targeted to persons with depression and serious mental illness. Examples are objectives related to increasing the proportion of homeless adults who get mental health services and to increasing the proportion of adults with depression or serious mental illness who get treatment. Brief hospital stays and inadequate community resources have resulted in an increased number of persons with serious mental illness living on the streets or in jail. Many of the persons in jail actually suffer from a mental illness. Some people arrested for nonviolent crimes could be better served if diverted from the jail system to a community-based mental health treatment program with linkage to mental health services. About half of the homeless persons in the United States have a serious mental illness or a substance abuse problem, and in 2019, 37,085 veterans were homeless (National Alliance to End Homelessness, 2019). Many people with severe mental disorders live in poverty because they lack the ability to earn or maintain a suitable standard of living. Even people who live with family caregivers or in supervised housing are at risk for inadequate services because the long-term care they require frequently depletes human and fiscal resources. An effective approach for helping persons with SMI is to partner with consumers to facilitate recovery through intensive case management (Fowler et al., 2018).

CASE STUDY

Two-year-old twins Reba and Tracy have had an eventful childhood. Their 16-year-old mother, Sheri, started prenatal care late in her pregnancy and delivered them at 35 weeks of gestation; they were small for gestational age. Sheri and the baby's father, Jeb, who was 21, had dropped out of high school; he used illegal drugs. The twins left the hospital at 2 weeks of age to live with Sheri at the Salvation Army apartments. Sheri's erratic and hostile behavior was impossible for her parents to tolerate. Her father was on disability compensation for extreme hypertension, and his elderly, bedridden mother lived in the mobile home as well.

Sheri, Jeb, and the twins were evicted from the Salvation Army when Sheri was found to be using drugs, so they moved in with some other young friends. By the time the twins were 15 months old, they showed clear signs of developmental delay. Tracy seemed not to see well, and Reba did not walk yet. Neither of the twins spoke an intelligible word, and neither was up to date on immunizations. With Sheri's permission, public health nurse Gina Smith talked with Sheri's parents about taking custody of the twins so that they might get the stability and care they needed. The grandparents agreed, and Sheri looked relieved when she moved the girls in with her parents. Sheri returned to living with friends.

Ms. Smith assessed the safety of the grandparents' mobile home for toddlers. She reviewed the normal milestones the girls should be attaining and taught the grandparents games they could play that would help the girls progress in their speech. She brought children's books from the local Book Buddies program for them to look at together. Normal nutritional needs for toddlers were reviewed. Within months, the girls started talking and gaining weight. Tracy got glasses, and Reba got physical therapy to help her learn to walk. With the help of the nurse and their grandparents, the twins began to thrive. Are there other actions that the nurse could take to provide comprehensive care to the grandparents who have now become the caregivers for these young twins?

Created by Deborah C. Conway, Assistant Professor (retired), School of Nursing, University of Virginia.

Nurses can provide important case management services, coordinate resources for consumers, and function as important members of assertive community treatment programs, which provide continuous assistance to persons with mental illness. Nurses by philosophy and training promote independent living and provide support and encouragement for persons to achieve a maximal level of wellness and function. Nurses recognize the importance of the mental health benefits of meaningful work that improves self-esteem and independence. Nursing interventions can be provided in shelters, soup kitchens, and other places in which homeless persons receive food and protection. In providing these nursing interventions, consider the nutritional value of the meals served in the shelters and soup kitchens. Would the food be appropriate for a person with diabetes, hypertension, or another chronic disease? If the person being housed in a shelter is mentally ill and needs to take medication regularly, will that be possible in terms of getting the medication and keeping it in a safe place?

Older Adults

According to the American Community Survey Reports, a service of the United States Census Bureau, "lower fertility and increased longevity have led to the rapid growth of the older population across the world and in the United States" (Roberts, Ogunwole,

Blakeslee, and Rabe, 2018, p. 1). "In 2015 among the 7.3 billion people estimated worldwide, 617.1 million (9 percent) were aged 65 and older. By 2030 it is estimated that 12% of the world's population or 1 billion people will be in this age group" (Roberts et al., 2018 and revised in 2019, p. 1). In the United States, the older population grew from 3.1 million in 1900 to 35.0 million in 2000, and this group was estimated in the 2016 ACS to be 49.2 million in the United States with more older females than males, 27.5 million compared to 21.8 million (Roberts et al., 2018). It is expected that the ethnic, racial, and cultural makeup of this group will become more diverse. The mental health and substance use (MH/SU) needs of this population often occur with other health problems, and this complicates treatment. The most prevalent of these conditions are depressive disorders and dementia-related behavioral and psychiatric symptoms. Compounding the problem is the fact that older people metabolize alcohol and drugs differently than their younger counterparts, and commonly used medications may alter physical or mental health problems and increase the person's risk for overdose. Although many older people maintain highly functional lives, others have mental health deficits associated with normal sensory losses related to aging, failing physical health, difficulty performing activities of daily living, and social deprivation or isolation. Life changes related to work roles and retirement often result in reduced social contacts and support. Other losses are associated with the death of a spouse, other family members, or friends. Reduced social networks and contacts brought about by these life events can influence mood and contribute to serious states of depression. Older adults were especially at risk for depression during the pandemic that began in 2020. Given their age, they were considered an at-risk population and were urged to stay home, socially isolate when they needed to leave home, and wear masks whenever they were out of the home and around other people. However, depression is not a normal part of aging. Given the losses of family, friends, and possibly their health that older individuals experience, it is important to differentiate between grief and major depression.

The depression rate among older adults is half that of younger people, but the presence of a physical or chronic illness increases rates of depression. Depression rates for older adults in long-term care either at home or in nursing homes range from 5% to 25% (Haigh et al., 2018). Alzheimer disease and vascular conditions can cause a severe loss of mental abilities with behavioral manifestations. Nearly half of those older than 85 years of age have symptoms of cognitive impairment severe enough to impair function. All of these conditions affect the mental health status of individuals and their family caregivers.

Older adults, because they may depend on others for care, are at risk for abuse and neglect. Healthy aging activities such as physical activity and establishing social networks improve the mental health of older adults. Older adults underuse the mental health system and are more likely to be seen in primary care or be recipients of care in institutions. The nurse can reach them by organizing health promotion programs through senior centers or other community-based settings. Many health-promoting activities beginning in 2020 were done remotely through the Internet in order to keep older

BOX 25.2 Examples of Sources of Information and Help for People With Mental Illness and Mental Health Problems

- National Alliance for the Mentally Ill: http://www.nami.org
- Alcoholics Anonymous: http://www.aa.org
- Al-Anon: http://www.al-anon.org
- Alzheimer's Association: http://www.alz.org
- American Anorexia/Bulimia Association: http://www.anad.org
- American Association of Suicidology: http://www.suicidology.org
- Anxiety Disorders Association of America: http://www.adaa.org
- Children and Adults with Attention Deficit Disorder: http://www.chadd.org
- Depression and Bipolar Support Alliance: http://www.dbsalliance.org
- Gamblers Anonymous: http://www.gamblersanonymous.org
- National Center for Post-Traumatic Stress Disorder: http://www.ptsd.va.gov
- National Center for Learning Disabilities: http://www.ncld.org
- International Obsessive-Compulsive Foundation: http://www.iocdf.org
- Overeaters Anonymous: http://www.oa.org
- Schizophrenics Anonymous: http://www.schizophrenia.com

adults engaged in the activities that they had previously attended in person. Most family caregivers are women who care for a spouse, an aging parent, or a child with a long-term disabling illness. These caregivers are also at risk for health disruption. The impact of caregiving has been studied in persons who care for those with chronic illness and in families of persons with schizophrenia. Caregivers of persons with severely disabling mental disorders often have their mental health threatened by lack of social support, the stigma of the disease, and chronic strain. During stressful life events such as these, it is important for caregivers to know how to manage the many competing demands in their lives. The need to meet competing demands accelerated during the COVID-19 pandemic when many male and female workers had to work at home, their children had to go to school at home, and there may have been adults or children in the home who needed special attention and care.

Activities to improve the mental health status of adults include public education programs, prevention approaches, and providing mental health services in primary care. An increasing number of these activities were moved to an online versus a face-to-face format beginning in 2020. Many national organizations designed for groups with specific problems have local chapters or information that can be accessed on the Internet (Box 25.2).

Cultural Diversity

As discussed in Chapter 7, health care providers need to understand the cultural differences among the various populations they serve. In particular, nurses need to know how various groups in the United States perceive mental health and mental illness and treatment services. These factors affect whether people seek mental health care, how they describe their symptoms, the duration of care, and the outcomes of the care received. Research has shown that various populations use mental health services differently. They may not seek mental health services in the formal system, they may drop out of care, or they may seek care at much later stages of illness, driving the service costs higher. Although all socioeconomic and cultural groups have mental health problems, low-income groups are at greater risk because they often lack resources for meeting basic physical and mental health needs.

The predominant minority populations in the United States are African Americans, Hispanics, Asian Americans and Pacific Islanders, Native Americans (including Native Alaskans), and Middle Eastern Americans. There is a great deal of diversity among these groups, as well as within each of these groups, because they are comprised of subgroups with unique cultural differences. Therefore it is important to avoid simplification and overgeneralization in discussions about the characteristics and problems of minorities. It is increasingly important to have competent interpreters if the health care provider does not speak the language of the patient or the family. Also, it is critical to conduct community assessments to determine unique characteristics and factors that contribute to mental health needs within specific aggregates of the population. The information presented here is intended to stimulate thinking and awareness for developing nursing activities in individual communities. Community assessments that include data about specific populations from organized agencies such as the Indian Health Service are important because assessment data guide the nurses' activities during all steps of the nursing process as well as when using the six essential cognitive skills of clinical judgment: recognize cues, analyze cues; prioritize hypotheses; generate solutions, take action, and evaluate outcomes. Nurses working within broad-based coalitions of consumers, families, other providers, and community leaders can help achieve the goals of accessible, culturally sensitive, and quality mental health services for all of our people.

LEVELS OF PREVENTION AND THE NURSE

It is important for nurses to understand levels of prevention related to poverty, homelessness, teen pregnancy, and mental illness. Nurses can influence political and social policies and programs such as those for affordable housing, community outreach services, preventive health services, and other assistance programs for their clients. It is difficult to separate services for these high-risk groups into primary, secondary, and tertiary levels of prevention because interventions can be assigned to more than one level. Affordable housing, for example, may qualify as primary prevention, but it could also be an important secondary or tertiary preventive intervention.

Examples of primary preventive services include affordable housing, housing subsidies, effective job-training programs, employer incentives, preventive health care services, multisystem case management, birth control services, safe-sex education, needle exchange programs, parent education, and counseling programs. As primary prevention for mental health problems, nurses can provide education about stress reduction techniques to seniors attending a health fair, and the health fair may be a virtual educational experience.

Secondary preventive activities are aimed at reducing the prevalence or pathological nature of a condition. They involve early diagnosis, prompt treatment, and limitation of disability. For example, these services might target persons on the verge of becoming high risk because of the threat of homelessness, as well as those who are newly homeless.

 LEVELS OF PREVENTION

Related to Community Mental Health

Primary Prevention: Prevent Disability
- Educate populations about mental health issues.
- Teach stress reduction techniques.
- Support and provide prenatal education.
- Provide support to caregivers.

Secondary Prevention: Limit Disability
- Conduct screenings to detect mental health disorders.
- Provide mental health interventions after stressful events.

Tertiary Prevention: Reduce Disability
- Provide health promotion activities to persons with serious and persistent mental illness.
- Promote support group participation for those with mental health disabilities.
- Advocate for rehabilitation and recovery services.

Examples include supportive and emergency housing, targeted case management, housing subsidies, soup kitchens and meal sites, and comprehensive physical and mental health services. When the COVID-19 pandemic occurred, many ways in which people received care were changed. There were drive-by or walk-up programs to provide food rather than in-person facilities.

Tertiary prevention efforts attempt to restore and enhance functioning. On a community level, these might include support of affordable housing, promotion of psychosocial rehabilitation programs, and involvement in advocacy groups for the mentally ill or homeless population. Tertiary prevention of homelessness includes comprehensive case management, physical and mental health services, emergency shelter housing, needle exchange programs, and drug and alcohol treatment. It is important to know about the social and political environment in which problems occur. Nurses can influence politicians and other policymakers at the federal, state, and local levels about the plight of vulnerable populations in their community.

ROLE OF THE NURSE

Nurses have a critical role in the delivery of health care to poor, homeless, mentally ill, and other high-risk people. To be effective, nurses need strong physical and psychosocial assessment skills, current knowledge of available resources, and an ability to convey respect, dignity, and value to each person. Nurses need to be able to work with their clients to promote, maintain, and restore health. Nurses must be prepared to look at the whole picture: the person, the family, and the community interacting with the environment. The assessment may take place in the home or in a community site. Visiting in the home provides a great deal of useful information about the family, their resources, support systems, and knowledge of common housekeeping and health issues.

QSEN   FOCUS ON QUALITY AND SAFETY EDUCATION FOR NURSES

Targeted Competency: Client-Centered Care—Recognize the client or designee as the source of control and full partner in providing compassionate and coordinated care based on respect for client's preferences, values, and needs.

Important aspects of client-centered care include the following:
- **Knowledge:** Describe how diverse cultural, ethnic, and social backgrounds function as sources of client, family, and community values.
- **Skills:** Provide client-centered care with sensitivity and respect for the diversity of human experience.
- **Attitudes:** Recognize personally held attitudes about working with clients from different ethnic, cultural, and social backgrounds.

Client-Centered Care Question:

Self-awareness is a key component of providing authentic, genuine client-centered care. To clarify their own values and perspectives about poverty, nurses should ask themselves the following questions about poverty and persons living in poverty:
- What do I believe to be true about being poor?
- What do I personally know about being poor?
- How have family and friends influenced my ideas about being poor?
- Have I ever personally been poor?
- How have media images of poor persons helped shape our images of poverty and poor persons?
- What do I feel when I see a hungry child? A hungry adult?
- Do I believe that people are poor because they just do not want to work? Or do I believe that society has a significant influence on one's becoming poor?
- What really causes poverty?
- What do I really think can be done to prevent poverty and homelessness?

Prepared by Gail Armstrong, ND, DNP, PhD, Professor and Assistant Dean of the DNP Program, Oregon Health Sciences University.

The following strategies are important to consider when working with at-risk individuals, families, and aggregates:
- **Create a trusting environment.** Trust is essential to the development of a therapeutic relationship. Many clients and families have been disappointed by their interactions with health care and social systems; they are now mistrustful and see little hope for change. By following through and doing what they say they will do, nurses can establish trusting relationships with clients. If the answer to a question is unknown, an appropriate response might be, "I don't know the answer, but I will try to find out. Let me make a few phone calls, and I will let you know Friday." Reliability helps build the foundation for a trusting relationship.
- **Show respect, compassion, and concern.** High-risk clients are defeated so often by life's circumstances that they may feel they do not deserve attention. Listen carefully, and empathize with clients to help them believe they are worthy of care. Clients respond well to nursing interactions that demonstrate respect; reflective statements typically convey acceptance and understanding of a situation.
- **Avoid making assumptions.** A comprehensive assessment helps in identifying underlying needs. When a young mother with three preschool children misses a clinic appointment, this does not mean that she does not care about her children's

health; she may not have transportation, one child may be sick, or she may be sick. Find out the reason for the absence, and help solve the problem.

- **Coordinate a network of services and providers.** The multiple and complex needs of high-risk clients make working with them challenging. Many services exist, but often the people who could benefit are unaware of their existence. Developing a coordinated network of providers involves conducting a thorough assessment of the service area to identify available federal, state, and local services. Where are the food banks? Where can you get clothing? What programs are available in the local churches and schools? How do people access these services? What are the eligibility requirements? How helpful are the people who work at the service agencies? What service is provided to eligible individuals and families? Nurses can identify these services and help link families with appropriate resources. In addition, a thorough assessment of available services in a nurse's service area can identify significant gaps in essential services. If gaps are identified, nurses can serve as case managers and work with other health care providers and with community members to advocate for necessary services. See Chapter 15 for information about the nursing role in case management. As seen in Fig. 25.6 the nurse working in community mental health may participate in developing educational groups and programs for consumers, families, and others provided either alone or in collaboration with other organizations.
- **Advocate for accessible health care services.** Poverty, homelessness, teen pregnancy, and mental illness can create barriers that prevent access to health care services. Nurses can advocate for accessible and convenient locations of health care services.
- **Focus on prevention.** Try to use every opportunity to provide preventive care and health teaching. Important health promotion (primary prevention) topics include child and adult immunization and education regarding sound nutrition, foot care, safe sex, contraception, and prevention of chronic illness. Screening for health problems such as TB, diabetes, hypertension, foot problems, and anemia is an important form of secondary prevention. Know what other screening and health promotion services are available in the target area, such as nutrition programs, job training programs, educational programs, housing programs, and legal services. All of these services may be included in a comprehensive plan of care. Younger sisters of pregnant teens are twice as likely to become pregnant themselves. Thus health teaching about sexuality issues when seeing the teens in the home or clinic can increase their knowledge and awareness.

- **Know when to walk beside the client and when to encourage the client to walk ahead.** This area is often difficult for the nurse to implement. Nursing interventions range from extensive care activities to minimal support. At times, nursing actions include providing encouragement and support or providing information. At other times, nurses may actually call a pediatrician to set up an appointment for a sick child and may call again to see that the appointment was kept. Nurses assess for the presence of strengths, problem-solving ability, and coping ability of an individual or family while providing information on where and how to gain access to services. For example, a local hospital may provide free mammograms for uninsured women. Women who qualify for this free service may not take advantage of it because they are afraid they may have breast cancer. Nurses can find out about this important service, inform the women of the service, teach them about the importance of preventive care, and assess and deal with fear and anxiety. The challenge for the nurse becomes choosing whether to schedule the appointments for the women or simply provide them with a referral sheet, knowing that many will not follow through. The choice is not clear, but the goal is to make a needed screening intervention available without taking away the woman's right to decide what to do for herself.
- **Develop a network of support for yourself.** Caring for high-risk populations is challenging, rewarding, and at times exhausting. It is important to find a source of personal strength, renewal, and hope. The people you encounter are often looking to you to maintain hope and provide encouragement. Discover for yourself what restores and encourages you. For some nurses it is poetry, music, painting, or weaving. For others it is a walk in a peaceful place, a weekend retreat, a good run, a workout at the gym, or meeting with other nurses who are engaged in the same work. Be attentive to your own needs, and create the time and space to restore your spirit.

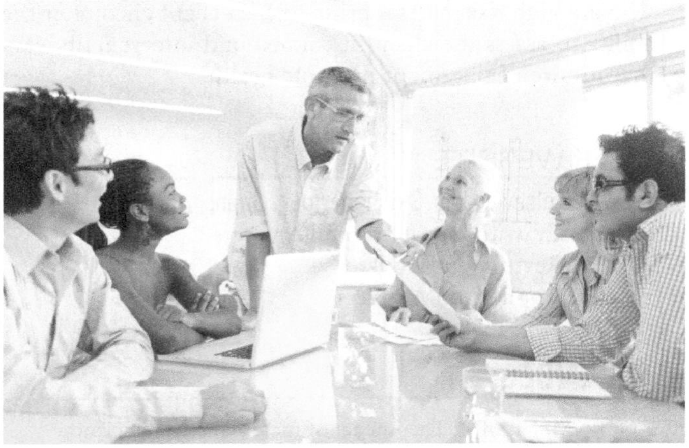

Fig. 25.6 Nurse Educator Teaching a Small Group of Clients. (Copyright Rawpixel Ltd, #489081731, iStock, Thinkstock.)

▶ APPLYING CONTENT TO PRACTICE

This chapter describes the role of the nurse who works with persons who are poor or who may be homeless, be a teen parent, or have serious mental illness. With each population, the role is diverse and complex, and relies on basic nursing knowledge as well as specific knowledge about the population. Providing effective nursing care in the community draws on many of the recommendations of nursing and public health groups. For example, the core competencies adopted by the Council on Linkages Between Academia and Public Health Practice (2014) include those related to assessment, policy development and program-planning skills, communication and cultural competency skills, and involvement with the community to provide services effectively. The Quad Council Coalition of Public Nursing Organizations (2018) further developed these skills and made clear application to nursing practice.

■ PRACTICE APPLICATION

A local youth-serving agency requested the assistance of a nurse in community health, Kristen Moore, in the implementation of a new high school–based program for pregnant and parenting teen girls. The primary goal of the program was to keep these teens in school through graduation. The secondary goal was to provide knowledge and skills about healthy pregnancy, labor and delivery, and parenting. After delivery, students enrolled in this program were paid for school attendance, and this money could be used to defray the costs of child care.

A nurse in community health was the ideal choice to conduct the educational sessions. The group met weekly during the lunch hour. These classes could also be taught electronically if students were doing online school. The curriculum that was developed had topics ranging from early pregnancy through the toddler years. Occasionally, Ms. Moore brought in outside speakers such as a labor and delivery nurse or an early intervention specialist.

She also met individually with each enrolled student to provide case management services. Ideally, she would ensure that each student had a health care provider for prenatal care, that each was visited at home by a nurse in community health, that each had enrolled in WIC and Medicaid, if eligible, and that both the pregnant teen and her partner knew about other parenting and support groups.

One educational session that was particularly interesting was the discussion about the postpartum period—the 6 weeks after delivery. There were many lively discussions about labor experiences, as well as some emotional discussions about the reality of coming home with a baby and changes in the relationship with the new mothers' male partners. Many girls benefited from understanding the normalcy of postpartum blues, but one young woman recognized that she had a more serious and persistent depression and privately approached the nurse for assistance.

At the end of the first school year, the dropout rate for pregnant and parenting teens was reduced by half, and preterm labor rates declined. The local school board and the local youth-serving agency joined together to provide financial support to continue this program for an additional 2 years. Ms. Moore was asked to expand the educational programs and interventions she had developed.

What are some directions in which the nurse could expand the program? List four.

Answers can be found on the Evolve website.

■ REMEMBER THIS!

- Poverty and homelessness affect the health status of people.
- To understand poverty, homelessness, teen pregnancy, and mental illness, consider your personal beliefs and attitudes, clients' perceptions of their condition, and the social, political, cultural, and environmental factors that influence the client's situation.
- Factors leading to the growing number of poor persons in the United States include decreased earnings, diminishing availability of low-cost housing, increases in the number of

households headed by women (women's incomes are traditionally lower than men's), inadequate education, lack of marketable job skills, welfare reform, and reduced Social Security payments to children.

- Poverty has a direct effect on health and well-being across the life span. Poor persons have higher rates of chronic illness, higher infant morbidity and mortality, shorter life expectancy, and more complex health problems.
- At present, the following groups often constitute the homeless in both rural and urban areas: families, single mothers, single women, recently unemployed persons, substance abusers, adolescent runaways, mentally ill individuals, and single men.
- Factors contributing to homelessness include an increase in the number of persons living in poverty, diminishing availability of low-cost housing, increased unemployment, substance abuse, lack of treatment facilities for mentally ill persons, domestic violence, and family situations causing children to run away.
- The complex health problems of homeless persons include inability to get adequate rest, exercise, and nutrition; exposure; infectious diseases; acute and chronic illness; infestations; trauma; and mental health problems.
- The provision of reproductive health care services to teens requires sensitivity to the special needs of this age group, including knowing about state laws concerning confidentiality and services for birth control, pregnancy, abortion, and adoption.
- Factors such as a history of sexual victimization, family dysfunction, substance use, and failure to use birth control can influence whether a young woman becomes pregnant.
- Adolescents, especially those who become pregnant, have special nutritional needs.
- The pregnant teen will need support during and after the pregnancy from the family and friends and from the father of the baby.
- Prevalence rates for mental health problems are high, and people are at risk for threats to mental health at all ages across the life span.
- Low-income and minority groups are often at increased risk for mental illness because they may lack access to services.
- Nurses have a critical role in the delivery of care to persons who are high risk. Nurses bring to each client encounter the ability to assess the client in context and intervene in ways that restore, maintain, or promote health.

EVOLVE WEBSITE

http://evolve.elsevier.com/Stanhope/foundations
- Case Study, with Questions and Answers
- NCLEX Review Questions
- Practice Application Answers

REFERENCES

Abu-Ouf NM, Jan MM: The impact of maternal iron deficiency and iron deficiency anemia on child's health, *Saudi Med J* 36(2): 146–149, 2015.

Alzheimer's Association: *Alzheimer's disease facts and figures 2020*, Retrieved August 2020-at http://www.alz.org.

American College of Obstetricians and Gynecologists: *ACOG strengthens LARC recommendations*, 2015. Retrieved August 2020 from: https://www.acog.org.

American College of Obstetricians and Gynecologists: *Frequently asked questions (FAQs),2020a*, Retrieved August 2020 at www.acog.org.

American College of Obstetricians and Gynecologists, *Nutrition during pregnancy*, 2020. www.acog.org.

American Psychiatric Association: *Diagnostic and statistical manual of mental disorders*, ed 5, Washington, DC, 2013, APA.

Angley M, Divney A, Magriples U, Kershaw T: Social support, family functioning and parenting competence in adolescent parents, *Matern Child Health J* 19(1):67–73, 2015.

Bassuk EL: Ending child homelessness in America, *Am J Orthopsychiatry* 80:496–504, 2010.

Boyd MA: Social change and mental health. In Boyd MA, ed.: *Psychiatric nursing: contemporary practice*, ed 5, Philadelphia, 2018, Lippincott Williams & Wilkins.

Centers for Disease Control and Prevention (CDC): *Social Determinants and Eliminating Disparities in Teen Pregnancy*, 2019. Retrieved August 2020 from: https://www.cdc.gov.

Centers for Disease Control and Prevention (CDC): *Reproductive Health: Teen Pregnancy, 2020a*. Retrieved August 2020 from: https://www.cdc.gov.

Centers for Disease Control and Prevention (CDC): *Youth Risk Behavior Surveillance — adolescent and school health, 2020b*, Retrieved November 2020 from: https://www.cdc.gov.

Charlton BM, Roberts AL, Rosario M, et al: Teen Pregnancy Risk Factors among Young Women of Diverse Sexual Orientations, *Pediatrics* 141(4):e20172278, 2018. Available at: http://pediatrics.aappublications.org.

Children's Defense Fund: *The State of America's Children 2020 Report*, 2020. Retrieved August 2020 from http://www.childrendefense.org.

Christian R, Mukarji-Connolly A: *A new Queer Agenda*, 2018. Retrieved from Scholar & Feminist Online: http://sfonline.barnard.edu/a-new-queer-agenda/whats-home-got-to-do-with-it-unsheltered-queer-youth/0/.

Cornforth T: *Healthy Eating for Pregnant Teens*. Very Well Family Organization, 2018. Retrieved July 2018 from: https://www.verywellfamily.com.

Council on Linkages Between Academic and Public Health Practice: *Core competencies for public health professionals*, Washington, DC, 2014, Public Health Foundation, Health Resources and Services Administration.

Cubanski J, Koma W, Damico A and Neuman T: *How many seniors live in poverty?* Kaiser Family Foundation, Issue Brief November 2018, Oakland CA.

Danawi H, Bryant Z, Hasbini T: Targeting unintended teen pregnancy in the US. *International Journal of Childbirth Education* 31(1):28–31, January 2016.

Dashow J: *New report on youth homeless affirms that LGBTQ youth disproportionately experience homelessness*, November 15, 2017. Retrieved from Human Rights Campaign: https://www.hrc.org/blog/new-report-on-youth-homeless-affirms-that-lgbtq-youth-disproportionately-ex.

Ethier KA, Kann L, McManus T: Sexual Intercourse Among High School Students—29 States and United States Overall, 2005-2015, *MMWR Morb Mortal Wkly Rep* 66:1393–1397, 2018.

Farrell T, Clyde A, Katta M, Bolland J: The impact of sexuality concerns on teenage pregnancy: a consequence of heteronormativity? *Cult Health Sex* 19(1):135–149, 2017.

Fowler D, Hodgkins J, French P, et al: Social recovery therapy in combination with early intervention services for enhancement of social recovery in patients with first-episode psychosis (SUPEREDEN3): a single-blind, randomized controlled trial, *Lancet Psychiatry*, 5(1):41–50, 2018.

Garwood SK, Gerassi L, Jonson-Reid M, Plax K, Drake B: More than poverty — teen pregnancy risk and reports of child abuse reports and neglect, *J Adolesc Health* 57(2):164–168, 2015.

Gerber L: Bringing home effective nursing care for the homeless, *Nursing*, 43:32-38, 2013.

Gregg D, Somers CL, Pernice FM, Hillman SB, Kernsmith P: Sexting rates and predictors from an urban Midwest high school, *J School Health* 88(6):423–433, 2018.

Guttmacher Institute: *Adolescent Sexual and Reproductive Health in the United States*, New York, 2019, Guttmacher Institute. Retrieved July 2020 from: https://www.guttmacher.org.

Haigh EAP, Bogucki OE, Sigmon ST, Blazer DG: Depression among older adults: A 20-year update on five common myths and misconceptions, *Am J Geriatr Psychiatry* 26(1):107–122, 2018.

Hallowell S, Froh E, Spatz D: Human milk and breastfeeding: an intervention to mitigate toxic stress. *Nurs Outlook* 65(1): 58-67, 2017.

Health Affairs: *Culture of health, housing and health: An overview of the literature*, Health Policy Brief, June 2018. Retrieved August 2020 from https://www.healthaffairs.org.

Healthy Children Organization (HCO): *Teen parents*, 2017, American Academy of Pediatrics. Retrieved June 2018 from: https://www.healthychildren.org.

Henry M, Watt R, Rosenthal L, Shivji A: *The 2017 Annual Homeless Assessment Report (AHAR) to Congress*, Washington, DC, 2017, US Department of Housing and Urban Development.

Macedo, AF: Neurobiology of mental illness from reductionism to integration, *Intern J of Clin Neurosci and Ment Health* 4(Suppl 3): S01, 2017.

Marvin-Dowle K, Kilner K, Burley VJ, Soltani H: Impact of adolescent age on maternal and neonatal outcomes in the Born in Bradford cohort, *BMJ Open* 8:e016258, 2018.

Massachusetts General Hospital (MGH): *Teen dads: the forgotten parent*, 2016. Retrieved July 2018 from: http://www.thefatherhoodproject.org.

McHugh MT, Kvernland A, Palusci V: An adolescent parents' programme to reduce child abuse, *Chld Abuse Review* 26(3):184–195, 2015.

Mechanic D, Olfson M: The relevance of the Affordable Care Act for improving mental health care, *Annu Rev Clin Psychol* 12: 515–542, 2016.

Merrill RM, Richards R, Sloan A: Prenatal maternal stress and physical abuse among homeless women and infant health outcomes in the United States, *Epidemiol Res Int* 2011:2011.

National Abortion and Reproductive Rights Active League (NARAL): *2019 Congressional Record on Choice*, Retrieved August 2020 at https://www.naral.org.

National Alliance to End Homelessness: *Resources overview: veteran homelessness*, Washington DC, 2018, National Alliance to End Homelessness.

National Alliance to End Homelessness: *How many veterans experience homelessness?* Washington DC, 2019, Retrieved August 2020 at https://www.endhomelessness.org.

National Alliance to End Homelessness: *Population at-risk: Homelessness and the COVID-19 crisis*, March 25, 2020, Retrieved August 2020 at https://www.enhomelessness.org.

National Coalition for the Homeless: Current state of *homelessness*, 2018. Retrieved August 2020 from http://www.Nationalhomeless.org.

National Coalition for the Homeless: *Health Care, 2019*. Retrieved from National Coalition for the Homeless: http://nationalhomeless.org.

National Institutes of Mental Health (NIMH), National Institutes of Health (NIH), US Department of Health and Human Services (USDHHS): *Any Anxiety Disorder*, Washington, DC, 2018, NIMH. Available at: https://www.nimh.nih.gov. Accessed July 2018.

National Network for Youth: *How many homeless youth are in America?* 2018. Retrieved from National Network for Youth: https://www.nn4youth.org/learn/how-many-homeless/.

Pandya A, Jan Myrick K: Wellness recovery program: a model of self-advocacy for people living with mental illness, *J Psychiatr Pract* 19:242–246, 2013.

Pascoe J, Wood D, Duffee J, Kuo A: *Mediators and adverse effects of child poverty in the United States*, Itasca, Illinois, 2016, American Academy of Pediatrics Committee on Psychosocial Aspects of Child and Family Health, Council on Community Pediatrics.

Pearlman SA: The Patient Protection and Affordable Health Care Act: impact on mental health services demand and provider availability, *J Am Psychiatric Nurses Assoc* 19:327–334, 2013.

Pirog MA, Jung H, Lee D: The changing face of teenage parenthood in the United States: evidence from NLSY79 and NLSY97, *Child Youth Care Forum* 47:317–342, 2017.

Restall A, Taylor RS, Thompson JM, et al: Risk factors for excessive gestational weight gain in a healthy, nulliparous cohort, *J Obes* 2014:148391, 2014.

Richards R, Merrill RM, Baksh L: Health behaviors and infant health outcomes in homeless pregnant women in the United States, *Pediatrics* 128:438–446, 2011.

Roberts AW, Ogunwole SU, Blakeslee L, Rabe MA: *The population 65 years and older in the United States: 2016*, American Community Survey Reports, October 2018 and reviewed in 2019, United States Census Bureau.

Roche M, Duffield C, Smith J, et al: Nurse-led primary health care for homeless men: a multimethods descriptive study, *Int Nurs Rev* 65:392–399, 2018.

Quad Council Coalition of Public Health Nursing Organizations: *Community/Public health nursing (C/PHN) competencies, 2018.* Retrieved August 2020 from www.achne.org.

Semega J, Kollar M, Crreamer J, and Mohanty A: US Census Bureau, Current Population Reports, P60-266(RV), *Income and Poverty in the United States, 2018*, US Government Printing Office, Washington, DC, 2020.

Stanford Center on Poverty & Inequality: *The poverty and inequality report: state of the union 2017*, Stanford, 2017, Pathways Magazine.

Substance Abuse and Mental Health Services (SAMHSA): *Key substance use and mental health indicators in the United States: results from the 2018 national survey on drug use and health, 2019*, Rockville, MD, SAMHSA.

Substance Abuse and Mental Health Services Administration (SAMHSA): *Mental health and substance use disorders*, 2020, Rockville, MD, SAMHSA.

US Bureau of Labor Statistics: *Consumer price index summary*, Washington, DC, 2020, US Department of Labor, Retrieved August 2020 at http://www.bls.gov.

US Department of Health and Human Services: *Healthy People 2030*, Washington, DC, 2020b, US Government Printing Office.

US Department of Health and Human Services: *Poverty Guidelines, 1/08/2020.* Washington DC, 2020a, Office of the Federal Register, Retrieved August 2020 at http://www.aspe.hhs.gov.

US Department of Health and Human Services (USDHHS): *Office of Adolescent Health: Trends in teen pregnancy and childbearing*, 2019. Retrieved August 2020 from: https://www.hhs.gov.

United States Interagency Council on Homelessness: *Homelessness in America: focus on veterans*, Washington, DC, 2018, USICH.

US Department of Housing and Urban Development, Office of Community Planning and Development, *The 2019 annual homeless assessment report (AHAR) to Congress, Part 1-point-in-time estimate of homelessness, January 2020*, Retrieved August 2020 at http://www.hudexchange.info.

Vázquez-Nava F, Vázquez-Rodriguez CF, Saldívar-González AH, et al: Unplanned pregnancy in adolescents: association with family structure, employed mother, and female friends with health-risk habits and behaviors, *J Urban Health* 91(1): 176–185, 2014.

Winkler P, Barrett B, McCrone P, Csémy L, Janoušková M, Höschl C: Deinstitutionalised patients, homelessness and imprisonment: systematic review, *Br J Psychiatry* 208(5):421–428, 2016.

World Health Organization: *Mental health. mhGAP Programme expands to include scalable psychological intervention*, May 20, 2016, at http://www.who.int.

World Health Organization: About social determinants of health, 2020. Retrieved August 2020 from http://www.who.int.

26

Alcohol, Tobacco, and Other Drug Problems in the Community

Mary Lynn Mathre and Amber M. Bang

OBJECTIVES

After reading this chapter, the student should be able to:

1. Describe attitudes about alcohol, tobacco, and other drug problems.
2. Differentiate among these terms: *substance use, abuse, dependence,* and *addiction.*
3. Discuss the differences among the major psychoactive drug categories of depressants, stimulants, marijuana, hallucinogens, and inhalants.
4. Explain the role of the nurse in primary, secondary, and tertiary prevention of alcohol, tobacco, and other drug problems as it relates to individual clients and their families.
5. Explain the effect of substance abuse on the community and on people within the community.

CHAPTER OUTLINE

KEY TERMS

Substance abuse is the leading national health problem, causing more deaths, illnesses, and disabilities than any other health condition. Considerable death and disability are caused by the use of alcohol, tobacco, and illicit drugs. The substance abuser not only is at risk for personal health problems but also may be a threat to the health and safety of family members, coworkers, and other members of the community. Substance abuse and addiction affect all ages, races, sexes, and segments of society. Tobacco use and substance abuse were two major topic areas in *Healthy People 2020* (US Department of Health and Human Services [USDHHS], 2010) and remain topics for *Healthy People 2030* (USDHHS, 2020a). *Healthy People 2030* discusses addictions under health conditions and has sections on drug and alcohol use and tobacco use under health behavior. Each section has specific goals. The phrase *alcohol, tobacco, and other drug (ATOD) problems* rather than *substance abuse* reminds us that alcohol and tobacco represent the major drugs of abuse when discussing substance abuse, drug addiction, or chemical dependency. This is a useful term. In 2013, when the American Psychiatric Association updated the Diagnostic and Statistical Manual, known as the DSM-5, the term, "substance use disorder (SUD)" was used. Both ATOD and SUD are used in the chapter.

SCOPE OF THE PROBLEM

ATOD abuse and addiction can cause multiple health problems for individuals. Factors that contribute to this abuse problem include lack of knowledge about the use of drugs, the emphasis on illicit drugs and law enforcement rather than the prevention and treatment of abuse and addiction of ATODs, overprescription; lack of quality control of illegal drugs; and punitive drug laws that label certain drug users as criminals, encouraging negative attitudes and stigma toward these persons.

Every culture has beliefs and attitudes toward ATOD. These attitudes are influenced by the way society categorizes drugs as either "good" or "bad." In the United States, good drugs are over-the-counter (OTC) drugs or those prescribed by a health care provider, although this makes them no less problematic or addictive. "Bad drugs" are the illegal drugs, and persons who use these drugs are considered criminals regardless of whether the drug has caused any problems. Americans rely heavily on prescription and OTC drugs to relieve (or mask) anxiety, tension, fatigue, and physical or emotional pain. Rather than learning holistic or alternative methods of coping, many people choose the "quick fix" and take pills to deal with their problems or negative feelings. Addicted persons are often viewed as immoral, weak-willed, or irresponsible, and others often think they should try harder to help themselves. Although alcoholism was recognized as a disease by the American Medical Association in 1954,

and drug addiction was recognized as a disease some years later, much of the public and many health care professionals do not consider alcoholics and addicted persons to be ill and in need of health care.

It is important for nurses to examine their attitudes toward ATOD use, abuse, and addiction before working with persons who have this health problem. In order to engage in therapeutic communication, nurses need to examine their own beliefs and realize that any drug can be abused, that anyone can develop drug dependence, and that drug addition can be successfully treated. The historical debate as to whether drug use and abuse is a public health problem or a criminal justice problem continues.

What, then, is SUD? The DSM-5 recognizes substance-related disorders that result from the use of 10 classes of drugs: alcohol; caffeine; cannabis; hallucinogens; inhalants; opioids; sedatives; hypnotics or anxiolytics; stimulants; tobacco; and other or unknown substances. There are 11 criteria used to diagnose a SUD. They are:

1. Taking the substance in larger amounts or for longer than you are meant to.
2. Wishing to decrease or stop taking the substance but not being able to do so.
3. Spending considerable time getting, using, or recovering from taking the substance.
4. Having cravings and urges to use the substance.
5. Not being able to perform at work, home, or school because of substance use.
6. Using even when it causes problems in relationships.
7. Giving up important activities because of substance use.
8. Using substances when it puts you in danger.
9. Continuing to use when you recognize that the substance is causing physical or psychological problems.
10. Developing tolerance, that is, needing increasing amounts of the substance to attain the desired effect.
11. Having withdrawal symptoms (Hartley, 2020).

The DSM-5 includes guidelines to determine how severe a SUD is: two or three symptoms–mild SUD; four or five–moderate SUD; and six or more–severe SUD or addiction (Addiction Policy Forum, 2020).

An important issue is the relationship between COVID-19 and substance use. It has been found that "Among the vulnerable populations (for COVID-19) are persons who smoke or vape, use opioids, or have a substance abuse disorder" (Volkow, 2020, p. 1). The reason is that persons who use substances may have compromised respiratory function, putting them at higher risk for contracting COVID-19. Specifically, COVID-19 is caused by severe respiratory syndrome coronavirus 2 (SARS-Co-V-2) (Wang, Kaelber, Xu, Volkow, 2020). There are many risks in the current pandemic to persons who abuse substances, such as housing instability and reduced access to health care and recovery support services. This is especially problematic for incarcerated persons since it is estimated that over half of the U.S. prisoners have a SUD, and prison populations are at higher risk for contracting the disease during a pandemic due to their close living quarters (Volkow, 2020).

The harm reduction model is a public health approach, and it recognizes the following:

- Addiction is a health problem.
- Any drug can be abused.
- Accurate information can help people make responsible decisions about drug use.
- People who have ATOD or SUD problems can be helped.

This approach accepts that psychoactive drug use is endemic, and it focuses on pragmatic interventions, especially education, to reduce the adverse consequences of drug use and get treatment for addicted persons. The United States has already taken a harm reduction approach with tobacco and alcohol. Educational campaigns have been used to inform the public about the health risks of tobacco use. Warnings have appeared on tobacco product labels since 1967 as a result of the Surgeon General's 1964 report on the dangers of smoking. In 1971, a ban on television and radio cigarette advertising was imposed. Cigarette smoking has decreased since that time. In January 2020, the US Surgeon General released the first report on smoking cessation in 30 years. As will be discussed in a later section of the chapter, smoking rates are at an all-time low; however, there is more work to be done to assist persons to quit smoking. In 2020, about 34 million Americans or 14% of the population smoked, and smoking remains the number one cause of preventable disease, death, and disability. According to the Surgeon General, "doctors could be doing more to help patients quit" (USDHHS, 2020b).

It is important to continue educating people about the dangers of SUD, to identify the causes of various health problems, and to plan realistic, nonjudgmental, holistic, and positive actions. The harm reduction model can be used effectively for these problems. To develop a therapeutic attitude, the nurse must realize that any substance can be abused, that anyone may develop dependence, and that addiction can be successfully treated.

Definitions

The terms *drug use* and *drug abuse* have virtually lost their usefulness because the public and government have narrowed the term *drug* to include only illegal drugs rather than including prescription, OTC, and legal recreational drugs. The acronym ATOD reminds us that the leading drug problems involve alcohol and tobacco and that new forms of abuse are being tried by youth and adults. The term *substance* broadens the scope to include alcohol, tobacco, legal drugs, and even foods and substances such as bath salts. **Substance use disorder** is the use of those substances identified by the American Psychiatric Association that threaten a person's health or impair social or economic functioning. The DSM-5 combines the previously used terms of substance abuse and substance dependence into a single disorder, Substance Use Disorder, which is measured on a continuum from mild to severe (American Psychiatric Association, 2013).

Drug dependence and drug addiction are often used interchangeably, but they are not synonymous. Drug dependence is a state of neuroadaptation (a physiological change in the central nervous system [CNS] and alterations in other systems caused by the chronic, regular administration of a drug). People who are dependent on drugs must continue using them to prevent symptoms of withdrawal. For example, when a person is given an opiate such as morphine on a regular basis for pain management, the morphine needs to be gradually tapered rather than abruptly stopped to prevent symptoms of withdrawal. Drug dependence is both psychological and physical. Psychological dependence includes feelings of satisfaction and a desire to repeat the drug experience or to avoid the discomfort of not having the drug. Craving and compulsion are part of this dependence. Physical dependence is seen when there is an abstinence effect. This effect results in physical changes that are uncomfortable.

Drug addiction is a pattern of abuse characterized by an overwhelming preoccupation with the use (compulsive use) of a drug and securing its supply and a high tendency to relapse if the drug is removed. Addicts may be both physically and psychologically dependent on a drug, and there may be a risk for harm and the need to stop drug use.

Alcoholism is an addiction to the drug called *alcohol*. Alcoholism and drug addiction are recognized as illnesses under a biopsychosocial model. Simply stated, the disease concept of addiction and alcoholism identifies them as chronic and progressive diseases in which a person's use of a drug or drugs continues despite problems it causes in any area of life—physical, emotional, social, economic, or spiritual.

PSYCHOACTIVE DRUGS

Although any drug can be abused, ATOD abuse and addiction problems generally involve psychoactive drugs. These drugs, which can alter emotions, are used for enjoyment in social and recreational settings and for personal use to self-medicate physical or emotional discomfort. Psychoactive drugs are divided into categories according to their effect on the CNS and the general feelings or experiences the drugs may induce. The Internet or a pharmacology text can provide detailed information on these drug categories (e.g., depressants, stimulants, hallucinogens). Often, if persons cannot obtain their drug of choice, another drug from the same category will be substituted. For example, a person who cannot drink alcohol may begin using a benzodiazepine as an alternative because both are CNS depressants.

Depressants lower the body's overall energy level, reduce sensitivity to outside stimulation, and, in high doses, induce sleep. Low doses of depressants may produce a feeling of stimulation caused by initial sedation of the inhibitory centers in the brain. In general, depressants decrease heart rate, respiration rate, muscular coordination, and energy while dulling the senses. Higher doses lead to coma and, if the vital functions shut down, death. Major categories include alcohol, barbiturates, benzodiazepines, and opioids.

People use stimulants to feel more alert or energetic. These drugs activate or excite the nervous system. An increase in alertness and energy results as the stimulant causes the nerve fibers to release noradrenaline and other stimulating neurotransmitters. However, these drugs do not give the person more energy; they only make the body expend its own energy sooner and in greater quantities than it normally would. Stimulants can be useful and have few negative effects if used carefully and appropriately. The body must be allowed time to replenish itself after the use of a stimulant. The cost for the "high" is the "down" state after the use of a stimulant—a feeling of sleepiness, laziness, mental fatigue, and possibly depression. Regular use of high doses can lead to physical dependence, and the withdrawal symptoms may include headaches, slowness, and occasional depression (Mayo Clinic staff, 2017). Many persons abusing stimulants begin a vicious cycle of avoiding the down feeling by taking another dose. They then become physically dependent on the stimulant to function. Common stimulants include nicotine, cocaine, caffeine, and amphetamines. There is a growing public health issue related to the use of energy drinks by children, adolescents, and young adults. Energy drinks are "beverages that contain caffeine, taurine, vitamins, herbal supplements, and sugar or sweeteners and are marketed to improve energy, weight loss, stamina, athletic performance, and concentration" (Seifert et al., 2011, p. 512). The sale of energy drinks is growing. Caffeine is their main ingredient, and they are different from sports drinks and vitamin waters. Caffeine causes coronary and cerebral vasoconstriction, relaxes smooth muscle, stimulates skeletal muscle, has cardiac effects, and reduces insulin sensitivity (Seifert et al., 2011). On the basis of an extensive review, Seifert et al. found that energy drinks have no therapeutic value and may put some children at risk for serious adverse health effects due to the high levels of caffeine. It should be noted that manufacturers claim that energy drinks are nutritional supplements, which shields them from the caffeine limits imposed on sodas and the safety testing and labeling required of pharmaceuticals (2011, p. 522).

Alcohol

Alcohol (ethyl alcohol, or ethanol) is the oldest and most widely used psychoactive drug in the world. In the *National Survey on Drug Use and Health—2018*, in the past month, about 139.8 million Americans aged 12 or older used alcohol; 16.6 million were heavy drinkers; and 67.1 million were binge drinkers. The percentage of adolescents aged 12 to 17 decreased between 2002 and 2018, yet 1 in 11 of them were past-month alcohol users (SAMHSA, 2019). Alcohol abuse contributes to illness in each of the top three causes of death in the United States: heart disease, cancer, and stroke.

Genetics and personal characteristics influence the development of alcohol use disorders. As much as 40% to 60% of risk variance in alcohol use disorders may be due to genetic factors. The incidence of alcohol abuse and dependence is higher in the biological children of people who have alcohol problems than in adoptive children (O'Malley and O'Malley, 2020a).

Alcohol abuse costs billions of dollars in lost productivity, property damage, medical expenses from alcohol-related illnesses and accidents, family disruptions, alcohol-related violence, and neglect or abuse of children. Chronic alcohol abuse has multiple metabolic and physiological effects on all organ systems. People who use excessive amounts of alcohol may also not eat an adequate diet and then may develop vitamin and other nutritional deficiencies. In addition to the nutritional effects of low folate, iron, and niacin levels, there may be gastrointestinal disturbances of the esophagus and stomach that can lead to inflammation and cancer. The liver and pancreas may be affected as well. Cardiovascular disturbances include cardiac dysrhythmias, cardiomyopathy, hypertension, atherosclerosis, and blood dyscrasias. CNS problems include depression, sleep disturbances, memory loss, organic brain syndrome, Wernicke-Korsakoff syndrome, and alcohol withdrawal syndrome. Neuromuscular problems include myopathy and peripheral neuropathy. There may be effects to the reproductive organs including decreased sex drive and, in men, enlarged breasts, smooth skin, and shrinking of the testes (O'Malley and O'Malley, 2018). Females who drink during pregnancy may have neonates with fetal alcohol syndrome (FAS) or fetal alcohol effects. Some of the metabolic disturbances include hypokalemia, hypomagnesemia, and ketoacidosis. Living in a household where one or both parents abuse alcohol can have significant effects on the children and their development, learning, and socialization.

Blood alcohol concentration (BAC) is determined by the concentration of alcohol in the drink, the rate of drinking, the rate of absorption (slower in the presence of food), the rate of metabolism, and a person's weight and sex. The amount of alcohol the liver can metabolize per hour is equal to about 0.25 oz of whiskey, 4 oz of wine, or 12 oz of beer.

How Much Is a Drink?

In the United States, a standard drink is one that contains about 14 g of pure alcohol, which is found in:
- 12 ounces of beer with about 5% alcohol content
- 5 ounces of wine with about 12% alcohol content
- 1.5 ounces of distilled spirits with about 40% alcohol content

The percent of "pure" alcohol, expressed here as alcohol by volume (alc/vol), varies within and across beverage types. Although the "standard" drink amounts are helpful for following health guidelines, they may not reflect customary serving sizes. A large cup of beer, an overpoured glass of wine, or a single mixed drink could contain much more alcohol than a standard drink (National Institute on Alcohol Abuse and Alcoholism: *Underage drinking*, 2020. Accessed at www.niaaa.nih.gov, June 2020).

Tolerance will develop with chronic consumption, and a person can reach a high BAC with minimal CNS effects. Women are more affected by alcohol than men because women have less alcohol dehydrogenase activity than men (except for males with chronic alcoholism). Because this enzyme detoxifies alcohol, a deficiency results in a higher bioavailability of alcohol. Consequently, females suffer the long-term effects of alcohol intake at much lower doses in a shorter time span. Women also tend to have smaller body sizes than men. Alcohol use in moderation may provide health benefits by providing mild relaxation and lowering the serum cholesterol. At-risk drinking is defined by the quantity and frequency of drinking which is: 14 drinks/week or 4 drinks per occasion for men; and 7 drinks/week or 3 drinks per occasion for women (O'Malley and

O'Malley, 2020a) Controlled drinking organizations such as Moderation Management (see http://www.moderation.org) provide guidelines for persons who want to have alcohol in their lives.

It is increasingly common to hear the term alcohol abuse disorder (AUD), a disease that causes: (1) craving–a strong need to drink; (2) loss of control–not being able to stop drinking once you have started; (3) negative emotional state–feeling anxious and irritable when you are not drinking (MedlinePlus, 2020). Some of the most effective treatments for AUD are rehabilitation programs, outpatient counseling, self-help groups, or medications (O'Malley and O'Malley, 2020a).

Tobacco

As mentioned, after three decades, the US Surgeon General released the 34th tobacco-related report. Major categories of findings are:

1. Smoking cessation is beneficial at any age. It improves health status and quality of life.
2. Smoking cessation reduces the risk of premature death; it can add as much as a decade to one's life.
3. Smoking leads to a large financial burden on smokers, health care systems, and society.
4. Smoking cessation reduces the risk for many adverse health effects, including reproductive health outcomes, cardiovascular diseases, chronic obstructive pulmonary disease, and cancer.
5. More than three out of five U.S. adults who have ever smoked cigarettes have quit.
6. There appears to be a higher prevalence of smoking in some groups.
7. Smoking cessation medications approved by the U.S. Food and Drug Administration (FDA) and given with behavioral counseling can be cost-effective cessation strategies.
8. Insurance coverage for treatment that is comprehensive, barrier-free, and widely promoted can lead to higher quit rates.
9. E-cigarettes: It is hard to make generalizations about their effectiveness for the cessation of cigarette smoking.
10. Smoking cessation can be increased by raising the price of cigarettes, adopting comprehensive smoke-free policies, implementing mass media campaigns, requiring pictorial health warnings, and maintaining comprehensive statewide tobacco control programs (USDHHS, 2020b). The Surgeon General's Report on Smoking Cessation is available in English, Spanish, Chinese, Korean, and Vietnamese, which makes the report accessible to many of the people living in the United States.

Nicotine, the active ingredient in the tobacco plant, is a toxic drug. To protect itself, the body quickly develops tolerance to the nicotine. If a person smokes regularly, tolerance to nicotine develops within hours, in contrast to days for heroin or months for alcohol. Pipes and cigars are less hazardous than cigarettes because the harsher smoke discourages deep inhalation. However, pipes and cigars increase the risk for cancer of the lips, mouth, and throat. There are large economic costs associated with the use of tobacco because of the diseases related to its use (Fig. 26.1).

Smoke can be inhaled directly by the smoker (mainstream smoke), or it can enter the atmosphere from the lighted end of the cigarette and be inhaled by others in the vicinity (sidestream smoke or secondhand smoke). Secondhand smoke contains higher concentrations of toxic and carcinogenic compounds than mainstream smoke and puts the people who are exposed to it at risk for serious illness. Smoking can cause cancer, heart disease, stroke, lung diseases, diabetes, and chronic obstructive pulmonary disease (COPD), including emphysema and chronic bronchitis. It also increases the risk for tuberculosis, certain eye diseases, and problems of the immune system, including rheumatoid arthritis, and it is a known cause of erectile dysfunction in males. Smokers tend to die 10 years earlier than nonsmokers (CDC, 2019). Secondhand smoke, which affects 58 million nonsmoking Americans, also causes stroke, lung cancer, and coronary heart disease in adults and places children who are exposed to secondhand smoke to increased risk of sudden infant death syndrome (SIDS), impaired lung function, acute respiratory infections, middle ear disease, and more frequent and severe asthma attacks. More than 16 million Americans are living with a disease caused by smoking.

From a global perspective, the World Health Organization (WHO) says that: (1) Tobacco kills up to half of its users, and this is 8 million people. (2) Approximately 80% of the world's 1.1 billion smokers live in low- and middle-income countries. (3) Tobacco kills more than 8 million people each year (2019). The costs of smoking are high ranging from the actual cost of the tobacco product to the lost human capital that results from tobacco-attributable morbidity and mortality. The WHO (2019) points out that in some countries, children from poor homes engage in tobacco farming to help support the family. This puts the children at risk for "green tobacco sickness," which is caused by the nicotine being absorbed into the skin when

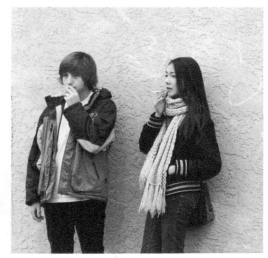

Fig. 26.1 Cigarette Smoking Poses Many Health Risks. (© 2012 Photos.com, a division of Getty Images. All rights reserved. Image #137167089.)

the children handle wet tobacco leaves. Around the world, it is important to teach youth the dangers of smoking and encourage them to not begin smoking.

Nicotine also is used as chewing tobacco or snuff. Marketed as "smokeless tobacco," a wad is put in the mouth, and the nicotine is absorbed sublingually. Higher doses of nicotine are delivered in the smokeless forms because the nicotine is not destroyed by heat. Nevertheless, this form is less addictive because nicotine enters the bloodstream less directly.

Electronic Nicotine Delivery Systems

This topic, because of its growing popularity, deserves its own section in the text. Electronic cigarettes (e-cigarettes) are known by a variety of names, and some look like regular cigarettes, cigars, or pipes. Some resemble pens, USB sticks, and other everyday items. They produce an aerosol by heating a liquid that often contains nicotine, flavoring agents, and other chemicals to help make the aerosol (Fig. 26.2) (Types of e-cigarettes, CDC, 2019). Users inhale the aerosol into their lungs. These cigarettes are not safe for youth, young adults, pregnant women, or adults who do not currently use tobacco products. People standing nearby can also breathe this aerosol into their lungs. It is important to consider what comprises the aerosols: nicotine; ultrafine particles that can be inhaled deep into the lungs; flavoring such as diacetyl, a chemical linked to a serious lung disease; volatile organic compounds, cancer-causing chemicals, and metals such as nickel, tin, and lead (CDC, 2020a).

The best approach to dealing with the deleterious effects of tobacco is for people to never use it. However, that is not always possible. The CDC recommends these strategies:

- Preventing young people from starting to use tobacco.
- Promoting quitting among adults and young people.
- Reducing exposure to secondhand smoke.
- Identifying and eliminating tobacco-related health disparities (National Center for Chronic Disease Prevention and Health Promotion, 2019).

A helpful resource is the CDC "Guide for Quitting Smoking," which has tips from former smokers. It is on the CDC website and was updated in June 2020.

- The WHO says that the following strategies have worked around the world to reduce the number of people who use to-

bacco: hard-hitting anti-tobacco mass media campaigns and pictorial health warnings get the attention of children and other vulnerable groups from beginning to use tobacco or to quit; bans on tobacco advertising; and tax increases (WHO, 2019).

EVIDENCE-BASED PRACTICE

Tobacco use continues to be a major public health problem in the United States. It is a leading cause of disability and premature death and disproportionately affects vulnerable populations and minority groups. While cigarette smoking is at an all-time low, the use of electronic cigarettes has increased. Teenagers are heavy users of electronic cigarettes, and this puts them at risk for tobacco dependence. Tobacco-related illnesses can be avoided by preventing the initiation of ever smoking. Nicotine is a highly addictive substance. Its potency is due to the mechanism of action in the body, especially the brain. The more nicotine consumption and the higher blood nicotine concentration, the more neurotransmitters that circulate. These neurotransmitters induce pleasurable effects for the tobacco user and encourage repetitive use. People who experience disproportionate rates of tobacco dependence and disease include but are not limited to: (1) adults between 25 and 44 who possess a high school education or less, (2) people who live at or below the poverty level; (3) people who are uninsured or on state Medicaid health plans; (4) members of ethnic and racial minority groups; (5) persons with disability or mental health illness; and (6) men and women who identify as gay, lesbian, or bisexual.

Nurse Use

Nurses, who are considered reliable sources of information, need to be informed about e-cigarettes and the potential dangers associated with them. The goal is to teach patients, families, caregivers, and community members about the detrimental effects of tobacco use. In addition to teaching and counseling, nurses can advocate for policy changes.

Fathi JT. Tobacco use: the current state of affairs and how nurses can help patients quit. *Online J Issues Nurs* September 30, 2020;25(3), Manuscript 1.

People who use e-cigarettes do not consider that they are smoking. Instead, they say they are vaping. Vaping users often have their own customs, traditions, and language. You can activate the e-cigarette device by pressing a button that "heats and aerosolizes the liquid in the cartridge containing a liquid, creating a vapor" (Antolin and Barkley, 2015, p. 60). Nicotine is dangerous. It is highly addictive, toxic to a developing fetus, and

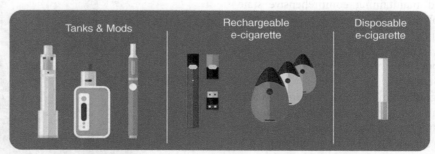

Fig. 26.2 Some E-Cigarettes Are Made to Look Like Regular Cigarettes, Cigars, or Pipes. Some resemble pens, USB sticks, and other everyday items. (From: Centers for Disease Control and Prevention. *Smoking and tobacco use: about electronic cigarettes (E-cigarettes)*. Last reviewed February 24, 2020. Accessed June 2020 at www.cdc.gov.)

harmful to the adolescent or young adult. Also, defective e-cigarette batteries have caused fires.

Nurses have a key role to play in assessing the use of e-cigarettes. They can then offer advice about the risks of smoking and vaping. Nurses also can direct youth and other e-cigarette users to the many websites that offer valuable information about the dangers of using e-cigarettes as well as ways to quit using e-cigarettes. For this reason, it is important that nurses have current information in an area that is changing rapidly. Fig. 26.2 illustrates the various forms in which e-cigarettes can be found.

Vaping increases the risk of contracting COVID-19. This is due to the fact that e-cigarettes affect the lungs and immune system, making the user more susceptible to COVID-19. The seriousness is increased when teens or other uses share the e-cigarettes. Halpers-Felsher, Folar, and Grosse (2020) found that people who vaped and smoked were five times more likely to develop COVID-19 symptoms, including coughs, fever, fatigue, and trouble breathing, than people who never smoked or vaped.

Caffeine

While caffeine is seldom considered a drug, it is a stimulant. With the growing number of coffee bars and the many different versions of caffeine-based products, it is important to recognize the contents of these items. A useful website is that of Caffeineinformer.com. The last update was in February 2020. Some of the topics included are:

- Calculate your personalized limits for any drink.
- Caffeine levels in drinks, food, and medications.
- Caffeine content in selected popular coffee brands.
- 20+ harmful effects of caffeine.

Cannabis (Marijuana)

Cannabis (*Cannabis sativa* or *C. indica*) is the most widely used illicit drug in the United States. The use of marijuana is growing in all adult ages, genders, and pregnant women. The risks of marijuana are not being discussed as much as in the past. Today's marijuana is stronger than ever before, and people can become addicted. The Substance Abuse and Mental Health Services Administration (SAMHSA) says "approximately 1 in 10 people who use marijuana will become addicted." The rate increases to 1 in 6 if the youth is under age 18 (SAMHSA, 2020a). Marijuana has several negative and long-term effects including: a decrease in permanent IQ for those who began to use at a young age; use can lead to depression, anxiety, suicide planning, and psychotic episodes; use affects athletic performance and driving and the development of a fetus.

In recent years, the amount of THC (tetrahydrocannabinol) has increased in the marijuana that is available, and this is the ingredient that gives the "high" sensation. The other component is cannabidiol (CBD); it is typically well tolerated and used in a variety of health conditions. Oils of CBD are increasingly popular, and it is important to know the efficacy of the supplier of CBD.

Side effects of marijuana use include dry and reddened eyes, increased appetite, dry mouth, drowsiness, and mild tachycardia. Adverse reactions include anxiety, disorientation, and paranoia. The use of marijuana as a medical treatment has not been approved by the U.S. FDA.

Opioids

The United States is experiencing a crisis of overdose deaths from opioids, including heroin, illicit fentanyl, and prescription opioids. Opioids are the number one cause of drug overdose deaths in the United States. In 2018, there were 46,800 deaths due to opioid overdose. This was a greater number of deaths than those due to motor vehicle crashes. Opioid addiction is referred to as opioid use disorder (OUD). Here are some startling facts about the incidence of OUD:

1. In 2015, the estimated cost of the opioid epidemic was $504 billion.
2. An estimated 1.7 million Americans have OUD related to opioid painkillers; 526,000 have heroin-related OUD.
3. Two million people in the United States, ages 12 or older, had OUD involving prescription opioids, heroin, or both in 2018 (SAMHSA, 2020b).
4. In 2018, 70% of the 46,802 U.S. drug overdose deaths involved an opioid (Wilson, Kariisa, Seth, Smith, and David, 2020).
5. While deaths involving opioids, prescription opioids, and heroin decreased by 2%, 13.5%, and 4.2%, deaths involving synthetic opioids increased 10%.

The illicit manufacturing of fentanyl has led to increased deaths. (Wilson et al., 2020). Opioids are primarily used for pain management by acting on opioid receptors on nerve cells to decrease pain and produce euphoria and drowsiness. Tolerance and physical dependence develop quickly. This requires tapering down in therapy to avoid withdrawal symptoms after several days' use (O'Malley and O'Malley, 2020b). Fentanyl is 50 times more potent than heroin and 100 times more potent than morphine. Other than fentanyl, there are two additional synthetic opioids: tramadol and fentanyl analogs.

The SAMHSA developed a Treatment Improvement Protocol (TIP). This document discusses the use of three Food and Drug Administration-approved medications to treat opioid use disorder: methadone, naltrexone, and buprenorphine, as well as other services and strategies to support recovery.

The key messages in the TIP are: (1) Addiction is a chronic, treatable illness; (2) General principles of good care for chronic diseases can guide OUD treatment; (3) Patient-centered care provides patients with information that helps them make better treatment decisions; (4) Choose your words carefully when talking with a person with OUD to avoid reinforcing prejudice, negative attitudes, or discrimination; (5) There is no "one size fits all" approach to OUD treatment; (6) Science demonstrates the effectiveness of medical care for OUD; (7) Remission and recovery do not occur only through medication; and (8) Medication for OUD can be combined with outpatient counseling, intensive outpatient treatment, inpatient treatment, or long-term, and it is useful to provide individualized psychosocial support when treating OUD persons with medications (SAMHSA, 2020b).

Heroin is one of the opioids, and the one most often used for recreational purposes. Opioids include the natural drugs found in the opium poppy, namely *opium, morphine,* and *codeine.* Opioids are synthetic drugs, such as heroin (semisynthetic), meperidine, methadone, oxycodone, and propoxyphene, which mimic the effects of natural opiates. The effectiveness of opioids for pain relief is being questioned. Previously, they were by far the most effective drugs for pain relief. Some studies have demonstrated that their use for chronic pain may worsen pain and functioning by increasing pain perception (Frieden and Houry, 2016). Even though there may be benefits to pain relief with the use of opioids, the risks of addiction and overdose must be considered. The CDC has issued a guideline about opioid prescribing that emphasizes patient care and safety. The CDC used a rigorous system process to develop the guidelines. The guidelines were based on three key principles: (1) "nonopioid therapy is preferred for chronic pain outside the context of active cancer, palliative, or end-of-life care," and nonpharmacological therapies can ameliorate chronic pain while posing substantially less risk to patients (e.g., exercise, weight loss, psychological therapies such as cognitive-behavioral therapy, interventions to improve sleep, and certain procedures); (2) when using opioids, use the lowest possible dose; and (3) exercise caution, and monitor patients closely (Frieden and Houry, 2016, pp 2–3).

Persons with OUD are especially susceptible to COVID-19 because this virus disproportionally affects socially marginalized persons with medical and psychiatric comorbid conditions, and these conditions often characterize persons who have OUD (Becker, Fiellin, 2020).

Cocaine

Cocaine is an expensive way to get high; it has powerful effects on the brain, heart, and emotions. Many users become addicted, and even occasional users run the risk of sudden death. Cocaine is a purified extract from the coca shrub found on the eastern slopes of the Andes region of South America. There are two main forms: (1) powdered, which dissolves in water and can be snorted or injected; and (2) crack, which is made by a chemical process that leaves it in a "freebase" form that is smoked. Young men between the ages of 18 and 25 are the biggest users of cocaine.

Cocaine users often describe a feeling of being "high," which includes an increased sense of energy and alertness, an elevated mood, and a feeling of supremacy. Other people feel irritable, paranoid, restless, and anxious. Signs of cocaine use include dilated pupils; high levels of energy and activity; and excited, exuberant speech. The immediate effects wear off in 30 to 120 minutes. In addition to effects on the brain, heart, and emotions, there can be effects on the lungs and respiratory system, GI tract, kidneys, and sexual function. After regular cocaine use for a period of time, withdrawal systems can include depression and anxiety, fatigue, difficulty concentrating, inability to feel pleasure, an increasing craving for the drug, and physical symptoms such as aches, pains, tremors, and chills (WebMD, 2019).

Amphetamines and Methamphetamines

Amphetamines are a class of stimulants similar to cocaine, but the effects last longer, and the drugs are cheaper. Amphetamines have a chemical structure similar to that of adrenaline and noradrenaline and are generally used to decrease fatigue, increase mental alertness, suppress appetite, and create a sense of well-being. They are popular among people who need to stay awake for long hours to work or study. They can be used to treat attention deficit hyperactivity disorder (ADHD) by changing the amounts of certain natural substances in the brain. This use of amphetamines should be carefully supervised by a health care provider (WebMD, n.d.)

Methamphetamines (meth) are easy-to-make street drugs that users swallow, smoke, snort, or inject. Like amphetamines, meth is a stimulant that creates an immediate high that fades quickly. Because of the fading, users may take the substance frequently, and this can lead to addiction. The physical effects are similar to those of cocaine and amphetamines. They include increased breathing, rapid heart rate, high blood pressure, and increased body temperature; with repeated use, meth users often lose weight, get skin sores, and have dental issues. Injecting the drug has all the same effects as any other drug injection.

PREDISPOSING AND CONTRIBUTING FACTORS

In addition to the specific drug being used, two other major variables influence the particular drug experience: set and setting. To understand various patterns of drug use and abuse by individuals, all three factors (i.e., drug, set, and setting) should be considered.

Set refers to the individual using the drug, as well as that person's expectations, including unconscious expectations, about the drug being used. A person's current health may alter a drug's effects from one day to the next. Some people are genetically predisposed to alcoholism or other drug addiction, and their chemical makeup is such that simply consuming the drug triggers the disease process. Persons with underlying mood disorders or other mental illness may try to self-medicate with psychoactive drugs. Sometimes their choice of drug exacerbates their symptoms; for example, a depressed person might consume alcohol and become more depressed.

Setting is the influence of the physical, social, and cultural environment within which the use occurs. Social conditions influence the use of drugs. The fast pace of life, competition at school or in the workplace, a frightening pandemic, and the pressure to accumulate material possessions are daily stressors. The advertising of pharmaceutical, alcohol, and tobacco companies entices people to use their products to feel and sleep better, to have more energy, or just as a "treat." Often people think that most of life's problems can be solved quickly and easily through the use of a drug. For some people, many of life's opportunities may seem out of reach. Rather than seeking relief through medical care, the use of psychoactive drugs may offer a way to numb the pain or escape from a hopeless reality. They also rely on alcohol or illicit drugs, which are more readily available. For some, dealing in illicit drugs may appear to be the only way to avoid a future of poverty and unemployment.

Genetic Factors in Addiction

Dependence on alcohol and other drugs often co-occurs. Evidence indicates that both disorders are, at least partially, influenced by genetic factors. Twin studies have been used to support this co-occurrence. Specifically, "a finding that the correlation between alcohol dependence in twin 1 and drug dependence in twin 2 is higher for identical (i.e., monozygotic) twins, who share 100% of their genes, than for fraternal (i.e., dizygotic) twins, who share on average only 50% of their genes, indicates that shared genes influence the risk of both alcohol and drug dependence" (Dick and Agrawal, 2008). It is complex to identify exactly which genes are likely to contribute to a person's susceptibility to alcohol and/or drug dependence. The environment is also a contributing factor. Some research indicates that addiction is 50% due to genetic factors and 50% to poor coping skills. Also, children of addicts are eight times more likely to develop an addiction than children of nonaddicts (Addictions and Recovery.org, 2017). The NIAAA has been funding the Collaborative Studies on Genetics of Alcoholism since 1989. The goal of these studies is to identify the specific genes that influence alcoholism (NIAAA, n.d.).

PRIMARY PREVENTION AND THE ROLE OF THE NURSE

Harm reduction, a primary care approach to substance abuse, focuses on health promotion and disease prevention. Primary prevention for ATOD problems includes (1) the promotion of healthy lifestyles and resiliency factors, and (2) education about drugs and guidelines for their use. Nurses can be effective in teaching, promoting, and facilitating people in choosing healthy options rather than reliance on drugs. This may entail adding these health-promoting actions to the use of prescription drugs or complementary remedies if the latter are consistent with the recommendations of the health care provider.

Specifically, you can teach clients to be assertive in their relationships with others and how to make better decisions by looking carefully at the pros and cons of each option and the related consequences. People may turn to medications, especially psychoactive drugs, when they experience persistent health problems such as difficulty sleeping, muscle tension, lack of energy, chronic stress, and mood swings. Nurses can help clients understand that medications may mask problems rather than solve them.

The lack of educational opportunities, job training, or both can contribute to socioeconomic stress and poor self-esteem, which can lead to drug use to escape the situation. These factors were apparent during the COVID-19 pandemic, when many people lost their jobs. Nurses can help clients identify community resources and solve problems to meet basic needs rather than avoid them. In addition to decreasing risk factors associated with ATOD/SUD problems, it is important to increase protective or resiliency factors. Prevention guidelines to teach parents and teachers how to increase resiliency in youths include the following strategies:

- Help them develop an increased sense of responsibility for their own success.
- Help them identify their talents.
- Encourage them to find ways to help society rather than believing that their only purpose in life is to be consumers.
- Provide realistic appraisals and feedback, stress multicultural competence, and encourage and value education and skills training.
- Increase cooperative solutions to problems rather than having competitive or aggressive solutions.

These skills also apply to adults. The objectives in *Healthy People 2030* provide guidance for ways to decrease the reliance on alcohol, drugs, and tobacco (USDHHS, 2020).

Drug Education

ATOD problems include more than abuse of psychoactive drugs. Today, more than 450,000 different drugs and drug combinations are available by prescription or over the counter. Nurses know about medication administration, the possible dangers of indiscriminate drug use, and the inability of drugs to cure all problems. Nurses can influence the health of clients by destroying the myth of good drugs versus bad drugs. This means (1) teaching clients that no drug is completely safe and that any drug can be abused, (2) helping persons learn how to make informed decisions about their drug use to minimize potential harm, and (3) teaching them to always tell their health care provider what supplements they are taking.

Drug technology is growing, and many people are learning how to safely use this technology. Harm reduction as a goal recognizes that people consume drugs and that they need to know about the use of drugs and the risks involved to make decisions about their drug use. Drug education should begin on an individual basis by reviewing the client's prescription medications.

? CHECK YOUR PRACTICE

You are working with a group of 18-year-old males who have recently completed a drug rehabilitation program. Your goal is to help them learn a new set of coping strategies other than the use of recreational drugs. Looking back at Chapter 14, which discusses health promotion, what would be some of the stress reduction strategies you would recommend? Are any of these strategies that you have tried for stress in your own life? You know that lack of sleep, improper diet, and lack of exercise contribute to many health complaints and may cause significant stress. Your goal is to provide stress-relieving strategies as an alternative to drug usage. Assisting clients to balance their need for rest, nutrition, and exercise on a daily basis can reduce these complaints. Nurses can provide useful information to groups, assisting in the development of community recreational resources or facilitating stress reduction, relaxation, or exercise groups. Nurses can help people learn about drug-free community activities. The How To box lists community activities in which the nurse may become involved.

What steps would you use in making a clinical judgment? How would you detect cues to what these young men need? In analyzing the cues, what would be your highest priority? What possible solutions or steps would you take to provide care to these youth? Once you have implemented your nursing steps, how would you evaluate the outcomes of your nursing practice?

Because a physician or nurse practitioner has prescribed the medication, clients often presume little risk is involved.

Is the client aware of any untoward interactions this drug may have with other drugs being used or with food? A common occurrence with drug users is taking drugs from different categories together or at different times to regulate how they feel. This practice is known as polysubstance use or abuse. For example, a person may drink alcohol when snorting cocaine to "take the edge off"; or some intravenous drug users combine cocaine with heroin (speedball) for similar reasons. Polysubstance use can cause drug interactions that can have addictive, synergistic, or antagonistic effects. Indiscriminate polysubstance abuse may lead to serious physiological consequences and can be complicated for the health care professional to assess and treat. It is important to encourage clients to ask questions about their drug use. The following list provides six key pieces of information that clients should obtain before taking a drug or medication to decrease the possible harm from unsafe medication consumption. They are:

- The chemical in the drug
- How and where the drug works in the body
- The correct dosage
- If there can be drug interactions, including those with herbal remedies
- If there are potential allergic reactions
- If there might be drug tolerance or if the drug might lead to physical dependence

Nurses can identify references and community resources available to provide the necessary information, and they can clarify the information. User-friendly reference texts and online resources are available that describe drug interactions among medications, other drugs (including alcohol, tobacco, marijuana, and cocaine), and other substances (food and beverages, including energy drinks) and that serve as excellent guides for nurses and their clients. See http://www.drugdigest.org for more information. There is a specific site for drug interactions on the drugdigest.org website. However, pharmacists are excellent sources of information related to drugs and the possible interactions. Clients should learn about and ask questions about their prescription medications and self-administered OTC products, including supplements, herbal remedies, and recreational drugs. Since many people take several alternative medications, it is helpful to keep a list and show your health provider who can consider any adverse interactions with your prescription or recommended OTC medications. This does not mean that nurses should encourage other drug use, but rather that the potential harm from self-medication can be reduced if clients have the necessary information to make more informed decisions. (See the Levels of Prevention box.)

Parents should seek information about their use of medications so they can act as role models for their children. It can be confusing for children and adolescents to be told to "just say no" to drugs when they see their parents or drug advertisements try to "quick fix" every health complaint, feeling of stress, anxiety, or depression with a medication. The simple "just say no" approach does not help young people for several reasons. First, children are naturally curious, and drug experimentation is often a part of normal development. Second, children from dysfunctional

---

LEVELS OF PREVENTION

Related to Abuse of Alcohol, Tobacco, and Other Drugs (Substance Abuse)

Primary Prevention

Provide community education to teach healthy lifestyles; focus on how to resist getting involved in the use of alcohol, tobacco, or drugs.

Secondary Prevention

Institute early detection programs in schools, the workplace, and other areas in which people gather to determine the presence of substance abuse.

Tertiary Prevention

Develop programs to help people reduce or end substance abuse.

---

homes may use drugs to get attention or to escape an intolerable environment. And finally, the "just say no" approach does not address the powerful influence of peer pressure.

Basic substance prevention programs for young people should combine efforts to increase resiliency factors with drug education. Nurses can serve as educators or as advisors to the school systems or community groups to ensure that all of these areas are addressed. Role playing is useful in teaching many of these skills.

QSEN FOCUS ON QUALITY AND SAFETY EDUCATION FOR NURSES

Targeted Competency: Informatics—Use information and technology to communicate, manage knowledge, mitigate error, and support decision making. Important aspects of informatics include the following:

- **Knowledge:** Identify essential information that must be available in a common database to support client care.
- **Skills:** Use information management tools to monitor outcomes of care processes.
- **Attitudes:** Value technologies that support clinical decision making, error prevention, and care coordination.

Informatics Question

You are taking over the role of the school nurse at a large regional high school. There has been a recent tragedy involving a senior from this high school drinking and driving with friends in the car, resulting in one student death and significant injury to the driver and another passenger. You have been asked to address the use of alcohol, tobacco, and other drugs (ATOD) at this high school.

1. What data will you collect to assess the scope of the ATOD problem at this school?
2. Who might be some key informants to interview? What information might they provide that would not be clear from quantitative statistics?
3. You decide that an alcohol and drug education class is needed in your school. What data should you gather to track over time to assess the effectiveness of this intervention?

SECONDARY PREVENTION AND THE ROLE OF THE NURSE

To identify substance use and plan appropriate interventions, nurses must assess each client individually. When SUD is identified, the nurse assists clients to understand the connection between their substance-use patterns and the negative consequences on their health, their families, and the community.

Assessing for Alcohol, Tobacco, and Other Drug Problems

The NIAAA published a clinician's guide for assessing health problems related to drinking. This free booklet, entitled "Helping Patients Who Drink Too Much: A Clinician's Guide," is available at http://www.niaaa.nih.gov/guide. This guide was developed in 2005, and it remains current. Self-assessment tools are available online at http://www.alcoholscreening.org and http://www.drugscreening.org. These screening tools are based on the Alcohol, Smoking, and Substance Involvement Screening Test (ASSIST) developed by the WHO, and the tools allow takers to get immediate anonymous feedback.

During health assessment, the nurse assesses for substance abuse problems, including both self-medication practices and recreational drug use. Thus, all relevant drug use history is collected and aids in the assessment of drug use patterns. Note any changes in drug use patterns over time. After obtaining a medication history, follow-up questions can determine whether problems exist. The following are examples:

- When using a prescription or OTC drug, is the client following the directions correctly?
- Has the client increased the dosage or frequency above the prescription level?
- Is the person using any prescribed psychoactive drugs? If yes, for how long, and what is the dosage?

When assessing self-medication and recreational or social drug use patterns, determine the reason the person uses the drug. Some underlying health problems (e.g., pain, stress, weight, insomnia) may be relieved by nonpharmaceutical interventions. The amount, frequency, and duration of use and the route of administration of each drug should be determined. To establish the presence of a substance abuse problem, determine whether the drug use is causing any negative health consequences or problems with relationships, employment, finances, or the legal system. The How To box lists examples of questions to ask to determine the presence of socioeconomic problems that are often secondary to substance abuse. If a pattern of chronic, regular, and frequent use of a drug exists, nurses should assess for a history of withdrawal symptoms to determine whether there is a physical dependence on the drug. A progression in drug use patterns and related problems warns about the possibility of addiction. Denial is a primary symptom of addiction. Methods of denial include the following:

- Lying about use
- Minimizing use patterns
- Blaming or rationalizing
- Intellectualizing
- Changing the subject
- Using anger or humor
- "Going with the flow" (i.e., agreeing that a problem exists and saying the behavior will change but not demonstrating any changes in behavior)

A problem should be suspected if the client becomes defensive or exhibits other behavior indicating denial when asked about alcohol or other drug use.

HOW TO ASSESS SOCIOECONOMIC PROBLEMS RESULTING FROM SUBSTANCE ABUSE

If the client admits to the use of alcohol, tobacco, or other drugs, ask the following questions:

- Do your parents, spouse, or friends worry or complain about your drinking or using drugs?
- Has a family member asked for help for your drinking or using drugs?
- Have you neglected family obligations as a result of drinking or using drugs?
- Have you missed work and/or does your boss complain about your drinking or using drugs?
- Do you drink or use drugs before or during work?
- Have you ever been fired or quit a job because of drinking or using drugs?
- Have you ever been charged with driving under the influence (DUI) or being drunk in public (DIP)?
- Have you ever had any other legal problems related to drinking and using drugs, such as assault and battery, breaking and entering, or theft?
- Have you had any accidents while intoxicated, such as falls, burns, or motor vehicle accidents?
- Have you spent your money on alcohol or other drugs instead of paying your bills (e.g., telephone, electricity, rent)?

Drug Testing

During the 1980s, preemployment or random drug testing in the workplace became a common practice. In drug testing, you can examine a person's urine, blood, saliva, breath (alcohol), or hair. Urine testing, the most common method, indicates only past use of certain drugs, not intoxication. You can identify a person who has used a certain drug in the recent past, but urine testing does not determine the degree of intoxication and the extent of performance impairment. Also, most drug-related problems in the workplace are related to alcohol, and alcohol is not always included in a urine drug screen. When is drug testing appropriate? Drug testing that follows documented impairment may help substantiate the cause of the impairment and serve as a backup rather than the primary screening method. It is also useful for recovering addicts. Part of their treatment is to abstain from psychoactive drug use; therefore, a urine test yielding positive results for a drug indicates a relapse.

Blood, breath, and saliva drug tests can indicate current use and amount. Any of these tests can help determine alcohol intoxication, and they are often used to substantiate suspected impairment. A serum drug screen to determine the specific drug ingested can be useful when an overdose is suspected. The testing of hair is gaining attention because the results can provide a long history of drug use patterns.

Alcohol and other drug testing should be used as a clinical and public health tool but not for harassment and punishment. For example, approximately 40% to 50% of people who are seen in trauma centers were drinking at the time of their injuries. Hence, it is recommended that breath alcohol testing be routinely done for persons admitted to the emergency department for traumatic injuries (Physicians and Lawyers for National Drug Policy, 2008).

Employee assistance programs (EAPs) are a beneficial service in many work settings. Often a sizable number of EAP clients have substance use problems because most adults with these problems are employed. EAP programs can identify health problems among employees and offer counseling or a referral to other health care providers as necessary. Such programs provide early identification of and intervention for substance abuse problems. They also offer services to employees to reduce stress and provide health care or counseling so that they may prevent substance abuse problems from developing. Nurses frequently develop and run these programs.

High-Risk Groups

Identifying high-risk groups helps nurses design programs to meet specific needs and mobilize community resources.

Adolescents

The younger a person is when beginning intensive experimentation with drugs, the more likely dependence will develop. Underage drinking is seen as the most serious drug problem for youth in the United States. Alcohol is the most widely used substance that is abused by youth. In 2018, it was found that by age 15, about 30% of teens had at least 1 drink and by age 18, about 58%. Also in 2018, 7.1 million young people ages 12 to 20 said they drank alcohol beyond "just a few sips in a month" (NIAAA, 2020). Underage drinking is dangerous because it causes many deaths and injuries, impairs judgment, increases the risk of physical and sexual assault, can lead to other problems, increases the risk of alcohol problems later in life, and interferes with brain development (NIAAA, 2020). The use of marijuana and the nonmedical use of prescription pain relievers are additional risk factors for adolescents.

Heavy drug use during adolescence can interfere with normal development. Note that *Healthy People 2030* objectives in the SU substance abuse category are directed toward reducing the use of drugs (see the *Healthy People 2030* box). Family-related factors (e.g., genetics, family stress, parenting styles, child victimization) and peer pressure may be the greatest variables that influence substance abuse among adolescents. The co-occurrence with psychiatric disorders (especially mood disorders) and behavioral problems is also associated with substance abuse among adolescents, leaving peer pressure as a less influential factor. Research suggests that successful social influence-based prevention programs may be driven by their ability to foster social norms that reduce an adolescent's social motivation to begin using ATOD.

♥ *HEALTHY PEOPLE 2030*

Objectives Related to Substance Abuse

- **SU-01:** Increase the proportion of people with a substance use disorder who got treatment in the past year.
- **SU-18:** Reduce the proportion of people who had opioid use disorder in the past year.
- **TU-16:** Increase Medicaid coverage of evidence-based treatment to help people quit using tobacco.

US Department of Health and Human Services. *Healthy People 2030.* Washington, DC; 2020, US Government Printing Office.

Older Adults

Worldwide, the number of older people is increasing. Alcohol abuse, and its associated disorders in the elderly, is a common and underrecognized occurrence. The disorders associated with the use of ATOD are a major cause of physical and psychological health problems. The social and physical changes that often accompany aging may increase a person's vulnerability to substance abuse. For example, the loss of loved ones, retirement, illness, lower levels of achievement, lack of mobility, having to move from one's home, juggling many roles, and being tired or sleep deprived may cause people to seek illicit drugs or self-medicate for anxiety and depression. This age group consumes more prescribed and OTC medications than any other age group. See the free public education brochure "As You Age . . . A Guide to Aging, Medicines and Alcohol" at a variety of websites, including www.fda.gov. The increased use of prescription drugs and alcohol causes slowed metabolic turnover of drugs, age-related organ changes, enhanced drug sensitivities, and a tendency to use drugs over long periods. Frequent use of multiple drugs contributes to greater negative consequences from drug use among older adults. Alcohol abuse may not be identified because its effects on cognitive abilities may mimic changes associated with normal aging or degenerative brain disease. Also, depression may be simply attributed to more frequent losses rather than the depressant effects of alcohol, and the older adult may subsequently receive medical treatment for depression rather than alcoholism. It is important for all persons who take medications to be knowledgeable about the drugs; it is especially important for older adults whose bodies respond differently to drugs and alcohol than younger people.

Injection Drug Users

In addition to the problem of addiction, injection drug users (IDUs) (i.e., those who self-administer intravenously or subcutaneously) are at risk for other health complications. Intravenous administration of drugs always carries a greater risk for overdose because the drug goes directly into the bloodstream. With illicit drugs, the danger is increased because the exact dosage is unknown and there may be fillers in the drug that could harm the user. Such fillers or other chemicals could be sugar, starch, or quinine, and these ingredients can cause negative consequences. Often, IDUs make their own solution for intravenous administration, and any particles present can result in complications from emboli.

Addicted persons often share needles. Contaminated needles can transmit hepatitis C and HIV infection and other bloodborne diseases. The risk of getting or transmitting HIV is high if an HIV-negative person uses injection equipment that someone with HIV has used. Needles, syringes, or other injection equipment may have blood in them. Blood can carry HIV, which can survive in a used syringe for up to 42 days. Abstinence is ideal but unrealistic for many addicts. Using the harm reduction model, the nurse should provide education on cleaning needles with bleach between uses; being careful to not get another person's blood on their hands or equipment; disposing equipment safely; and needle exchange programs to decrease the spread of the virus. Studies indicate that needle exchange programs have not increased injection drug abuse but have increased the number of people entering treatment programs. Many communities have syringe services programs (SSPs), and people can get free sterile needles and syringes and safely dispose of used ones (CDC, 2020b).

Drug Use During Pregnancy

Most drugs can negatively affect a fetus. Thus, the use of any drug during pregnancy should be discouraged unless medically necessary. *Healthy People 2030* objectives address this issue under the Pregnancy and Childbirth area. The objectives for this issue are found in this area under Drug and Alcohol Use. Fetal alcohol syndrome is considered the leading preventable birth defect, causing mental and behavioral impairment. Heavy drinking is becoming less of a problem for pregnant women due to the available information on the results of drinking during pregnancy; tobacco remains a problem. Symptoms of depression and anxiety are often prevalent during pregnancy and influence a woman's decision to use alcohol or other substances. In some states, pregnant women who are using illicit drugs are reported to child protective services because of the potential harm to the fetus.

Use of Illicit Drugs

The strategy of "just say no" to drugs is both simplistic and misleading. Indiscriminate use of "good" drugs has caused more health problems from adverse reactions, drug interactions, dependence, addiction, and overdoses than the use of "bad" drugs. The black market associated with illicit drug use puts otherwise law-abiding citizens in close contact with criminals, prevents any quality control of the drugs, increases the risk for AIDS and hepatitis secondary to needle sharing, and hinders health care professionals' accessibility to the abuser or addict. The lack of quality control (i.e., unknown strength and purity) can cause unexpected overdoses or secondary effects of the impurities. Unsafe administration (contaminated needles) leads to local and systemic infections. The high cost of drugs on the black market leads to crime to support the addiction. Young people are the most likely group to use illicit drugs.

Codependency and Family Involvement

Drug addiction is often a family disease. One in four Americans experiences family problems related to alcohol abuse. People close to the addicted person often develop unhealthy coping mechanisms to continue the relationship. This behavior is known as codependency, a stress-induced preoccupation with the addicted person's life, leading to extreme dependence and excessive concern for the addict. Strict rules typically develop in a codependent family to maintain the relationships, such as don't talk, don't feel, don't trust, don't lose control, and don't seek help from outside the family.

Codependents try to meet the addicted person's needs at the expense of their own. Codependency may underlie medical complaints and emotional stress seen by health care providers such as ulcers, skin disorders, migraine headaches, chronic colds, and backaches. When the addicted person refuses to admit the problem, the family continues to adapt to emotionally survive the stress of the addict's irrational, inconsistent, and unpredictable behavior. Family members consequently develop roles that tend to exaggerate normal family roles, and they cling irrationally to these roles, even when they are no longer functional. One of the most significant roles a family member may assume is that of an enabler. Enabling is the act of shielding or preventing the addict from experiencing the consequences of the addiction. As a result, the addict does not always understand the cost of the addiction and thus is "enabled" to continue to use. Although codependency and enabling are closely related, a person does not have to be codependent to enable. Anyone can be an enabler—a police officer, a supervisor or coworker, and even a drug treatment counselor. Health care professionals can be enablers when they fail to address the negative health consequences of drug use with the addicted person.

The nurse can help families recognize the problem of addiction and help them confront the addicted member in a caring manner. Regardless of whether the addicted family member is agreeable to treatment, family members should be given guidance about the resources and services available to help them cope more effectively. The nurse can help identify treatment options, counseling assistance, financial assistance, support services, and (if necessary) legal services for the family members. Children of ATOD abusers or addicts are themselves at a greater risk for developing an addiction and must be targeted for primary prevention. A useful website is the National Institute on Drug Abuse at http://www.drugabuse.gov. See the Drug Facts series, which covers a range of topics, including prescription and OTC medications, spice (synthetic marijuana), and commonly abused prescription drugs. Also, look at http://www.drugabuse.gov which is the website for the National Institute on Drug Abuse. This site has a variety of useful resources. The SAMHSA national helpline is useful also: 800-662-HELP (4357), as is the CDC helpline at 800-QUITNOW. *Healthy People 2030* has a section on addictions under Health Conditions, a section on drug and alcohol use under Behaviors, and a section on tobacco use. Each section has specific goals as their national health targets.

TERTIARY PREVENTION AND THE ROLE OF THE NURSE

The nurse is in a key position to help the person who has a SUD and his or her family. The nurse's knowledge of community resources and how to mobilize them can significantly influence the quality of care clients receive.

Detoxification

Detoxification is the clearing of one or more drugs from the person's body and managing the withdrawal symptoms. Depending on the particular drug and the degree of dependence, the time required may range from a few days to several weeks. Because withdrawal symptoms vary (depending on the drug used) and range from uncomfortable to life-threatening, the setting for and management of withdrawal depend on the drug used. Stimulants or opiates may produce withdrawal symptoms that are uncomfortable but not life-threatening. Detoxification from these drugs does not require direct medical supervision, but medical management of the withdrawal symptoms increases the comfort level. On the other hand, drugs such as alcohol, benzodiazepines, and barbiturates can produce life-threatening withdrawal symptoms. These clients should be under close medical supervision during detoxification and should receive medical management of the withdrawal symptoms to ensure a safe withdrawal. Of those who develop delirium tremens from alcohol withdrawal, 15% may not survive despite medical management; therefore, close medical management is initiated as the blood alcohol level begins to fall. A general rule in detoxification management is to wean the person off the drug by gradually reducing the dosage and frequency of administration. Thus, a person with chronic alcoholism could be safely detoxified by a gradual reduction in alcohol consumption. In practice, however, the switch to another drug, usually a benzodiazepine, often offers a safer withdrawal from alcohol as well as an abrupt end to the intoxication from the drug of choice. For example, chlordiazepoxide (Librium) is commonly used for alcohol detoxification. Outpatient or home detoxification for persons requiring medical detoxification for alcohol withdrawal can be a cost-effective treatment. Nurses can monitor and evaluate the client's health status in the home environment to reduce the risk for medical complications related to alcohol withdrawal and to provide encouragement and support for the client to complete the detoxification.

Addiction Treatment

Addiction treatment differs from the management of negative health consequences of chronic drug abuse, overdose, and detoxification. Addiction treatment focuses on the addiction process. The goal is to help clients view addiction as a chronic disease and assist them to make lifestyle changes to halt the progression of the disease. According to the disease theory, addicted persons are not responsible for the symptoms of their disease; they are, however, responsible for treating their disease. People 12 years of age and older seek treatment for addictions.

Most treatment facilities are multidisciplinary because the intervention strategies require a wide range of approaches. Their programs involve interactions among the addict, family, culture, and community. Strategies include medical management, education, counseling, vocational rehabilitation, stress management, and support services. The key to effective treatment is to match individual clients with the interventions most appropriate for them.

For those addicted individuals unwilling or unable to completely abstain from psychoactive drugs, other medications can assist them in abstaining from their drug of choice. Methadone maintenance programs are used to treat heroin and other opioid addictions. Methadone, when administered in moderate or high daily doses, produces a cross-tolerance to other opioids, thereby blocking their effects and decreasing the craving for heroin. The advantages of methadone are that it is long acting and effective orally, does not produce a "high," is inexpensive, and has few known side effects. The oral use of methadone offers a solution to the danger of the spread of HIV infection and other blood-borne infections that commonly occur among needle-sharing addicts. Although not recognized as a cure for heroin (or other opiate) addiction, methadone maintenance is a harm reduction intervention because it reduces deviant behavior and introduces addicted persons to the health care system (Volkow et al., 2014).

Recovery from addiction requires a lifetime commitment and may include periods of relapse. The addicted person must realize that modern medicine has not found a cure for addiction; therefore, returning to drug use may ultimately reactivate the disease process.

Long-term residential programs, also called *halfway houses,* can help ease the person recovering from an addiction back into society. These facilities provide continued support and counseling in a structured environment for persons needing long-term assistance in adjusting to a drug-free lifestyle. The residents are expected to secure employment and take responsibility for managing their financial obligations.

Outpatient programs are similar in the education and counseling offered, but they allow the clients to live at home and continue to work while undergoing treatment. This method is effective for persons in the earlier stages of addiction who feel confident that they can abstain from drug use and who have established a strong support network.

Most programs include family counseling and education. In addition, specific programs address the needs of various populations such as adolescents, women during pregnancy, specific ethnic groups, gays and lesbians, and health care professionals.

CASE STUDY

Ryan Swabbs, MSN, works at a drug rehabilitation center and provides individual and group counseling for clients who are in the process of controlling or stopping their drug addiction. Tonya Lamburg is a 16-year-old mother of a 2-year-old son who currently lives with his grandmother. Ms. Lamburg entered the drug rehabilitation center with the goal of ending her problem with the use of alcohol and cocaine. Mr. Swabbs is assigned to her case.

At their first meeting, Mr. Swabbs assesses Ms. Lamburg's level of drug abuse and readiness for change. Ms. Lamburg has been at the center for 1 week and has not used any drugs since checking in. She said that she has repeatedly tried to quit alcohol and cocaine "cold turkey" but started to feel "bad and shaky" and went back to using to stop the withdrawal symptoms. "I have no money. I cannot pay for food for my baby. Everything goes to pay for booze or to get high," said Ms. Lamburg. "I dropped out of school when I got pregnant. Everywhere I try to work I get fired. I decided to get help when I saw my baby get into my coke stash. I do not want my boy to die. I do not want to die." If you were the nurse working with Ms. Lamburg, what steps would you take to help her succeed in meeting her goal of becoming drug-free? What would your first goal be? Depending on her response, what might your next steps be?

Smoking Cessation Programs

In 2018, over half of the adult cigarette smokers in the United States had made a quit attempt in the past year. In that same year, more than 7 out of 100 people who tried to quit succeeded. Between 2012 and 2018, the CDC estimates that more than 16.4 million smokers attempted to quit, and one million succeeded using the Tips program. The Tips information on the CDC website offers useful information to guide nurses in referring patients to this tool (CDC, 2019). Nearly 35 million Americans try to quit smoking each year. Fewer than 10% of those who try to quit on their own are able to stop for a year; those who use an intervention are more likely to be successful. Interventions that involve medications and behavioral treatments appear most promising (USDHHS, 2014). For example, nicotine replacement therapy can be used to help smokers withdraw from nicotine while focusing their efforts on breaking the psychological craving or habit. Four types of nicotine replacement products are available. Nicotine gum and skin patches are available OTC, and nicotine nasal spray and inhalers are available by prescription. These products are about equally effective and can almost double the chances of successfully quitting. Other treatments include smoking cessation clinics, hypnosis, and acupuncture. The most effective way to get people to stop smoking and prevent relapse involves multiple interventions and continuous reinforcement, and most smokers require several attempts at cessation before they are successful. Many resources are available on smoking cessation and support groups. Two useful helplines are: (1) SAMHSA National Helpline at 1-800-622-help (4357). In the first quarter of 2018, the Helpline received an average of 68,683 calls per month. It is a free, confidential service available in English or Spanish. (2) CDC has this helpline:1-800-QUITNOW.

Support Groups

The founding of Alcoholics Anonymous (AA) in 1935 began a strong movement of peer support to treat a chronic illness. AA groups have developed around the world. Their success has led to the development of other support groups such as the following:

- Narcotics Anonymous (NA) for persons with narcotic addiction
- Pills Anonymous for persons with polydrug addictions
- Overeaters Anonymous
- Gamblers Anonymous

AA and NA help addicted people develop a daily program of recovery and reinforce the recovery process. The fellowship, support, and encouragement among AA members provide a vital social network for the person recovering from an addiction.

Al-Anon and Alateen are similar self-help programs for spouses, parents, children, or others involved in a painful relationship with an alcoholic (Nar-Anon for those in relationships with persons with narcotic addictions). Al-Anon family groups are available to anyone who has been affected by involvement with an alcoholic person. The purposes of Alateen include providing a forum for adolescents to discuss family stressors, learn coping skills from one another, and gain support and encouragement from knowledgeable peers. Adult Children of Alcoholics (ACOA) groups are also available in most areas to address the recovery of adults who grew up in alcoholic homes and are still carrying the scars and retaining dysfunctional behaviors. Many of these support groups offer assistance in person, online, or in visual and audio online meetings.

For some persons, the AA program places too much emphasis on a higher power or focuses too much on the negative consequences of past drinking. Women for Sobriety, a program by women for women, focuses on rebuilding self-esteem, a core issue for many women with alcoholic problems. See http://www.womenforsobriety.org for additional information.

THE NURSE'S ROLE

Many people with SUD become lost in the health care system. If satisfactory care is not provided in one agency or the waiting list is months long, the person may give up rather than seeking alternative sources of care. The nurse who knows the client's history, environment, and support systems and the local treatment programs can offer guidance to the most effective treatment modality. See the Center for Substance Abuse Treatment (CSAT) for information on the SAMHSA website at http://www.samhsa.gov for a variety of print and video materials for professionals on helping persons with substance abuse problems. CSAT promotes the availability and quality of substance abuse treatments that are community based for use by individuals and families. SAMHSA also describes three steps to accessing care and five signs of quality treatment, SAMHSA, n,d,) Brief interventions by health care professionals who are not treatment experts can be effective in helping ATOD abusers and addicted persons change their risky behavior. Brief interventions may convince the ATOD abuser to reduce substance consumption or follow through with a treatment referral (SAMHSA, 2011). Box 26.1 describes six elements commonly included in brief interventions, using the acronym FRAMES. Strategies used with clients can vary depending on their readiness for change. Understanding the stages of change listed in Box 26.2 and recognizing which stage a client is in are important factors for determining which interventions and programs may be most helpful to the client (DiClemente et al., 2004). After the client has received treatment, the nurse can coordinate aftercare referrals and follow up on the client's progress. The nurse can provide additional support in the home as the client and family adjust to changing roles and the stress involved with such changes. The nurse can support addicted persons who have relapsed by reminding them that relapses may well occur but that they and their families can continue to work toward recovery and an improved quality of life.

BOX 26.1 Brief Interventions Using the FRAMES Acronym

- **Feedback.** Provide the client direct feedback about the potential or actual personal risk or impairment related to drug use.
- **Responsibility.** Emphasize personal responsibility for change.
- **Advice.** Provide clear advice to change risky behavior.
- **Menu.** Provide a menu of options or choices for changing behavior.
- **Empathy.** Provide a warm, reflective, empathetic, and understanding approach.
- **Self-efficacy.** Provide encouragement and belief in the client's ability to change.

Modified from Bien TH, Miller WR, Tonigan JS. Brief interventions for alcohol problems: a review. *Addictions* 1993;88:315.

BOX 26.2 Stages of Change

Precontemplation

At this stage, the person does not intend to change in the foreseeable future. The person is often unaware of any problem. Resistance to recognizing or modifying a problem is the hallmark of precontemplation.

Contemplation

At this stage, the individual is aware that a problem exists and is seriously thinking about overcoming it but has not yet made a commitment to take action. The nurse can encourage the individual to weigh the pros and cons of the problem and the solution to the problem.

Preparation

Preparation was originally referred to as decision making. At this stage, the individual is prepared for action and may reduce the problem behavior but has not yet taken effective action (e.g., cuts down the amount of smoking but does not abstain).

Action

At this stage, the individual modifies the behavior, experiences, or environment to overcome the problem. The action requires considerable time and energy. Modification of the target behavior to an acceptable criterion and significant overt efforts to change are the hallmarks of action.

Maintenance

In this stage, the individual works to prevent relapse and consolidate the gains attained during action. Stabilizing behavior change and avoiding relapse are the hallmarks of maintenance.

Modified from DiClemente CC, Schlundt D, Gemmell L. Readiness and stages of change in addiction treatment. *Am J Addictions* 2004;13:103–20.

▶▶ APPLYING CONTENT TO PRACTICE

Using the tools of primary, secondary, and tertiary prevention with individuals, families, and communities for whom alcohol and other drug use is an issue incorporates both public health and public health nursing guidelines and competencies. Specifically, the core competencies of the Council on Linkages Between Academia and Public Health Practice (2014) begin by identifying the analytic and assessment skills needed by public health professionals. The 14 skills in this competency category are used in providing services to the population described in this chapter. For example, you begin by describing "factors affecting the health of a community (e.g., equity, income, education, environment)" (p. 5) in Skill one: Analytical/Assessment Skills and then examine the remaining skills to plan your intervention.

▌ PRACTICE APPLICATION

Jane Doe, a female RN, is a home health case manager in a large, low-income housing area in her local community. She designs care plans and coordinates health care services for clients who need health care at home. She makes the initial visits to determine the level and frequency of care needed and then acts as supervisor of the volunteers and aides who perform most of the day-to-day care. Single-parent families are the norm, and drug dealing is commonplace in this housing area.

Ms. Doe made a home visit to Anne Smith, a 26-year-old mother of three who takes care of her 62-year-old maternal grandfather, Mr. Jones, who is recovering from cardiac bypass surgery. Mr. Jones has a history of smoking two packs per day for almost 40 years. Since his surgery, he has decreased to one pack per day, but he refuses to quit. He had a history of alcohol dependence, reportedly consuming up to a fifth of liquor per day, and a history of withdrawal seizures. Four years ago, Mr. Jones went through alcohol detoxification, but he refused to stay at the facility for continued treatment, stating he could stay sober on his own. Since that time, he has had several binge episodes, but Ms. Smith says he has not been drinking since the surgery. A widower for 5 years, Mr. Jones now lives with his granddaughter and her children.

Ms. Smith is a widow and has two sons, ages 3 and 9 years, and a daughter, age 5 years. The oldest son's father is an alcoholic who is currently incarcerated for manslaughter while driving under the influence of alcohol, and the father of her two youngest children was killed by a stray bullet in a cocaine bust 3 years ago. She and her husband had smoked crack cocaine for several months, but both stopped when she became pregnant with their youngest child and remained cocaine-free. She has been angry at the system and frightened of police officers ever since the drug raid in which her husband was killed. Other residents were also hurt, and less than $500 worth of cocaine was found three apartments away from hers.

Ms. Smith does not consume alcohol, but she smokes one to two packs of cigarettes per day. She quit smoking during her pregnancies but restarted soon after each birth.

A. What type of interventions can the nurse provide for Mr. Jones regarding his smoking?

B. How can the nurse help Ms. Smith cope with the potential risk for Mr. Jones continuing to drink when he progresses to more independence?

C. How can Ms. Doe help Ms. Smith with her cigarette smoking?

D. Knowing that there is a genetic link to alcoholism and being aware of the high rate of drug problems in the housing area, how can Ms. Doe help prevent Ms. Smith and her children from developing substance abuse problems?

E. What are the most significant problems related to the drug laws, and what can Ms. Doe do to help make the environment safer and more nurturing?

Answers can be found on the Evolve website.

▌ REMEMBER THIS!

- Substance use disorder is a leading national health problem linked to numerous forms of morbidity and mortality.
- Harm reduction is a new approach to ATOD/SUD problems; it deals with substance abuse primarily as a health problem rather than a criminal problem.
- All persons have ideas, opinions, and attitudes about drugs that influence their actions.
- Social conditions such as a fast-paced life, excessive stress, and the availability of drugs influence the incidence of substance abuse.
- New forms of substance abuse are growing, including the use of electronic cigarettes and energy drinks. Nurses need to be familiar with these substances and their effects.

- Primary prevention for substance abuse includes education about drugs and guidelines for use, as well as the promotion of healthy alternatives to drug use either for recreation or to relieve stress.
- Nurses can play a key role in developing community prevention programs.
- Secondary prevention depends heavily on the careful assessment of the client's use of drugs. Such assessment should be part of all basic health assessments.
- High-risk groups include pregnant women, young people, older adults, intravenous drug users, and illicit drug users.
- Drug addiction is often a family problem, not merely an individual problem.
- Codependency describes a companion illness to the addiction of one person in which the codependent member is addicted to the addicted person.
- Brief interventions by a nurse can be an effective part of treatment.
- Nurses are in ideal roles to assist with tertiary prevention for both the addicted person and the family.

EVOLVE WEBSITE

http://evolve.elsevier.com/Stanhope/foundations
- Case Study, with Questions and Answers
- NCLEX Review Questions
- Practice Application Answers

REFERENCES

Addiction Policy Forum: *Navigating treatment and addiction: A guide for families,* August 2020, Retrieved November 2020 at http://www.addictionpolicy.org.

Addictions and Recovery.org: *The genetics of addiction,* June 18, 2017, Author.

American Psychiatric Association: *Diagnostic and statistical manual of mental disorders* (5th ed), 2013, Washington, DC, American Psychiatric Association.

Antolin VM, Barkley TW: Electronic cigarettes: what nurses need to know. *Nursing* 45(11):60–64, 2015.

Becker WC, Fiellin DA: When epidemics collide: Coronavirus Disease 2019 (COVID-19) and the opioid crisis, *Annals of Internal Medicine, 2020,* retrieved November 2020 at http://www.Annals.org.

Centers for Disease Control and Prevention, *Smoking & tobacco use: fast facts,* Revised November 15, 2019, accessed February 19, 2020 at www.cdc.gov.

Centers for Disease Control and Prevention, *Smoking & tobacco use: about electronic cigarettes (E-cigarettes),* February 24, 2020a, Accessed at www.cdc.gov June 2020.

Centers for Disease Control and Prevention: *Injection drug use and HIV risk,* Last reviewed February 6, 2020b, Accessed June 2020 at www.cdc.gov.

Council on Linkages Between Academic and Public Health Practice: *Core competencies for public health professionals,* Washington, DC, 2014, Public Health Foundation, Health Resources and Services Administration.

Dick DM, Agrawal A: The genetics of alcohol and other drug dependence, *Alcohol Research and Health* 31(2):111–118, 2008.

DiClemente CC, Schlundt D, Gemmell L: Readiness and stages of change in addiction treatment, *Am J Addictions* 13:103–120, 2004.

Fathi JT: Tobacco use: The current state of affairs and how nurses can help patients quit, *The Online Journal of Issues in Nursing,* 25(3), Manuscript 1, September 30, 2020.

Frieden TR, Houry D: Reducing the risks of relief–the CDC Opioid-prescribing guideline, *N Engl J of Med* downloaded from nejm.org on March 29, 2016. Vol 374:1501–1504, April 21, 2016.

Halpers B, Felsher-Folar P, and Grosse M: CoVID-19 risk up to 7 times higher for young vapers, cited in Health Day, August 11, 2020, Health Day News. From the *Jl of Adolescent Health,* August 11, 2020.

Hartley E: DSM 5 Criteria for substance abuse disorders, *Verywell mind.* March 21, 2020,

Mayo Clinic Staff: *Caffeine: how much is too much?* Rochester, MN, March 2, 2017, Mayo Clinic. Retrieved July 2020 from www.mayoclinic.org.

Medline Plus: *Alcohol use disorder (AUD),* Accessed June 2020 at https://medline plus.gov/alcoholusedisorderaud.htm.

National Center for Chronic Disease Prevention and Health Promotion: *Tobacco use,* Centers for Disease Control and Prevention, last reviewed March 18, 2019, www.cdc.gov. Accessed June 2020.

National Institute on Alcohol Abuse and Alcoholism: *Alcohol facts and statistics,* Accessed June 2020 from www.niaaa.nih.gov.

National Institute on Alcohol Abuse and Alcoholism: *Genetics of alcohol use disorder.* Retrieved June 30, 2020, from https://www.niaaa.nih.gov.

National Institute on Alcohol Abuse and Alcoholism: *Underage drinking, 2020,* Retrieved from www.niaaa.nih.gov, June 2020.

O'Malley GF, O'Malley R: *Alcohol toxicity and withdrawal,* In Merck Manual online 2018, Retrieved June 2020 from www.merckmanuals.com.

O'Malley GF and O'Malley R: *Alcohol use disorders and rehabilitation,* In Merck Manual online 2020a, Retrieved June 2020.

O'Malley GF and O'Malley r: *Opioid use disorder and rehabilitation,* In Merck Manual online 2020b, Retrieved November 2020.

Physicians and Lawyers for National Drug Policy: *Policy priorities: summary,* 2008. Retrieved July 2020 from http://www.plndp.orgl.

Seifert SM, Schaechter JL, Hershorin EG, Lipshultz SE: Health effects of energy drinks on children, adolescents, and young adults, *Pediatrics* 127(3): 511-528, 2011.

Substance Abuse and Mental Health Services Administration: *Finding quality treatment for substance disorders,* n.d. Accessed February 2020 at www/store.samhsa.gov.

Substance Abuse and Mental Health Services Administration: *Screening, Brief Intervention and referral to Treatment (SBIBT) in Behavioral Healthcare,* January 4, 2011. Available at www.samhsa.gov. Accessed June 2020.

Substance Abuse and Mental Health Services Administration: *Key substance use and mental health indicators in the United States,* Results from the 2018 National Survey on Drug use and Health, 2019, Retrieved June 2020 from www.samhsa.gov/data/.

Substance Abuse and Mental Health Services Administration: *National helpline,* Last updated November 6, 2019, Accessed at www.samsha.gov, February 2020.

Substance Abuse and Mental Health Services Administration: *Learn about marijuana risks,* 2020a, Accessed June 2020 at www.samhsa.gov.

Substance Abuse and Mental Health Services Administration: *TIP 63: Medications for opioid use disorder,* 2020b, Accessed May 6, 2020, at www.store.samhsa.gov.

US Department of Health and Human Services: *Healthy People 2020,* Washington, DC, 2010, US Government Printing Office.

US Department of Health and Human Services: *Healthy People 2030,* Washington, DC, 2020a, US Government Printing Office.

US Department of Health and Human Services: *The health consequences of smoking—50 years of progress: a report of the Surgeon General*, Atlanta, GA, 2014, USDHHS, CDC, National Center for Chronic Disease Prevention and Health Promotion.

US Department of Health and Human Services. *Smoking Cessation: A Report of the Surgeon General–Executive Summary.*2020b, Atlanta, GA: US Department of Health and Human Services, Centers for Disease Control and Prevention, National Center for Chronic Disease Prevention and Health Promotion, Office on Smoking and Health, 2020.

Volkow ND, Frieden TR, Hyde PS, et al.: Medical-assisted therapies—tackling the opioid overdose epidemic. *N Engl J Med* 370: 2063–2066, 2014.

Volkow ND: Collision of the COVID-19 and addiction epidemics, *Annals of Internal Medicine,* published online April 2, 2020, at Annals.org.

Wang QQ, Kaelber DC, Xu R, Volkow ND: COVID-19 risk and outcomes in patients with substance use disorders: analyses from electronic health records in the United States, *Springer Nature,* Published online, September 14, 2020, Retrieved November 2020 from http://www.nature.com.

WebMD: *Street drugs: know the facts and risks.* Reviewed 2019. Retrieved June 2020 from http://www.webmd.com.

WebMD: *Attention deficit hyperactivity disorder,* n.d. Reviewed 12/4/19 by Jennifer Casaretla, Accessed June 2020 at www.webmd.com.

Wilson N, Karlisa M, Seth P, Smith H IV, Davis NL: *Drugs and opioid-involved overdose deaths—United States, 2017-2018, MMWR Morb Mort Wkly Rep 2020: 69: 290-297.*

World Health Organization: *Tobacco: key facts,* July 26, 2019, www.who.int. Accessed June 2020.

27

Violence and Human Abuse

Jeanne L. Alhusen, Gerard M. Jellig, and Jacquelyn C. Campbell

OBJECTIVES

After reading this chapter, the student should be able to:

1. Discuss the scope of the problem of violence in American communities, and describe at least three factors in most communities that encourage violence and human abuse.
2. Identify at least three factors existing in communities that are considered risk factors for violence.
3. Define the four general types of child abuse: neglect, physical, emotional, and sexual.
4. Discuss the dynamics and signs of female abuse by male partners.
5. Describe the growing community health problem of elder abuse.
6. Analyze the nursing role in working with survivors of violence.
7. Discuss forensic nursing and its relationship to public health nursing.
8. Describe a public health approach for the prevention of violence.

CHAPTER OUTLINE

KEY TERMS

Violence is a pervasive public health, social, and developmental threat. It is the leading cause of death and disability that disproportionately affects youth, low-income populations, and people of color. In 2017, suicide was the second leading cause of death for persons aged 10 to 14, 15 to 19, and 20 to 24, and homicide ranked third for persons aged 15 to 19 and 20 to 24 (Curtin and Heron, 2019). Nearly 45,000 suicides and 19,362 homicides occurred in the United States in 2016 (Decker, Wilcox, Holliday, Webster, 2018). Community violence, intimate partner violence, and sexual violence (collectively called "interpersonal violence" and suicide are the most and severe forms of violence. According to Decker et al., "Community violence refers to violence that occurs between strangers, friends, or acquaintances, and it typically takes place outside of residual dwellings. It includes physical fighting and assault with or without the use of firearms and other weapons" (p. 655). "Intimate partner violence includes physical, sexual, or psychological harm, including stalking, caused by a current or former partner or spouse" and "Sexual violence refers to sexual activity when consent is not obtained or not given freely" (Decker et al., p. 655). Suicide in contrast is self-directed violence.

For many forms of nonfatal violence including child maltreatment, youth violence, intimate partner violence, sexual violence, elder abuse and homicides, progress has been made. However, the burden to individuals, families and communities remains high (Sumner, Mercy, & Dahlberg et al., 2015). It should also be noted that one cannot perfectly determine the incidence of these forms of violence. People may not seek health or social service assistance when they are victims of violence. The victims may be young, embarrassed, afraid, or unaware of how to seek help. Victims often think that if they leave the abuser they will have no other place to live and no other form of support.

COVID-19 increased the cases of intimate partner violence and child abuse. Many adults and children were forced to stay home to work and go to school due to the virus. "COVID-19 has caused major economic devastation, disconnected many from community resources and support systems, and created widespread uncertainty and panic. Such conditions may stimulate violence in families where it did not exist before and worsen situations in homes where mistreatment and violence has been a problem" (SAMHSA, 2020). Given the effects of the COVID-19 pandemic, it is important to consider the cost to society that results from intimate partner violence and child abuse.

Nurses are uniquely qualified to develop community responses to violence, to influence public policy, and to provide individuals, families and communities with the necessary resources to mitigate violence and its consequences. This chapter examines violence as a public health problem and identifies nursing actions.

The Division of Violence Prevention within the Centers for Disease Control and Prevention (CDC, 2020a) developed "The public health approach to violence prevention." This is a step-by-step approach that is applicable in any community. The questions asked using this approach are: Where does the problem begin? How could we prevent it from occurring? Implementing this approach requires participation from many people, organizations and systems. The steps are:

1. Identify the problem: Collect data to determine the "who," "what," where," "when," and "how." This is an epidemiological approach.
2. Identify the risk factors. Why does one person or one community experience violence, and another does not?
3. Develop and test prevention strategies and share this information with others.
4. Disseminate and implement the strategies in step 3. See Fig. 27.1 for a depiction of this model.

The Centers for Disease Control and Prevention (CDC) has many resources available on its website. For example, there are fact sheets on the CDC site for violence prevention related to adverse

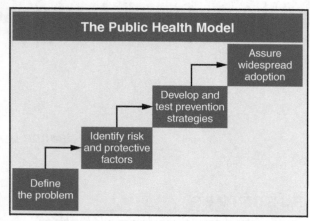

Fig. 27.1 Public Health Approach to Violence Prevention. (From https://www.cdc.gov/violenceprevention/about/publichealthapproach.html.)

childhood experiences (ACEs), child abuse and neglect, elder abuse prevention, prevention of firearm violence, interpersonal partner violence, sexual and youth violence. Visit http://www.cdc.gov for guides and information that were updated in 2018. In 2014, the World Health Organization (WHO) published its "Global Status Report on Violence Prevention," which is the first report of its kind to assess national efforts that address interpersonal violence, namely child maltreatment, youth violence, intimate partner and sexual violence, and elder abuse worldwide (WHO, 2014a). This report included data from 133 countries. Violence is a major cause of premature mortality and lifelong disability, and violence-related morbidity is a significant factor in health care costs. The *Healthy People 2030* box lists three of the objectives for reducing violence in communities (USDHHS, 2020a).

HEALTHY PEOPLE 2030

Objectives for Reducing Violence

- **IVP-03:** Reduce the number of your adults who report 3 or more adverse childhood experiences.
- **IVP-D04:** Reduce intimate partner violence.
- **IVP-12:** Reduce gun carrying among adolescents.

From US Department of Health and Human Services: *Healthy People 2030*, 2020a. Available at http://health.gov/healthypeople.

SOCIAL AND COMMUNITY FACTORS INFLUENCING VIOLENCE

The ultimate goal is to stop violence before it begins. As seen in step two of the CDC approach to violence prevention, it is essential to identify the factors that protect individuals or place them at high risk for experiencing or perpetrating violence. Many factors in a community can support or minimize violence. Changing social conditions, multiple demands on people, economic conditions, pandemics and the subsequent social isolation, job losses or working at home, remote school meetings rather than in person, and social institutions influence the level of violence and human abuse. Rates of violence vary by geographic location, density of population, age group, sex, race, and ethnicity (Sumner et al., 2015).

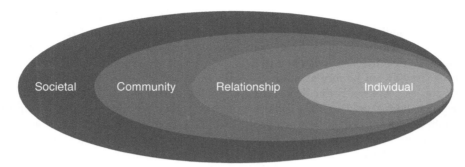

Fig. 27.2 Socioecological Model: A Framework for Prevention. (From http://www.cdc.gov/violence prevention).

The CDC used a four-level socioecological model to aid in understanding the complex interplay among the individual, relationship, community and societal factors. At each level, there are varied factors that increase a person's risk for violence or that serve as protective measures. However, the presence of risks does not guarantee violence. Neither do protective factors eliminate the risk of violence. The overlapping rings within the model illustrate how factors at one level influence factors at another level. It is important in order to prevent violence to act across multiple levels of the model simultaneously (CDC, 2020b). See Fig. 27.2 for a diagram of the model. The following section discusses selected factors that can influence violence.

Individual

The first level identifies biological and personal history factors that may increase the likelihood of a person becoming a victim or perpetrator of violence. In addition to the risk factors above, others include education, substance use, a history of abuse including witnessing abuse, and mental health disorders.

Relationship

The second level of the model examines how close social relationships including those with peers, intimate partners, and family members increase one's risk for violent victimization and perpetration of violence. For example, the risk for violence is increased in a woman and one or more children living with an abuser. Also, adolescents are more likely to engage in violent behavior when their peers accept this behavior (Garthe et al., 2017).

Community

The third level of this model refers to the community and includes settings such as schools, workplaces, and neighborhoods. Regarding neighborhoods, it is important to consider if there is a high level of mobility, low level of cohesiveness and affiliation with neighbors, high population density, highly built environment with few green areas for games and recreation, or drug traffic. Factors that increase peoples' and communities' resilience to violence include:

- Coordination of resources and support services among community agencies.
- Access to mental health and substance abuse treatment services.
- Support and connectedness, including to one's community, family, peers, and school.

As mentioned, in the community it is important to fully understand risk factors for violence in the workplace, schools, and the media. Is the workplace one that tolerates verbal abuse? How do the schools deal with bullying? To what extent does the media focus on violent acts versus acts of support and caring for others? Is the community one of high density where there is limited personal space either inside the home or outside? What is the level of unemployment? Are there jobs if people are able and willing to work? How do youth socialize and interact? Are there community recreation facilities that support team sports or ad hoc play? To what extent do the youth find their peer group in a gang rather than at sports, arts, or church peer groups?

Societal

The fourth and final level of the ecological model examines the broader societal factors that influence rates of violence. These include factors that contribute to a culture that accepts violence, those that reduce inhibitions against violence, and those that both create and perpetuate disparities between different segments of society. Other factors are "health, economic, educational and social policies that help maintain economic or social inequalities between groups in society" (CDC, 2020b).

According to Sumner et al. (2015, p. 8), "Violence is higher in communities where there are limited economic opportunities; where there are high concentrations of poor and unemployed people; where people move frequently; and where there are limited public, mental health, and social services available to residents and fewer civic and voluntary associations." It is important to know about the community in which you are providing services to individuals, families, and the community in general.

VIOLENCE AGAINST INDIVIDUALS OR ONESELF

The potential for violence against individuals (e.g., murder, robbery, rape, assault) or oneself (e.g., suicide) is directly related to the level of violence in the community. Persons living in areas with high rates of crime and violence are more likely to become victims than those in more peaceful areas. The major categories of violence addressed in this chapter are described in terms of the scope of the problem in the United States and the underlying dynamics.

Homicide

Homicide is defined as a death resulting from the use of force against another person when a preponderance of evidence indicates that force was intentional (Parks, 2014). Although homicide rates have decreased over the last 20 years, homicide rates in the United States are still alarming. The Uniform Crime Report uses the term "murder" rather than homicide. The FBI's Uniform Crime Report (UCR) Program defines murder and non-negligent manslaughter as "the wilful non-negligent killing of one human being by another" (US Department of Justice, 2019). Their data is based on police investigation. In 2018 the UCR estimated that there were 16,214 murders in the United States: this was a 6.2% decrease from the 2017 estimate. Interestingly, of the estimated number of murders in the United States in 2018, 46.2% were in the South; 22.0% in the Midwest, 19.9% in the West, and 11.9% in the Northeast. The following category of homicides in *Health, United States* are listed by age group and are based on data recorded on death certificates for 2017:

Age	Number of Homicides
5–14	332
15–24	4905
25–44	8839
45–64	4019

None were reported in the 65 years and older category (National Center for Health Statistics, 2019). A friend, acquaintance, or family member commits the majority of homicides. Therefore, the prevention of homicide is at least as much an issue for the public health system as for the criminal justice system.

A large percentage of homicides are caused by the use of firearms. Research has demonstrated that a higher proportion of household gun ownership at the state level is associated with statistically significant increased rates of nonstranger total firearm homicides. However, there is not a statistically significant relationship between household gun ownership and stranger homicides (Siegel et al., 2014). Firearm injuries are a serious public health problem. In 2018, there were 39,740 firearm-related deaths in the United States, and more people suffer nonfatal firearm-related injuries than the number who die. Males account for 85% of all victims of firearm fatalities and 88% of nonfatal firearm injuries (CDC, 2020c) (Fig. 27.3).

These statistics do not account for the significant morbidity associated with interpersonal violence. For every person who dies as a result of violence, many more are injured and suffer lasting physical, sexual, and mental health sequelae.

An alarming aspect of family homicide is that children may witness the murder or find the body of a family member (Lysell et al., 2016). No automatic follow-up or counseling of these children occurs through the criminal justice or mental health system in most communities. These children are at great risk for mental disorder, self-harm, substance use, and completed suicide if older than 18 years of age (Lysell et al., 2016).

The underlying dynamics of homicide within families vary greatly from those of other murders. Women are nine times more likely to be killed by an intimate partner than a stranger. The intimate partner may be a husband, boyfriend, same-sex partner, or ex-partner (Campbell et al., 2007). The top risk factor for intimate partner homicide (IPH) is previous domestic violence; other risk factors are access to guns, estrangement, threats to kill and threats with a weapon, nonfatal strangulation, and a stepchild in the home if the victim is a female (Campbell et al., 2007). Other risk factors are violent crime convictions in general and major mental disorder (Lysell et al., 2016).

Thus, the prevention of family homicide involves working with abusive families. In a study of IPH of women, 75% of the women who were killed by a husband, boyfriend, or ex-partner had been seen in a health care setting during the year before the homicide (Nannini et al., 2008). Nurses have a duty to warn family members of the possibility of homicide when severe abuse is present, just as they warn them of the hazards of smoking. Other nursing care issues are discussed further in the section on family violence and abuse.

Assault

The death toll from violence is staggering, yet the physical injuries and emotional costs of assault are equally important issues in both the acute health care system and the community. Violent crime rates, which had been declining for several years, reversed direction in 2018. The 2018 National Crime Victimization Survey (MCVS) found that the number of violent crime victims was higher in 2018 than in 2015. This increase over a 3-year period in victims age 12 or older was due to increased numbers of victims

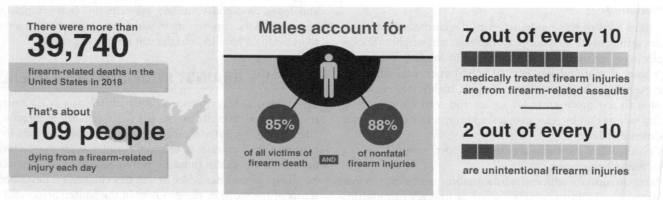

There were more than
39,740
firearm-related deaths in the United States in 2018

That's about
109 people
dying from a firearm-related injury each day

Males account for

85% of all victims of firearm death AND **88%** of nonfatal firearm injuries

7 out of every 10
medically treated firearm injuries are from firearm-related assaults

2 out of every 10
are unintentional firearm injuries

Fig. 27.3 Firearm Violence Prevention. (From https://www.cdc.gov/violenceprevention/firearms/fastfacts.html.)

of rape or sexual assault, aggravated assault, and simple assault. Specifically, the number of violent crime victims age 12 or older grew from 2.7 million in 2015 to 3.3 million in 2018 (Morgan and Ouderkerk, 2019). According to the Bureau of Justice Statistics (Morgan and Ouderkerk, 2019), the "offender was of the same race or ethnicity as the victim in 70% of violent incidents involving black victims, 62% involving white victims, 45% of those involving Hispanic victims, and 24% of those involved Asian victims" (p.1).

Aggravated assault is reported to police more often than simple assault or rape, but all assault types are underreported (Truman and Langston, 2015). The greatest risk factor for an individual's victimization through violence is age, and youths are at significantly higher risk. Whereas more males than females are victims of homicide and assault, women are more likely to be victimized by a relative, especially a male partner. Both females and males suffer injuries as victims of intimate partner violence. Sometimes the difference between a homicide and an assault is only the response time and the quality of emergency transport and treatment facilities. The same community measures used to address homicide can be used to combat assault. Also, nurses often see assaulted persons in home health care with long-term health problems such as head injuries, spinal cord injuries, and stomas from abdominal gunshot wounds. In addition to physical care, nurses must address the emotional trauma of a violent attack. They can help victims talk through their traumatic experience to try to make some sense of the violence and refer them for further counseling if anxiety, sleeping problems, or depression persists after the assault.

Sexual Violence and Rape

Sexual violence is forcing a person to take part in a sexual act when the person does not consent, and includes rape (attempted and completed), sexual coercion, being made to penetrate a perpetrator, unwanted sexual contact experiences, and unwanted sexual noncontact experiences (e.g., being flashed or made to view sexually explicit media) (Breiding et al., 2014). Based on data from the Bureau of Justice Statistics National Crime Victimization Survey, the rate of rape or sexual assault increased from 1.4 incidents per 1000 persons age 12 or older in 2017 to 2.7 per 1000 in 2018 (Morgan and Ouderkerk, 2019). The survey determined that the number of violent crime victims age 12 or older increased from 2015 to 2018 from 2.7 to 3.3 million and was driven by increases in the number of victims of rape or sexual assault, aggravated assault, and simple assault (p. 1). From 2017 to 2018, rates of violent victimization increased for persons living in households with the lowest and highest incomes. The age groups with the highest rates were persons ages 12 to 17 years and 19 to 24 years (Morgan and Ouderkerk, 2019).

Rape on college campuses has some unique characteristics, such that the White House established the Task Force to Protect Students from Sexual Assault in 2014 (Krebs et al., 2016). Sexual assault prevention is a discussion in freshman orientation at most if not all universities. However, freshmen are busy adjusting to life away from home, classes, and new friends, and they often do not pay close attention to the safety measures they are being taught. Also, the availability of alcohol compounds the situation. Primary prevention is the first step. That is, teach people they need to be aware, to understand what they are seeing and experiencing, and to take steps toward maintaining their safety. In fact, one in four college women will be a victim of sexual assault; of these assaults, 60% will be perpetrated by an acquaintance of the victim, heavy episodic drinking will increase the chance of being raped eight-fold (One in Four USA, 2016), and fewer than 5% of all incidents will be brought to the attention of administrators or authorities. Campbell et al. (2017) found that female undergraduates were more likely to be victimized than graduate students, and the vast majority of students who experienced sexual violence were victimized when they were incapacitated due to intoxication or asleep. Nonheterosexual students are more likely to be victimized than heterosexual students (Krebs et al., 2016). Sexual violence can affect health by causing both physical injuries and emotional harm. Physical injuries can be cuts, scratches, bruises, or welts or more serious injuries such as broken bones, internal bleeding, chronic pain, stomach problems, sexually transmitted diseases (STDs), unwanted pregnancies, and head trauma. The emotional pain can lead to trauma symptoms such as flashbacks, panic attacks, trouble sleeping, eating disorders, and depression (Black et al., 2011; Sumner et al., 2015). Victims may engage in negative health behaviors such as smoking, abusing alcohol or drugs, or engaging in risky sexual behaviors.

Also be alert for signs of date and marital rape. Rape victims seldom offer sensitive information unless you specifically ask for it and make it clear that confidentiality will be upheld (WHO, 2014b). Dating violence includes sexual violence, physical violence, psychological aggression, and stalking, and can take place in person or electronically such as by texting or posting sexual pictures of a partner online (CDC, 2020d). These four forms of violence also apply to intimate partner violence. Psychological aggression refers to the use of verbal and nonverbal communication with the intent to harm another person mentally, emotionally, or as a form of exerting control. Stalking is repeated, unwanted attention and contact by another person that causes fear or concern for one's own safety or that of someone close to the victim (CDC, 2020d). During 2019, nearly 1 in 11 female teens and 1 in 15 male teens reported experiencing physical dating violence; 1 in 9 female and 1 in 36 male high school students reported sexual dating violence; and 26% of women and 15% of men experienced intimate partner violence for the first time before age 18 (CDC, 2020d). Teen victims of dating violence are more likely to be depressed or anxious and do poorly in school. They may take part in unhealthy behaviors such as using drugs, tobacco, and alcohol; think about suicide; and have antisocial behaviors such as lying, stealing, bullying, or hitting others (CDC, 2020d). The CDC has developed a toolkit entitled, *Dating Matters: Strategies to Promote Healthy Teen Relationships* to stop teen dating violence before it starts. It focuses on 11- to 14-year-olds. See www.cdc.gov/violenceprevention/datingmatters.

For reported rapes, cities constitute higher risk areas than do rural areas, and the hours between 8 pm and 2 am, the weekends, and the summer are the most critical times. In about 50% of rapes, the victim and the offender meet on the street, whereas in other cases, the rapist either enters the victim's home or somehow entices or forces the victim to accompany him. The majority of rapists are known to the victim.

Prevention of rape, like that of other forms of human abuse, requires a broad-based community focus for educating both the community as a whole and key groups such as police, health care providers, educators, and social workers. Prevention should begin early by promoting healthy, respectful relationships in families so that children learn that interactions should be based on respect and trust, and conflict resolution should occur without using violence. These same forms of communication should be reinforced in schools and social organizations. It is also important to address the beliefs, attitudes, and messages that are sent that may condone sexual violence, stalking, and IPV. Violence should be recognized as being deep rooted, and as having social and economic causes.

It is also important to be aware of cultural differences related to sexual violence, including rape. Cultural and social norms influence behavior, including violence. For example, the use of violence to solve conflicts or as part of child rearing can be a risk factor for interpersonal violence. Children learn to accept the use of violence when they see corporal punishment, violence in the family, or violence in the media or other settings. Examples of cultural and social norms that support violence would include beliefs that men have a right to control or discipline women through physical means, which can lead to IPV and sexual exploitation of girls. Other factors would be the belief that violence is a private affair, which might prevent the victims from speaking out (WHO, 2014a). Also, societies that tolerate higher rates of acute alcohol intoxication report stronger associations between alcohol use and violence than societies in which alcohol is used more moderately.

A first step in intervening in the incidence of rape and treatment of rape survivors is to change and clarify misconceptions about rape and victims of rape. Rape is a crime of violence, not a crime of passion. The underlying issues are hostility, power, and control rather than sexual desire. The defining issue is lack of consent of the victim. When a woman or man refuses any sexual activity, that refusal means "no." People have the right to change their mind, even when they seemed initially agreeable. Pressure from physical contact, threats, or deliberate inducement of drug or alcohol intoxication is a violation of the law. The myths that women say "no" to sex when they really mean "yes" and that the victims of rape are culpable because of the way they dress or act must end. On college campuses, attitudes toward acquaintance or date rape are slow to change. Also, one of the risk factors for teen dating violence that applies to instances on college campuses is the use of alcohol.

People react to rape differently, depending on their personality, past experiences, background, and support received after the trauma. Some cry, shout, or discuss the experience. Others withdraw and are afraid to discuss the attack. During the immediate and follow-up stages, victims may blame themselves for what has happened. When working with rape victims, help them identify the issues behind self-blame. Fault should not be placed on survivors; they should be taught to take control, learn assertiveness, and think they can take specific actions to prevent future rapes. Survivors need to talk about what happened and to express their feelings and fears in a nonjudgmental atmosphere. Nonjudgmental listening is important. In any psychological trauma, the right to privacy and confidentiality is crucial. Victims should be given privacy, respect, and assurance of confidentiality; told about health care procedures conducted immediately after the rape; given a complete physical examination by a trained nurse examiner (i.e., sexual assault or forensic nurse examiner); and linked with proper resources for ease of reporting. Other suggestions for sexual violence prevention are outlined in "STOP SV: A Technical Package to Prevent Sexual Violence" (Basile et al., 2016).

When a person is admitted to a hospital with traumatic injuries, they should be evaluated to determine the forensic nature of the injuries (Sheridan and Nash, 2009). Nurses often provide continuous care once the victim enters the health care system. Because many victims deny the event once the initial crisis has passed, a single-session debriefing should be completed during the initial examination. Specially trained providers should conduct the physical assessment, examination, and debriefing. In most states, nurses trained in sexual assault examination (sexual assault nurse examiner [SANE] nurses, a subspecialty of forensic nursing) perform the physical examination in the emergency department to gather evidence (e.g., hair samples, skin fragments beneath the victim's fingernails, evidence from pelvic examinations using colposcopy) for criminal prosecution of sexual assault. This crucial nursing intervention often takes time and allows the nurse to begin communication with the victim (Campbell et al., 2011). Nurses' evidence is credible and effective in court proceedings (Campbell et al., 2014). These nurses often have experience in emergency and trauma services and can analyze wound patterns and the physiological response to injury. The nurse who works in the forensic area often provides a key link between the investigative process, health care, and the court (Campbell et al., 2014). Campbell and colleagues (2014) created a toolkit that outlines how SANE nurses can work within their communities to increase sexual assault reporting by victims, a historically challenging issue.

There are specific actions that nurses should take when they work with victims. It is essential that they carefully collect evidence in a systematic manner. For example, when cutting the shirt off a person who has been shot in the chest, be sure to avoid cutting through the bullet hole in the shirt. Instead, cut to the side of the hole to protect the point of origin of the bullet for later criminal investigation. The most common types of evidence are clothing, bullets, bloodstains, hairs, fibers, and small pieces of material, such as fragments of metal, glass, paint, and wood. Also, DNA provides key information in the analysis of sexual assault. When nurses treat victims of rape, it is important to do so in a manner that preserves evidence for the victim.

Rape is a situational crisis for which advance preparation is rarely possible. Therefore, nurses need to help victims cope with the stress and disruption of their lives caused by the attack. Counseling focuses on the crisis and the fears, feelings, and issues involved. Nurses can help survivors learn how to regroup personal forces. If posttraumatic stress disorder (PTSD) has developed, professional psychological or psychiatric treatment is indicated.

Many rape victims need follow-up mental health services to help them cope with the short-term and long-term effects of the crisis. The time after a rape is one of disequilibrium, psychological breakdown, and reorganization of attitudes about the safety of the world. Common, everyday tasks often tax a person's resources. Many individuals forget or fail to keep appointments. Nurses can make appropriate referrals and obtain permission from the victim to remain in contact through telephone conversations, which allows for ongoing assessment of the victim's needs and opportunities to intervene when needed.

The best way to prevent sexual violence is to stop it before it begins. The CDC advocates strategies such as (1) promoting social norms that protect against violence; (2) teaching skills to prevent sexual violence; (3) providing opportunities to empower girls and women; (4) creating protective environments; and (5) supporting victims/survivors to lessen harm (Basile et al., 2016).

Human Trafficking

Human trafficking is a significant public health issue globally, including in the United States. Human trafficking is an umbrella term that includes activities involved in recruiting, harboring, transporting, or providing an individual for forced service or commercial sex acts through the use of force, deception or coercion (United Nations Office on Drugs and Crime, 2019). "It occurs when a trafficker uses force, fraud, or coercion to compel another person to engage in commercial sex or any form of labor against his or her will. A child under age 18 engaged in commercial sex is a victim of sex trafficking even if the youth's participation is not forced or coerced" (USDHHS, Administration for Children and Families [USDHHS, ACF], 2020b). Due to the secretive nature of human trafficking, accurate prevalence estimates are difficult to obtain, yet an estimated 50,000 women and children may be trafficked into the United States each year (Siskin and Sun, 2013). In 2018 the National Human Trafficking Hotline reported a total of 41,088 contacts via phone calls, texts, webchats, webforms and emails. Tragically, there was a 25% increase in cases from 2017 to 2018. The three top types of trafficking in 2018 were sex (7859); labor (1249); sex and labor (637) and 1202 cases not specified (Human trafficking hotline.org 2018. Human trafficking is the fastest growing and one of the most lucrative crimes in the United States. Thus it is imperative that nurses and other health care professionals are trained in the identification, care, and supports needed for these individuals (United Nations Office on Drugs and Crime, 2019).

Human trafficking affects all races, ages, and genders; yet, women and children under the age of 18 are at heightened risk. Children are often targeted due to their earning potential, with runaway and homeless youth at greatest risk (United Nations Office on Drugs and Crime, 2019). The majority of individuals experiencing human trafficking in the United States are women or girls, and the majority of these individuals are forced into the sex service industry (United Nations Office on Drugs and Crime, 2019).

Most trafficked individuals will come in contact with a health care provider, often through the emergency department setting, for treatment of an illness or injury at some point during their captivity. Yet, they are seldom appropriately identified as victims of trafficking (Peters, 2013). Victims are not likely to identify themselves as such for a number of reasons including fear of captor, distrust of available support systems (e.g., medical, legal, social services), uncertainty about available supports, unfamiliarity with regional language or culture, or feelings of shame about their situation (Becker and Bechtel, 2015).

Victims of human trafficking will often present to the health care system accompanied by their trafficker, who may identify themselves as a family member or trusted support person. The trafficker may be male or female, and may appear to be supportive, caring, and sympathetic to the individual (Becker and Bechtel, 2015). Thus, identifying trafficked individuals may be difficult, but there are "red flags" in their presentation that can be useful. A "family member" or "friend" who doesn't allow the individual to answer the health care provider's questions or consistently answers for them should raise suspicion. The individual may appear to be reluctant in describing symptoms or the events leading up to the presenting complaint; they may be vague in their responses or report inconsistencies in their responses. Individuals may not be able to provide a home address, have no identification documents, and may be unaware of the city or state in which they are receiving services.

The signs and symptoms of trafficking are multifaceted and may occur in isolation or in combination. Physical symptoms may include, but are not limited to, unexplained bruises, burns, lacerations, bite marks, vaginal or anal tearing, sexually transmitted infections, unintended pregnancy, nutritional deficits, and substance use disorder (De Chesnay, 2013; Isaac et al., 2011; Richards, 2014). With regard to mental health issues, victims of human trafficking are at increased risk for depression, PTSD, suicidal ideation, or suicide attempts (Richards, 2014).

Caring for a potential victim of human trafficking requires a trauma-informed, nonjudgmental manner. The goal of the interaction should be to create a safe space and support empowerment. It is important for the health care provider to interview the patient alone, thereby facilitating disclosure. Explaining that it is routine practice in a particular health care setting to interview patients alone may decrease suspicion in the captor. However, if it is difficult to obtain a one-on-one interview, it can be helpful to accompany the patient to a restroom or to a private setting for a particular reason, such as the laboratory or x-ray. If the victim does not speak English, it is critical to use a professional interpreter to assure accuracy in the assessment.

Although there are no validated screening questions for human trafficking. Nurses can ask:

- Can you come and go from your home (or job) whenever you please?
- Has anyone at home or work ever physically harmed you?
- Have you been threatened for trying to leave your job?
- Is anyone forcing you to do things you do not want to do?
- Do you have to ask permission to eat, sleep, or use the bathroom?
- Are there locks on your doors and windows that keep you from leaving?

- Have you ever been denied food, water, sleep, or medical care?
- Has anyone ever threatened your family?
- Has anyone taken away your identification papers or cards? (Crane, 2013)

If the health care provider suspects that a patient is a victim of human trafficking, it is essential to engage the assistance of a social worker or victim advocate early in the patient's care. For patients under the age of 18, a call to the state's child protective services agency is necessary. If the health care provider thinks that the patient is in immediate danger, law enforcement should be contacted. If the patient is not believed to be in immediate danger, the health care provider should notify the patient prior to engaging law enforcement on their behalf. Involving the patient may improve trust and facilitate disclosure by the victim.

There are a number of resources available for providing care to victims of human trafficking. The National Human Trafficking Resource Center hot line (1-888-373-7888) is available to anyone with a suspicion of trafficking. It is toll free, available 24 hours/day, and available in 180 languages. The Center can provide guidance on interview questions as well as indicators of potential trafficking. Importantly, it can provide access to safety resources including shelters, as well as other critical safety resources. Another helpful resource is https://polarisproject.org. This site includes an interactive map of the United States with updated listings of local organizations and resources for victims, as well as state laws regarding human trafficking.

Human trafficking is a significant issue in the United States. The physical and mental health sequelae for victims of trafficking are significant and sustained. It is critical that health care providers recognize the warning signs, acknowledging that engagement with the health care system may be one of the few opportunities for victims to escape their situations. An understanding of this issue and supports available is key to saving lives. See "Human trafficking of children" at https://www.childwelfare.gov/topics/preventing/ for information on "What to do if you suspect a child is a victim of human trafficking."

Suicide

Suicide is a large and growing public health problem. From 2008 to 2017, suicide ranked as the 10th leading cause of death for all ages in the United States. Using the National Violent Death Reporting System, the age-adjusted suicide rate increased 33% from 10.5 per 100,000 people to 14.0 between 1999 and through 2017. During this time period rates for males, females, and persons living in the most rural and most urban counties increased (Hedegaard, Curtin, and Warner, 2018). In 2018, there were more than 48,000 deaths by suicide, and this is 1 death in every 11 minutes. Suicide affects all age groups. It is the second leading cause of death for people 20 to 34 years of age; the fourth for those 35 to 54 years old, and the eighth for people 55 to 64 years of age. Suicide varies by race/ethnicity, and is highest in non-Hispanic American Indian/Alaska Native and non-Hispanic White populations. Other groups that have disproportionate rates of suicide include veterans, other military personnel, and workers in construction and the arts, design, entertainment, sports, and media fields (CDC, 2020e).

Affluent and educated people often have higher rates of suicide than do economically and educationally disadvantaged people. The exceptions are Native Alaskan and American Indian populations, who are often poor and yet commit suicide in alarming numbers. The presence of a gun in the home is an important risk factor for both suicide and homicide (Miller and Hemenway, 2008).

In 2017, suicide was the second leading cause of death in persons between the ages of 10 and 24 (Curtin and Heron, 2019). The most frequent ways in which violent deaths occur are by firearms, hanging, strangulation and suffocation, or poisoning. Precipitating factors are IPV and mental or physical health problems. When people commit suicide their family and friends often experience shock, anger, guilt, and depression. Also, the economic toll is large due to lifetime medical and work-loss costs alone. People who attempt suicide and survive may have serious and costly injuries (CDC, 2020e). Suicide risk is higher among people who have experienced violence, including bullying, child or sexual abuse, depression, and other mental disorders (CDC, 2020e).

The majority of individuals who complete suicide have visited a health care provider in the prior month; therefore, nurses and other health care providers need to screen and intervene for at risk individuals. Nurses can aid in reducing suicide and in caring for victims at the community, family, and individual level. On a community level, nurses can be involved in a coordinated response for suicide prevention and the care of people who attempt suicide. Nurses can assist in developing policies and protocols for suicide prevention across the life span. Care may focus on family members and friends of suicide victims. Survivors often feel angry toward the dead person, yet may turn the anger inward. Likewise, survivors often question their own liability for the death. The impact of suicide can affect family, friends, coworkers, and the community. Survivors may find it hard to deal with their feelings toward the dead person. It may be difficult for them to concentrate, and they may limit their social activities because their friends and family may be unable to talk about the suicide. Nurses can help survivors cope with the trauma of the loss and make referrals to a counselor or support groups. The CDC has a collection of strategies designed to prevent or reduce suicide. It is entitled "Preventing suicide: A technical package of policy, programs, and practices" and is available on their website.

FAMILY VIOLENCE AND ABUSE

Family violence, including sexual, emotional, and physical abuse, causes significant injury and death. These three forms tend to occur together as part of a system of coercive control. Generally, family violence is violence of the most powerful against the least powerful. As mentioned earlier in the chapter, intimate partner violence (IPV) is defined as physical, sexual, or psychological harm caused by a former or current intimate partner, and is a significant public health problem. In terms of psychological harm, it includes stalking and psychological aggression. These terms are described in the chapter's section on sexual violence. In the 2015 Intimate Partner data brief, about 1 in 4 women and 1 in 10 men experience sexual violence, physical violence, and/or stalking by an intimate partner and reported this during their lifetime; that translates to 43.6 million women and 37.3 million men who experienced sexual violence, physical violence, and/or stalking by an intimate partner during their lifetime. An estimated 1 in 18 or 6.6 million women and about 1 in 20 or 5.8 million men experienced sexual violence, physical violence, or stalking by an intimate partner during the 12 months prior to the survey (Smith, Zhang, Basile et al., 2018). As with heterosexual IPV, dynamics of power and control caused by race, gender expression, ability, immigration status, age, and class are methods of control in same-sex IPV (National Coalition of Anti-Violence Programs, 2017). LGBTQ people face more barriers to seek help than non-LGBTQ people.

Recognizing the battered child or spouse in the emergency department is relatively simple after the fact. It is unfortunate that by the time medical care is sought, serious physical and emotional damage may have already occurred. Nurses are in a key position to predict and deal with abusive tendencies. By understanding factors contributing to the development of abusive behaviors, nurses can identify abuse-prone families and can assist them to describe their abuse in a nonthreatening environment.

Development of Abusive Patterns

To help abusive families, nurses need to understand that the factors that characterize people who become involved in family violence include upbringing, living conditions, and increased stress. Of these factors, the one most predictably present is previous exposure to some form of violence. As children, abusers were often beaten or saw siblings or parents beaten. They learned that violence is a way to manage conflict. Both men and women who witnessed abuse as children were more likely to abuse their children. Financial solvency and support tended to decrease the incidence of child abuse (Zimmerman and Mercy, 2010). Childhood physical punishment teaches children to use violent conflict resolution as adults. A child may learn to associate love with violence because a parent is usually the first person to hit a child. Children may think that those who love them also are those who hit them. The moral rightness of hitting other family members thus may be established when physical punishment is used to train children, especially when it is used more than occasionally. These experiences predispose children ultimately to use violence with their own children.

As well as having a history of child abuse themselves, people who become abusers tend to have hostile personality styles and be verbally aggressive. They often learn these behaviors from their own childhood experiences. Their parents may have set unrealistic goals, and when the children failed to perform accordingly, they were criticized, demeaned, punished, and denied affection. Additionally, parents who are at risk for child abuse tend to be young, single, have many children who are dependent on them, substance abuse issues, mental health problems, and low income (Fortson et al., 2016). These children grow up feeling unloved and worthless. They may want a child of their own so that they will feel love.

To protect themselves from feelings of worthlessness and fear of rejection, abused children form a protective shell and may become hostile and distrustful of others. The behavior of potential abusers reflects a low tolerance for frustration, emotional instability, and the onset of aggressive feelings with minimal provocation. Because of their emotional insecurity, they often depend on a child or spouse to meet their needs of feeling valued and secure. When an adult's needs are not met by others, they may become overly critical of the child. Critical, resentful behavior and unrealistic expectations of others lead to a vicious cycle. The more critical these people become, the more they are rejected and alienated from others. Abusive individuals often think the target of their hostility is "out to get" them. For example, a parent might think or say that an infant deliberately kept him or her awake all night. We know that infants do not intentionally keep parents awake. Rather, infants cry for reason of their own, not to annoy and inconvenience others.

A perceived or actual crisis may precede an abusive incident. Because a crisis reinforces feelings of inadequacy and low self-esteem, multiple events may occur in a short time to precipitate abusive patterns. Unemployment, marital strains, or an unplanned pregnancy can set off violence. The daily hassles of raising young children, especially in an economically strained household, intensify an already stressed atmosphere for which an unexpected and difficult event provokes violence. Stressful life events, poverty, and the number of small children in the home are often associated with family violence. Crowded living conditions can precipitate abuse. Several people living in a small space increases tensions and reduces privacy. Tempers flare as a result of the constant stimulation from others. Social isolation reduces social support and can decrease a family's ability to cope with stress and lead to abuse. Social isolation, working, and going to school at home during the COVID-19 pandemic created risk factors for abuse. It was also a time when individuals and families were unable to go to their needed clinical visits or have the same level of home health visits as at other times.

Frequent moves disrupt social support systems, are associated with an increased stress level, and tend to isolate people, at least briefly. Mobility can have a serious negative effect on the abuse-prone family. These families do not readily initiate new relationships. They rely on the family for support. Resources may be unfamiliar or inaccessible to them. Because frequent moving may be both a risk factor for abuse and a sign of an abusive family trying to avoid detection, nurses should assess such families carefully for abuse.

Types of Family Violence

Family violence may not be limited to one family member; thus, nurses who detect child abuse should also suspect other forms of family violence. When older adult parents report that their (now adult) child was abused or has a history of violence toward others, the nurse should recognize the potential for elder abuse. Physical abuse of women may be accompanied by sexual abuse, both inside and outside the marital relationship. Severe wife abusers may commit other acts of violence, especially child abuse. Also, when one child is abused, others may be physically, sexually, or emotionally abused. Families who are verbally aggressive in conflict resolution (e.g., using name calling, belittling, screaming, yelling) are more likely to be physically abusive. Although the various forms of family violence are discussed separately, they should not be thought of as totally separate phenomena. No member of the family is guaranteed immunity from abuse and neglect.

Child Abuse

Child abuse and neglect are major public health problems, and such adverse childhood experiences (ACEs) can have long-term negative effects on the child. The four common types of child abuse and neglect are:

- Physical abuse—intentional use of physical force that can result in physical harm , that is, hitting, kicking, shaking, burning, or other shows of force against a child.
- Sexual abuse—pressuring or forcing a child to engage in sexual acts, that is, fondling, penetration and exposing a child to other sexual acts.
- Emotional abuse—behaviors that harm a child's self-worth or emotional well-being, that is, name calling, shaming, rejection, withholding love, and threatening.
- Neglect—failure to meet a child's basic physical and emotional needs, that is, housing, food, clothing, education and access to health care (CDC, 2020f).
- Trafficking—in which a commercial sexual act is induced by force, fraud, or coercion, or in which the person induced to perform such act has not attained 18 years of age (USDHHS, ACF, 2020b, p 37).

In 2018, nearly 1770 children died of abuse and neglect in the United States, and at least 1 in 7 children experienced child abuse and neglect the previous year. During 2018 there were 678,000 victims of child abuse and neglect, and children in their first year of life have the highest rate of being victims. Girls have slightly higher rates (9.6 per 1000) than boys, who have rates of 8.7 per 1000 people (USDHHS, ACF, 2020a). Children who live in poverty are five times more likely to be abused and neglected than children with higher socioeconomic resources. The lifetime economic burden of child abuse and/or neglect is about the same as that of stroke and type 2 diabetes. The perpetrator is the person responsible for the abuse or neglect, and more than four-fifths are between the ages of 18 and 44; more than half are female; and the three highest percentage groups are White (49.6%), African American (20.6%), and Hispanic (19.3%). The majority of perpetrators (77.5%) are a parent of the victim (USDHHS, ACF, 2020a).

Many children are exposed to violence, not only as victims, but also as witnesses, and being a witness can lead to mental health issues and aggressive behavior (Child Trends Data Bank, 2016). Also, children living in homes in which violence takes place between their parents are more likely to be abused themselves. Risk factors for children who are abused include parental factors such as limited family economic resources, lack of social support, parental domestic violence, and problems with substance abuse. Some of the risk factors are identified in Box 27.1.

The presence of child abuse signifies ineffective family functioning. Abusive parents who recognize their problem are often

---

BOX 27.1 Determining Risk Factors for Child Abuse

Ask the following questions or observe the following behaviors to determine whether risk factors are present.

1. Are the parents unemployed?
2. Do the parents have the financial resources to care for a child?
3. Is there a support network that is willing to offer assistance?
4. Do one or both parents have a history of child abuse?
5. Is a parent a victim or perpetrator of intimate partner violence?
6. Do the parents have knowledge about child development?
7. Do one or both parents have problems with substance abuse?
8. Are the parents overly critical of the child?
9. Are the parents communicative with each other and the nurse?
10. Does the mother of the child seem frightened of her partner?
11. Does the child suffer from recurrent injuries or unexplained illnesses?

Data from Rodriguez CM: Personal contextual characteristics and cognitions: predicting child abuse potential and disciplinary style. *J Interpers Viol* 25:315–335, 2010; US Department of Health and Human Services, Administration for Children and Families, Administration on Children, Youth and Families, Children's Bureau: *Child maltreatment 2014*, Retrieved from http://www.acf.hhs.gov/programs/cb/research-data-technology/statistics-research/child-maltreatment, 2016; Zimmerman F, Mercy JA: A better start: child maltreatment prevention as a public health priority. *Zero Three* 30:4–10, 2010.

---

reluctant to seek assistance because of the stigma attached to being considered a child abuser. Children may be victims of abuse because they are small and relatively powerless. In many families, only one child is abused. Parents may identify with this particular child and be especially critical of the child's behavior. In some cases, the child may have certain qualities, such as looking like a relative, being handicapped, trying to resist the violence, or being particularly bright and capable or strong willed, that provoke the parent. Often, in families in which child abuse occurs, there is an explicit or covert threat to children other than the one who is most severely abused. Thus other children may have conflicting feelings of both guilt and relief, and the targeted child is often coerced into silence by threats toward the sibling(s).

Parents with low social support, a tendency toward depression, multiple economic stressors, and a history of abuse are at risk for abusing their children (Fortson et al., 2016). Abusive parents often have unrealistic expectations of a child's developmental abilities. They tend to have little involvement with and show minimal warmth toward their child (Child Welfare Information Gateway, 2019). Parents who abuse their children use physical discipline more frequently, often in the form of physical punishment and verbal abuse (Wilkins et al., 2014). The nurse can teach normal parental behavior and also address the underlying emotional needs of the parents. They need to teach forms of parental control other than physical punishment. These parents often experience pain and poor emotional stability and need intervention as much as their children. The How To box lists some of the behavioral indicators of potentially abusive parents.

HOW TO IDENTIFY POTENTIALLY ABUSIVE PARENTS

The following characteristics in couples expecting a child constitute warning signs of actual or potential abuse:

- Denial of the reality of the pregnancy, for example, refusal to talk about the impending birth or to think of a name for the child
- An obvious concern or fear that the baby will not meet some predetermined standard, for example, sex, hair color, temperament, or resemblance to family members
- Failure to follow through on the desire for an abortion
- An initial decision to place the child for adoption and a change of mind
- Rejection of the mother by the father of the baby
- Family experiencing stress and numerous crises so that the birth of a child may be the last straw
- Initial and unresolved negative feelings about having a child
- Lack of support for the new parents
- Isolation from friends, neighbors, or family
- Parental evidence of poor impulse control or fear of losing control
- Contradictory history
- Appearance of detachment
- Appearance of misusing drugs or alcohol
- Shopping for hospitals or health care providers
- Unrealistic expectations of the child
- Verbal, physical, or sexual abuse of the mother by the father, especially during pregnancy
- Child is not the biological offspring of the husband or the mother's current boyfriend
- Excessive talk of needing to "discipline" children and plans to use harsh physical punishment to enforce discipline

CASE STUDY

As nurse Marie Mason was preparing to visit a newborn and her mother, Vicki Jones, she was told that two other children had been removed from Ms. Jones's care in the past by Child Protective Services. During the initial visit and all other visits, Ms. Mason would unclothe the baby and assess her growth and development, as well as look for bruises or abrasions. Ms. Mason gained the mother's trust during her weekly visits, and for the first month thought all was progressing well. The father of the baby, Max, was often present, and he appeared to care for the child. Although the grandmother lived in the apartment at night, she spent her days at a treatment center for the mentally ill.

When the infant was 2 months of age, the nurse noticed that Ms. Jones did not support the infant's head despite her explanations that the baby needed that. Also, the mother advanced the baby's diet to include pureed canned fruits and meats well ahead of what had been advised. Ms. Jones, who had type 2 diabetes mellitus, also ate erratically and failed to test her own blood sugars. She was overweight but said she had been losing weight because she was only eating take-out Chinese food once a day. Ms. Mason set small goals with Ms. Jones each week, such as adding an easy, nutritious breakfast to her diet and testing her blood sugar at least once per day.

When the baby was 3 months of age, Ms. Jones told Ms. Mason that she had told Max not to come back because he had spoken harshly of her mother. On further questioning, she said that she was afraid Max would hurt her and that he had slapped her on occasion. There was also a new man who seemed to be living in the house and was clearly fond of Ms. Jones and her child.

Created by Deborah C. Conway, Assistant Professor (retired), School of Nursing, University of Virginia.

CHECK YOUR PRACTICE

The case study illustrates many of the signs of a potentially abusive pattern. Looking back at the case, note that the nurse did the following: carefully examined the baby during each visit to detect any signs of abuse; used role modeling to demonstrate how to hold the baby and to show that babies are to be held in a careful way; and helped the mother set small goals for her own diet to maintain her diabetes in better control. What else did the nurse do that had a positive effect? Although signs of active abuse were not noted in the case, there were signs of neglect as a result of limited knowledge. What could the nurse do in future visits to help this family not become abusive? What community resources might be considered, such as parenting classes or groups for mothers? Are there role models for good parenting who live near Ms. Jones and who might be lay helpers with this family?

Now apply the six steps in the clinical judgment schema to this case study. First, list all the cues you find that might indicate an abusive pattern. Then analyze the cues and begin to establish priorities for the actions you could take. Identify what potential solutions you would anticipate if you acted on your highest ranked action. Last, cite what you would expect your possible solution to be for intervening in potential abuse.

When child abuse is discovered, the child is often placed in a foster home. Unfortunately, quality foster care is not available for all abused children. Abused children generally want to return to their parents, and most agencies try to keep natural families together as long as it is safe for the child. Nurses often monitor a family in which a formerly abused child is returned from foster care. Clinical judgment and close collaboration with social services are essential. The nurse must ensure the safety of the child while working with the parents in an empathetic way. The nurse's goal is to enhance their parenting skills, not to be viewed as yet another watchdog. Remember also that abusive parents may try to replace a child who has been removed by the courts because of abuse. This is a normal response to the grief of losing a child. Rather than regarding another pregnancy as a sign of continued poor judgment or pathological behavior, the pregnancy can be perceived by the nurse as an opportunity for intensive intervention to prevent the abuse of the expected child. Generally, the parents are eager to avoid further problems if they are enlisted as partners in the project.

Indicators of child abuse. Nurses need to recognize the physical and behavioral indicators of abuse and neglect. Child abuse ranges from violent physical attacks to passive neglect. The children suffer physical injuries, including cuts, bruises, burns, and broken bones; they may also be beaten, burned, kicked, or shaken. Passive neglect may result in malnutrition or other problems. Abuse is not limited to physical maltreatment but includes emotional abuse such as yelling at or continually demeaning, shaming, rejecting, withholding love from, threatening, and criticizing the child. Maltreatment can cause stress that can disrupt early brain development and, at extreme levels, can affect the development of the nervous and immune systems. Abused children are then at higher risk for adult health problems, including alcoholism, depression, substance abuse, eating disorders, obesity, sexual proximity, smoking, suicide, and some chronic diseases (Child Welfare Information Gateway, 2019a).

Children at risk for child maltreatment are (1) those who have young parents who may lack experience with children and who have unrealistic expectations; (2) those in families struggling with poverty, unstable housing, divorce, or unemployment; (3) those who have parents who abuse drugs or alcohol; (4) those who have parents who have themselves had childhood trauma; (5) those with parents who are isolated and do not have a supportive partner, family, or community (USDHHS, ACF, 2020b).

Emotional abuse is "any pattern of behavior that impairs a child's emotional development or sense of self-worth, including constant criticism, threats, and rejection" (USDHHS, ACF, 2020b). Children who are abused or who witness domestic violence can suffer developmentally; adolescents may run away from home as a direct result of domestic violence, abuse of substances, or become depressed (Fletcher, 2010). To recognize actual or potential child abuse, be alert to these signs: (1) an unexplained injury; (2) on the skin burns, old or recent scars, ecchymosis, soft tissue swelling, or human bites; (3) recent or healed fractures; (4) subdural hematomas; (5) trauma to the genitalia; (6) whiplash caused by shaking children; (7) dehydration or malnourishment without obvious cause; (8) giving inappropriate food or drugs; (9) evidence of poor general care including poor hygiene, dirty clothes, unkempt hair, or dirty nails; (10) unusual fear of the nurse or others; and (11) being referred to as a "bad" child.

Physical symptoms of stress from physical, sexual, or emotional abuse may include hyperactivity, withdrawal, overeating, dermatological problems, vague physical complaints, and exacerbation of stress-related physical problems, such as asthma, stuttering, enuresis (bladder incontinence), and encopresis (bowel incontinence). Sadly, bedwetting is often a trigger for further abuse, which creates a particularly vicious cycle. When a child displays physical symptoms without clear physiological origin, ruling out the possibility of abuse should be part of the nurse's assessment process. See "Long-term consequences of child abuse and neglect" by Child Welfare Information Gateway (2019b) which is an office of the United States Children's Bureau for a detailed list of physical, psychological, behavioral, and social consequences of abuse and neglect. Fig. 27.4 depicts the results of the federal research on Adverse Childhood Experiences (ACE). The ACE Pyramid represents the conceptual framework for the ACE Study. The ACE Study has uncovered how ACEs are strongly related to development of risk factors for disease and well-being throughout the life course (CDC, 2020g).

Child Neglect

Neglect is the failure to meet a child's basic needs, including those for housing, food, clothing, education, and access to health care (USDHHS, ACF, 2020b). The two categories of child neglect are physical and emotional. Physical neglect is defined as failure to provide adequate food, proper clothing, shelter, hygiene, or necessary medical care. Physical neglect is most often associated with extreme poverty. In contrast, emotional neglect is the omission of basic nurturing, acceptance, and caring essential for healthy personal development. These children are largely ignored or in many cases treated as nonpersons. Such neglect usually affects the development of self-esteem. It is difficult for a neglected child to feel a great deal of

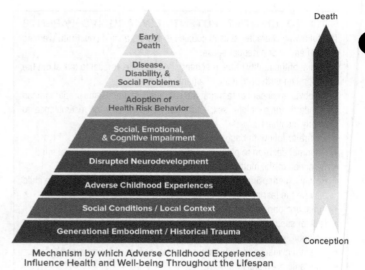

Fig. 27.4 The Adverse Childhood Experiences (ACE) Pyramid. (From https://www.cdc.gov/violenceprevention/about/publichealthapproach.html.)

self-worth because the parents have not demonstrated that they value the child. Neglect is more difficult to assess and evaluate than abuse because it is subtle and may go unnoticed. It is not directly related to poverty and occurs across the socioeconomic spectrum of families. Astute observations of children, their homes, and the way in which they relate to their caregivers can provide clues of neglect.

Sexual Abuse

Child abuse also includes sexual abuse. Child sexual abuse is a major public health problem. About 1 in 4 girls and 1 in 13 boys in the US experience sexual abuse at some time in their childhood (American Academy of Child and Adolescent Psychiatry [AACAPP], 2020). According to RAINN (Rape Abuse and Incest National Network, 2020), every 73 seconds, an American is sexually assaulted. However, the good news is that the rate of sexual violence has fallen by more than a half since 1993. In 2016, 1.2 people out of 1000 were sexually abused. The majority of sexual assaults occur at or near the victim's home. The majority of child sexual abuse is committed by someone the child or the family knows. Child sexual abuse within the home is often perpetrated by a parent, stepparent, sibling or another relative. Outside the home, the perpetrator might be a friend, neighbor, childcare person, teacher, or stranger (AACAP, 2020). The long-term effects of sexual abuse include emotional and psychological reactions with the most common being depression, posttraumatic stress disorder, drug addiction, sexual disorders, and suicidal behaviors later in life. The child may be threatened by the abuser and afraid to tell anyone about the abuse (AACAP, 2020; RAINN, 2020). Signs and symptoms of PTSD include: intrusion (memories), avoidance, negative alterations in cognition and mood, and hyperarousal (Betts, 2020). Betts (2020) lists several useful assessment tools, the use of pharmacotherapy, and an interprofessional approach to treating PSTD in children.

Father-daughter incest is the type of incest most often reported; however, mothers do engage in child sexual abuse. In recent years more males have discussed their experiences of child sexual abuse. Many cases of parental incest go unreported because victims fear punishment, abandonment, rejection, or family disruption if they acknowledge the problem. Incest occurs in all races, religious groups, and socioeconomic classes. Although incest is receiving greater attention because of mandatory reporting laws, too often its incidence remains a family secret.

Because nurses are often involved in helping women deal with the aftermath of incest, it is crucial to understand the typical patterns and the long-term implications. In a typical pattern of paternal incest, the daughter involved is usually about 9 years of age at the onset and is often the oldest or only daughter. The father or stepfather seldom uses physical force. He most likely relies on threats, bribes, intimidation, or misrepresentation of moral standards, or he exploits the daughter's need for human affection.

Nurses must be aware of the incidence, signs and symptoms, and psychological and physical trauma of incest. Symptoms of sexual abuse include pain, bleeding, redness, or swelling in the anal or genital area; age-inappropriate sexual play with toys, self, or others; and age-inappropriate knowledge of sex (USDHHS. ACF, 2020a.). Adolescents may display inappropriate sexual activity or truancy or may run away from home. Running away is usually considered a sign of delinquency; however, an adolescent who runs away may be using a healthy response to a violent family situation. Therefore the assessment should include a thorough inquiry about sexual and physical abuse at home and an appropriate physical examination. It is also important to remember that the absence of physical evidence does not mean that sexual violence such as rape did not occur (WHO, 2015).

Intimate Partner Abuse

Intimate partner violence (IPV) is "abuse or aggression that occurs in a close relationship," and this can refer to both current and former spouses and dating partners (CDC, 2019a). IVP can be threatened, attempted or completed physical, sexual, or emotional abuse, and can also include financial abuse. As mentioned earlier in the chapter, IPV includes four types of behavior: physical or sexual violence; stalking, and psychological aggression. In 2018 in the United States over 1 in 3 women experienced contact sexual violence, physical violence, and/or stalking by an intimate partner during their lifetime (Smith, Zhang, Basile et al., 2018). Intimate partner sexual assault and rape are used as a form of power and control to intimidate and demean victims (National Coalition Against Domestic Violence, 2017). Neither the term wife abuse nor the term spouse abuse takes into account violence in dating or cohabiting relationships or violence in same-sex relationships. The abuse of female partners has the most serious community health ramifications because of the greater prevalence, the greater potential for homicide (Campbell, 2007), the effects on the children in the household, and the more serious long-term emotional and physical consequences (American College of Obstetricians and Gynecologists [ACOG], 2012).

The majority of IVP is directed toward women. Lesbian, gay, bisexual, transgender, queer (LGBTQ) people typically follow similar dynamics as heterosexual IPV and have similar outcomes. As with heterosexual IVP, dynamics of power and control caused by race, gender expression, ability, immigration status, age, and class are methods of control (National Coalition of Anti-Violence Programs, 2017).

Victims of child abuse and individuals who saw their mothers being battered are at risk for using violence toward an intimate partner, whether one is male or female. However, using evidence of a violent childhood to identify women at risk for abuse is less useful, because abuse cannot be predicted on the basis of characteristics of the individual woman. The violent background of an abusive male, combined with his tendencies to be possessive, controlling, and extremely jealous, is most predictive of abuse (CDC, 2019b). The CDC site on violence prevention has an extensive list of risk factors for IPV perpetration (CDC, 2019b). Substance abuse is also associated with battering, although it cannot be said to cause the violence.

Signs of abuse. Battered women often have bruises and lacerations of the face, head, and trunk of the body. Attacks are often carefully inflicted on parts of the body that can easily be disguised by clothing, such as breasts, abdomen, upper thighs, and back (Sheridan and Nash, 2009). Ranging from physical restraint to murder, the American College of Obstetricians and Gynecologists (ACOG) (2012) lists these forms of physical abuse: hitting, kicking, punching, slapping, strangling, shaking, confining, burning, freezing, pushing, tripping, scratching, cutting, biting, pinching, throwing things, or hiding medications. Emotional, psychological, and verbal abuse include coercion, manipulation, isolation, intimidation, mocking or criticizing, humiliating, lying, screaming, threatening, or using menacing forms of nonverbal behavior (ACOG, 2012). Financial abuse is seen when a partner limits the other person's access to money as a method of control.

Once abused, women tend to exhibit low self-esteem and depression (Humphreys and Campbell, 2010). Few are able to come right out and ask for help, which means that the nurse needs to communicate honestly, openly, and with sensitivity. Complete any screening in a quiet, private setting; do not ask anyone who accompanies the woman to translate or explain; it is best to have no one else present during the interview; and remember that any person accompanying the victim might be an abuser.

When a woman has a black eye or bruises about the mouth, ask, "Who hit you?" rather than, "What happened to you?" The latter implies that the nurse is neither knowledgeable nor comfortable with violence, and this may prompt the woman to fabricate a more acceptable cause of her injury.

Abused women have more physical health problems than other women, specifically chronic headaches, palpitations, sleep and appetite disturbances, chronic pelvic pain, urinary frequency and/or urgency, irritable bowel syndrome and other abdominal symptoms, sexual dysfunction, and recurrent vaginal infections (ACOG, 2012). Ask, "When did this happen?" Also ask, "Where did this happen?" Write up what the person actually said using quotation marks, and make note of grooming, posture, and mannerisms (WHO, 2015).

Abuse as a process. Ford-Gilboe et al. (2011) identified a process of response to battering in which the woman's emotional and behavioral reactions change. Initially she tries to minimize the seriousness of the situation. The violence usually starts with a slight shove in the middle of a heated argument. Most couples argue and disagree, and some fight. When there is any physical aggression, both the man and the woman tend to blame the incident on something external such as a particularly stressful day at work or drinking too much. The male partner usually apologizes for the incident, and as with any problem in a relationship, the couple tries to improve the situation. Although marital counseling may be useful at this early stage, it is generally contraindicated at all other stages because of the risk to the woman's safety. Unfortunately, abuse tends to escalate in frequency and severity over time, and the man's remorse tends to lessen. The risk is such that women who try to leave an abusive relationship are at significant risk for homicide (Campbell, 2007).

Because women often feel responsible for the success of a relationship, they may try to change their behavior to end the violence. They may even blame themselves for infuriating their spouse. Women who blame themselves for provoking the abuse are more likely to have low self-esteem and be depressed than those who do not blame themselves. Some women experience a moral conflict between their need to leave an abusive relationship and their sense that it is their responsibility to maintain the relationship. Women find that no matter what they do, the violence continues. During this period, the woman tries to hide the violence because of the stigma attached. She tries to placate her spouse and feels she is losing her sense of self. She is often concerned about her children, whether she leaves or stays. Some women literally fear for their lives and those of their children. She fears that her partner will try to kill her, the children, or both if she attempts to leave. This fear may be justified. She may kill herself or her abuser to escape because she sees no other way out (Campbell, 2007). Because of the severity of the abuse, a woman may flee to a shelter to obtain physical safety for herself and her children (WHO, 2013). As a woman tries to leave, the risk for homicide increases. In the United States, 39% of homicides of women are committed by an intimate partner (Catalano, 2013). Often the woman thinks she will die if she stays or leaves the relationship. A nurse encountering a family in which there is severe abuse needs to consider the safety of the woman and her children as the priority. The woman will need an order of protection, a legal document specifically designed to keep the abuser away from her. The abuser may ignore the order of protection. The woman will also need help in getting to a safe place, such as a wife abuse shelter in a location that the abuser cannot find. At the very least, the woman must design a carefully thought-out plan for escape and arrange for a family member, friend, neighbor or an adolescent child to call the police when another violent episode occurs.

Short-term help for women in abusive relationships can often be found. Many women, however, have identified a dearth of long-term and family-oriented services. Unfortunately, financial constraints sometimes factor into the decision-making process of whether to remain in abusive relationships. The high cost of attorney fees to obtain equitable divorces or child custody is a factor many women face when leaving these relationships.

An alternative to ending the relationship is for the male partner to attend a program for batterers. These programs are most effective if they are court mandated and if the perpetrator's underlying values about women are addressed, as well as his violence, and if the perpetrator is held accountable. Abused women need affirmation, support, reassurances of the normalcy of their responses, accurate information about shelters and legal resources, and brainstorming about possible solutions. These needs can be met by other women in similar situations and by professionals such as nurses. Women should not be pushed into actions that they are not ready to take. Also consider cultural factors that influence the way in which women respond to IPV, and use this information to design the intervention.

After the abusive relationship has ended, a period of recovery ensues. This includes a normal grief response for the relationship that has ended and a search for meaning in the experience. Thus a formerly battered woman who is feeling depressed and lonely after the relationship has ended is exhibiting a normal response for which support is needed.

Nurses need to assess for intimate sexual abuse in which the battered woman is forced into sexual encounters. Often women who have come to emergency departments because of abuse have also been sexually abused. These women are at risk for STDs and mental health problems (ACOG, 2012). Therefore like intimate partner violence in the past, marital rape remains a private issue. There is also an alarming incidence of date rape, the dynamics of which may parallel marital rape. Adolescent boys are more likely to perpetrate sexual dating violence than are girls. Young women who have been victims of dating violence experience low self-esteem, depression, anger, irritability, and physical health problems (CDC, 2020d).

To assess for sexual assault, the question, "Have you ever been forced into sex you did not wish to participate in?" should be used in all nursing assessments to see if marital rape, date rape, or rape of a male has occurred (WHO, 2014b). If you observe signs of IPV, other questions to ask include:

- Is someone hurting you?
- Are you frightened of your partner?
- Did someone you know do this to you?

Battering during pregnancy has serious implications for the health of both women and their children. These women are at risk for spontaneous abortion, premature delivery, delivery of low–birth-weight infants, substance abuse during pregnancy, and depression (ACOG, 2012). Abuse before pregnancy often precedes abuse during pregnancy. A man's control of contraception, a form of abusive controlling, may lead to unintended pregnancy and subsequent abuse. In addition, a man's refusal to use a condom places a woman at an increased risk for STDs, including infection with HIV (ACOG, 2012). Infants whose mothers were battered are often at high risk for child abuse. All pregnant women should be assessed for abuse at each prenatal care visit, and postpartum home visits should include assessment for child abuse and partner abuse.

A form of IPV that is often overlooked is strangulation. Strangulation "is a violent and deadly act" and it may not leave visible evidence until hours or days after the incident (McCarthy and Stagg, 2020, p. 25). Victims often are hesitant to report the strangulation because they fear they will not be believed since there may not be visible signs. Sexual assault increases the risk for nonfatal strangulation (NFS). Subjective data that may indicate possible strangulation include neck or throat pain; discomfort or difficulty swallowing or talking; vocal changes; shortness of breath; loss of consciousness; memory loss; dizziness; feeling faint; blurry vision; involuntary urination or defecation; and tinnitus (McCarthy and Stagg, 2020). Nurses should suspect NFS if the client has neurological symptoms such as seizures, stroke symptoms, concentration and recall difficulties, or agitation. Physical signs may include linear abrasions; bruising on the upper neck, chin, or face; subconjunctival hemorrhage; conjunctivae petechiae; neck swelling or neck tenderness upon palpation. McCarthy and Stagg (2020) provide information about a danger assessment tool as well as resources if you suspect NFS.

EVIDENCE-BASED PRACTICE

McCabe and colleagues (2016) conducted a study to test whether partner communication about HIV and/or alcohol intoxication influenced reductions in IPV in a culturally specific HIV risk-reduction intervention group for Hispanic women called SEPA (*Salud* [health], *Educación* [education], *Promoción* [promotion], *y* [and] *Autocuidado* [self-care]). There were five SEPA sessions, covering sexually transmitted disease/HIV prevention, partner communication, condom negotiation/use, and IPV. SEPA reduced IPV and alcohol intoxication, and improved partner communication compared with controls in a randomized trial with 548 adult US Hispanic women, split into a SEPA group and a control group.

Results indicated that SEPA prevented deterioration in partner communication about HIV, which reduced the likelihood of IPV. Communication strategies leading to fewer relationship conflicts worked to reduce male-to-female IPV, which in turn reduced female-to-male IPV.

Nurse Use

Because IPV does not occur solely at an individual level, it is important for nurses to understand how to assist patients to develop healthy communication practices around issues like safe sex and IPV. The study results suggest that IPV prevention/reduction strategies can be combined with preexisting health promotion/disease prevention programs, hopefully leading to effective and inexpensive ways of addressing the health of Hispanic women, families, and communities.

Data from McCabe BE, Gonzalez-Guarda RM, Peragallo NP, et al.: Mechanisms of partner violence reduction in a group HIV-risk intervention for Hispanic women. J Interpers Violence 31:2316–2337, 2016.

Abuse of Older Adults

Elder abuse is growing as a form of family violence. **Elder abuse** "is an intentional act or failure to act that causes a risk of harm to an older adult." An older adult is considered to be a person age 60 or older (CDC, 2020h). The WHO defines elder abuse as a "single or repeated act, or lack of appropriate action, occurring within any relationship where there is an expectation of trust, which causes harm or distress to an older person" (WHO, 2020). Abuse, including neglect and exploitation, is thought to affect about 1 in 10 elders who live at home (CDC, 2020h). The WHO estimated in 2020 that 1 in 6 people 60 years or older experienced a form of abuse in community settings in the past year, and rates of abuse are also high in nursing homes and long-term care facilities (WHO, 2020). Like spouse abuse and child abuse, most cases of elder abuse go unreported because

the elder is afraid to tell police, friends, or family about the violence (CDC, 2020h). As with other forms of human abuse, elder maltreatment can be physical when the person is hit, kicked, pushed, slapped, or burned, or sexual when the elder is forced to take part in a sexual act against his or her will or when the elder cannot consent. Emotional abuse includes behaviors to demean or affect the elder's self-esteem, such as name-calling, scaring, embarrassing, destroying property, or not letting the person see family or friends. Neglect occurs when the basic needs for food, housing, clothing, and medical care are not met, and in abandonment, the caregiver leaves the elder and no longer provides care for him or her. In financial abuse, the elder's money, property, or assets are misused (CDC, 2020h). Elders also may be abused by the following actions of caregivers:

- Rough handling that can lead to bruises and bleeding into body tissues because of the fragility of elders' skin and vascular systems. It is often difficult to determine whether the injuries of elders result from abuse, falls, or other natural causes. Careful assessment through both observation and discussion can help determine the cause of injuries.
- Imposing unrealistic toileting demands.
- Ignoring special needs and previous living patterns.
- Giving food that the older person cannot chew or swallow or that is contraindicated because of dietary restrictions or social or cultural preferences.
- Giving medication to induce confusion or drowsiness so that the elders will be less troublesome, will need less care, or will allow others to gain control of their financial and personal resources.

The most common form of psychological abuse is rejection or simply ignoring older adults, indicating that they are worthless and useless to others. Elders may subsequently regress and become increasingly dependent on others, who tend to resent the imposition and demands on their time and lifestyles. The pattern becomes cyclical; as the person becomes more regressed, the level of dependence increases. Furthermore, the past accomplishments and present abilities of the older person may not be consistently acknowledged, causing the person to feel even less capable. There are several precipitating factors for elder abuse. The elder may be a physical, emotional, or financial burden on the caregiver, leading to frustration and resentment. Or the elder may have previously been the abuser. The abuser may be an acquaintance, close or extended family member, caregiver, or stranger. Children who have lived in abusive households learn that behavior. All elders should be assessed for abuse. This is especially true for confused and frail elders. These illnesses place a high burden on the caregiver, with subsequent caregiver depression. Living with and providing care to a confused elder is difficult. The around-the-clock tasks often exhaust family members. In addition, clients with Alzheimer's disease may become verbally and even physically aggressive as a result of their illness, which may trigger retaliatory violence. Family stress increases as members work harder to fulfill their other responsibilities in addition to meeting the needs of the elder.

When families plan to care for an older family member at home, nurses must help them fully evaluate that decision and prepare for the stressors that will be involved. A plan for regular respite care is essential. Strategies for the primary and secondary prevention of elder abuse include victim support groups, senior advocacy volunteer programs, and training for providers working with elders.

Elderly people need to retain as much autonomy and decision-making ability as possible. Nurses have many ways to detect elder abuse, and they have the skills and responsibility for discovering it, giving treatment, and making referrals. Many families who care for elderly members exhaust their resources and coping ability. Nurses can help them find new sources of support and aid.

The CDC (2020h) recommends the following actions to prevent elder abuse before it begins:

1. Listen to older adults and their caregivers to understand their challenges and provide support.
2. Report abuse or suspected abuse to Adult Protective Services.
3. Educate yourself and others about ways to recognize and report elder abuse.
4. Learn how the signs of elder abuse differ from the normal aging process.
5. Check in often on adults who may have few friends and family members.
6. Provide overburdened caregivers with support and help from friends, family, or local relief care groups; adult day care programs; counseling; and outlets intended to promote emotional well-being.

NURSING INTERVENTIONS: VIOLENCE AND ABUSE

Primary prevention begins with a community approach that incorporates strategies from criminal justice, education, social services, community advocacy, and public health to prevent violence. Refer back in the chapter to the socioecological model with its prevention framework that includes individual, relationship, community and societal factors. For each type of violence, the CDC has developed a technical resource package that provides guidance to health care providers. Some communities have used the following:

- School-based curricula that teach children and youth how to cope with anger, stress, and frustration and that also teach communication and mediation skills.
- Family programs that teach parents how to more effectively respond to their children.
- Preschool programs that help children develop intellectual and social skills.
- Public education programs to educate communities about different forms of violence and ways to get help and intervene. This is especially important with the social unrest in many communities.
- Home visit programs designed to prevent child abuse and neglect for at-risk families.
- Lobbying for passage of legislation to outlaw physical punishment in schools and marital rape.

Strong community sanctions against violence in the home, as well as high levels of community cohesion, can reduce levels of abuse (Wilkins et al., 2014). Nurses can work with advocate groups to make sure police and other community workers deal with assault within marriage as swiftly, surely, and severely as assault between strangers. Nurses can encourage others to intervene when they see children who are hit when in a store or other public place, notice that an elder is not being properly cared for, see a youth beat up or verbally bully a classmate, or hear a neighbor hitting someone in the home. However, whenever a person intervenes in a violent episode, the safety of the one who is intervening should clearly be kept in mind.

QSEN   FOCUS ON QUALITY AND SAFETY EDUCATION FOR NURSES

Targeted Competency: Teamwork and Collaboration—Function effectively within nursing and interprofessional teams, fostering open communication, mutual respect, and shared decision making to achieve quality client care. Important aspects of teamwork and collaboration include the following:

- **Knowledge:** Recognize the contributions of other individuals and groups in helping the client/family achieve health goals.
- **Skills:** Assume the role of team member or leader based on the situation.
- **Attitudes:** Respect the unique attributes that members bring to a team, including variations in professional orientations and accountabilities.

Teamwork and Collaboration Question:

If you learned after careful assessment of your community that family violence is a significant community health problem, what plan of action could you take to intervene? Remember that the goal is to promote health. Are there other individuals in the community whose collaboration you could enlist? Might there be insights and assistance that could be offered by leaders in church organizations, educators in schools, primary care providers, or social workers? Outline a plan of action with objectives, timetables, implementation strategies, and evaluation plans for intervening in family violence in your community. Include the unique contributions of other team members.

Prepared by Gail Armstrong, ND, DNP, MS, PhD, Professor and Assistant Dean of the DNP Program, Oregon Health and Sciences University.

Second, people can take measures to reduce their vulnerability to violence by improving the physical security of their homes and learning personal defense measures. Nurses can encourage people to keep windows and doors locked, trim shrubs around their homes, and keep lights on during high-crime periods. Neighbors may informally agree to monitor one another's property and safety.

Unfortunately, handguns are far more likely to kill family members than intruders (Azrael et al., 2018). Firearm accidents are a leading cause of death for young children, and handguns kept in the home are easy to use in moments of extreme anger with other family members or in extreme depression. The majority of homicides between family members and most suicides involve a handgun. Nursing assessments should include a question about guns kept in the home. The family should be made aware of the risk that a handgun holds for family members. If the family thinks that keeping a gun is necessary, safety measures should be taught, such as keeping the gun unloaded and in a locked compartment, keeping the ammunition separate from the gun and also locked away, and instructing children about the dangers of firearms. Lobbying for handgun-control laws is a primary prevention effort that can significantly decrease the rate of death and serious injury caused by handguns in the United States.

Identification of risk factors is an important part of primary prevention used by nurses who work with clients in a variety of settings. Although abuse cannot be predicted with certainty, several factors influence the onset and support the continuation of abusive patterns. Factors to include in an assessment for individual or family violence, or for potential family violence, are illustrated in Fig. 27.5. Factors to be included when assessing a community for violence are shown in Box 27.2.

As seen in the Levels of Prevention box and in Box 27.3, primary prevention of violence can take place through community, family, and individual interventions. Nurses, in their work in schools, community groups, employee groups, daycare centers, and other community institutions, can foster healthy developmental patterns and identify signs of potential abuse. Nurses may participate in media campaigns that identify risk factors for abuse or in developing after-school programs and late-night programs to support youth in using their energies toward positive goals and developing a constructive support network. Nurses can strengthen families by serving as role models and teaching parenting skills in a class, clinic or home visit such as diapering, feeding, quieting, holding, rocking, and nonphysical disciplining. The Nurse-Family Partnership (NFP)

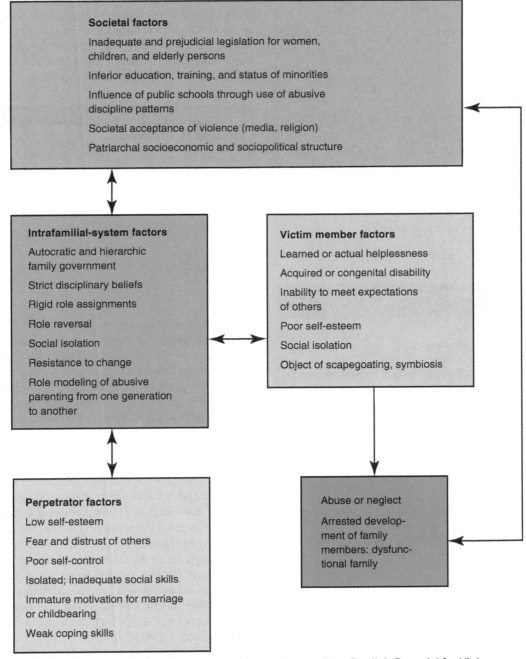

Fig. 27.5 Factors to Include When Assessing an Individual's or Family's Potential for Violence.

BOX 27.2   Assessing for Violence in a Community Context

Individual Factors
- Signs of physical abuse (e.g., abrasions, contusions, burns)
- Physical symptoms related to emotional distress
- Developmental and behavioral difficulties
- Presence of physical disability
- Social isolation
- Decreased role performance within the family and on the job or decreased school-related activities
- Mental health problems such as depression, low self-esteem, and anxiety
- Fear of intimacy with others
- Substance abuse

Familial Factors
- Economic stressors
- Presence of some form of family violence
- Poor communication
- Problems with child rearing
- Lack of family cohesion
- Recurrent familial conflict
- Lack of social support networks
- Poor social integration into the community
- Multiple changes of residence
- Access to guns
- Homelessness

Community Characteristics
- High crime rate
- High levels of unemployment
- Lack of neighborhood resources and support systems
- Lack of community cohesiveness

BOX 27.3   Prevention Strategies for Violence

Individual and Family Levels
- Assess during routine examination (secondary)
- Assess for marital discord (secondary)
- Educate on developmental stages and the needs of children (primary)
- Counsel for at-risk parents (secondary)
- Teach parenting techniques (primary)
- Assist with controlling anger (secondary)
- Treat for substance abuse (tertiary)
- Teach stress-reduction techniques (primary)

Community Level
- Develop policy
- Conduct community resource mapping
- Collaborate with the community to develop systematic responses to violence
- Develop a media campaign
- Develop resources such as transition housing and shelters

provides intensive prenatal and postnatal home visits, ideally to the child's second birthday. Home visits are delivered by registered nurses to low-income first-time mothers, and has been shown to reduce the rate of child maltreatment (Eckenrode et al., 2017).

When abuse occurs, nurses can initiate secondary prevention measures to reduce or terminate further abuse. Both developmental and situational crises present opportunities for abusive situations to develop. Nurses can help form groups to assist battered women. Nurses can work closely with shelters in identifying the needs of individuals who seek sanctuary from abusive situations. Nurses can also develop screening practices in the health care arena (Alhusen et al., 2013).

On a family level, nurses can help family members discuss problems and seek ways to deal with the tension that led to the abusive situations. Injured persons must be temporarily or permanently placed in a safe location. Secondary preventive measures are most useful when potential abusers recognize their tendency to be abusive and seek help. For children, there is often a need for 24-hour child protection services or caregivers who can take care of the child until the acute family or individual crisis is resolved. Respite care is extremely important in families with frail elderly family members. Telephone crisis lines can be used to provide immediate emergency assistance to families.

LEVELS OF PREVENTION

Related to Violence

Primary Prevention
Strengthen the individual and family by teaching parenting skills.

Secondary Prevention
Reduce or end abuse by early screening; teach families how to deal with stress and how to have fun and enjoy recreation.

Tertiary Prevention
When signs of abuse are evident, refer the client to appropriate community organizations.

Effective communication with abusive families is important. Typically, these families do not want to discuss their problems, and many are embarrassed to be involved in an abusive situation. Often feelings of guilt are present. Effective communication must be preceded by an attitude of acceptance. It is often difficult for nurses to value the worth of an individual who willfully abuses another. The behavior, not the person, should be condemned.

In addition, not all families know how to have fun. Nurses can assess how much recreation is integrated into the family's lifestyle. Through community assessment, nurses know what resources and facilities are available and how much they cost. Families may need counseling about the value of recreation and play in reducing tension and appropriately dealing with aggressive impulses.

Although it may be difficult to form a trusting relationship with abusive families, nurses can engage in tertiary prevention by acting as a case manager and coordinating the other agencies and activities involved. Principles of giving care to families who are experiencing violence include the following:
- Intolerance for violence
- Respect and caring for all family members

- Safety as the first priority
- Absolute honesty
- Empowerment

Abusers frequently fear they will be condemned for their actions, so it is often difficult to make and maintain contact with abusive families. Although nurses convey an attitude of caring and concern for them, families may doubt the sincerity of this concern. They may avoid being home at the scheduled visit time because of fear of the consequences of the visit or an inability to believe that anyone really wants to help them. If the victim is a child, parents may fear that the nurse will try to remove the child. Nurses are mandatory reporters of child abuse, even when only suspected, in all states. They are also mandatory reporters of elder abuse and abuse of other physically and cognitively dependent adults, as well as of felony assaults of anyone in most states. The mandatory reporting laws also protect reporters from legal action on cases that are never substantiated. Even so, physicians and nurses are sometimes reluctant to report abuse. They may be more willing to report abuse in a poor family than in a middle-class one, or they may think that an older adult or child is better off at home than in a nursing home or foster home. Referral to protective service agencies is a way to get help, rather than an automatic step toward removal of the victim or toward criminal justice action. Families should be included in any reporting so they can have input. Absolute honesty about what will be reported to officials, what the family can expect, what the nurse is entering into records, and what the nurse is feeling is essential.

To further assist the family, the nurse needs to recognize and capitalize on the violent family's strengths, as well as to assess and deal with its problems. The nurse must use a nurse-family partnership rather than a paternalistic or authoritarian approach. Families often can generate many of their own solutions, which tend to be more culturally appropriate and individualized than those the nurse generates in isolation. Victims of direct attacks need information about their options and resources and reassurance that abuse is unfortunately rather common and that they are not alone in their dilemma. They also need reassurance that their responses are normal and that they do not deserve to be abused. Continued support for their decisions must be coupled with nursing actions to ensure their safety.

Referral is an important component of tertiary prevention. Nurses should know about available community resources for abuse victims and perpetrators. Examples of community resources are listed in Box 27.4. If attitudes and resources are inadequate, it is often helpful to work with local radio and television stations and newspapers to provide information about the nature and extent of human abuse as a community health problem. This also helps acquaint people with available services and resources. Frequently, people do not seek services early in an abusive situation because they simply do not know what is available to them. Ideally, a program or plan for abused people begins with a needs assessment to identify potential clients and to determine how to effectively serve this group. Nurses can help get programs started and provide public education.

BOX 27.4 Common Community Services

- Child Protective Services
- Child Abuse Prevention programs
- Adult Protective Services
- Parents Anonymous
- Wife abuse shelter
- Program for children of battered women
- Community support group
- 24-hour hotline for crisis intervention or counseling. These crisis hotlines may offer a variety of counseling services or only target one type of crisis. They are available at national and local levels.
- Legal advocacy or information
- State coalition against domestic violence
- Batterer treatment
- Victim assistance programs
- Sexual assault programs

» APPLYING CONTENT TO PRACTICE

According to the Quad Council Coalition of Public Health Nursing (2018) and the American Public Health Association (Krisberg, 2020), public health nurses must collaborate in partnership with communities to assess and identify community needs; plan, implement, and evaluate community-based programs; and assist in the setting of policy that will contribute to the needs of the community in relationship to all types of interpersonal violence. The Quad Council competencies in the analytic assessment domain direct nurses to conduct thorough health assessments of individuals, families, communities, and populations and to develop diagnoses for the population being assessed. Public health nurses can help the community in many ways, as described throughout this chapter.

▮ PRACTICE APPLICATION

Mrs. Smith, a 75-year-old bedridden woman, consistently became rude and combative when her daughter, Mary, attempted to bathe her and change her clothes each morning. During a home visit, Mary told the nurse, Mrs. Jones, that she had gotten so frustrated with her mother on the previous morning that she had hit her. Mary felt terrible about her behavior. She stressed that her mother's incontinence made it essential that she be kept clean; her clothes had to be changed every day for her own safety and physical well-being.

A. How should Mrs. Jones respond to this disclosure?
B. What specific nursing actions should be taken?
C. What ongoing services does the nurse need to provide?
Answers can be found on the Evolve website.

▮ REMEMBER THIS!

- Violence and human abuse are not new phenomena, but they are growing public health concerns.
- People in the United States are frustrated by increasing levels of violence.
- Nurses and other workers in the community can evaluate and intervene in community and family violence.

- To intervene effectively, nurses must understand the dynamics of violence and human abuse.
- Factors influencing violence include changing social conditions, economic conditions, polarization of groups, population density, community facilities, and institutions within a community.
- Violence and abuse of family members can happen to any family member: spouse, elder, child, or physically or mentally compromised person.
- Human trafficking is a growing public health problem.
- People who abuse family members were often abused themselves; they react poorly to real or perceived crises. Other factors that characterize the abuser are the way the person was raised and the unique character of that person. Cultural factors should be considered when abuse is suspected.
- Child abuse can be physical, emotional, or sexual. Incest is a particularly destructive form of child abuse.
- Spouse abuse is usually wife abuse. It involves physical, emotional, and frequently, sexual abuse within a context of coercive control. It usually increases in severity and frequency and can escalate to homicide of either partner.
- Nurses can identify potential victims of family abuse because they see clients in a variety of settings, such as schools, businesses, homes, and clinics. Treatment of family abuse includes primary, secondary, and tertiary prevention and therapeutic intervention.
- COVID increased the incidence of family violence.

WHAT WOULD YOU DO?

1. Read in the local newspaper or online to determine what are the most common forms of violence in your community. Based on what you learn, what would be a beneficial form of primary prevention that public health nurses could implement?
2. If you learned, after a careful assessment of your community, that family violence is a significant community health problem, what plan of action could you take to intervene? Remember that the goal is to promote health. Outline a plan of action with objectives, timetables, implementation strategies, and evaluation plans for intervening in family violence in your community. Who else might need to be involved to intervene in this health problem?
3. What resources are available in your community for victims of violence?
   a. Interview a person who works in an agency that seeks to aid victims of violence.
   b. What is the role of the agency? Do its services seem adequate? Who is eligible? Is there a waiting list? What is the fee scale? Is the care culturally competent?

EVOLVE WEBSITE

http://evolve.elsevier.com/Stanhope/foundations
- Case Study, with Questions and Answers
- NCLEX® Review Questions
- Practice Application Answers

REFERENCES

American Academy of Child and Adolescent Psychiatry: *Sexual abuse*, 2020. Retrieved November 2020 at http://www.aacap.org.

Alhusen JL, Lucea M, Bullock L. et al.: Intimate partner violence and adverse neonatal outcomes among urban women, *J Pediatr*, 16:3:471-478, 2013.

American College of Obstetricians and Gynecologists: Intimate partner violence, Committee opinion No. 518, *Obstet Gynecol* 119:412–417, 2012.

Azrael D, Cohen J, Salhi C, et al.: Firearm storage in gun-owning households with children: results of a 2015 national survey, *J Urban Health* 95:295-304, 2018.

Basile KC, DeGue S, Jones K, et al.: *STOP SV: A technical package to prevent sexual violence*, Atlanta, 2016, National Center for Injury Prevention and Control, Centers for Disease Control and Prevention.

Becker HJ, Bechtel K: Recognizing victims of human trafficking in the pediatric emergency department, *Pediatr Emerg Care* 2: 144-147, 2015.

Betts KJ: Children and post traumatic stress disorder, *American Nurse Journal*, 15(5):52-55, 2020.

Black MC, Basile KC, Breiding MJ, et al.: *The national intimate partner and sexual violence survey (NISVA): 2010 summary report*, Atlanta, 2011, National Center for Injury Prevention and Control, Centers for Disease Control and Prevention.

Breiding MJ, Smith SG, Basile KC, et al.: Prevalence and characteristics of sexual violence, stalking, and intimate partner violence victimization, National Intimate Partner and Sexual Violence Survey, United States, 2011, *MMWR* 63:1-18, 2014.

Campbell JC: *Assessing dangerousness: violence by batterers and child abusers*, 2nd ed., New York, 2007, Springer.

Campbell JC, Glass N, Sharps PW et al.: Intimate partner homicide: review and implications of research and policy, *Trauma Violence Abuse*, 8:246-269, 2007.

Campbell R, Greeson M, Patterson D: Defining the boundaries: How sexual assault nurse examines (SNEs) balance patient care and law enforcement collaboration, *J Forensic Nurs* 10:208- 216, 2011.

Campbell R, Townsend SM, Shaw J, et al.: Evaluating the legal impact of sexual assault nurse examiner programs: An empirically validated toolkit for practitioners, *J Forensic Nurs*10:208-216, 2014.

Campbell JC, Sabari B, Budhathoki C, et al.: Unwanted sexual acts among university students: correlates of victimization and perpetration, *J Interpers Violence*, Published online October 2017.

Catalano S: *Intimate partner violence: attributes of victimization, 1993-2011*, Washington, DC, 2013, Bureau of Justice Statistics. Retrieved July 2016 from http://www.bjs.gov/content/pub/pdf/ipvav9311.pdf.

Centers for Disease Control and Prevention: *Preventing intimate partner violence*, Atlanta, 2019a. Retrieved July 2020 from http://www.cdc.gov/violenceprevention.

Centers for Disease Control and Prevention: *Risk and protective factors for perpetration*, Atlanta, 2019b, Retrieved July 2020 from http://www.cdc.gov/violenceprevention.

Centers for Disease Control and Prevention: *The public health approach to violenceprevention*, 2020a, Retrieved July 2020 at www.cdc.violenceprevention.

Centers for Disease Control and Prevention: *The social-ecological model: A framework for prevention*,. Atlanta, 2020b, Retrieved July 2020 from http://www.cdc.gov/violenceprevention.

Centers for Disease Control and Prevention: *Firearm violenceprevention*, Atlanta, 2020c, Retrieved November 2020 from http://www.cdc.gov/violenceprevention.

Centers for Disease Control and Prevention: *Preventing teen dating violence,* 2020d, Atlanta, Retrieved July 2020 from http://www.cdc.gov/violenceprevention.

Centers for Disease Control and Prevention: *Preventing suicide,* Atlanta, 2020e. Retrieved July 2020 from http://www.cdc.gov/violenceprevention.

Centers for Disease Control and Prevention: *Preventing child abuse & neglect,* Atlanta, 2020f. Retrieved July 2020 from http://www.cdc.gov/violenceprevention.

Centers for Disease Control and Prevention: *About the CDC-Kaiser ACE study.* Atlanta, 2020g. Retrieved July 2020 from http://www.cdc.gov/violenceprevention.

Centers for Disease Control and Prevention: *Preventing elder abuse,* Atlanta, 2020h, Retrieved July 2020 from http://www.cdc.gov/violenceprevention.

Child Welfare Information Gateway: *What is child abuse and neglect? Recognizing the signs and symptoms,* Washington, DC: US Department of Health and Human Services, Children's Bureau, 2019a.

Child Welfare Information Gateway: *Long term consequences of child abuse and neglect,* Washington, DC, 2019b, US Department of Health and Human Services, Children's Bureau.

Child Trends: Children's exposure to violence, 2016, Accessed July 2020 at: https://www.childtrends.org/?indicators=childrens-exposure-to-violence.

Crane P: A Human trafficking toolkit for nursing intervention. In: De Chesnay M: Sex Trafficking: A clinical guide for nurses. New York, 2013, Springer.

Curtin SC, Heron M: Death rates due to suicide and homicide among persons aged 10-24, United States, 2000-2017, NCHS Data Brief, No 352, Hyattsville, National Center for Health Statistics, 2019.

De Chesnay M: *Sex trafficking: A clinical guide for nurses.* New York, 2013, Springer.

Decker MR, Wilcox HC, Holliday CN, et al.: An integrated public health approach to interpersonal violence and suicide prevention and response, *Public Health Rep,* 133(Suppl 1): 65S-79S, 2018.

Eckenrode J, Campa MI, Morris PA, et al.: The prevention of child maltreatment through the Nurse Family Partnership Program: Mediating effects in a long-term follow-up study, *Child Maltreatment* 22:92–99, 2017.

Fletcher J: The effects of intimate partner violence on health in young adulthood in the United States, *Soc Sci Med* 70:130–135, 2010.

Ford-Gilboe M, Varcoe C, Wuest J, et al.: Intimate partner violence and nursing practice. In Humphreys J, Campbell JC, editors: *Intimate partner violence and nursing practice,* New York, 2011, Springer.

Fortson BL, Klevens J, Merrick MT, et al.: *Preventing child abuse and neglect: A technical package for policy, norm, and programmatic activities,* Atlanta, 2016, National Center for Injury Prevention and Control, Centers for Disease Control and Prevention.

Garthe RC, Sullivan TN, McDaniel MA: A meta-analytic review of peer risk factors and adolescent dating violence, *Psychol Violence* 7:45–57, 2017.

Hedegaard H, Curtin SC, Warner M: *Suicide mortality in the United States,* 1996-2017, NCHS Data Brief, No 330, Hyattsville, National Center for Health Statistics, 2018.

Humphreys JC, Campbell JC: *Family violence and nursing practice,* New York, 2010, Springer.

Isaac R, Solak J, Giardino A: Health care providers' training needs related to human trafficking: Maximizing the opportunity to effectively screen and intervene. *J Appl Res Child* 2:1-32, 2011.

Krebs C, Lindquist C, Berzofsky M, et al.: *Campus Climate Survey Validation Study final technical report,* Washington, DC, January 2016, Bureau of Justice Statistics. R&DP-2015:04, NCJ 249545.

Krisberg K: Are the 10 essential public health services out of date? Review underway, *The National's Health* 49(10):1-16, January 2020.

Lysell, H, Dahlin M, Langstrom N, et al.: Killing the mother of one's child: Psychiatric risk factors among male perpetrators and offspring consequences, *J Clin Psychiatry* 77:342–347, 2016.

McCabe BE, Gonzalez-Guarda RM, Peragallo NP, et al.: Mechanisms of partner violence reduction in a group HIV-risk intervention for Hispanic women, *J Interpers Violence* 31:2316–2337, 2016.

McCarthy J, Stagg D: Strangulation: A silent but deadly form of intimate partner violence, *Am J Nurs,* 15(2):24-27, 2020.

Miller M, Hemenway D: Guns and suicide in the United States, *N Engl J Med* 359:989–991, 2008.

Morgan RE, Oudekerk BA: Criminal victimization, 2018, US Department of Justice, NCJ, September 2019.

Nannini A, Lazar J, Berg C, et al.: Physical injuries reported on hospital visits for assault during the pregnancy-associated period, *Nurs Res* 57:144–149, 2008.

National Center for Health Statistics,: *Healthy United States, 2018,* Hyattsville, 2019, Accessed July 2020 at www.cdc.gov.

National Human Trafficking Hotline, 2018 Statistics, Accessed July 2020 at www.humantraffickinghotline.org.

National Coalition of Anti-Violence Programs: *A crisis of hate: A mid-year report on Lesbian, Gay, Bisexual, Transgender and Queer Hate Violence Homicides.* 2017, Retrieved May 2018 from: http://avp.org/wp-content/uploads/2017/08/NCAVP-A-Crisis-of-Hate-Final.pdf.

National Coalition Against Domestic Violence, *Domestic violence and sexual assault,* 2017. Retrieved August 10, 2017 from http://ncadv.org/files/Domestic%20and%20Abuse%20NCADV.pdf.

One in Four USA: *Sexual assault statistics.* Retrieved July 2016 from http://www.oneinfourusa.org/statistics.php.

Parks SE, Johnson LL, McDaniel DD, et al.: Surveillance for violent deaths—National Violent Death Reporting System, 16 States, 2010, *MMWR Surveill Summ* 63:1–33, 2014.

Peters K: The growing business of human trafficking and the power of emergency nurses to stop it, *J Emerg Nurs* 39:280-288, 2013.

Quad Council Coalition of Public Health Nursing Organizations: *Community/public health nursing competencies,* Public Health Foundation, Washington DC, 2018.

RAINN: *Recovering from sexual violence,* 2020, Retrieved July 2020 at RAINN: Rape, Abuse and Incest National Network.

Richards T: Health implications of human trafficking. *Nurs Womans Health* 18:155-162, 2014.

Sheridan DJ, Nash KR: Acute injury patterns of intimate partner violence victims, *Trauma Violence Abuse* 8:281–289, 2009.

Siegel M, Negussie Y, Vanture S, et al.: The relationship between gun ownership and stranger and nonstranger firearm homicide rates in the United States, 1981-2010, *Am J Public Health* 104:1912–1919, 2014.

Siskin A, Sun WL: Trafficking in persons: US policy and issues for Congress. Washington, DC: Congressional Research Service, 2013.

Smith SG, Zhang X, Basile KC, et al.: *The National Intimate Partner and Sexual/violence Survey (NISVS):* 2015 Data Brief-Updated Research. Atlanta: National for Injury Prevention and Control, Centers for Disease Control and Prevention, 2018.

Sumner SA, Mercy JA, Dahlberg LL, et al.: Violence in the United States, *JAMA* 314(5):478-488, 2015.

Truman JL, Langston L: *Criminal victimization 2014,* Washington, DC, August 2015, Bureau of Justice Statistics. NCJ 248973.

United Nations Office on Drugs and Crime: Human trafficking, 2019. Retrieved from: https://www.unodc.org/unodc/en/human-trafficking/what-is-human-trafficking.html.

US Department of Health and Human Services: *Healthy People 2030 Objectives*, Washington, DC, 2020a, Office of Disease Prevention and Health Promotion, USDHHS.

US Department of Health and Human Services, Administration for Children and Families, Administration on Children, Youth and Families, Children's Bureau: *Child maltreatment 2018*, 2020b. Retrieved July 2020 from http://www.acf.hhs.gov/programs/cb/research-data-technology/statistics-research/child-maltreatment.

US Department of Health and Human Services, Administration for Children and Families, Administration on Children, Youth and Families, Children's Bureau, Chapter 4: *Protecting children, Understanding child abuse and neglect*, 2020c Accessed July 2020 at www.acfhhs.gov/programs.ch.

US Department of Health and Human Services, Administration for Children and Families, Administration on Children, Youth and Families, Children's Bureau, *Human trafficking*, 2020d, Accessed July 2020 at www.acfhhs.gov.programs.

US Department of Justice Uniform Crime Report, *Crime in the United States, 2018*, Accesssed July 2020 at www.ucr.fbi.gov.

Wilkins N, Tsao B, Hertz M, et al.: *Connecting the dots: an overview of the links among multiple forms of violence*, Atlanta, 2014, National Center for Injury Prevention and Control, Centers for Disease Control and Prevention. Oakland, Prevention Institute.

World Health Organization: *Global status report on violenceprevention 2014*, Geneva, 2014a, WHO. Retrieved July 2016 from http://www.who.int/violence_injury_prevention/violence/status_report/2014.

World Health Organization: *Elder abuse: key facts*, Accessed July 2020 at who.int.

World Health Organization: *Health care for women subjected to intimate partner violence or sexual violence: A clinical handbook*, Geneva, 2014b, WHO.

World Health Organization: *Strengthening the medico-legal response to sexual violence*, Geneva, 2015, WHO.

Zimmerman F, Mercy JA: A better start: child maltreatment prevention as a public health priority, *Zero Three* 30:4–10, 2010.

28

Nursing Practice at the Local, State, and National Levels in Public Health

Lois A. Davis

OBJECTIVES

After reading this chapter, the student should be able to:

1. Define public health, the public health system, public health nursing, and local, state, and national roles.
2. Identify trends in public health nursing.
3. Describe examples of public health nursing roles.
4. Assess the emerging public health issues that specifically affect public health nursing.
5. Describe the principles of partnerships.
6. Identify educational preparation of public health nurses and competencies necessary to practice.

CHAPTER OUTLINE

KEY TERMS

All of public health involves partnerships. Public health programs are designed with the goal of improving a population's health status. They go beyond the administration of health care to include the following:

- Community health assessment
- Community level interventions
- Analysis of health statistics
- Public education
- Outreach
- Case management
- Advocacy
- Recordkeeping
- Professional education for providers
- Disease surveillance and investigation
- Emergency preparedness and response
- Compliance with regulations for some institutions, agencies, and school systems
- Follow-up of population health problems

The following are examples requiring follow-up care:

- Persons with active, untreated tuberculosis
- Pregnant women who have not kept prenatal visits
- Parents of underimmunized children
- Families or individuals diagnosed with COVID-19

Public health programs are frequently implemented by the development of partnerships or coalitions with other providers, agencies, and groups in the location being served. Nurses are involved in these activities in various ways, depending on the public health agency (local, state, federal) and the identified needs. The Community-Campus Partnerships for Health (CCPH) defines partnerships as "a close mutual cooperation between parties having common interests, responsibilities, privileges and power" (CCPH Board of Directors, 2018). A nurse may be the facilitator of the partnership or a member of the partnership representing the agency for which he or she works. Box 28.1 explains the principles of partnerships.

Public health is not a branch of medicine; it is an organized community approach designed to prevent disease, promote health, and protect populations. It works across many disciplines and is based on the scientific core of epidemiology (Institute of Medicine [IOM], 2003; Friis and Sellers, 2021). Nurses in public health work with multidisciplinary teams of people both within the public health areas and in other human services agencies. A critical partnership that shapes public health in the United States is the interaction of local, state, and federal agencies.

BOX 28.1   Principles of Partnership

Community-Campus Partnerships for Health (CCPH) involved its members and partners in developing the following "principles of good practice" for community partnerships:

- The Partnership forms to serve a specific purpose and may take on new goals over time.
- The Partnership agrees upon mission, values, goals, measurable outcomes, and processes for accountability.
- The relationship between partners in the Partnership is characterized by mutual trust, respect, genuineness, and commitment.
- The Partnership builds upon identified strengths and assets but also works to address needs and increase capacity of all partners.
- The Partnership balances power among partners and enables resources among partners to be shared.
- Partners make clear and open communication an ongoing priority in the Partnership by striving to understand each other's needs and self-interests and developing a common language.
- Principles and processes for the Partnership are established with the input and agreement of all partners, especially for decision making and conflict resolution.
- There is feedback among all stakeholders in the Partnership, with the goal of continuously improving the Partnership and its outcomes.
- Partners share the benefits of the Partnership's accomplishments.
- Partnerships can dissolve and, when they do, need to plan a process for closure.
- Partnerships consider the nature of the environment within which they exist as a principle of their design, evaluation, and sustainability.
- The Partnership values multiple kinds of knowledge and life experiences.

From Community-Campus Partnerships for Health (CCPH) Board of Directors: *Position Statement of Authentic Partnerships.* Community-Campus Partnerships for Health, 2013. Available at https://ccph.memberclicks.net/principles-of-partnership. Accessed May 13, 2015.

ROLES OF LOCAL, STATE, AND FEDERAL PUBLIC HEALTH AGENCIES

In the United States the local-state-federal partnership includes federal agencies, the state and territorial public health agencies, and the approximately 3200 local public health agencies (ASTHO, 2020). The interaction of these agencies is critical to effectively use precious resources—financial and personnel—and protect and promote the health of populations. Nurses working in all of these agencies work together to identify, develop, and implement interventions that will improve and maintain the nation's health.

Federal public health agencies develop regulations that implement policies formulated by Congress and provide a significant amount of funding to state and territorial health agencies to do the following:

- Provide public health activities
- Survey the nation's health status and health needs
- Set practices and standards
- Provide expertise that facilitates evidence-based practice
- Coordinate public health activities that cross state lines
- Support health services research

The US Department of Health and Human Services (USDHHS) and the Environmental Protection Agency (EPA) are the federal agencies that most influence public health activities at the state and local levels. The USDHHS includes the Centers for Disease Control and Prevention (CDC); the Health Resources and Services Administration (HRSA); the Agency for Healthcare, Research, and Quality (AHRQ); and the US Food and Drug Administration (FDA). The USDHHS is the agency that facilitates development of the nation's *Healthy People* objectives (USDHHS, 2020).

Each of the states and territories has a single identified official state public health agency that is managed by a state health commissioner. The structure of state public health agencies varies. Some states require that the state health commissioner be a physician. A growing number of states do not limit the position to physicians but rather, require specific public health experience. California, Maryland, Iowa, Oregon, Washington, and Michigan are examples of states that focus on public health experience as a requirement for the state health commissioner position. This allows for the appointments of nurses and other professionals to this position. State public health agencies are responsible for monitoring health status and enforcing laws and regulations that protect and improve the public's health. These agencies receive funding from federal agencies for the implementation of public health interventions. The following are examples:

- Communicable disease programs
- Maternal and child health programs
- Chronic disease prevention programs
- Injury prevention programs

The agencies distribute federal and state funds to the local public health agencies to implement programs at the community level, and they provide oversight and consultation for local public health agencies. State health agencies also delegate some public health powers, such as the power to quarantine, to local health officers.

Local public health agencies have responsibilities that vary depending on the locality, but they are the agencies that are responsible for implementing and enforcing local, state, and federal public health codes and ordinances and providing essential public health programs to a community. The goal of the local public health department is to safeguard the public's health and improve the community's health status. The health department's authority is delegated by the state for specific functions (Box 28.2). As with state health departments, some states require that local health directors be physicians, whereas others focus on public health experience (National Association of County and City Health Officials [NACCHO], 2014). For example, public health nurses in Maryland, Washington, Wisconsin, and California hold local health director positions. The duties of local health departments vary depending on the state and local public health codes and ordinances and the responsibilities assigned by the state and local governments. Usually, the local public health department provides for the administration, regulatory oversight, public health, and environmental services for a geographic area.

The majority of local, state, and federal public health agencies will be involved in the following:

- Collecting and analyzing vital statistics
- Providing health education and information to the population served
- Receiving reports about and investigating and controlling communicable diseases
- Protecting the environment to reduce the risk to health
- Providing some health services to particular populations at risk or with limited access to care (local public health agencies, guided by state and federal policies and goals and community needs)
- Planning for and responding to natural and human-made disasters and emergencies
- Identifying public health problems for at-risk and high-risk populations
- Conducting community assessments to identify community assets and gaps
- Partnering with other organizations to develop and implement responses to identified public health concerns

Nurses in public health work for local, state, and federal agencies. They work in partnership with each other, other public health staff, other governmental agencies, and the community to fulfill the functions of providing some health services to individuals, families, and groups who may have limited access to health care. They also engage in case finding to identify persons at risk for disease and those being lost to the health care system.

Other public health agency staffs include the following:

- Physicians
- Nutritionists
- Environmental health professionals
- Health educators
- Various laboratory workers
- Epidemiologists
- Health planners
- Paraprofessional home visitors
- Outreach workers

Examples of community-based organizations include the following:

- The United Way
- The American Red Cross
- Free clinics
- Head Start programs
- Daycare centers
- Community health centers
- Hospitals
- Senior centers
- Advocacy groups
- Churches
- Academic institutions
- Businesses

Other government agencies include the fire and emergency services departments, law enforcement agencies, schools, parks and recreation departments, and elected officials. Changes in

---

BOX 28.2 Local Public Health Agency Functions

The following are selected standards by essential public health services, performed by local public health agencies:

Essential Public Health Service 1: Monitor Health Status to Identify Community Health Problems
- Obtain data that provide information on the community's health.
- Develop relationships with local providers and others in the community who have information on reportable diseases and other conditions of public health interest and facilitate information exchange.
- Conduct or contribute expertise to periodic community health assessments in order to develop a comprehensive picture of the public's health.
- Integrate data with other health assessment and data collection efforts conducted by the public health system.
- Analyze data to identify trends and population health risks.

Essential Public Health Service 4: Mobilize Community Partnerships to Identify and Solve Health Problems
- Engage the local public health system in an ongoing, strategic, community-driven, comprehensive planning process to identify, prioritize, and solve public health problems; establish public health goals; and evaluate success in meeting the goals.
- Promote the community's understanding of, and advocacy for, policies and activities that will improve the public's health.
- Develop partnerships to generate interest in and support for improved community health status, including new and emerging public health issues.

Essential Public Health Service 7: Link People to Needed Personal Health Services and Ensure the Provision of Health Care When Otherwise Unavailable
- Engage the community to identify gaps in culturally competent, appropriate, and equitable personal health services, including preventive and health promotion services, and develop strategies to close the gaps.
- Support and implement strategies to increase access to care and establish systems of personal health services, including preventive and health promotion services, in partnership with the community.
- Link individuals to available, accessible personal health care providers.

From National Association of County and City Health Officials: *Operational Definition of a Functional Local Health Department,* 2014. Available at http://www.naccho.org. Accessed August 23, 2014.

local, state, and federal governments affect public health services, and nursing has to develop strategies for dealing with these changes. To meet the changing needs of a community, nurses must identify public health concerns and work in programs to provide needed services.

HISTORY AND TRENDS OF PUBLIC HEALTH

A person born today can expect to live 30 years longer than a person born in 1900. Medical care accounts for 5 years of that increase, but public health is responsible for the additional 25 years through prevention efforts brought about by changes in social policies, community actions, and individual and group changes in behavior (USDHHS, 2020). Historically, nurses working in public health were valued by and important to society and functioned in an autonomous setting. They worked with populations and in settings that were not of interest to other health care disciplines or groups. Much public health service was delivered to the poor and to women and children, who did not have political power or voice. During the course of the 20th century, public health responsibilities expanded beyond communicable disease prevention, occupational health, and environmental health programs to include reproductive health, chronic disease prevention, and injury prevention activities.

As a result of Medicaid managed care, many public health agencies were no longer providing personal health care services. Public health agencies began to shift emphasis from a focus on primary health care services to a focus on core public health activities such as the investigation and control of diseases and injuries, population health assessment, community health planning, and involvement in environmental health activities. As the 20th century came to a close, genetics, newly emerging communicable diseases, preventing bioterrorism and violence, and handling and disposing of hazardous waste were emerging as additional public health issues (CDC, 2011; Schneider, 2017).

The IOM (2003) identified the following seven priorities for public health in the 21st century:
- Understand and emphasize the broad determinants of health.
- Develop a policy focus on population health.
- Strengthen the public health infrastructure.
- Build partnerships.
- Develop systems of accountability.
- Emphasize evidence-based practice.
- Enhance communication.

In supporting the 2003 IOM priorities, the National Academy of Medicine (NAM) released *Public Health 3.0: A Call to Action for Public Health to Meet the Challenges of the 21st Century* and recommended actions for public health as follows:
- Public health leaders should take on the role of chief health strategists in their communities.
- Health departments should work with private and public stakeholders in their communities to form partnerships to guide health initiatives.
- Accreditation of public health departments by the Public Health Accreditation Board (PHAB) should be encouraged and supported to assure all citizens are served by a nationally accredited health department.
- Timely, reliable, and actionable data should be accessible to communities, and clear metrics should be developed to document success of public health's practice to guide, focus, and assess the impact of prevention initiatives, which include targeting the social determinants of health and enhancing health equity.
- Public health funding should be enhanced and substantially modified by using innovative funding models to expand financial support for both infrastructure and community level work (NAS/NAM, 2017).

Public health activities at the beginning of the 21st century were shaped by the September 11, 2001, airplane attacks on the World Trade Center and the Pentagon and the plane crash into a field in Pennsylvania, in which thousands were murdered. However, public health activities at the federal, state, and local levels were even more dramatically affected by a series of anthrax exposures that occurred shortly after the airplane attacks. In addition to anthrax exposures in Florida and New York, a month after the plane attacks, thousands of workers at the Brentwood Post Office and the Senate Building in Washington, DC were exposed to an especially virulent strain of anthrax from a contaminated letter. The anthrax exposures alerted policymakers to the weakening public health infrastructure required to respond to bioterrorism events. These exposures required public health nurses to rapidly establish mass medication distribution clinics, while also responding to frightened calls from community members and requests for information from the media.

At the beginning of the 21st century, resources for communicable disease services had already decreased as surveillance and containment activities and protection of water and food supplies produced decreasing rates of communicable disease. As the 21st century arrived, nurses in public health were faced with issues such as unprecedented influenza, tetanus, and childhood vaccine shortages and emerging infections that competed with bioterrorism activities for resources. As an example, in 2009 an outbreak of H1N1 occurred in the United States that led to President Barack Obama to declare the outbreak a national emergency, and in 2015 and 2016 the emergence of the Ebola and Zika viruses in the United States alerted the public to how ill prepared the country was to deal with public health concerns. Then in 2020 came the COVID-19 pandemic, which further underscored how ill prepared the United States was to deal with public health concerns and how the United States basically dismissed the scientists who could provide direction to control the pandemic.

During the 20th century, public health nurses were a major force in the nation, achieving immunization rates that accounted for the dramatic decrease in measles. In 1996 nearly 900,000 fewer cases of measles were reported than in 1941 (CDC, 2019). However, the general public was not informed about how this immunization activity was accomplished or about its effect on improving health and lowering health care cost. For public health services to receive adequate funding, it is necessary for the public and the government to be aware of the benefits provided to a community by nurses. A prime example of emerging infectious diseases in the 21st century is severe acute respiratory syndrome (SARS), caused by a virus, which brought illness and death to many in 2003. The disease spread quickly from China to other countries, being transported by airline passengers traveling internationally. The same means of transportation is a prime cause of other infectious diseases such as the Ebola, Zika, and COVID-19 viruses.

Scope, Standards, and Roles of Nursing in Public Health

In 1920, C. E. A. Winslow defined public health as "the science and art of preventing disease, prolonging life and promoting health and efficiency through organized community effort" (Morrow and Pirani, 2022, p. 15). This definition is still used in public health textbooks because it focuses on the relationship between social conditions and health across all levels of society. Nursing practice in public health focuses on the individuals, families, and groups in areas in which nurses live, work, and play. Nurses educated as public health nurses work with communities and populations.

Additional knowledge, skills, and aptitudes are necessary for a nurse to go beyond focusing on the health needs of the individual to focusing on the health needs of populations (see Chapter 1). This additional knowledge distinguishes the public health nurse from other nurses who are practicing in the community setting.

A variety of settings and a diversity of perspectives are available to nurses interested in developing a career in public health. Nurses working at the federal, state, and local levels integrate community involvement and knowledge about the entire population with clinical understandings of the health and illness experiences of individuals and families in the population. They translate and articulate the health and illness experiences of diverse, often vulnerable individuals and families in the population to health planners and policymakers, and they help members of the community to voice their problems and aspirations. Nurses are knowledgeable about multiple strategies for intervention, focusing primarily on those for the family and the individual. They translate knowledge from the health and social sciences to individuals and population groups through targeted interventions, programs, and advocacy. Nurses are directly engaged in the interdisciplinary activities of the core public health functions of assessment, assurance, and policy development. In any setting, the role of the nurse focuses on the prevention of illness, injury, or disability and on the promotion and maintenance of the health of populations (American Nurses Association, 2013; American Public Health Association, Public Health Nursing Section, 2013). Public health nurses deliver services within the framework of ever-constricting resources coupled with emerging and complex public health issues. This requires the efficient, equitable, and evidence-based use of resources. The National Public Health Performance Standards Program (CDC, 2018), a federal, state, and local partnership, has developed evaluation instruments that can be used to collect and analyze data on the programs provided through state and local public health

systems. The instruments link with the 10 essential services of public health that define the core functions of public health (see Chapter 1).

Nurses make a significant difference in improving the health of a community by monitoring and assessing critical health status indicators such as the following:
- Immunization levels
- Communicable diseases
- Infant mortality

On the basis of their assessment and in partnership with the community, nurses advocate for evidence-based interventions to respond to negative health status indicators. Nurses provide the link for people who need personal health services and ensure health care when it is needed and not available elsewhere (PHAB, 2019).

A shift in the focus of public health from being the primary care provider of last resort to developing partnerships to meet the health promotion and disease prevention needs of populations in a community has raised concerns about available health care for the uninsured and underinsured. The nurse's role in this ongoing shift in health care delivery is still being developed for many agencies. Nurses retain responsibility for ensuring that all populations have access to affordable, quality health care services. They accomplish this by the following:
- Providing clinical preventive services to certain high-risk populations
- Establishing programs and services to meet special needs
- Recommending clinical care and other services to clients and their families in clinics, homes, and the community
- Providing referrals through community links to needed care
- Participating in community provider coalitions and meetings to educate others and identify service centers for community populations
- Providing clinical surveillance and identification of communicable disease

Case management at the community level is a renewed effort in nursing. Through case management activities, nurses link persons with needed health care providers (see Chapter 15).

Uninsured individuals seek services on a sliding payment scale from sources such as university clinics, public hospital clinics, neighborhood health centers, or one of the variety of free clinics. Nurses serve as a bridge between these populations and the resource needs for this at-risk group by approaching health care providers on behalf of individuals seeking medical or health services and keeping the needs of this population on the political agenda. Frequently, low-income populations or populations with multiple chronic illnesses lack the knowledge and skills to negotiate the complex health care system. This population needs the following:
- Education and training in identifying their problems
- Approaches to self-care
- Illness prevention strategies
- Lifestyle choices that will have an effect on their health

The nurse understands the barriers these populations confront, such as transportation and difficulty understanding and following health care provider instructions.

Although vulnerable populations have always benefited from nursing services, the populations that are most acutely in need of public health services have changed dramatically over the past two decades. Of particular concern are the number of young women and their partners who are substance abusers and have risky behaviors that put their pregnancy or children at high risk for injury or abuse. Nurses at the federal, state, and local levels have developed innovative, collaborative approaches to prepare staff to work effectively with this population.

The population and public health are benefiting from the passing of the Affordable Care Act (2010). The Affordable Care Act provides for the Prevention Fund for an expanded and sustained national investment in prevention and public health programs that will improve health and help to restrain the rate of growth in private- and public-sector health care costs. The law provides for many preventive services to be free so that health care issues can be caught early or totally prevented. The senior members of the population and children receive free preventive services, Medicaid coverage has been expanded, more access to home health and community services is available (Key Features of the Affordable Care Act, 2014: see Chapter 3).

 LEVELS OF PREVENTION

Approaches Related to Nurses and Public Health

The health of the American public has improved on many fronts over the past decades—from decreasing incidence of lung cancer in men to large reductions in the number of childhood lead poisoning cases.

However, many diseases and illnesses are increasing in frequency. Although the reasons for these increases are often unknown, to the extent that the causes are recognized or suspected, preventive measures are desirable. Public health focuses on prevention of disease and health promotion rather than the diagnosis and treatment of diseases.

Prevention activities are typically categorized by the following three definitions:

1. Primary prevention—intervening before health effects occur, through measures such as
   - Vaccinations
   - Altering risky behaviors (poor eating habits, tobacco use)
   - Banning substances known to be associated with a disease or health condition
2. Secondary prevention—screening to identify diseases in the earliest stages before the onset of signs and symptoms through measures such as
   - Mammography
   - Regular blood pressure testing
3. Tertiary prevention—managing disease post diagnosis to slow or stop:
   - Disease progression through measures such as
     - Chemotherapy
     - Rehabilitation
     - Screening for complications

CDC: *Picture of America*. 2017, USDHHS, Washington, DC. Can be accessed at www.USA.gov.

Local Prevention Strategies for Public Health Nurses

Community level prevention strategies support individual prevention efforts. Social community actions can be particularly effective in bringing about changes that prevent or reduce environmentally related illness and disease. Strategies that can be used range from community education to neighborhood awareness strategies. Zoning laws can be changed to provide incentives for the creation of bike paths or that reduce the number or density of liquor stores by local governments for the benefit of a community. Information sharing between neighborhood associations, faith communities, community-based organizations, and other local groups can help to achieve public health outcomes.

State Prevention Strategies for Public Health Nurses

States are important partners in promoting both local and federal prevention efforts and in establishing prevention strategies through their own initiatives. For example, through inspections and regulations, illness and statewide diseases can be prevented at food service establishments, swimming pools, hazardous waste disposal sites, and other locations. State-sponsored efforts can also be involved in supporting health screening programs, antismoking campaigns, and health education. States can and do partner with federal agencies and states to assist in implementation of programs such as the CDC's Childhood Lead Poisoning Prevention Program and the CDC's National Heart Disease and Stroke Prevention Program.

National Prevention Strategies for Public Health Nurses

National prevention activities involve initiatives, regulatory programs, and policies that establish nationwide programs to reduce both the presence of and exposure to harmful agents in the environment (e.g., the Clean Water Act, National Tobacco Control Program, National Asthma Control Program). Many agencies are involved in activities that either directly or indirectly reduce public exposure. The USDHHS, which includes the CDC and the US Food and Drug Administration; the EPA; the Department of Housing and Urban Development (HUD); and the US Department of Agriculture (USDA) all participate in prevention efforts.

What Can Public Health Nurses Do?

Nurses, either individually or through groups or professional organizations, can work to influence policy and legislation to improve the health of the public. They can mobilize neighborhoods and communities; establish or work with coalitions and networks; and work with others to change internal practices and policies of agencies and institutions. Nurses can educate health care providers and other professionals about policies or needed change. Nurses can also promote community education on ways to improve health outcomes. Professional organizations and individuals working with legislators can influence and/or suggest changes in the national prevention strategies (CDC: *Picture of America*. Washington, DC, 2017, USDHHS. Can be accessed at www. USA.Gov).

ISSUES AND TRENDS IN PUBLIC HEALTH NURSING

The discovery and development of antibiotics in the 1940s, coupled with immunization programs and improvements in sanitation, contributed to the decrease in infectious disease–related morbidity and mortality during the 20th century (CDC, 2011; Rosen, 2015). Issues facing public health nurses in the 21st century include the following:

- Increasing rates of drug resistance to community-acquired pathogens
- Social issues such as welfare reform
- Racial and ethnic disparities in health outcomes
- Behaviorally influenced issues (e.g., chronic diseases, violence in society, substance abuse)
- Emergency preparedness activities
- Emerging infections
- Unequal access to health care

Nurses must keep abreast of the issues that affect all of society. Assessments need to be changed to include the factors that affect the populations they serve.

For example, a major 21st-century public health challenge is emerging infections resulting from drug-resistant organisms. The widespread, often inappropriate use of antimicrobial drugs has resulted in a loss of effectiveness for some community-acquired infections, such as gonorrhea, pneumococcal infections, and tuberculosis (TB), and increasing rates of drug resistance in community-acquired pathogens such as *Streptococcus pneumonia, Escherichia coli,* and *Salmonella* species. The nurse can influence this trend by objecting to inappropriate use of antibiotics by providers and educating individuals, families, health care providers, and the community about the dangers of misuse and overuse of antibiotics (CDC, 2018).

Social issues such as welfare and health insurance reform will influence a population's ability to obtain preventive health services, either because of providers not accepting government-sponsored health care coverage or because the low-wage jobs they take do not allow time off for health care.

When child care is an issue for a mother receiving welfare, who is returning to work, effects on the individual, family, community, and population must be considered. Nurses assess the problem and determine what is wrong with a system that forces parents to go to work so they can be removed from welfare rolls but does not provide for child care. The question to be answered by a nurse is "What will it take to change the system?"

Partnerships and collaboration among groups are much more powerful in making change than the individual client and nurse working alone. As another example, the depressed, nonfunctional mother in need of counseling is a significant public health concern because the needs of the mother, children, and family are not being met. Frequently, the problem may not be obvious to the health professional who sees this woman for the first time. Nurses have special preparation to help them both identify the individual's problem and look at its effects on the broader community. In this example, consider the following:

- The children may grow to be adults with mental health problems.
- The mental health services of the community services will need to be able to handle the increase in this population.
- Children may become violent adults, resulting in a need for more correction facilities.
- Mothers may need additional mental health services.
- Children may be absent from school often and may not be able to contribute to society.
- Adults may be nonproductive in the workplace because absence from school leads to lack of skills.
- Often, one problem of the single individual places great burdens on the community.

The IOM (2002) reports that disparities in health care treatment account for some of the gaps in health outcomes between racial and ethnic groups. This report found that minority groups receive lower-quality health care than do White people, regardless of insurance status, income, and severity of the condition. This report is supported by the National Healthcare Quality and Disparities Report (Agency for Healthcare Research and Quality [AHRQ], 2011). The report indicates that access to health care did not improve for most racial and ethnic groups in the years 2002 through 2008, leading up to enactment of the Patient Protection and Affordable Care Act of 2010. The data contained in the National Healthcare Disparities Report and the companion National Healthcare Quality Report predate the Patient Protection and Affordable Care Act; however, some provisions in the new health care law are improving health care quality and addressing health care disparities. The USDHHS Action Plan to Reduce Health Disparities, announced in April 2011, outlines goals and actions to reduce health disparities among racial and ethnic minorities, building on important efforts made possible by the Patient Protection and Affordable Care Act and other ongoing initiatives. The Action Plan was updated in 2015 with plans for implementation (AHRQ, 2011 & 2015).

Public health nurses work as case managers and at the policy level to promote equal access to health care, including health literature and spoken services that reflect the community in which the services are being delivered. The nurse working directly as a case manager or in a clinic setting can promote culturally and linguistically appropriate services by partnering with other community agencies, such as interpreter services. Equal access to health care can be facilitated by identifying and alerting the community to gaps in services available in the community. For example, some communities may appear to have an adequate number of pediatricians to meet the community's needs. However, a community assessment may reveal that the community is home to a high number of children who rely on Medicaid as payment for services or to families whose primary language is not English. Matching this information with the pediatrician population may reveal that none of the pediatricians accept Medicaid as payment for services or that they all deliver services in English only.

EDUCATION AND KNOWLEDGE REQUIREMENTS FOR PUBLIC HEALTH NURSES

The Association of Community Health Nursing Educators states that the educational preparation of public health nurses should be at least a baccalaureate degree. Those who have associate degrees are encouraged to seek further degrees because of the increasing complexity of better care delivery in public health.

The Council on Linkages Between Academia and Public Health Practice (2001, 2010, 2014, 2020) examined a decade of work to identify a list of core public health competencies that represent a set of skills, knowledge, and attitudes necessary for the broad practice of public health. In 2020, the Council was in process of updating the competencies. These capture the crosscutting competencies necessary for all providers who work in public health, including nurses, physicians, environmental health specialists, health educators, and epidemiologists. The competencies are applied (at the three skill levels of *aware, knowledgeable,* and *proficient*) to three job categories of entry level, supervisors/managers, and senior managers/CEOs. In addition to having the core public health competencies, public health nurses have specialized competencies, as described in the *Scope and Standards of Public Health Nursing Practice* (American Nurses Association, 2013). The core public health competencies are divided into the following eight domains:

1. Analytic assessment skills
2. Basic public health sciences skills
3. Cultural competency skills
4. Communication skills
5. Community dimensions of practice skills
6. Financial planning and management skills
7. Leadership and systems thinking skills
8. Policy development and program planning skills

Many of these core public health competencies are provided by nurses who have learned these skills in the workplace while gaining knowledge through years of practice. Rapid changes in public health are providing a challenge to nurses in that neither the time nor the staff is available to provide as much on-the-job training as is needed to learn and upgrade skills and knowledge of staff. Nurses with baccalaureate or master's degrees are needed to provide a strong public health system (see Chapter 1).

NATIONAL HEALTH OBJECTIVES

Since 1979 the US Surgeon General has worked with local, state, and federal agencies, the private sector, and the US population to develop health objectives for the nation. These objectives are revisited every 10 years. State health departments play a key role in implementing the *Healthy People* objectives. New partnerships develop related to specific goals. Communities may develop coalitions to address selected objectives based on community needs to include all of the local community stakeholders, such as social services, mental health, education, recreation, government, and businesses.

HEALTHY PEOPLE 2030

The following selected national health objectives relate to the public health infrastructure. The overarching goal is to make sure public health agencies at all levels have the necessary infrastructure for key public health services.

- **PHI-R08:** Explore financing of the public health infrastructure
- **PHI-R05:** Monitor the education of the public health workforce
- **PHI-R04:** Monitor and understand the public health workforce
- **PHI-03:** Increase the number of tribal public health agencies that are accredited
- **PHI-02:** Increase the proportion of local public health agencies that are accredited

From US Department of Health and Human Services: *Healthy People 2030: National health promotion and disease prevention objectives,* Washington, DC, 2020, USDHHS. Accessed at healthypeople.gov/2030/.

The following are some *Healthy People 2030* Immunization and Infectious Disease areas of focus:
- Vaccine-preventable infectious diseases
- Sexually transmitted diseases (STDs)
- Pneumococcal infections
- TB NOTE: you have deleted this twice. hope it is spelled out someplace in the text.
- Health care–associated infections

To help clients reduce their risk for acquiring a communicable disease, nurses provide clients with instructions on the use of barrier methods of contraception and information on the hazards of multiple sexual partners and street drug use. Getting a complete sexual history on all clients coming to the health department for services takes special skills but is essential to determine the behaviors that have brought the client to the local health department. Abstinence as a birth control method can be addressed with all populations. Education of young persons before they become sexually active has helped to reduce the incidence of some STDs in this population.

FUNCTIONS OF PUBLIC HEALTH NURSES

Nurses in public health have many functions, depending on the needs and resources of an area (Fig. 28.1). Advocate is one of the many roles of the nurse. As an advocate, the nurse collects, monitors, and analyzes data and discusses with the client which services are needed and whether the client is an individual, a family, or a group. The nurse and the client then develop the most effective plan and approach to take, and the nurse helps the client to implement the plan so the client can become more independent in making decisions and obtaining the services needed.

Case manager is a major role for nurses. Nurses use the nursing process of assessing, planning, implementing, and evaluating outcomes to meet clients' needs. Clear and complex communications are frequently an important component of case management. Other health and social agency participants may not be familiar with the home and community living conditions that are known to the nurse. It is the nurse who has been there and seen the living conditions and who can tell the story for the client or assist the individual or family with the telling of their story. Case managers assist clients in identifying and

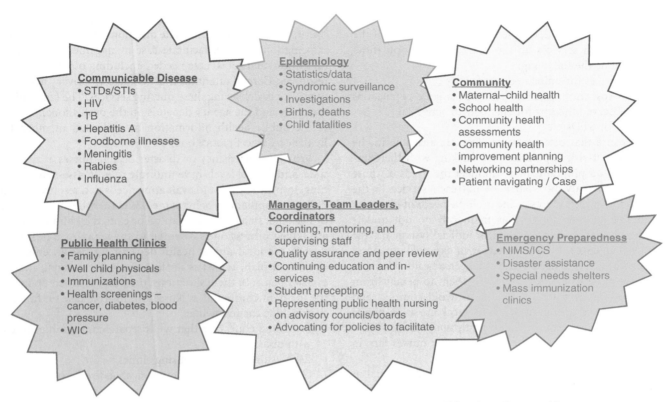

Communicable Disease
- STDs/STIs
- HIV
- TB
- Hepatitis A
- Foodborne illnesses
- Meningitis
- Rabies
- Influenza

Epidemiology
- Statistics/data
- Syndromic surveillance
- Investigations
- Births, deaths
- Child fatalities

Community
- Maternal–child health
- School health
- Community health assessments
- Community health improvement planning
- Networking partnerships
- Patient navigating / Case

Public Health Clinics
- Family planning
- Well child physicals
- Immunizations
- Health screenings – cancer, diabetes, blood pressure
- WIC

Managers, Team Leaders, Coordinators
- Orienting, mentoring, and supervising staff
- Quality assurance and peer review
- Continuing education and in-services
- Student precepting
- Representing public health nursing on advisory councils/boards
- Advocating for policies to facilitate

Emergency Preparedness
- NIMS/ICS
- Disaster assistance
- Special needs shelters
- Mass immunization clinics

Fig. 28.1 Public Health Nursing Roles. *HIV,* Human immunodeficiency virus; *ICS,* Incident Command System; *NIMS,* National Incident Management System; *STD,* sexually transmitted disease; *STI,* sexually transmitted infection; *TB,* tuberculosis; *WIC,* Women, Infants, and Children. Source: (Prepared by Lois Davis, RN, MSN, MA, public health clinical instructor, University of Kentucky College of Nursing, Lexington, KY.)

obtaining the services they need the most at the least cost. For example, a nurse may go into the home to visit a new mother and baby. On assessment, the nurse may find that the mother needs help in finding a new job, child care, a pediatrician, and in finding health insurance. The nurse helps the mother in the following ways:

- Assists with prioritizing the problems
- Helps to make a plan for resolving the problems
- Contacts other agencies on behalf of the mother when needed
- Follows up with the mother to see if the problems are being resolved
- Follows up with the agencies, such as social services, to make certain the mother's request to enroll her children in the state Children's Health Insurance Program has been honored

Nurses are a major referral resource. They maintain current information about health and social services available within the community. They know what resources will be acceptable to the client within the social and cultural norms for that group. The nurse educates clients to enable them to use the resources and to learn self-care. Nurses refer to other services in the area, and other services refer to the nurse for care or follow-up. For example, the mother and new baby may be referred to the nurse for postnatal care with postpartum home visit follow-up.

Assessor of literacy is a large part of nursing in public health. Many individuals are limited in their ability to read, write, and communicate clearly. The nurse has to be culturally

sensitive and aware of the specific areas of unique problems of clients, such as financial limitations that may in turn limit educational opportunities. Frequently, when persons go to a physician's office, clinic, or hospital, they are clean and neatly dressed. The assumption is made that when they nod at the health care provider, it means that they understand what has been said. This is frequently not the case, but the client is embarrassed to admit that he or she does not understand what has been said. Being illiterate does not mean a person is mentally slow. It is important for the nurse to follow up on the many contacts the individual or family has with medical, social, and legal services to clarify what is understood and to find answers to the questions that have not been asked by the client or answered by the services.

The nurse is an educator, teaching to the level of the client so that the information received is information that can be used. Patience and repetitions over time are necessary to develop trust and enable the client to use the relationship with the nurse for more information. As educator, the public health nurse identifies community needs (e.g., playground safety, hand hygiene, pedestrian safety, safe-sex practices) and develops and implements educational activities aimed at changing behaviors over time.

Although not as frequently as in the past, nurses in public health are direct primary caregivers in many situations, both in the clinic and in the community. Where the nurse provides primary care is determined by community assessment and is usually in response to an identified gap to which the private sector is unable to respond, coupled with an assessment of the effect of the gap in services on the health of the population. Examples include the following:

- Prenatal services for uninsured women
- Free or low-cost immunization services for targeted populations
- Directly observed therapy for clients with active TB
- Treatment for STDs

Nurses ensure that direct care services are available in the community for at-risk populations by working with the community to develop programs that will meet the needs of those populations. Currently, no system of outreach service in the medical models of care addresses the multiple needs of high-risk populations. High-risk populations frequently do not understand the medical, social, educational, or judicial system and the professional languages, codes of behavior, or expected outcomes of these services. Clients need a case manager, a health educator, an advocate, and a role model to enable them to benefit from these services and to teach them how to avoid complex and expensive problems in the future. The local nurse in public health fills these roles and many more for this population. These are examples of the difficult clinical issues that nurses face in making ethical and professional decisions.

The nurse's role in public health is unique and essential in many situations. Access to homes gives the nurse information that usually cannot be gathered in the hospital or clinic setting. The nurse learns to ask intimate questions creatively and to seek information that will facilitate case management and provide the clinical and social care needed, including other community resources. Careful attention must be paid to privacy and confidentiality in delivering these nursing services. The credibility of the nurse and the agency depends on the professional handling of the public health information by each staff member. (See Evidence-Based Practice box)

When an emergency or disaster occurs, nurses at the local, state, and federal levels have multiple roles in assessment, planning, implementing, and evaluating needs and resources for the different populations being served. Whether the disaster is local or national, small or large, natural or caused by humans, nurses are skilled professionals essential to the team. As a health care facility, the local public health department has an emergency operations plan, as well as a role in the local, regional, and state disaster plans. In these situations, the nurse is called upon to be the incident commander. Nurses in this role take on functions that include the following:

- Providing education that will prepare communities to cope with disasters
- Establishing mass-dispensing clinics
- Conducting enhanced communicable disease surveillance
- Working with environmental health specialists to ensure safe food and water for disaster victims and emergency workers
- Serving on the local emergency planning committee

Their presence may be required in other regions of the state or country to provide official nursing duties in a time of crisis, such as a hurricane, that requires a lengthy period of recovery. Each governmental jurisdiction has an emergency plan. The public health agency is expected to provide planning and staffing during a disaster. These local emergency preparedness plans may be multigovernmental, which requires coordination among communities.

EVIDENCE-BASED PRACTICE

The Kentucky Health Access Nurturing Development Services (HANDS) program is a voluntary home visiting program targeting first-time pregnant mothers or parents with infants (up to 3 months old), who may have challenges such as low income, single parenthood, or substance abuse problems, or have been victims of abuse or domestic violence. HANDS is designed to facilitate positive pregnancy and child health outcomes and maximize child growth and development, as well as prevent child maltreatment and improve family functioning. A trained paraprofessional or professional home visitor, such as a public health nurse or social worker, conducts prenatal and postnatal home visits with parents, performs assessments, provides parenting information, problem-solving techniques, parenting skill development; and addresses basic needs.

An analysis compared a group of 2253 prenatal mothers who were referred to the HANDS program and received at least one home visit, with a group of 2253 demographically similar mothers who did not participate in HANDS. HANDS participants had lower rates of preterm delivery and low birth weight infants. HANDS participants also were significantly less likely to have a substantiated report of child maltreatment compared with controls. Participants in the HANDS program also had an increase in adequate prenatal care and a reduction in maternal complications during pregnancy. An additional conclusion showed pregnancy outcomes improved as the number of prenatal home visits increased. The rate of preterm births among those receiving seven or more prenatal home visits was 9.4% lower than the statewide rate.

Nurse Use

HANDS program participation appears to result in significant improvements in maternal and child health outcomes, most specifically for those receiving seven or more prenatal home visits. As a statewide, large-scale home visiting program, this has significant implications for the continued improvement of maternal and child health outcomes in Kentucky (Williams et al., 2017).

CHECK YOUR PRACTICE

As a nurse in the local health department, you have been asked to be the incident commander for a recent outbreak of COVID-19 in the community. What would you do? See if you can apply these steps to this scenario. (1) Recognize the cues, looking at available data about rates of COVID-19 in the state and your community; (2) analyze the cues looking at the numbers of cases in this population and what it means to be the incident commander for this population; (3) state several and prioritize the hypotheses you have stated; (4) generate solutions for each hypothesis; (5) take action on the number one hypothesis you think best reflects the best approach to testing the community population to determine community spread; and (6) evaluate the outcomes you would expect as a result of the work you will do as the incident commander.

Essential and unique roles for nurses in public health exist in the area of infectious and communicable disease control. Nursing skills are necessary for education, prevention, surveillance, and outbreak investigation. Nurses can do the following:

- Find infected individuals
- Notify contacts

- Refer to other health providers or agencies for care
- Administer tests and treatments when available
- Educate the individual, family, community, professionals, and populations
- Act as advocate for the clients
- Use state-of-the-art resources to reduce or control the rate of the disease in the community

The infectious and communicable disease role is one of the most important roles for nursing during disasters, including the COVID-19 pandemic of 2020. The following are a few examples of past disasters and the responses. During the September 11, 2001, airplane attacks on the World Trade Center in New York, nurses at the federal, state, and local levels immediately implemented active enhanced surveillance activities. Information about communicable diseases seen at the local level was passed on to the state public health agency and finally to the CDC. At each step, the data were analyzed for evidence of unusual disease trends.

It is important for nurses in public health to practice confidentiality when they have knowledge about an individual or family communicable disease outbreak, community-level problem, or any special knowledge obtained in the public health work setting.

When October 2001 alerts from the CDC began presenting information about a photo editor in Florida who had been hospitalized with inhalation of anthrax, nurses in public health and hospital infection control practitioners throughout the nation increased activity. Public health response to disasters requires that resources be redirected temporarily from other programs while maintaining programs that will prevent additional outbreaks. Therefore nurses not normally involved in communicable disease activities can be shifted to this function. The exposures resulting from the anthrax-tainted letters presented unprecedented public health challenges. The Washington, D.C. anthrax exposures resulted in thousands of possible work-related exposures, five cases of inhalation anthrax in the region, and two deaths over a period of months. Public

health at the federal, state, and local levels was looked to for coordinated leadership and answers to a situation in which experience was limited and answers were uncertain. Although infectious/communicable disease control is a core public health service, the role of public health as incident commander in a widespread public health emergency is a new role. The following were issues to be addressed:

- How to conduct mass testing or treatment in response to a bioterrorism event
- Which jurisdiction is in charge
- How to communicate unclear information to the public
- Who should take antibiotics, if available, and for how long
- Resolving this rapidly across jurisdictional and agency lines

The anthrax exposures are typical of the nature of public health emergencies. They unfold as the communicable disease moves through communities.

Nurses in public health are essential partners in disaster drills. In Virginia, an electrical company has a nuclear plant that requires annual multijurisdictional disaster drills. These disaster planning and practice sessions are an opportunity for local nurses to get to know other agencies' representatives and to let them know what nursing can offer. Because nurses are out in the communities and have assessment skills, they are essential in evaluating how the disaster was handled and in making suggestions about how future events might be managed. To be most effective as disaster responders, nurses have to be a part of the team *before* an emergency. Knowing what type of disaster is likely to occur in a community is essential for planning. Types of disasters vary from place to place, but there is a history of past events and how they were handled, as well as resources and training from regional, state, and federal agencies. Nurses can help to educate the public about the individual responsibilities and preparations that can be in place for both the person and the community. Nurses at the local, state, and federal levels work in partnership to accomplish each function.

QSEN FOCUS ON QUALITY AND SAFETY EDUCATION FOR NURSES

Public Health Nursing at Local, State, and National Levels

Targeted Competency: Teamwork and Collaboration—Function effectively within nursing and interprofessional teams, fostering open communication, mutual respect, and shared decision making to achieve quality patient care. Important aspects of teamwork and collaboration include the following:

- **Knowledge:** Describe scopes of practice and roles of health care team members.
- **Skills:** Integrate the contributions of others who play a role in helping client/family to achieve health goals.
- **Attitudes:** Respect the unique attributes that members bring to a team, including variations in professional orientations and accountabilities.

Teamwork and Collaboration Question

Your state has recently been awarded funding from the Centers for Disease Control and Prevention to prevent the spread of viral hepatitis through increased testing, improving access to care, and strengthening surveillance to detect viral hepatitis transmission and disease. You are a staff nurse for the local Public Health Department and currently serve on the Infectious Disease Prevention

(IDP) committee. The IDP committee has been given the responsibility to determine how to best use this new funding to effectively meet the objectives of the grant. Consider the following:

- As a staff nurse for the local Public Health Department, what is your role in addressing this initiative within the community? How would your role change if you were a public health nurse working at the state health department?
- In addition to nursing, give examples of other professionals who likely serve on the IDP committee with you. Describe the role of each professional on this committee.
- Identify local and state organizations in your community that you would recommend that the IDP committee collaborate with to develop and implement a response to identified issues.
- Through this grant, your state is addressing several objectives in the *Healthy People 2030* focus area of Immunization and Infectious Diseases. Go to the *Healthy People 2030* website and identify which specific objectives would apply to this initiative.

Prepared by Lisa Turner, PhD, RN, PHCNS-BC, Assistant Professor, Berea College Nursing Program, Berea, Kentucky.

APPLYING CONTENT TO PRACTICE

This chapter focuses on the role of the nurse in public health in local, state, and national health initiatives. The history of public health has changed throughout the decades, and the nurse is currently involved in keeping the community and clients safe from emerging infectious diseases and is more focused on managing disasters. There is an increasing expansion of the functions of public health as well as the roles of the nurse in public health. Not only does the nurse function as a case manager, referral source, assessor, educator, advocate, and role model to the community and provide direct-care services that may not otherwise be available but now also serves as an incident commander for urgent and emergent situations in the community. Education for the public health nurse is key to assisting the nurse in performing these functions. The competencies needed by the nurse in public health are discussed in each of the previous chapters.

PRACTICE APPLICATION

A retirement community in a small town reported to the local health department 24 cases of severe gastrointestinal illness that had occurred among residents and staff of the facility during the past 24 to 36 hours. It was determined that the ill clients became sick within a short, well-defined period and that most recovered within 24 hours without treatment. The communicable disease outbreak team, composed of nurses, public health physicians, and an environmental health specialist, was called to respond to this possible epidemic.

How should they respond to this situation?

A. Call the Centers for Disease Control and Prevention, and ask for help with surveillance.
B. Send all the ill persons in the retirement community to the hospital.
C. Evaluate the agent, host, and environment relationships to determine the cause of the problem.
D. Close the dining room, and find another source to provide food to the residents.

Answers can be found on the Evolve website.

REMEMBER THIS!

- Local public health departments are responsible for implementing and enforcing local, state, and federal public health codes and ordinances while providing essential public health services.
- The goal of the local health department is to safeguard the public's health and improve the community's health status.
- Nursing in community health is the practice of promoting and protecting the health of populations using knowledge from nursing and social and public health sciences.
- Public health is based on the scientific core of epidemiology.
- Marketing of nursing in public health is essential to inform both professionals and the public about the opportunities and challenges of populations in public health care.
- A driving force behind nursing changes is the economy and the increase in managed care.
- Nurses need ongoing education and training as public health changes.

- Some of the roles in which nurses function are advocate, case manager, referral source, counselor, primary care provider, educator, outreach worker, incident commander, and disaster responder.
- Nurses have an important role in helping with local disasters, including planning, staffing, and evaluating events.

EVOLVE WEBSITE

http://evolve.elsevier.com/Stanhope/foundations
- Case Study, with Questions and Answers
- NCLEX Review Questions
- Practice Application Answers

REFERENCES

Agency for Healthcare Research and Quality: *National healthcare quality and disparities report and 5th anniversary update on the national quality strategy,* Rockville, 2011 & 2015, AHRQ. Retrieved from http://www.ahrq.gov.

American Nurses Association: *Public health nursing: scope and standards of practice,* Silver Spring, 2013, ANA.

American Public Health Association, Public Health Nursing Section: *The definition and practice of public health nursing: a statement of public health nursing section,* Washington, DC, 2013, APHA.

Association of State and Territorial Health Officers. United States Federal, State, Local and Territorial Public Health Organizations. 2020, Arlington, Virginia.

Centers for Disease Control and Prevention: *Ten public health achievements of first decade of 21st century,* Atlanta, 2011, CDC. Retrieved from http://www.cdc.gov.

Centers for Disease Control and Prevention: *National public health performance standards program (NPHPSP),* Atlanta, 2018, CDC. Retrieved from http://www.cdc.gov

Center for Disease Control and Prevention: National Update on Measles Cases and Outbreaks, *MMWR* 2019. Available at: CDC. gov. https://www.cdc.gov. .

Centers for Disease Control and Prevention: *Picture of America. 2017,* USDHHS, Washington DC. Can be accessed at www.USA.Gov

Community Campus Partnerships for Health Board of Directors: Position Statement of Authentic Partnerships. 2018.Retrieved from https//ccph.health.org.

Council on Linkages Between Academia and Public Health Practice: *Core competencies for public health professionals,* Washington, DC, 2001, Public Health Foundation.

Council on Linkages Between Academia and Public Health Practice: *Tier 1, tier 2, and tier 3 core competencies for public health professionals,* Washington, DC, 2010, Public Health Foundation. Retrieved from http://www.phf.org .

Council on Linkages Between Academia and Public Health Practice: *Core competencies for public health professionals,* Washington, DC, 2014, PHF. Retrieved from http://www.phf.org.

Council on Linkages Between Academia and Public Health Practice: *Core competencies for public health professionals,* Washington, DC, 2020, PHF.

Friis RH, Sellers TA: *Epidemiology for Public Health Practice,* 6th ed., Sudbury, 2021, Jones and Bartlett.

Institute of Medicine: *Unequal Treatment: Confronting Racial and Ethnic Disparities in Health Care,* Washington, DC, 2002, National Academies Press.

Institute of Medicine: *The Future of Public Health in the 21st Century,* Washington, DC, 2003, National Academies Press.

Morrow CB, Pirani S: *Turnock's Public Health: What It Is and How It Works,* 7th ed., Sudbury, 2022, Jones and Bartlett.

National Academies of Sciences, Engineering, and Medicine, Health and Medicine division: *Public Health 3.0: A Call to Action for Public Health to Meet the Challenges of the 21st Century,* 2017. Retrieved from: https://nam.edu.

National Association of County and City Health Officials: *Operational Definition of a Functional Local Health Department,* 2014. Available at http://www.naccho.org. Accessed August 23, 2014.

Public Health Accreditation Board: *Public Health Accreditation Standards, 2019.* Available at: http://www.phaboard.org/. Accessed Nov 2020.

Rosen G: *History of Public Health,* Baltimore, 2015, John S Hopkins University Press.

Schneider MJ: *Introduction to Public Health,* 5th ed., Burlington, 2017, Jones & Bartlett Learning.

US Department of Health and Human Services: *Healthy People 2030,* 2020. Available at: http://www.healthypeople.gov .

US Department of Health and Human Services: *The ACA Prevention and Public Health FUND,* 2014. Retrieved from HHS.gov, 2014.

Williams C, Cprek S, Asaolu I, et al.: Kentucky Health Access Nurturing Development Services Home Visiting Program Improves Maternal and Child Health, *Maternal & Child Health Journal* 21(5):1166–1174, 2017.

29

The Faith Community Nurse

Lisa M. Zerull

OBJECTIVES

After reading this chapter, the student should be able to:

1. Define the role of the nurse in the faith community and holistic health promotion, disease prevention, and spiritual care.
2. Differentiate between spirituality and religiosity.
3. Examine the historical roots of the faith community and nursing.
4. Discuss scope and standards of practice for the nurse within the faith community.
5. Apply the nursing process in a faith community to assess, implement, and evaluate programs for healthy congregations.

CHAPTER OUTLINE

KEY TERMS

DEFINITIONS IN FAITH COMMUNITY NURSING

Nursing within the faith community is defined by the American Nurses Association (ANA) as a specialized practice of professional nursing that focuses on the intentional care of the spirit as well as the promotion of whole-person health and the prevention or minimization of illness within the context of a faith community and the wider community (ANA/HMA, 2017).

With the 2005 revision of the *Scope and Standards of Practice*, the nurse title changed from parish nurse to faith community nurse (ANA/HMA, 2005). The new title was more inclusive of diverse faith traditions and in response to international considerations (ANA/HMA, 2017). Parish nurse was the original title chosen by Granger Westberg in the 1980s as a theological choice because it connoted service to the congregation and the wider community within a geographical area. A congregation also refers to a variety of faith institutions, including churches, synagogues, temples, and mosques or other faith-based organizations (ANA/HMA, 2017; Mattern, 2016). The word parish can mean *congregation* and *geographical area served by a congregation*. Additional titles for nurses working out of faith communities include parish nurse, congregational nurse, health ministry nurse, crescent nurse, or health and wellness nurse (ANA/HMA, 2012).

The nurse in the faith community is a licensed registered nurse "with well-developed clinical and interpersonal skills, a strong personal religious faith, and a desire or felt call to serve the needs of a faith community" (O'Brien, 2017). With additional education in spiritual care of self, individuals, and groups, the nurse works out of the congregational setting. It is expected that the professional registered nurse possesses competence in practice resulting from his or her application of knowledge, skills, and experience, functions with a deep understanding of the faith community's traditions, and fully integrates *care of the spirit* with care of the body and mind (ANA/HMA, 2017; O'Brien, 2017). The assumptions that underlie this specialty are as follows:

1. Health and illness are human experiences.
2. Health is the integration of the spiritual, physical, psychological, and social aspects of the health care consumer to create a sense of harmony with self, others, the environment, and a higher power.
3. Health may be experienced in the presence of disease or injury.
4. The presence of illness does not preclude health nor does optimal health preclude illness.
5. Healing is the process of integrating the body, mind, and spirit to create wholeness, health, and a sense of well-being when the health care consumer's illness is not cured.

QSEN FOCUS ON QUALITY AND SAFETY EDUCATION FOR NURSES

The Nurse in the Faith Community

Targeted Competency: Quality Improvement—Use data to monitor the outcomes of care processes and use improvement methods to design and test changes to continuously improve the quality and safety of health care systems. Important aspects of safety include:

- **Knowledge:** Describe approaches for changing processes of care.
- **Skills:** Design a small test of change in daily work (using an experiential learning method such as plan-do-study-act).
- **Attitudes:** Value measurement and its role in good patient care.

Quality Improvement Question
You are a paid nurse within a faith community at a busy urban church that partners with a regional hospital on a transitional care project to decrease readmission rates for chronically ill older adults. Transitional care within the faith community is defined as *care provided by a nurse working out of the faith community to support the patient's experience of transition from one level of care to another* (Ziebarth, 2016). An alarmingly high percentage of your congregation is over the age of 65 and challenged with chronic diseases of congestive heart failure (CHF) and type 2 diabetes.

As the nurse, you obtained additional training in transitional care at the local hospital and developed a relationship with the discharge planning team.

Accepting one or two referrals every 6 months, you work closely with the discharge planning team and the referred individual to create the best plan of care. Beginning interventions include a holistic assessment; medication and diabetes management review with teach-back; signs and symptoms of acute exacerbations of chronic disease; and spiritual care interventions requested by the individual such as healing presence, prayer, or scripture reading. You also accompanied the individual to primary care provider appointments for clarification of information. You want to evaluate the effectiveness of these interventions.

Step 1: What is the problem or issue that the nurse providing the transitional care addresses?

Step 2: Identify both short-term and long-term goals for transitional care.

Step 3: How would you document the specific program outcomes?

Step 4: Are there best practices that might inform your whole-person care interventions or your collaboration with the local hospital and discharge planning team?

Step 5: How would you evaluate the short-term and long-term goals of the transitional care program?

Faith communities are organizations of groups, families, and individuals who share common values, beliefs, religious doctrine, and faith practices that influence their lives, such as a church, homeless shelter, synagogue, temple, or mosque, and that function as a patient system, providing a setting for nursing practice (ANA/HMA, 2017). Faith communities are found all over the world wherever individuals gather for the common purpose of worship, fellowship, the giving and receiving of love, grace, and hope, as well as the invitation, not obligation, to participate in the rites and rituals of a faith tradition (Fig. 29.1). Some common examples include baptism, devotions, communion, reading of scripture, prayer, and singing.

Health ministries are visible activities, programs, and rituals of faith organized around health and healing of the congregation's membership and offered by the nurse, clergy, layperson, or community resource. Health ministries may be informal or more specifically planned and encompass a gamut of activities, including home visitation, providing meals for families in crisis or upon return home after hospitalization, quilting circles, grief support groups, and support for spiritual, emotional, and physical needs are addressed for healing purposes (Fig. 29.2) to name a few (Church Health Center, 2018; Patterson, 2012, 2013).

According to the ANA *Scope and Standards of Practice* for all nurses (ANA/HMA, 2012), spiritual care is part of all nursing practice and acknowledges a person's sense of meaning and purpose in life, which may or may not be expressed through formal religious beliefs and practices. It is also described as a distinct type of care defined by acts of listening, compassionate presence, open-ended questions, prayer, use of religious objects, talking with clergy, guided visualization, contemplation, meditation, conveying a benevolent attitude, or instilling hope (O'Brien, 2017). Spiritual care is helping the client make meaning out of

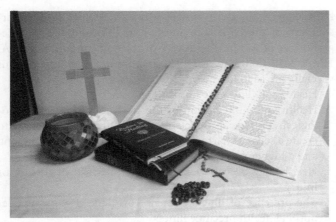

Fig. 29.1 Religious Symbols, Images, Rituals, and Sacred Places Are Significant to Ministry.

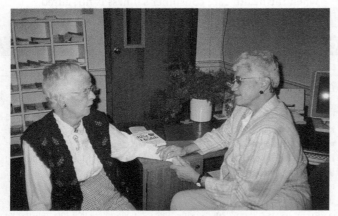

Fig. 29.2 A Nurse Provides Support for Spiritual, Emotional, and Physical Needs.

his or her experience or find hope (Ziebarth, 2016). Unique to the faith community as a specialty practice for nurses is the primary focus on care of the spirit, with *spirit* defined as the core of a person's being. Box 29.1 provides a detailed listing of the core interventions for care of the spirit performed by the nurses. Spiritual care is much different from religious care. Whereas religious care stems from the doctrine, rites, and rituals of a specific denomination or set of beliefs, spiritual care is unique to the individual's purpose in life, the fulfilling of that purpose, and living it wholeheartedly. Intentional spiritual care is invited, expected, and appreciated by the faith community members.

Holistic or whole-person care relates to the relationship between body, mind, and spirit in a constantly changing environment and involves caring for the soul in a special kind of engagement that goes beyond seeing the physical patient but includes observation of the entire patient (Dossey and Keegan, 2016). The nurse, supported by members of the congregation, assesses, plans, implements, and evaluates holistic care programs. The process of operationalizing holistic care is enhanced by an active wellness committee or health cabinet composed of congregation members or congregants who may or may not be health professionals (e.g., doctors, therapists, social workers) and who are fully engaged in health ministry (Patterson, 2003; Westberg, 1990). An active wellness committee provides leadership and influence throughout the faith community; ideas come not from one individual but are generated out of a committee structure (McNamara, 2006; Patterson, 2003; Westberg, 1990). The nurse uses the collective knowledge and skills of this collaborative group to provide comprehensive and effective services. The outcome is a caring congregation that understands the strong link between faith and health and supports healthy, spiritually fulfilling lives.

BOX 29.1   Nursing Interventions Classification Core Interventions for Faith Community

- Abuse Protection Support
- Active Listening
- Anticipatory Guidance
- Caregiver Support
- Coping Enhancement
- Crisis Intervention
- Culture Brokerage
- Decision-Making Support
- Emotional Support
- Environmental Management: Community
- Family Integrity Promotion
- Family Support
- Forgiveness Facilitation
- Grief Work Facilitation
- Guilt Work Facilitation
- Health Care Information Exchange
- Health Education
- Health Literacy Enhancement
- Health System Guidance
- Hope Inspiration

- Humor
- Listening Visits
- Medication Management
- Presence
- Referral
- Religious Addiction Prevention
- Religious Ritual Enhancement
- Relocation Stress Reduction
- Self-Care Assistance: IADL
- Socialization Enhancement
- Spiritual Growth Facilitation
- Spiritual Support
- Surveillance
- Sustenance Support
- Teaching: Group
- Teaching: Individual
- Telephone Consultation
- Touch
- Values Clarification

IADL, Instrumental activities of daily living.
From Bulechek G, Dochterman J, Butcher H, et al.: Core interventions for nursing specialty areas: faith community nursing. In *Nursing interventions classification (NIC)*, 7th ed., St. Louis, 2018, Elsevier.

PERSPECTIVES ON NURSING IN THE FAITH COMMUNITY

The nurse within the faith community, previously called parish nursing, is a recognized nursing specialty practice, yet is frequently overlooked when creative strategies are needed for improving the health of individuals and the larger community. This is not surprising when only 11.7% of nurses reported receiving adequate spiritual care training as part of their nursing education, yet 92.4% of nurses feel strongly that spiritual care is a legitimate part of the profession (Delgado, 2015). Nurses often confuse religious practice or religiosity with spirituality and may neglect patients' spiritual needs (O'Brien, 2017). Whereas religiosity relates to "a person's beliefs and behaviors associated with a specific religious tradition or denomination" (O'Brien, 2017), spirituality is "an individual's attitudes and beliefs related to transcendence (God) or to the non-material forces of life and nature" (O'Brien, 2017). Thus additional education in spiritual care is needed to distinguish between the two and to provide the nurse with an understanding of the faith community (Delgado, 2015).

Registered nurses working out of a faith community or congregation establish close relationships with individuals, families, and, often, the larger community to coordinate programs and services that significantly affect health, healing, and wholeness (ANA/HMA, 2017; Butler and Diaz, 2017; Callaghan, 2016; Gotwals, 2018; Laming and Stewart, 2016; Young, 2016; Ziebarth, 2015, 2016). Nurses balance knowledge and skill in their role to facilitate the faith community as it becomes a caring place—a place that is a source of health and healing for its members. Many nurses are drawn to practice within the faith community because it encourages the expression of spirituality as a part of health and healing. Others are drawn to this specialty practice out of vocational calling (O'Brien, 2017).

Nurses address health concerns of individuals, families, and groups of all ages (Callaghan, 2015). Like other communities, the members of faith communities experience the following:

- Birth
- Death
- Acute and chronic illness
- Growth and development
- Stress
- Dependency concerns
- Challenges from life transitions
- Decisions regarding healthy lifestyle choices

Serving as good stewards of resources, nurses encourage partnering with public health agencies as well as lay and professional church leaders to arrive at creative responses to health issues and to develop health-promoting and spiritually healing activities. The nurse serves the faith community by focusing on the needs of the individual parishioner and the overall faith community with special attention given to spiritual care support.

HISTORY OF NURSING WITHIN THE FAITH COMMUNITY

Nursing within the faith community has its historical roots in the Judeo-Christian tradition with early biblical references to women providing care to the sick and persons in need. For centuries, Catholic sisters and Protestant women, specially trained as nurses, have promoted health and cared for the sick, the poor, the fallen, and the unbelieving (Doyle, 1929; Fliedner, 1870). Likewise, parish nurses, now called nurses within the faith community, have followed this same tradition for more than three decades by working out of the congregation to promote whole-person health—ministering to body, mind, and spirit of parishioners from the time of birth through the end of life.

In 1984, the concept of parish nursing was introduced to churches in the Chicago, Illinois area by Lutheran chaplain Granger Westberg (1913–1999) as way of expanding existing health ministries and providing another link between faith and health (Box 29.2). Westberg described parish nursing as a way for the church to reclaim its traditional role in healing (1990). Having previous experience with setting up holistic health centers out of churches, Westberg fully understood that hospitals and physicians deal with illness, yet there is a need for preventive medicine and wellness in the community, and churches fit right in (1990). He also recognized that it was nurses who could have the largest impact on the delivery of whole-person care within a congregation, using the nurse's broad background of health promotion, education, spiritual care, and social work (Westberg, 1985).

By 1984, Westberg partnered with Lutheran General Hospital (Park Ridge, Illinois—now known as Advocate Health) on a pilot project within six Chicago-area churches (Zurull and Solari-Twadell, 2020). These partnerships established the first institutionally based, paid parish nurse program between a health system and churches in the United States (Westberg and McNamara, 1987).

As the contemporary parish nurse movement grew, information was spread by advocates of whole-person health. This resulted in the establishment of a Resource Center (International Parish Nurse Resource Center [IPNRC]) in 1986 to provide information, printed literature, and news of emerging parish nurse programs across the United States, both paid and unpaid. Through the collaborative efforts of the health system, educators, and the IPNRC, a foundational course was designed to provide basic education to prepare nurses in parish nursing.

The need of a membership organization for a growing number of parish nurses served as a catalyst for the founding of the Health Ministries Association (HMA) in 1989. The HMA provided networking and communications for nurses along with others active in health ministry. Through HMA's leadership, the ANA recognized parish nursing as a professional nursing specialty in 1997 with the first scope and standards of practice published in 1998 (ANA/HMA 2017). The title of parish nurse was changed to the nurse in the faith community with the 2005 revisions to the scope and standards reflective of the need to be inclusive of nurses in all faith traditions (ANA/HMA 2005). Another milestone was reached in 2014 when the American Nurses Credentialing Center (ANCC) released a nurse specialty certification for these nurses; however, due to low applicant volumes combined with administrative costs, the certification was discontinued after 3 years (ANCC, 2017).

BOX 29.2   Timeline of Evolution of Nursing in the Faith Community

- 1983 pilot program with a nurse running a wellness clinic out of the congregation setting—Our Saviour Lutheran Church, Tucson, AZ.
- 1984 Parish Nurse Program partnership begun with six congregations and Lutheran General Hospital, Park Ridge, IL.
- 1986 Lutheran General Hospital establishes a Parish Nurse Resource Center to share information about health ministry and parish nursing with others.
- 1987 First Westberg Parish Nurse Symposium is held and Granger Westberg publishes book *The Parish Nurse*. Parish Nurse Resource Center becomes the *National* Parish Nurse Resource Center.
- 1989 Health Ministries Association began in Iowa.
- 1991 Marquette University offers 8-day parish nurse education program titled the *Wisconsin Model*, a curriculum later modified to become the *Foundations of Faith Community Nursing* course.
- 1995 Lutheran General merges with Evangelical Health Systems Corporation to create Advocate Health Care. National Parish Nurse Resource Center becomes the *International* Parish Nurse Resource Center.
- 1997 American Nurses Association recognizes parish nursing as a specialty practice.
- 1998 ANA/HMA publish first Scope and Standards for parish nursing. Parish Nurse Preparation Curriculum is published.

- 1999 Parish Nurse Coordinator Curriculum is published. Death of Granger Westberg (July 1913–February 1999).
- 2002 IPNRC transfers assets from Advocate Health System, Chicago, IL, to Deaconess Foundation, St. Louis, MO.
- 2004 World Forum for Faith Community Nursing is formed with 22 members from Australia, Canada, South Korea, Swaziland, and United States.
- 2005 ANA/HMA revised and published scope and standards. Nurse title changed from parish nurse to faith community nurse.
- 2011 IPNRC transfers assets from Deaconess Foundation, St. Louis, MO, to the Church Health Center, Memphis, TN. The 25th Annual Westberg International Parish Nurse Symposium is held.
- 2012 ANA/HMA publish second edition *Faith Community Nurse Scope and Standards*.
- 2014 American Nurses Credentialing Center (ANCC) launches faith community nursing certification through portfolio. *Foundations of Faith Community Nursing* curriculum revised.
- 2016 IPNRC renamed Westberg Institute. The 30th anniversary of the Annual Westberg International Parish Nurse Symposium held in Chicago, IL.
- 2017 ANA/HMA publish third edition *Faith Community Nurse Scope and Standards*. ANCC ends FCN certification by portfolio.
- 2018 Thirty-one countries active with faith community nursing.

ANA, American Nurses Association; *FCN*, faith community nurse; *HMA*, Health Ministries Association; *IPNRC*, International Parish Nurse Resource Center.

Another key contributor to this focus in nursing is the IPNRC, whose name was changed to Westberg Institute in 2016 for a variety of reasons (Campbell, 2016). First was to honor the contemporary nurse role in the faith community, also to honor the founder, Granger Westberg, and to support its parent organization Church Health's branding for planning future marketing strategies (Campbell, 2016). Throughout the resource center's history, the focus has remained on the provision and promotion of quality education, research, and support through curriculum, resources, and continuing education opportunities.

Today, nurses working in faith communities continue to be recognized as in a specialty practice by the ANA, complete with scope and standards to guide nursing practice and an ever-increasing body of research and evidence-based practice literature. There are more than 17,000 nurses working in faith communities across the United States and in at least 31 countries around the world such as Australia, Canada, New Zealand, Germany, and Swaziland. The number of nurses with the faith community designation is a conservative estimate based on the number of nurses who report taking foundation courses. It also does not reflect the numbers of nurses who provide some form of health ministry to congregations without formal education in the specialty area (Daniels, 2018). The faith community continues to evolve as a nursing specialty practice area offering creative strategies for whole-person health.

RATIONALE FOR FAITH COMMUNITY AS A VIABLE PUBLIC (POPULATION) HEALTH MODEL FOR NURSING

The health care delivery system is challenged to work within parameters of tighter financial constraints while addressing patients' complex health concerns and also responding to federal mandates for expensive automated systems (i.e., electronic health records) that span the continuum of care. Nurses are well positioned to provide lower cost and holistic community-based care for vulnerable and underserved populations as well as collaborate with other care providers (McLean and Habicht, 2016; Young, 2016; Ziebarth, 2016).

Fragmented care and inadequate caregiver training and availability are problems for the disenfranchised, underserved, and uninsured, as well as for economically well-situated and better-educated persons. Families are challenged to seek the best ways to meet the multiple demands of young children, teens, and aging parents, whether living in metropolitan, suburban, or rural areas.

Consumer demand for involvement in health care decisions continues to increase, and society emphasizes individual responsibility for health. Simultaneously, consumers have increased interest in their own well-being and have expressed needs for health information to be available in a variety of formats (McLean and Habicht, 2016). In addition to consumer interest and a heightened awareness of responsibility for one's own health, health care providers and managed care systems have found it financially advantageous for individuals to remain healthy and minimize unnecessary access to care. Consumers struggle to cope with the challenges of rising costs of care, decreasing reimbursement, and the complex health system demands on individuals and families.

It is important to differentiate the unique practice of nurses within the faith community from other community-focused specialty practices. These nurses share many similarities with home health, hospice, and public health nursing—promoting health in the community setting where people live, work, play, and attend school and churches; however, while these nurses focus on the whole-person health approach, they emphasize the care of the spirit. Nursing care is shaped and guided by the faith community's traditions, rites, and rituals.

A primary focus of all nurses in the last few decades has been to coordinate care and to link health care providers, groups, and community resources as the client tries to understand complicated health plans. Negotiating with individuals, agencies, and community partnerships within the complex maze of the broader health care environment demands a knowledgeable and seasoned professional. Nurses are aware of the necessity of collaborative practices and the formation of partnerships to care for groups and individuals across the life span. These nurses recognize the need for identifying strategies to address health promotion and disease prevention at all levels. They advocate for healthy lifestyle choices in exercise, nutrition, substance use, and stress management. Nurses realize that information and guidance must be available via media, in schools, workplaces, faith communities, and residential neighborhoods. Nurses partner with others such as faculty in academic settings, health care institutions, and federal agencies as they serve populations in faith communities to help improve health outcomes (Opalinski et al., 2017; Power et al., 2016; Young and Smothers, 2018; Ziebarth, 2016).

NURSING PRACTICE IN THE FAITH COMMUNITY

Similar to public health nurses in the United States, nurses working with faith communities identify the need for health promotion services across the life span, particularly in underserved urban and rural areas. Nurses are adept at creatively addressing gaps in the delivery of service. The congregation provides an ideal setting of care for congregants to benefit from health counseling and health promotion services at all levels of prevention. The following provides an overview of levels of prevention for older adult health.

Nursing services emphasize whole-person health promotion and disease prevention within a supportive and caring faith community. Nurses acknowledge the inner strength and spirituality of persons and groups to enhance healing. Nurses draw on knowledge and skills with communication, negotiation, collaboration, and leadership. Working with the congregation as the population group, nurses attempt to include in the wellness programs those persons who are less vocal or visible in the community of faith. The spiritual dimension of health is optimized by complementing pastoral care with nursing care.

Profile of the Nurse in the Faith Community

The practice of the nurse is governed by:
1. the Nurse Practice Act of the state in which the nurse practices
2. *Nursing: Scope and Standards of Practice* (ANA, 2015a)
3. *Faith Community Nursing: Scope and Standards of Practice* (ANA/HMA, 2017)
4. *Code of Ethics with Interpretive Statements* (for nurses) (ANA, 2015b)

LEVELS OF PREVENTION
Older Adult Health

Primary Prevention
- Encourage a variety of activities of individual and group interest and discourage extended inactivity.
- Encourage healthy snacks and meals for older adult gatherings and activities.
- Initiate a walk for fun program (e.g., Walk to Emmaus).
- Host a community health fair offering resources related to whole-person health.

Secondary Prevention
- Provide health assessment and counseling during home visits for health promotion after a hospitalization.
- When making home visits, identify safety concerns and make suggestions such as eliminating throw rugs, decreasing clutter, decreasing use of extension cords, and moving heat sources from flammable products such as oxygen.
- Using an attitudinal/behavioral risk survey, identify factors influencing identified poor health behaviors.

Tertiary Prevention
- Collaborate closely with ministerial team about sessions that deal with overweight and advantages of maintaining a healthy weight, and support stress management and improved quality-of-life sessions.
- Follow up and monitor health care provider's plan of care for older adults challenged with chronic diseases such as diabetes, hypertension, and depression; provide education, support, and spiritual care.
- Discuss in gatherings of older adults who have mental health issues the need for loving, caring friends and the support needed for improving mental health and overall well-being.

Requirements for the nurse include the following (ANA/HMA, 2017; Westberg Institute, 2018):
1. An active registered nurse license in the state in which he or she practices
2. Minimum diploma or associate degree in nursing; however, a minimum of baccalaureate degree in nursing preferred
3. Completion of an educational course to prepare for this nursing specialty practice (and ministry)
4. Experience in public/population health nursing experience preferred
5. Specialized knowledge of the spiritual beliefs and practices of the faith community served
6. Reflection of personal spirituality maturity in his or her practice
7. Being organized, flexible, a self-starter, and a good communicator

Variation in the depth and breadth of nursing practice results from the nurse's education, experience, practice setting, and populations cared for by the nurse.

Because many nurses practice within their own faith community congregation, they are considered to be a known and trusted resource. By virtue of this relationship, congregants access the services of the nurse with a high comfort level and awareness that information shared will be kept confidential by the professional nurse. Nurses in faith communities are aware of the beliefs, faith practices, and level of spiritual maturity of the members served and link these with health and healing.

Many of these nurses function in a part-time capacity and serve as salaried or unpaid staff. Some nurses are responsible for providing services for several faith communities, whereas others engage with a faith community as part of a full-time commitment in other capacities. For example, a nurse might be employed part-time as a public health nurse and part-time with a faith community. Alternatively, a nurse employed full-time in an acute care setting may spend time serving in an unpaid capacity working in a faith community with a group of other nurses. Depending on the practice model, the nurse has a narrowly defined or a wider realm of responsibility. The nurse's practices may be integrated into a health care system or into practices that collaborate with related professional practice areas such as health departments or colleges of nursing. Health care systems sometimes employ nurse coordinators for faith communities. The coordinator facilitates different arrangements with several faith communities of varying backgrounds (Solari-Twadell and Brown, 2020).

The advanced practice nurses increase in numbers in working in the faith community, They have a variety of arrangements within the faith community. An evaluation of the practice trends used within the faith community is necessary. Nursing must be accountable and responsive to those being served, as well as to those who provide opportunities to serve.

The following goals for a faith community are clearly defined in the 2017 scope and standards for practice (ANA/HMA, 2017):

1. The protection, promotion, and optimization of health and abilities of the congregants
2. The prevention of illness and injury and facilitation of healing The nurse works to alleviate suffering through the diagnosis, referral, and treatment.
3. Advocate for all persons in the context of the values, beliefs, and practices of the congregation

Characteristics of the Nursing Practice in the Faith Community

Since the early 1990s, five characteristics have been identified as central to the philosophy of faith community nursing by nursing educators and practitioners (Solari-Twadell and Ziebarth, 2020):

1. The spiritual dimension is central to the practice. Nursing embodies the physical, psychological, social, and spiritual dimensions of clients into professional practice. Although parish nursing includes all four, it focuses on intentional and compassionate care, which stems from the spiritual dimension of all humankind.
2. The roots of the role balance both knowledge and skills of nursing, using nursing sciences, the humanities, and theology. The nurse combines nursing functions with pastoral care functions. Visits in the office, home, hospital, or nursing home often involve prayer and may include a reference to scripture, symbols, sacraments, and liturgy of the faith community represented by the nurse. The values and beliefs of the faith community are integral to the supportive care given. Nurses also assist with worship services as appropriate within the faith community.
3. The focus of the specialty is the faith community and its ministry. The faith community is the source of health and

healing partnerships, which result in creative responses to health and health-related concerns. Partnerships may be among individuals, groups, and health care professionals within the congregation. They may also be among various congregations or community agencies, institutions, or individuals. Partnerships also evolve as the congregation visualizes its health-related mission beyond the walls, stones, and steeples of its own place of worship.

4. The services of the nurse emphasize the strengths of individuals, families, and communities. As congregations realize the need for care and to care for one another, their individual and corporate relationship with their Creator is often enhanced. This provides additional coping strength for future crisis situations within the family and community.
5. Health, spiritual health, and healing are considered an ongoing, dynamic process. Because spiritual health is central to well-being, influences are evident in the total individual and noted in a healthy congregation. Well-being and illness may occur simultaneously; spiritual healing or well-being can exist in the absence of cure.

❓ CHECK YOUR PRACTICE

At the conclusion of the worship service, you notice a long-time member of the congregation sitting alone in a back pew with her head down. Mrs. E is an 84-year-old widow whose husband died 1 month ago. She is well known to you, as you visited the couple's home many times over the course of his lengthy battle with cancer. She is visibly sad and withdrawn from other congregants leaving the sanctuary. You do not know if she wants to be left alone or desires the healing presence of the nurse who ministers to this faith community. What should you do? See if you can apply these steps to this scenario. (1) Recognize the cues, looking at available resources about signs of grief; (2) analyze the cues, looking at Mrs. E. and the changes in her behavior; (3) state several and prioritize the hypotheses you have stated to best deal with Mrs. E's current situation; (4) generate solutions for each hypothesis; (5) take action on the number one hypothesis you think best reflects the best approach to helping Mrs. E. through this process; and (6) evaluate the outcomes you would expect as a result of your interventions with Mrs. E.

Nurse Interventions and Programs Used in the Faith Community

Nurses provide care to individuals, families, congregations, and populations across life, regardless of ethnicity, lifestyle, gender, sexual orientation, or creed.

The practice includes the culture of the population and the geographic community. The nurse incorporates faith and health, uses the nursing process in providing services to the faith community, and facilitates collaborative health ministries as an important component of the practice.

One of the first tasks of a new nurse is to explore the social demographics and identify the health needs of the congregation (O'Brien, 2017). This is accomplished by selecting a congregational health needs survey available online or in print for public use (Durbin et al., 2013). In collaboration with the ministry team, the nurse determines actionable priorities and then applies his or her knowledge, skills, and experience to plan health promotion and spiritual care initiatives. Often, due to limited congregational resources, the nurse must conduct a resource assessment to determine feasibility when matching need with time and financial resources.

The following set of questions helps determine what is possible to consider in advance of carrying out health promotion projects (Solari-Twadell, et al 2020):

1. What resources are needed?
2. What resources are available?
3. Which of the available resources are accessible to the nurse for the accomplishment of a specific effort or project?
4. Can the work of the project or program be accomplished with what is available and accessible?

Several images of the nurse in faith community practice highlight varying settings and professional activities. Central to all interactions is intentional care of the spirit and the healing presence of the nurse. Healing presence and prayer are frequently offered in most interactions. Bulletin board displays are helpful to promote health topics of interest in hallways with high visibility. Blood pressure screenings offer therapeutic touch as well as assessment for cardiac status, social health, and overall well-being as the individual spends time with the nurse. Informal pew-side consultations take place after worship when individuals ask health-related questions or request resource or referral information. Young families require comprehensive support with diverse needs related to age, supportive relationships, child care support, and parenting (Fig. 29.3). The health educator role requires creative and differing teaching strategies for the nurse based on the ages of individuals or groups being taught.

Nurses may organize an annual health fair, inviting community partners and service agencies to share resources and promote health ministries to parishioners of all ages (Fig 29.4). Hospital and institutional care visits provide spiritual and emotional support when unexpected illness and health crisis may challenge coping skills and raise questions about faith and denominational theology (Fig. 29.5).

In congregations with older adults, an organized bereavement/grief support group for widows and widowers may or may not be led by the nurse. Depending on social ministries in place, the nurse may interface with homeless persons accessing congregational resources of food or financial support. Other interventions, services, or programs provided by the nurse are determined by taking into consideration specific congregation needs—the mission, vision, and strategic plan of the congregation matched with the knowledge, skills, and experience as well as time availability of the nurse.

As one of the trusted members of the pastoral care staff, the nurse will find it helpful to develop ease in inquiring about a person's spiritual journey. Assessments, whether physical or spiritual, are used to gather data for planning nursing care. Because care of the spirit is central to nursing in the faith community, spiritual assessment instruments are useful tools and applicable to diverse populations (Puchalski, 2018). One widely used spiritual assessment tool is constructed with sample questions and the acronym FICA:

F-Faith or beliefs: What are your spiritual beliefs? Do you consider yourself spiritual? What things do you believe in that give meaning to life?

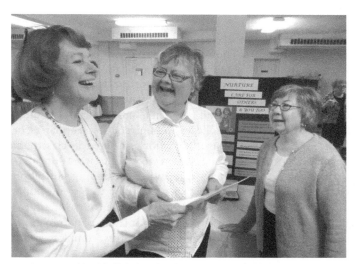

Fig. 29.4 Health Fair for the Congregation and Community.

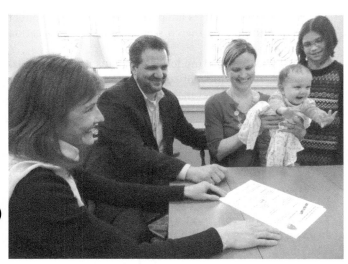

Fig. 29.3 Offering Education and Support to Families.

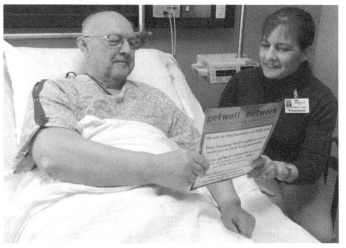

Fig. 29.5 Hospital Visitations Include Care of the Spirit.

I-Importance and influence: Is faith/spirituality important to you? How has your illness and/or hospitalization affected your personal practices/beliefs?

C-Community: Are you connected with a faith center in the community? Does it provide support/comfort for you during times of stress? Is there a person/group/leader who supports/assists you in your spirituality?

A-Address: What can I do for you? What support/guidance can health care provide to support your spiritual beliefs/practices? (Puchalski, 2018).

In addition to assessment data, history of family relationships and past association with faith communities provides background information. The nurse needs to be comfortable with questions that lead parishioners to expand on their faith beliefs. Compassionate, careful listening involves being still, reflecting, and being intentionally in the present. Being sensitive to the differing needs of personal spirituality during various points along life's journey is important to consider while guiding persons through the spiritual assessment. The nurse then also helps individuals share necessary information about spirituality needs with other health care providers and clergy as appropriate.

Education for Nurses in the Faith Community

The registered nurse choosing to serve a faith community in a formal role should obtain additional education in the nursing specialty practice, recognizing that most undergraduate nurse programs offer limited content on spiritual care. A variety of educational programs and curricula are available through health care institutions, colleges and universities, seminaries, or faith-based denominations. Education is offered in classroom or online formats, and ranges from weekend to week-long curricula, which may or may not award continuing education contact hours. Academic courses awarding 3 to 6 credit hours of study are also available. Depending on the course or education sponsor, additional content may include denomination-specific topics, regional community resources, complementary therapies, and transitional care, to name a few.

The most widely used continuing education curriculum around the world is published by the Westberg Institute, supported by Church Health in Memphis, Tennessee. Guided by the Scope and Standards for Faith Community Nursing and incorporating the latest evidence in research and practice, the curriculum provides comprehensive education organized around four core values of spiritual formation, professionalism, whole-person health, and community (Church Health Center, 2014). A list of available courses using this curriculum is found at https://westberginstitute.org (Box 29.3).

Ongoing education for these nurses may be obtained locally, regionally, or internationally.

Advanced practice opportunities also enrich a specialty practice. Master's-prepared nurses (with specialization in congregational leadership, congregational health, public health nursing, or holistic nursing) and nurse practitioners have found niches in faith communities. Universities and seminaries have developed creative and unique partnerships to provide educational opportunities for faculty and students at the undergraduate and graduate levels.

BOX 29.3 Westberg Institute Curriculum for Two Courses—Foundations and the Coordinator/Advanced

- **The Foundations Course** offers topics within content areas to include theology of health and healing; the nurse's role in spiritual care; use of prayer; the history, philosophy, and models of care; advocacy; assessment; beginning your ministry; working with a congregation; care coordination; communication and collaboration; documentation, ethical and legal issues; family violence; grief and loss; healing and wholeness; health promotion; and self-care (Westberg Institute, 2020).
- **The Coordinator/Advanced Course** is designed to build on the Foundations Course and offers administrative and program management content. The Advanced Course equips the nurse with the tools necessary to coordinate a group of nurses within a congregation or a larger regional or denomination-based network.

Formal educational preparation and continuing education options must continue to include the basics and enrichment courses in nursing practice, research, theology, and pastoral care (see the following How To box). In addition, the specialty practice nurse benefits from updates in the areas of public health, medicine, technology, and sensitivity awareness with the lesbian/gay/bisexual/transgender/queer (LGBTQ) community or bariatric population. Enhancing collaboration, negotiation, and coordination skills, as well as consultation, leadership, and research skills, is essential. Nurses in faith communities accept responsibility for ongoing professional education within nursing and ministry arenas (ANA/HMA, 2017).

Models of Nursing applied to the Faith Community

Consideration is given to the organizational mission of the faith community along with the influencing factors of economics, infrastructure, available personnel, and willingness of stakeholders to take some risks. Four primary models are found in practice. The models are differentiated by employer and remuneration wherein the nurse is paid or unpaid.

- A paid institutional model is supported by a health care institution (e.g., hospital, health department, or long-term care facility) where nurses are paid (salary or hourly) either by the institution or a shared salary with the congregation over time.
- An unpaid institutional model, where an institution provides soft support in the form of continuing education and spiritual development; however, the nurse is not paid a salary and is governed by the congregation, which budgets for some expenses such as mileage and health education materials. Many nonprofit hospitals provide soft support to a faith network as a partnership for promoting wellness to residents in the community and to meet requirements for tax-exempt status (Butler and Diaz, 2017).
- The paid congregational model, where the nurse is governed and paid by the congregation with no contractual support from any sponsoring health care institution.
- The unpaid congregational model, where the nurse is governed by the congregation with no contractual support

from any sponsoring health care institution. When unpaid, the nurse may negotiate financial support for expenses such as gas/mileage, postage, and health promotion literature.

Pros and cons exist for each model. Paid nurses tend to work more hours, more fully develop the role, and provide a stronger presence within the congregation than the unpaid nurse. In all models, nurses work closely with health care professionals, pastoral care and health ministry staff, and lay volunteers.

The pursuit of faith community nursing as a specialty practice has been somewhat hindered by the larger number of unpaid nurses practicing a few hours per week or preferring to serve in a volunteer yet professional role. The ongoing question of pay is similar to the evolution of paid congregational staff for youth education and music ministry. The trend for older nurses to call themselves faith community nurses "after retirement" also sends the message of a volunteer ministry versus a professional

nurse engaged in a specialty practice of nursing. Yet as nurses wanting to do more in their churches can attest, financial constraints of smaller churches have prevented the creation of a paid position or increasing hours from part-time to full-time status. Regardless of the selected model, the nurse uses knowledge, skills, and experience to promote whole-person health of body, mind, and spirit. The ideal outcome is a caring congregation that supports healthy, spiritually fulfilling lives.

Holistic Health Care

Holistic health practices emphasize nurses' and clients' commitment to optimal wellness. Such practices focus nurses and clients on seeking the meaning of wellness for the individual or situation, and on considering options from an array of therapies. Harmony between the physical, emotional, psychological, and spiritual self is sought. In addition to sharing backgrounds and functions similar to those of public health nursing, nursing in the faith community also parallels and benefits from commonalities and distinct practices of holistic nursing. Regardless of specialty or practice setting, nurses who practice in a holistic manner acknowledge wholeness as more than the sum of the individual parts (Dossey et al., 2016). The philosophy of holistic nursing practice (also a specialty in nursing) embraces concepts of presence, healing, and holism. The interconnectedness of body, mind, and spirit is basic to holistic nursing and is embedded in the practice of other nursing specialties nurses. Like faith community nursing, holistic nursing emphasizes wholeness of persons across the life span.

Nurses working with faith communities and holistic nurses share the skill of creating a healing environment (Dossey et al., 2016). Listening coupled with intentional compassion is basic to effective interventions. Selected interventions that are often used in both specialties of nursing are prayer, meditation, counseling, guided imagery, health promotion guidance, journaling, therapeutic touch, healing presence, and massage.

ISSUES RELATED TO NURSING PRACTICE IN FAITH COMMUNITIES

As a specialty practice of nursing, the nurse in the faith community must be alert to issues of accountability to populations served, as well as to those who entrust the nurse with the responsibility to serve a designated population. Because the role involves professional, legal, ethical, theological, and relational issues, the nurse will need to review, understand, and apply all professional parameters involved. The potential for conflicts can be reduced by the following:

- Negotiations with the pastoral staff, congregations, institutions, and the wider community must be involved in job description preparation and program planning.
- Provision of care for individuals and groups is documented and remains confidential.
- Issues such as privacy, confidentiality, group concerns, access, and record management must be discussed with the pastoral staff or the contracting agency at the outset of any program agreement.
- Discussions of health promotion activities may include the individual, the family, and the leadership within the faith community.

Professional Issues

A position description is a necessary tool for defining the nurse's practice. The description should accurately reflect the qualifications, skills, accountabilities, and responsibilities of the position. Annual and periodic evaluations of the nurse and the practice, as well as assessments and evaluations of services needed, are certainly indicated. Evaluations should include input from self, peer, congregational staff, and institutional evaluations as applicable for constructive feedback and to enhance practice.

Professional appraisal, or a portfolio, is becoming a standard in nursing practice and therefore is needed. The appraisals guide the nurse's professional development as well as program development. Because the scope of the nursing practice is broad and focuses on the independent practice, the nurse must consider a wide variety of topics to be used in the appraisal, such as the following:

- Position descriptions
- Professional liability
- Professional educational
- Experiential preparation
- Collaborative agreements
- Ability to work with lay volunteers as well as practicing and retired professionals

Abiding by the professional nursing code is understood and must be reflected in the appraisal. The nurse must also be assessed in the application of skills related to the polity, expectations, and mission of the particular faith community.

The nurse is required to be the following:

- Knowledgeable about lines of authority and channels of communication in the congregation and in the collaborative institutions
- Well acquainted with the personnel committees of the congregation
- An advocate for well-being to highlight justice issues in local and national legislation
- A contributor of information to policymakers about the implications for health and well-being for the parish and the local and global communities
- An active participant in political activities that contribute to spiritual growth and healthy functioning

Documentation Issues

An ongoing challenge for nurses is documenting care provision and reporting trends and outcomes. Extracting meaningful data from traditional, handwritten notes is cumbersome and labor intensive, and paper records were not designed with the accountable care requirements of today's health care system (Mayernik, 2013). Technology offers an alternative option to paper records. With advances in electronic health records, both online and stand alone databases are widely available, though often at considerable expense that prevents many smaller faith communities from using them. As a nursing specialty practice, it is imperative that nurses document care to maintain and enhance quality of preparation and services offered, engage in evidence-based practice, network within professional organizations, and become involved in outcomes-oriented research. According to the American Nurses Association Scope and Standards of Practice for Faith Community Nurses (2017), documentation should contribute to the quality of nursing practice and be kept confidential and secure while also being easily retrievable for those with permission to access.

Legal Issues

Although the provision of nursing care in the congregational setting carries lower risk for litigation than other settings, nurses engage in autonomous practice and may be involved in a legal suit. Within the legal system, the courts find no difference in the actions of nurses working in a hospital versus an alternative setting because both must adhere to the same standards of practice (ANA/HMA, 2017). Therefore it is strongly recommended that the nurse carry individual malpractice insurance. In addition, the nurse must maintain an active nursing license, abide by the laws and regulations set forth by the state's nurse practice act, and adhere to the ANA's Scope and Standards for Registered Nurses and for specialty nurse practice (ANA, 2015a; ANA/HMA, 2017). Additional legal concerns pertain to institutional contractual agreements, health records management, release of information, and volunteer liability. Resources to address legal issues of faith community practice include the community's legal consultant, the position statements for faith community nursing practice, and guidelines of any institutional partner (ANA/HMA, 2017).

As required by law, nurses advocate for individuals and groups. The nurse is also expected to identify and report cases of neglect, abuse, and illegal behaviors to the appropriate legal sources. The nurse appropriately refers members to pastoral or community resources if the scope of the problem is not within the professional realm of the nurse. Referral is also indicated if conflict between nurse and parishioner is such that no further progress is possible. The nurse who has a positive relationship that values open dialogue with the pastoral team will be supported in efforts to select the most appropriate community resource for clients.

Financial Issues

Most congregations are dependent on the contributions of their members and often operate with a limited budget for operations, salaries, and expenses. While larger congregations can support larger budgets and expanded ministries, smaller congregations are often challenged to meet expenses for operations and clergy salary. Thus there may not be sufficient funds available for a paid faith community nurse. Regardless of paid status, the faith community nurse is challenged to be creative in identifying sustainable financial support for programs as well as in finding low-cost or free resources. Considerations for planning budget may include educational and promotional materials, equipment, travel expenses, postage, continuing education, and malpractice insurance. Money, time, and human resources may limit what services or programs are offered within a faith community. Nonetheless, as evidenced by the literature, nurses can offer much to a congregation in the form of assessment, screening, health promotion, and healing presence (Alexander and Branstetter, 2017; Callaghan, 2016; Laming and Stewart, 2016; Meyer and Holland, 2016).

Future Growth

These nurses can develop comprehensive, population-focused practices. They may also implement programs at beginning levels of population-based practices to ensure comprehensive care for individuals and families. The continuing challenge for nurses, other health care providers, and the communities will be to garner government, foundation, and private funding, and combine it with support from volunteer activities, family involvement, and community groups to create the unique mix needed for each community. Nurses are asked to partner with community members where they live, work, attend school, and gather for worship; to closely partner with these same members to advocate for those who are powerless; to identify health and health-related needs; to detect and address those needs to prevent costly use of the health care system; and to be closely aligned with those who can implement visionary policy that improves health care for community members across the life span.

Uncovering and understanding the intricacies of the work of these nurses is a difficult task because minimal research on the outcomes of nursing interventions within faith communities has been conducted (Callaghan, 2016). The following How To box provides a general guide to program evaluation. Comprehending the distinctiveness of the role of the nurse is important to the maturation of the specialty because it allows for a clear recognition of the work done (Solari-Twadell and Ziebarth, 2020).

HOW TO EVALUATE PROGRAM OUTCOMES IN FAITH COMMUNITIES

Nurses plan and provide health-promotion and disease-prevention activities within faith communities. The following model for program development and evaluation is useful in the creation of high-quality and cost-effective programs:

Step 1: What problem or issue is the program designed to address? Be specific about the problem as it guides the search for evidence-based information.

Step 2: Identify program partnerships such as regional faith communities, hospitals, chronic disease management centers.

Step 3: Identify both short- and long-term goals. The goals help prioritize what needs to be documented, tracked, and reported.

Step 4: Document the specific program outcomes. This may include numbers of attendees, participation rates, desired changes in measurements, and any unexpected outcomes.

Step 5: Develop and implement the interventions for the program, as determined by best practices, to achieve the goals identified in Step 4.

Step 6: Evaluate the short- and long-term goals and the specific program outcomes. Share the outcome results with individuals or in aggregate form to the faith community.

Step 7: Disseminate findings to other nurses in faith communities at local, national, and international levels.

Data from Callaghan DM: Implementing faith community nursing interventions to promote healthy behaviors in adults. *IJFCN* 2(1), 2016. Available at https://digitalcommons.wku.edu.

NATIONAL HEALTH OBJECTIVES AND FAITH COMMUNITIES

Healthy People 2030 provides evidence-based national objectives for improving the health and well-being of all Americans. The *Healthy People 2030* indicators support individuals of all ages and families, communities, and other settings to make informed decisions retain a high quality of life free of preventable diseases, and create environments or access to settings that promote health. Faith communities offer an ideal setting for health promotion and have long-held positions of esteem and influence in communities and where strong partnerships can be established with health care institutions and community agencies.

Recognizing that older adults are one of the fastest-growing age groups in the community, including baby boomers (adults born between 1946 and 1964), congregations with large numbers of older adults present special needs for the faith community nurse to address in order to improve the health and well-being of this vulnerable population (see *Healthy People 2030* box).

 HEALTHY PEOPLE 2030

Objectives Related to Older Adult Health in Faith Communities

- **OA-01:** Increase the proportion of older adults with physical or cognitive health problems who get physical activity.
- **OA-02:** Reduce the proportion of older adults who use inappropriate medications.
- **OA-03:** Reduce the rate of emergency department visits due to falls among older adults.
- **OA-04:** Reduce the rate of pressure ulcer-related hospital admissions among older adults.
- **OA-05:** Reduce the rate of hospital admissions for diabetes among older adults.
- **OA-06:** Reduce the rate of hospital admissions for pneumonia among older adults.
- **OA-07:** Reduce the rate of hospital admissions for urinary tract infections among older adults.

From U.S. Department of Health and Human Services: *Healthy People 2030*. HHS, 2020. Available at https://health.gov/healthypeople.

EVIDENCE-BASED PRACTICE

Researchers wondered what interventions by nurses within faith community (FCNs) are used most frequently with other adults and how FCNs contribute to successful aging. The researcher clarified that successful aging included "good health and an active life, with lower risk of disease and disability and high mental and physical functioning." A secondary analysis of deidentified cumulative qualitative data from the Henry Ford Macomb Hospital Faith Community Nursing/Health Ministries Documentation and Reporting System was completed. Data from five networks, comprised of 169 faith communities in Illinois, Michigan, Nebraska, and Indiana, were used. Descriptive statistics were used to describe the overall sample characteristics. Analysis showed that more than 60% of clients receiving care from FNCs were age 66 and older, with the 66 to 80 age range identified as the largest group. Group education/information activities were the most frequently provided group activity, with nutrition education being the most popular out of a list of 31 topics. Exercise/activity support groups, healthy lifestyle support groups, and blood pressure screenings were other frequent interventions by FCNs. Among individual interactions, conversations regarding spiritual/emotional/rational (SER) issues and health/wellness issues occurred most often. Active listening was the most frequently occurring intervention, followed by individual interventions of presence, prayer, and touch/hug.

Nurse Use

Faith community nurses provide vital services to older adults to promote health and educate about disease prevention. Increased collaboration between health care institutions, government, and faith communities could provide the supports needed to increase the number of FCNs to support older adults and lessen the burden on traditional health care settings.

Hixson LB, Loeb SJ: Promoting successful aging through faith community nursing. *J Christ Nurs* 35(4):242–249, 2018.

APPLYING CONTENT TO PRACTICE

In a span of more than 30 years, nursing in parish/faith community went from pilot project to recognition as a nursing specialty practice complete with scope and standards. Screening, monitoring, wellness education, and referrals to appropriate services are combined with a spiritual component of care to promote health and healing and fulfill the church's historic role in health and healing. Ongoing research documents favorable outcomes associated with intentional holistic health promotion to individuals, groups, and faith communities. Successful nurse networks, whether institutional or congregation-based models, continue to be established in the United States and around the world. Careful examination of the nurses' work in the faith community provides the opportunity for leaders in nursing and health policy to identify successful strategies that could improve the health and well-being of a community.

This chapter described individual, group, and population health out of the congregational setting. The faith community is instrumental in providing the structure, place, and resources, and may intentionally seek out the vulnerable and marginalized to receive support from other community or denominational organizations closely aligned with mission and outreach activities for a common purpose. The organizations may include a health care institution, a child care or adult daycare center, an immigrant community, a homeless shelter, an amusement park, a crisis center, a preschool, or local public schools. Depending on desired outcomes, the nurse combines knowledge, skills, and experience in collaboration with others to make a difference for a larger population.

To illustrate, a faith community partners with a hospital, the local agency on aging, and a retirement community to promote older adult health. Key stakeholders gather for discussions on priorities identified from a community needs assessment completed by the hospital. The stakeholders also review suggested prevention and services objectives for older adult health from *Healthy People 2030*. The group considers baseline data and identifies desired outcomes. From discussions, activities and programs are planned, drawing from the collective human and financial resources. In this example, the nurse works with hospital staff to coordinate screenings and health promotion programs held in the congregation setting and at various locations using a mobile health vehicle. Participating older adults requested additional services such as medication reviews and educational health talks on topics of depression, advance directives, and Medicare enrollment benefits. Successful disease management programs for diabetes and congestive heart failure were extended beyond the walls of the hospital into the community to reach a larger population. Data for hospital readmission within 30 days were reviewed with the faith community nurses to identify creative strategies to reduce future readmissions. All services were evaluated for content and quality, as well as to track, trend, and report outcomes. As with most collaborative initiatives, more was accomplished through partnership with the congregation, and the faith community nurse was instrumental in bringing the partners together.

PRACTICE APPLICATION

The nursing process is a method that can be used for program planning and evaluation in the faith community setting. Such an approach involves congregants and faith community nurses in a dynamic endeavor to jointly learn about the members' individual health status, as well as that of the faith community, local community, and broader geographic community. The faith community nurse programs are derived in various ways. Initially, the impetus for these programs developed from an unmet health need, from members' concern about caring for vulnerable individuals or groups within the congregation, or from committee recommendations related to health and wellness issues.

Which of the following activities is most likely to increase the interest and involvement of the faith community's members?
A. Writing a contract for the services of the nurse and developing a program for the congregants
B. Exploring the faith community's environment
C. Offering a multiple-week Bible study on the topics of health, healing, and wholeness
D. Gathering information on leaders and valued activities in the congregation through focus groups of pastoral staff
E. Conducting a congregational health needs assessment survey
F. Holding a health fair
G. Attending a regional faith community nursing network meeting.
Answers can be found on the Evolve website.

REMEMBER THIS!

- Nurse services respond to health, healing, and wholeness within the context of the faith community. Although the emphasis is on health promotion and disease prevention across the life span, the central focus of practice is on the "intentional care of the spirit."
- Spiritual care is different from religious care and is an expected and welcomed component of nursing care.
- Note that spiritual assessment and care can also be provided outside of a congregational setting in the larger community. The nurse from the faith community may work in other settings of retirement communities, faith-based amusement parks, senior centers, food pantries, and day shelters.
- Faith community nursing evolved from the historical roots of healing traditions in faith communities; early public health nursing efforts with individuals, families, and populations in the community; and more recently, the professional practice of nursing.
- The nurse partners with the congregational wellness committee and volunteers to plan programs that address health-related concerns within faith communities.
- The usual functions of the nurse include health counseling and teaching for individuals and groups, facilitating linkages and referrals to congregation and community resources, advocating and encouraging support resources, and providing spiritual care.
- Nurses collaborate to plan, implement, and evaluate health promotion activities considering the faith community's beliefs, rituals, and polity. *Healthy People 2030* objectives and health indicators offer effective frameworks for health ministry efforts of wellness committees and basic partnering for programs.
- Nurses in congregational or institutional models enhance health ministry programs of faith communities when carefully chosen partnerships are formed within the congregation, with other faith communities, and with local health and social community organizations.
- Nurses working within faith communities must obtain foundational and ongoing educational and skill preparation to be accountable to those served.
- These nurses document care interventions offered to individuals and groups, in addition to tracking and reporting

program statistics and outcomes to validate and sustain the professional practice.

- The nurse may offer additional resources to hospitals and health systems challenged to reduce 30-day hospital readmissions.
- Nurses are encouraged to consider innovative approaches to creating caring communities. These may be in individual faith communities; among several faith communities in a single locale, regionally, or internationally; or in partnership with other organizations and institutions.
- To sustain oneself as a nurse who provides spiritual care to support individuals, families, and communities in the healing and wholeness process, the nurse must be intentional about self-care, spiritual formation, and renewal.

EVOLVE WEBSITE

http://evolve.elsevier.com/Stanhope/community/
- Answers to Practice Application
- Case Study

REFERENCES

Alexander L, Branstetter ML: General nutrition knowledge and perceived stress in a rural female faith community, *Int J Faith Community Nurs* August 2017. Retrieved from https://digitalcommons.wku.edu.

American Nurses Association: *Holistic nursing: scope and standards of practice*, 2nd ed, Silver Spring, 2013, ANA.

American Nurses Association: *Nursing: scope and standards of practice*, 3rd ed., Silver Spring, 2015a, ANA.

American Nurses Association: *Code of Ethics with Interpretive Statements (for nurses)*, 2015b. Retrieved from https://www.nursingworld.org.

American Nurses Association and Health Ministries Association (ANA/HMA): *Scope and standards of practice of parish nursing practice*, Washington DC, 2017, American Nurses Publishing.

American Nurses Association and Health Ministries Association (ANA/HMA): *Faith community nursing: scope and standards of practice*, Silver Spring, 2005, ANA.

American Nurses Association and Health Ministries Association (ANA/HMA): *Faith community nursing: scope and standards of practice*, 2nd ed., Silver Spring, 2012, ANA.

American Nurses Association and Health Ministries Association (ANA/HMA): *Faith community nursing: scope and standards of practice*, 3rd ed., Silver Spring, 2017, ANA.

American Nurses Credentialing Center: *Faith community nurse certification no longer available*, October 2017, Retrieved from http://www.nursecredentialing.org.

Bulechek G, Dochterman J, Butcher H, et al.: Core interventions for nursing specialty areas: faith community nursing. In *Nursing interventions classification (NIC)*, 7th ed., St. Louis, 2018.

Butler S, Diaz C: *Nurses as Intermediaries in the Promotion of Community Health: Exploring their Roles and Challenges*, 2017. Retrieved from https://www.brookings.edu.

Callaghan DM: Implementing faith community nursing interventions to promote healthy behaviors in adults, *Int J Faith Community Nurs* February 2016. Retrieved from https://digitalcommons.wku.edu.

Callaghan DM: The development of a faith community nursing intervention to promote health across the life span, *Int J Faith Community Nurs* July 2015. Retrieved from https://digitalcommons.wku.edu.

Campbell KP: IPNRC becomes the Westberg Institute, *Perspectives* 15(2):1, 2016.

Centers for Disease Control and Prevention: *Chronic Diseases and Health Promotion*, June 28, 2017. Retrieved from http://www.cdc.gov.

Church Health Center: *Foundations in faith community nursing-participant*, Memphis, 2014.

Church Health Center: FCNS active around the world, *Perspectives* 17(2):8–9, 2018.

Church Health Center: Health promoters lead congregations into healing, *Church Health Reader* 3(1):14, 2013.

Crisp CL: Faith, hope and spirituality: supporting parents when their child has a life-limiting illness, *J Christ Nurs* 33(1), 2016.

Daniels M: Faith community nursing—It can appear a small thing, but then ...! *Perspectives* 15(2):12–13, 2018.

Delgado C: Nurses' spiritual care practices: becoming less religious, *J Christ Nurs* 32(2):116–122, 2015.

Dossey BM, Keegan L: *Holistic nursing: A handbook for practice*, 7th ed., Burlington, 2016, Jones & Bartlett Learning.

Doyle A: Nursing by religious orders in the United States: part VI—Episcopal sisterhoods 1845–1928, *Am J Nurs* 29(12): 1466–1484, 1929.

Durbin NLR, Cassimere M, Howard C, et al: *Faith community nurse coordinator manual: a guide to creating and developing your program*, Memphis, TN, 2013, Church Health Center.

Fliedner T: *Some account of the deaconess work in the Christian church.* Kaiserswerth, Germany, 1870, Sam Lucas, p 26.

Gotwals B: Self-efficacy and nutrition education: a study of the effect of an intervention with faith community nurses, *J Relig Health* February 2018. Retrieved from https://link.springer.com.

Hixson LB, Loeb SJ: Promoting successful aging through faith community nursing. *J Christ Nurs*, 35I(4): 242-249, 2018.

Johnson EJ, Testerman N, Hart D: Teaching spiritual care to nursing students: an integrated model, *J Christ Nurs* 31(2):94–199, 2014.

Laming E, Stewart A: Parish nursing: an innovative community service, *Nurs Stand* 30(46):46–51, 2016.

Mattern LA: A day in the life of a wellness nurse at a retirement community, *Home Healthcare Now [serial online]* November/December 2016. Retrieved from https://www.nursingcenter.com.

Mayernik D: Faith community nursing in the accountable care era: documentation of interventions demonstrates improved health outcomes, *Perspectives* 12(3):6–7, 2013.

Meyer JL, Holland BE: Health coaching in faith-based community diabetes education, *Int J Faith Community Nurs* 2(1), 2016. Retrieved from http://digitalcommons.wku.edu.

McLean E, Habicht L: Perceptions of advance care planning among latino adults in the community setting, *Creat Nurs* 22(2): 106–113, 2016.

McNamara JW: *Health & wellness: what your faith community can do*, Cleveland, 2006, Pilgrim Press.

O'Brien ME: *Spirituality in nursing: standing on holy ground*, ed 6, Sudbury, 2017, Jones and Bartlett.

Opalinski A, Dyess SM, Stein N, Saiswick K, Fox V: *Broadening Practice Perspective by Engaging in Academic-Practice Collaboration: A Faith Community Nursing Exemplar*, August 2017. Retrieved from https://digitalcommons.wku.edu.

Patterson DL: *The essential parish nurse*, Cleveland, 2003, The Pilgrim Press.

Patterson D: *Get my people going: On a journey toward wellness,* Memphis, TN, 2012, Church Health Center.

Patterson D: Top ten ways to improve the health of a congregation, *Church Health Read* 3(1):5, 2013.

Power R, Toone AR, Deal B: Nurse educator perceptions of faith-based organizations for service-learning, *Nursing Faculty Publications and Presentations* Paper 18, 2016.

Puchalski C: *FICA Spiritual History Tool of the George Washington Institute for Spirituality and Health,* 2018. Retrieved from https://smhs.gwu.edu.

Solari-Twadell PA, Brown, AR: Integration of faith community nursing into health care systems: stimulating community-based quality care strategies. In: Solari-Twadell PA, Ziebarth DJ, eds.: *Faith community nursing: an international specialty practice changing the understanding of health,* Switzerland, 2020, Springer Nature, p. 213-226.

Solari-Twadell PA, Ziebarth DJ, editors: *Faith community nursing: an international specialty practice changing the understanding of health,* Switzerland, 2020, Springer Nature.

Solari-Twadell PA, Ziebarth DJ: Research agenda in faith community nursing. In Solari-Twadell PA, Ziebarth DJ, editors: *Faith community nursing: an international specialty practice changing the understanding of health,* Switzerland, 2020, Springer Nature, p. 231-356.

US Department of Health and Human Services: *Healthy People 2030.* HHS, 2020. Available at https://health.gov/healthypeople.

Westberg GE: *Presentation on 12 September 1985, Westberg Collection,* Loyola University at Chicago University Archives, Box 1, folder 3, 1.

Westberg GE: *The parish nurse: providing a minister of health for your congregation,* Minneapolis, 1990, Augsburg Press.

Westberg GE, McNamara JW: *The parish nurse: How to start a parish nurse program in your church,* Park Ridge, IL, 1987, Parish Nurse Resource Center.

Westberg Institute: *Position paper: Faith community nursing (FCN): Direct care or "hands-on" practice and glucose testing,* Memphis, 2018, Church Health.

Westberg Institute: *About the institute,* 2020. Retrieved from westberginstitute.org.

Young S, Urban parish nurses: a qualitative analysis of the organization of work in community-based practices, *J Nurs Educ Pract* 6(2):19–26, 2016.

Young S, Smothers: Partnership for faith community nurse practice: a model of nursing faculty practice within a faith community, *Perspectives* 17(1):4–5, 2018.

Zerull LM: FCNs active around the world, *Perspectives* 17(2), Church Health: 8–9, 2018.

Ziebarth D: Factors that lead to hospital readmissions and interventions to reduce them: moving toward a faith community nursing intervention, *Int J Faith Community Nurs,* Spring, 2015. Retrieved from https://digitalcommons.wku.edu/.

Ziebarth DJ: *Transitional care interventions as implemented by faith community nurses,* Dissertation, Philadelphia, 2016, LWW Journals.

Ziebarth D, Campbell KP: A transitional care model: using faith community nurses, *J Christ Nurs* 33(2):112–118, 2016.

30

The Nurse in Public Health, Home Health, Palliative Care, and Hospice

Karen S. Martin and Kathryn H. Bowles

OBJECTIVES

After reading this chapter, the student should be able to:

1. Compare different practice models for home- and community-based services.
2. Summarize the basic roles and responsibilities of public health, home health, hospice, and palliative care nurses.
3. Differentiate the professional standards and educational requirements for nurses in public health, home health, hospice, and palliative care.
4. Describe the three components of the Omaha System.
5. Recognize how nurses in public health, home health, hospice, and palliative care use best practices, evidence-based practice, and quality improvement strategies to improve the care they provide.
6. Cite examples of trends and opportunities in public health, home health, hospice, and palliative care involving technology, informatics, and telehealth.

CHAPTER OUTLINE

KEY TERMS

Public health, home health, hospice, and palliative care nursing are rapidly expanding specialties under the broad umbrella of public health, community-oriented, and population-focused practice. When nurses practicing these specialties provide comprehensive assessment, planning, intervention, and evaluation services, they contribute to the total health of the general public, as noted on the first page of this book and Chapter 1. Two additional nurse-led models are summarized in this chapter, the Nurse-Family Partnership (NFP) and transitional care. Although the practice of these nurses is very diverse, evidence-based practice should be the goal.

For the purposes of this chapter, public health, home health, hospice, and palliative care nursing refer to a wide variety of practice settings and holistic services typically provided to clients of all ages by these nurses in their residences, noninstitutional settings, and some institutional settings. In general, public health and home health providers offer intermittent, skilled supportive care, treatments, and/or assistance with activities of daily living so that elders and others who are ill or have disabilities remain safe and avoid unnecessary hospitalization. Hospice and palliative care services are intended to provide comfort and meet physical, emotional, and spiritual needs of all ages. Hospice services are provided at end of life and do not include curative treatment, according to Medicare rules. In contrast, palliative care is a wider range of services, is not limited to the days or weeks prior to end of life, and may include curative treatment.

A number of agencies have agreements with diverse settings, including residential and acute care facilities, so that nurses provide services in locations in addition to clients' homes. These additional settings include:

- Community or senior centers
- Libraries
- Corrections facilities, and
- Work sites.

As will be described later, public health, home health, hospice, and palliative care nurses and their interprofessional colleagues are employed by diverse organizations such as public health departments and voluntary, hospital-based, and proprietary organizations. It is very important to note that an organization's name does not predict the types of programs and services provided.

Numerous references in this chapter describe research, finances, client personal preference, and new technology suggesting that the home is the optimal location for diverse health and nursing services (Ansberry, 2018; Buhler-Wilkerson, 2002; Gao, Maganti, and Monsen, 2017; Gorski, 2017; Marrelli, 2018a; Milone-Nuzzo and Hollars, 2017; NFP, 2017; National Hospice and Palliative Care Organization [NHPCO], 2018; Reddy, 2018; Wright, 2018). Client residences include houses, apartments, trailers, boarding and care homes, hospice houses, assisted living facilities, shelters, and cars. Home health, hospice, and palliative services are provided by formal caregivers who include:

- Nurses
- Social workers
- Physical and occupational therapists
- Home health aides

- Licensed practical nurses
- Chaplains
- Physicians and others.

Because of the nature of the practice, a team approach and interprofessional collaboration are required. The specific disciplines involved vary with the program, the intensity of the client and family's needs, the location of the program and home, and reimbursement, if required.

The Triple Aim model for health care was published in 2008 (Berwick, Nolan, and Whittington, 2008). However, the primary concepts of the model have been the foundation and core values of public health, home health, and related community-based services from their inception:

- Improve the health of populations
- Enhance the experience of care for individuals, and
- Reduce the per capita cost of health care.

The Triple Aim is a good strategy to encourage health promotion, prevention, and healthier lifestyles regardless of the program or setting, although all illness, including chronic illness, cannot be prevented or cured. Although a related concept, population health, is older than the Triple Aim, the term was not widely used in this country until more recently. Population health is the health status of a population of individuals, including the distribution of health status within the group (Kindig and Stoddart, 2003). According to Storfjell, Winslow, and Saunders (2017), nurses must become a well-utilized population health resource and full partner in bringing solutions to the national high-cost/poor-health dilemma.

Access to other health care professionals, resources, and equipment is very different when home and institutional care settings are compared. Many nurses find public health, home health, hospice, and palliative practice very rewarding because they observe the impact of their services and practice with a high degree of autonomy. Nurses who make home visits need to have good:

- Organizational skills
- Communication skills
- Critical thinking skills
- Documentation skills, and
- Understanding of ever-changing reimbursement regulations.

Essential characteristics of these nurses include:

- Competence
- Integrity
- Adaptability
- Good judgment, and
- Creativity.

Public health, home health, hospice, and palliative nurses need to watch for risks in the physical environment and to be savvy about their own safety as well as the safety of their clients. The Agency for Healthcare Research and Quality (AHRQ, 2017) provides rich resources about client and patient safety. It is important to stay alert and change the plan of action quickly if trouble arises when using cars or public transportation, and when inside, entering, or leaving clients' residences (Marrelli, 2018a; Milone-Nuzzo and Hollars, 2017; Schoon, Porta, and Schaffer, 2018). The terms client versus patient are distinguished by who makes the decision to receive services and how much control they have over the services provided. The client has more control while the patient, who has opportunity to make some decisions, has less control.

When entering a residence, the public health, home health, hospice, or palliative care nurse is a guest and needs to earn the trust of the family and establish a partnership with the client and family. It is essential that clients and families are involved in making decisions for home-based services to be efficient and effective; this team approach may be referred to as consumer engagement.

Family is defined by the individual client and includes any caregiver or significant other who assists the client with care at home. Family caregiving involves:

- Transportation
- Helping clients meet their basic needs, and
- Providing care such as personal hygiene, meal preparation, medication administration, and simple as well as complex treatments.

Clients and family caregivers nowadays provide many aspects of care in the home that were previously provided in hospitals or in home by professional caregivers. Care can be confusing, challenging, stressful, burdensome, and frightening for family caregivers; many are not well prepared for their new roles. Clients need to be monitored regularly, and some require 24-hour care. Many family caregivers need assistance to identify diverse support services that enable them to provide care while maintaining their own physical and emotional health (Ansberry, 2018; Chow and Dahlin, 2018; Diefenbeck, Klemm, and Hayes, 2017; Gao et al., 2017; Gasper et al., 2018; Gorski, 2017; Izumi, 2017; Marrelli, 2018a; Milone-Nuzzo and Hollars, 2017; NHPCO, 2018; Reddy, 2018; Wright, 2018).

HOME HEALTH CARE

Evolution of Home Health Care

Home health care provided by formal caregivers in the United States originated in the 19th century. In many communities, the initial programs evolved into nonprofit visiting nurse agencies and health departments. The movement expanded rapidly in the United States, resulting in the formation of 71 home health agencies prior to 1900 and 600 organizations by 1909. Additional historical details are described in Chapter 2 and other publications (Buhler-Wilkerson, 2002; Donahue, 2011).

Home health services were included as a major benefit when Medicare and Medicaid legislation was passed in 1965 and implemented in 1966. (See Chapter 5, Economic Influences.) Both resulted in significant changes nationally. During the next 30 years, the number of Medicare-certified agencies grew rapidly as a result of the aging population and prospective payment legislation that decreased the length of hospital stays. This trend changed when the Balanced Budget Act of 1997 was enacted, changing the home health payment system from a fee-for-service model to prospective payment based on a standardized assessment completed at admission. Between 2004 and 2015, the number of agencies grew by more than 60%, a dramatic increase. However, since 2015, the number of

agencies is declining, possibly due to an intentional consolidation of agencies by the Centers for Medicare and Medicaid Services (CMS) to make oversight easier (Holly, 2020; MedPAC, 2018; US Census Bureau, 2017; Wright, 2018).

Description of Home Health Care

Home health care is a broad concept and approach to services and is at the top of the list of the fastest-growing service-providing industries in this country (Bureau of Labor Statistics [BLS], 2020). It includes a focus on primary, secondary, and tertiary prevention; the primary focus can involve aggregates, similar to those provided by other population-focused nurses. (See the Levels of Prevention box.) Initiatives involving primary and secondary prevention have always been important to home health care.

📋 LEVELS OF PREVENTION

Home Health

Primary Prevention
The nurse (1) administers seasonal and newer strains of flu vaccine or (2) provides case management interventions so clients obtain the vaccines at convenient locations.

Secondary Prevention
The nurse monitors clients in their homes for early signs of new health problems to initiate prompt treatment. When the nurse works collaboratively with the physician and/or nurse practitioner, effective interventions can be provided. An example is monitoring clients for medication side effects.

Tertiary Prevention
The nurse provides instruction about dietary modifications and insulin injections to clients with new diagnoses of diabetes. Clients and their families implement the therapeutic plan to identify signs of infection, prevent complications, and maintain the highest possible level of health and self-care.

Home health nursing is "a specialty area of nursing practice that promotes optimal health and well-being for patients, their families, and caregivers within their homes and communities. Home health nurses use a holistic approach aimed at empowering patients/families/caregivers to achieve their highest levels of physical, functional, spiritual, and psychosocial health. Home health nurses provide nursing services to patients of all ages and cultures and at all stages of health and illness, including end of life" (American Nurses Association [ANA], 2014). Home health nurses include generalist nurses, public health nurses, clinical nurse specialists, and nurse practitioners. They and their interprofessional team members provide diverse services to target populations such as:

- New parents
- Clients recovering from injuries, acute illness, and surgery
- Frail elders
- Clients managing disabilities, and
- Chronic health problems.

Some home health agencies include wellness programs, health fairs, school nurses, communicable disease prevention, and other programs that are similar to those offered by public health departments.

Home health nurses and their team members help clients and their families achieve improved health and independence in a safe environment. In addition to nursing care, the following are available to those who are Medicare eligible:

- Physical therapy
- Occupational therapy
- Speech and language pathology
- Home health aides, and
- Medical social services.

Skilled nursing care and skilled nursing services are the Medicare terms that describe the duties of the registered nurse, refer to the requirement of professional nursing judgment, and include diverse assessment, teaching, case management, and other interventions (CMS, 2016, 2018a, 2018b). Assessment involves environmental, psychosocial, physiologic, and health-related behaviors and concerns, and interventions are categorized as teaching, guidance, and counseling; treatments and procedures; case management; and surveillance (Martin, 2005; Monsen, 2018; Omaha System, 2019a).

According to MedPAC (2020), approximately 3.4 million individuals received Medicare-certified home health services in 2018 that were reimbursed by the CMS. The majority of home health clients were 65 years and older; more were women than men; and many had diagnoses of circulatory disease, diabetes, neurologic conditions, and depression (CMS, 2016; MedPAC, 2018).

Home health agencies can be divided into five general categories (Box 30.1 and Fig. 30.1) (Fazzi, 2018; MedPAC, 2018).

Although agencies vary by programs offered, size, administration, ownership, organization, and board structures, they

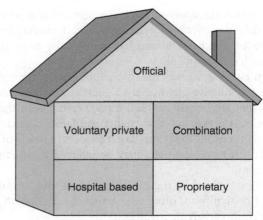

Fig. 30.1 Types of Home Health Agencies.

must meet ever-changing licensure, certification, and accreditation regulations established by national and state groups. The primary source of those regulations is the CMS (CMS, 2017b, 2018a, 2018b, 2019). To be Medicare-certified and reimbursed, the CMS requires that home health agencies, including all five agency categories, complete a rigorous certification process, follow the rules of the Conditions of Participation (CoPs), and provide intermittent skilled professional services (CMS, 2017b).

The CoPs are lengthy, complex, and subject to change. Home health nurses must be well informed about Medicare regulations to determine the visit frequency and timing based on their clients' conditions, and communicate with physicians. Frequently, clients and their families ask nurses to help them understand their Medicare benefits.

HOSPICE AND PALLIATIVE CARE

Evolution of Hospice and Palliative Care

Hospice care was introduced in the United States in the 1970s by Florence Wald, often referred to as the mother of the hospice movement. Before establishing the Connecticut Hospice in 1974, Dr. Wald collaborated with Dame Cicely Saunders, a British nurse, physician, and social worker who founded St. Christopher's Hospice in England in 1967 (ANA/Hospice and Palliative Nurses Association [HPNA], 2014; Wright, 2018; Zerwekh, 2006). During the same era, Dr. Elisabeth Kübler-Ross, a physician, published *On Death and Dying* (1969), a book that was widely read by the public and health care professionals. Dr. Ross described the inhumanity of a death-denying society such as the United States, the need to provide sensitive end-of-life care and involve clients in choices, and an emphasis on the quality of life (ANA/HPNA, 2014; Perry and Parente, 2017; Zerwekh, 2006).

Medicaid reimbursement for hospice care began in 1980 and Medicare in 1983; reimbursement determines many aspects of the programs, including the types and length of services. Services not covered by Medicare may be covered by other insurance plans or charitable organizations.

Because the time of death is difficult to predict and many people in this country are reluctant to acknowledge a terminal

---

BOX 30.1   Descriptions of Home Health Agencies

- Official or public health agencies receive tax revenue and are operated by state, county, city, or other local government units, such as health departments. Typically, official agencies also offer well-child clinics, immunizations, health education programs, and home visits for preventive health care.
- Voluntary and private agencies are nonprofit home health agencies and usually receive some funds from United Way, donations, and endowments. Currently, there are approximately the same number of voluntary and private agencies. Visiting Nurse Associations, for example, are usually freestanding, voluntary, nonprofit organizations governed by a board of directors, and usually financed by earnings, donations, and tax-deductible contributions. Sometimes they are categorized with combination agencies because of their similar characteristics.
- Combination agencies have characteristics of both governmental and voluntary agencies. The number of combination agencies continues to decrease, although some are large agencies.
- Hospital-based agencies grew rapidly during the 1970s and 1980s, when the advent of diagnosis-related groups led to earlier hospital discharges and Medicare reimbursement was encouraging. Since then, some hospitals and their home health agencies separated because of changes in reimbursement and other pressures.
- Proprietary agencies are freestanding, for-profit agencies that are required to pay taxes. Many are part of large chains. Proprietary agencies now dominate the industry and represent approximately 80% or more of all agencies. Almost all new providers are proprietary agencies.

prognosis, hospice care often begins late in the disease process. Barriers and stigmas continue to be associated with hospice for some clients, families, and physicians. Because they equate hospice with hopelessness and giving up, they are reluctant to consider hospice. A number of the same people are receptive to the concept of palliative care and will accept those services (Buch and Nies, 2019; CMS, 2018b; Gasper et al., 2018; Marrelli, 2018b; NHPCO, 2018; Perry and Parente, 2017; Stober, 2017; Wright, 2018; Zerwekh, 2006).

In 1987, the first comprehensive, integrated palliative care program was established in the United States at the Cleveland Clinic. The focus was specialized care for those living with signs and symptoms and the stress of serious illness. Similar palliative care programs originated earlier in England (Etkind et al., 2017). In 1999, the Robert Wood Johnson Foundation (RWJF) funded the Center to Advance Palliative Care (CAPC) to stimulate the development of high-quality palliative care programs in hospitals and other health care settings. In 2010, the CAPC convened a consensus panel to establish criteria for palliative care assessment components at hospital admission and during the hospital stay (CAPC, 2018; Weissman and Meier, 2011). Assessment items include:

- Recent history of the illness
- Pain and symptom assessment
- Patient-centered goals of care, and
- Transition of care plans.

The goal is to help clinicians identify those individuals and their families who need palliative care.

Description of Hospice and Palliative Care

Hospice and palliative care are similar and, yet, very different. Similarities that are described throughout this chapter include:

- A client-focused/consumer engagement approach
- Holistic
- Evidence-based practice
- Emphasis on ethics
- Communication skills
- Interprofessional collaboration
- Care coordination
- Focus on transitions of care
- Caregiving skills that include symptom management, pain relief, and comfort.

The differences are primarily related to reimbursement requirements in this country and include the length of care and frequency and intensity of services (Box 30.2).

Palliative care is a broad term occurring over a longer period of time, and hospice is a subset with a short time period. The HPNA developed an illustration referred to as the Trajectories of Palliative Care and included it in their 2014 publication (ANA/HPNA, 2014). The title of the illustration is palliative care and represents an extended continuum of chronic serious illness to acute serious illness during which stabilization and exacerbations may occur. Services and treatment vary during this time. The continuum encompasses three segments: a longer segment that is referred to as diagnosis, limited signs and symptoms, and increasing severity of signs and symptoms; a relatively short period of hospice care and death; and a period of bereavement care for family members.

> **BOX 30.2** **The Goals of Hospice and Palliative Care Services**
>
> - The goal of the hospice movement is to humanize the end-of-life experience. For hospice services, physicians need to indicate that clients have 6 months or fewer to live, and clients acknowledge that they have a terminal prognosis and select care that is comfortable, not life-extending.
> - In contrast, the goal of palliative care is quality of life, and palliative services are not restricted based on disease or disease progress. Palliative services may be appropriate for those with a serious, complex illness regardless if they are expected to recover fully, live with a chronic illness for an extended time, or experience serious disease progression (ANA/HPNA, 2014; CMS, 2019; 2018a, 2018b; Chow and Dahlin, 2018; Etkind et al., 2017; Perry and Parente, 2017; Slipka and Monsen, 2018; US Census Bureau, 2017).

The HPNA is an umbrella organization that represents hospice and palliative nurses and other members of the team employed in home-based organizations as well as acute and long-term care, outpatient, and other settings (ANA/HPNA, 2014, 2017). The organization's mission is to advance expert care during serious illness; it is based on four pillars of education, advocacy, leadership, and research. Nurses who are members of hospice and palliative care teams "provide evidence-based physical, emotional, psychosocial, and spiritual or existential care to individuals and families experiencing life-limiting, progressive illness" (ANA/HPNA, 2014). The definition of hospice focuses on comfort for individuals and their families at the end of life and does not include curative treatment. The HPNA did not define their specialty in their new 2014 publication, but instead, endorsed the definition of the National Consensus Project of Palliative Care (NCP) definition. "Palliative care means patient and family-centered care that optimizes quality of life by anticipating, preventing, and treating suffering. Palliative care throughout the continuum of illness involves addressing the physical, intellectual, emotional, social, and spiritual needs and [facilitating] patient autonomy, access to information, and choice" (NCP, 2013; NCP, 2018).

Both the interprofessional hospice and palliative care teams work closely together to provide comprehensive care in partnership with clients and their families. The teams include:

- Nurses
- Physicians
- Social workers
- Therapists
- Chaplains
- Counselors
- Aides
- Pharmacists
- Volunteers

The need for employees and volunteers is increasing dramatically (BSL, 2020). Most agencies and team members consider conferences and continuing education essential to develop and renew their skills involving topics such as advance care planning, end-of-life comfort measures, new medications and treatments, therapeutic communication, compassion fatigue, spirituality, complex family dynamics, and cultural awareness. Working with clients who are dying involves unique emotional stress; hospice and palliative care programs usually address the team's well-being as well as that of the clients and families (ANA/HPNA, 2014, 2017; Buch and Nies, 2019; Diefenbeck et al., 2017; Hinds et al., 2005; Izumi, 2017; NHPCO, 2018; Slipka and Monsen, 2018; Wright, 2018; Zerwekh, 2006).

Clients and their families and friends are at the center of the hospice and palliative care teams and will be involved in advance care planning, symptom and medication management, personal care, and the use of supplies. Death produces intense emotions even when family members have prepared for it. Bereavement services that are part of hospice involve attending the funeral or other services for the deceased client, and contact at anniversaries of death, holidays, and the client's birthday for 13 months after the client's death. Hospice organizations usually offer support group opportunities for families or refer them to support groups in the area.

Palliative care has no specific federal designation as a specialty; rather, it exists as a consultative discipline delivering a philosophy of care. Palliative care programs in hospitals have been growing steadily. Palliative care clinicians must meet certain regulatory requirements when they practice in home health or other community agencies (ANA/HPNA, 2014).

Hospice is a formalized, funded program in hospice and home health agencies with extensive data. For that reason, it is the focus of the following paragraphs. Initially, cancer was the primary diagnosis of most clients in hospice programs. More recently, cancer is the diagnosis of approximately 20% to 30% of hospice clients, and dementia, cardiac and circulatory, neurologic, respiratory, and other end-stage diseases make up 70% to 80% of the diagnoses (NHPCO, 2018). More than one million clients received Medicare-certified hospice services in 2017, with an average stay of 87.8 days (MedPAC, 2018). The average length of stay will rise if home health nurses and others provide information about end-of-life hospice care to clients and families and if hospice becomes more widely accepted by the public. Most agencies are educating their nurses to recognize clients in need of hospice or palliative care and have discussions with clients and families as a strategy to decrease the hospice stigma that results in late referrals or missed opportunities. Even when nurses, physicians, and others discuss quality of life and encourage the transition from palliative services to hospice, clients and/or families may continue in denial and not accept hospice until the last several days of life. Late referrals resulting in brief hospice stays make it difficult for the hospice team to provide comprehensive, expert, cost-effective services to clients and families. For many in this country, death is not viewed as a normal or natural part of the life cycle (Buch and Nies, 2019; Izumi, 2017; Marrelli, 2018b; NHPCO, 2018; Perry and Parente, 2017; Wright, 2018; Zerwekh, 2006).

Hospice providers can be divided into four general categories. Freestanding facilities are the most common, followed by home health agencies and hospital-based facilities. Skilled nursing facilities are the least common. Many freestanding facilities are for-profit providers, similar to home health agencies (NHPCO, 2018).

After the client acknowledges a terminal prognosis and selects comforting care rather than life-extending or curative care, hospice organizations coordinate services in partnership with the client and family and provide financial case management.

Hospice is the only Medicare benefit that includes medications, medical equipment, 24-hour/7-day-a-week access to care, and support for family members after death. Authorization by physicians is required for the certification periods (CMS, 2018c, 2019; Perry and Parente, 2017).

Hospice programs are usually operated and staffed as independent entities or corporations even when they are part of a larger organization because of the specialized nature of the practice and the complex Medicare regulations and financial requirements. Similar to home health, hospice nurses must be familiar with regulations and financial requirements; however, the Outcomes and Assessment Information Set (OASIS) is not a requirement for hospice programs as it is for home health.

Medicare, Medicaid, the US Department of Veterans Affairs (VA), managed care, private insurance, and private donations fund most hospice services. Medicare provides the most funds. Hospice services account for approximately 6% of the total Medicare budget, approximately twice as much as home health services (CMS, 2016, 2018b, 2019; NHPCO, 2018).

Home Care of Dying Children

"The death of a child alters the life and health of others immediately and for the rest of their lives" (Hinds et al., 2005, p. S70). The needs of dying children and their families are unique because of the degree of emotional impact and because the young are not expected to die or predecease their parents. Nurses need to recognize the child's physical, cognitive, psychosocial, and spiritual development as well as the family's dynamics, cultural heritage, and spiritual beliefs. That recognition is essential to provide appropriate pain management, assist the child and family to communicate with each other, advocate for their needs in the community, and provide case management and continuity of care (Hinds et al., 2005; Kaye et al., 2015; Levine et al., 2017; Weaver et al., 2016).

Bereavement programs as described for hospice programs are especially important for families who have lost a child. Parents, grandparents, and siblings can participate in a variety of support groups offered by the hospice program or other bereavement organizations (Levine et al., 2017; Weaver et al., 2016).

ADDITIONAL NURSE-LED MODELS

The NFP and transitional care are focused on interprofessional collaboration as well as care coordination, critical thinking, best practices, and evidence-based practice. Best practices suggest using credible, established evidence from a variety of sources including research, experience, and expert clinicians; evidence-based practice suggests increased emphasis on programs of research that demonstrate consistently good outcomes (Melnyk and Fineout-Overholt, 2019; Melnyk and Gallagher-Ford, 2015). With both models, nurses have essential roles in the provision of care, documentation of services, program development and

HOW TO USE A HOSPICE APPROACH TO CARE IN ANY SETTING

The hospice philosophy of care means providing comfort measures to individuals before death and support for their families before and after death. Individuals may be any age. Death may occur in the individual's home, a hospital setting, or an uncontrolled setting such as the community. How does one adapt nursing care in any situation? What basic skills can professional caregivers use that can be applied in any situation or setting? How do professional caregivers adapt to the death of a hospice client, inpatient death, or a sudden, unexpected death where, for example, many people have died as a result of a natural disaster or a terrorist act?

- Be prepared. Consider your own philosophy of death so that you can assist others without distraction when that time comes.
- Cultures vary in their beliefs about and responses to death. Know the differences in cultural responses so that you can effectively help people in their time of need.
- Death events cannot be totally controlled, even in a hospice environment where the eventual death has been illustrated to family and friends and the dying individual before the death. Expect the unexpected and take cues from the client and the loved ones regarding their needs.
- Shock, disbelief, and crisis reactions occur even with prepared hospice deaths. Ask family and caregivers what they need; provide them with the basics such as food or blankets; provide comfort; if it is not contraindicated, provide the family/friends with personal effects or mementos of the individual; give sensitive, caring support. Sit with them and listen.

Modified from Mistovich JJ, Karren KJ: *Prehospital emergency care*, 10th ed., Upper Saddle River, 2014, Pearson Education; Mistovich JJ, Karren, KJ: *Prehospital emergency care*, 11th ed., Upper Saddle River, 2018, Pearson Education.

management, outcome measurement and effectiveness analysis, and public education.

Nurse-Family Partnership

The NFP was initiated in 1977 by a researcher, David Olds, and a nurse, Harriet Kitzman; it is probably the best-known and most well-funded nurse home visit specialty program in the United States (Enoch et al., 2016; NFP, 2017; Olds et al., 1997). The Partnership is a network of nurses, families, and policy makers. Nurses receive extensive orientation and provide structured education and case management during regularly scheduled home visits to pregnant women; visits continue until the children's second birthday. The goals of the program are to improve pregnancy outcomes, child health and development, and economic self-sufficiency of the families.

Transitional Care

As a result of a fragmented health care system, increasing complexity of client care, and rising costs, transitional care has gained much needed attention in this country and internationally (Meadows et al., 2014). Transitional care is defined as "a set of actions designed to ensure the coordination and continuity of health care as clients transfer between different locations and different levels of care in the same location" (Parry et al., 2008). Challenges to quality care originate from a lack of depth, accuracy, and timeliness of information received from the referring site; the need for complex medication reconciliation; and difficulties with communication and coordination among community-based providers.

Transitional care programs that involve home health have emerged as low- and high-intensity interventions that include, but vary from, traditional home health interventions. Low-intensity interventions provided by the nurse include coaching, telephone follow-up, and specific disease management programs. High-intensity transitional care programs are designed for populations who have complex or high-risk health problems and usually provided by advanced practice nurses. Outcomes achieved with the Transitional Care Model consistently show cost savings and improvements in clinical and quality outcomes for clients receiving the intervention compared with usual care (Naylor et al., 2013, 2016, 2017). The most common outcome across all populations is a consistent reduction in readmissions to a hospital.

? CHECK YOUR PRACTICE

You are working with a home health agency that is interested in defining the populations they serve. You have been asked to suggest an approach to accomplish this task. What approach would you suggest and how can you help with the task? What would you do? See if you can apply these steps to this scenario. (1) Recognize the cues, looking at available data, like reports developed by the agency where the population data can be found; (2) analyze the cues, looking at the numbers of clients in various age groups, ethnicity, locations, and diagnoses; (3) state several and prioritize the hypotheses you have stated; (4) generate solutions for each hypothesis; (5) take action on the number one hypothesis you think best offers the plan that will define the populations; and (6) evaluate the outcomes you would expect as a result of the work you will do to define the populations.

POPULATION HEALTH

Population health is the health status of a population of individuals, including the distribution of health status within the group, as mentioned early in this chapter and in Chapter 1. The field or emerging specialization of population health includes health status, determinants of the population's health, and policies and interventions that link those two (Kindig and Stoddart, 2003). After the concepts of the Triple Aim were widely embraced, population health began appearing more frequently in practice, education, research, health care literature, and the public press. The speed increased when CMS and private insurers began to move away from fee-for-service reimbursement and toward value-based care. An example of a population health approach will be described in the Medication Management section later in this chapter.

SCOPE AND STANDARDS OF PRACTICE

Nursing is a theory and practice-based profession that incorporates art and science. Examples of nursing, family, and systems theories are mentioned and summarized in other chapters of this book. Chapter 7 focuses on cultural diversity and includes many references. Chapter 9 addresses evidence-based practice; the concept is addressed frequently in this chapter, and one example is included. Several chapters of this book describe the Quad Council Coalition's (2018) eight domains of practice; those domains are linked to information in this chapter in the Applying Content to Practice box.

The nursing process is the theoretical framework used by the ANA, which notes that the nursing process is the essential methodology by which client goals are identified and achieved. Their scope and standards publications, including those for public health, home health nursing, and palliative nursing, are organized according to the nursing process and contain two sections: the Standards of Care and the Standards of Professional Performance (ANA, 2013, 2014; ANA/HPNA, 2014). Publications include the six steps of the nursing process: assessment, diagnosis, outcomes identification, planning, implementation, and evaluation. The steps are linked to standards and more specific measurement criteria that are stated in behavioral objectives. The standards address:

- Quality of care
- Performance appraisal
- Critical thinking skills
- Education
- Collegiality
- Ethics
- Collaboration
- Research, and
- Resource use.

OMAHA SYSTEM

The Omaha System was initially developed to operationalize the nursing process and provide a practical, easily understood, computer-compatible, quantifiable guide for daily use in diverse community settings. It is the only ANA-recognized terminology developed inductively by and for nurses who practice in the community. It is primarily used by home health agencies (Omaha System, 2019b).

As early as 1970, the staff and administrators of the Visiting Nurse Association (VNA) of Omaha, Nebraska, began addressing nursing practice, documentation, and information management concerns. At that time, no systematic nomenclature or classification of client problems existed that could be used with a problem-oriented record system, and practitioners were not using computers. These realities provided the incentive for initiating research.

During the next 20 years, the VNA of Omaha staff conducted four extensive, federally funded Omaha System development, reliability, validity, and usability research projects. The result of the research was the Problem Classification Scheme, the Intervention Scheme, and the Problem Rating Scale for Outcomes. These three components of the Omaha System were designed to be used together, be comprehensive, relatively simple, hierarchical, multidimensional, and computer compatible.

As depicted in Fig. 30.2, the Omaha System conceptual model is based on the dynamic, interactive nature of the nursing or problem-solving process, the practitioner-client relationship, and concepts of diagnostic reasoning, critical thinking, and quality improvement. The client as an individual, a family, or a community appears at the center of the model; this location shows the many ways the Omaha System can be used and the essential partnership between clients and practitioners. Most nurses and other clinicians employed in community settings

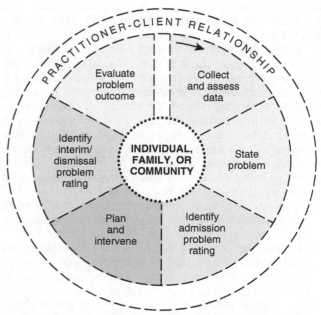

Fig. 30.2 Omaha System Model of the Problem-Solving Process. (From Martin KS: *The Omaha System: a key to practice, documentation, and information management*, reprinted, 2nd ed., Omaha, 2005, Health Connections Press.)

recognized that partnership was essential from the beginning of their employment. The outer circle is the practitioner-client relationship.

The Omaha System was intended for use by nurses and all members of the health care delivery team. The goals of the research were:

1. To develop a structured and comprehensive system that could be both understood and used by members of various disciplines.
2. To foster collaborative practice.

Therefore the Omaha System was designed to guide practice decisions, sort and document pertinent client data uniformly, and provide a framework for an agency-wide, multidisciplinary clinical information management system capable of meeting the daily needs of clinicians, managers, and administrators (Eardley et al., 2018; Martin, 2005; Martin and Kessler, 2017; Monsen et al., 2018; Omaha System, 2018a; Quad Council Coalition, 2018). See the tools in Appendix B.4 for the Omaha System Problem Classification Scheme with Case Study Application.

An alphabetical list of 75 targets or objects of action and one "other" appear at the second level. Client-specific information generated by clinicians is at the third level. The Intervention Scheme provides the terms for care plans and services. It enables clinicians to describe, quantify, and communicate their practice, including improving or restoring health, describing deterioration, or preventing illness.

GUIDELINES FOR NURSES

Nursing practice is based on education, experience, and evidence. Because home health and hospice and palliative care nurses usually work with clients and their families in their homes, they must

> **BOX 30.3 Guidelines for Public Health, Home Health, and Hospice Practice in a Home Visit; and for Other Noninstitutional Settings**
>
> - Review client data, including the referral from the intake department, hospital discharge summary, orders, and plan of care to become familiar with the client's history, purpose of the visit, and expectations.
> - Contact the client or family by calling the telephone number listed on the referral information to obtain agreement for the visit, schedule the day and time, and discuss the address.
> - Gather agency and Medicare forms, a nursing bag, cellular phone or pager, portable computing device, teaching materials, and supplies; understand the client's location; follow the agency policy when checking out for the visit.
> - Observe the neighborhood for resources and safety when approaching the client's home.
> - Greet the client/family to begin developing a positive, appropriate professional relationship; involve them as much as possible during the visit and postvisit activities.
> - Obtain signatures and complete needed forms.
> - Provide care by completing a comprehensive assessment, identifying client problems, providing interventions, and evaluating client outcomes. Interventions may include teaching, guidance, and counseling; treatments and procedures; case management; and surveillance (Martin, 2005).
> - Discuss the plan of care with the client and family during informal or formal conferences; modify as needed.
> - Document some or all of the visit details in the home, preferably while using a portable computing device and an electronic health record (EHR).
> - Discuss the next visit as well as follow-up activities and referrals.
> - Proceed to the next scheduled visit after checking in, according to the agency policy.
> - Complete remaining visit documentation, submit forms, coordinate referrals to other community resources, and communicate with agency colleagues, the referral source, physicians, and others as appropriate. Obtain revised orders if needed.
> - Revisit to reassess the client and provide care.

develop skills to conduct home visits efficiently, effectively, and safely, including (Box 30.3):

- A positive attitude about client-centered care, the nurse-client partnership, and consumer engagement
- Critical thinking skills
- Effective care coordination requires familiarity with community resources.
- Knowledge and skills involving medications, treatments, documentation, and equipment are necessary.

Clinical Example From Community-Focused Practice

The example describes an innovative and collaborative community-focused program developed in Tucson, Arizona, by the Pima County Health Department and the Pima County Public Library. Since this program was initiated, other communities have involved nurses in their libraries (Innes, 2012; RWJF, 2013, 2018). The Pima County Public Library requested that the health department hire a social worker to increase safety and a welcoming environment in five high-risk libraries. Concerns included loitering, behavioral health concerns, encampment, and abandonment. Many patrons were homeless and/or had chronic diseases that were not being managed. Children and elders were left at the library by family members while they completed errands or went to work.

After a careful analysis, the decision was made by the Public Health Nursing Division Manager and the Health Department and Library management staff to hire one full-time public health nurse in January 2012, a first in this country. It was decided that a nurse could better meet the identified needs of the patrons and library staff. In addition to increasing safety and a welcoming environment, a goal was to coordinate with community resource agencies to provide nutritious snacks for children and reduce hunger concerns.

During the first year, the program expanded to include five public health nurses working in six high-risk libraries. They made 180 visits to the libraries and had 2181 patron encounters. Client problems and clinician interventions were documented. The most frequently identified problems were health care supervision, nutrition, circulation, hearing, personal care, and cognition. The nurses instructed the library staff on communicable disease prevention topics. During the first year, calls made to the police and 911 were reduced by 6% and calls to 911 for medical emergencies were reduced by 20%.

In the second year, the program expanded to 13 library sites, including 2 bookmobile sites serving rural communities. Student nurses assisted the public health nurses as they completed community assessments and tailored services to the needs of each library. Working with library patrons, nurses completed 3746 encounters and 1160 assessments; 1420 health education sessions; and 192 referrals for services. They also provided health education to 76 library staff members. During the third year, nurses provided diverse health education and services to patrons. Services include assistance applying for public or private insurance, diabetes education, flu vaccine, and health education for library staff.

Using the Omaha System and an automated documentation system to capture community-level data had numerous benefits. Included were communication between the nurses and between the nurses and their health department; an evidence-based approach to practice; a standardized method of assessment, care planning, services, and evaluation; and a process that generated accurate and consistent data capable of conversion to information and useful reports.

LINKAGES IN THE PRACTICE SETTING

There are no limits to the diversity of clients who live in the community, their problems, and their strengths; the interventions that nurses provide; and the client outcome data that are generated. Although many examples are diverse, as can be seen in the practice application, they represent a small fraction of the actual roles and responsibilities of public health, home health, hospice, and palliative care nurses.

The fundamental principles of professional practice are:

1. A holistic approach to the steps of the nursing or problem-solving process
2. Consumer engagement or a partnership with clients as unique individuals, families, and communities
3. Focus on outcomes

The following sections of the chapter are designed to increase the reader's understanding about the links between systematic best practices, evidence-based practice, and other aspects of the public health, home health, hospice, and palliative milieu. The typical nurse will not be involved with the theme of each section daily but will over a period of months.

Setting short- and long-term goals provides criteria for evaluation and increases continuity of care and the potential for improved outcomes. Research has shown that goals set with the client rather than for the client are more successful regarding self-motivation, adherence, and attainment (Curtis et al., 2018; Zhang et al., 2015).

Outcome and Assessment Information

The Outcomes and Assessment Information Set (OASIS) measures outcomes for quality improvement and client satisfaction with care. Funded by the CMS and the RWJF, OASIS underwent extensive testing and is required for use by Medicare-certified home health agencies (Marrelli, 2018b).

Completion of the OASIS provides a systematic, comparative measurement of client outcomes at two or more points in time. The completed OASIS improves communication about the clients' conditions among the agency's clinicians, other agency staff, and external groups; improves reimbursement; and demonstrates improved, cost-effective client outcomes as a result of home health services. OASIS also provides data for calculating the agency's reimbursement for a particular client's episode and promotes a standardized approach to assessment within the home care industry (Fig. 30.3) (CMS, 2020). OASIS results are publicly reported by CMS on Home Health Compare to provide comparisons of agency performance on select OASIS items such as improvement in managing daily activities and pain, treating symptoms, and preventing unplanned hospitalization (Medicare, n.d.).

The OASIS has had several revisions to improve its comprehensiveness, ease of use, reliability, and validity. The current version, OASIS-C2, was implemented on January 1, 2017, and the OASIS-D collection became available in January of 2019 to meet requirements within the IMPACT Act of 2014 (CMS, 2018c). Major sections include functional, physical, and service-related items, each followed by a list of choices or fill-in-the-blanks (CMS, 2017b).

The OASIS is a complex and important component of home health practice. While providing care in the home, a nurse or therapist (physical, occupational, or speech and language) collects and completes the OASIS with the client and their caregivers at the start of care, after hospitalization, at the 60-day recertification date following admission, at discharge, or if transferred to a facility. It is important for clinicians to complete the OASIS accurately and consistently to reflect a client's actual status and integrate the OASIS with other portions of the agency's comprehensive assessment. They or their colleagues compare initial data to future versions, as do Medicare surveyors and reimbursement reviewers. Final data from the OASIS must be submitted to CMS electronically.

The OASIS offers a challenging assignment for those who provide direct care, and one that requires extensive orientation and review. In many agencies, nurse experts serve as compliance officers to help ensure accurate and consistent completion. Not only is evidence of the quality of care related to OASIS but so is agency reimbursement and a publicly available comparison of their client outcomes to those of other agencies. Agencies may receive sanctions or be denied payment by CMS for services provided based on claims data, audits, or surveys that reflect responses on OASIS. More recently, agencies have received Additional Development Requests (ADRs) generated by CMS. ADRs require agencies to submit extensive verification that the services they provided were essential; if verification is not adequate, agencies must initiate a legal appeal or return funds to CMS.

Target areas for emphasis on OASIS mirror clients' health challenges identified by nurses and home health agencies. Included are diabetic foot care, fall prevention, depression intervention, pain, pressure ulcers, safety, medication management, and infection control. Although all target areas are important, the latter two are of special concern to many nurses employed in hospice and palliative programs, as well as diverse public health and other health care settings; they are summarized next.

Medication Management

Medication management is an important component of home health practice. The goal is to assist clients and family caregivers to become independent and reliable in managing medication administration at home, and prevent adverse drug events, side effects, inadequate symptom control, and hospitalizations. However, home health clients experience many challenges, including the complexity of their chronic conditions, impaired cognitive status, inadequate coordination of their medical care, drug-drug interactions and side effects of medications, and cost.

Home health nurses expect to spend considerable time with medication reconciliation and management. They address medications during the initial and subsequent home visits. Unlike clients in residential settings, home health clients may or may not have all of their medications, may not take them as ordered, and may not store them appropriately. When nurses ask to see medications, they are often given a box or bag that

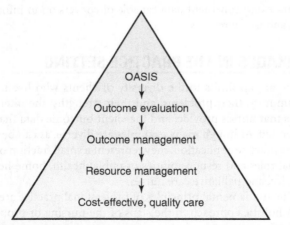

Fig. 30.3 The Outcome Paradigm. *OASIS*, Outcome and Assessment Information Set. (From Centers for Medicare and Medicaid Services: *Outcome-based quality improvement (OBQI) manual*, Baltimore, 2012, CMS. pp. 2.4, 2.10.)

includes current medications and ones that are extremely outdated, discontinued, or prescribed for other family members.

Many tools are available in addition to those specific for home health nurses to assess and manage medication administration. Teaching clients to use a medication organizer for oral medications is frequently an initial intervention. However, that alone does not ensure that medications will be taken appropriately; subsequent teaching, return demonstrations, and surveillance are essential. Often the medication administration is complex, with multiple drugs, in repeated dosages throughout the day, by various routes of administration.

A population health approach to medication management, for example, might be for providers to screen the medication regimen of all heart failure patients for complexity and polypharmacy. They would then work with their interdisciplinary partners (physicians and pharmacists) to simplify the medication regimen. This is also an area in need of further research and innovation.

Nurses must also understand the impact of medication management on the client and seek clients' perspectives, voices, and needs around medication adherence and management (Zullig and Hayden, 2017). Self-efficacy, or the person's belief in their ability to manage their medications, is associated with medication adherence (Huang, Shiyanbola, and Smith, 2018). In addition, clients and caregivers need comprehensive materials about medication benefits, interactions, and side effects as well as the steps they should take to communicate that information to others (Roux et al., 2018). Materials need to be simple, understandable, and in the appropriate language. Clients who cannot read need graphic materials.

Another growing medication-related challenge is the management of opioid medications and overdose risk in home and community settings. Clinicians must be aware of addiction issues; know how to safely administer an antidote or direct its administration by others; and teach clients and caregivers how to safely administer, store, and dispose of narcotics (McAuley, Munro, and Taylor, 2018). Home care agencies have policies on the safe disposal of narcotics and other pharmaceutical products. Proper disposal is important for client, child, and environmental safety, and the nurse has a role in teaching safe disposal by the client. The US Food and Drug Administration (FDA) provides guidance on where and how to dispose of unused medicines through drug take-back programs or self-disposal through the trash or down the sink or toilet (FDA, 2020). Under current law, unless there is local legislation that allows disposal, home health and hospice staff are not legally permitted to handle or destroy controlled substances in the home. Pending legislation regarding the disposal of unused medication will permit disposal by clinicians if passed (National Association for Home Care and Hospice [NAHC], 2018).

Infection Prevention

Infection prevention is an important priority in home health and hospice practice. Infection prevention usually focuses on wound care and invasive devices such as urinary and intravenous catheters as well as chest, tracheostomy, gastrostomy, and other tubes. Preventing infection by promoting appropriate

vaccinations such as flu and pneumonia is also a priority. Most importantly, nurses need to assume that every client is potentially infected or colonized with an organism that can be transmitted, and recognize that all blood and body secretions may contain transmissible agents. They need to be familiar with the infectious process, research evidence and best practices, bag technique, personal protective equipment, cleaning equipment, medical waste management, and infection control programs. Nurses need to practice sound technique during every client encounter (see How To box).

HOW TO PROMOTE INFECTION PREVENTION STANDARDS

The practice of standard precautions means that all blood and body fluids must be treated as potentially infectious. Standard precautions are implemented to prevent exposure and infection of family caregivers and health care providers.

- Hand hygiene is the single most important practice in preventing infections. Hand hygiene should be performed before and after providing client care, and before and after preparing food, eating, feeding, or using the bathroom.
- Use extreme care to prevent injuries when handling needles, scalpels, and razors. Do not recap, bend, break, or remove needles from syringes before disposal. Discard needles and syringes in puncture-resistant containers made of plastic or metal and dispose of them as directed by agency policy or community guidelines.
- Wear barrier precautions such as gloves, masks, eye covering, and gowns when contact with blood and body fluids is expected. Use masks in combination with eye protection to eliminate contact with respiratory secretions or sprays of blood or body fluids during invasive respiratory procedures or wound irrigations.
- Use aseptic technique with all sterile injection equipment.
- Double-bag and discard soiled dressings or other materials contaminated with body fluids in polyethylene garbage bags.
- Clean kitchen counters, dishes, and laundry with warm water and detergent after use. Clean bathrooms with a household disinfectant.
- For clients with multidrug-resistant organisms, limit the amount of nondisposable equipment brought into the home; use disposable stethoscopes, etc., when possible.

Nurses need to become familiar with evidence-based practice literature specific to infection prevention. Nurses are increasingly called upon to have a role in antibiotic stewardship (Carter et al., 2018; CDC, 2020). Guidelines exist for long-term care but not for community-based care, providing an opportunity for nursing leadership in this area (Centers for Disease Control and Prevention [CDC], 2020). The CDC offers a variety of materials, including guidelines to prevent the most frequent infections (CDC, 2018). In 2014, the American Society for Parenteral and Enteral Nutrition (ASPEN) published a comprehensive set of recommendations about parenteral nutrition safety, and a publication by Ayers et al. (2014) is another good resource.

ACCOUNTABILITY AND QUALITY MANAGEMENT

Evidence-Based Quality/Performance Improvement

All providers, whether they are within community-based settings, hospitals, long-term care, or private practices, are accountable to their clients, reimbursement sources, and professional standards. Accountability is directly linked to quality or the degree to which health services for individuals, families, and communities increase the likelihood of desired health outcomes and are consistent with current professional knowledge.

Most public health, home health, hospice, and palliative care providers have a long history of evaluating the quality of care they provided to their clients. Often, agencies use a systematic, triangulated approach in their pursuit of excellence that includes:

- Hiring qualified personnel
- New employee orientation
- Mentoring programs
- Case conferences
- Supervisory shared visits
- Record audits
- Utilization reviews
- Quality studies
- Client satisfaction surveys
- In-service education
- Recognition for outstanding performance
- Annual evaluations.

Some agencies became accredited as a way to distinguish themselves from other providers.

The sophistication of quality and performance improvement strategies used in home health, hospice, and palliative care has dramatically improved in recent years. Changes were prompted by the interest in research-based practice that has evolved into programs of research and evidence-based practice, use of computers and the Internet, guidelines developed by the National Quality Forum (2020), and the mandate from Medicare to use the OASIS and Outcome-Based Quality Improvement (OBQI). Nurses should have access to current research literature, know how to critique that research, and apply it to their practice.

Evaluating the quality of care professionally and legally should be done in many ways, but documentation is of special significance. The steps of the nursing process must be documented and include communication with team members, physicians, and community resources. It is through the clinical record that nurses demonstrate that they are delivering quality care and identifying strategies to improve the quality of care.

Outcome-Based Quality Improvement

Outcome measurement and cost control are the focus of the CMS Outcome-Based Quality Improvement (OBQI) program. Their definition of outcomes is:

(1) Health status changes between two or more time points, where the term *health status* encompasses physiologic, functional, cognitive, emotional, and behavioral health

(2) Changes that are intrinsic to the client

(3) Positive, negative, or neutral changes in health status; and

(4) Changes that result from care provided or natural progression of disease and disability, or both (CMS, 2012).

Data from OASIS-C2 are part of the two-stage CMS OBQI framework to produce various reports. The first stage, outcome analysis, enables an agency to compare its performance to a national sample, note factors that may affect outcomes, and identify final outcomes that show improvement in or stabilization of a client's condition. Comparing agency data and trends with a national sample is also known as benchmarking, an analysis process that has been used by many businesses but is relatively new to health care. The second stage, known as outcome enhancement, enables the agency to select specific client outcomes and determine strategies to improve care. Reports include agency-client–related characteristics (case mix), potentially avoidable events (adverse event outcomes), and end-result and utilization outcomes.

Accreditation

Public health, home health, and hospice providers may, per requirements, participate in several different continuous quality improvement options. They may choose to meet the accreditation standards of one of the following groups and complete the Medicare survey according to their guidelines:

- The Joint Commission
- The Community Health Accreditation Partner
- The Accreditation Commission for Health Care
- The Public Health Accreditation Board (PHAB)

If providers do not seek accreditation, Medicare surveyors will conduct regular reviews. In 2007, the PHAB was established to offer national public health accreditation. Because some home health and hospice programs are integrated with health departments, they will participate in public health accreditation (PHAB, 2020).

After an agency applies for accreditation, a lengthy self-study must be completed that addresses all aspects of the agency's operation, and an accreditation team schedules a site visit. All three accrediting organizations review agencies' organizational structure, compliance with Medicare CoP, care provided during home visits and documentation of those visits, and the outcomes of client care with a focus on improved health status. Site visitors accompany nurses and other clinicians on home visits to observe the steps of the problem-solving process in action. To maintain accreditation, agencies must follow guidelines and undergo periodic reviews. Some futurists predict that accreditation may become a requirement for licensure of all home health agencies.

PROFESSIONAL DEVELOPMENT AND COLLABORATION

Education, Certification, and Roles

Nurses working in public health, home health, hospice, and palliative care come from a variety of educational and practice backgrounds. They should be educated to function at a high level of competency so that they can be relied on not only by their professional colleagues but also by the community. They have diverse roles and responsibilities in their practice settings; autonomy is a fundamental characteristic that was mentioned earlier in this chapter. Nurses are responsible for basing their practice on research evidence. A growing number of public health, home health, hospice, and palliative care nurses are conducting research; some are members of interprofessional research teams. Their studies add to the body of knowledge for evidence-based practice, especially when the focus is on outcomes of care. The application of existing evidence and generation of new research must be priorities to increase the quality and cost effectiveness of care (ANA, 2014; ANA/HPNA, 2014). A high-quality resource is the Alliance for Home Health Quality and Innovation (AHHQI), a not-for-profit organization focused on leading and sponsoring research and education on the value home health provides to clients and the entire US health system (AHHQI, 2020).

The educational preparation of the 177,790 nurses employed in home health agencies varies greatly (BLS, 2020b). According to the ANA (2014), a baccalaureate degree in nursing should be the minimum requirement for entry into professional practice, and the Home Health Nursing Scope and Standards states that completion of a baccalaureate degree is the appropriate and preferred educational preparation. Roles for nurses include:

- Care management and coordination of care
- Education
- Advocacy
- Administration
- Supervision
- Quality improvement.

The nurse with a baccalaureate degree functions in the role of a generalist, providing skilled nursing and coordinating care for a variety of clients. Nurses with graduate degrees are prepared for roles as clinical specialists, nurse practitioners, researchers, administrators, or educators. Educational programs are increasing to prepare nurses for advanced practice roles in home health. As home health continues to expand, the need for specialized nurse clinicians will also increase to meet the highly technological and complex care needs of individuals, families, and communities.

The HPNA offers many conferences, certification examinations, and credentialing (ANA/HPNA, 2014). There are approximately 15,000 credentialed registered hospice and palliative nurses. Licensed registered nurses may qualify for two levels of specialty practice certification that are differentiated by education, complexity of practice, and performance of certain nursing functions. Like home care, generalists provide direct care, function as educators, case managers, nurse clinicians, administrators, and other roles. The roles of the advanced practice nurse in hospice and palliative care include:

- Expert clinician
- Leader and facilitator of interprofessional teams
- Educator
- Researcher
- Consultant
- Collaborator
- Advocate
- Case manager
- Administrator.

Interprofessional Collaboration

Typically, public health, home health, hospice, and palliative care nurses are members of interprofessional teams. The primary goal of the team is to help populations and individual clients achieve their maximum level of health, self-care, and independent functioning in a safe environment. Medicare regulations,

---

BOX 30.4 Factors for Successful Interprofessional Collaboration

Knowledge
1. Understand how the group process can be used to achieve group goals.
2. Understand problem solving.
3. Understand role theory.
4. Understand what other professionals do and how they view their roles.
5. Understand the differences between client levels of acuity across levels of care, including acute care, home care, ambulatory care, and long-term care.

Skills
1. Use principles of group process effectively.
2. Communicate clearly and accurately.
3. Communicate without using the profession's jargon.
4. Express self clearly and concisely in writing.

Attitudes
1. Feel confident in role as a professional.
2. Trust and respect other professionals.
3. Share tasks with other professionals.
4. Work effectively toward conflict resolution.
5. Be flexible.
6. Adopt an attitude of inquiry.
7. Be timely.

---

professional organizations, and state licensing boards influence team composition and functions.

Box 30.4 illustrates successful interprofessional collaboration that depends on the knowledge, skills, and attitudes of each team member. When team members work collaboratively in partnership with clients, families, volunteers, and community resources, the plan of care can be implemented effectively and reinforced by all. Although each team member has a specific responsibility, any overlap in responsibilities can be beneficial for reinforcement. Team members communicate through email, phone calls, video calls, and face-to-face case conferences to review the plan of care, client progress, and team effectiveness (Marrelli, 2018a; Martin, 2005; Milone-Nuzzo and Hollars, 2017; Wright, 2018). Nurses often serve as team leaders or care managers, in part because nursing service may be the client's primary need. Larger agencies may expand their nursing services to include wound and ostomy, intravenous, psychiatric/mental health, nurse practitioner, and other nursing specialists.

Physicians are an integral part of interprofessional teams; they submit initial and interim orders and review and sign the initial and updated plan of care. Many agencies hire a physician on a part-time basis or have an agreement with a physician who serves as a voluntary consultant. Because state laws are changing rapidly, nurse practitioners are increasingly involved and may have responsibilities similar to physicians. In addition, agencies may have specialized services such as podiatrists, pharmacists, registered dietitians, respiratory therapists, music therapists, psychologists, and chaplains.

The services of physical therapists, occupational therapists, speech and language pathologists, social workers, and home health aides are available in most agencies. They may be employed by the agency or hired through contractual agreements. Their roles are summarized as follows.

- Physical therapists: Provide maintenance and preventive and restorative treatment that includes strengthening muscles, restoring mobility, controlling spasticity, gait training, and teaching active and passive resistance exercises.
- Occupational therapists: Focus on upper extremities to restore muscle strength and mobility for functional skills and performance of activities of daily living.
- Speech and language pathologists: Evaluate speech and language abilities, develop a plan of care, and teach clients to improve their communication involving speech, language, or hearing.
- Social workers: Help clients and families to manage social, emotional, and environmental factors that affect their well-being through identification and referral to appropriate community resources.
- Home health aides: Provide personal care and assist with activities of daily living under the supervision of nurses or physical therapists. Home health aides or homemakers may also help with light housekeeping, laundry, meal preparation, and shopping.

LEGAL, ETHICAL, AND FINANCIAL ISSUES

The potential for human error as well as illegal and unethical activity exists in every health care organization. Examples of Medicare fraud and abuse in home health and hospice include inappropriate use of services, excessive payments to administrative staff or owners, "kickbacks" for referrals, and billing for visits and/or medical supplies that are not authorized or not provided. In addition, the complex regulations of CMS are difficult to understand and have not been interpreted consistently by Medicare surveyors.

Nurses are confronted with legal and ethical issues regularly. They need to be familiar with the living will, power of attorney for health care, and do-not-resuscitate documents. In addition, they need to be informed about local, state, and federal regulations that govern their profession and nursing license, and those that govern their employers. They need to be alert for potential problems or violations and identify solutions in a proactive manner. The privacy guidelines of the Health Insurance Portability and Accountability Act of 1996 ensure protection of clients' personal health information, include provisions about informed consent, and allow clients full access to their health care records (US Department of Health and Human Services [USDHHS], 2017).

Nurses are expected to follow professional, legal, and ethical standards to deliver care to clients, develop trusting relationships, act as client advocates, and help clients and families to increase their self-advocacy skills. Because these responsibilities can produce tension, nurses need to recognize their personal values and biases to make certain they do not interfere with those of clients and families. Nurses should continually reassess client and family needs to avoid inappropriate use and overuse of services.

The safety of clients who live alone as well as family caregiver neglect and/or abuse are ethical concerns. If the clients' needs are greater than what reimbursement allows, nurses need to talk to the clients, their families, and agency personnel to consider alternatives. In addition, many agencies have established ethics committees to assist with ethical dilemmas.

Reimbursement for home health, hospice, and palliative care is complex and tenuous. Medicare, state and local governments, Medicaid, and managed care are the principal funding sources for home health and hospice (NHPCO, 2016). If clients meet the eligibility criteria for the CoP, Medicare is used as their primary payment source. When clients no longer meet those criteria and still require care, their services may be reimbursed by Medicaid, private insurance, donations, or the agency's United Way and other special needs funds. As mentioned earlier, value-based purchasing programs with bundled payments are the newest innovations in reimbursement models to affect community-based care. These innovations make partnering with acute care and other referral sources even more important, and effective collaboration among the interprofessional team is critical to achieve positive outcomes.

Nurses who work in public health, home health, hospice, and palliative care are more involved than most other nurses with financial aspects of care. Nurses and their social work colleagues must be well informed about services available in the communities and those that are covered by Medicare and other funding sources, and recognize how tenuous those funding sources are. Clients and families often ask for help to understand decisions about care and the numerous notices and bills that they receive. Nurses participate directly in decisions about the frequency, length, and type of client services, and their documentation needs to accurately support those decisions (Irani et al., 2018). Nurses must be knowledgeable about the reimbursement of medical supplies and should discuss problematic situations with clients, families, and agency personnel.

TRENDS AND OPPORTUNITIES
National Health Objectives

Because nurses are working with clients and families in the home and community, they are in a position to promote the achievement of some of the key *Healthy People 2030* objectives. The nurse can assess the client's status related to key objectives, identify available resources and gaps to meet client needs, and coordinate care with other providers and community agencies. They can participate in numerous population-level projects and campaigns.

The *Healthy People 2030* box highlights objectives relevant to home health and hospice nurses. Note that many objectives relate to lifestyle issues. With appropriate health education, referral to community resources, and follow-up, there is a potential to reduce morbidity and mortality and decrease chronic disabilities. Nurses can make important contributions on one-to-one and population-focused levels.

HEALTHY PEOPLE 2030

Examples of National Health Objectives for the Year 2030

- **C-01:** Reduce the overall cancer death rate
- **C-11:** Increase proportion of cancer survivors who are living 5 years or longer after diagnosis
- **CKD-01:** Reduce the proportion of adults with chronic kidney disease
- **HAI-D01:** (Developmental) Reduce inappropriate antibiotic use in outpatient settings
- **HDS-01:** Improve cardiovascular health in adults
- **HDS-05:** Increase control of high blood pressure in adults
- **0-02:** Reduce hip fractures among older adults

From U.S. Department of Health and Human Services: *Healthy People 2030*, 2020. Available at http://health.gov/healthypeople.

Organizational and Professional Resources

It is increasingly important for nurses to be involved in political, economic, and regulatory issues at the local, state, and national levels before they affect practice and services to clients. Joining organizations, reviewing the Internet, networking with colleagues, reading professional literature, and serving on expert panels provide opportunities to become informed and influence decisions.

Technology, Informatics, and Telehealth

Technology

Advances in technology, informatics, and telehealth are pervasive in health care and nursing practice. They are changing the ways in which care is provided. Many home health and hospice nurses have developed specialized technical skills in the following: wound management, parenteral nutrition, chemotherapy, intravenous therapy for hydration and antibiotics, intrathecal pain management, ventilators, ventricular assist devices, and apnea monitors. As mentioned earlier in the chapter, clients and family caregivers must learn to complete procedures and manage equipment frequently. It is the responsibility of the nurse and fellow team members to determine if such procedures and equipment can be used safely; when the answer is yes, team members must provide sufficient education, demonstrations, and monitoring so that care continues safely and effectively. Advances in technology, informatics, and telehealth are not replacements for nurses, but team members are tools to improve the quality and effectiveness of their practice. The tools are evolving rapidly, influencing community-based practice, and transforming home health operations.

Nursing Informatics

Nursing informatics (NI) is defined as the "science and practice (that) integrates nursing, its information and knowledge, with information and communication technologies to promote the health of people, families, and communities worldwide" (Nelson and Staggers, 2018). NI is one of the most important new tools for nurses in all settings as they face urgent information management challenges, including the need for timely, reliable, and valid quantified data and information about clients, the services they receive, and their outcomes of care (Eardley et al., 2018; Monsen, 2018). They also need verbal and automated methods to communicate with other nurses and health care providers wherever they are in the community.

Now that electronic data sets are more available and can be linked to national claims data and other rich sources of health information to form large data sets, data science is a growing methodology nurse scientists may use to capitalize on this resource (Carroll, 2019). Public health, home health, and hospice are ripe with opportunities for data science research, especially when standardized data sets are used for clinical operations (Monsen et al., 2018).

The sharing of information from one health care setting or provider to another is critical for community-based care, especially as clients make the transition between hospital and home. Safe, high-quality care is dependent on the sharing of information, goals of care, and care plans. Health information exchanges (HIEs) support this need and are growing in number and functionality. HIEs give care providers access to patient records from hospitals, emergency departments, skilled nursing facilities, and laboratories across the state, saving valuable time and costs associated with searching paper records, faxing, making phone calls, or re-collecting information.

Public health and other community-based practitioners play an important role in identifying critical information needed to conduct care and to communicate with clients, families, interprofessional team members, policy makers, and payers. They also must support the development and seek the purchase of certified EHRs that meet documentation and interoperability standards and meaningful use criteria.

Increasingly, individuals and families served by public health, home health, hospice, and palliative care nurses have information technology skills. They may use the Internet frequently and be well informed about diagnoses, treatments, and medications. They may also use smartphones, other mobile devices, and social media. Nurses need to inquire about their clients' skills rather than make assumptions based on their age or other factors.

Telehealth

Telehealth supports long-distance health care, client and professional health-related education, and public health and health administration using electronic information, medical devices, and telecommunications technologies (Schlachta-Fairchild et al., 2018). The technology used varies to include live videoconferencing, the Internet, store-and-forward imaging, streaming media, satellite, wireless communications, and plain old telephone systems. Telehealth equipment and program components include telephone triage and advice, and biometric telemonitoring equipment to measure vital signs, weight, cardiac function, and point-of-care diagnostics. The system may or may not include video technology for live interaction (Schlachta-Fairchild et al., 2018).

Telemonitoring is increasingly being used with infants, women with high-risk pregnancies, and adults with various health problems, including mental health. Smart homes are emerging to help the older adult to "age in place" (Adler, 2020). Sensors can monitor activities and detect adverse events such as a fall or lack of movement and trigger a call for help. Medication management devices remind clients to take their medications, dispense medications, and send alerts to providers if devices are not accessed as expected (Marek et al., 2013). The next generation of devices is taking advantage of handheld devices such as smartphone and tablet technologies, making telemonitoring even more ubiquitous.

Specific details about barriers and facilitators for sustainable tele-homecare programs are described in the Evidence-Based Practice box (Radhakrishnan et al., 2016).

EVIDENCE-BASED PRACTICE

Performing a systematic review of the literature, researchers sought to identify the barriers and facilitators for sustainability of tele-homecare programs implemented by home health nursing agencies for chronic disease management. They searched for English-language articles on home telehealth in the CINAHL, PubMed/MEDLINE, PsychInfo, Web of Science, and Cochrane Reviews databases published from January 1996 to December 2013. Data extraction using PRISMA guideline and quality appraisal using the Mixed Methods Appraisal Tool (MMAT) were completed on relevant empirical studies, as well as thematic analysis across the studies to synthesize knowledge. Sixteen studies met the inclusion criteria. The sustainability of tele-homecare programs was found to be influenced by home health nurses' and patients' perceptions on effectiveness of tele-homecare programs to achieve clinical and behavioral outcomes;

the degree to which tele-homecare programs are tailored to patient-centered factors and needs; the role played by tele-homecare programs in nurse-patient or interprofessional communication and relationships; the organizational culture and process within home health agencies; and quality of the tele-homecare technology.

Nurse Use

Tele-homecare programs can help with chronic disease management. Home health nursing agencies can help such programs realize their potential for chronic disease management by training their nurses on how to best utilize the programs, tailoring programs to individual patient circumstances, and investing in high quality tele-homecare technology.

From Radhakrishnan K, Xia B, Berkley A, Kim M: Barriers and facilitator for sustainability of tele-homecare programs: a systematic review, *Health Serv Res* 51(1):48–75, 2016.

QSEN FOCUS ON QUALITY AND SAFETY EDUCATION FOR NURSES

Targeted Competency: Client-Centered Care—Recognize the client or designee as the source of control and full partner in providing compassionate and coordinated care based on respect for client's preferences, values, and needs.

Important aspects of client-centered care include:

- **Knowledge:** Demonstrate comprehensive understanding of the concepts of pain and suffering, including physiologic models of pain and comfort.
- **Skills:** Elicit expectations of client and family for relief of pain, discomfort, or suffering.
- **Attitudes:** Recognize that client expectations influence outcomes in management of pain or suffering.

Client-Centered Care Question

Visit a community-based hospice or palliative care unit. Spend time observing the care provided in this setting.

1. How is care provided in this setting different from care you have seen in the acute care setting? In the home health setting?
2. Notice how nurses and nursing assistants assess pain in this environment.
3. Discuss with the nurses how they address concerns around pain and suffering with clients and families in this environment. How do nurses evaluate clients' and families' expectations around pain?
4. Discuss with the nurses differences in care approaches between a community-based hospice or palliative care versus care approaches for home hospice and palliative care. Is there additional education that is required for the client and family, because the family often provides some aspects of care for home hospice and palliative care?

Prepared by Gail Armstrong, ND, DNP, MS, PhD, Professor and Assistant Dean/DNP program, Oregon Health and Sciences University

---

≫ APPLYING CONTENT TO PRACTICE

Public health, home health, hospice, and palliative care continue to evolve with changing national policies and innovations. The need for nurses prepared to practice in these specialties is growing as the public becomes more interested in prevention, the population ages, chronic illness increases, and more care is delivered in the community. Practice will become ever more complex and diverse as individuals live longer with multiple chronic conditions and they and their families are more engaged in their care and request more choices and personalized care. Practice in this challenging environment requires a strong educational background, critical thinking skills, and a commitment to lifelong learning. The autonomy afforded by community-based practice requires strong interpersonal, communication, technological, and clinical skills. It is a good time to celebrate the past, embrace the present, and look forward to the future.

The individuals, families, and communities served by public health, home health, palliative, and hospice nurses are described throughout this chapter, as are the knowledge, skills, and attitudes of nurses who function well in those settings. The descriptions are evident in the text, clinical examples, boxes/figures/tables, references, and other parts of the chapter. The competencies in this chapter are congruent with the following core competencies of the Quad Council Coalition's Domains of Public Health Nursing (2018): (1) assessment of analytic skills, (2) policy development and program planning skills, (3) communication skills, (4) cultural competency skills, (5) community dimensions of practice skills, (6) public health sciences skills, (7) financial planning and management skills and planning skills, and (8) leadership and systems thinking skills. Students and new graduates cannot be expected to have developed all of these skills when they begin to practice (Milone-Nuzzo and Hollars, 2017; Schoon et al., 2018, Smith, 2017a, 2017b; Wright, 2018). However, as nurses proceed in their career development and gain valuable work experience, they will progress along the novice to expert continuum.

PRACTICE APPLICATION

The home visit is the hallmark of public health nursing, home health, palliative care, and hospice. When a nurse enters a client's home, he or she is a guest and must recognize that the services offered can be accepted or rejected. The first visit sets the stage for success or failure. The initial assessment of the client, the support system, and the environment is critical.

A. What strategies would the nurse consider to develop a trusting relationship during the first visit?

B. What would be the most important elements to assess in the home environment?

C. What should the nurse include in the client contract?

D. How can the nurse assess the preferred learning style?

Answers can be found on the Evolve website.

REMEMBER THIS!

- Public health, home health, hospice, and palliative care nursing practice provided in the client's home differ from care in institutional settings. The home setting affects practice in unique ways, including establishing trust, developing care partnerships (consumer engagement), selecting interventions, collecting outcomes and data, ensuring client safety, and promoting quality.

- Family members, including caregivers and significant persons who provide assistance and/or care, are essential members of the health care team.

- Home health has its roots in public health nursing, with an emphasis on health promotion, illness prevention, and caring for people in their communities.

- Home health and hospice practice and reimbursement changed when they became major Medicare benefits.

- Models of care are described in this chapter: public health, home health, hospice, palliative care, Nurse-Family Partnership, and transitional care. All nurses should become familiar with these models to inform clients, their families, and their communities about options and educate providers who are potential referral sources.

- Medicare-certified home health and hospice agencies are divided into various types of administrative and organizational structures. However, many aspects of nursing practice are the same in the various types.

- Standards of public health, home health, and hospice/palliative care nursing practice originate from the ANA in partnership with specialty organizations and encourage adoption of evidence-based practice.

- Consistently demonstrating professional competency is essential for public health, home health, hospice, and palliative care nurses.

- Interprofessional collaboration is inherent in public health, home health, hospice, and palliative care.

- The Omaha System is unique in that it is the only comprehensive vocabulary developed initially by and for nurses practicing in the community.

- The Omaha System is designed to enhance practice, documentation, and information management. These areas are of concern to community health educators and students as well as clinicians and administrators.

- Interprofessional clinicians employed in Medicare-certified home health agencies use OASIS-C2 at designated intervals; it is the outcome measurement tool mandated by the Centers for Medicare and Medicaid Services' Conditions of Participation.

- Evidence-based quality/performance improvement is important in all home health and hospice agencies.

- Exciting trends and opportunities are pervasive in public health, home health, hospice, and palliative care. Many nurses are developing skills using technology, informatics, and telehealth; a commitment to lifelong learning is necessary.

EVOLVE WEBSITE

http://evolve.elsevier.com/Stanhope/community/
- Answers to Practice Application
- Case Study
- Glossary
- Review Questions

REFERENCES

Addler SE: *Today's Smart Home Tech Can Help You Age in Place,* AARP, January 9, 2020. Retrieved from: https://www.aarp.org/home-family/personal-technology/info-2020/future-smart-home-devices.html.

Agency for Healthcare Research and Quality (AHRQ): *Patient Safety Measure Tools and Resources,* 2017. Retrieved from http://www.ahrq.gov.

Alliance for Home Health Quality and Innovation (AHHQI): *About the Alliance,* 2020. Retrieved from http://ahhqi.org/about/.

American Nurses Association (ANA): *Home health nursing: scope and standards of practice,* 2nd ed., Silver Spring, 2014, Nursesbooks.org.

American Nurses Association (ANA): *Public health nursing: scope and standards of practice (ebook),* 2nd ed., Silver Spring, 2013, Nursesbooks.org.

American Nurses Association, Hospice and Palliative Nurses Association (ANA/HPNA): *Palliative nursing: scope and standards of practice—an essential resource for hospice and palliative nurses,* Silver Spring, 2014, Nursesbooks.org.

American Nurses Association, Hospice and Palliative Nurses Association (ANA/HPNA): *Call for Action: Nurses Lead and Transform Palliative Care,* 2017. Retrieved from https://bit.ly/2Lut4vb.

Ansberry C: U.S. is running out of caregivers, *Wall St J* 10(7):21–22, 2018.

Ayers P, Adams S, Boullata J, et al.: A.S.P.E.N. parenteral nutrition safety consensus recommendations, *JPEN J Parenter Enteral Nutr* 38:296–333, 2014.

Berwick DM, Nolan TW, Whittington J: The Triple Aim: care, health, and cost, *Health Aff (Millwood)* 27:759–769, 2008.

Buch CL, Nies MA: Home health and hospice. In Nies MA, McEwen M, eds.: *Community/public health nursing: promoting the health of populations,* 7th ed., St. Louis, 2019, Elsevier, pp. 674-690.

Buhler-Wilkerson K: No place like home: a history of nursing and home care in the U.S., *Home Health Nurse* 20:641–647, 2002.

Bureau of Labor Statistics (BLS): *Employment Projections,* 2019-2029, 2020a. Retrieved from https://www.bls.gov/emp/.

Bureau of Labor Statistics (BLS): *Occupational Employment and Wages, May 2019*, 2020b. Retrieved from https://www.bls.gov/oes/current/oes291141.htm.

Carroll W: Putting the 'N' in STEM: A call for nurse data scientists. *Online Journal of Nursing Informatics (OJNI)*, 23(2), 2019.

Carter EJ, Greendyke WG, Furuya EY, et al: Exploring the nurses' role in antibiotic stewardship: a multisite qualitative study of nurses and infection preventionists, *Am J Infect Control* 46(5):492–497, 2018.

Center to Advance Palliative Care (CAPC): *Growth of Palliative Care in U.S. Hospitals: 2018 Snapshot*, 2018. Retrieved from https://media.capc.org.

Centers for Disease Control and Prevention (CDC): *Healthcare-Associated Infections*, 2018. Retrieved from https://www.cdc.gov.

Centers for Disease Control and Prevention (CDC): *The Core Elements of Antibiotic Stewardship for Nursing Homes*, 2020. Retrieved from https://www.cdc.gov.

Centers for Medicare and Medicaid Services (CMS): *Outcome-Based Quality Improvement (OBQI) Manual*, 2012. Retrieved from https://www.cms.gov.

Centers for Medicare and Medicaid Services (CMS): *2016 CMS Statistics*, 2016. Retrieved from https://www.cms.gov.

Centers for Medicare and Medicaid Services (CMS): *Outcome and Assessment Information set OASIS-C2 Guidance Manual*, 2017b. Retrieved from https://www.cms.gov.

Centers for Medicare and Medicaid Services (CMS): *Home Health Providers*, 2018a. Retrieved from https://www.cms.gov.

Centers for Medicare and Medicaid Services: *Hospice*, 2018b. Retrieved from https://www.cms.gov.

Centers for Medicare and Medicaid Services (CMS): *IMPACT Act Spotlights and Announcements*, 2018c. Retrieved from https://www.cms.gov.

Centers for Medicare and Medicaid Services (CMS): *Hospice Payment System*, 84 FR 38484, 2019. Retrieved from https://www.cms.gov.

Chow K, Dahlin C: Integration of palliative care and oncology nursing, *Semin Oncol Nurs* 34(3):192–201, 2018.

Curtis JR, Downey L, Back AL, et al.: Effect of a patient and clinician communication-priming intervention on patient-reported goals-of-care discussions between patients with serious illness and clinicians: a randomized clinical trial, *JAMA Intern Med* 178(7):930–940, 2018.

Diefenbeck CA, Klemm PR, Hayes ER: "Anonymous meltdown": content themes emerging in a nonfacilitated, peer-only, unstructured, asynchronous online support group for family caregivers, *Comput Inform Nurs* 35:630–638, 2017.

Donahue MP: *Nursing, the finest art*, 3rd ed., St. Louis, 2011, Elsevier.

Eardley DL, Krumwiede KA, Secginli S, et al: The Omaha System as a structured instrument for bridging nursing informatics with public health nursing education: a feasibility study, *Comput Inform Nurs* 36:275–283, 2018.

Enoch MA, Kitzman H, Smith JA, et al: A prospective cohort study of influences on externalizing behaviors across childhood: Results from a nurse home visiting randomized controlled trial, *J Am Acad Child Adolesc Psychiatry* 55:376–382, 2016.

Etkind SN, Bone AE, Gomes B, et al.: How many people will need palliative care in 2040? Past trends, future projections and implications for services, *BMC Med* 15:102, 2017.

Fazzi: *Home Health & Hospice Data*, 2018. Retrieved from https://www.fazzi.com.

Gao G, Maganti S, Monsen KA: Older adults, frailty, and the social and behavioral determinants of health, *Big Data Inf Anal* 2: 191–202, 2017.

Gasper AM, Magdic K, Ren D, Fennimore L: Development of a home health-based palliative care program for patients with heart failure, *Home Healthc Now* 36:84–92, 2018.

Gorski LA: Infection prevention concepts. In Gorski LA, ed.: *Fast facts for nurses about home infusion therapy: the expert's best-practice guide in a nutshell*, New York, 2017, Springer Publishers, pp. 27–42.

Hinds PS, Schum L, Baker JN, Wolfe J: Key factors affecting dying children and their families, *J Palliat Med* 8(Suppl 1):S70–S78, 2005.

Holly R: The number of Medicare-certified home health agencies is dwindling. *Home Health Care News*, July 19, 2020. Retreived from: https://homehealthcarenews.com/2020/07/the-number-of-medicare-certified-home-health-agencies-is-dwindling/.

Huang YM, Shiyanbola OO, Smith PD: Association of health literacy and medication self-efficacy with medication adherence and diabetes control, *Patient Prefer Adherence* 12:793–802, 2018.

Innes, S.: Library nurses look after those in need, Arizona Daily Star, Tucson, AZ, 2012, Retrieved from https://tucson.com.

Irani E, Hirschman KB, Cacchione PZ, Bowles KH: Home health nurse decision-making regarding visit intensity planning for newly admitted patients: a qualitative descriptive study, *Home Health Care Serv Q* 37(3):211–231, 2018.

Izumi S: Advance care planning: the nurse's role, *Am J Nurs* 117: 56–61, 2017.

Kaye EC, Rubenstein J, Levine D, Baker JN, Dabbs D, Friebert SE: Pediatric palliative care in the community, *CA Cancer J Clin* 65:316–333, 2015.

Kindig D, Stoddart G: What is population health? *Am J Public Health* 93:380–383, 2003.

Kübler-Ross E: *On death and dying*, New York, 1969, McMillan.

Levine DR, Mandrell BN, Sykes A, et al.: Patients' and parents' needs, attitudes, and perceptions about early palliative care integration in pediatric oncology, *JAMA Oncol* 3:1214–1220, 2017.

Marek KD, Stetzer F, Ryan PA, et al: Nurse care coordination and technology effects on health status of frail older adults via enhanced self-management of medication: Randomized clinical trial to test efficacy, *Nurs Res* 62;269–278, 2013.

Marrelli TM: *Handbook of home health standards: quality, documentation, and reimbursement*, 6th ed., Venice, 2018a, Marrelli & Associates.

Marrelli TM: *Hospice and palliative care handbook: quality, compliance, and reimbursement*, 3rd ed., Venice, 2018b, Marrelli & Associates.

Martin KS: *The Omaha System: a key to practice, documentation, and information management,* reprinted, 2nd ed., Omaha, 2005, Health Connections Press.

Martin KS, Kessler PD: The Omaha System: improving the quality of practice and decision support. In Harris MD, editor: *Handbook of home health care administration*, 6th ed., Burlington, 2017, Jones & Bartlett, pp 235–248.

McAuley A, Munro A, Taylor A: "Once I'd done it once it was like writing your name": lived experience of take-home naloxone administration by people who inject drugs, *Int J Drug Policy* 58:46–54, 2018.

Meadows CA, Fraser J, Camus S, Henderson K: A system-wide innovation in transition services: transforming the home care liaison role, *Home Health Nurse* 32:78–86, 2014.

Medicare: *What is Home Health Compare?* n.d. Retrieved from https://www.medicare.gov.

Medicare Payment Advisory Commission (MedPAC): *Hospice Services*, 2018. Retrieved from http://www.medpac.gov.

Medicare Payment Advisory Commission (MedPAC): *Report to the Congress: Medicare Payment Policy*, 2020. Retrieved from http://www.medpac.gov/.

Melnyk BM, Fineout-Overholt E: *Evidence-based practice in nursing and healthcare: a guide to best practice*, ed 4, Philadelphia, PA, 2019, Wolters Kluwer.

Melnyk BM, Gallagher-Ford L: Implementing the new essential evidence-based practice competencies in real-world clinical and academic settings: moving from evidence to action in improving healthcare quality and patient outcomes, *Worldviews Evid Based Nurs* 12(2):67–69, 2015.

Milone-Nuzzo P, Hollars ME: Transitioning nurses to home care. In Harris MD, editor: *Handbook of home health care administration*, ed 6, Burlington, MA, 2017, Jones & Bartlett, pp 455–466.

Mistovich JJ, Karren KJ, Hafen B: *Prehospital emergency care*, ed 10, Upper Saddle River, NJ, 2014, Pearson Education.

Mistovich JJ, Karren KJ: *Prehospital emergency care*, ed 11, Upper Saddle River, NJ, 2018, Pearson Education.

Monsen KA: *Intervention effectiveness research: quality improvement and program evaluation*, Cham, Switzerland, 2018, Springer.

Monsen KA, Kelechi TJ, McRae ME, Mathiason MA, Martin KS: Nursing theory, terminology, and big data: data-driven discovery of novel patterns in archival randomized clinical trial data, *Nurs Res* 67:122-132, 2018.

National Association for Home Care & Hospice (NAHC): *NAHC Supports Bill to Permit Disposal of Unused Hospice Meds in the Home*, 2018. Retrieved from https://www.nahc.org.

National Consensus Project for Quality Palliative Care (NCP): *Clinical practice guidelines for quality palliative care*, ed 3, Pittsburgh, PA, 2013, Author.

National Consensus Project for Quality Palliative Care (NCP): *2018 Clinical practice guidelines for quality palliative care*, ed 4, Pittsburgh, PA, 2018, Author.

National Hospice and Palliative Care Organization (NHPCO): *Facts and Figures Hospice Care in America Revised*, 2018. Retrieved from https://www.nhpco.org.

National Quality Forum: *About Us*, 2020. Retrieved from http://www.qualityforum.org.

Naylor MD, Bowles KH, McCauley KM, et al: High-value transitional care: translation of research into practice, *J Eval Clin Pract* 19:727–733, 2013.

Naylor MD, Hirschman KB, Hanlon AL, et al: Effects of alternative interventions among hospitalized, cognitively impaired older adults, *J Comp Eff Res* 5(3):259–272, 2016.

Naylor MD, Shaid EC, Carpenter D, et al: Components of comprehensive and effective transitional care, *J Am Geriatr Soc* 65(6):1119–1125, 2017.

Nelson R, Staggers N: *Health informatics: an interprofessional approach*, ed 2, St. Louis, MO, 2018, Elsevier.

Nurse-Family Partnership (NFP): *Annual Report 2017*, 2017. Retrieved from https://www.nursefamilypartnership.org.

Olds DL, Eckenrode J, Henderson CR Jr, et al: Long-term effects of home visitation on maternal life course and child abuse and neglect: fifteen-year follow-up of a randomized trial. *JAMA* 278:637–643, 1997.

Omaha System: *Intervention Scheme* 2019a. Retrieved from www.omahasystem.org.

Omaha System: *Welcome to the Omaha System Web site!* 2019b. Retrieved from www.omahasystem.org.

Parry C, Mahoney E, Chalmer SA, Coleman EA. Assessing the quality of transitional care further applications of the care transitions measure, *Medical Care, 3*: 317–322, 2008.

Perry KM, Parente CA: Integrating palliative care into home care practice. In Harris MD, editor: *Handbook of home health care administration*, ed 6, Burlington, MA, 2017, Jones & Bartlett, pp 767–782.

Public Health Accreditation Board (PHAB): *Welcome to PHAB*, 2020. Retrieved from http://www.phaboard.org.

Quad Council Coalition: *Community/Public Health Nursing Competencies*, 2018. Retrieved from http://quadcouncilphn.org.

Radhakrishnan K, Xia B, Berkley A, Kim M: Barriers and facilitator for sustainability of tele-homecare programs: a systematic review, *Health Research and Educational Trust, 51*(1): 48-75, 2016.

Reddy S: A tech test to keep seniors in their homes longer, *Wall St J*, A12, July 26, 2018.

Robert Wood Johnson Foundation:(RWJF): Public Health NUrses bringing care to libraries, 2013, Retrieved from https://www.rwjf.org.

Robert Wood Johnson Foundation (rwJF): Creating a shared vision to help restore Atlantic City,2018, Retrieved fromwww.rwjf.org.

Roux P, Pereira F, Santiago-Delefosse M, Verloo H: Medication practices and experiences of older adults discharged home from hospital: a feasibility study protocol, *Patient Prefer Adherence, 12*: 1055-1063, 2018.

Schlachta-Fairchild L, Rocca M, Cordi V, et al: Telehealth and applications for delivering care at a distance. In Nelson R, Staggers N, editors: *Health informatics: an interprofessional approach*, ed 2, St. Louis, MO, 2018, Elsevier, pp 131–152.

Schoon P, Porta C, Schaffer M: *Population-based public health nursing clinical manual: the henry street model for nurses*, ed 3, 2018, Sigma Theta Tau International.

Slipka AF, Monsen KA: Toward improving quality of end-of-life care: encoding clinical guidelines and standing orders using the Omaha System, *Worldviews Evid Based Nurs* 15:26–37, 2018.

Smith LS: Cultural competence: a nurse educator's guide, *Nursing* 47:18–21, 2017a.

Smith LS: Cultural competence: a guide for nursing students, *Nursing* 47:18–20, 2017b.

Stober M: Palliative care in home health: a review of the literature, *Home Healthc Now* 35:373–377, 2017.

Storfjell JL, Winslow BW, Saunders JSD: *Catalysts for Change: Harnessing the Power of Nurses to Build Population Health in the 21st Century*, 2017. Retrieved from https://www.rwjf.org.

U.S. Census Bureau: *Profile American Facts for Features*. CB17-FF 08, April 10, 2017. Retrieved from https://www.census.gov.

U.S. Department of Health and Human Services (USDHHS): *Healthy People 2030*, 2020. Retrieved from http://health.gov/healthypeople.

U.S. Department of Health and Human Services (USDHHS): *HIPAA for Professionals*, 2017. Retrieved from https://www.hhs.gov.

U.S. Food & Drug Administration (FDA): *Where and How to Dispose of Unused Medicines*, 2020. Retrieved from https://www.fda.gov.

Weissman DE, Meier DE: Identifying patients in need of a palliative care assessment in the hospital setting: a consensus report from the Center to Advance Palliative Care, *J Palliat Med* 14:17–23, 2011.

Wright E: Clients receiving home health and hospice care. In Rector C, editor: *Community and public health nursing*, ed 9, Philadelphia, PA, 2018, Wolters Kluwer, pp 1166–1189.

Weaver MS, Heinze KE, Bell CJ, et al: Establishing psychosocial palliative care standards for children and adolescents with cancer and their families: an integrative review, *Palliat Med* 3:212–223, 2016.

Zerwekh JV: *Nursing care at the end of life: palliative care for patients and families*, Philadelphia, PA, 2006, F.A. Davis.

Zhang KM, Dindoff K, Arnold JM, Lane J, Swartzman LC: What matters to patients with heart failure? The influence of non-health-related goals on patient adherence to self-care management, *Patient Educ Couns* 98(8):927–934, 2015.

Zullig LL, Hayden B: *Engaging Patients to Optimize Medication Adherence*, 2017. Retrieved from https://catalyst.nejm.org.

31

The Nurse in the Schools

Erin G. Cruise

OBJECTIVES

After reading this chapter, the student should be able to:

1. Discuss the history of school nursing and describe, compare, and contrast the professional standards and scope of practice of school nursing with those of public health nursing.
2. Differentiate the roles, responsibilities, and activities of school nurses from those of nurses in other settings.
3. Describe various frameworks and models that provide the foundation for school nursing practice.
4. Discuss common health problems of children and adolescents seen in the school setting and the school nurse's support of education for children with illness and disabilities.
5. Assess the nursing care given in schools in the context of primary, secondary, and tertiary levels of prevention.
6. Identify future trends in school nursing.

CHAPTER OUTLINE

KEY TERMS

School nursing is a specialty practice focused on providing health care and illness prevention to school-age children with the goal of facilitating their participation in educational opportunities (American Nurses Association [ANA] & National Association of School Nurses [NASN], 2017). School nursing services are provided to individuals within the school setting, including children, staff, and teachers. School nursing is also population focused, utilizing many of the concepts of public health nursing to prevent illness and injury and to stop the spread of disease within the school, family, and community. While school nursing has required a comprehensive approach to health care and health promotion since its inception, the practice continues to evolve and increase in complexity (Wolfe, 2019a). School nurses provide leadership and coordinate health and safety programs in their schools and communities.

According to the National Center for Education Statistics, there were an estimated 56.4 million school children in 2020 (Institute of Education Sciences [IES]: National Center for Education Statistics [NCES], 2020). Of these, 35.3 million attended preschool, elementary, and middle public schools and 15.4 million were in grades 9 through 12. Enrollment was predicted to be an additional 5.7 million students attending private schools. School nurses provide care to these children in all school settings, as well as in their homes, correctional settings, hospitals, and during field trips, athletic competitions, and other extracurricular events (ANA & NASN, 2017).

US public and private schools employ about 3.7 million teachers as well as other adult school administrators and staff such as administrative assistants, custodians, food service workers, and bus drivers ([IES: NCES], 2020). In addition to care for children, school nurses are often asked to provide health services for these adult school staff members. This requires school nurses to have expertise in a wide variety of adult health care issues, including nutrition, medication, communicable diseases, and chronic illness (Wolfe, 2019a).

This chapter discusses the history of school nursing and examines the evolving roles and activities of school nurses in modern times. Frameworks for evidence-based school nursing practice will be explained, as well as professional scope and standards of the specialty. The impact of federal regulations on the education of children and the practice of school nursing will be investigated. This chapter will also assess the relationship of public health nursing and school nursing. Different types of school health services will be examined, and the levels of care required for a variety of children's health problems most commonly found in schools will be discussed. The chapter ends with a discussion of the ethical dilemmas that may arise for school nurses, and the future of nursing in the schools is predicted for ever-changing communities.

HISTORY OF SCHOOL NURSING

Origins of School Nursing

The history of school nursing began with the earliest efforts of nurses to care for people in the community. The following discussions present a timeline of events.

- In the late 1800s in England, the Metropolitan Association of Nursing provided medical examinations for children in the schools of London.
- By 1892, nurses in London were responsible for checking the nutrition of the children in the schools (Rosen and Fee, 2015).
- In 1897, nurses in New York City schools began to identify ill children. They then excluded these children from classes so that other children would not be infected (Houlahan, 2018).
- Many states had laws in the late 1800s mandating that within the schools, nurses would teach about the abuse of alcohol and narcotics (Sharma, 2017).

In the early 1900s in the United States, the main health problem in the community was the spread of infectious diseases. On October 1, 1902, in New York City, Lillian Wald's Henry Street Settlement nurses began going into homes and schools to assess children. At first, these public health nurses were in only four schools, caring for about 10,000 children. They made plans to identify children with lice and other infestations and children with infected wounds, tuberculosis (TB), and other infectious diseases (Houlahan, 2018; Ruel, 2014).

The need for school nurses was immediately recognized by the health care community.

- By 1910, Teachers College in New York City added a course on school nursing to their curriculum for nurses.
- In 1916 a school superintendent requested that a public health nurse be sent to the schools to care for children of immigrants (Houlahan, 2018).
- By the 1920s, school nurse teachers were employed by most municipal health departments.
- In the 1940s the nurses were employed mostly by the school districts directly.
- The nurses in the 1940s also provided home nursing and health education for the children and their parents (Houlahan, 2018).

After World War II and into the 1950s, as a result of the increased use of immunizations and antibiotics, the number of children with communicable diseases in schools decreased.

- School nurses then turned their attention to screening children for common health problems and for vision and hearing problems.
- School nurses were less likely to teach health concepts in the children's classrooms and more likely to consult with teachers about health education (Houlahan, 2018).
- There was an increased emphasis on employee health, and school nurses began screening teachers and other school staff for health problems (Galemore et al., 2016).
- In the 1960s there was an upsurge in the call for higher levels of education for school nurses.
- A position paper delivered at the 1960 (ANA) convention called for a Bachelor of Science degree in nursing as the minimum educational preparation for school nurses.

Table 31.1 gives the highlights of school nursing history over the last century.

Federal Legislation Affecting School Nursing Practice

Community involvement in health in schools was a major thrust in the 1970s and 1980s.

TABLE 31.1 High Points In School Nursing History

Decade	Major Events in School Nursing
1890s	English and American nurses are used in schools to examine children for infectious diseases and to teach about alcohol abuse.
1900s	Henry Street Settlement in New York City sends nurses into schools and homes to investigate children's overall health.
1910s	School nursing course added to Teachers College nursing program. School nursing spreads throughout the country.
1920s and 1930s	School nurses are employed by community health departments.
1940s	School districts employ school nurses.
1950s	Children are screened in schools for common health problems.
1960s	Educational preparation for school nurses is debated.
1970s	School nurse practitioner programs began. Increased emphasis put on mental health counseling in schools.
1980s	Children with long-term illness or disabilities attend schools. Introduction of *School Nursing: Scope and Standards of Practice* by ANA and NASN.
1990s	School-based and school-linked clinics are started. Total family and community health care is offered.
2000s	School nurses give comprehensive primary, secondary, and tertiary levels of nursing care. *The Framework for 21st Century School Nursing Practice* is adopted.

Data from Apple R: School health is community: school nursing in the early twentieth century in the USA, *Hist Educ Rev* 46(2):136–149, 2017; Wolfe L: Historical perspectives of school nursing. In Selekman J, Shannon RA, Yonkaitis CF, editors: *School nursing: a comprehensive text*, ed 3, Philadelphia, 2019b, F.A. Davis Company, pp. 2–16.

- Counseling and mental health services were added to the responsibilities of school nurses, who began to directly teach children concepts of health.
- Children were no longer just being screened for illnesses (Loschiavo, 2015).
- Because of federal laws that required schools to make accommodations for handicapped children, medically fragile children were attending schools, often for the first time.

One of these laws, Public Law (PL) 93-112, Section 504 of the Rehabilitation Act, required that public schools and other entities receiving federal funding could not be discriminated against and children could not be denied the benefits of an education (US Department of Education Office for Civil Rights [DOE-OCR], 2010). This was an important step in helping all children enjoy a normal educational experience. This law was followed by PL 94-142, Education for All Handicapped Children Act, which required that children with disabilities have services provided for them in schools (Yonkaitis & Shannon, 2017). This law was amended several times over the next decade, increasing eligibility for services to children ages birth to 21 years and providing financial incentives to states for early intervention programs. States were also encouraged to provide transition to work and adult life programs for disabled children as they aged out of the school system (Halbert & Yonkaitis, 2019).

After the passing of the Americans with Disabilities Act (ADA) in 1992, PL 105-17, Individuals with Disabilities Education Act (IDEA) was passed in 1997 (Halbert & Yonkaitis, 2019). Both of these laws required that more children be allowed to attend schools. Schools had to make allowances for children's special needs, which included ensuring that their school experience was in balance with their health care needs by developing individualized education plans (IEPs) and individualized health plans (IHPs). That meant that more children with human immunodeficiency virus (HIV), acquired immunodeficiency syndrome (AIDS), chronic illnesses, or mental health problems were in the classrooms and needed more attention from the school nurse (Halbert & Yonkaitis, 2019). IDEA was renamed the Individuals with Disabilities Education Improvement Act (IDEIA) in 2004 and extended coverage till the child turns 22 (Gibbons et al., 2013). The No Child Left Behind Act (PL 107-110) of 2001 requires a healthy environment in schools, which also affects children who have health problems. In 2015 the No Child Left Behind Act (NCLB) was revised, creating the new law, PL 114-95, Every Student Succeeds Act (ESSA) (US Congress, 2015). NCLB required that accommodations be made to promote academic achievement for children with disabilities and those living in poverty, having limited English proficiency (LEP), or who were homeless (US Department of Education (USDOE), 2020). ESSA strengthens and clarifies these requirements but also includes regulations requiring that states must allocate a percentage of their federal funds toward activities that support safe and healthy students (USDOE, 2020).

The Child Nutrition Act (CNA) was originally passed in 1964 to combat malnutrition and hunger among disadvantaged children and pregnant women. This law funds the National School Lunch Program, breakfast and summer food programs in schools and preschools, and food supplements for pregnant and breastfeeding women and their preschool children (US Congress, 2010). The Act also establishes minimum standards for nutrition content of meals, requires decreased student access to non-nutritious foods on school grounds, and the inclusion of nutrition education, physical activity, and school wellness programs. This law has been reauthorized every five years, with the last reauthorization in 2010 as the Healthy, Hunger-Free Kids Act (HHFK) (US Congress, 2010). By continuing to reauthorize the CNA in its various iterations, Congress and presidents have acknowledged the importance of nutrition in promoting child health, which in turn improves children's ability to engage in educational opportunities. The HHFK Act expired in 2015 due to differences between the House and Senate on policy, including nutrition standards (Food Research and Action Center, 2018). However, the HHFK/CNA programs continue as permanent law so long as Congress continues to fund them.

Health information of students in schools is protected under both the Family Education Rights and Privacy Act (FERPA) of 1974 and the Health Insurance Portability and Accountability Act (HIPAA) of 1996. FERPA covers educational records of any child in an educational setting that receives federal funding from the US Department of Education (Brous, 2019). This includes

TABLE 31.2 Federal Legislation Affecting School Nursing

Law	Effect on School Nurses and Children
1954: Desegregation of schools; 1964: Civil Rights Act	Schools can no longer be segregated by race. Expanded civil rights open the door for children with disabilities to attend schools.
1973: PL 39-112, Section 504 of Rehabilitation Act	Children cannot be excluded from schools because of a handicap. The school must provide health services that each child needs.
1975: PL 94-142, Education for All Handicapped Children Act	All children should attend school in least restrictive environment. Requires school district's committee on handicapped to develop individualized education plans (IEPs) for children.
1992: Americans with Disabilities Act	Persons with disabilities cannot be excluded from activities.
1997: PL 105-17, Individuals with Disabilities Education Act (IDEA) with updates in 2004	Educational services must be offered by schools for all disabled children from birth through age 22 years.
2001: No Child Left Behind Act of 2001 (NCLB); 2015 Every Student Succeeds Act (ESSA)	NCLB requires all children must receive standardized education in a healthy environment. ESSA includes provisions for health and safety in schools.
2004: Child Nutrition and WIC Reauthorization Act of 2004	Every local education agency (LEA) participating in federal school meal programs must establish a local school wellness policy.
2010: Healthy, Hunger-Free Kids Act of 2010	Reform of the National School Lunch Program and National School Breakfast Program through increased funding and setting policy on nutritional quality of foods served on school grounds. Also opens eligibility requirements to improve access to the free and reduced-price lunch program.

WIC, Women, Infants, and Children program.
Data from Halbert L, Yonkaitis CF: Federal laws protecting students with disabilities. In Selekman J, Shannon RA, Yonkaitis CF, editors: *School nursing: a comprehensive text*, ed 3, Philadelphia, 2019, F.A. Davis Company, pp. 154–171; US Department of Education: *The Every Student Succeeds Act: P.L. 115-224*, 2018; US Department of Education, Office for Civil Rights: *Free appropriate public education for students with disabilities: requirements under section 504 of The Rehabilitation Act of 1973*, 2010.

student health records maintained by all public schools and many private schools in the United States.

School nurses should stay abreast of laws and regulations that affect their practice and the health of the children in their care. Knowing these legal requirements can help them advocate for students and their rights to a healthy and safe school environment.

Table 31.2 summarizes the effects of these laws on school nurses and schoolchildren.

STANDARDS OF PRACTICE FOR SCHOOL NURSES

The professional organization for school nurses is the National Association of School Nurses (NASN), headquartered in Washington, DC. The mission of the NASN is "To optimize student health and learning by advancing the practice of school nursing" (NASN, 2020a, para.1). NASN advances school nursing practice through education, state and national conferences, access to legal and school health resources, lobbying efforts on behalf of children and school nurses, and establishment of the *School Nursing: Scope and Standards of Practice,* which were most recently updated in 2017 (ANA & NASN, 2017). These standards "are professional expectations that guide the practice of school nursing" (ANA & NASN, 2017). They delineate the roles, activities, ethical requirements, and standards of professionalism and practice for which school nurses are held accountable to the public.

Within the *Scope and Standards of Practice,* the *Standards of Practice* follow the nursing process: assessment, diagnosis, outcomes identification, planning, implementation, and evaluation. The *Standards of Professional Performance for School Nursing*

describe the professional competencies that school nurses are responsible for. These include:

- Ethical practice
- Ensuring confidentiality of student health information
- Cultural competence
- Effective communication and interprofessional collaboration
- Continuing education to ensure current, quality, and evidence-based nursing practice
- Ongoing self-evaluation
- Appropriate and responsible utilization of resources
- School health services program management and policy development with accountability for student health
- Leadership within the school health program and community (ANA & NASN, 2017)

EDUCATIONAL AND LICENSURE CREDENTIALS OF SCHOOL NURSES

The practice of school nursing is highly complex and requires a great deal of autonomy and clinical judgment. Experts in the field of pediatrics and school health recommend that school nurses have a minimum licensure of RN and a minimum education level of bachelor's degree in nursing (BSN) for entry into the school nursing specialty (AAP, 2016; NASN, 2016). The American Nurses Association (2013) asserts that public health nursing requires a minimum of a BSN to practice. Because school nurses care for groups of children and school personnel whose health issues may affect the greater community population, this practice is considered to be a type of public health nursing (NASN, 2016).

The NASN also recommends school nurse certification, which requires training beyond that provided in most bachelor's degree preparation (NASN, 2016). While individual states may have various requirements or pathways for certification of school nurses, certification at the national level requires licensure as an RN and a bachelor's degree in a health-related field, not necessarily nursing (National Board for Certification of School Nurses, 2018). Despite these recommendations, school nurses across the United States vary widely in their educational preparation for assuming this critical role.

School nurses in some schools may be advanced practice nurses (APNs) who specialize in caring for children. These APNS may be clinical nurse specialists or nurse practitioners with specialization in pediatrics, family nursing, school nursing, or public health nursing (ANA & NASN, 2017). Some of these APNs are providing school health services at the conventional level, or they may be providing primary care services in school-based clinics (Resha, 2019). Having APNs provide primary care may improve access to health care for families who lack a provider or health insurance, as well as minimize barriers such as transportation for families without a vehicle or employer restrictions on parents leaving work. These advanced practice nurses may be certified by professional organizations such as the ANA or their own professional organization. Most hold master's degrees in nursing (ANA & NASN, 2017).

Just as with educational and certification requirements, there is little consistency in the minimal requirements for years or types of work experience for newly hired nurses across the United States. While it is common that school nurses come to the field with prior nursing experience, it is possible for newly graduated nurses to work in the schools, depending on the entry criteria of their state and local health departments and schools.

ROLES AND FUNCTIONS OF SCHOOL NURSES

School nurses function in many roles within their practice. They serve as educators, counselors, consultants, case managers, and direct caregivers to children and school staff. They must coordinate the health care of many students in their schools with the health care that the children receive from their personal health care providers.

In order to ensure that school nurses can provide safe and effective care for their students, the *Healthy People 2030* Objective AH-R08 recommends an increase in the proportion of secondary schools with a full-time registered nurse (US Department of Health and Human Services, 2020). However, as of 2016, only 10.9% of schools have a required minimum school nurse-to-student ratio (CDC, 2016). The NASN (2020b) supports increasing the proportion of schools served by full-time school nurses and states that "every student needs direct access to a school nurse so that all students have the opportunity to be healthy, safe, and ready to learn" (para. 10). Only one-third of schools in the United States require a full-time nurse, and fewer than 80% of school districts employed school nurses as of 2016, a decline of 14% since 2000 (CDC, 2016).

School Nurse Roles
Direct Caregiver

The school nurse functioning in the role of direct caregiver is expected to give immediate nursing care to ill or injured children or school staff members. While many people envision the school nurse caregiver role as providing minor interventions such as bandages and ice packs, nothing could be further from the truth in the majority of US schools (Anderson et al., 2017). Whenever a child comes into the clinic, the school nurse must first assess the seriousness of their complaint or symptoms and then determine possible causes. Some causes are obvious, such as an injury from a fall, and some less so, such as respiratory symptoms, which could be due to communicable disease, allergies, etc. The school nurse intervenes to alleviate symptoms, provide first aid in the event of an injury, stabilize the child in an emergency situation, provide ongoing care for chronic illnesses, such as diabetes or asthma, and prevent the spread of communicable diseases (AAP, 2016). Many children now attend school with even more complex medical needs, requiring procedures such as intermittent catheterization, tube feeding, tracheostomy suctioning and care, and ventilator management (Shannon & Minchella, 2015; Toothaker & Cook, 2018). Some children's care needs are so time consuming, they require the assignment of a personal or private duty nurse during the school day. This nurse assumes care for that child alone, rather than the entire student body.

Although most school nurses are in public or private schools and give care only during school hours, the nurse in boarding schools, summer camps, and detention centers provides nursing care to children 24 hours a day and seven days a week. In these residential programs, children live on the premises and may only go home for vacations or not at all if they are incarcerated. In some settings, the nurse also lives at the school and may be on call at all times. School nurses in these residential settings can impact students' academic outcomes by partnering with administrators, teachers, and families to promote a healthy school environment, adequate rest, good nutrition, regular physical activity, and comprehensive, high-quality health care services (Wernette & Emory, 2017). The nurse makes many of the health care decisions for the child and has a referral system to contact parents or guardians and other health care providers, such as physicians and psychological counselors, if needed.

Health Educator

The school nurse in the health educator role may be asked to teach children both individually and in the classroom. School nurses may provide education about disease process and management to parents and children, especially if they don't understand instructions from the primary provider (Anderson et al., 2017). School nurses provide health education to groups of children about injury and communicable disease prevention, dental hygiene, puberty, substance abuse, and nutrition, among others (AAP, 2016; Rebmann et al., 2018). They may be required by state or local school board policies to teach specific subjects or develop health education based on the needs of the school and parent requests.

Case Manager

The school nurse is expected to function as a case manager, helping coordinate the health care for children with complex health problems (AAP, 2016). School nurses may collaborate with the family, teachers, and administrators to ensure that health care services promote the child's ability to learn and participate in the academic environment to the greatest extent possible. Care may be provided in the schools by physical therapists, occupational therapists, speech therapists, or other health care providers during the school day. The nurse may need to develop health care plans for children that clearly explain procedures and treatments needed for their conditions, as well as provide referrals and reports to other health care providers about children's response to treatments and interventions provided in the school (ANA & NASN, 2017).

Consultant

The school nurse is the person best able to provide health information to school administrators, teachers, and parent-teacher groups. As a consultant, the school nurse can provide professional information about proposed changes in the school environment and their impact on the health of the children. The nurse can also recommend changes in the school's policies or engage community organizations to help make the children's schools healthier places (Schaffer et al., 2016). This is a population-level role for the school nurse; the population consists of all children, families, staff, and the surrounding community.

Counselor

School nurses are reported to spend nearly one-third of their time assisting students with mental health needs (Government Accountability Office, as cited in Bohnenkamp et al., 2015). School nurses are familiar and trusted members of the school community. Children often see the nurse as a safe person in whom they may confide about problems such as bullying, physical abuse, substance abuse, grief, and suicidal thoughts. School nurses should always be alert to the potential for such problems when children come to their clinic, especially those who visit frequently with vague complaints or frequent requests to go home (Bohnenkamp et al., 2015). It is important for nurses to be honest with the child about the need to report dangerous situations to their parents, school officials, social services, and/or legal authorities. The nurse should emphasize that the child's confidentiality and privacy are central and reporting is only done as needed to protect them from harm.

Community Outreach

When participating in community outreach, nurses can be involved in community health fairs or festivals in the schools, using that opportunity to promote health through education, screenings, and immunization programs. They may be able to engage local providers, such as dentists and ophthalmologists, to provide free screenings at the school (Schaffer et al., 2016). School nurses should collaborate with area schools of nursing to provide clinical experiences for nursing students, as well as involve those future nurses in providing various health promotion and education events for the children. School nurses should

attend meetings of parent-teacher associations, so they get to know the families of their students and offer education on health concerns these families raise. Attendance at school board meetings may also provide school nurses with opportunities to be seen as experts available to answer questions about school health needs, as well as concerned and engaged members of the school community.

Nurses can participate in coalitions focused on addressing a multitude of school and community health concerns from bullying and violence prevention to poverty and teenage pregnancy (Shaffer et al., 2016). They may be able to engage community faith-based and service organizations in providing food and other supplies for children living in poverty. Some school nurses coordinate weekend backpack food relief for children who only eat regularly on school days.

Researcher

Research on school nursing practice and impact has grown steadily over the past couple of decades. Current, ongoing research can be found on school nursing practice, staffing and workloads, educational preparation and professional development of school nurses, and the use of evidence-based practice for a host of health conditions addressed by school nurses (NASN, 2020b; NASN 2020c; Willgerodt et al., 2018). School nurses are responsible for providing nursing care that is based on solid, evidence-based practice. School nurses can, and should, be involved in research as participants by completing surveys and questionnaires from reputable researchers and professional organizations (NASN, 2020c). School nurses may also function as researchers if they are properly educated to conduct ethical and scientifically founded research, provide human subject protections if applicable, and obtain institutional review board approval from their school system or an affiliated health care or educational institution.

EVIDENCE-BASED PRACTICE

An integrative review of the literature examined the influence of school nurses on academic outcomes such as absenteeism, missed class time, grades, and test scores. The researcher reviewed English-language, peer-reviewed studies between 2002 and 2018 identified from CINAHL, PsycINFO, PubMed: MEDLINE, ERIC, and Educators Reference Complete. Sixteen articles met the inclusion criteria of the review. The findings suggest that the presence of a school nurse is associated with reduced absenteeism and missed class time, but not with academic achievement. Case management, infection prevention, and school nurse evaluation of illness were all school nurse interventions that demonstrated improved attendance and class time. More research, using more rigorous study designs, is needed to evaluate the impact of school nurses on educational outcomes.

Nurse Use

This study indicates that school nurses may make an impact on some educational outcomes due to the presence of the student and improved class time. As such, these findings can be used to advocate for more nurses in the schools and increasing resources for school nurses.

McKinley Yoder C: School nurses and student academic outcomes: an integrative review, *J Sch Nurs*. 36(1):49–60, 2019.

SCHOOL HEALTH SERVICES

School health services vary in their scope throughout the United States. However, there are common parts to the programs.

CHECK YOUR PRACTICE

While working as a student in school health, you have been asked to participate in the development of a school health program for your community that emphasizes the development of healthy schools. What would you do? See if you can apply these steps to this scenario. (1) Recognize the cues, looking at available resources that define a healthy school, plus look at data that shows the number of "healthy schools" in your school system and your community; (2) analyze the cues, looking at the numbers of children in this population served by "healthy schools; (3) state several and prioritize the hypotheses you have stated; (4) generate solutions for each hypothesis; (5) take action on the number one hypothesis you think best reflects the impact of a school health-healthy schools program; and (6) evaluate the outcomes you would expect as a result of your participation in this project

Federal School Health Programs

The federal government, through the coordination of the CDC, with an emphasis on the health of the population of children and the school community, developed the Healthy Schools initiative, which utilizes the Whole School, Whole Community, Whole Child (WSCC) model as a framework that school health programs are encouraged to follow (CDC, 2019a) (Fig. 31.1).

CDC Healthy Schools provides funding, training, and other resources that support schools in promoting health and adopting the components of the WSCC framework. CDC Healthy Schools provided more than $15 million to the nation's schools in 2019 with the goals of eliminating health disparities, providing evidence-based health education and services, and utilizing epidemiologic surveillance and research to prevent chronic disease and decrease the spread of communicable disease (CDC, 2019b).

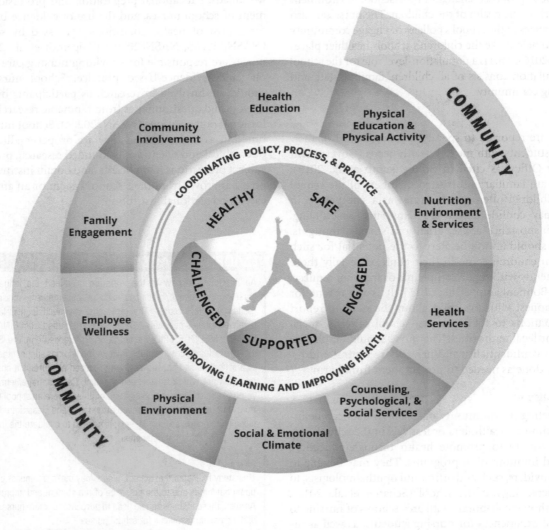

Fig. 31.1 WSCC Model for School Health Practice. *WSCC,* Whole School, Whole Community, Whole Child. (Available at https://www.cdc.gov.)

School Health Policies and Practices Study 2016

Since 1994, the School Health Policies and Practices Study (SHPPS) has been conducted periodically (at least every 6 years) in all 50 states and the District of Columbia to evaluate the 10 components of the WSCC model. The study also measures progress in achieving *Healthy People* (CDC, 2016).

The 2016 study found that the number of school districts with arrangements for school-based or off-site health centers to provide health services such as primary care, dental services, or counseling/mental health services to students decreased significantly in recent years. This is concerning because school-based health centers (SBHCs) provide a variety of health services to children who may not have access to other community resources (Price, 2017). Having these services located at the school allows children to receive timely care and decreases time missed from class. Children whose health problems are not addressed may not be able to take full advantage of academic opportunities (Price, 2017). Having services on site may also help parents avoid missing work in order to take their children to an off-site provider. Some employers do not allow time off for such activities. School nurses can more easily assist families to get health care for their children when an SBHC is available.

According to the SHPPS (CDC, 2016), most students in the United States were found not to be participating in the recommended 60 minutes a day of physical activity. Fewer than half of school districts had an indoor air quality (IAQ) management program, though more than 75% had policies requiring regular inspections of ventilation, heating and cooling systems, and other aspects of building integrity that could promote mold growth and other environmental contamination within school buildings. On the positive side, the SHPPS found that around 80% of districts prohibited all tobacco use, including vaping and e-cigarettes, by students, employees, or visitors during the school day or at school events (CDC, 2016). Furthermore, a majority of school districts have enhanced security and safety measures in their schools, instituted disaster/crisis preparedness plans, and established programs to prevent bullying and address issues related to aggressive behaviors.

SCHOOL NURSES AND *HEALTHY PEOPLE 2030*

Many *Healthy People 2030* proposed objectives are directed toward the health of children. In addition, several point directly at the care that nurses give to children in the schools. The *Healthy People 2030* box lists the objectives that involve school-age children. The goal is to promote physical health and well-being for children and adolescents, with objectives related to schools providing safe and supportive environments, healthy foods, health education, and physical education. They can also offer access to health care and mental health services and help students manage chronic conditions. Nurses can accomplish the goals and objectives using the three levels of prevention, as discussed next.

HEALTHY PEOPLE 2030

Objectives Related to School Health and School Nursing

- **AH-04:** Increase the proportion of students participating in the School Breakfast Program
- **AH-D03:** Reduce the proportion of public schools with a serious violent incident
- **AH-R06:** Increase the proportion of schools requiring students to take at least 2 health education courses from grade 6 to 12
- **AH-R08:** Increase the proportion of secondary schools with a full-time registered nurse
- **ECBP-D01:** Increase the proportion of middle and high schools that provide case management for chronic conditions
- **EH-D01:** Increase the proportion of schools with policies and practices that promote health and safety
- **EMC-D06:** Increase the proportion of children and adolescents who get preventive mental health care in school

From US Department of Health and Human Services: *Healthy People 2030.* HHS, 2020. Available at https://health.gov/healthypeople.

THE LEVELS OF PREVENTION APPLIED IN SCHOOLS

The three levels of prevention—primary, secondary, and tertiary—have always been a part of health care in the schools (Duff, 2019). Primary prevention provides health promotion and education to prevent health problems in children. Secondary prevention includes the screening of children for various illnesses, monitoring their growth and development, and caring for them when they are ill or injured. Tertiary prevention in the schools is the continued care of children who need long-term health care services, along with education within the community (Fig. 31.2).

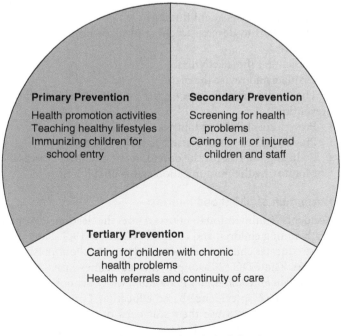

Fig. 31.2 Prevention Levels in Schools.

Primary Prevention in Schools

Primary prevention encompasses activities that are intended to prevent the development of illness, disease, and injury in those who are currently healthy (Duff, 2019). The strategies for achieving primary prevention are health promotion and implementation of measures that protect people from agents that may cause disease or injury.

Health education is the most commonly used approach in health promotion. Historically, health teaching was considered "the fundamental basis of all school health work" (Struthers, as cited in Duff, 2019). The school nurse may have the opportunity to go into the classroom to teach health promotion concepts, such as handwashing or dental hygiene skills. This is population-level primary prevention.

School nurses also provide individual education to children who come to the school clinic for various health concerns or questions. Individual education about disease prevention may also be provided to school employees and parents (Duff, 2019).

HOW TO TEACH YOUNG CHILDREN IN SCHOOL

When teaching children in preschools and elementary schools:
- Keep the lesson to no more than 10 min.
- Use a lot of examples, pictures, and stuffed animals in the talk.
- Always remember the developmental stage of the children when teaching them.

School nurses use the nursing process while they care for children in the schools. In their primary prevention efforts, they do the following:
- Assess children and families to determine their level of knowledge about health issues.
- Find out whether children are at risk for preventable problems.
- Analyze the assessment findings.
- Make plans to develop teaching plans or health promotion activities.
- Implement these activities.
- Evaluate and revise the plan.

The school nurse focuses on the following areas of primary prevention:
- Preventing childhood injuries
- Preventing substance abuse behaviors
- Reducing the risk for the development of chronic diseases
- Monitoring the immunization status of children.

Prevention of Childhood Injuries

Accidents (unintentional injuries) are the leading cause of death among children and teenagers (CDC, 2019c). The school nurse educates children, teachers, and parents about preventing injuries. The CDC (2019c) provides guidelines in its *National Action Plan for Child Injury Prevention,* which school nurses can utilize to develop evidence-based educational programs to encourage children to use their seat belts or bicycle helmets to prevent injuries. Other classes can be on crossing the street, water safety, and fire safety. The school nurse, as a trusted health care provider at school, is able to quickly give information to help prevent injuries from occurring, since most injuries are preventable (Rebmann et al., 2018).

School nurses also provide health promotion to prevent playground injuries, which number over 200,000 injuries to children under age 14 per year (CDC, 2019d). School nurses can utilize guidelines published by the US Consumer Product Safety Commission (2015) to assess their school playgrounds for equipment safety.

School sports also have the potential to cause injuries to children. The school nurse is often involved in deciding with parents and coaches on how to best prevent injuries when children are engaged in athletic activities (Rebmann et al., 2018). School nurses can also promote the use of helmets and knee pads and work with communities to provide safe places, such as skateboard parks, for children to engage in these activities. Educating parents, children, and school personnel on safety measures to prevent any type of injury can decrease the incidence of these injuries, as well as decrease emergency department visits (Bandzar et al., 2018; Salam et al., 2016). This makes the entire community safer and decreases health care costs for all.

Substance Abuse Prevention Education

Primary prevention interventions by the school nurse include educating children and adolescents about the effects of tobacco, drugs, and alcohol on their bodies. School nurses should start early with education of children about the negative effects of street drugs (such as marijuana, cocaine, crack, and heroin), tobacco, and alcohol on their bodies and how to avoid them (NASN, 2020d).

Despite the overall decrease in use of substances, misuse of some illegal and legal drugs has remained steady or increased. Providers are seeing an increase in the use of "club drugs" such as lysergic acid (LSD), ketamine, gamma hydroxybutyrate (GHB), Rohypnol, and Ecstasy (MDMA). The school nurse can provide instruction about the serious side effects of Ecstasy, especially that it causes a very high body temperature that can lead to death. Marijuana and alcohol use have leveled off in recent years rather than decreasing, as with many other substances. Researchers postulate that this is related to easier accessibility of these substances to youth, especially with the legalization of marijuana in many states and marketing of these substances as safe and enjoyable by their powerful lobby groups (Substance Abuse and Mental Health Services Administration [SAMHSA], 2019). Students may find these substances in their homes being used by their parents. In the past decade, the abuse of opioids has reached epidemic proportions. Teaching children about the dangers of all drugs is an important responsibility of the school nurse. In addition, the school nurse can teach parents and other members of the community about the risks of substance use, ways to secure their own prescriptions and model safe use of legal substances, and how to recognize warning signs of substance abuse in their children so that early intervention can occur. Increasing everyone's awareness of these dangerous trends may lead to a decrease in abuse of those substances that is on the rise in the United States and subsequently improve the overall health of the population (NASN, 2020d).

Disease Prevention Education

The nurse has the opportunity to teach children healthy lifestyles to reduce their risk of disease later in life. For example, children can be taught ways to reduce their risk of becoming obese by teaching and reinforcing healthy nutrition and exercise. Health education may also include ways to promote cardiovascular health, oral health, and prevent the spread of communicable diseases. The school nurse should collaborate with teachers to create evidence-based health education plans.

Getting health promotion information to the parents of the children is often a challenge for the school nurse. There are many ways to increase accessibility of health information, such as providing a website or newsletter that parents can read outside of school hours without interfering with their work schedules. School nurses may consider presenting information during a parent-teacher association meeting. They could survey families for health issues they have questions or concerns about and arrange a guest speaker if the nurse is not well versed on the topic. Providing babysitters, food, and transportation to these meetings could remove barriers for families with low incomes and long workdays. By educating parents and children, the school nurse is able to promote the health of not only the schoolchildren but also the community.

Vaccinations for Schoolchildren

All states have laws that require that children receive immunizations, or vaccinations, against communicable diseases before they attend school (CDC, 2017). School nurses must be up to date on the latest laws on immunizations for children in their own state and actively educate parents about the benefits of vaccinating their children. The CDC (2017) provides recommendations for vaccinations, but it is up to each individual state to determine which immunizations are required for enrollment and attendance at a school or childcare facility. Vaccine requirements and exemptions laws vary from state to state (CDC, 2017). Depending on the state's law, children may be prevented from enrolling in or attending school if they have not had the required immunizations or have not provided the required paperwork for exemptions (either for medical, religious, or philosophical/conscientious belief reasons) (CDC, 2017). Some parents may request that their child be exempted from the required immunizations because of their belief that not all immunizations are good for their children, for medical reasons, or for religious or philosophical reasons (NASN, 2020e). The school nurse should be aware of the laws in the state regarding acceptable reasons for immunization exemption. At the same time, the nurse has the opportunity to teach parents and the rest of the community about the overall benefits to society and to their children from the use of immunizations (NASN, 2020e).

For children entering kindergarten, most state-required vaccinations include diphtheria, pertussis, and tetanus (the DTaP series); measles, mumps, and rubella (the MMR series); polio; and others. Chapters 11 and 12 have a more complete discussion of communicable diseases and immunizations in children.

The school nurse must keep a complete file of all of the children's vaccination records in order to meet the state's laws. These files will contain the following:

- Student's name
- Date of birth
- Address
- Telephone number
- Parents'/guardians' names
- Contact information
- Primary health care provider's name, telephone number, and address
- All the vaccinations with the dates the child received booster shots

This makes it easier for the school nurse to find out which children still need immunizations or boosters or, in the event of a vaccine-preventable disease outbreak, to notify parents about the signs and symptoms of the disease, when to seek care, and the potential need to keep their children home from school until the outbreak is resolved.

The HIPAA of 1996 requires that all health information be private. The USDHHS published a statement in 2008 that protected health information may be shared between school nurses and primary providers when needed to make decisions about treatment of children in the schools (USDHHS, 2008).

Because children are prevented from attending school if they have not had the required shots, the school nurse must make every effort to find missing data in the immunization record.

- The nurse must contact the parents to get the immunization history for the child.
- Written notes should be sent to each child's home at least one year before each new immunization is needed so that the parents have time to get the child to his or her health care provider for the shots.
- If the parents or guardians do not speak English, these notes will need to be translated into the family's language.
- If the parents have lost the information that gives the child's immunization history, they should be encouraged to contact their physician or nurse practitioner to get it.

Many problems with children not being immunized or having incomplete vaccination records may arise in families who have moved a great deal, such as those serving in the armed services or experiencing homelessness, or those who do not have a regular physician. The parents may have no idea whether the child has even received the recommended or required vaccines. Some parents are not aware that since the implementation of the Affordable Care Act, insurance is required to pay for certain preventive care, including childhood immunizations (Hahn, 2016). Families may also believe that if they do not have health insurance, they will have to pay for their children's immunizations out of pocket, which can be expensive. Certain low-income families without health care insurance may qualify for federal programs that provide free immunizations to children (CDC, 2017). Most states have their own programs to fund childhood immunizations, many through state and local public health departments, so school nurses will want to become familiar with what their state provides.

School nurses can also play an important role in immunizing children against seasonal flu. The CDC (2020b) recommends that everyone six months of age and older receive an annual seasonal influenza vaccination, especially children younger than five years of age and all children with chronic medical conditions. Vaccination against influenza should begin as soon as that season's vaccine becomes available (CDC, 2020b). School nurses may administer the influenza vaccine to children at the school or work with the local public health department to do so, with the parents' permission. This has the potential to promote health within the entire community, as well as decrease costs and missed work time for parents (NASN, 2018a).

Secondary Prevention in Schools

Because secondary prevention involves early intervention for children when they need health care, this is the largest responsibility for the school nurse (Duff, 2019). This includes caring for ill or injured students and school employees. It also involves screening and assessing children and referral to appropriate health agencies or providers. The school nurse uses the nursing process during secondary prevention activities. When an ill or injured child comes to the school's health office, the nurse must immediately assess the child for the degree of illness or injury.

Children seek out the school nurse for a variety of different needs:

- Headaches
- Stomachaches
- Diarrhea
- Anxiety over being separated from the parents
- Cuts, bruises, or other injuries

In addition, children may seek reassurance from the school nurse or even appear to hide in the nurse's office. This may be a result of harassment or bullying from other children in the school (Jakubowski & Perron, 2019).

Once the assessment data are gathered, the nurse determines the course of action and follows it through the implementation and evaluation phases. This occurs for direct care as well as for screening children for other health problems. If assessment indicates the child has a health problem, the school nurse continues to follow the nursing process to intervene within his or her scope of practice or to refer the child to providers who can provide the most appropriate health care.

Nursing Care for Emergencies in the School

Events that occur in or near schools may cause a crisis for children, teachers, and staff. The school nurse must have an emergency plan in place so that a routine can be followed when emergencies occur. Disaster planning in the schools include preparing for (Rebmann et al., 2016):

- Natural disasters (such as fire or severe weather)
- Manmade disasters (such as school shooting or structure collapse)
- Health condition emergencies (such as asthma attack or seizure)

The NASN recommends that school nurses provide leadership to schools in all phases of emergency preparedness and management (NASN, 2019a). The following summarizes the NASN's recommendations of the role of the school nurse during each phase of disaster planning (NASN, 2019a):

- Prevention/Mitigation: perform an ongoing assessment to identify hazards
- Preparedness: serve on planning groups, establish emergency response plans, provide training to school personnel

---

> **BOX 31.1   Dealing With a Disaster: Responsibilities of the School Nurse**
>
> - Provide triage.
> - Communicate with emergency medical personnel.
> - Assess the school community for the presence of shock and stress.
> - Recommend reduced television viewing of the disaster.
> - Provide grief counseling.
> - Communicate with the children, parents, and school personnel.
> - Follow up with assessment of children for anxiety, depression, regression, and post-traumatic stress disorder.

Modified from Sharron RA, Guilday P: Emergency and disaster preparedness and response for schools. In Selekman J, Shannon RA, Yonkaitis CF, editors: *School nursing: a comprehensive text*, ed 3, Philadelphia, 2019, F.A. Davis Company, pp. 457–479.

- Response: perform triage, coordinate the first-aid response team, provide direct hands-on care to victims, act as a counselor to help everyone cope with the emotional aspects of this serious event (Box 31.1)
- Recovery: provide direct support, act as liaison between community resources and those in need; school may become an emergency shelter for community at large

The US Department of Education et al. (2013) recommended that all schools have crisis plans in place to help the children, teachers, parents, and community cope with the sudden event. Crisis teams are prepared to help everyone respond quickly to the crisis, to ensure the safety of the school, and to follow up on the effects of the crisis on the members of the school (NASN, 2019a). The crisis plan developed included an administrative policy made either for the entire school district or, if the schools are large, for each individual school. The plan included the names of the persons on the crisis team: the superintendent of the school district, the school nurse, the guidance counselor, the school psychologist or social worker, teachers, police or school security, clergy from the community, and parents. Plans to obtain and share information could be made quickly (US Department of Education et al., 2013).

The nurse can help the crisis team make a checklist for everyone to follow that explains what to do in every possible crisis situation. Then, at the end of the crisis, the crisis team will want to take time to counsel all of the people who helped in the crisis, including the teachers, emergency personnel, and parents, as well as the children. That way, everyone can talk about the crisis. The crisis plan should be reviewed every year to see what parts of the plan need updating. Drills take place to act out the plan to see how it works and how it can be revised to make it more workable (NASN, 2019a; US Department of Education et al., 2013).

Individualized emergency plans are made for all students who may have a health problem that could result in an emergency situation in the school (NASN, 2019a). This plan could be for a:

- Child with food allergies (e.g., to peanuts)
- Child who has sensitivity to insect bites that could result in anaphylactic shock
- Child with a chronic illness, such as asthma, diabetes, or hemophilia

The individualized emergency plan should include:

- The student's medical history
- List of medications
- Location of emergency medication
- List of personnel trained to administer emergency medication

It is important that the school nurse communicate with school personnel about students requiring emergency medication to ensure quick access to emergency medications at all times.

The nurse may not always be at the school and the emergency may have to be handled by a teacher, administrator, secretary, custodian, or coach (US Department of Education et al., 2013). Therefore all emergency procedures must be clearly spelled out and easily accessible to anyone in the school. Along with the procedures and an emergency manual written or obtained by the school nurse, an injury or illness log should be available for personnel to fill out so that there is an accurate record of what happened. Along with this form, procedures for notifying the parents or legal guardians about the emergency are explained. Information must be provided to parents about any actions taken for the child and where the child was sent if transfer to a hospital or other medical agency was required (NASN, 2019a). Good communication with parents is important to decrease their anxiety and assist them in reuniting with their children. School nurses are uniquely qualified to provide this information because they may have ongoing relationships with parents due to providing day-to-day care for their children.

Because the school nurse may have to give nursing care to a child or adult in respiratory or cardiac arrest, the nurse must have current certification in cardiopulmonary resuscitation (CPR) and the use of the automated external defibrillator (AED), which should be available to all school nurses. All 50 states have passed laws requiring that public gathering places have AEDs available, some requiring them in the schools (AED Brands, 2019). Other education in the area of emergency response would also be helpful to the school nurse, including pediatric advanced life support (PALS) or emergency nursing for pediatrics (ENPC) certification (Sharron & Guilday, 2019).

Emergency Equipment in the School Nurse's Office

The school nurse needs a great deal of equipment to deal with emergencies in the school. These needs are based on the guidelines of the NASN (Sharron & Guilday, 2019). The school office will need to have basic emergency items on hand. Additional equipment may be obtained if a nurse is present in the school every day (Box 31.2). Various sizes of these items are needed since children may be of different ages in the school. Another recommended item for the nurse's office includes an epinephrine auto injector kit (EpiPen Auto-Injector) in case a child goes into anaphylactic shock after exposure to an allergen (Wahl et al., 2015). This should be locked in a medication cabinet because of the needle in the kit. The school nurse will need to teach other school personnel how to use the EpiPen Auto-Injector in an emergency (Wahl et al., 2015).

Gloves to meet standard precautions guidelines and a telephone available for calling emergency personnel and parents are essential. Next to the telephone, paper and pen should be

---

BOX 31.2 Emergency Items for Schools With and Without a School Nurse Present

Supplies for Schools WITHOUT a School Nurse Present

- Accessible keys to locked supplies
- Accessible list of phone resources
- Automated external defibrillator (AED) if school meets the AHA guidelines
- AED supplies stored with AED (razor, alcohol pads, dry towel, scissors, electrode pads)
- Biohazard waste bags
- Blunt scissors
- Clock with a second hand
- CPR-trained staff on-site when students are on the premises
- Disposable blankets
- Emergency cards on all staff
- Emergency cards on all students
- Established relationship with local EMS personnel
- Eye protection (full peripheral glasses or goggles, face shield)
- Ice (not cold packs)
- Individual care plans/emergency plans for students with specialized needs
- First aid tapes
- Nonlatex gloves
- One-way resuscitation mask
- Cell phone or other two-way communication device
- Posters with CPR/abdominal or chest thrusts instructions
- Refrigerator or cooler
- Resealable plastic bags

- School-wide emergency operations/response plan
- Sharps container
- Soap and source of water/hand sanitizer for hand and wound cleansing
- Source of oral glucose (i.e., frosting gel, glucose tablets, juice box)
- Splints
- Names of staff who have received basic first aid training
- Variety of bandages and dressings
- Water source/normal saline for wound/eye irrigation

Additional Supplies for Schools with a School Nurse Present

- C-spine immobilizers of different sizes
- Glucose monitoring device[a]
- Medications
- Albuterol
- Epinephrine (auto injector preferred)
- Oxygen
- Nebulizer
- Penlight
- Self-inflating resuscitation device in two sizes (500 mL and 1 L) with appropriate sized masks to meet needs of population being served
- Stethoscope
- Sphygmomanometer and cuffs in pediatric, adult regular, and adult large sizes
- Suction equipment (minimal source, does not have to be electric, i.e., bulb suction or v-vac type device)

AHA, American Heart Association; *CPR*, cardiopulmonary resuscitation; *EMS*, emergency medical services.
[a]Committee acknowledges challenges with maintenance and expense of test strips. Monitoring of machine must also be in compliance with CLIA (Clinical Laboratory Improvement Amendments).

available so that instructions from the emergency personnel can be written down (Sharron & Guilday, 2019). The AED should be located in a central location in the school for easy access in an emergency. It should not be locked in the nurse's office but available for school staff to obtain in case the nurse is off site that day.

Giving medication in school. The school nurse, as part of secondary prevention, may be responsible for giving medications to children during the school day (NASN, 2017a). These may include (NASN, 2017a):

- Prescribed medications
- Over-the-counter medications that parents have asked the school's nurse to give (such as cold remedies)
- Vitamins

In all instances, the nurse should collaborate with school district administration to develop a series of medication administration policies and guidelines that allow children to receive care they need to perform well in school while following the laws and nurse practice act of the state. As part of the assessment of the health history and needs of children enrolled in the school, the school nurse should inquire of parents whether the child is taking any medications (NASN, 2017a). A current, signed parental consent form, with primary care provider's approval and directions, must be provided before administering medication to any student (NASN, 2017a). HIPAA requires that all of this information be kept confidential, but the consent form should include permission for the school nurse to discuss the medication and treatment plan with the prescribing provider to ensure the safety of the child (Brous, 2019). Nurses may also need to request permission to discuss the medication with the child's teachers so they are aware of potential side effects or adverse reactions and can alert the nurse immediately if there are any problems.

- The prescribed drug must have the original prescription label on it and be in the original container to decrease the risk of errors and securely stored (Maughan, McCarthy, et al., 2017).
- Over-the-counter medications should also be stored securely in their original and labelled containers.
- A current medication (drug) book should be in the nurse's office so that it can be consulted for information.

The school nurse should also have a means of contacting a pharmacist to ask questions regarding the medication if needed.

Delegation. Some states allow school nurses to delegate medication administration to unlicensed assistive personnel (UAP) or to a licensed practical nurse (NASN, 2017a). There are several benefits and challenges associated with delegation in the school setting. On the positive side, delegation allows services to be provided in the absence of a school nurse, which is especially helpful if a nurse is covering multiple schools (NASN, 2019b). Also, delegation allows children with more complex medical needs to attend school more safely, as UAPs can be trained to provide one-on-one care for some procedures. The challenge with delegation is ensuring the UAPs receive adequate training and regular supervision and monitoring of the UAP (NASN, 2019b). Delegation

can be done safely in the school environment provided the nurse has clear policies and procedures to follow, understands the "Five Rights of Delegation," understands the scope of practice and procedures allowed to be delegated under the state's nurse practice act, and has a trusting relationship with the UAP and school administrators (NASN, 2019b).

QSEN FOCUS ON QUALITY AND SAFETY EDUCATION FOR NURSES

Targeted Competency: Safety—Safety minimizes risk of harm to patients and providers through both system effectiveness and individual performance. Important aspects of safety include:

- **Knowledge:** Describe factors that create a culture of safety (such as open communication strategies and organizational error reporting systems).
- **Skills:** Communicate observations or concerns related to hazards and errors to patients, families, and the health care team.
- **Attitudes:** Value own role in preventing errors.

Safety Question

Imagine you are working as a nurse in an elementary school. Due to budget cuts, you are only at the school two days a week. Juan, a student in the third grade, is newly diagnosed with asthma and will have an inhaler at school for emergencies. Your state allows nurses to delegate the administration of inhaler medications to unlicensed personnel. You decide to delegate the administration of Juan's emergency inhaler to his classroom teacher, Mr. Smith. What steps would you take to ensure you safely delegated this medication?

Answer

First, you would need to establish open communication between Mr. Smith and yourself. After providing the initial medication training, you should maintain open communication by checking in with Mr. Smith on a regular basis to assess his knowledge and comfort level in administering Juan's inhaler. Second, in the event that Mr. Smith gives Juan a dose from the inhaler, have a system in place to document when and why the medication was given. Emphasize the importance of such documentation to avoid medication errors/overdose and to track Juan's health condition and response to treatment. Periodically review the records to ensure that everything was documented correctly and that the medication was given for appropriate reasons. Last, in the event of a medication error, report to the proper authorities, evaluate the circumstances that led to the error, and determine what can be done differently to prevent future errors. In some circumstances, delegation may need to be withdrawn if it is determined that Mr. Smith is not capable of properly and safely administering Juan's medication.

Assessing and Screening Children at School

Children should receive screening for vision, hearing, height and weight, oral health, TB, and scoliosis in the schools (Duff, 2019). For each of these areas, the school nurse must keep a confidential record of all of the screening results for the children in the school according to HIPAA requirements. In addition, each state has different laws regarding screenings requirements, and the nurse will need to be aware of these laws.

Screening for TB in schoolchildren is required in several states prior to school entry (Duff, 2019). It may be difficult to administer screening at school because the nurse cannot read the Mantoux test, or the TST test, until three days after it is administered. Often nurses are part-time and may not be at the school on the day the child's test needs to be read. In some states, school nurses are required to participate in a training program to read the tests. It may be more efficient to have children screened for TB at their pediatrician's office or the local health department or prior to admission to the school (Galemore, Kirnel, & Tedder, 2019). If the school nurse is trained to read the test, he or she sends the results to the health clinic for follow-up. If the site is positive, it is possible the child has been exposed to TB and needs further health screening, including a chest x-ray, and treatment. A determination will need to be made about whether the child has active TB and could have spread it to other children or staff at school. In that case, the health department must be notified so that screening and prophylactic medications can be administered to all exposed individuals (Galemore, Kirnel, & Tedder, 2019).

The school nurse can also screen children and adolescents for hypertension, or high blood pressure. Children who develop high blood pressure are more likely to have this condition in adulthood (Jackson et al., 2018). Identifying and treating hypertension early can prevent many serious, long-term health conditions.

Physical examinations prior to participation in a school sport are required by all 50 states (Johnson et al., 2018). While students may also obtain these physicals from their primary provider, an urgent care clinic, or a community health center, some children may not have access to a regular physician or other primary health care provider because they are uninsured or the agency is not open during hours that parents are off from work. School nurses can assist by arranging for sports physicals at school, conducting part of the screenings within their scope of practice, and monitoring or assisting with the portions of these examinations being done by the school's physician or nurse practitioner. The school nurse's presence during these screenings can facilitate health education, case findings, and referrals to community resources or specialists for health problems (Johnson et al., 2018). School nurses may arrange for dentists to provide group oral health screenings in the schools. In some states, school nurses may be able to conduct these screenings and refer children to a dentist for follow-up of suspected problems with oral health.

Screening Children for Pediculosis (Lice)

School nurses are frequently called upon to screen children in their schools for pediculosis or lice infestation. Many myths abound related to risks of transmission of head lice, leading to unnecessary panic and exclusion of children from school, despite the fact that pediculosis is frequently misdiagnosed even by experienced nurses and primary care providers (NASN, 2020f). Lice do not spread disease, even though they may cause irritating symptoms, such as itching, sleep disturbance (due to itching), and sores from scratching (Cummings, Finlay, & MacDonald, 2018).

Children determined to have lice or lice eggs in their hair miss an average of four days per school year in schools with "no-nit" (no lice eggs) policies. Besides the loss to children of academic opportunity, such absenteeism costs schools

hundreds of millions of dollars in annual funding and parents thousands of dollars in lost wages and treatment expenses per occurrence (NASN, 2020f). NASN, AAP, the Harvard School of Public Health, and the CDC recommend against no-nit policies because it is impossible for nits to be transmitted from one person to another. Nits firmly adhere to the hair shaft when they are laid by the louse, making them unlikely to come off without significant effort to remove them. Lice require human hosts to live, so if they fall off and are not deposited on a person's head within 24 hours, they will die. Nits require the warmth of the human body to hatch. The idea that lice are a sign of poverty and poor hygiene is also a myth. Lice are found in all socioeconomic groups and are just as likely to be seen in clean hair as unwashed.

Due to the inaccuracy of results, the lack of impact on the incidence of head lice in a school, and the significant loss of educational time, the NASN, AAP, and CDC recommend against routine screening for head lice or after a case has been identified (NASN, 2020f).

- There is significant risk of violation of privacy rights when conducting a classroom screening.
- The stigma and shame associated with even false identification of head lice and subsequent exclusion from school can be emotionally and socially devastating for students and caregivers (NASN, 2020f).
- Frequent or incorrect use of pediculosis treatments, especially in misdiagnosed children, can have side effects from localized irritation of the scalp, eyes, and skin to allergic reactions and neurological repercussions in susceptible persons.

The following are responsibilities of the school nurse (NASN, 2020f):

- Provide accurate health education to the school community about the etiology, transmission, assessment, and treatment of head lice.
- Advocate for school policy that is more caring and less exclusionary (i.e., elimination of "no-nit" school policies).
- Implement intervention strategies that are student centered.
- Support the current treatment recommendations of the AAP and CDC.
- Participate in research that evaluates the effectiveness of head lice policies and educational programs.

Identification of Child Abuse or Neglect

The school nurse is mandated by state laws to report suspected cases of child abuse or neglect. These laws differ from state to state, and the nurse should be aware of the particular requirements for reporting in each state.

A nurse who identifies a child who may be abused or receives information from a teacher or other staff member that leads to the belief that a child has been abused must contact the appropriate legal authorities and the school's principal. A confidential file should be made about the incident. However, the nurse should let the government authorities, usually the state or county child protection department, look into the suspected case. In all cases, the child should be protected from harm, and those who have no right to know that child abuse or neglect is suspected should not be given any information.

Communicating With Health Care Providers

The school nurse often makes an assessment of a child that requires referral to the child's family physician or other health care provider. The findings from these assessments must be communicated accurately to the child's parent and the provider (Brous, 2019). The nurse must be able to disseminate the information quickly and accurately to the child's parents. Again, HIPAA privacy rules must be followed (ASTHO, 2015).

HOW TO DEVELOP GOOD RELATIONSHIPS WITH FAMILIES

School nurses need to have good relationships with families. The school nurse can make this possible by doing the following:

- Being visible at school events.
- Sending home invitations for parents and guardians to call the nurse at any time.
- Inviting parents to visit the school health office.
- Calling parents or guardians to ask about ill children.
- Offering to help families cope with children who have long-term illnesses.
- Acting as a referral source for families with health care needs.
- Including parents and members of the community in health education activities.

One way to do this is to write a detailed report about the findings. This information can be given to the child to take home to the parents, but there may also be issues related to parental literacy (de Buhr & Tannen, 2020). If the concern is not an emergency, the best way to communicate with parents may be to speak to them directly by phone or meet with them if they come to pick up their child at the end of the day. If the nurse expresses concern for the child's well-being, most parents will appreciate this personal interaction (Selekman, Chewey, Cogan, & Conway, 2019). Explain to the parents why the child needs to see the physician or nurse practitioner and that the child will be bringing the information home that day so they can ask the child for it at the end of the day. Verbal explanations will help in the case of low health literacy, as well as give the parent the opportunity to ask questions. The nurse may also pick up on the need for assistance during the conversation and can refer the family to community resources if they do not have a primary care provider.

Efforts to Prevent Suicide and Other Mental Health Problems

Among teenagers, more than 17% have considered suicide and more than 8% have actually attempted to take their own lives (SAMHSA, 2017). Suicide is caused by complex interactions of multiple factors, such as social and environmental problems, gender identity confusion, academic problems, mental illness, bullying, and exposure to violence (Steele, Thrower, Noroian, & Saleh, 2018). Protective factors for suicide prevention include strong family relationships, supportive religious connections, and interest in hobbies and other activities.

Suicide prevention must be addressed by school nurses, who can do the following:

- Lead educational programs within the schools to emphasize coping strategies and stress management techniques for children and adolescents who have problems and to teach about the risk factors.
- Teach faculty members to look for the risk factors.
- Help organize a peer assistance program to help teenagers cope with school stresses.

Students who are expressing feelings associated with suicide risk or threaten suicide at school must be taken seriously. They should be asked directly if they are contemplating suicide, referred to mental health services within the school, encouraged to talk about their feelings, denied access to any methods of self-harm, and monitored for increasing symptoms and other risk factors (NIMH, 2017). Many states require that schools notify parents if children express intent to harm themselves. Students threatening to commit suicide should be immediately removed from any situation that is contributing to their despair. While the parents are being called, the nurse and available mental health professionals in the school should monitor and assess the student for having already made their attempt using medications or other method and if so, call for immediate emergency first responders.

In the unfortunate instance that a student commits suicide, the school nurse is called upon to help the school population, both students and teachers, cope with the death. Grief counseling should be set up and coordinated by the school nurse, usually in collaboration with guidance counselors and school administrators. In addition, further assessments can be made regarding the suicide potential among the deceased teenager's friends, since suicide clusters have been noted.

Other mental health problems may affect students. Adolescents may have early signs of mental or emotional problems such as behavioral problems in class or severe class or test anxiety. Families may be in crisis, which can translate into problems for their children. Sometimes, children with mental health issues come to the school nurse with somatic complaints and nothing can be found on assessment (Bohnenkamp et al., 2015). The nurse should be alert to the possibility that the child is experiencing emotional problems, hunger, or family problems in such cases and investigate further to find the source of the complaints.

Children who are homeless have special problems. Because these children do not have a stable address, they may have moved frequently from school to school. Children whose parents are addicted to drugs or alcohol can also benefit from support from the school nurse, such as referrals to mental health counselors. The lack of a stable environment may increase chances that children will develop a mental or emotional problem (Bohnenkamp et al., 2015). The school nurse should be an advocate for these children and their families.

Violence at School

Results of the 2015 National Youth Risk Behavior Survey demonstrated that 6% of students were threatened with a weapon at school, 6% stayed home from school due to fears of violence, and 23% were in a physical fight at school (Flynn et al., 2018). Hundreds of students reported carrying a weapon onto school grounds, and nearly two-thirds of schools reported the occurrence of at least one violent crime during the previous school year. In the past several years, there has been an increase in school shootings by students or other attackers against other students and teachers.

Bullying is at the center of attention among child and adolescent advocates. In 2015, about 20% of US high school students experienced bullying while on school property and 16% were bullied online ("cyberbullying") (NASN, 2018b). Bullying is defined as repetitious, unwanted, aggressive behavior intended to cause harm to another. Students with disabilities, academic problems, and speech impairments, as well as those who are lesbian, gay, bisexual, transgender, or questioning (LGBTQ) are most frequently targeted. Physical injury, social and emotional distress, suicide attempts, and even death can result from bullying. Affected students may come to the school nurse complaining of psychosomatic illnesses, such as headaches and stomachaches, due to bullying (NASN, 2018b). The school nurse needs to be knowledgeable about bullying, take students' concerns seriously, and work to protect them from aggression. School nurses should provide leadership to implement bullying prevention strategies in their schools and communities, such as increased supervision and anti-bullying policies. In an effort to reduce the prevalence of bullying, 49 states now have anti-bullying laws (USDHHS, 2018).

The school nurse's primary goal is to prevent violence from occurring and prioritize the safety of everyone on the school's campus (Flynn et al., 2018). Interventions that the nurse can implement to prevent violence include:

- Facilitate student connectedness to the school community.
- Engage parents in school activities that promote connections with their children, and foster communication, problem solving, limit setting, and monitoring of children.
- Support activities and strategies to help establish a climate that promotes and practices respect for others and for the property of others.
- Support policies of zero tolerance for weapons on school property, including school buses.
- Advocate for adult monitoring in the hallways between classes and at the beginning and end of the school day, and the assignment of staff to monitor the playground, cafeteria, and school entrances before and after school.
- Serve as positive role models, developing mentoring programs for at-risk youth and families.
- Educate students and their parents about gun safety (Flynn et al., 2018; NASN, 2018b).

If violence occurs, the school nurse should do the following:
- Coordinate emergency response until rescue teams arrive;
- Provide nursing care for injured students;
- Apply crisis intervention strategies that help de-escalate a crisis situation and help resolve the conflict;
- Identify and refer those students who require more in-depth counseling services; and
- Participate in crisis intervention teams (Sharron & Guilday, 2019)

By helping identify the student who might be considering school violence or by teaching students and teachers about these warning signs in students, the school nurse may be able to help prevent violent actions through education and follow-up

of children who need help. The US federal government has many agencies and resources that can help school nurses develop programs in their schools (US Department of Education et al., 2013).

Tertiary Prevention in Schools

Using the nursing process, the school nurse gives nursing care related to tertiary prevention when working with children who have long-term or chronic illnesses or special needs. The goal of tertiary prevention is to assist children to return to their highest level of function possible after injury or illness, as well as to prevent complications (Duff, 2019). As prevalence of chronic conditions such as asthma and diabetes increases among children, today's school nurse faces a school population that is more medically diverse than ever seen in the past (Shannon & Minchella, 2015; Toothaker & Cook, 2018; Wolfe, 2019a). The school nurse should be part of the team that develops an IEP for students with long-term health needs that may affect their learning abilities and needs. The nurse's responsibilities include the following:

- The nurse must have information about child's medications that need to be given during school hours.
- The nurse must know if child needs any type of procedure, such as tracheostomy suctioning or intermittent catheterization, or therapy during the school day, such as physical or occupational therapy (Shannon & Minchella, 2015; Toothaker & Cook, 2018).
- The nurse must know if the child has a hearing or vision problem.
- The nurse must ask the teacher to seat the child in the best place in the classroom so the child can see or hear better.

If a child is in a wheelchair or uses crutches, federal regulations may require that the school building itself accommodates the child's ability to get around the school and use the restrooms. It is the responsibility of the nurse to tell the school's administrators about any needs such as these.

Children With Allergies

Food and insect allergies that result in anaphylaxis are being diagnosed more frequently (Pistiner & Mattey, 2017). Anaphylaxis is a severe allergic reaction that occurs quickly and can be life-threatening. In 2019, 16.7% of high school students reported having to avoid foods due to the risk of allergy (CDC, 2020c). Milk, eggs, fish, shellfish, wheat, soy, peanuts, and tree nuts account for most serious allergic reactions in the United States (CDC, 2020d). Insect allergies may be to stinging insects, such as bees and wasps; household pests, such as cockroaches and dust mites; or biting insects, such as bedbugs and some flies (Asthma and Allergy Foundation of America, 2015).

The school nurse must take a leadership role in coordinating care for these students. The school nurse must develop a plan for preventing exposure to a known allergen and responding to an allergy emergency, collaborating with the student, the student's parents, and school personnel to determine the best plan of action (NASN, 2015). The school nurse must provide annual training to school personnel who are involved with the student

(NASN, 2015). Most states have laws that allow students to carry emergency medication and, if developmentally appropriate, self-administer as needed (NASN, 2014c). Some states allow trained unlicensed assistive personnel to administer the emergency medication if the student is unable to do so and a nurse is not available. The school nurse must provide annual training to school personnel who are involved with the student or possibly responding to an emergency reaction (Pistiner & Mattey, 2017).

Children With Asthma

Asthma is the leading cause of children being absent from school because of a chronic illness (Cicutto et al., 2017). Children may be hospitalized with an asthma attack or they may have just returned home from the hospital. Time missed from class, either for treatment or because of absenteeism, can interfere with a child's educational progress. Asthma can also be caused by allergic triggers that affect children in the school. The following are possible culprits (CDC, 2018):

- Chalk dust from the blackboards
- Molds or mildew in the school
- Dander from pets that live in some classrooms

There may also be concerns about the quality of the air in the school building because many doors are shut. Indoor air pollution within schools can occur as a result of materials used in art class, woodworking, or cooking, perfumes and other scented body products, air fresheners, exhaust fumes from buses and delivery vehicles that idle near open doors or ventilation systems, outdated ventilation systems and those lacking proper maintenance, radon, mold, and secondhand smoke (US Environmental Protection Agency [EPA], 2020). The school nurse should keep track of the indoor air quality (IAQ) of the school and student complaints potentially related to IAQ so that school administrators have data about what can affect the children. Surveillance of the numbers of asthma and allergy exacerbations will help the school nurse recognize potential problems. Fig. 31.3 contains the questions developed by the EPA that the school nurse should answer regarding the air quality of the school.

The nurse uses tertiary prevention when helping children who have asthma. This includes:

- Administering or helping children use their inhalers or other asthma rescue medications (Cicutto et al., 2017)
- Teaching administrators, teachers, children, and parents about asthma and ways to reduce allergens in the classroom (Asthma and Allergy Foundation of America, 2015)
- Advocating for a transition to safer cleaning solutions and assess safe storage as part of regular school IAQ inspections

Children With Diabetes Mellitus

Diabetes is one of the most prevalent chronic diseases in children and adolescents, and its long-term impact and the cost of treatment make it vitally important to be addressed by school nurses (Miller et al., 2016). While most children are diagnosed with type 1 diabetes, in the last couple of decades, type 2 diabetes (formerly known as adult-onset diabetes) has been reported among US children and adolescents with increasing frequency (Miller et al., 2016). Case management and coordination of

care are critical roles for the school nurse in caring for diabetic students (Siminerio, 2015). The school nurse must work with students' primary care provider, parents, and school personnel to establish a plan of care for managing diabetes. This includes methods of monitoring blood glucose levels and administering insulin or other medications during the school day, as well as how to respond in the event of hyperglycemic or hypoglycemic reactions (Siminerio, 2015). Emergency medications, such as glucagon, should be readily available, and staff involved with the student should be trained to administer them in case the nurse is not present in the school during an emergency. Special nutritional needs also need to be discussed with parents, teachers, and cafeteria staff. There may be significant challenges getting the child's nutritional restrictions met due to the institutional nature of most school food services and lack of education of staff about nutrition-related health concerns. The family, school nurse, and other school personnel may benefit from consultation and/or training by a diabetes educator or registered dietitian/nutritionist (Siminerio, 2015).

Children With Autism or Autism Spectrum Disorder

"Autism, or autism spectrum disorder (ASD), refers to a broad range of conditions characterized by challenges with social skills, repetitive behaviors, speech and nonverbal communication" (Autism Speaks, 2020, para. 1). Autism may also be associated with medical problems such as gastrointestinal disorders and seizures. Because most children are expected to attend some school regardless of their illness, children with autism are legally entitled to attend public schools (DOE-OCR, 2010). Children with autism are more likely to experience fragmented services leading to unmet health care needs, as well as difficulty with school accommodations for their medical, sensory, social, and educational challenges (Russell & McCloskey, 2016). Parents caring for children with special needs such as autism report a sense of guilt, emotional strain, financial hardship, social isolation, and marital difficulties. They expressed dissatisfaction and frustration with providers and schools for not collaborating with the family to meet their child's needs (Russell & McCloskey, 2016). Because many children with autism have communication problems, the school nurse can advocate for the child and collaborate with the parents to learn the most effective ways to determine and meet the child's needs. The nurse can give the child prescribed medications for mood or prevention of seizures. The nurse may recommend the use of sign language, picture boards, or other types of communication devices that are used by the child. In addition, the nurse can teach the parents about autism. The nurse can also help parents work with others in the health care system, such as speech-language therapists and developmental specialists, so that the child can have a positive learning experience at school (Ibesaine, 2018).

Children With Attention-Deficit/Hyperactivity Disorder

In 2016, there were an estimated 6.1 million children ages 2 to 17 diagnosed with ADHD in the United States (CDC, 2020a). Of these, two-thirds had another mental health or behavioral problem. Children with ADHD often have trouble sitting still,

Health Officer/School Nurse

This checklist discusses three major topic areas:
Student Health Records Maintenance
Public Health and Personal Hygiene Education
Health Officer's Office

Instructions:
1. Read the IAQ *Backgrounder*.
2. Read each item on this Checklist.
3. Check the diamond(s) as appropriate or check the circle if you need additional help with an activity.
4. Return this checklist to the IAQ Coordinator and keep a copy for future reference.

Name: _____

Room or Area: _____

School: _____

Date Completed: _____

Signature: _____

MAINTAIN STUDENT HEALTH RECORDS

There is evidence to suggest that children, pregnant women, and senior citizens are more likely to develop health problems from poor air quality than most adults. Indoor Air Quality (IAQ) problems are most likely to affect those with preexisting health conditions and those who are exposed to tobacco smoke. Student health records should include information about known allergies and other medically documented conditions, such as asthma, as well as any reported sensitivity to chemicals. Privacy considerations may limit the student health information that can be disclosed, but to the extent possible, information about students' potential sensitivity to IAQ problems should be provided to teachers. This is especially true for classes involving potential irritants (e.g., gaseous or particle emissions from art, science, industrial/vocational education sources). Health records and records of health-related complaints by students and staff are useful for evaluating potential IAQ-related complaints.

Include information about sensitivities to IAQ problems in student health records
• Allergies, including reports of chemical sensitivities.
• Asthma.
◇ Completed health records exist for each student.
◇ Health records are being updated.
O Need help obtaining information about student allergies and other health factors.

Track health-related complaints by students and staff
• Keep a log of health complaints that notes the symptoms, location and time of symptom onset, and exposure to pollutant sources.
• Watch for trends in health complaints, especially in timing or location of complaints.
◇ Have a comprehensive health complaint logging system.
◇ Developing a comprehensive health complaint logging system.
O Need help developing a comprehensive health complaint logging system.

Recognize indicators that health problems may be IAQ
• Complaints are associated with particular times of the day or week.
• Other occupants in the same area experience similar problems.
• The problem abates or ceases, either immediately or gradually, when an occupant leaves the building and recurs when the occupant returns.
• The school has recently been renovated or refurnished.
• The occupant has recently started working with new or different materials or equipment.
• New cleaning or pesticide products or practices have been introduced into the school.
• Smoking is allowed in the school.
• A new warm-blooded animal has been introduced into the classroom.
◇ Understand indicators of IAQ-related problems.
O Need help understanding indicators of IAQ-related problems.

HEALTH AND HYGIENE EDUCATION

Schools are unique buildings from a public health perspective because they accommodate more people within a smaller area than most buildings. This proximity increases the potential for airborne contaminants (germs, odors, and constituents of personal products) to pass between students. Raising awareness about the effects of personal habits on the well-being of others can help reduce IAQ-related problems.

Obtain *Indoor Air Quality: An Introduction for Health Professionals*
• Contact IAQ INFO, 800-438-4318.
◇ Already have this EPA guidance document.
◇ Guide is on order.
O Cannot obtain this guide.

Inform students and staff about the importance of good hygiene in preventing the spread of airborne contagious diseases
• Provide written materials to students (local public health agencies may have information suitable for older students).
• Provide individual instruction/counseling where necessary.
◇ Written materials and counseling available.
◇ Compiling information for counseling and distribution.
O Need help compiling information or implementing counseling program.

Provide information about IAQ and health
• Help teachers develop activities that reduce exposure to indoor air pollutants for students with IAQ sensitivities, such as those with asthma or allergies (contact the American Lung Association [ALA], the National Association of School Nurses [NASN], or the Asthma and Allergy Foundation of America [AAFA]). Contact information is also available in the IAQ Coordinator's Guide.
• Collaborate with parent-teacher groups to offer family IAQ education programs.
• Conduct a workshop for teachers on health issues that covers IAQ.
◇ Have provided information to parents and staff.
◇ Developing information and education programs for parents and staff.
O Need help developing information and education program for parents and staff.

Establish an information and counseling program regarding smoking
• Provide free literature on smoking and secondhand smoke.
• Sponsor a quit-smoking program and similar counseling programs in collaboration with the ALA.
◇ "No Smoking" information and programs in place.
◇ "No Smoking" information and programs in planning.
O Need help with a "No Smoking" program.

HEALTH OFFICER'S OFFICE

Since the health office may be frequented by sick students and staff, it is important to take steps that can help prevent transmission of airborne diseases to uninfected students and staff (see your IAQ Coordinator for help with the following activities).

Ensure that the ventilation system is properly operating
• Ventilation system is operated when the area(s) is occupied.
• Provide an adequate amount of outdoor air to the area(s). There should be at least 15 cubic feet of outdoor air supplied per occupant.
• Air filters are clean and properly installed.
• Air removed from the area(s) does not circulate through the ventilation system into other occupied areas.
◇ Ventilation system operating adequately.
O Need help with ventilation-related activities.

☐ **No Problems to Report.** I have completed all the activities on this checklist, and I do not need help in any areas.

Fig. 31.3 Environmental Protection Agency Indoor Air Quality Checklist. (From U.S. Environmental Protection Agency: *School and child care-based asthma education programs*, 2010. Available from http://www.epa.gov.)

may be forgetful, have difficulty focusing on tasks or instructions, and may exhibit poor impulse control. Causes are unknown, though children exposed to environmental toxins, such as lead, and those with brain injury, prematurity, and low birth weight are more likely to be diagnosed with ADHD. School nurses may administer medications at school and may need to monitor the child for adverse reactions (Heuer & Williams, 2016). Due to their difficulty focusing, children with ADHD may need reminders to take their medications. Some medications can decrease appetite, so the school nurse can partner with parents and teachers to ensure that children do not experience nutritional deficits. Because of the behaviors common in children with ADHD, school personnel may become frustrated with them. The school nurse must advocate for the child, work with him or her to facilitate behavioral and time management skills, and encourage good communication with parents, providers, and school personnel (Heuer & Williams, 2016). Referral to mental health providers within or outside the school may be needed if the child's behaviors interfere with their ability to function and learn.

Children With Special Needs in the Schools

As discussed earlier in this chapter, children may attend school who need (Toothaker & Cook, 2018):

- Urinary catheterization
- Dressing changes
- Peripheral or central line intravenous catheter maintenance
- Tracheotomy suctioning
- Gastrostomy or other tube feedings
- Intravenous medication

The school nurse may supervise a health aide or personal care nurse who is assigned to the child to assist with complex nursing needs. In all these cases, the school nurse provides tertiary care to maintain the child's health. The nurse has the skills needed to assess the child's well-being. In addition, the nurse may have to teach another person in the school how to care for the child in case the nurse is not in the building when the child needs help (NASN, 2019b). It is the responsibility of the school nurse to keep up to date with the latest health care information through in-service and continuing education programs, as well as regularly reading journals in the fields of pediatrics and school nursing.

Children with HIV or AIDS attend school and may require care from the school nurse to manage their illness and prevent complications. Because of privacy and confidentiality laws, the school nurse may not even know that the child has this disease. In some cases, the nurse may be directly notified of the child's HIV status either by the parents or physician or may suspect the diagnosis due to HIV medications being administered during the school day (Selekman & Ness, 2019). In all cases, the nurse must maintain confidentiality. This means that information cannot be released to anyone, including teachers, other health professionals, other students, or staff.

School nurses should ensure that universal precautions are practiced by all personnel handling blood or body fluids of anyone at school. Most school districts are required to provide employees with bloodborne pathogens training and protective equipment under Occupational Safety and Health Administration (OSHA) (2011) regulations. These precautions can protect employees from exposure to HIV, as well as other bloodborne diseases such as hepatitis B and C.

- As part of regular health education in the school, the school nurse can provide education about HIV/AIDS prevention and risks to the children, school employees, and community (Rasberry et al., 2017).
- The school nurse should also be part of the school health advisory committee to develop an HIV/AIDS health curriculum that teaches about HIV/AIDS prevention and transmission so that children know how to protect themselves and are not afraid to go to school with children who have the disease.
- Continuing education programs can be useful to teach the teachers and parents about the disease.

Children With DNAR Orders

As part of tertiary prevention, the school nurse cares for children with highly complex conditions and terminal diseases who attend school. The numbers of children receiving only palliative care is rising (NASN, 2018c). These children benefit from participation in school activities, socialization with their peers, and following a daily routine. The IDEIA, as discussed earlier in this chapter, requires that children be allowed to attend school in the "least restrictive environment" (DOE-OCR, 2010). Therefore children with terminal illnesses may have do-not-attempt-resuscitation orders (DNAR orders) at school, and some may die at school, though this is not common (NASN, 2018c). DNAR orders are signed by the parents and the physician according to their state's law.

The AAP's committees on school health and bioethics reaffirmed a set of guidelines to help school health providers and the schools decide what to do when a child with a DNAR order attends the school (AAP, 2010/2016).

- A formal request to the school and the school board from the parents and physician is a must regarding the written DNAR order.
- The school nurse should be involved in discussions regarding when to use the DNAR order.
- The decision not to do anything for a dying child, and how to function if the child were to suddenly face death, can be emotionally and ethically difficult.

As an advocate for the child and family, school nurses should coordinate ongoing communication with parents, providers, school staff, and administrators well in advance of such an event (NASN, 2018c).

When a child dies in school, the nurse is responsible for helping the children who witnessed the death. The nurse becomes a grief counselor and helps the children and teachers cope with the death. Further education about death and dying given by the school nurse would also help the school community cope with death in the schools (NASN, 2018c).

Homebound Children

Even though the laws regarding disabled persons state that all children should go to school, some children cannot. Instead, they may be taught in the home or in another institutional setting such as the hospital. In these situations, the school nurse functions as follows:

- Should be a liaison between the child's teacher, physician, school administrators, parents, and any nurses and other health care providers caring for the child in the home regarding the child's needs (Shannon & Minchella, 2015).
- Helps these individuals make up the child's IEP so that it is appropriate for the child and does not remove necessary learning from the plan
- Allows the child to go to school when he or she is able
- Coordinates the child's health care needs and classes

Pregnant Teenagers and Teenage Mothers at School

Many teenage girls who are pregnant attend school. Therefore the school nurse may provide ongoing care to the mother as well as coordination of care outside the school system, including visits to the physician or nurse practitioner and assistance with setting up home school until the teen is released from medical restrictions following birth. Although this may appear to be primary prevention, it is tertiary prevention because adolescent pregnancies are considered to be high risk. Teen fathers may also require advocacy from the school nurse if they are involved with their child's care.

CONTROVERSIES IN SCHOOL NURSING

School nursing has evolved into a complex health care role, and some areas of the field still cause controversy, such as providing education on family planning and providing birth control to students in the schools where it is allowed. Although differences in opinion exist relating to sex education, reproductive services, and screening for sexually transmitted diseases in the schools, the literature supports a comprehensive approach to sexual health education (NASN, 2017b). The school nurse should educate community members, the school board, teachers, parents, and students about the benefits of different types of services in the schools to the health of students and school personnel.

ETHICS IN SCHOOL NURSING

The school nurse may be faced with ethical issues in the schools, such as the following:

- A child may have a DNAR order that the parents wish to be used if the child dies at school (see earlier text), but following the DNAR order may be against the nurse's personal beliefs.
- Perhaps a girl asks the nurse where she can get an abortion and wishes to talk to the school nurse about how she feels, but the nurse is against abortions.
- A teenager asks for emergency contraception, which conflicts with the nurse's religious beliefs or the nurse is not allowed to provide with his or her scope of practice, state laws, or school district regulations.

In these cases, as in any other setting, the nurse must give nursing care to the student client according to the *School Nursing: Scope and Standards of Practice* (ANA & NASN, 2017) and the state's nurse practice act. However, if the nurse feels so strongly that he or she cannot work with the situation, another school nurse should be called for help, or the student should be referred to other health providers who can give the care the student needs. Care should never be denied or ignored; referral is a good option.

FUTURE TRENDS IN SCHOOL NURSING

The future of school nursing is strong. The amount of health care being given in the schools is increasing. In the future, school nursing may coordinate primary health care and specialist consultations for students in rural areas with limited access to care. Telecommunication may also be utilized to teach health education or to facilitate care coordination and make meetings more accessible for collaboration with other school nurses (NASN, 2017c). Online resources are listed in Table 31.3. The school nurse is responsible for keeping up with the latest changes in health care and health practice so that the health of children in the schools can be enhanced by new trends in health care.

The National Association of School Nurses is looking to the future through development of the *Framework for 21st Century School Nursing Practice* (Maughan et al., 2018). This framework (Fig. 31.4) was developed by the NASN board of directors and an advisory group including school nurses and school nurse leaders. This framework integrates various models and principles that have been utilized to guide school nursing practice through the years. As the health needs of children become more complex and expectations of schools and parents grow, this framework " . . . provides guidance for the practicing school nurse to reach the goal of supporting student health and academic success by contributing to a healthy and safe school environment" (Maughan et al., 2018).

TABLE 31.3 Online Resources for School Nurses

Organization	Internet Address
The American Academy of Child and Adolescent Psychiatry	http://www.aacap.org
American Academy of Pediatrics	http://www.aap.org
National Association of School Nurses	http://www.nasn.org
Center for Health and Health Care in the Schools	http://www.healthinschools.org
National Youth Violence Prevention Centers	https://www.cdc.gov
US Department of Education Emergency Preparedness	https://www.fema.gov
Healthy Schools Network	http://www.healthyschools.org
US Environmental Protection Agency	https://www.epa.gov

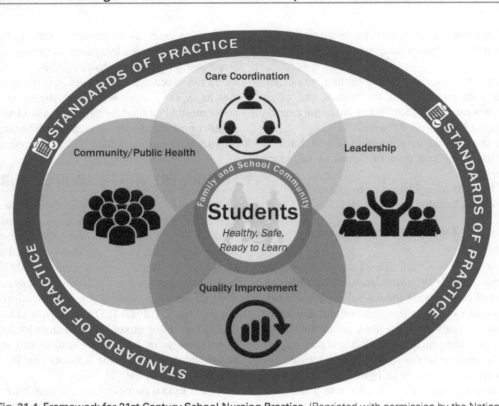

Fig. 31.4 Framework for 21st Century School Nursing Practice. (Reprinted with permission by the National Association of School Nurses. Available at https://www.nasn.org/nasn/nasn-resources/professional-topics/framework.)

APPLYING CONTENT TO PRACTICE

School nurses play a primary role in the development and implementation of the CDC's WSCC model components. These components are described below and addressed throughout this chapter. The emphasis in this program design is working with the school as a population or community. This plan has 10 parts (CDC, 2020e):

- Physical education and physical activity—The CDC recommends that schools follow the national comprehensive physical activity framework, which includes support for regular physical activity during and outside of the school day, coordination with community, families, and school staff, and a curriculum throughout the child's school career that teaches health behaviors, sportsmanship, and other important skills related to health. Teachers of this curriculum should be licensed and certified in physical education.
- Nutrition environment and services—The entire school environment should promote healthy eating, which has been shown to support student learning. Information on nutrition and diet should be taught to all children. In addition, schools should provide healthy food choices for students in their meal programs (both breakfast and lunch). School nutrition staff should be educated to prepare food in ways that are both healthy and appetizing to encourage nutritious eating habits among staff and students. Nutrition staff should also be trained annually on safe food handling practices to decrease the risk of communicable disease outbreaks. Vending machines, school celebrations, and concession stands should offer healthy choices, following the Smart Snacks in Schools initiative, or be off limits to children, especially during the school day. School employees, including school nurses, should model healthy eating behavior.
- Health education—This component includes teaching children about how to stay healthy and how to avoid becoming ill or being injured. The health education should be offered in a planned, sequential, K-12 curriculum that

addresses all dimensions of health, following the National Health Education Standards.
- Health services—School health services should be designed to prevent illness, promote health, and intervene in the event of illness or injury of students and school staff. Specifically, the schools can provide services to ensure access or referral to primary care, prevent and control communicable disease, provide emergency care for illness or injury, and provide educational and counseling opportunities for promoting and maintaining health across all settings. Health services should be provided by qualified professionals, including school nurses.
- Counseling, psychological, and social services—This component emphasizes prevention and intervention to meet the needs of students in the areas of behavioral and mental health. School counselors, psychologists, and social workers should be qualified to provide guidance for children and their family, to alleviate barriers for children with learning needs, and provide referrals to community mental health and social services when needed.
- Physical environment—The physical environment includes the school building and grounds, as well as environmental influences within and outside of the school that may impact the health of school staff and students. Indoor air quality, safe handling and use of chemicals (including pesticides and cleaning supplies), temperature and noise levels, and lighting are all addressed under this component. This component also addresses violence and crime prevention in the schools.
- Social and emotional school climate—This component encompasses a safe and supportive environment for students and staff. A supportive environment fosters healthy growth and development, as well as academic achievement and healthy relationships among students.
- Employee wellness—Nurses often provide health care for teachers and other staff members in the schools. Staff can ask nurses about their health and obtain health education at school during their workday. This component also

covers worksite safety for employees. Nurses should be familiar with OSHA guidelines for personal protective equipment, bloodborne pathogen prevention education, and healthy school environment (available from www.osha.gov). Healthy school employees are less likely to miss work and to be more productive, thereby reducing costs of finding replacements and decreasing health insurance costs for everyone.
- Community involvement—The school health program should contact families and community leaders to find out what health services are needed the most and how they can work together to emphasize health education, promote health in the school and community, and thereby support student learning. Coalition building

with school community partners is an important role for the school nurse, as discussed earlier in this chapter.
- Family engagement—Families should be made to feel welcome in the school. Their support is critical to the health and learning of their children. Families can provide support for adequate, safe, and high-quality school health services by educating their school board representatives about children's health needs and parents' expectations for health care during the school day. Families should feel confident that privacy will be protected so they can comfortably share health and social information, as well as bring supplies and medications that may be needed to support their children's health at school.

CDC, Centers for Disease Control and Prevention; *WSCC,* Whole School, Whole Community, Whole Child.

PRACTICE APPLICATION

The elementary school principal has notified the school nurse that Melissa and John, 8-year-old twins who receive daily physical therapy for mild cerebral palsy, have transferred to the school. The nurse must comply with federal laws related to providing education and services to all children with disabilities.

A. What nursing responsibilities should the school nurse carry out?
B. What factors must be considered when the nurse coordinates the IEP and IHP plans?
C. How will this situation impact other children at school?
D. What is the central focus of Melissa's and John's education? *Answers can be found on the Evolve website.*

REMEMBER THIS!

- School nurses provide health care for children and families.
- In the early 1900s school nurses screened children for infectious diseases and educated families on prevention and treatment.
- School nursing practice has grown in complexity, becoming more holistic and adhering to professional practice standards.
- The NASN is the professional organization for school nurses.
- School nurses have varying educational levels depending on state laws.
- The US government supports school-based health centers, school-linked programs, and full-service school-based health centers.
- *Healthy People 2030* has objectives to enhance the health of children in schools and increase the number of nurses working in the schools.
- Primary prevention in schools includes health promotion and education to prevent childhood injuries, disease, and substance abuse.
- The school nurse monitors the children for all of their state-mandated immunizations for school entry.
- HIPAA privacy rules regarding the health information of children apply in schools.
- Secondary prevention involves screening children for illnesses and providing direct nursing care.
- School nurses develop plans for emergency care in the schools.

- Giving medications to children in the school must be monitored carefully to prevent errors.
- School health nurses are mandated reporters of suspected cases of child abuse and/or neglect.
- Disaster-preparedness plans should be set up for all schools with the school nurse as a member of the crisis response team.
- Tertiary prevention includes caring for children with long-term health needs, such as asthma, diabetes, and disabling conditions.
- School nurses carry out catheterizations, suctioning, gastrostomy feedings, and other complex clinical skills in schools.
- Some ethical dilemmas in the schools are related to women's health care.
- Some school nurses utilize telecommunications to coordinate health care for children and their families.

EVOLVE WEBSITE

http://evolve.elsevier.com/Stanhope/community/
- Answers to Practice Application
- Case Study
- Review Questions

REFERENCES

AED Brands: *AED State Laws & Legislation,* 2019. Retrieved from https://www.aedbrands.com.

American Academy of Pediatrics (AAP), Council on School Health: Role of the school nurse in providing school health services, *Pediatrics* 137(6):1–6, 2016.

American Academy of Pediatrics (AAP), Council on School Health and Committee on Bioethics: Honoring do-not-attempt-resuscitation requests in schools, *Pediatrics* 125(5):1073–1077, 2010/reaffirmed 2016.

American Nurses Association: *Public Health Nursing: Scope and Standards of Practice,* ed 2, Silver Spring, 2013, Author.

American Nurses Association and National Association of School Nurses (ANA & NASN): *School nursing: scope and standards of practice,* ed 3, Silver Spring, 2017, Authors.

Anderson LJW, Schaffer MA, Hiltz C, O'Leary SA, Luehr RE, Yoney EL: Public health interventions: School nurse practice stories, *J Sch Nurs* 34(3):192–202, 2017.

Apple RD: School health is community: School nursing in the early twentieth century in the USA, *His Educ Rev* 46(2):136–149, 2017.

Association of State and Territorial Health Officials (ASTHO): *Public health and schools toolkit: Public health access to student health data: authorities and limitations in sharing information between schools and public health agencies (Issue Brief)*, 2015. Retrieved July 2016 from http://www.astho.org/Programs/Preparedness/Public-Health-Emergency-Law/Public-Health-and-Schools-Toolkit/Public-Health-Access-to-Student-Health-Data/.

Asthma and Allergy Foundation of America: *Insect Allergies,* 2015. Retrieved from http://www.aafa.org.

Autism Speaks: *What is Autism?* 2020. Retrieved from https://www.autismspeaks.org.

Bandzar S, Funsch DG, Hermansen R, Gupta S, Bandzar A: Pediatric hoverboard and skateboard injuries, *Pediatrics* 141(4):e20171235, 2018.

Bohnenkamp JH, Stephan SH, Bobo N: Supporting student mental health: The role of the school nurse in coordinated school mental health care, *Psychol Sch* 52(7):714–727, 2015.

Brous E: The law and school nursing practice. In Selekman J, Shannon RA, Yonkaitis CF, editors: *School nursing: a comprehensive text*, ed 3, Philadelphia, 2019, F.A. Davis Company, pp. 136-153.

Centers for Disease Control and Prevention (CDC): *Results from the School Health Policies and Practices Study,* 2016. Retrieved from https://www.cdc.gov.

Centers for Disease Control and Prevention (CDC): *School Vaccination Requirements and Exemptions,* 2017. Retrieved from https://www.cdc.gov.

Centers for Disease Control and Prevention (CDC): *Controlling Asthma in Schools,* 2018. Retrieved from https://www.cdc.gov.

Centers for Disease Control and Prevention (CDC): *About CDC Healthy Schools,* 2019a. Retrieved from https://www.cdc.gov.

Centers for Disease Control and Prevention (CDC): *Healthy Schools: How CDC helps students get a healthy start,* 2019b. Retrieved from https://www.cdc.gov.

Centers for Disease Control and Prevention (CDC): *National Action Plan for Child Injury Prevention,* 2019c. Retrieved from https://www.cdc.gov.

Centers for Disease Control and Prevention (CDC): *Playground Safety,* 2019d. Retrieved from https://www.cdc.gov.

Centers for Disease Control and Prevention (CDC): *Data and Statistics about ADHD,* 2020a. Retrieved from https://www.cdc.gov.

Centers for Disease Control and Prevention (CDC): *Key Facts about Seasonal Flu Vaccine,* 2020b. Retrieved from https://www.cdc.gov.

Centers for Disease Control and Prevention (CDC): *1991-2019 High School Youth Risk Behavior Survey Data,* 2020c. Available at http://yrbs-explorer.services.cdc.gov/. Accessed on 10/25/2020.

Centers for Disease Control and Prevention (CDC): *Food Allergies in School,* 2020d. Retrieved from https://www.cdc.gov.

Centers for Disease Control and Prevention (CDC): *Whole School, Whole Community, Whole Child,* 2020e. Retrieved from https://www.cdc.gov.

Cicutto L, Gleason M, Haas-Howard C, Jenkins-Nygren L, Labonde S, Patrick K: Competency-based framework and continuing education for preparing a skilled school health workforce for asthma care: the Colorado experience, *J Sch Nurs* 33(4):277–284, 2017.

Cummings C, Finlay JC, MacDonald, NE: Head lice infestations: a clinical update, *Pediatric & Child Health, 23*(1): e18-e24, 2018.

De Buhr E, Tannen A: Parental heath literacy and health knowledge, behaviors and outcomes in children: a cross-sectional survey, *BMC Public Health, 20*:1096, 2020.

Duff CL: Frameworks and models for school nursing practice. In Selekman J, Shannon RA, Yonkaitis CF, editors: *School nursing: a comprehensive text*, ed 3, Philadelphia, 2019, F.A. Davis Company, pp. 51-74.

Food Research and Action Center: *Child Nutrition Reauthorization (CNR),* 2018. Retrieved from http://www.frac.org.

Flynn K, McDonald CC, D'Alonzo BA, Tam V, Wiebe DJ: Violence in rural, urban, and suburban schools in Pennsylvania, *J Sch Nurs* 34(4):263–269, 2018.

Galemore CA, Bowlen B, Combe LG, Ondeck L, Porter J: Whole school, whole community, whole child—calling school nurses to action, *NASN School Nurse* 31(4):216–223, 2016.

Galemore C, Kirnel L, & Tedder G: Health promotion and screenings for school-age children. In Selekman J, Shannon RA, Yonkaitis CF, editors: *School nursing: a comprehensive text*, ed 3, Philadelphia, 2019, F.A. Davis Company, pp. 282-312.

Gibbons, LJ, Lehr K, Selekman J: Federal laws protecting children and youth with disabilities in the schools. In Selekman J, editor: *School nursing: a comprehensive text,* ed 2, Philadelphia, 2013, FA davis, pp. 257-283.

Hahn J: The Affordable Care Act at the 6 Yr. mark: A policy update, *Virginia Nurses Today* 24(3):6–7, 2016.

Halbert L, Yonkaitis CF: Federal laws protecting students with disabilities. In Selekman J, Shannon RA, Yonkaitis CF, editors: *School nursing: a comprehensive text*, ed 3, Philadelphia, 2019, F.A. Davis Company, pp. 154-171.

Houlahan B: Origins of school nursing, *J Sch Nurs* 34(3):203–210, 2018.

Heuer B, Williams S: Collaboration between PNPs and school nurses: Meeting the complex medical and academic needs of the child with ADHD, *J Pediatr Health Care* 30(1):88–93, 2016.

Ibesaine L: What do health visitors and school nurses know about the health needs of children with autism? *J Health Visit, 6*(4), 2018.

Institute of Education Sciences: National Center for Education Statistics: *Fast Facts: Back to School Statistics,* 2020, Author. Retrieved from https://nces.ed.gov.

Jackson SL, Zhang Z, Wiltz JL, Loustalot F, Ritchey MD, Goodman AB, Yang Q: Hypertension among youths – United States, 2001-2016. *MMWR Morb Mortal Wkly Rep, 67*: 758-762, 2018.

Jakubowski T, Perron T: Students with common health complaints. In Selekman J, Shannon RA, Yonkaitis CF, editors: *School nursing: a comprehensive text*, ed 3, Philadelphia, 2019, F.A. Davis Company, pp. 335-366.

Johnson KE, Morris M, McRee AL: Full coverage sports physicals: School nurses' untapped role in health promotion among student athletes, *J Sch Nurs* 34(2):139–148, 2018.

Loschiavo J: *Fast facts for the school nurse: school nursing in a nutshell*, ed 2, New York, 2015, Springer Publishing Company.

Maughan ED, Bobo N, Butler S, Schantz S: Framework for 21st century school nursing practice, *NASN School Nurse* 31(1): 45–53, 2018.

Maughan ED, McCarthy AM, Hein M, Perkhounkova Y, Kelly MW: Medication management in schools: 2015 survey results, *J Sch Nurs* 1–12, 2017.

Miller GF, Coffield E, Leroy Z: Prevalence and costs of five chronic conditions in children, *J Sch Nurs* 32(5):357–364, 2016.

National Association of School Nurses (NASN): *Clinical conversations for food allergy management,* 2015, Silver Spring. Retrieved from https://www.nasn.org/programs/educational-initiatives/conversations-food-allergy.

National Association of School Nurses (NASN): *Education, Licensure, and Certification of School Nurses* (Position statement), 2016,

Silver Spring: Beshears V, Clark E, Lambert P. Retrieved from https://www.nasn.org.

National Association of School Nurses (NASN): *Medication administration in schools* (Position Statement). 2017a, Silver Spring: Hinkson E, Mauter E, Wilson L, Johansen A, Maughan E. Retrieved from https://www.nasn.org.

National Association of School Nurses (NASN): *Sexual Health Education in Schools* (Position Statement), 2017b, Silver Spring: Kern L, Emge G, Reiner K, Rebowe D. Retrieved from https://www.nasn.org.

National Association of School Nurses (NASN): *The Role of School Nursing in Telehealth* (Position Statement), 2017c, Silver Spring: Haynie KM, Lindahl B, Simons-Major K, Meadows L, Maughan ED. Retrieved from https://www.nasn.org.

National Association of School Nurses (NASN): *School-Located Vaccination* (Position Statement), 2018a, Silver Spring: Fiorivant, M, Ward C. Retrieved from https://www.nasn.org

National Association of School Nurses (NASN): *Bullying and Cyberbullying—Prevention in Schools* (Position Statement), 2018b, Silver Spring: Wheeler, J. M., Ward, C., Rebowe D. Retrieved from https://www.nasn.org.

National Association of School Nurses (NASN): *Do not Attempt Resuscitation—The Role of the School Nurse* (Position Statement), 2018c, Silver Spring: Begley C, Cowan T, Crowe D, Allsbrook P, Graf K. Retrieved from https://www.nasn.org.

National Association of School Nurses (NASN): *Emergency Preparedness* (Position Statement), 2019a, Silver Spring: Allsbrook P, Begley C, Graf K. Retrieved from https://www.nasn.org.

National Association of School Nurses (NASN): *Nurse delegation in the school setting* (Position Statement), 2019b, Silver Spring: Reiner KL, Bartholomew K. Retrieved from www.nasn.org.

National Association of School Nurses (NASN): *About: NASN*, 2020a, Author. Retrieved from https://www.nasn.org.

National Association of School Nurses (NASN): *School Nurse Workload: Staffing for Safe Care:* (Position *Statement*). 2020b, Silver Spring: Rau W, Jameson B, midon C, Thronton J, Wilson W, Maughan E, Combe L. Retrieved from https://www.nasn.org.

National Association of School Nurses (NASN): *Research Priorities: NASN Research Priorities* 2020-2021. 2020c, Author. Retrieved from https://www.nasn.org.

National Association of School Nurses (NASN): *Naloxone Use in the School Setting* (Position Statement), 2020d, Silver Spring: Levasseur S, Nelson L, Crowe D, Major, K. Retrieved from https://www.nasn.org.

National Association of School Nurses (NASN): *Immunizations* (Position Statement), 2020e, Silver Spring: Griffin C, Barker P, McDermott E, Meadows L, Peiffer C. Retrieved from https://www.nasn.org.

National Association of School Nurses (NASN): *Head Lice Management in the School Setting* (Position Statement), 2020f, Silver Spring: Kern L, Wetzel CS, Kerley K, Elliot K, Bailey S. Retrieved from https://www.nasn.org.

National Board for Certification of School Nurses: *Eligibility to Take the NCSN Exam,* 2018, Author. Retrieved from https://www.nbcsn.org.

National Institute of Mental Health: *Suicide Prevention*, 2017. Retrieved from https://www.nimh.nih.gov.

Occupational Safety and Health Administration: *OSHA's Bloodborne Pathogens Standard,* OSHA Fact Sheet, 2011. Retrieved from https://www.osha.gov.

Pistiner M, Mattey B: A universal anaphylaxis emergency care plan: introducing the new allergy and anaphylaxis care plan from the American Academy of Pediatrics, *NASN Sch Nurse* 32(5): 283–286, 2017.

Price OA: Strategies to encourage long-term sustainability of school-based health centers, *Am J Med Res* 4(1):61–83, 2017.

Rasberry CN, Liddon N, Adkins SH: The importance of school staff referrals and follow-up in connecting high school students to HIV and STD testing, *J Sch Nurs* 33(2):143–153, 2017.

Rebmann T, Elliott MB, Artman D, VanNatta M, Wakefield M: Impact of an education intervention on Missouri K-12 school disaster and biological event preparedness, *J Sch Health* 86(11): 794–802, 2016.

Rebmann T, Weaver NL, Elliott MB, DeClue RW, Patel NJ, Schulte L: Factors related to injury prevention programming by Missouri school nurses, *J Sch Nursg* 34(4):292–300, 2018.

Resha C: Standards of school nursing practice. In Selekman J, Shannon RA, Yonkaitis CF, editors: *School nursing: a comprehensive text*, ed 3, Philadelphia, 2019, F.A. Davis Company, pp. 31-50.

Rosen G, Fee E: *A history of public health*, Baltimore, 2015, Johns Hopkins University Press.

Ruel SR: Lillian Wald, *Home Healthcare Nurse* 32(10):597–600, 2014.

Russell S, McCloskey CR: Parent perceptions of care received by children with an autism spectrum disorder, *J Pediatr Nurs* 31(1):21–31, 2016.

Salam RA, Arshad A, Das JK, et al.: Interventions to prevent unintentional injuries among adolescents: A systematic review and meta-analysis, *J Adolesc Health* 59(Suppl 4):S76–S87, 2016.

Schaffer MA, Anderson LJ, Rising S: Public health interventions for school nursing practice, *J Sch Nurs* 32(3):195–208, 2016.

Selekman J, Chewey L, Cogan R, Conway S: School nurse collaboration with the community. In Selekman J, Shannon RA, Yonkaitis CF, editors: *School nursing: a comprehensive text*, ed 3, Philadelphia, 2019, F.A. Davis Company, pp. 116-135.

Selekman J, Ness M: Students with chronic conditions. In Selekman J, Shannon RA, Yonkaitis CF, editors: *School nursing: a comprehensive text*, ed 3, Philadelphia, 2019, F.A. Davis Company, pp. 480-499.

Shannon RA, Minchella L: Students requiring personal nursing care at school: Nursing care models and a checklist for school nurses, *NASN Sch Nurse* 30(2):76–80, 2015.

Sharma M: *Theoretical foundations of health education and health promotion*, ed 3, Burlington, 2017, Jones and Bartlett Learning.

Sharron RA, Guilday P: Emergency and disaster preparedness and response for schools. In Selekman J, Shannon RA, Yonkaitis CF, editors: *School nursing: a comprehensive text*, ed 3, Philadelphia, 2019, F.A. Davis Company, pp. 457-479.

Siminerio LM: Diabetes education and support, *NASN Sch Nurse* 30(6):320–321, 2015.

Steele IH, Thrower N, Noroian P, Saleh FM: Understanding suicide across the lifespan: A United States perspective of suicide risk factors, assessment, & management, *Journal of Forensic Sciences,* 63(1): 162-171, 2018.

Substance Abuse and Mental Health Services Administration: *Suicide Prevention*, 2017. Retrieved from https://www.samhsa.gov.

Substance Abuse and Mental Health Services Administration: *Substance Misuse Prevention for Young Adults.* Publication No. PEP19-PL-Guide-1 Rockville: National Mental Health and Substance Use Policy Laboratory. Substance Abuse and Mental Health Services Administration, 2019.

Toothaker R, Cook P: A review of four health procedures that school nurses may encounter, *NASN Sch Nurse* 33(1):19–22, 2018.

US Congress: *Public Law 111-296: Healthy Hunger Free Kids Act*, 2010. Retrieved from https://www.congress.gov.

US Congress: *Public Law 114-95: Every Student Succeeds Act*, 2015. Retrieved from https://www.congress.gov.

US Consumer Product Safety Commission: *Public playground safety handbook*, 2015, Author. Retrieved from https://www.cpsc.gov.

US Department of Education (USDOE): *Every Student Succeeds Act*, 2020. Retrieved from www.ed.gov.

US Department of Education, Office for Civil Rights: *Free appropriate public education for students with disabilities: requirements under section 504 of the rehabilitation Act of 1973*, 2010, Author. Retrieved from https://www2.ed.gov.

US Department of Education (USDOE), US Department of Health and Human Services, US Department of Homeland Security, US Department of Justice, Federal Bureau of Investigation, & Federal Emergency Management Agency: *Guide for developing high-quality school emergency operations plans*, 2013. Retrieved from https://ed.gov.

US Environmental Protection Agency: *Indoor air quality tools for schools action kit*, 2020. Retrieved from https://www.epa.gov.

US Department of Health and Human Services: *Stopbullying.gov: Laws & policies*, 2018, Author. Retrieved from https://www.stopbullying.gov.

US Department of Health and Human Services (USDHHS): *Health information privacy: FAQ*, 2008, Author. Retrieved from https://www.hhs.gov.

US Department of Health and Human Services: *Healthy People 2030.* HHS, 2020. Available at https://health.gov/healthypeople.

Wahl A, Stephens H, Ruffo M, Jones AL: The evaluation of a food allergy and epinephrine autoinjector training program for personnel who care for children in schools and community settings, *J Sch Nurs* 31(2):91–98, 2015.

Wernette MJ, Emory J: Student bedtimes, academic performance, and health in a residential high school. *J Sch Nurs* 33(4): 264–268, 2017.

Willgerodt MA, Brock DM, Maughan ED: Public school nursing practice in the United States, *J Sch Nurs* 34(3):232–244, 2018.

Wolfe L: The profession of school nursing. In Selekman J, Shannon RA, Yonkaitis CF, editors: *School nursing: a comprehensive text*, ed 3, Philadelphia, 2019a, F.A. Davis Company, pp. 17-30.

Wolfe L: Historical perspectives of school nursing. In Selekman J, Shannon RA, Yonkaitis CF, editors: *School nursing: a comprehensive text*, ed 3, Philadelphia, 2019b, F.A. Davis Company, pp. 2-16.

Yonkaitis CF, Shannon RA: The role of the school nurse in the special education process: Part 1: student identification and evaluation, *NASN School Nurse* 32(3):179–184, 2017.

32

The Nurse in Occupational Health

Bonnie Rogers

OBJECTIVES

After reading this chapter, the student should be able to:

1. Describe the nursing role in occupational health.
2. Discuss current trends in the US workforce.
3. Use the epidemiologic model to explain work–health interactions using examples of work-related illness, injuries, and hazards.
4. Complete an occupational health history.
5. Recognize the differing functions of the Occupational Safety and Health Administration (OSHA) and the National Institute for Occupational Safety and Health (NIOSH).
6. Describe an effective disaster plan in occupational health.

CHAPTER OUTLINE

KEY TERMS

In America, work is viewed as important to one's life experiences, and most adults spend about one-third of their time at work (Rogers, 2019). Work—when fulfilling, fairly compensated, healthy, and safe—can help build long and contented lives and strengthen families and communities. No work is completely risk free, and all health care professionals should have some basic knowledge about workforce populations, work and related hazards, and methods to control hazards and improve health.

Important developments are occurring in occupational health and safety programs designed to prevent and control work-related illness and injury and to create environments that foster and support health-promoting activities. Occupational health nurses have performed critical roles in planning and delivering worksite health and safety services, which must continue to grow as comprehensive and cost-effective services. In addition, the continuing increase in health care costs and the concern about health care quality have prompted the inclusion of primary care and management of non–work-related health problems in the health services' programs. In some settings, family services are also provided.

Health at work is an important issue for most individuals for whom the nurse provides care. With many individuals spending so much time working, the workplace, regardless of setting, has significant influence on health and can be a primary site for the delivery of health promotion and illness prevention. The home, the clinic, the nursing home, and other community sites, such as the workplace, will become the dominant areas where health and illness care will be sought.

This chapter describes the nurse's role in occupational health—working with employees and the workforce population. The focus is on the knowledge and skills needed to promote the health and safety of workers through occupational health programs, recognizing work-related health and safety, and the principles for prevention and control of adverse work–health interactions. The prevalence and significance of the interactions between health and work underscore the importance of including principles of occupational health and safety in nursing practice. The types of interactions and the frequent use of the general health care system for identifying, treating, and preventing occupational illnesses and injuries require nurses to use this knowledge in all practice settings. The epidemiologic triangle is used as one model for understanding these interactions, as well as risk factors, and effective nursing care for promoting health and safety among employed populations.

DEFINITION AND SCOPE OF OCCUPATIONAL HEALTH NURSING

Adapted from the American Association of Occupational Health Nurses (AAOHN) (2016a), occupational and environmental health nursing is the specialty practice that provides for and delivers health and safety programs and services to workers, worker populations, and community groups. The practice focuses on the promotion and restoration of health, prevention of illness and injury, and protection from work-related and environmental hazards. Occupational and environmental health nurses (OHNs) have a combined knowledge of health and business that they blend with health care expertise to balance the requirement for a safe and healthful work environment with a "healthy bottom line."

The foundation for occupational and environmental health nursing is research-based. Recognizing the legal context for occupational health and safety, this specialty practice derives its theoretical, conceptual, and factual framework from a multidisciplinary base including, but not limited to:

- Nursing science
- Medical science
- Public health sciences such as epidemiology and environmental health

- Occupational health sciences such as toxicology, safety, industrial hygiene, and ergonomics
- Social and behavioral sciences
- Management, administration, and financial principles

Guided by an ethical framework made explicit in the AAOHN *Code of Ethics* (2016b), OHNs encourage and enable individuals to make informed decisions about health care concerns. Confidentiality of health information is integral and central to the practice. OHNs are advocates for client(s), fostering equitable and quality health care services and safe and healthy environments in which to work.

HISTORY AND EVOLUTION OF OCCUPATIONAL HEALTH NURSING

Nursing care for workers began in 1888 and was called industrial nursing. A group of coal miners hired Betty Moulder, a graduate of the Blockley Hospital School of Nursing in Philadelphia (now Philadelphia General Hospital), to take care of their ailing coworkers and families (AAOHN, 1976). Ada Mayo Stewart, hired in 1885 by the Vermont Marble Company in Rutland, Vermont, is often considered the first industrial nurse. Riding a bicycle, Miss Stewart visited sick employees in their homes, provided emergency care, taught mothers how to care for their children, and taught healthy living habits (Felton, 1985). In the early days of occupational health nursing, the nurse's work was family centered and holistic.

Employee health services grew rapidly during the early 1900s as companies recognized that the provision of worksite health services led to a more productive workforce. At that time, workplace accidents were seen as an inevitable part of having a job. However, the public did not support this attitude, and a system for workers' compensation arose that remains today (McGrath, 1945).

Industrial nursing grew rapidly during the first half of the twentieth century. Educational courses were established, as were professional societies. By World War II there were about 4000 industrial nurses (Brown, 1981). The American Association of Industrial Nursing (AAIN) (now called the American Association of Occupational Health Nurses) was established as the first national occupational nursing organization in 1942. The aim of the AAIN was to improve industrial nursing education and practice and to promote interprofessional collaborative efforts (Rogers, 1988).

Passage of several laws in the 1960s and 1970s to protect workers' safety and health led to an increased need for occupational health nurses. In particular, the passing of the landmark Occupational Safety and Health Act in 1970, which created the Occupational Safety and Health Administration (OSHA) and the National Institute for Occupational Safety and Health (NIOSH), discussed later in this chapter, resulted in a great need for nurses at the worksite to meet the demands of the many standards being implemented. Under OSHA, the Act focuses primarily on protecting workers from work-related hazards. NIOSH focuses on education and research. In 1988 the first occupational health nurse was hired by OSHA to provide technical assistance in standards development, field consultation, and occupational health nursing expertise. In 1993 the Office of Occupational Health Nursing was established within the agency. In 1998, the AAOHN adopted the concept of environmental health as a significant component of the practice field. To this end, AAOHN has incorporated the term "environmental," as in OHN, in its documents and publications. In 1999, AAOHN published its first set of competencies in occupational health nursing, and established the AAOHN Foundation to support education, research, and leadership activities in occupational health nursing. Role expansion includes environmental health, total worker health, and forging sustainable relationships in the community to better improve worker health.

ROLES AND PROFESSIONALISM IN OCCUPATIONAL HEALTH NURSING

As US industry has shifted from agrarian to industrial to highly technological processes, the role of the occupational health nurse has continued to change. The focus on work-related health problems now includes the spectrum of human responses to multiple, complex interactions of biopsychosocial factors that occur in community, home, and work environments. The customary role of the occupational health nurse has extended beyond emergency treatment and prevention of illness and injury to include the promotion and maintenance of health, overall risk management, care for the environment, efforts to reduce health-related costs in businesses, and total worker health. The interprofessional nature of occupational health nursing has become more critical as occupational health and safety problems require more complex solutions. The occupational health nurse frequently collaborates closely with multiple disciplines and industry management, as well as with representatives of labor.

Occupational health nurses constitute the largest group of occupational health professionals. The most recent national survey of registered nurses (RNs) indicated that there were about 11,000 RNs and 1700 advanced practice registered nurses (APRNs) specializing in occupational health nursing (Health Resources and Services Administration, 2020). Occupational health nurses hold positions as nurse practitioners, clinical nurse specialists, managers, supervisors, consultants, educators, and researchers, and many occupational health nurses are employed in single-managed occupational health nurse units in a variety of businesses. The occupational health nursing role requires the nurse to adapt to an organization's needs as well as to the needs of specific groups of workers.

The professional organization for occupational health nurses is the American Association of Occupational Health Nurses. The AAOHN's mission is comprehensive. It supports the work of the occupational health nurse and advances the specialty. The AAOHN also does the following:

- Promotes the health and safety of workers
- Defines the scope of practice and sets the standards of occupational health nursing practice
- Develops the code of ethics for occupational health nurses with interpretive statements
- Promotes and provides continuing education in the specialty

- Advances the profession through supporting research
- Responds to and influences public policy issues related to occupational health and safety

The AAOHN (2016a) provides the Standards of Occupational and Environmental Health Nursing Practice to define and advance practice and provide a framework for practice evaluation. The AAOHN Code of Ethics lists eight code statements based on the goal of OHNs to promote worker health and safety (AAOHN, 2016b). Both documents can be obtained from the AAOHN at http://www.aaohn.org.

Occupational health nurses have many roles, such as (Rogers, 2019):

- Clinician
- Case manager
- Coordinator
- Manager
- Nurse practitioner
- Corporate director
- Health promotion specialist
- Educator
- Consultant
- Researcher

The majority of occupational health nurses work as solo clinicians, but additional roles are being included increasingly in the specialty practice. In many companies, the occupational health nurse has assumed expanded responsibilities in job analysis, safety, and benefits management. Many occupational health nurses also work as independent contractors and consultants or have their own businesses that provide occupational health and safety services to industry. Specializing in the field is often a requirement.

Ethical conflict is nothing new in occupational and environmental health nursing practice. Traditional concerns about confidentiality of employee health records, hazardous workplace exposures, issues of informed consent, risks and benefits, and dual-duty conflicts (workers versus management) are now married with newer concerns of genetic screening, worker literacy and understanding, work organization issues, and untimely return to work (Rogers, 2019). With the current changes in health care delivery and the movement toward managed care, occupational health nurses will need increased skills in primary care, health promotion, and disease prevention. The aim of the occupational health nurse will be to devote much attention to keeping workers and, in some cases, their families healthy and free from illness and worksite injuries.

Academic education in occupational health and safety is generally at the graduate level. Certification in occupational health nursing is provided by the American Board for Occupational Health Nurses (ABOHN). However, ABOHN offers two basic certifications: the COHN (Certified Occupational Health Nurse) and COHN-S (Certified Occupational Health Nurse–Specialist). Eligibility for the COHN requires licensure as an RN, whereas the COHN-S requires RN licensure plus a baccalaureate degree. Certification is achieved through experience, continuing education, professional activities, and examination. Those interested in certification can view the requirements on the ABOHN website (www.abohn.org).

WORKERS AS A POPULATION AGGREGATE

The population of the United States is expected to increase by 79 million people by 2060 (Vespa, Medina, & Armstrong, 2018). In 2030, the Baby Boomer generation will all be older than 65 years and by 2034 the number of older adults is expected to outnumber children for the first time in US history. The Bureau of Labor Statistics (BLS, 2018) data showed total workforce projection to increase by 7.4% from 2016 to 2026, with workers aged 65 to 74 experiencing the fastest growth rate.

By 2024, the BLS projects the labor force will grow to 164 million civilian wage and salary workers employed in the United States (Toossi & Torpey, 2017). More than 91% of those who are able to work outside of the home do so for some portion of their lives. These statistics do not indicate the number of individuals who may be at risk of exposure to work-related health hazards plus exposure to diseases existing in the workforce such as COVID-19. Although some individuals may currently be unemployed or retired, they continue to bear the health risks of past occupational exposures. The number of affected individuals may be even larger, as work-related illnesses like COVID-19 are found among spouses, children, and neighbors of exposed workers. In addition, more than seven million individuals reported that they work multiple jobs which increases the amount of exposure to work-related illnesses for workers and families (BLS, 2018). As an example of the effects of COVID-19 on business and industries, IBIS World reported in July 2020, that the disease had impacted sectors across countries including Australia, Canada, Germany, New Zealand, the UK, and the United States.

The categories of work-related cutbacks, shutdowns, or closure include:

- Mining
- Utilities
- Construction
- Manufacturing
- Wholesale trade
- Retail trade
- Transportation and warehousing
- Information
- Finance and insurance
- Education
- Professional, scientific, and technical services
- Real estate and rental and leasing
- Health care
- Accommodation and food services
- Arts, entertainment, and recreation
- Administrative and support services
- Public administration and safety
- Personal services
  Updates can be found at www.ibisworld.com

Americans are employed in diverse industries that range in size from one to tens of thousands of employees. Types of industries, to name a few, include the following:

- Traditional manufacturing (e.g., automotive and appliances)
- Service industries (e.g., banking, health care, and restaurants)
- Agriculture
- Construction
- High-technology firms, such as computer chip manufacturers
  Although some industries are noted for the high degree of hazards associated with their work (e.g., manufacturing, mines, construction, and agriculture), no worksite is free of occupational health and safety hazards. as can be seen by the list of worldwide businesses and industries above. The larger the company, the more likely it is that there will be health and safety programs for employees. Smaller companies are more apt to rely on external community resources to meet their needs for occupational health and safety services.

Characteristics of the Workforce

The US workplace has changed rapidly over time (BLS, 2018):

- Jobs in the economy continue to shift from manufacturing to service.
- Longer hours, compressed workweeks, shift work, reduced job security, and part-time and temporary work are realities of the modern workplace.
- New chemicals, materials, processes, and equipment are developed and marketed at an ever-increasing pace.
- As the population increases, the US workforce is expected to grow as well and will become older and more racially diverse.
- Major changes in the working population are reflected in the increasing numbers of women, older individuals, and those with chronic illnesses who are part of the workforce.
  Because of changes in the economy, extension of life span, legislation, and more working women, the proportion of the employed population that these three groups represent will probably continue to grow.

Characteristics of Work

There has been a dramatic shift in the types of jobs held by workers. Following the evolution from an agrarian economy to a manufacturing society and then to a highly technological workplace, in the past, the greatest proportion of paid employment was in the following occupations:

- Trade
- Transportation
- Utilities
  As the nature of work has changed, it has been accompanied by many new occupational hazards, such as complex chemicals, nanotechnology, nonergonomic workstation design (requiring the adaptation of the workplace or work equipment to meet the employee's health and safety needs), and many issues related to work organization such as job stress, burnout, and exhaustion. In addition, the emergence of a global economy with free trade and multinational corporations presents new challenges for health and safety programs that are culturally relevant.

Work–Health Interactions

The influence of work on health, or work–health interactions, is shown by statistics on illnesses, injuries, and deaths associated with employment (see discussion of COVID-19 above).

As reported by the Census of Fatal Occupational Injuries (CFOI) (BLS, 2019a), there were 5250 fatal work injuries recorded in the United States in 2018, a 2% increase from the 5147 fatal injuries reported in 2017. This is the fourth consecutive increase in annual workplace fatalities and the second time more than 5000 fatalities have been recorded by the CFOI since 2008. The fatal injury rate was to 3.5 per 100,000 workers, the second highest rate since 2010. Fatal work injuries from falls, slips, or trips decreased 11% to 791, the lowest total since 2013. Unintentional overdoses from the nonmedical use of drugs or alcohol while on the job increased 12%, from 272 to 305, noting an annual increase for 6 years in a row.

Employers reported 3.5 fatal work injuries per 100,000 workers in 2017 (BLS, 2019a). Occupational injuries alone are reported to cost over $100 billion in lost wages and lost productivity, administrative expenses, health care, and other costs. This figure does not include the cost of occupational diseases. These figures are often described as the "tip of the iceberg," because many work-related health problems go unreported. However, even the recorded statistics are significant in describing the amount of human suffering, financial loss, and decreased productivity associated with workplace hazards. In 2018, there were 2.8 million nonfatal workplace injuries and illnesses, resulting in days away from work with a median of 8 days absent (BLS, 2019b).

The high number of work injuries and illnesses can be drastically reduced. In fact, significant progress has been made in improving worker protection since Congress passed the 1970 Occupational Safety and Health Act. For example, vinyl chloride–induced liver cancers and brown lung disease (byssinosis) from cotton dust exposure have been almost eliminated. Reproductive disorders associated with certain glycol ethers have been recognized and controlled. Fatal work injuries have declined substantially through the years.

The US workplace is rapidly changing and becoming more diverse. Major changes are also occurring in the following areas:
- The way work is organized
- Increased shift work
- Reduced job security
- Part-time and temporary work
- New chemicals, materials, processes, and equipment (such as nanotechnology and fermentation processes in biotechnology) continue to be developed and marketed at an accelerating pace, creating new work-related hazards.

APPLICATION OF THE EPIDEMIOLOGIC MODEL

The Epidemiologic Triangle can be used to understand the relationship between work and health (Fig. 32.1). The reader is referred to Chapter 10, Epidemiology, for a fuller description.

With a focus on the health and safety of the employed population, the host is described as any susceptible human being. Because of the nature of work-related hazards, nurses must assume that all employed individuals and groups are at risk of being exposed to occupational hazards. The agents, factors associated with illness and injury, are occupational exposures that are classified as biological, chemical, enviromechanical, physical,

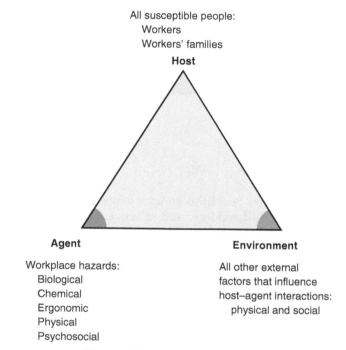

Fig. 32.1 The Epidemiologic Triangle.

or psychosocial (Box 32.1). The environment includes all external conditions that influence the interaction of the host and agents. These may be workplace conditions such as:
- Temperature extremes
- Crowding
- Shift work
- Inflexible management styles

The basic principle of epidemiology is that health status interventions for restoring and promoting health are the result of complex interactions among these three elements. To understand these interactions and to design effective nursing strategies for dealing with them in a proactive manner, nurses must look at how each of these elements influences the others.

BOX 32.1   Categories of Work-Related Hazards

Biological and infectious hazards—Infectious/biological agents, such as bacteria, viruses, fungi, or parasites, that may be transmitted via contact with infected clients or contaminated body secretions/fluids to other individuals

Chemical hazards—Various forms of chemicals, including medications, solutions, gases, vapors, aerosols, and particulate matter, that are potentially toxic or irritating to the body system

Enviromechanical hazards—Factors encountered in the work environment that cause or potentiate accidents, injuries, strain, or discomfort (e.g., unsafe/inadequate equipment or lifting devices, slippery floors, workstation deficiencies)

Physical hazards—Agents within the work environment, such as radiation, electricity, extreme temperatures, and noise, that can cause tissue trauma

Psychosocial hazards—Factors and situations encountered or associated with one's job or work environment that create or potentiate stress, emotional strain, or interpersonal problems

From Rogers B: *Occupational health nursing: concepts and practice.* 2003.

Host

Each worker represents a host within the worker population group. Certain host factors are associated with increased risk of adverse response to the hazards of the workplace. These include (Rogers, 2019):

- Age
- Gender
- Health status
- Work practices
- Ethnicity
- Lifestyle factors

For example, the population group at greatest risk for experiencing work-related accidents with subsequent injuries is new workers with less than 1 year of experience on the current job. Most nonfatal injuries and illnesses involving days away from work occur among new workers (the highest percentages were in mining [44%]; agriculture, forestry, and fishing [43%]; construction [41%]; and wholesale and retail trade [34%]). Thirty-five percent of injury and illness cases with days away from work occurred among workers with 5 or fewer years of service with their employer (BLS, 2017b). The host factors of age, gender, and work experience combine to increase this group's risk of injury because of characteristics such as risk taking, lack of knowledge, and lack of familiarity with the new job.

Older workers may be at increased risk in the workplace because of diminished sensory abilities, the effects of chronic illnesses, and delayed reaction times.

Another population group that may be very susceptible to host factors in the workplace are women in their childbearing years because of the following:

- Hormonal changes during these years
- Increased stress of new roles and additional responsibilities
- Transplacental exposures
- This group's responses to potential toxins

In addition to these host factors, there may be other, less well-understood individual differences in response to occupational hazard exposures. Even if employers maintain exposure levels below the level recommended by occupational health and safety standards, 15% to 20% of the population may have health reactions to the "safe" low-level exposures (Levy et al., 2017). This group has been termed *hypersusceptible*. A number of host factors appear to be associated with this hypersusceptibility:

- Light skin
- Malnutrition
- Compromised immune system
- Glucose-6-phosphate dehydrogenase deficiency
- Serum alpha-1 antitrypsin deficiency
- Chronic obstructive pulmonary disease
- Sickle cell trait
- Hypertension

Individuals who have known hypersusceptibility to chemicals that are respiratory irritants, hemolytic chemicals, organic isocyanates, and carbon disulfide may also be hypersusceptible to other agents in the work environment (Levy et al., 2017). Although this has prompted some industries to consider preplacement screening for such risk factors, the associations between these individual health markers and hypersusceptible response are unclear.

Agent

Work-related hazards, or agents (see Box 32.1), present potential and actual risks to the health and safety of workers in the millions of business establishments in the United States. Any worksite commonly presents multiple and interacting exposures from all five categories of agents. Table 32.1 lists some of the more common workplace exposures, their known health effects, and the types of jobs associated with these hazards.

Biological Agents

Biological agents are living organisms whose excretions or parts are capable of causing human disease, usually by an infectious process. Biological hazards are common in workplaces such as health care facilities and clinical laboratories, where employees are potentially exposed to a variety of infectious agents, including viruses, fungi, and bacteria. Of particular concern in occupational health is the infectious agent transmitted by humans (e.g., from client to worker or from worker to worker) in a variety of work settings. Bloodborne and airborne pathogens represent a significant class of exposures for US health care workers at risk. Occupational transmission of bloodborne pathogens (including the hepatitis B and C viruses and the human immunodeficiency virus [HIV]) occurs primarily by means of needlestick injuries as well as through exposures to the eyes or mucous membranes (Centers for Disease Control and Prevention [CDC], 2019).

While the number of cases and reports of tuberculosis (TB) has decreased in the United States, transmission of TB within health care settings (especially multidrug-resistant TB) continues as a major public health problem (Schwartz, Price, Pratt, & Langer, 2020). Since 1989 outbreaks of this type of TB have been reported in hospitals, and some workers have developed active drug-resistant TB. In addition, among workers in health care, social service, and correctional facilities who work with populations at increased risk of TB, hundreds have experienced tuberculin skin test conversions. Reliable data are lacking on the extent of possible work-related TB transmission among other groups of workers at risk for exposure.

Many workers in these settings were employed as maintenance workers, security guards, aides, or cleaning people, who were not well protected from inadvertent exposure. Education should be provided to all health care workers, including those not having direct client care, in the proper handling and disposal of potentially contaminated linens, soiled equipment, and trash containing contaminated dressings or specimens (Schwartz et al., 2020).

Chemical Agents

More than 300 billion pounds of chemical agents are produced annually in the United States. Of the about 2 million known chemicals in existence, less than 0.1% have been adequately studied for their effects on humans. Of those chemicals that have been linked to carcinogens, about half test positive as animal carcinogens. Most chemicals have not been studied epidemiologically to determine the effects of exposure on

TABLE 32.1 Selected Job Categories, Exposures, and Associated Work-Related Diseases and Conditions

Job Categories	Exposures	Work-Related Diseases and Conditions
All workers	Workplace stress	Hypertension, mood disorders, cardiovascular disease
Agricultural workers	Pesticides, infectious agents, gases, sunlight	Pesticide poisoning, "farmer's lung," skin cancer
Anesthetists	Anesthetic gases	Reproductive effects, cancer
Automobile workers	Asbestos, plastics, lead, solvents	Asbestosis, dermatitis
Butchers	Vinyl plastic fumes	"Meat wrappers' asthma"
Caisson workers	Pressurized work environments	Caisson disease ("the bends")
Carpenters	Wood dust, wood preservatives, adhesives	Nasopharyngeal cancer, dermatitis
Cement workers	Cement dust, metals	Dermatitis, bronchitis
Ceramic workers	Talc, clays	Pneumoconiosis
Demolition workers	Asbestos, wood dust	Asbestosis
Drug manufacturers	Hormones, nitroglycerin, etc.	Reproductive effects
Dry cleaners	Solvents	Liver disease, dermatitis
Dye workers	Dyestuffs, metals, solvents	Bladder cancer, dermatitis
Embalmers	Formaldehyde, infectious agents	Dermatitis
Felt makers	Mercury, polycyclic hydrocarbons	Mercurialism
Foundry workers	Silica, molten metals	Silicosis
Glass workers	Heat, solvents, metal powders	Cataracts
Hospital workers	Infectious agents, cleansers, radiation	Infections, latex allergies, unintentional injuries
Insulators	Asbestos, fibrous glass	Asbestosis, lung cancer, mesothelioma
Jack-hammer operators	Vibration	Raynaud phenomenon
Lathe operators	Metal dusts, cutting oils	Lung disease, cancer
Office computer workers	Repetitive wrist motion on computers	Tendonitis, carpal tunnel syndrome, tenosynovitis, eye strain

humans (Levy et al., 2017). As a consequence of general environmental contamination with chemicals from work, home, and community activities, a variety of chemicals have been found in the body tissues of the general population.

In many workplaces, significant exposure to a daily, low-level dose of workplace chemicals may be below the exposure standards but may still create a potentially chronic and perhaps cumulative assault on workers' health. Predicting human responses to such exposures is further complicated because multiple chemicals often combine and interact to create a new chemical agent. Human effects may be associated with the interaction of these agents rather than with a single chemical. Another concern about occupational exposure to chemicals is reproductive health effects. Workplace reproductive hazards have become important legal and scientific issues. Toxicity to male and female reproductive systems has been demonstrated from exposure to common agents such as lead, mercury, cadmium, nickel, and zinc, as well as in antineoplastic drugs. Because data for predicting human responses to many chemical agents are inadequate, workers should be assessed for all potential exposures and cautioned to work preventively with these agents. High-risk or vulnerable workers, such as those with a latex allergy—a widely recognized health hazard—should be carefully screened and monitored for optimal health protection (Levy et al., 2017). To accurately assess and evaluate the exposure and recommend changes for abatement, it is essential that the nurse have a good understanding of the basic principles of toxicology, including routes of exposure (i.e., inhalation, skin absorption, and ingestion), dose-response relationships, and differences in effects (i.e., acute versus chronic toxicity).

Enviromechanical Agents

Enviromechanical agents are those that can potentially cause injury or illness in the workplace. They are related to the work process or to working conditions, and they can cause postural or other strains that can produce adverse health effects when certain tasks are performed repeatedly. Examples are repetitive motions, poor or unsafe workstation-worker fit, slippery floors, cluttered work areas, and lifting heavy loads. Severity of illness or injury can be estimated from the number of days away from work.

In 2018 (BLS, 2019b), sprains and strains, bruises/contusions, cuts/lacerations, fractures, and multiple injuries accounted for more days away from work than for all types of injury and illness. Back pain/injury is one of the most common and significant musculoskeletal problems in the world. Although the exact cost of back disorders is unknown, the estimates are staggering and in the billions per year. Regardless of the estimate used, the problem is large both in health and economic terms. The research on these hazards, related human responses, and prevention is evolving. The most productive strategy in preventing these exposures is redesigning the workplace and the work machinery or processes.

Physical Agents

Physical agents are those that produce adverse health effects through the transfer of physical energy. Commonly encountered physical agents in the workplace include the following:

- Temperature extremes
- Vibration
- Noise
- Lasers
- Radiation
- Electricity

For example, vibration, which accompanies the use of power tools and vehicles such as trucks, affects internal organs, supportive ligaments, the upper torso, and the shoulder girdle structure.

Localized effects are seen with handheld power tools; the most common is Raynaud phenomenon. The control of worker exposure to these agents is usually accomplished through engineering strategies such as eliminating or containing the hazardous agent. In addition, workers must use preventive actions, such as practicing safe work habits and wearing personal protective equipment when needed. Examples of safe work habits include taking appropriate breaks from environments with temperature extremes and not eating or smoking in radiation-contaminated areas. Personal protective equipment includes the following:

- Hearing protection
- Eye guards
- Protective clothing
- Devices for monitoring exposures to agents, such as radiation

Psychosocial Agents

Psychosocial agents are conditions that create a threat to the psychological and/or social well-being of individuals and groups (Rogers, 2019). A psychosocial response to the work environment occurs as an employee acts selectively toward the environment in an attempt to achieve a harmonious relationship. When such a human attempt at adaptation to the environment fails, an adverse psychosocial response may occur. Work-related stress or burnout has been defined as an important problem for many individuals (Rogers, 2019). Responses to negative interpersonal relationships, particularly those with authority figures in the workplace, are often the cause of vague health symptoms and increased absenteeism. Epidemiologic work in mental health has pointed to environmental variables such as these in the incidence of mental illness and emotional disorder.

The psychosocial environment includes characteristics of the work itself, as well as the interpersonal relationships required in the work setting and shift work. About 10% of US workers do some form of shift work that has the potential to lead to a variety of psychological and physical problems, including exhaustion, depression, anxiety, and gastrointestinal disturbance (BLS, 2018).

Strategies to minimize the adverse effects of shift work are beneficial. For example, a rotating shift allows the employee to move through a cycle of working the day shift, then the evening shift, and then the night shift over the course of several weeks, with the goal of the workforce sharing the stress of the least desirable shifts. Job characteristics such as low autonomy, poor job satisfaction, and limited control over the pace of work have been associated with an increased risk of heart disease among clerical and blue-collar workers.

Interpersonal relationships among employees and coworkers or bosses and managers are often sources of conflict and stress. Another aspect is organizational culture. This refers to the norms and patterns of behavior that are sanctioned within a particular organization. Such norms and patterns set guidelines for the types of work behaviors that will enable employees to succeed within a particular firm. The following are examples (Burke, 2018):

- Following organizational norms for working overtime
- Expressing constructive dissatisfaction with management
- Making work a top priority

These factors and the employee's response to them must be assessed if strategies for influencing the health and safety of workers are to be effective.

Nonfatal violence in the health care worker's workplace is a serious problem that is underreported. Much of the study of health care worker violence has been in psychiatric settings; however, reports in other areas such as the emergency department have been provided. Risk factors associated with this type of violence must be identified and strategies implemented to reduce the risk (Rogers et al., 2017).

Environment

Environmental factors influence the occurrence of host-agent interactions and may direct the course and outcome of those interactions. The physical environment involves the geological and atmospheric structure of an area and the source of such elements as water, temperature, and radiation, which may serve as positive or negative stressors. Although aspects of the physical environment (e.g., heat, odor, ventilation) may influence the host-agent interaction, the social and psychological environment can be equally important (Merrill, 2021).

New environmental problems continue to arise, such as an increase in industrial wastes and toxins and indoor and outdoor environmental pollution, which present opportunities for significant health threats to the working and general population. The social aspects of the environment encompass the economic and political forces affecting society and its health. This includes factors such as the following:

- Sanitation and hygiene practices
- Housing conditions
- Level and delivery of health care services
- Development and enforcement of health-related codes (e.g., occupational health and safety, pollution)
- Employment conditions
- Population crowding
- Literacy
- Ethnic customs
- Extent of support for health-related research
- Equal access to health care

In addition, addictive behaviors such as alcohol and substance abuse and various forms of psychosocial stress may be an outgrowth of negative social environments. Consider an employee who is working with a potentially toxic liquid. Providing education about safe work practices and fitting the employee with protective clothing may not be adequate if the work must occur in a very hot and humid environment. As the worker becomes uncomfortable in the hot clothing, protection may be compromised by rolling up a sleeve, taking off a glove, or wiping the face with a contaminated piece of clothing. If the norms in the workplace condone such work practices (e.g., "Everyone does it when it's too hot"), the interventions that address only the host and agent will be ineffective; strategies to address the environment itself must be considered, such as cooling fans or minimization of exposure through job rotation.

The epidemiologic triangle can be used as the basis for planning interventions to restore and promote the health of workers. These efforts are influenced by society and by organizational activities related to occupational health and safety (Rogers, 2019).

The occupational environment, within the context of the social environment, is represented by the workplace and work setting and the interactive effects of this environment on the worker. The nurse must consider the hazards and threats posed by this environment and the commitment of the employer to providing a safe and healthful workplace through use of preventive strategies and controls (e.g., engineering, substitution) (Rogers, 2019) (see Evidence-Based Practice box).

EVIDENCE-BASED PRACTICE

The aim of this qualitative descriptive study was to describe and explore sleep-related and safety decision-making among truck drivers. Flyers and sampling of truck drivers who were available at a site was used to recruit participants. Semi-structured interviews were done and an analysis of themes was completed to create descriptions of participants' experiences. The sample consisted of 10 Caucasian males, with an average of 22 years' truck-driving experience. Four themes emerged: sentinel events, driver characteristics, relationships, and company-level factors. The study found that both internal and external factors likely influence sleep and safety decisions and that personal relationships with others, such as family members, and professional relationships with company dispatchers were important influences among participants.

Nurse Use

During encounters with truck drivers, occupational health nurses should assess sleep quality and quantity and review healthy sleep hygiene strategies. Nurses should also promote company policies that support healthy sleep among truck drivers.

Modified from Heaton K, Mumbower R, Childs G: Sleep and safety decision-making among truck drivers, *Workplace Health & Safety*, online publication, 2020. https://doi.org/10.1177/2165079920950255

ORGANIZATIONAL AND PUBLIC EFFORTS TO PROMOTE WORKER HEALTH AND SAFETY

Promotion of worker health and safety is the goal of occupational health and safety programs (Friis, 2016). These programs are offered primarily by the employer at the workplace, but the range of services and the models for delivering them have been changing dramatically over the past few years. In addition to specific services, legislation at the federal and state levels has had a significant effect on efforts to provide a healthy and safe environment for all workers. Under the Occupational Safety and Health Act and because of increased public concern about worker health and safety, companies are cited for not meeting minimal occupational health and safety standards. Criminal charges have been filed against business owners when preventable work-related deaths occurred. These events have redirected an emphasis on preventive occupational health and safety programming.

Unless OSHA-regulated exposures are identified, business firms are not required to provide occupational health and safety services that meet any specified standards. With few exceptions, there is no legal recourse for specific services or level of personnel provided by employers to protect worker health and safety. Therefore the range of services offered and the qualifications of the providers of occupational health and safety vary widely across industries. An important stimulus for health and safety programs is avoiding cost that can be attributed to the effectiveness of prevention services, as well as the need to support occupational health and safety and health promotion at the worksite.

On-Site Occupational Health and Safety Programs

Optimally, on-site occupational health and safety services are provided by a team of occupational health and safety professionals. The following are core members of this team:
- Occupational health nurse
- Occupational physician
- Industrial hygienist
- Safety professional

In addition, more and more ergonomists are playing an important role in the occupational health and safety team. The largest group of health care professionals in business settings is occupational health nurses; therefore the most frequently seen model is that of the one-nurse unit. This nurse collaborates with a community physician or occupational medicine physician who provides consultation and accepts referrals when medical intervention is needed. The collaboration may occur primarily through telephone contact, or the physician may be under contract with the company to spend a certain amount of on-site time each week. As companies grow, they are likely to hire the following:
- Additional nurses
- Safety professionals
- Industrial hygienists
- Physicians, usually on a part-time or consultant basis
- Employee assistance counselors
- Physical therapists
- Health educators
- Physical fitness specialists
- Toxicologists

An increasingly popular option is to contract some health, safety, and industrial hygiene work to external providers. The largest firms often have corporate occupational health and safety professionals who set policy and participate in company decision making at the corporate level. These professionals work with the nurses employed at the individual sites within

BOX 32.2 Scope of Services Provided Through an Occupational Health and Safety Program

- Health/medical surveillance
- Workplace monitoring/surveillance
- Health assessments
- Preplacement
- Periodic, mandatory, voluntary assessments and services
- Transfer of clients/services
- Retirement/termination
- Executive
- Return to work
- Health promotion
- Health screening
- Employee assistance programs
- Case management
- Primary health care for workers and dependents
- Worker safety and health education related to occupational hazards
- Job task analysis and design
- Prenatal and postnatal care and support groups
- Safety audits and accident prevention
- Workers' compensation management
- Risk management, loss control
- Emergency preparedness
- Preretirement counseling
- Integrated health benefits programs

the company. Depending on the needs of the company and the workers, additional professionals may be on the occupational health and safety team.

The services provided by on-site occupational health programs range from those focused only on work-related health and safety problems to a wide scope of services that includes primary health care (Box 32.2). Increasingly employers supporting health promotion programs are offering employees incentives to stay healthy, such as gym memberships, on-site exercise facilities, or massage therapists during work hours.

In industries that have exposures regulated by law, certain programs are required, such as respiratory protection or hearing conservation. The ability of a company to offer additional programs depends on the following:

- Employee needs
- Management's attitudes and understanding about health and safety
- Acceptance by the workers
- Economic status of the company

A significant increase in the number of health promotion and employee assistance programs offered in industry has occurred over the past few years. Health promotion programs focus on lifestyle choices that cause risks to health (e.g., job stress, obesity, smoking, stress responses, or lack of exercise) (O'Donnell, 2017). Employee assistance programs are designed to address personal problems (e.g., marital/family issues, substance abuse, or financial difficulties) that affect the employee's productivity. Since such efforts are cost effective for businesses, they should continue to increase.

Similar types of occupational health and safety programs are available on a contractual basis from community-based providers. These may be offered by free-standing occupational health clinics, health maintenance organizations, hospitals, emergency clinics, and other health care organizations. In addition, consultants in each discipline work in the private sector (self-employed, in group practice, or in insurance companies) and in the public sector (in local and state health departments or departments of labor and industry). These services may be provided on-site, delivered at a specific location in the community, or offered through a mobile van that visits companies. These multiple resources have increased the options for companies that need occupational health and safety services, and they have also broadened the employment opportunities for health and safety professionals.

NURSING CARE OF WORKING POPULATIONS

The nurse is often the first health care provider seen by an individual with a work-related health problem. Consequently, nurses are in key positions to intervene with working populations at all levels of prevention (see the Levels of Prevention box).

LEVELS OF PREVENTION
Occupational Health

Primary Prevention
Nurse provides education on use of personal protective equipment in the workplace to prevent injury/exposure.

Secondary Prevention
Nurse screens for hearing loss resulting from noise levels in the plant.

Tertiary Prevention
Nurse works with chronic diabetic workers to ensure appropriate medication use and blood glucose screening to avoid lost workdays.

The occupational health nurse practices all levels of prevention (Rogers, 2019). Delivery of primary prevention services to employees is directed toward promoting health and averting a problem. In the occupational health setting, the purpose of health promotion is to maintain or enhance the well-being of individuals or groups of employees, and the company in general. This may include programs designed to enhance coping skills or good nutrition and knowledge about potential health hazards both inside and outside of the workplace.

Health protection (i.e., taking primary prevention measures) is designed to eliminate or reduce the risk of disease in order to prevent the development of an illness or injury. Walk-throughs by the occupational health nurse and/or other team members to identify workplace hazards are aimed at health protection.

Specific protection programs or interventions often require active participation on the part of the employee. Participation in an immunization program, employment of personal protective equipment such as respirators or gloves, and cessation of smoking are examples of specific health protection measures.

Secondary prevention occurs after a disease process has already begun. It is aimed at early detection, prompt treatment, and prevention of further limitations. For employees, early detection involves health surveillance and periodic screening to identify an illness at the earliest possible moment in its course, and elimination or modification of the hazard-producing situation. Interventions aimed at disability limitation are intended to prevent further harm or deterioration, and they include referral for counseling and treatment of an employee with an emotional or mental health problem whose work performance has deteriorated, as well as removal of workers from heavy-metal exposure who manifest neurological symptoms.

Tertiary prevention is intended to restore health as fully as possible and assist individuals to achieve their maximum level of functioning. Rehabilitation strategies such as return-to-work programs after a heart attack or limited duty programs after a cumulative trauma injury are examples of tertiary prevention.

Worker Assessment

The initial step of assessment involves the traditional history and physical assessment, emphasizing exposure to occupational hazards and individual characteristics that may predispose the client to the increased health risk of certain jobs. The occupational health history is an indispensable component of the health assessment of individuals (Rogers et al., 2017) (see Appendix B.3). Because work is a part of life for most people, including an occupational health history in all routine nursing assessments is essential. Many workers in the United States do not have access to health care services in their workplaces, yet it is not unusual to find health care providers in the community who have little or no knowledge about workplaces or expertise in occupation-related illnesses and injuries. Because of the large number of small businesses that do not have the resources for maintaining on-site health care, injured and ill workers are first seen in the public and private health care sector (e.g., in clinics, emergency departments, physicians' offices, hospitals, health maintenance organizations, and ambulatory care centers). Nurses are often the first-line assessors of these individuals and perhaps the only contact for education about self-protection from workplace hazards.

Identifying workplace exposures as sources of health problems may influence the client's course of illness and rehabilitation and may also prevent similar illnesses among others with potential for exposure (Levy et al., 2017). Including occupational health data into client assessments begins with recognizing the possible relationship between health and occupational factors. The next step is to integrate into the history-taking procedure some routine assessment questions that will provide the data necessary to confirm or rule out occupationally induced symptoms.

Symptoms of hazardous workplace exposures may be indicated by vague complaints involving any body system. These complaints are often similar to common medical problems. The occupational health histories should include the following points:

- A list of current and past jobs the client has held
- Questions about exposures to specific agents and relationships between the symptoms and activities at work
- Job titles
- History of exposures
- Other factors that may influence the client's susceptibility to occupational agents (e.g., lifestyle history such as smoking, underlying illness, previous injury, or disabling condition)

Questions about the employee's occupational history can be included in existing preplacement assessment tools. The more complete the data collected, the more likely the nurse is to notice the influence of work–health interactions. All employees should be questioned about their employment history. To describe only a current status of "retired" or "housewife" may lead to the omission of needed data. The nurse should be aware that not all workers are well informed about the materials with which they work or about potential hazards. For this reason, the nurse must develop basic knowledge about all of the types of jobs held by clients and the possible hazards associated with them. Because there is an increased likelihood of multiple exposures from other environments such as the home and the community that may interact with workplace exposures, the nurse should extend the questioning to include this information.

Identifying work-related health problems should be an integrated focus of any assessment effort. A systematic approach for evaluating the potential for workplace exposures is the most effective intervention for detecting and preventing occupational health risks. Preplacement exams help ensure that your prospective employee can safely perform the job they are applying for. Because of this, preplacement exams are an important part of the onboarding process—especially for physically intensive jobs.

Fig. 32.2 shows one short assessment tool that can be incorporated into routine history taking. Similar questions can be included in the assessment of workers' spouses and dependents, who may receive secondhand or indirect exposure to occupational hazards.

During these health assessments, the nurse has the opportunity to teach about workplace hazards and prevention measures the worker can use. At the same time, the nurse is obtaining information that will be valuable in optimizing the fit between the job and the worker. Such assessments may be done as follows:

- During preplacement examinations before the client begins a job
- On a periodic basis during employment

I.   Present Job

A.   What is your job title? _____

B.   What do you do for a living? _____

C.   How long have you had this job? _____

D.   Describe the specific tasks of this job: _____
_____

E.   What product or service is produced by the company where you work? _____
_____

F.   Are you exposed to any of the following on your present job?

Metals	Radiation	Stress
Vapors, gases	Vibration	Others: _____
Dusts	Loud noise	
Solvents	Extreme heat or cold	

G.   Do you feel you have any health problems that may be associated with your work?
If yes, describe: _____
_____

H.   How would you describe your satisfaction with your job? _____
_____

I.   Have any of your coworkers complained of illness or injuries that they associate with their job?
If yes, describe: _____
_____

II. All Past Work

Starting with your first job, please provide the following information:

Job title	Years held	Description of work	Exposures	Injuries/illnesses	Personal protection equipment used

III. Other Exposures

A.   Do you have any hobbies that involve exposure to chemicals, metals, or any of the other agents mentioned before? If yes, describe: _____

B.   Are any other members of your household exposed to any of the substances listed above? If yes, describe:
_____

C.   Do you live near any factories, dump sites, or other sources of pollution? If yes, describe: _____
_____

Fig. 32.2 Occupational Health History Form.

- When a work-related health problem or exposure becomes apparent
- When an employee is being transferred to another job with different requirements and exposures
- At termination
- At retirement

The goal of these assessments is to identify agent and host factors that could place the employee at risk and to determine prevention steps that can be taken to eliminate or minimize the exposure and potential health problem.

When the health data from such assessments are considered collectively, the nurse may determine some patterns in risk factors associated with the occurrence of work-related injuries and illnesses in a total population of workers. For example, a nurse practitioner in a clinic noted a dramatic increase in the number of dermatitis cases among her clients. When she looked at factors in common among these individuals, she determined that they all worked at a company with solvent exposure commonly associated with dermal irritations. She worked with the union and the company to assess the environment/agent exposure to the employees and design mitigation strategies. This nursing intervention led to a safer work environment and a decrease in dermatitis in this population group. Such an approach can be used at the company, industry, and community levels. The initial collection of data and the questioning about workplace exposures are vital steps for any intervention.

Workplace Assessment

The nurse may conduct a similar assessment of the workplace itself. The purpose of this assessment, known as a worksite walk-through or survey, is to learn about the following (Rogers et al., 2017):

- Work processes and the materials
- Requirements of various jobs
- Presence of actual or potential hazards
- Work practices of employees

Fig. 32.3 shows a brief outline that can be used to guide a worksite assessment.

More complex surveys are performed by industrial hygienists and safety professionals when the purpose of the walk-through is environmental monitoring using sampling techniques or a safety audit. However, most occupational health nurses have developed expertise in these areas and include such tasks as part of their functions. For all health care providers who assess workers, this information makes an important database. In addition, for the on-site health care provider, worksite walk-throughs assist the professional in developing rapport with and being seen as a credible worker among the employees.

A worksite survey begins with an understanding of the type of work that occurs in the workplace. All business organizations are classified within the North American Industry Classification System (NAICS) with a numerical code. This code, usually a two- to four-digit number, indicates a company's product and therefore the possible types of occupational health hazards that may be associated with the processes and materials used by its employees. NAICS codes are used to collect and report data on businesses. For example, illness and injury rates of one company are compared with the rates of other companies of similar size with the same code to determine whether the company is having an excess of illness or injury. By knowing the NAICS code of a company, a health care professional can access reference books that describe the usual processes, materials, and by products of that kind of company.

The nurse will want to review the work processes and work areas by jobs or locations in the workplace. These preliminary data provide clues about what hazards may be present and an understanding of the types of jobs and health requirements that may be involved in a particular industry. A description of the work environment is next and provides an overall picture of general appearances, physical layout, and safety of the environment. Are safety signs posted and readable where needed? Is there clutter or dampness on the floor that could cause slips or falls?

A description of the employee group is necessary information to understand the demographics and the work distribution in the company. Knowing about shift work and productivity can be helpful in pinpointing potential stressors. Human resources' management and corporate commitment to health and safety are needed to develop a supportive culture for effective and efficient programming. Reviewing the status of policies and procedures and assessing opportunities for input into improving service are important to establish the organization's strength in occupational health and safety management. Gathering data about the incidence and prevalence of work-related illnesses and injuries and the cost patterns for these conditions provides useful epidemiologic trend data and helps target high-cost areas. The types of occupational safety and health services and programs are important to know. This will show whether required

Name of company: _____ Date: _____

Address: _____

Telephone: _____

Parent company (if any): _____

Location of corporate offices: _____

SIC code: _____

The Work:

Major products: _____

Major processes and operations, raw materials, by products: _____

_____

Type of jobs: _____

_____

Potential exposures: _____

_____

Work Environment

General conditions: _____

Safety signs: _____

Physical environment: _____

Worker Population

Employees

Total number: _____ Number in production: _____ Others: _____

% Full-time: _____ % Men: _____ % Women: _____

% First shift: _____ % Second shift: _____ % Third shift: _____

Age distribution: _____

% Unionized: _____ Names of unions: _____

Human Resources Management

Corporate commitment to health

Personnel

Policies/procedures

Input/surveys/committees

Recordkeeping

Health Data

Work-related illnesses, injuries, deaths per annum: _____

OSHA recordable: _____ Workers' Compensation: _____

Other: _____ Most frequent complaints: _____

Average number of monthly calls to the health unit: _____

Absenteeism rate: _____

Occupation Health and Safety Services

Examinations

Employee assistance

Treatment of illness/injury

Health education

Physical fitness, health promotion activities

Mandatory programs

Safety audits

Environmental monitoring

Health risk appraisal

Screenings

Health promotion

Control Strategies

Engineering

Work practice

Administrative

Personal protective equipment

Fig. 32.3 Worksite Assessment Guide. *OSHA,* Occupational Safety and Health Administration; *SIC,* Standard Industrial Classification.

programs are being offered and includes health promotion and disease prevention strategies.

Finally, examining control strategies that are effective in eliminating or reducing exposure is important in determining risk reduction. Engineering controls can reduce worker exposure by modifying the exposure source, such as putting needles in a puncture-proof container (see the How To box).

HOW TO ASSESS A WORKER AND THE WORKPLACE

Assessing the worker for a work-related problem is a critical practice element. You need to do the following:

- Complete general and occupational health history taking with emphasis on workplace exposure assessment, job hazard analysis, and list of previous jobs.
- Conduct a health assessment to identify agent and host factors that interact to place workers at risk.
- Identify patterns of risk associated with illness/injury.

Assessing the work environment is necessary to determine workplace exposures that create worker health risk. You need to do the following:

- Understand the work being done.
- Understand the work process.
- Evaluate the work-related hazards.
- Gather data about incidence/prevalence of work-related illness/injuries and related hazards.
- Conduct a walk-though of the work environment.
- Examine prevention and control strategies in place for eliminating exposures.

Finally, examining control strategies that are effective in eliminating or reducing exposure is important in determining risk reduction. Control strategies follow a hierarchical approach. Engineering controls can reduce worker exposure by modifying the exposure source, such as putting needles in a puncture-proof container. Work practice controls include good hygiene and proper waste disposal and housekeeping. Administrative controls reduce exposure through job rotation, workplace monitoring, and employee training and education. Finally, personal protective control is the last resort and requires the worker to actively engage in strategies for protection such as use of gloves, masks, and gowns to prevent exposures (Rogers et al., 2017).

The more information that can be collected before the walk-through, the more efficient the process of the survey will be. After the survey is conducted, the nurse can use the information with the aggregate health data to evaluate the effectiveness of the occupational health and safety program and to plan future programs.

HEALTHY PEOPLE 2030 DOCUMENT RELATED TO OCCUPATIONAL HEALTH

In an attempt to meet the goal of attaining high-quality, longer lives free of preventable disability, injury, and premature death for Americans, health promotion and protection strategies are proposed to address the needs of large population groups such as the American workforce. As part of the *Healthy People 2030* document (USDHHS, 2020), occupational safety and health objectives were identified to promote good health and well-being among workers, including the elimination and reduction of elements in occupational environments that cause death, injury, disease, or disability. In addition, this document promotes the minimizing of personal damage from existing occupationally related illness.

 HEALTHY PEOPLE 2030
Objectives Related to Occupational Health

- **ECBP-D03:** Increase the proportion of worksites that offer an employee health promotion program
- **ECBP-D04:** Increase the proportion of worksites that offer an employee physical activity program
- **ECBP-D05:** Increase the proportion of worksites that offer an employee nutrition program
- **OSH-01:** Reduce deaths from work-related injuries
- **OSH-02:** Reduce work-related injuries resulting in missed workdays
- **OSH-04:** Reduce pneumoconiosis deaths
- **OSH-05:** Reduce work-related assault
- **OSH-06:** Reduce new cases of work-related hearing loss

Data from US Department of Health and Human Services (USHHS): *Healthy People 2030.* HHS, 2020. Available at https://health.gov/healthypeople.

LEGISLATION RELATED TO OCCUPATIONAL HEALTH

The occupational health and safety services provided by an employer are influenced by specific legislation at federal and state levels. Although the relationship between work and health has been known since the second century (Ramazzini, 1713), public policy that effectively controlled occupational hazards was not enacted until the 1960s. The Mine Safety and Health Act of 1968 was the first legislation that specifically required certain prevention programs for workers. This was followed by the Occupational Safety and Health Act of 1970, which established two agencies, OSHA and NIOSH, each with discrete functions (Box 32.3) to carry out the Act's purpose of ensuring "safe and healthful working conditions for working men and

---

BOX 32.3 Functions of Federal Agencies Involved in Occupational Safety and Health

Occupational Safety and Health Administration (OSHA)

- Determines and sets standards and permissible exposure limits (PELs) for hazardous exposures in the workplace
- Enforces the occupational health standards (including the right of entry for inspection)
- Educates employees and employers about occupational health and safety
- Develops and maintains a database of work-related injuries, illnesses, and deaths
- Monitors compliance with occupational health and safety standards

National Institute for Occupational Safety and Health (NIOSH)

- Conducts research and reviews findings to recommend exposure limits for occupational hazards to OSHA
- Identifies and researches occupational health and safety hazards
- Educates occupational health and safety professionals
- Distributes research findings relevant to occupational health and safety

From US Department of Health and Human Services, National Institute for Occupational Safety and Health: *National Occupational Research Agenda.* Cincinnati, 2018, USDHHS.

women" (Public Law 91-596, 1970). The reader is also referred to Chapters 3 and 5, the Affordable Care Act, for additional information on employer mandates.

In the context of the Occupational Safety and Health Act, OSHA, a federal agency within the US Department of Labor, was created to develop and enforce workplace safety and health standards and regulations on workers' exposure to potentially toxic substances, enforcing these at the federal and state levels. Specific standards and information about compliance can be obtained from federal, regional, and state OSHA offices, which can be found on the OSHA website.

The National Institute for Occupational Safety and Health (NIOSH) was established by the Occupational Safety and Health Act of 1970 and is part of the Centers for Disease Control and Prevention (CDC). In 1996 NIOSH and its partners unveiled a 10-year National Occupational Research Agenda (NORA), a framework to guide occupational safety and health research into the following decade. The NIOSH agency identifies, monitors, and educates about the incidence, prevalence, and prevention of work-related illnesses and injuries and examines potential hazards of new work technologies and practices (USDHHS/NIOSH, 2018). Subsequently, the NORA has been updated and is focused on targeted sectors to reduce the still significant toll of workplace illness and injury.

Many standards have been established by OSHA and promulgated to protect worker health. One example is the Hazard Communication Standard. This standard is based on the premise that while working to reduce and eliminate potentially toxic agents in the work environment, an important line of defense is to provide the work community with information about hazardous chemicals in order to minimize exposures. The Hazard Communication Standard, which was first established in 1983, requires that all worksites with hazardous substances inventory their toxic agents, label them, and provide information sheets, called safety data sheets (SDSs), for each agent. In addition, the employer must have in place a hazard communication program that provides workers with education about these agents. This education must include agent identification, toxic effects, and protective measures. Numerous standards have been established by OSHA for specific chemicals and programs. A standard familiar to all health care professionals is the *Bloodborne Pathogens Standard.*

Workers' compensation acts are important state laws that govern financial compensation to employees who suffer work-related health problems. These acts vary by state, and each state sets rules for the reimbursement of employees with occupational health problems for medical expenses and lost work time associated with the illness or injury. Workers' compensation claims and the experience-based insurance premiums paid by industry have been important motivators for increasing the health and safety of the workplace.

DISASTER PLANNING AND MANAGEMENT

Although disaster planning and management have been functions of occupational health and safety programs, this is an area of legislation that affects businesses and health professionals.

The legislation of the Superfund Amendment and Reauthorization Act (SARA) requires that written disaster plans be shared with key resources in the community, such as fire departments and emergency departments. Concern about disasters—such as the terrorist attacks on the World Trade Center and Pentagon on September 11, 2001; the methyl isocyanate leak in Bhopal, India; effects of hurricanes such as Katrina and Sandy; or the community exposure to chemicals at Times Beach, Missouri, and exposure to radiation from crippled nuclear plants in Japan—has mandated more attention to disaster planning.

In occupational health, the goals of a disaster plan are to prevent or minimize injuries and deaths of workers and residents, minimize property damage, provide effective triage, and facilitate necessary business activities. A disaster plan requires the cooperation of different personnel within the company and community. The nurse is often a key person on the disaster planning team, along with safety professionals, physicians, industrial hygienists, the fire chief, and company management. The potential for disaster (e.g., explosions, floods, fires, leaks) must be identified, and this is best achieved by completing an exhaustive chemical and hazard inventory of the workplace. The SDS and plant blueprints are critical for correctly identifying substances and work areas that may be hazardous. Worksite surveys are the first step to completing this inventory. The reader is also referred to Chapter 16 on the public health nurse (PHN) and disaster management.

Effective disaster plans are designed by those with knowledge of the work processes and materials, the workers and workplace, and the resources in the community. Specific steps must be detailed for actions to be put in place by specific individuals in the event of a disaster. The written plan must be shared with all who will be involved. Employees should be prepared in first aid, cardiopulmonary resuscitation, and fire brigade procedures. Plans must be clear, specific, and comprehensive (i.e., covering all shifts and all work areas) and must include activities to be conducted within the worksite and those that require community resources. Transportation plans, fire response, and emergency response services should be coordinated with the agencies that would be involved in an actual disaster. The disaster plan, emergency and safety equipment, and the first response team's abilities should be tested at least annually with a drill. Practice results should be carefully evaluated, with changes made as needed.

Hospitals and other emergency services, such as fire departments, should be involved in developing the disaster plan and should receive a copy of the plan and a current hazard inventory. It is imperative that the plan and hazard inventory be periodically updated. The occupational health nurse or another company representative should provide emergency health care providers with updated clinical information on exposures and appropriate treatment. It should never be presumed that local services will have current information on substances used in industry. Representatives of these agencies should visit the worksite and accompany the nurse on a worksite walk-through so that they are familiar with the operations.

In disaster planning, the nurse is often assigned or assumes the responsibility for coordinating the planning and implementing efforts, working with appropriate key people within the company and in the community to develop a workable, comprehensive plan. Other tasks include providing ongoing communication to keep the plan current; planning the drills; educating the employees, management, and community providers; and assessing the equipment and services that may be used in a disaster.

In the event of a disaster, the nurse should play a key role in coordinating the response. Principles of triage may be used as the response team determines the extent of the disaster and the ability of the company and community to respond. Post disaster nursing interventions are also critical. Examples include identifying the ongoing disaster-related health needs of workers and community residents, collecting epidemiologic data, and assessing the cause and the necessary steps to prevent a recurrence.

▷ APPLYING CONTENT TO PRACTICE

This chapter emphasizes the roles and functions of the nurse in occupational health. This dynamic specialty practice is broad and is founded in public health practice, supporting a model of health promotion, risk reduction, protection, and illness prevention. The occupational health nurse must have interprofessional skills and linkages to provide the most effective care and service. The epidemiological model is applied to occupational health and considers the host, agent, and environmental issues that may result in injury or illnesses. The goal is to assess the workplace to prevent injuries or illnesses where possible. In applying the model the nurse uses the nursing process and considers the impact of the workforce characteristics, the characteristics of the work, and work–health interaction in order to work toward a healthy and safe environment. Thus it is important to assess both the worker and the workplace to build this environment. Occupational health nursing has a rich history in the profession, beginning in the 1800s. The roles and functions of the occupational health nurse are many, and the education and certification of the nurse are considered as the nurse seeks a position as an occupational health nurse.

Occupational health nursing is a broad, dynamic specialty practice. The Public Health Foundation provides the basis for practice, supporting a health promotion and protection and prevention model. The occupational health nurse must have interprofessional skills and linkages to provide the most effective care and service. Occupational health nurses are involved in all levels of prevention in their practice.

▮ PRACTICE APPLICATION

An insurance company recently renovated its claims processing office area and fitted the workstation with new computers. The company's occupational health nurse noticed an increase in visits to the health unit for complaints of headaches, stiff neck muscles, and visual disturbances consistent with computer usage.

To conduct a complete investigation of this problem, the nurse assessed the workers, the agent (computer), previously existing potential agents, and the work environment. Interventions focused on designing the health hazard out of the work process, if possible. In the present example, the first level of intervention was to refit the workstation for better worker use of the computer.

Minimizing the possible hazards of the agent involved recommendations for desks, chairs, and lighting designs that would accommodate the individual worker and allow shielding of the monitor. The nursing interventions included strengthening the resistance of the host by prescribing appropriate rest breaks, eye exercises, and relaxation strategies. Recognizing that previous cervical neck injury or impaired vision may increase the risk of adverse effects from computer work, the nurse would include assessment for these factors in employees' preplacement and periodic health examinations.

For the environmental concerns, the nurse educated the manager about the health risks of paced, externally controlled work expectations and recommended alternatives.

This case is an example of which of the following?
A. The application of the occupational health history
B. A worksite assessment or walk-through
C. A work–health interaction
D. The use of the epidemiologic triangle in exploring occupational health problems

Answers can be found on the Evolve website.

▮ REMEMBER THIS!

- Occupational health nursing is an autonomous practice specialty.
- The scope of occupational health nursing practice is broad, including worker and workplace assessment and surveillance, case management, health promotion, primary care, management/administration, business and finance skills, and research.
- The workforce and workplace are changing dramatically, requiring new knowledge and new occupational health services.
- The type of work has shifted from primarily manufacturing to service and technological jobs.
- Workplace hazards include exposure to biological, chemical, enviromechanical, physical, and psychosocial agents.
- The Occupational Safety and Health Act of 1970 states that workers must have a safe and healthful work environment.
- The interprofessional occupational health team consists of the occupational health nurse, occupational medicine physician, industrial hygienist, and safety specialist.
- Work-related health problems must be investigated and control strategies implemented to reduce exposure.
- Control strategies include engineering, work practice, administration, and personal protective equipment.
- The Occupational Safety and Health Administration enforces workplace safety and health standards.
- The National Institute for Occupational Safety and Health is the education and research agency that provides grants to investigate the causes of workplace illness and injuries.
- Workers' compensation acts are important laws that govern financial compensation of employees who suffer work-related health problems.
- The occupational health nurse should play a key role in disaster planning and coordination.
- Academic education in occupational health nursing is generally at the graduate level.

EVOLVE WEBSITE

http://evolve.elsevier.com/Stanhope/community/

- Answers to Practice Application
- Case Study
- Review Questions

REFERENCES

American Association of Occupational Health Nurses: *The nurse in industry*, New York, 1976, AAOHN.

American Association of Occupational Health Nurses: *Standards of occupational and environmental health nursing practice*, Chicago, 2016a, AAOHN.

American Association of Occupational Health Nurses: *Code of ethics*, Chicago, 2016b, AAOHN.

Brown M: *Occupational health nursing*, New York, 1981, MacMillan.

Bureau of Labor Statistics: *Labor force statistics for current population*, Washington, DC, 2018, US Department of Labor.

Bureau of Labor Statistics: *National census of fatal occupational injuries in 2018 News Release*. USDL-19-2194. December 17, 2019a. Retrieved from https://www.bls.gov.

Bureau of Labor Statistics: *Employer-Reported Workplace Injury and Illnesses – 2018 News Release*, USDL-19-1909. November 7, 2019b. Retrieved from https://www.bls.gov.

Burke WW: *Organizational change: theory and practice*, Thousand Oaks, 2018, SAGE Publicatins.

Centers for Disease Control and Prevention (CDC): *Stop Sticks Campaign*, 2019. Retrieved from https://www.cdc.gov.

Felton J: The genesis of American occupational health nursing, part 1, *Occup Health Nurs* 33:615, 1985.

Friis RH: *Occupational health and safety for the 21st century*, Burlington, 2016, Jones and Bartlett Learning.

Health Resources and Services Administration: *Characteristics of the US nursing workforce with patience care responsibilities: resources for epidemic and pandemic response*, 2020. US Department of Health and Human Services, Bureau of Health Workforce,

National Center for Health Workforce Analysis. Retrieved from http://bhw.hrsa.gov.

Heaton K, Mumbower R, Childs G: Sleep and safety decision-making among truck drivers, *Workplace Health & Safety*, online publication, 2020. https://doi.org/10.1177/2165079920950255

Levy BS, Wegman DH Baron SL, Sokas RK: *Occupational health: recognizing and preventing occupational disease*, Philadelphia, 2017, Lippincott Williams & Wilkins.

McGrath B: Fifty years of industrial nursing, *Public Health Nurs* 37: 119, 1945.

Merrill RM: *Introduction to epidemiology*, ed 8, Burlington, 2021, Jones & Bartlett Learning.

O'Donnell M: *Health promotion in the workplace*, Troy, 2017, Art & Science of Health Promotion Institute.

Public Law 91-596: *The occupational safety and health act*, Washington, DC, 1970, US Department of Labor.

Quad Council Coalition Competency Review Task Force: Community/ Public Health Nursing Competencies, 2018.

Ramazzini B: *De Morbis Artificum [Diseases of Workers], 1713,* Translated by Wright WC, Chicago, 1940, University of Chicago Press.

Rogers B: Perspectives on occupational health nursing, *AAOHN J* 36:100–105, 1988.

Rogers B, Randolph S, Mastroianni K: *Occupational health nursing guidelines for primary clinical conditions*, ed 5, Beverly, 2017, OEM Press.

Rogers B: Occupational Health Nursing: *Concepts and Practice*. In Press, 2019.

Schwartz NG, Price SF, Pratt RH, Langer AJ: Tuberculosis – United States, 2019, *MMWR Morb Mortal Wkly Rep, 69*: 286-289, 2020. Toossi M, Torpey E: *Older Workers: Labor Force Trends and Career Options*, 2017. Retrieved from https://www.bls.gov.

US Department of Health and Human Services: *Healthy people 2030*, HHS, 2020. Available at https://health.gov/healthypeople.

US Department of Health and Human Services, National Institute for Occupational Safety and Health (USDHHS/NIOSH): *National Occupational Research Agenda*. Cincinnati, 2018, USDHHS.

Vespa J, Medina L, Armstrong DM: *Demographic turning points for the United States: population projects for 2020 to 2060*. US Census Bureau Current Population Reports P25-1144. 2018. Retrieved from https://www.census.gov.

APPENDIX A   GUIDELINES FOR PRACTICE

A.1: *The Health Insurance Portability and Accountability Act* (HIPAA): What Does It Mean For Public Health Nurses?

A.2: Living Will Directive

APPENDIX B   ASSESSMENT TOOLS

B.1: Community Assessment Model

B.2: Comprehensive Occupational And Environmental Exposure History

APPENDIX C   ESSENTIAL ELEMENTS OF PUBLIC HEALTH NURSING

C.1: Examples of Public Health Nursing Roles and Implementing Public Health Functions

C.2: American Nurses Association Standards of Practice and Professional Performance For Public Health Nursing

C.3: Minnesota Department of Health Public Health Interventions Wheel

APPENDIX D   HEPATITIS INFORMATION

D.1: Summary Description of Hepatitis A-E

D.2 Recommendations For Prophylaxis of Hepatitis A

D.3: Recommendations For Postexposure Prophylaxis For Contacts of Patients Positive For HBsAg are as Follows

Guidelines for Practice

A.1 *The Health Insurance Portability and Accountability Act (HIPAA): What Does It Mean For Public Health Nurses?*

Public Health Nursing Practice: Definition—the synthesis of nursing and public health theory applied to promoting and preserving the health of populations. The practice focuses on the community as a whole and on the effect of the community's health status (resources) on the health of individuals, families, and groups. The goal is to prevent disease and disability and promote and protect the health of the community as a whole.

EXPLANATION

- Federal privacy standards were created by the US Department of Health and Human Services (USDHHS) to protect patients' medical records and other health information provided to health plans, doctors, hospitals, and other health care providers.
- These standards took effect on April 14, 2003.
- The *Health Insurance Portability and Accountability Act* sought to reduce the cost of and improve the delivery of health care through the standardization of electronic transactions and the elimination of inefficient paper forms.

PRIVACY RULE

- Protects the confidentiality of individually identifiable health information, whether it is on paper, in computers, or communicated orally.
  - Protected health information (PHI) is the name for this individually identifiable health information.
  - Limits the ways that health plans, pharmacies, hospitals, and other covered entities can use patients' personal medical information.

PATIENT PROTECTIONS

- Patients should be able to see, obtain copies of, and make corrections to their medical records.
- Patients should receive a notice from health care providers regarding how their personal medical information may be used by them and their rights under the privacy regulation. Patients can restrict this use.
- Limits have been set on how health care providers can use individually identifiable health information. Doctors, nurses, and other providers can share information needed to treat a patient. For purposes other than medical care, personal health information generally may not be used.
- Pharmacies, health plans, and other covered entities must obtain an individual's authorization before disclosing patient information for marketing purposes.

PUBLIC HEALTH SERVICES AND PROTECTED HEALTH INFORMATION

Overview: Although protection of health information is important, PHI is used for the public good by health officials to identify, monitor, and respond to disease, death, and disability among populations. Examples of ways PHI is used include public health surveillance, program evaluation, terrorism preparedness, outbreak investigations, direct health services, and public health research. Public health authorities have taken precautions in the past to protect the privacy of individuals and will continue to do so under HIPAA. The privacy rule, however, still permits PHI to be shared for important public health purposes.

PERMITTED PROTECTED HEALTH INFORMATION DISCLOSURES TO A PUBLIC HEALTH AUTHORITY WITHOUT AUTHORIZATION

- Reporting of disease, injury, and vital events
- Conducting public health surveillance, investigations, and interventions
- Reporting child abuse or neglect to a public health or other government authority legally authorized to receive such reports
- Reporting to a person subject to the jurisdiction of the US Food and Drug Administration (FDA) concerning the quality, safety, or effectiveness of an FDA-related product or activity for which that person has responsibility
- To a person who may have been exposed to a communicable disease or may be at risk for contracting or spreading a disease or condition, when legally authorized to notify the person as necessary to conduct a public health intervention or investigation
- To an individual's employer, under certain circumstances and conditions, as needed for the employer to meet the

requirements of the Occupational Safety and Health Administration, Mine Safety and Health Administration, or similar state law

HEALTH INSURANCE PORTABILITY AND ACCOUNTABILITY ACT AND NURSING RESEARCH

Definitions

Covered entity: A health plan, a health care clearinghouse, or a health care provider who transmits any health information in electronic form.

Individually Identifiable Health Information (IIHI): Information about an individual regarding his or her physical or mental health, the provision of health care, or the payment for the provision of health care and that identifies the individual.

- It is the covered entity's obligation not to disclose the information improperly when a researcher seeks data that includes PHI.

A covered entity can disclose IIHI for research purposes under any of the following conditions:

1. The IIHI pertains only to deceased persons.
2. The IIHI can be examined for reviews preparatory to research if it is not removed from the covered entity.
3. Information that has been deidentified can be disclosed; this information is no longer considered IIHI and thus is not covered by HIPAA.
4. Data must be disclosed as part of a limited data set if the researcher has a data use agreement with the covered entity.
5. The researcher has a valid authorization from the research subject to disclose IIHI.
6. An institutional review board or privacy board has waived the authorization requirement.

Creating Data

Researchers may also be creating IIHI. If the researcher is part of a covered entity, any PHI obtained by any means is covered by HIPAA, and the researcher and his or her institution are bound by HIPAA regulations. Most universities with nursing schools will be hybrid entities (i.e., some parts of the university are a covered entity and some are not). Researchers should check their institution's policies.

Disclosing Data

Nurse researchers should be aware that sharing data with colleagues and students may constitute disclosures of IIHI and they should conform to HIPAA regulations. In this case, the researcher is the holder of the IIHI and can disclose it only under appropriate conditions:

1. Patients agree to specific disclosures in the initial authorization.
2. Former patients sign an additional authorization.
3. An institutional review board or privacy board waives the need for authorization.
4. The holder allows the colleague to review the data to prepare a research protocol if the colleague takes no information away.
5. A holder enters the data in a limited data set and signs a data use agreement with the recipient.
6. A holder deidentifies the data and shares it freely.

From Begley EB, Ware JM, Hexem SA, et al: Personally identifiable information in state laws: Use, release, and collaboration at health departments, *Am J Public Health* 107(8):1272–1276, 2017. doi:10.2105/AJPH.2017.303862; Bernstein AB, Sweeney MH: Public health surveillance data: legal, policy, ethical, regulatory, and practical issues, *MMWR Suppl* 61(03):30–34, 2012. Available at: https://www.cdc.gov/mmwr/preview/mmwrhtml/su6103a7.htm?s_cid%3Dsu6103a7_x (accessed July 2017); Centers for Disease Control and Prevention: HIPAA privacy rule and public health, *MMWR* 52 (S-1):1–12, 2003. Available at: http://www.cdc.gov/mmwr/preview/mmwrhtml/su5201a1.htm (accessed July 2017); Goldstein ND, Sarwate AD: Privacy, security, and the public health researcher in the era of electronic health record research, *Online J Public Health Inform*, 8(3):e207, 2016; Institute of Medicine: Beyond the HIPAA privacy rule: enhancing privacy, improving health through research, Washington, DC, 2009, National Academies Press; Jacobson PD, Wasserman J, Botoseneaunu A, et al: The roles of law in public health preparedness: Opportunities and challenges, *J Health Politics Policy Law* 37(2):297–328, 2012; Olsen DP: HIPAA privacy regulations and nursing research, *Nurs Res* 52:344–348, 2003; US Department of Health and Human Services: Health information privacy: public health. Washington, DC, 2003, USDHHS, available at: http://www.hhs.gov/ocr/privacy/hipaa/understanding/special/publichealth/index.html (accessed July 2017).

A.2 Living Will Directive

Living Will Directive

My wishes regarding life-prolonging treatment and artificially provided nutrition and hydration to be provided to me if I no longer have decisional capacity, have a terminal condition, or become permanently unconscious have been indicated by checking and initialing the appropriate lines below. By checking and initialing the appropriate lines, I specifically:

Designate _____ as my health care surrogate(s) to make health care decisions for me in accordance with this directive when I no longer have decisional capacity. If _____ refuses or is not able to act for me, I designate _____ as my health care surrogate(s).

Any prior designation is revoked.

If I do not designate a surrogate, the following are my directions to my attending physician. If I have designated a surrogate, my surrogate shall comply with my wishes as indicated below:

_____ Direct that treatment be withheld or withdrawn, and that I be permitted to die naturally with only the administration of medication or the performance of any medical treatment deemed necessary to alleviate pain.

_____ DO NOT authorize that life-prolonging treatment be withheld or withdrawn.

_____ Authorize the withholding or withdrawal of artificially provided food, water, or other artificially provided nourishment or fluids.

_____ DO NOT authorize the withholding or withdrawal of artificially provided food, water, or other artificially provided nourishment or fluids.

_____ Authorize my surrogate, designated above, to withhold or withdraw artificially provided nourishment or fluids, or other treatment if the surrogate determines that withholding or withdrawing is in my best interest; but I do not mandate that withholding or withdrawing.

In the absence of my ability to give directions regarding the use of life-prolonging treatment and artificially provided nutrition and hydration, it is my intention that this directive shall be honored by my attending physician, my family, and any surrogate designated pursuant to this directive as the final expression of my legal right to refuse medical or surgical treatment, and I accept the consequences of the refusal.

If I have been diagnosed as pregnant and that diagnosis is known to my attending physician, this directive shall have no force or effect during the course of my pregnancy.

I understand the full import of this directive and I am emotionally and mentally competent to make this directive.

Signed this _____ day of _____, 20____.

Signature and address of the grantor.

_____

In our joint presence, the grantor, who is of sound mind and eighteen (18) years of age, or older, voluntarily dated and signed this writing or directed it to be dated and signed for the grantor.

_____

Signature and address of witness.

_____ Signature and address of witness.

OR

_____

_____ County

Before me, the undersigned authority, came the grantor who is of sound mind and eighteen (18) years of age, or older, and acknowledged that he voluntarily dated and signed this writing or directed it to be signed and dated as above.

Done this _____ day of _____, 20____.

_____

Signature of Notary Public or other.

_____

Date commission expires.

Execution of this document restricts withholding and withdrawing of some medical procedures. Consult State Revised Statutes or your attorney.

B.1 Community Assessment Model

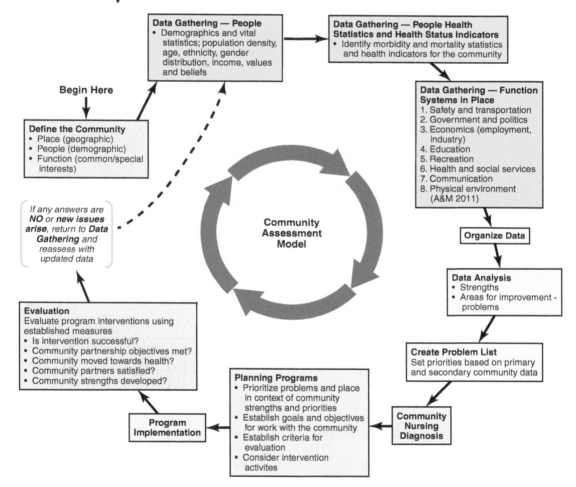

Using the figure above, the first step of the community assessment is to define the community. To do this, geographic boundaries, the population within the boundaries, the purpose of the assessment, and a data collection plan will be identified. Census blocks or tracts and geopolitical boundaries such as city or county lines will allow for collection of consistent data about the region under study. Included in "place" is the type of terrain or environment, the climate, the history of the area, and its size. The population is the next identifier. How does your assessment define those within the community? Are they members of a specific group or the population in general? What data are available for the assessment and where will you seek your sources? In essence, the identification of the community's members comprises the "client" within these boundaries.

What is the local history? Who were the original settlers and how has the community developed over time? Is it an area of growth or decline? Are original families still living in the area or has the early population been replaced? History can reveal a lot about customs and mores that could influence the health of the community.

From Stanhope M, Lancaster L: *Public health nursing: Population-centered health care in the community*, 9th ed. St. Louis, 2016, Elsevier.

599

B.2 Comprehensive Occupational and Environmental Exposure History

Exposure History Form

Part 1. Exposure Survey   Name: _____ Date: _____

Please circle the appropriate answer.   Birth date:_____ Sex (circle one): Male   Female

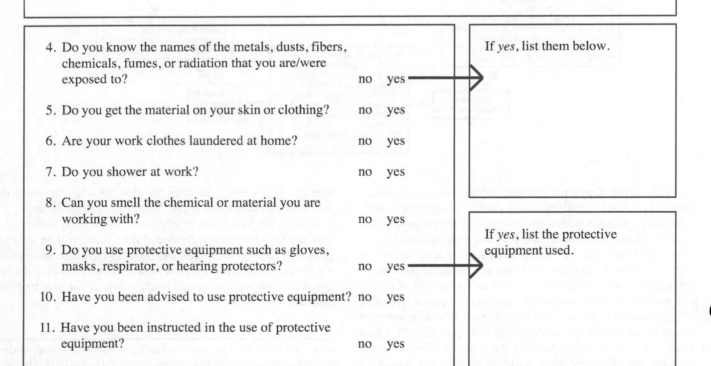

1. Are you currently exposed to any of the following?

metals	no	yes
dust or fibers	no	yes
chemicals	no	yes
fumes	no	yes
radiation	no	yes
biologic agents	no	yes
loud noise, vibration, extreme heat or cold	no	yes

2. Have you been exposed to any of the above in the past?   no   yes

3. Do any household members have contact with metals, dust, fibers, chemicals, fumes, radiation, or biologic agents?   no   yes

---

If you answered *yes* to any of the items above, describe your exposure in detail—how you were exposed, to what you were exposed. If you need more space, please use a separate sheet of paper.

---

4. Do you know the names of the metals, dusts, fibers, chemicals, fumes, or radiation that you are/were exposed to?   no   yes   →   If *yes*, list them below.

5. Do you get the material on your skin or clothing?   no   yes

6. Are your work clothes laundered at home?   no   yes

7. Do you shower at work?   no   yes

8. Can you smell the chemical or material you are working with?   no   yes

9. Do you use protective equipment such as gloves, masks, respirator, or hearing protectors?   no   yes   →   If *yes*, list the protective equipment used.

10. Have you been advised to use protective equipment?   no   yes

11. Have you been instructed in the use of protective equipment?   no   yes

12. Do you wash your hands with solvents?   no   yes

13. Do you smoke at the workplace?   no   yes   At home?   no   yes

14. Are you exposed to secondhand tobacco smoke at the workplace?   no   yes   At home?   no   yes

15. Do you eat at the workplace?   no   yes

16. Do you know of any coworkers experiencing similar or unusual symptoms?   no   yes

17. Are family members experiencing similar or unusual symptoms?   no   yes

18. Has there been a change in the health or behavior of family pets?   no   yes

19. Do your symptoms seem to be aggravated by a specific activity?   no   yes

20. Do your symptoms get either worse or better at work?   no   yes
                at home?   no   yes
                on weekends?   no   yes
                on vacation?

21. Has anything about your job changed in recent months (such as duties,   no   yes
procedures, overtime)?

22. Do you use any traditional or alternative medicines?   no   yes

23. Have you or your child ever eaten nonfood items such as paint, plaster, dirt,   no   yes
and/or clay?

If you answered *yes* to any of the questions, please explain.

Part 2. Work History
A. Occupational Profile

Name: _____

Birth date: _____ Sex: Male Female

The following questions refer to your current or most recent job:

Job title: _____ Describe this job: _____

Type of industry: _____ _____

Name of employer: _____ _____

Date job began: _____ _____

Are you still working in this job? yes   no   _____

If *no*, when did this job end? _____ _____

Fill in the table below listing all jobs you have worked, including short-term, seasonal, part-time employment, and military service. Begin with your most recent job. Use additional paper if necessary.

Dates of Employment	Job Title and Description of Work	Exposures*	Protective Equipment

*List the chemicals, dusts, fibers, fumes, radiation, biologic agents (i.e., molds or viruses) and physical agents (i.e., extreme heat, cold, vibration, or noise) that you were exposed to at this job.

Have you ever worked at a job or hobby in which you came in contact with any of the following by breathing, touching, or ingesting (swallowing)? If *yes*, please check the circle beside the name.

○ Acids	○ Chloroprene	○ Methylene chloride	○ Styrene
○ Alcohols (industrial)	○ Chromates	○ Nickel	○ Talc
○ Alkalies	○ Coal dust	○ PBBs	○ Toluene
○ Ammonia	○ Dichlorobenzene	○ PCBs	○ TDI or MDI
○ Arsenic	○ Ethylene dibromide	○ Perchloroethylene	○ Trichloroethylene
○ Asbestos	○ Ethylene dichloride	○ Pesticides	○ Trinitrotoluene
○ Benzene	○ Fiberglass	○ Phenol	○ Vinyl chloride
○ Beryllium	○ Halothane	○ Phosgene	○ Welding fumes
○ Cadmium	○ Isocyanates	○ Radiation	○ X-rays
○ Carbon tetrachloride	○ Ketones	○ Rock dust	○ Other (specify)
○ Chlorinated naphthalenes	○ Lead	○ Silica powder	
○ Chloroform	○ Mercury	○ Solvents	

B. Occupational Exposure Inventory   *Please circle the appropriate answer.*

1. Have you ever been off work for more than 1 day because of an illness related to work?   no   yes

2. Have you ever been advised to change jobs or work assignments because of any health problems or injuries?   no   yes

3. Has your work routine changed recently?   no   yes

4. Is there poor ventilation in your workplace?   no   yes

Part 3. Environmental History   *Please circle the appropriate answer.*

1. Do you live next to or near an industrial plant, commercial business, dump site, or nonresidential property?   no   yes

2. Which of the following do you have in your home?
   Please circle those that apply.

Air conditioner	Air purifier	Central heating (gas or oil?)	Gas stove
Fireplace	Wood stove	Humidifier	Electric stove

3. Have you recently acquired new furniture or carpet, refinished furniture, or remodeled your home?   no   yes

4. Have you weatherized your home recently?   no   yes

5. Are pesticides or herbicides (bug or weed killers; flea and tick sprays, collars, powders, or shampoos) used in your home or garden, or on pets?   no   yes

6. Do you (or any household member) have a hobby or craft?   no   yes

7. Do you work on your car?   no   yes

8. Have you ever changed your residence because of a health problem?   no   yes

9. Does your drinking water come from a private well, city water supply, or grocery store?

10. Approximately what year was your home built?_____

11. Does your food come from somewhere other than a grocery store?   no   yes

---

If you answered *yes* to any of the questions, please explain.

From the US Department of Health and Human Services Agency for Toxic Substances and Disease Registry: *ATSDR Case Studies in Environmental Medicine Taking an Exposure History,* Course WB 2579, 2015. Available at https://www.atsdr.cdc.gov/csem/csem.asp?csem=33&po=9 (accessed July 2017).

Essential Elements of Public Health Nursing

C.1 Examples of Public Health Nursing Roles and Implementing Public Health Functions

This document is intended to clearly present the role of public health nurses in one state. Nurses are members of multidisciplinary public health teams in a changing health care environment. The following matrices present the role of public health nursing in one state. The following definitions were used to develop these matrices.

Essential Elements of public health and nursing are considered the three pillars or building blocks for the public health infrastructure. These are assessment, assurance, and policy development. There are 10 essential services to be provided to support the public health infrastructure:

1. **Monitor** health status to identify community health problems.
2. **Diagnose and investigate** health problems and health hazards in the community.
3. **Inform, educate, and empower** people about health issues.
4. **Mobilize** community partnerships to identify and solve health problems.
5. **Develop policies and plans** that support individual and community health efforts.
6. **Enforce** laws and regulations that protect health and ensure safety.
7. **Link** people to needed personal health services and assure the provision of health care when otherwise unavailable.
8. **Assure** a competent public health and personal health care workforce.
9. **Evaluate** effectiveness, accessibility, and quality of personal and population-based health services.
10. **Research** for new insights and innovative solutions to health problems.

Public Health Function is defined as a broad public health activity needed to ensure a strong, flexible, accountable public health infrastructure. It may require a multidisciplinary team to carry out.

Public Health Nurse Role is the activity the public health nurse is responsible for, either alone or as a member of a team, to accomplish the stated public health functions (essential elements). This can be the public health nurse at the local level or at the state level. The nurse participates in these functions depending upon the level of education of the nurse. The nurse also adheres to the scope and standards of public health nursing practice (ANA, 2013)—see discussion in C.2.

State Role is what public health nurses need from the state level to do their jobs (e.g., policy, aggregate data, training). This refers to any Central Office program or staff, not just nurses.

A process can be implemented that would involve all public health nurses in a state. Although the timeline to completion may be lengthened when nurses at local and state levels are participating, it will ensure that the final document represents a consensus developed through creative open dialog.

From American Public Health Association: *Ten essential public health services*, Washington, DC, 2017, available at: https://www.apha.org/about-apha/centers-and-programs/quality-improvement-initiatives/national-public-health-performance-standards-program/10-essential-public-health-services (accessed July 2017), and CDC, National Public Health Performance Standards Program, Atlanta, 2015, available at: https://www.cdc.gov/nphpsp/ (accessed July 2017).

This is how one state might have defined and described the application of the standards to public health nursing (PHN) practice.

Standard 1: Conduct Community Assessment: Systematically collect and make available health-related data for the purpose of identifying and responding to community- and state-level public health concerns for conducting epidemiological and other population-based studies.

Public Health Function	PHN Roles	State Roles
Develop frameworks, methodologies, and tools for standardizing data collection and analysis and reporting across all jurisdictions and providers.	• Provide, review, and comment on proposed methodologies and tools for data collection. • Field test tools and methods.	• Collaborate with professional organizations and academic and governmental institutions to develop and test tools and methods. • Provide educational opportunities in areas of and use of tools. • Work with local level agencies to standardize definitions, data collected, etc., across jurisdictions and among all stakeholders (schools, community-based organizations, and private providers). • Provide aggregated data to the local level in a timely and accurate manner. • Provide census tract–level aggregated data to the local level.

Standard 2: Population Diagnosis and Priorities: The public health nurse analyzes the assessment data to determine the population diagnoses and priorities.

Public Health Function	PHN Roles	State Roles
Collect and analyze data.	• Collaborate with the community to identify population-based needs and gaps in service. • Analyze data and needs, knowledge, attitudes, and practices of specific populations. • Identify patterns of diseases, illness, and injury and develop or stimulate development of programs to respond to identified trends.	• Provide national and state comparisons to be used with local data to obtain trends and assist localities in documenting need, progress, etc., to attain standard outcomes.

Standard 3: Outcomes Identification: The public health nurse identifies expected outcomes for a plan that is based on population diagnoses and priorities.

Public Health Function	PHN Roles	State Roles
Promote competency in public health issues throughout the health delivery system. Collect data.	• Provide educational and technical assistance in areas such as case management and appropriate treatment and control of communicable diseases to the community. • Participate in data collection with a target population. • Ensure that the data collection system supports the objectives of programs serving the community by participating in the design and operation of data collection systems. • Collect data via surveys, polls, interviews, and focus groups that will enable assessment of the community's perception of health status and understanding of how the system works and how to obtain needed services.	• Develop appropriate regulatory, educational, and technical assistance programs. • Provide technical assistance and training to local health departments for local forecasting and interpretation of data. • Work with localities (health districts, private providers, and other state and local agencies) to develop standard data elements and definitions across jurisdictions and among all stakeholders, especially for consistency in coding of population-based data. • Identify data collection and analytic issues related to monitoring the impact of health system changes such as costs and benefits of record linkage, strategies for ensuring confidentiality, and strategies for analyzing trends in health within a broader social and economic context. • Advocate for uniform data collection from all managed care plans so that outcomes and health trends can be analyzed and tracked, and sentinel events reported.

Continued

Standard 3: Outcomes Identification—cont'd

Public Health Function	PHN Roles	State Roles
Analyze data to ensure the accurate diagnosis of health status, identification of threats to health, and assessment of health service needs.	• Participate in a systematic approach to convert data into information that will identify gaps in service at the local and state level and will lead to action. • Monitor health status indicators to identify emerging problems and facilitate community-wide responses to identified problems. • Facilitate data analysis as part of a local collaborative effort.	• Develop a systematic, integrated, statewide approach to converting data into information that directs action. • Ensure that resources to analyze data, such as hardware and software, are available at the local level. • Work with localities (health districts, private providers, other state and local agencies) to address issues related to variable access to technology, confidentiality issues. • Educate and train currently employed public health nurses in areas of epidemiology and population-based services.
Monitor health status indicators for the entire population and for specific population groups and/or geographic areas.	• Identify target populations that may be at risk for public health problems such as communicable diseases and unidentified and untreated chronic diseases. • Conduct surveys or observe targeted populations such as preschools, child care centers, and high-risk census tracks to identify health status. • Monitor health care utilization of vulnerable populations at the local and regional level.	• Develop methodology for identification, measurement, and analysis of key indicators of health care utilization of vulnerable populations.
Monitor and assess availability, cost effectiveness, and outcomes of personal and population-based health services.	• Identify gaps in services (e.g., a neighborhood with deteriorating immunization rates may indicate a lack of available primary care services). • Ensure that all receive the same quality of care, including comprehensive preventive services. • Monitor the impact of health system reforms on vulnerable populations. • Evaluate the effectiveness and outcomes of care. • Plan interventions based on the health of the overall population, not just for those in the health care system. • Identify interventions that are effective and replicable.	• Develop analyses that demonstrate the cost effectiveness of investment in public health services. • Develop protocols and technical assistance for ensuring accountability of Medicaid-managed care plans and other government-funded plans for service delivery and overall health status of their covered populations. • Identify standard theoretical, methodological, and measurement issues that are specific to population subgroups for monitoring the impact of health system changes on vulnerable populations.
Disseminate information.	• Disseminate information to the public on community health status, including how to access and use the services appropriately. • Disseminate information to other health care providers regarding gaps in services or deteriorating health status indicators.	• Ensure a mechanism for public accountability of performance and outcomes through public dissemination of information and, in particular, ensure that underservice, a risk inherent in capitated plans, is measurable through available data. • Ensure that information is provided to communities, local health departments, managed care plans, and other appropriate state agencies.

Standard 4: Planning: The public health nurse develops a plan that reflects best practices by identifying strategies, action plans, and alternatives to attain expected outcomes.

Public Health Function	PHN Roles	State Roles
Develop programs that prevent, contain, and control the transmission of diseases and danger of injuries (including violence).	• Provide community-wide preventive measures in the form of health education and mobilization of community resources. • Ensure isolation/containment measures when necessary. • Ensure adequate preventive immunizations. • Implement programs that control the transmission of diseases and danger of injuries during disasters.	• Work with local jurisdictions to develop tools such as videos, PSAs, and/or posters that local jurisdictions can use. • Work with local jurisdictions to develop disaster plans for the control of the transmission of diseases and danger of injuries during disasters. • Facilitate state-level partnerships that promote health, healthy lifestyles, and wellness (individual and family).

Standard 4: Planning—cont'd

Public Health Function	PHN Roles	State Roles
Develop regulatory guidelines for the prevention of targeted diseases.	• Implement regulatory measures. • Implement OSHA Guidelines for Bloodborne Pathogens and the Prevention of the Transmission of TB in Health Care Settings. • Serve as a clearinghouse or source of information.	• In partnership with localities, develop regulatory guidelines.
Develop methods/tools for the collection and analysis of health-related data (occurrence of mortality and morbidity relating to both communicable and chronic diseases, injury registries, sentinel event establishment, environmental quality, etc.).	• Provide reporting guidelines and consultation regarding disease prevention, diagnosis, treatment, and follow-up of cases/contacts to physicians and institutions (emergency department, university and secondary school student health, prisons, industries, etc.). • Conduct/participate in community needs assessments to determine customer/provider knowledge deficits and perceptions of need. • Provide education to individuals, providers, targeted populations, etc., in response to knowledge deficits, disease outbreaks, toxic waste emissions, etc. • Provide individual follow-up/case management of communicable diseases that are transmitted by air, water, food, and fomites (TB, hepatitis A, salmonella, and Staphylococcus, etc.).	• Develop standard methodology and tools for the collection and analysis of health-related data. • Provide training in the area of data collection and analysis. • Evaluate activities and outcomes of interactions. • Work in partnership with localities to develop programs based on data analysis needs.
Develop programs that promote a safe environment in the home.	• Provide childhood lead poisoning screenings and follow-up. • Teach clients to inspect homes for safety violations and toxic substances and to practice safe behaviors; assist families to access/use available resources/safety devices. • Assess/teach regarding safe food selection, preparation, and storage. • Train/supervise volunteers/auxiliary personnel in the performance of the above tasks. • Teach families that all men, women, and children have a right to a safe environment free of physical and mental abuse.	• Provide consultation and technical assistance to state and local organizations regarding laws and regulations that protect health and ensure safety. • In partnership with localities, develop and evaluate educational programs.
Develop programs that promote a safe environment in the workplace.	• Provide consultation in the implementation of OSHA regulations relating to occupational exposure to diseases. • Provide educational programs related to healthy lifestyles (smoking cessation, back protection, etc.). • Ensure provision of screenings for individuals to determine baselines and the occurrence of infectious diseases and preventable deterioration of health and function: hearing, back soundness, lung capacity, RMS indicators, PPDs, etc. • Assist in policy/practice development to address the prevention of the above. • Provide immunizations.	• Monitor and assist localities to implement prevention activities. • Assist localities in developing and evaluating educational programs. • Monitor outcomes of screening activities and evaluate interventions.
Develop programs that promote a safe environment in the school setting.	• Provide consultations on the implementation of OSHA regulations relating to occupational exposure to diseases. • Provide educational programs related to healthy lifestyles (smoking cessation, etc.). • Ensure provision of screenings for students to determine baselines and the occurrence of infectious disease and preventable deterioration of health and function. • Assist in policy/practice development to address prevention of the above. • Provide immunizations.	• Develop guidelines that ensure accountability in meeting standards set forth. • Ensure that policy is developed to protect children in the school environment. • Monitor the immunization status of children and provide immunizations during outbreaks and evaluate activities.

Continued

Standard 4: Planning—cont'd

Public Health Function	PHN Roles	State Roles
Develop programs that promote a safe environment in the community.	• Identify population clusters exhibiting an unhealthy environment; provide consultation/group education regarding preventive measures. • Participate in the development of local disaster plans to ensure provision of safe water, food, air, and facilities. • Respond in time of natural disasters such as floods, tornadoes, and hurricanes. • Participate in developing plans for shelter management during disasters, especially "Special Needs" shelters that may require nursing staff.	• In times of disaster, facilitate the availability of resources across jurisdictions. • Have a statewide plan. • Ensure that localities have developed plans to protect the public in time of national and/or other disasters. • Coordinate efforts statewide. • Assist localities in responding. • Evaluate efforts.
Develop and issue standards that guide regulations and program development, and mandate policy.	• Survey worksites, schools, institutions, etc., for compliance to regulations that protect health and ensure safety.	• Develop a systematic evaluation tool for the collection of data to measure trends.
Develop protocols to ensure accountability of all health care providers, public and private.	• Provide technical assistance, i.e., interpretation, implementation, and evaluation processes.	• Assist localities in developing standards to mandate accountability.
Provide in-service to all providers of health care services.	• Share and implement knowledge gained in in-services.	• Provide consultation/technical assistance to localities.

Standard 5 encompasses the elements of implementation, coordination, health education and health promotion, consultation, and regulatory activities. Each element is described and the table that follows integrates and applies these five elements.

Standard 5: Implementation: The public health nurse implements the identified plan by partnering with others.

Standard 5A: Coordination: The public health nurse coordinates programs, services, and other activities to implement the identified plan.

Standard 5B: Health Education and Health Promotion: The public health nurse employs multiple strategies to promote health, prevent disease, and ensure a safe environment for populations.

Standard 5C: Consultation: The public health nurse provides consultation to various community groups and officials to facilitate the implementation of programs and services.

Standard 5D: Regulatory Activities: The public health nurse identifies, interprets, and implements public health laws, regulations, and policies.

Public Health Function	PHN Roles	State Roles
Promote informed decision making of residents about things that influence their health on a daily basis.	• Exert influence through contact with individuals and community groups. • Accept and issue challenges concerning healthy lifestyles to all contacts. • Reinforce and reward positive informed decisions made for healthy lifestyles.	• Develop and monitor standards to determine changes in behavior.
Promote effective use of media to encourage both personal and community responsibility for informed decision making.	• Be a resource for the community. • Gather data and address findings as appropriate. • Work with community groups to promote accurate information for healthy lifestyles through the media. • Utilize current information and other agencies' resources to maximize information accessible to the public.	• Assist localities to provide current information to community organizations and other state organizations. • Serve as a resource for localities and work with media.
Develop a public awareness/marketing campaign to demonstrate the importance of public health to overall health improvement and its proper place in the health delivery system.	• Provide education to special groups, e.g., local politicians, school boards, PTAs, churches, civic groups, and news media, regarding the benefits of preventive health.	• Develop training activities to assist localities in marketing.
Develop public information and education systems/programs through partnerships.	• Provide educational sessions/programs to the public regarding the components of healthy lifestyles. • Access grants/other funding sources to promote healthy lifestyle decisions (e.g., cervical and breast cancer prevention; bike helmets, hypertension). • Provide/promote teaching for individuals and families at every opportunity (home, clinic, community settings).	• Assist localities in developing and evaluating educational programs. • Assist localities in funding. • Hold regional/state training sessions. • Evaluate outcomes and plan ongoing educational systems/programs.

Standard 5D: Regulatory Activities—cont'd

Ensure accessibility to health services that will improve morbidity, decrease mortality, and improve health status outcomes.

- Provide family-centered case management services for high-risk and hard-to-reach populations that focus on linking families with needed services.
- Improve access to care by forming partnerships with appropriate community individuals and entities.
- Increase the influence of cultural diversity on system design and on access to care, as well as on individual services rendered.
- Ensure that translation services are available for the non-English-speaking populations.
- Participate in ongoing community assessment to identify areas of concern and need for rules.
- Provide outreach services that focus on preventing epidemics and the spread of disease, such as tuberculosis and sexually transmitted diseases.
- Provide direct services for specific diseases that threaten the health of the community and develop programs that prevent, contain, and control the transmission of infectious diseases.

- Provide funds in cooperation with the locality.
- Ensure policy development that includes case management and is culturally sensitive.
- Provide adequate ongoing continuing education for the staff (especially in areas common to all localities).
- Participate in state-level contract development to ensure that contracts with health plans require and include incentives for health plans to offer and deliver preventive health services in the minimum benefits package.
- Educate financing officials about the roles of public health both in performing core public health services and in ensuring access to personal health services.

Provide direct services for specific diseases that threaten the health of the community and develop programs that prevent, contain, and control the transmission of infectious diseases.

- Plan, develop, implement, and evaluate:
  Sexually transmitted disease services
  Communicable disease services
  HIV/AIDS services
  Tuberculosis control services
- Develop and implement guidelines for the prevention of the above targeted diseases.

- Establish standards/criteria for personal health care.
- Work with local health departments to assist in developing infrastructure and management techniques to facilitate recordkeeping and appropriate financial monitoring and tracking systems, which enable local health departments to enter into contractual arrangements for preventive health and primary care services.

Provide health services, including preventive health services, to high-risk and vulnerable populations (e.g., the uninsured working poor), and in geographic areas in which primary health care services are not readily accessible or available in a privatized setting.

Provide leadership to stimulate the development of networks or partnerships that will ensure the availability of comprehensive primary health care services to all, regardless of the ability to pay.

Initiate collaboration with other community organizations to ensure the leadership role in resolving a public health issue.

- Provide coordination, follow-up, referral, and case management as indicated.
- Integrate supportive services, such as counseling, social work, and nutrition, into primary care services.
- Assess the existing community medical capacity for referral and follow-up.
- Advocate for improved health.
- Disseminate health information.
- Build coalitions.
- Make recommendations for policy implementation or revision.
- Facilitate resources that manage environmental risk and maintain and improve community health.
- Provide information for a community group working on impacting policy at the local, state, or federal level.
- Use results of community health assessments to stimulate the community to develop a plan to respond to identified gaps in service.

- Continue to work at the state and local level to build primary and preventive health services capacity, particularly in traditionally underserved areas, to ensure availability to providers and primary care sites essential to primary care access.
- Facilitate the establishment and enhancement of statewide high-quality, needed health services.
- Administer quality improvement programs.

- Use information-gathering techniques of assessment to assist policy/legislature activities to develop needed health services and functions that require statewide action or standards.
- Recommend programs to carry out policies.

Standard 6: Evaluation: The public health nurse evaluates the health status of the population.

Public Health Function	PHN Roles	State Roles
Ensure ongoing prevention research relating to biomedical and behavioral aspects of health promotion and prevention of disease and injury.	• Develop outcome measures. • Identify research priorities for target communities and develop and conduct scientific and operations research for health promotion and disease/injury prevention.	• Provide training in the area of measuring program effectiveness.
Implement pilot or demonstration projects.	• Develop and implement linkages with academic centers, ensuring that clients and populations participating in research projects benefit as a result of the research.	• Support evaluations and research that demonstrate the benefits of public health, as well as the consequences of failure to support public health interventions.

The above was adapted and excerpted from the work of Diane B. Downing and the Virginia Public Health Nurses, 2013 by Marcia Stanhope.

C.2 American Nurses Association Standards of Practice and Professional Performance for Public Health Nursing

THE STANDARDS OF PRACTICE FOR PUBLIC HEALTH NURSING

Standard 1: Assessment: The public health nurse collects comprehensive data pertinent to the health status of populations.

Standard 2: Population Diagnosis and Priorities: The public health nurse analyzes the assessment data to determine the population diagnoses and priorities.

Standard 3: Outcomes Identification: The public health nurse identifies expected outcomes for a plan specific to the population or situation.

Standard 4: Planning: The public health nurse develops a plan that prescribes strategies and alternatives to attain expected outcomes.

Standard 5: Implementation: The public health nurse implements the identified plan.

Standard 5A: Coordination of Care: The public health nurse coordinates care delivery.

Standard 5B: Health Teaching and Health Promotion: The public health nurse employs multiple strategies to promote health and a safe environment.

Standard 5C: Consultation: The public health nurse provides consultation to influence the identified plan, enhance the abilities of others, and effect change.

Standard 5D: Prescriptive Authority: Not applicable

Standard 5E: Regulatory Activities: The public health nurse participates in applications of public health laws, regulations, and policies.

Standard 6: Evaluation: The public health nurse evaluates the progress toward attainment of outcomes.

STANDARDS OF PROFESSIONAL PERFORMANCE FOR PUBLIC HEALTH NURSING

Standard 7: Ethics: The public health nurse practices ethically.

Standard 8: Education: The public health nurse attains knowledge and competence that reflect current nursing practice.

Standard 9: Evidence-Based Practice and Research: The public health nurse integrates evidence and research findings into practice.

Standard 10: Quality of Practice: The public health nurse contributes to quality nursing practice.

Standard 11: Communication: The public health nurse communicates effectively in a variety of formats in all areas of practice.

Standard 12: Leadership: The public health nurse demonstrates leadership in the professional practice setting and the profession.

Standard 13: Collaboration: The public health nurse collaborates with the population, and others in the conduct of nursing practice.

Standard 14: Professional Practice Evaluation: The public health nurse evaluates her or his own nursing practice in relation to professional practice standards and guidelines, relevant statutes, rules, and regulations.

Standard 15: Resource Utilization: The public health nurse utilizes appropriate resources to plan and provide nursing and public health services that are safe, effective, and financially responsible.

Standard 16: Environmental Health: The public health nurse practices in an environmentally safe, fair, and just manner.

Standard 17: Advocacy: The public health nurse advocates for the protection of the health, safety, and rights of the population.

C.3 Minnesota Department of Health Public Health Interventions Wheel

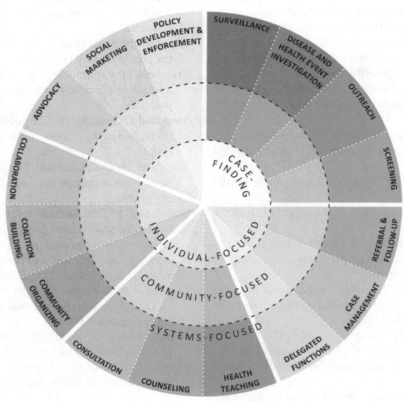

PUBLIC HEALTH INTERVENTIONS

(POPULATION-BASED)

Minnesota Department of Health Public Health Intervention Wheel. (Used with permission from Keller LO, Strohschein S, Lia-Hoagberg B, et al.: Population-based public health interventions: Practice-based and evidence-supported, part I. *Public Health Nurs* 21:453–468, 2004.)

DEFINITION OF POPULATION-BASED PRACTICE

Population-Based Practice

1. **Focuses on entire populations**

   A **population** is a collection of individuals who have one or more personal or environmental characteristics in common.[1]

   A **population-of-interest** is a population that is essentially healthy but which could improve factors that promote or protect health.

   A **population-at-risk** is a population with a common identified risk factor or risk exposure that poses a threat to health.

Population-based practice always begins with identifying everyone who is in the population-of-interest or the population-at-risk. It is not limited to only those who seek service or who are poor or otherwise vulnerable.

2. **Is grounded in an assessment of the population's health status**

   Population-based practice reflects the priorities of the community. Community priorities are determined through an assessment of the population's health status and a prioritization process.

3. **Considers the broad determinants of health**

   Population-based practice focuses on the entire range of factors that determine health rather than just personal health risks or disease. Health determinants include income and social status, social support networks, education, employment and working conditions, biology and genetic endowment, physical environment, personal health practices and coping skills, and health services.

---

[1]Williams, CA, Highriter ME: Community health nursing: population focus and evaluation, *Public Health Rev* 7(3-4):197-221, 1978.

4. Emphasizes all levels of prevention

Prevention is anticipatory action taken to prevent the occurrence of an event or to minimize its effect after it has occurred.[2] Not every event is preventable, but every event does have a preventable component. Primary prevention promotes health or keeps problems from occurring; secondary prevention detects and treats problems early; tertiary prevention keeps existing problems from getting worse. Whenever possible, population-based practice emphasizes primary prevention.

---

[2]Turnock, BJ: Public health: what it is and how it works, 5th ed. Burlington, 2012, Jones & Bartlett Learning.

5. Intervenes with communities, systems, individuals, and families

Population-based practice intervenes with communities, with the systems involving the health of communities, and/or with the individuals and families that comprise communities. Community-focused practice changes community norms, attitudes, awareness, practices, and behaviors. Systems-focused practice changes organizations, policies, laws, and power structures of the systems that affect health. Individual/family-focused practice changes knowledge, attitudes, beliefs, values, practices, and behaviors of individuals (identified as belonging to a population), alone or as part of a family, class, or group. Interventions at each level of practice contribute to the overall goal of improving population health status.

PUBLIC HEALTH INTERVENTIONS WITH DEFINITIONS

Public Health Intervention	Definition
Surveillance	Describes and monitors health events through ongoing and systematic collection, analysis, and interpretation of health data for the purpose of planning, implementing, and evaluating public health interventions. (Modified from *MMWR*, 1988.)
Disease and other health event investigation	Systematically gathers and analyzes data regarding threats to the health of populations, ascertains the source of the threat, identifies cases and others at risk, and determines control measures.
Outreach	Locates populations-of-interest or populations-at-risk and provides information about the nature of the concern, what can be done about it, and how services can be obtained.
Screening	Identifies individuals with unrecognized health risk factors or asymptomatic disease conditions in populations.
Case finding	Locates individuals and families with identified risk factors and connects them with resources.
Referral and follow-up	Assists individuals, families, groups, organizations, and/or communities to identify and access necessary resources in order to prevent or resolve problems or concerns.
Case management	Optimizes self-care capabilities of individuals and families and the capacity of systems and communities to coordinate and provide services.
Delegated functions	Directs care tasks that a registered professional nurse carries out under the authority of a health care practitioner as allowed by law. Delegated functions also include any direct care tasks that a registered professional nurse entrusts to other appropriate personnel to perform.
Health teaching	Communicates facts, ideas, and skills that change knowledge, attitudes, values, beliefs, behaviors, and practices of individuals, families, systems, and/or communities.
Counseling	Establishes an interpersonal relationship with a community, a system, family, or individual intended to increase or enhance their capacity for self-care and coping. Counseling engages the community, a system, family, or individual at an emotional level.
Consultation	Seeks information and generates optional solutions to perceived problems or issues through interactive problem solving with a community, system, family, or individual. The community, system, family, or individual selects and acts on the option best meeting the circumstances.
Collaboration	Commits two or more persons or organizations to achieve a common goal through enhancing the capacity of one or more of the members to promote and protect health. (Modified from Henneman EA, Lee J, Cohen J: Collaboration: a concept analysis, *J Advan Nurs* 21:103–109, 1995.)
Coalition building	Promotes and develops alliances among organizations or constituencies for a common purpose. It builds linkages, solves problems, and/or enhances local leadership to address health concerns.
Community organizing	Helps community groups to identify common problems or goals, mobilize resources, and develop and implement strategies for reaching the goals they collectively have set. (Modified from Minkler M, editor: *Community organizing and community building for health*, New Brunswick, 1997, Rutgers University Press.)

Public Health Intervention	Definition
Advocacy	Pleads someone's cause or acts on someone's behalf, with a focus on developing the community, system, individual, or family's capacity to plead their own cause or act on their own behalf.
Social marketing	Utilizes commercial marketing principles and technologies for programs designed to influence the knowledge, attitudes, values, beliefs, behaviors, and practices of the population-of-interest.
Policy development	Places health issues on decision makers' agendas, acquires a plan of resolution, and determines needed resources. Policy development results in laws, rules and regulations, ordinances, and policies.
Policy enforcement	Compels others to comply with the laws, rules, regulations, ordinances, and policies created in conjunction with policy development.

THREE LEVELS OF PUBLIC HEALTH PRACTICE

Public health interventions are population based if they consider all levels of practice. This concept is represented by the three inner rings of the model. The inner rings of the model are labeled community-focused, systems-focused, and individual/family-focused.

A population-based approach considers intervening at all possible levels of practice. Interventions may be directed at the entire population within a community, the systems that affect the health of those populations, and/or the individuals and families within those populations known to be at risk.

Levels	Definition
Population-based **community-focused** practice	Changes community norms, community attitudes, community awareness, community practices, and community behaviors. They are directed toward entire populations within the community or occasionally toward target groups within those populations. Community-focused practice is measured in terms of what proportion of the population actually changes.
Population-based **systems-focused** practice	Changes organizations, policies, laws, and power structures. The focus is not directly on individuals and communities but on the systems that affect health. Changing systems is often a more effective and long-lasting way to affect population health than requiring change from every individual in a community.
Population-based **individual-focused** practice	Changes knowledge, attitudes, beliefs, practices, and behaviors of individuals. This practice level is directed at individuals, alone or as part of a family, class, or group. Individuals receive services because they are identified as belonging to a population-at-risk.

From Section of Public Health Nursing, Minnesota Department of Health: *Public Health Interventions*, 2001, available at http://www.health.state.mn.us/divs/opi/cd/phn/docs/0301wheel_manual.pdf.

D.1 Summary Description of Hepatitis A-E

HEPATITIS A (HAV)

Description: A viral liver disease that can cause mild to severe illness and that is transmitted by ingesting contaminated food or water or through direct contact with an infected person. It is transmitted via the fecal-oral route. Most people with HAV recover and have lifetime immunity.

Risk Factors: Consuming contaminated food or water, especially during international travel; direct contact with an infected person; sexual contact with a person who has HAV infection; men having sex with men; use of illegal drugs, injected or not injected; homelessness; occupational exposure; close contact with an international adoptee; having a clotting factor disorder such as hemophilia.

Symptoms: Loss of appetite; headache; malaise; fatigue; nausea; vomiting; fever; jaundice; abdominal pain; diarrhea; dark urine; clay-colored stools.

Precautions: Strict handwashing, especially by food handlers; avoiding the risk factors.

Prevention: Hepatitis A vaccine.

HEPATITIS B (HBV)

Description: A viral infection that attacks the liver and can cause both acute and chronic disease; is spread from blood, semen, or other body fluids from an infected person.

Risk Factors: Exposure to human blood; lives with an infected person; injects drugs or shares needles, syringes, or other injection equipment; has multiple sex partners; men having sex with men or has a sex partner infected with HBV; is an infant born to an infected mother; is on hemodialysis; or has a needle-stick injury, tattoo, piercing, or exposure to infected blood or body fluids.

Symptoms: Jaundice; poor appetite; nausea; vomiting; stomach or joint pain; fatigue; gray-colored stools; dark urine.

Precautions: Vaccinate: all infants, unvaccinated children <19 years; people at risk for infection by sexual exposure or by percutaneous or mucosal exposure to blood; who have hepatitis C virus infection, chronic liver disease, HIV, or who are incarcerated; international travelers to counties with high or intermediate levels of endemic HBV; and people with hepatitis C virus infection.

Prevention: Hepatitis B vaccine.

HEPATITIS C

Description: A virus that can cause both acute and chronic illness ranging from mild to severe; is a major cause of liver cancer; is a blood-borne virus; all adults, pregnant women, and people with risk factors should get tested for hepatitis C. People with Hepatitis C may not have symptoms, and there is no vaccine.

Risk Factors: Drug injections and sharing equipment; exposure to human blood, including transfusions, organ transplants, or giving birth; hemodialysis; multiple sex partners or sex with an infected person; heavy alcohol use; health care exposures; sharing personal items such as razors, glucose monitors, nail clippers, toothbrushes, or other items that could come in contact with blood; living with a person with hepatitis B infection.

Symptoms: Same as hepatitis B infection.

Precautions: Avoid engaging in the risk factors.

Prevention of Spread: No vaccine is available; practice safe sex; have only one sex partner; routine screening of blood from donors.

HEPATITIS D

Description: A virus that requires hepatitis B virus (HBV) for its replication; is spread from blood or other body fluids from an infected person. Hepatitis D can be acute or chronic and can cause death. There is no vaccine.

Risk Factors: Injection drug users; hemophilia clients; birth to an infected mother; sex with infected partner; contact with blood from or the open sores of an infected person; occupational exposure to blood or blood-contaminated body fluids.

Symptoms: Same as hepatitis B infection.

Precautions: Avoid all risk factors, including avoiding sexual contact with injection drug users; do not use needles used by others; and use proper sterilization procedures in institutions.

Prevention of Spread: Vaccination with HBV vaccine can protect people from HDV infection; individual screening for HBV; and blood screening for HBV and HDV.

HEPATITIS E

Description: HEV is found in the stool of an infected person. It is usually acute and does not typically cause chronic disease.

Risk Factors: Ingestion of contaminated fecal material; international travelers; pregnant women; persons in Asia, the Middle East, Africa, and Central America as are people who live in crowded camps or temporary housing.

Symptoms: Same as Hepatitis B.

Precaution: Avoid contaminated water.

Prevention of Spread: No current vaccine, so take precautions.

Data are from the Centers for Disease Control and Prevention: *Viral Hepatitis*, 2020, Links to Hepatitis A, B, C, D, and E.

World Health Organization, *Hepatitis A, B, C, D, and E,* 2020, http:// www.who.int.

See also: National Institutes of Health (NIH): *Viral hepatitis A though E and Beyond,* 2020, http://www.niddk.nih.gov.

D.2 Recommendations for Prophylaxis of Hepatitis A

In 2020 the Advisory Committee on Immunization Practices (ACIP) issued new recommendations.

"The following ACIP recommendations are new, updated, or no longer recommended:

- Vaccination of all children and adolescents aged 2 to 18 years who have not previously received Hep A vaccine (i.e., children and adolescents are recommended for catch-up vaccination)
  - Vaccination of all persons aged ≥1 year infected with human immunodeficiency virus (HIV)
  - Vaccination of persons with chronic liver disease, including but not limited to persons with hepatitis B virus (HBV) infection, hepatitis C virus (HCV) infection, cirrhosis, fatty liver disease, alcoholic liver disease, autoimmune hepatitis, or an alanine aminotransferase (ALT) or aspartate aminotransferase (AST) level persistently greater than twice the upper limit of normal
  - Vaccination of pregnant women who are identified to be at risk for HAV infection during pregnancy (e.g., international travelers, persons who use injection or noninjection drugs [i.e., all those who use illegal drugs], persons who have occupational risk for infection, persons who anticipate close personal contact with an international adoptee, or persons experiencing homelessness) or for having a severe outcome from HAV infection (e.g., persons with chronic liver disease or persons with HIV infection)
  - Vaccination during hepatitis A outbreaks of persons aged ≥1 year who are at risk for HAV infection (e.g., persons who use injection or noninjection drugs [i.e., all those who use illegal drugs], persons experiencing homelessness, or men having sex with men (MSM) or who are at risk for severe disease from HAV (e.g., persons with chronic liver disease or who are infected with HIV)
  - Vaccination in settings providing services to adults in which a high proportion of persons have risk factors for HAV infection (e.g., health care settings with a focus on those who use injection or noninjection drugs [i.e., all those who use illegal drugs], group homes, and nonresidential day care facilities for developmentally disabled persons)
  - Vaccination of persons who receive blood products for clotting disorders (e.g., hemophilia) is no longer recommended.

"New CDC clinical guidance is provided for the vaccination of the following: infants aged 6 to 11 months traveling outside the United States, persons aged >40 years, persons with immunocompromising conditions, and persons with chronic liver disease planning on traveling, persons with HIV infection, pregnant women, postexposure prophylaxis and vaccination during outbreaks" (p. 2). See this reference for further details on the new or updated CDC recommendations.

The ACIP made these recommendations about adults at risk for HAV infection or for severe disease if they contracted the infection. These groups needed to be vaccinated:

1. International travelers from developed countries who travel to countries with a high or intermediate level of HAV. Specifically travelers at risk include tourists, non-immune immigrants and their children who travel back to visit in their home country, military personnel, missionaries and people who work or study abroad (p. 6)
2. Men who have sex with men
3. Persons who use injection or non-injection drugs (p. 7)
4. Persons with occupational risk for exposure, such as those who work in labs containing HAV or work with nonhuman primates
5. Persons who anticipate close personal contact with an international adoptee
6. Homeless persons or those living in group settings or are incarcerated
7. Persons with HIV or chronic liver disease (pp. 7–8)
8. Older people (p. 9)

Groups at settings with low risk for Hepatitis A:

1. Persons with blood clotting disorders
2. Food service establishments
3. Child care centers, schools, and health care institutions
4. Public works systems and workers exposed to sewage (p. 10)

Vaccines containing HAV antigen that are licensed in the United States are the single-antigen vaccines Havrix and Vaqta and the combination vaccine Twinrix (containing both HAV and HBV antigens).

Source: Nelson NP, Weng MK, Hofmeister MG, et al. Prevention of hepatitis A virus infection in the United States: recommendations of the advisory committee on immunization practices, 2020. *MMWR Recomm Rep*, 69 (No. RR-5):1–38, 2020.

D.3 Recommendations for Postexposure Prophylaxis for Contacts of Patients Positive for HBsAg are as Follows

- Perinatal exposure—HBIg* plus HBV vaccine at the time of birth (90% effective)
- Sexual contact with an acutely infected patient—HBIg plus HBV vaccine
- Sexual contact with a chronic carrier—HBV vaccine
- Household contact with an acutely infected patient—None
- Household contact with an acutely infected person resulting in known exposure—HBIg, with or without HBV vaccine
- Infant (age <12 months) primarily cared for by an acutely infected patient—HBIg, with or without HBV vaccine

HBIg is hepatitis B immune globulin and provides immediate, shorter term protection against hepatitis B infection: *HealthLinkBC:*. healthlinkbc.ca, 2016.

Samji NS: What are recommendations for post exposure hepatitis B virus (HBV) prophylaxis? *Medscape Nurses*, 2017, http://www.medscape.com. (Accessed November 2020).

Note: Page numbers followed by "*f*" refer to illustrations; page numbers followed by "*t*" refer to tables; page numbers followed by "*b*" refer to boxes.